Psychiatry in Law/
Law in Psychiatry

Second Edition

Psychiatry in Law/ Law in Psychiatry

Second Edition

RALPH SLOVENKO

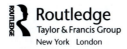

Routledge
Taylor & Francis Group
New York   London

Routledge
Taylor & Francis Group
711 Third Avenue,
New York, NY 10017

Routledge
Taylor & Francis Group
2 Park Square,
Milton Park, Abingdon,
Oxfordshire OX14 4RN

First issued in paperback 2014

Routledge is an imprint of the Taylor and Francis Group, an informa business

© 2009 by Taylor & Francis Group, LLC

ISBN 978-0-415-99491-0 (hbk)
ISBN 978-1-138-87296-7 (pbk)

Library of Congress Cataloging-in-Publication Data

Slovenko, Ralph.
    Psychiatry in law/law in psychiatry / Ralph Slovenko. -- 2nd ed.
        p. cm.
    Includes bibliographical references and indexes.
    ISBN 978-0-415-93365-0 (hardbound : alk. paper)
     1. Forensic psychiatry--United States. 2. Psychiatrists--Legal status, laws, etc.--United States. I.
Title.
     [DNLM: 1. Forensic Psychiatry--United States. W 740 P635pc 2009]

KF8965.S59 2009
614'.1--dc22   2008023713

Visit the Taylor & Francis Web site at
http://www.taylorandfrancis.com

and the Routledge Web site at
http://www.routledge.com

In memory

Dr. James A. Knight
Dr. Harold I. Lief
Dr. C.B. Scrignar

Beloved friends and colleagues

Contents

Preface

The interplay of law and psychiatry has changed markedly during the 20th century. Before World War II the interplay was mainly the penetration by psychiatry into law, but after the war it has been primarily the other way. The practice of psychiatry is no longer unfettered as it once was. In the case of both the penetration by psychiatry into law and the penetration by law into psychiatry, there are swings of the pendulum, but whatever the vagaries of the day, there is one constant. The state—through elected officials, judges, legislators, and administrators—determines when, where, and why psychiatry and law interact.

From the dawn of civilization deviant behavior has been explained in one of three ways: stupidity, sin, and sickness—involving educators, the clergy, lawyers and judges, and physicians, with each discipline using its own techniques of persuading, preaching, punishing, and prescribing. The decline in the influence of family and religion has led to a more prominent role of law and medicine, especially psychiatry, in the resolution of human conflict and controversy. Psychiatry has increasingly replaced the church as the refuge of the troubled. Psychiatrists have been called the new secular priests.

Most notably, there has been a lawyerization, as well as psychiatrization, of the country since the early 1960s. The interplay of law and psychiatry has prompted mental health professionals to become aware of legal issues and the legal profession to become aware of psychiatric issues, so much so that at times the mental health professional sounds like a lawyer and the lawyer sounds like a mental health professional.

As a discipline, the law is divided into a number of categories, including crimes, torts, contracts, property, and domestic relations. Psychiatry plays a role in all of these categories. In criminal law, *mens rea*, that is, a guilty mind, is an essential element. Much of the law of torts rests upon the negligence of the individual sought to be found liable. Under the law of contracts, the contracting parties must have a "meeting of the minds." The validity of testamentary disposition of property is largely based on the mental competency of the testator at the time the will is formulated.

The conceptual center of law and psychiatry has long been criminal responsibility, and it remains so, but practically speaking, psychiatrists (and psychologists) participate in many other types of cases. The infiltration of psychiatry into law may be broadly catalogued into matters of credibility, culpability, competency, compensation, and custody. In other words, the intermix of psychiatry in law includes problems of a witness's credibility, the culpability of the accused, a defendant's competency to stand trial, the imposition and carrying out of the death penalty, the individual's competency to make a will or contract or to take care of one's self or one's property, the compensation of injured persons, and the custody of children. Although the interplay of psychiatry in law is not limited to those areas, they constitute the major part of forensic work.

Conversely, law has played a role in the practice of psychiatry. The growing intervention of law in psychiatry has been fueled by criticism of psychiatry from both inside and outside the profession. According to civil libertarians, the primary reason underlying the recent movement to restrict coercive psychiatry is that the benevolent motive—to help the disturbed who are in distress—is not achieved by mental hospitalization, major tranquilizers, electroshock therapy, behavior modification, or psychosurgery. They put forward two additional arguments against involuntary hospitalization: first, that the mental health system, like other social service systems, has an inherent conflict of interest, as it is responsive to those it employs as well as to its consumers; and second, that there is no moral basis to deprive a harmless, disturbed person of physical freedom for the sake of unwanted treatment by substituting a psychiatrist's decision for that of the disturbed person. As a result of these criticisms, criminal justice procedures and standards, as opposed to psychiatric professional standards, are now applied in civil commitment procedures.

Some say that physicians no longer have the best interest of patients at heart. Since 1960, civil libertarians have been challenging benevolence as a mask for intrusion and have been establishing legal rights for their clients. Legislation has been enacted—some say to enlarge the market for lawyers—that provides for the establishment of legal services for the mentally ill and developmentally disabled persons and for residents in private and public mental hospitals and in community facilities. Even more upsetting to the psychiatric profession is a sudden shift of emphasis away from self-regulation toward external governmental control. Psychiatry is now called, in the words of Dr. Jonas Rappeport, the "belegaled" profession; it is the most regulated profession.

The United States is a litigious society, and as a consequence the law has had significant impact on the practice of psychiatry. Some examples of the impact are hospitalization of the mentally ill, right to treatment, right to refuse treatment, malpractice, confidentiality, and informed consent. Similarly, psychiatry has significantly impacted the law. Some examples of this relationship include criminal responsibility, competency to stand trial, sentencing, posttraumatic stress disorder, child custody, and contractual and testamentary capacity. *Psychiatric News*, the biweekly publication of the American Psychiatric Association, might be called *Psychiatric Legal News*, as much of its content is about psychiatry and law.

The law-related issues most frequently raised by psychiatrists fall into three major areas: (1) malpractice (risks of particular drugs or other forms of therapy, commitment and voluntary hospitalization, liability for acts of others, treatment without informed consent, insurance coverage, suicide, and duty to warn); (2) business-related matters; and (3) confidentiality and privilege.

Once an arcane subject matter, the interplay of psychiatry and law since about 1960 has emerged from an elective seminar to a topic of national prominence. There has been a substantial increase in lawyer involvement and litigation in this area, essentially due to the financial support by public, private, and charitable organizations. Perhaps indicative of this relatively recently developed interest of the legal profession in problems of law as related to mental disorder is the inclusion for the first time of a special topic, "mental health," in the *Sixth Decennial Digest*, the digest of court cases. A monthly summary of reported state and federal court decisions relating to mental health, *Mental Health Court Digest*, is prepared especially for mental health agencies and personnel. Beginning in 1963, the American Bar Association has published a bimonthly, *Mental & Physical Disability Law Reporter*. In 1961, the American Bar Foundation, prompted by its parent organization, the American Bar Association, published *The Mentally Disabled and the Law*, which surveyed and evaluated how the law had seen fit to foster and regulate the relationship between those with mental impairments and those who treat them.

During the past quarter century, a substantial body of literature as well as case law on psychiatry and law has developed. In particular, the decisions of Chief Justice Warren Burger of the U.S. Supreme Court and Chief Judge David L. Bazelon of the District of Columbia Circuit Court of Appeals, which figure prominently in any collection of cases, and the publications of Dr. Karl Menninger and Dr. Thomas Szasz have stimulated discussion regarding the role of the psychiatrist in the legal process. Their untraditional and pioneering views are provocative and have reached a wide audience, including television viewers. For many students, it is Szasz's writings that prompt registration or discussion in law–psychiatry courses. One might take issue with these writings, but they will certainly be found interesting.

Also during the past quarter century, a number of extended programs of study and research and a number of professional organizations in law and the behavioral sciences have developed.

Paralleling the broadening of the scope of psychiatric residency training programs to include community problems, concern about curriculum relevance has prompted law schools to seek breadth and depth in legal education. Foundations have made substantial grants to a number of law schools to establish interdisciplinary teaching and research in law and the behavioral sciences.

At the initiative of Dr. Jonas R. Rappeport along with Dr. Robert Sadoff, the American Academy of Psychiatry and the Law (AAPL) was founded in 1969 and now has a membership of some 2,000 psychiatrists. The American Psychology–Law Society (AP–LS) was founded in 1968 and it too has rapidly grown in membership. There are chapters of AAPL throughout the United States, with the first district branch organized by Dr. Richard Rosner. The goal of AAPL and AP–LS is to teach forensic issues. Then, too, there are the American College of Forensic Psychiatry, American College of Forensic Psychology, and the International Academy of Law and Mental Health. The American Academy of Forensic Sciences has a section on forensic psychiatry. In 1976, the American Board of Forensic Psychiatry was established.

These associations publish specialized journals on law and psychiatry or psychology. They include the *Journal of the American Academy of Psychiatry and the Law, American Journal of Forensic Psychiatry, International Journal of Law and Psychiatry, Journal of Forensic Sciences,* and *Law and Human Behavior.* Then, too, there are *Behavioral Sciences and the Law; Journal of Psychiatry and Law; Psychology, Public Policy, and Law;* and the *Hastings Center Report.* In addition, law reviews published by law schools present symposia or feature articles on law and psychiatry. Several casebooks on law and psychiatry have been published for law school use. As a by-product, they stir up wide interest.

Time and again, the disappointment that many psychiatrists have experienced regarding the direction that clinical psychiatry has taken largely determined by constraints imposed by the insurance industry and compounded by an unholy alliance (they say) between psychiatrists and the pharmaceutical industry have prompted many to seek refuge in forensic psychiatry. The MacArthur Foundation has given millions of dollars in support of research on mental health and the law.

This book stems from my two-volume *Psychiatry in Law/Law in Psychiatry* published in 2002. Since that time, much has transpired in the field of law and psychiatry. This volume includes 11 new chapters and most others are revised or updated. It omits nine chapters and the appendices from the two-volume edition. The new regulations that went into effect in 2003 of the Emergency Medical Treatment and Active Labor Act (EMTALA) are discussed in the chapter on failure to treat. The Health Insurance Portability and Accountability Act (HIPAA) is discussed in Chapter 30 on breach of confidentiality.

As in the two-volume edition, this book is designed to serve three principal purposes. First, it is intended to serve as a course textbook for psychiatric residents and law students, and as a basic reference source for the psychiatrist or lawyer who is only occasionally confronted with problems in law and psychiatry. Second, it is designed to assist those practitioners who regularly work in this area by suggesting new approaches and by providing material to assist them in preparing and documenting their cases. Third, it is intended to provide a critical exposition of many of the practices and basic premises of the terrain of law and psychiatry.

Introduction

THE INTERMIX OF PSYCHIATRY AND LAW

In the United States, the 20th century has been called "the age of psychiatry." During this time discussions about human behavior have been framed in the vocabulary of psychiatry, so it is not surprising that psychiatry impacts the law. The late Associate Justice Tom C. Clark of the United States Supreme Court observed, "Psychiatry is beyond a doubt wedded to the effective administration of justice."[1] Was he overly optimistic? As in every relationship, the intermix of psychiatry and law has had hills and valleys both in setting out legal policy and in resolving particular cases.

With the advent of Freudian psychiatric theory in the early part of the 20th century, psychological principles emphasizing unconscious motivation and determinism challenged and influenced society's views toward deviant behavior. Many crimes were redefined as mental health problems. The use or abuse of alcohol or drugs was labeled a disease, like asthma or diabetes. Sex offenders came to be known as "sexual psychopaths" and were confined in special institutions. Prevailing psychological concepts of child development infiltrated child custody cases. Juvenile misbehavior was classified as a problem of delinquency or neglect and received the special attention of juvenile courts.

About two centuries ago, the state began to take over many of the functions of the church. Then, with the decline in the influence of religion, law and psychiatry played a more prominent role in the resolution of human conflict and controversy. (Islam is surging, however, as is fundamentalism and Orthodox Judaism among young people.) Psychiatry has replaced—or at least infiltrated—religion, which had been the foundation of law.[2] The very word *sin* has disappeared from our vocabulary and has been replaced by psychiatric terminology. Such changes affect the way we think because we do so in words. The conversion of major church buildings into restaurants and centers of psychotherapy—as seen in many places—is a visible answer to Dr. Karl A. Menninger's question: "Whatever became of sin?" in a book by that title.[3] Hymns and hallelujahs have been replaced by jazz, rock and roll, and punk music. Over a century ago, Anton Chekhov, the celebrated writer who was also a physician, wrote, "[I]f mankind really learns to alleviate its sufferings with pills and drops, it will completely abandon religion and philosophy, in which it has hitherto found not merely protection from all sorts of trouble, but even happiness."[4]

Following World War II, the impact of psychiatry and psychology was so total as to leave no area of American society unaffected. Psychologists and psychiatrists became known figures in most communities, in the media, and in virtually every corner of popular culture. A visitor from Mars, lacking familiarity with psychiatry, would make little sense of much of contemporary America. Freud's popularizers succeeded in placing his theories, however imperfectly understood, in the public domain. For about half a century after Freud's visit to the United States in 1911, Freudian psychoanalysis permeated the American psyche. His theories were seized upon, popularized, and bastardized (Figure I.1). Freud's theories even appeared in the comic strips (Lucy in Charles Schulz's popular "Peanuts" provided psychiatric care for 5¢). Freud's cultural

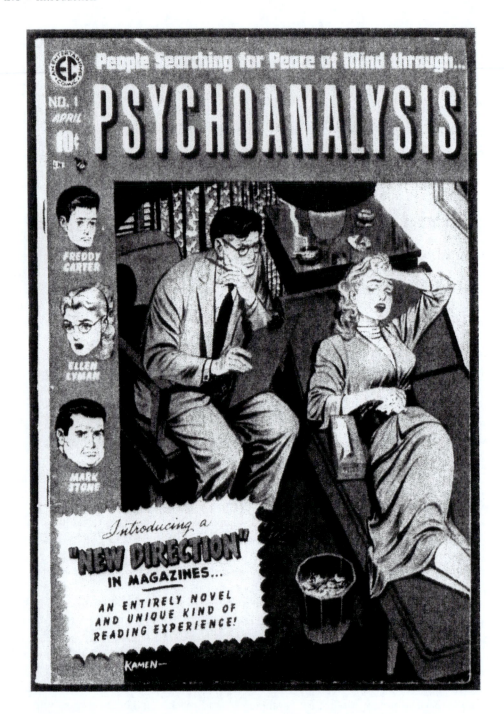

Figure I.1 Psychoanalysis pervades mass culture

status was most succinctly stated by the poet W.H. Auden: "To us he is no more a person/Now but a whole climate of opinion."[5] That phenomenon led the eminent sociologist Philip Rieff to speak in the 1950s of the "tyranny of psychology" and later, in 1966, to publish an influential analysis of American culture titled *The Triumph of the Therapeutic*. In that now classic book he observed that "psychological man" has replaced "Christian man" as the dominant character type in our society.[6]

In the years preceding World War I, there was considerable interest in Europe—especially in Germany—in the psychology of testimony. In 1906, Sigmund Freud delivered to a law class at the University of Vienna a lecture titled "Psychoanalysis and the Ascertaining of Truth in Courts of Law," in which he said:

> There is a growing recognition of the untrustworthiness of statements made by witnesses, at present the basis of so many judgments in Courts of Law; and this has quickened in all of you, who are to become judges and advocates, an interest in a new method of investigation, the purpose of which is to lead the accused person to establish his own guilt or innocence objectively. This method is of a psychological and experimental character and is based upon psychological research; it is closely connected with certain views, which have only recently been propounded in medical psychology.[7]

The task of the judge, Freud claimed, is the same as the task of the therapist: He must discover the hidden psychic material. "To do this," Freud said, "we have invented various methods of detection, some of which lawyers are now going to imitate." Yet he cautioned: "It is necessary to consider [the] points of difference in the psychological situation in the two cases."

Was Freud, while cautious, naive in his assumption that psychoanalysis has something to offer in ascertaining the truth in courts?[8] Freud failed his examination in medical jurisprudence—his only academic failure—but he was not naive about the law. At one time he seriously considered the study of law instead of medicine, perhaps because of the discrimination and persecution that he had endured. When, in 1938, he was exiled from his country, he carried a manuscript on Moses, the supreme lawgiver of the Jewish people. He was intensely interested in law and criminal behavior, but apart from his lecture on psychoanalysis and the ascertainment of truth, he was exceedingly pessimistic about the possible application of psychoanalysis to the legal process.

In 1924, Colonel McCormick of the *Chicago Tribune* offered Freud $25,000 or anything he named to come to Chicago to "psychoanalyze" Nathan Leopold and Richard Loeb, presumably to demonstrate that they should not be executed for the murder they had committed. Having heard that Freud was ill, McCormick was prepared to charter a special liner so that Freud could travel undisturbed by other company. In a letter to George Seldes of the *Chicago Tribune* who had extended the invitation on behalf of McCormick, Freud responded: "In reply I would say that I cannot be supposed to be prepared to provide an expert opinion about persons and a deed when I have only newspaper reports to go on and have no opportunity to make a personal examination. An invitation from the Hearst Press to come to New York for the duration of the trial I have had to decline for reasons of health."[9]

At the time of the case, psychology in the United States had moved to a position of considerable authority. The publications of American professors of psychology multiplied rapidly, so much so that by the 1920s psychology was the only science in which America surpassed Europe. In the 1920s, Freudian theory, as well as behaviorism, began to dominate the ethos of the country and books that popularized psychology appeared regularly on the list of American bestsellers. The public wondered how two brilliant teenagers from wealthy and cultured Chicago homes could in cold blood arbitrarily select a young boy, Loeb's cousin, an acquaintance for murder. Would psychology or psychiatry have the answer?

Leopold and Loeb were friends and lovers. For the thrill of it, they planned to commit the "perfect murder." They confessed to the killing and their motivation. In the sentencing phase of the trial, the prominent attorney Clarence Darrow called three psychiatrists who subscribed to a medicalizing ideology—Bernard Glueck, William Healy, and William Alanson White; all three hoped to expand the influence of psychiatry in the courtroom and to deny the role of free will. They shifted focus of the case from the sociopathy of Leopold and Loeb to the ordinariness of abnormal male behavior in the wake of a World War where youths of the same age learned to kill without conscience.

It has been suggested that if the case had occurred in Germany, Austria, or France, the Jewish identity of the criminals would undoubtedly have provided the most acceptable explanation for decadence because continental psychologists tended to contrast the Aryan and the Jewish psyches. In the United States, despite the rising anti-Semitism of the early and mid-1920s, the Jewishness of Leopold and Loeb was not newsworthy; on the contrary, the press sympathetically emphasized the essential similarity of the Leopold and Loeb families to those of other Americans.[10] Likely, their Jewishness was not mentioned because the victim was also Jewish.

Even more pessimistic than Freud about the application of psychoanalysis to the legal process, Theodore Reik of the Freudian circle wrote that psychoanalysis has no contribution to make to evidence of guilt in a particular case, as it is concerned with mental (inner) reality rather than material (outer) reality.[11]

In any event, not long after Freud's lecture, Hugo Munsterberg, a professor of psychology at Harvard who had emigrated from Germany, in a book titled *On the Witness Stand* suggested that prospective witnesses be tested for reliability in experimental situations before their testimony could be accepted in court. He severely criticized the legal profession for its failure to apply psychological principles to the evaluation of testimony.[12]

John Wigmore, whose name is synonymous with the law of evidence, quickly took Munsterberg to task. In an article in 1909, satirically cast in the form of a lawsuit against Munsterberg for defamation of the legal profession, Wigmore asked: "[W]here are the exact and precise experimental and psychological methods of ascertaining and measuring the testimonial certitude of witnesses?" Tell us, Wigmore urged, about the methods that might be applicable to judicial practice. Wigmore pleaded ignorance to the exactness and practical utility of these wonderful methods that the legal profession had persisted in rejecting or ignoring.[13]

Though he mocked Munsterberg, Wigmore did not rule out hope that science might one day help the law distinguish truth from falsehood. In 1923, in the second edition of his monumental *Treatise on the Anglo-American System of Evidence*, he asserted, "If there is ever devised a psychological test for the valuation of witnesses, the law will run to meet it." Indeed, he had come to believe that science was on the verge of making such a test practicable. Guilty knowledge left a trace as surely as a fingerprint, he wrote.[14]

Not until the spectacular trial of Alger Hiss, in the early 1950s, did the issue of psychiatric evaluation of a witness again attract much attention. Hiss, chairman of the Carnegie Foundation for Peace and the fair-haired boy of the Democratic Party, was accused by Whittaker Chambers of having passed secrets to Communists in the 1930s. The fate of the Democratic Party was at stake, Senator Joe McCarthy having charged it with 20 years of treason. Dr. Carl Binger, a renowned Harvard psychiatrist, testified that Chambers, the principal government witness, was a "psychopath with a tendency toward making false accusations." Binger testified that his opinion was based on "personal observation of Mr. Chambers at the first trial for five days and one day at this trial" and that he had "read plays, poems, articles, and book reviews by Mr. Chambers and books he had translated from German." Binger was the author of what the Hiss defense called the "theory of unconscious motivation." He claimed that Chambers's accusations were rooted in an obsession with Hiss that began in the mid-1930s when the two men had briefly known each other.[15] On cross-examination, however, Binger's testimony that Chambers was a "psychopathic liar" was discredited, and to this day that cross-examination, a high point of the Hiss trial, is used as a model in trial advocacy programs. The case also appears in every evidence casebook used in law schools. Supporting Binger's belief in Hiss's innocence, psychoanalyst

Meyer A. Zeligs, in a 476-page book, surmised that a latent homosexual relationship prompted Chambers to falsely accuse Hiss,[16] but that contention apparently convinced no one other than psychoanalysts. A near avalanche of books has supported Chambers.[17]

In the 1930s and 1940s, Jerome Frank, judge on the United States Court of Appeals, Second Circuit, and a professor of evidence at the Yale Law School, had spoken of judging in psychoanalytic terms. The likelihood of unconscious wishes and reactions affecting the behavior of judges so concerned him that he suggested in one book that every judge "should undergo something like a psychoanalysis."[18] In an earlier book he sought to demonstrate that the law often functions as an unconscious parent symbol.[19] Indeed, it was his belief that many of the public's mistaken ideas and exaggerated expectations concerning the law—including the idea that the law is or ought to be completely definite, entirely predictable, and capable of coping with practically every conceivable controversy—mirrored the displacement of unconscious ideas and expectations of childhood regarding the father onto the law. Likewise, he believed that attacks on the law (including the rejection of the law) reflected the unconscious directing of father-oriented hostility and disappointment onto the law.

At Yale University, psychiatrist Lawrence Z. Freedman, together with political scientist Harold D. Lasswell, founded Yale's study unit in psychiatry and law. Freedman was chairman of the unit from 1953 to 1960, at which time he moved to the University of Chicago. In the 1950s and early 1960s, Freedman took part in formulating the test of criminal responsibility of the American Law Institute (ALI), which expanded the *M'Naghten* test to include the impact of mental illness not only on cognition, but also on control. The rule reads as follows: "A person is not responsible for criminal conduct if at the time of such conduct as a result of mental disease or defect he lacks substantial capacity either to appreciate the criminality [wrongfulness] of his conduct or to conform his conduct to the requirements of the law." The ALI test proved to be a popular one, with a majority of the country's jurisdictions adopting it over the next two decades, but soon after the insanity acquittal of John Hinckley in 1982, the federal government and many states removed the volitional prong. Today only about 20 states recognize volitional impairment as a basis for an insanity defense. An obituary about Freedman was captioned: "Lawrence Freedman, 85, Dies; Peered Into Killers' Psyches."[20] In 1980, he had testified for the defense in the murder trial of John Wayne Gacy, who was later executed for the murders of 33 men and boys. He subsequently used his investigations into the psychological backgrounds of killers to build profiles of would-be presidential assassins for the Secret Service.

To return to the 1960s, it was in 1967 that Jay Katz, a psychoanalyst on the Yale law faculty; Joseph Goldstein, a law professor also at Yale who was steeped in psychoanalysis; and Alan M. Dershowitz of Harvard Law School collaborated in producing an 822-page collection of readings in legal and psychoanalytic thought for use by law students.[21] The study of psychiatry and law became a seminar or course in many law schools, though it has not become a subject on the bar examination. In 1968, Dr. Andrew S. Watson, a professor of psychiatry and a professor of law at the University of Michigan, published *Psychiatry for Lawyers*, which has a foreword by David L. Bazelon, Chief Judge of the U.S. Court of Appeals, District of Columbia. Watson urged lawyers to explore the contributions behavioral science may be able to make to the legal system. In his book he presented an outline of human behavior and development, and related this to some of the problems of the law.[22]

In recent years two prominent psychiatrists, Alan A. Stone and Paul S. Appelbaum, who have written and lectured extensively on psychiatry and law, were elected to the presidency of the American Psychiatric Association. They have cautioned psychiatrists regarding assessment of dangerousness and informed consent, and they have pondered over the ethics of forensic psychiatry. Thomas Gutheil and Phillip Resnick over the years have presented well-attended courses in psychiatry and law. Dr. Paul McHugh, past chairman of the Johns Hopkins Department of

Psychiatry, while not usually known as a forensic psychiatrist, has testified frequently and, along with Dr. Harold I. Lief and Professor Frederick Crews, has been at the forefront in challenging the "revival of memory" of childhood sexual abuse and multiple personality.[23]

For many years psychological notions have played an important role in child custody disputes. In the early 1970s, Anna Freud, Sigmund Freud's daughter, came to Yale University to join law professor Joseph Goldstein and Dr. Albert Solnit of the Department of Psychiatry in writing about child custody. They suggested that a decision on custody be made quickly (because of the child's perspective of time) and that when a decision had been made on placement with one parent, there should be no court-required visitation with the other parent. In those situations in which a court order is necessary for the visitation, they said, the visitation is more likely to be unfavorable to the child's development. They believed the court to be too blunt an instrument to rule on the vagaries of child rearing.[24] Most lawyers would argue, however, that leaving the control of visitation to the custodial parent would all too often result in the termination of visitation; even more, they say, the children would be the victims of a continuing feud between the parents. No state adopted the proposal. On the other hand, their recommendations on factors that should be considered in awarding custody have been studied and followed by judges and legislators.

In all criminal cases the cardinal question to be answered pertains to motivation. The same criminal act can be the result of self-defense, of negligence, or of intent; therefore, the motivation of the perpetrator is what decides society's reaction to the act. Allegedly, the psychiatric expert can aid the court in ascertaining the motivation. It has been said that if Freud's thesis that behavior is determined by both conscious and unconscious motivation is true, the offender will be able to offer only a partial explanation of what he did and why he did it; he cannot account for his often decisive unconscious motivations.[25] In the essay "Criminality from a Sense of Guilt," Freud suggested that guilt feelings may originate from repressed antisocial cravings, and that those cravings and feelings may often be the chief determinants of criminal acts.[26] In other words, a sense of guilt may precede rather than follow a criminal act. According to this theory, the individual who is punished for his transgressions is relieved temporarily from the unconscious sense of guilt. The theory explains why so many offenders commit inept crimes and practically invite apprehension. It explains "suicide by cop" where an individual induces a police officer to shoot.

Extending Freud's thesis, Dr. Franz Alexander went on to become one of the first from a psychoanalytic frame of reference to challenge existing legal methods of dealing with offenders. With a Berlin lawyer, Hugo Staub, he studied a series of cases in which they suspected unconscious motivations as predominant factors. Their thesis was published in 1929 in *The Criminal, the Judge and the Public*.[27] They did not, however, set out a road map on how to implement their theory in the legal system.

Carrying forward the work begun by Alexander, Dr. Karl A. Menninger (who had been analyzed by Alexander) wrote about man's self-destructiveness in *Man Against Himself* (1938). Menninger was renowned as dean of American psychiatry. In this book, which he later called his best, Menninger wrote, "In the end each man kills himself in his own selected way, fast or slow, soon or late. We all feel this, vaguely; there are so many occasions to witness it before our eyes. The methods are legion, and it is these [that] attract our attention. Some of them interest surgeons, some of them interest lawyers and priests, some of them interest heart specialists, some of them interest sociologists."[28]

Menninger compared people to tightrope walkers who try to reach and keep a balance. In his book *The Vital Balance* (1963),[29] which he wrote shortly before undertaking *The Crime of Punishment* (in which I had a hand), he set forth his view of "mental illness," to wit, the persistent failure to cope with internally or externally induced stresses. Every individual, constantly exchanging with his or her environment, tries to make the best bargain possible with it, considering its threats, demands, opportunities, and dangers. To end a crisis, from birth trauma to an ingrown toenail, one needs an "anticrisis" in order to achieve that vital balance, or "homeostasis," to use a biological term. Overstresses may build beyond ordinary control and threaten to upset internal balances. Sometimes an assist from one's family or friends, pastor, or physician may reduce the tensions. Sometimes the assistance is food or drugs. It is often purely happenstance what the manifestation of the imbalances is called and what type of help the individual receives—medical, legal, social, or pastoral. The commission of a criminal act, Menninger suggested, may be the result of an endeavor to achieve that vital balance.

In *The Crime of Punishment* (1968),[30] Menninger set out and elaborated his lifelong view that "all the crimes committed by the jailed criminals do not equal in total social damage that of the crimes committed against them."[31] He decried the shame of prisons. He circulated his manuscript among the staff at the Menninger Foundation soliciting a title; the result was a play on Dostoevsky's *Crime and Punishment*, but the choice gave rise to the impression that Menninger ignored individual responsibility or subverted the rule of law. The book got much publicity, some favorable, some not. It was said: "He doesn't want to punish anyone." "He wants to let all the criminals out on the street." Those charges bewildered him. In fact, he urged that everyone, whether epileptic or delusional, or whatever the unconscious motivation, be held responsible for his acts. As Menninger put it, "It was *his* act; who else's? It was not mine." He thought the law was confused in requiring a "voluntary act" and "*mens rea*." He advocated that *everyone* be held accountable for his or her behavior, but that the disposition be tailored to the individual case, just as in medicine. He did not consider the implications of unfettered discretion of the decision maker on the rule of law.

Menninger urged that psychiatrists be excluded from testifying at trial. Their place is not in the courtroom, he maintained, but rather, after the case has been tried, their role should be to carry out an examination and render a report setting out the potentialities of the offender, his liabilities, and the possible remedies. With Menninger as the motivating force, the Kansas State Reception and Diagnostic Center was established in 1961, its purpose to "provide a thorough and scientific examination and study of all felony offenders of the male sex sentenced by the courts … to state penal institutions so that each such offender may be assigned to a state penal institution having the type of security (maximum or minimum) and programs of education, employment, or treatment designed to accomplish a maximum of rehabilitation for such offender."[32]

In order to implement the purpose of the center, it being concerned only with postsentence evaluation, Kansas enacted a law giving the trial judge the unusual authority to modify a sentence after its imposition, so as to take into account the center's report.[33] The trial judge could modify a sentence within 120 days after its imposition and grant probation. Because the court could reduce but not increase the original sentence following the center's report, there was a tendency in initial sentencing to impose the maximum. The convicted person was selected by the court to be sent to the center for a maximum 60-day period of evaluation, (the center could not evaluate all offenders), and during this time the inmate usually tried to con the examiner, putting on acts of subservience. Operation of the center cost approximately five times more per inmate than prison, a fact that some legislators found difficult to justify. The center was closed in 1997, as were other state institutions during the 1990s.

A postsentence examination often comes too late. By that time, the offender has already been evaluated by the police, the district attorney, and the judge or jury. In effect, examination by the clinic is a fourth evaluation, so it should come as no surprise that most of the recommendations made at this time suggested that the offender be kept in custody. Moreover, the type of person referred by the judge was usually one who was an annoyance to him (*e.g.*, bad check writers). Initiation of the psychiatric examination was thus left to the judge who was generally unfamiliar with the symptoms of mental disorders, and recommendations made by the staff at the center were often impractical. The examining psychiatrist tended to be unfamiliar with the institutions to which the inmate could be sent and so was not in a position to make recommendations that could be realistically carried out.

The concept of a court clinic or forensic center had its origin in 1909, when William Healy began his pioneer work in Cook County Juvenile Court in Chicago. At first, the idea spread quickly, and in the early 1920s clinics were established either informally or by legislative act in a number of cities. However, the trend lagged during the war and postwar years. Then too, the more recent sentencing guidelines and mandatory minimum sentences give a lesser role to evaluation in the posttrial phase of a criminal proceeding. The guidelines focus on the nature of the offense, with little attention paid to the nature of the actor. The exercise of discretion in considering the actor's mental state or capacity now occurs almost entirely in the pretrial and trial stages of prosecution. A psychodynamic formulation in a report by a forensic examiner to an attorney, expressed in ordinary language, may assist in the settlement of a case—over 96% of criminal cases are plea bargained, and about the same number of civil cases are settled. Over 70% of acquittals by reason of insanity result from plea bargaining.[34] More or less, a psychiatric evaluation of an accused person may influence alternative sentencing, mitigation of sentence, or plea bargaining.

In 1929, two committees, one representing the American Bar Association and the other representing the American Psychiatric Association, met to draft a position statement that advocated that every criminal and juvenile court have a psychiatric service to assist the court in the disposition of offenders. It resulted in the creation of clinics or forensic centers. The clinics or forensic centers that were established can be subsumed in either one or more of the following categories:

1. To conduct pretrial examinations to determine either the fitness of the defendant to stand trial or the legal responsibility of the defendant for the crime committed.
2. To carry out treatment and restoration of functions.
3. To conduct presentence examinations and prepare a report that the judge may use to determine the proper sentence or treatment for the offender.
4. To conduct postsentence examinations that may be for either of two purposes: preparation of a psychiatric history and recommendations for the treatment of the offender at the institution or penitentiary, to whichever he is sent; or recommendations as to the proper course of therapy to be allowed, if needed, when the offender is placed on probation.

In the past decade or two, treatment-oriented courts have developed in a number of jurisdictions. These special jurisdiction courts—called drug courts or mental health courts—mandate and monitor treatment. They are designed to apply a rehabilitative philosophy to certain types of cases. The assumption is that treatment and other types of problem-solving responses are more appropriate than punishment or institutionalization for certain types of individuals. Failure to comply with a treatment program results in a penal sanction or civil commitment.[35]

We may recall that in 1954, in the case of a housebreaker named Monte Durham, Judge David L. Bazelon ruled the trial inadequate because it had not permitted the expert witness to present his full testimony.[36] By asking whether the crime was the "product" of a mental disease or defect, the *Durham* rule gave more leeway for psychiatrists and others to tell the jury about the defendant. In the place of the *M'Naghten* rule, which focused on the impact of mental illness on an understanding of the nature and quality of an act, Bazelon formulated the Durham rule: "An accused is not criminally responsible if his unlawful act was the product of mental disease or defect." The phrase "mental disease or defect" was not modified by functional criteria as in

M'Naghten and, as a result, the courts had difficulty in dealing with the term. As the Durham rule did not ask whether the accused appreciated that the act was wrong, as under *M'Naghten*, it would be irrelevant in the case of a command hallucination whether the command came from God or the devil. According to the grapevine, Dr. Andrew Watson assisted Bazelon in the writing of the opinion.

An expansion of the insanity defense, Bazelon said, serves "to alert the community to the root causes of crime"—poverty and social degradation.[37] Harvard law professor Alan Dershowitz, who at one time clerked for Bazelon, has written that Bazelon wanted to open up the insanity test "to the urban poor whose crimes were the product of their upbringing, social conditions, and other deprivations."[38] Bazelon himself grew up in harsh poverty, and although he overcame his circumstances, he always identified with the poor and downtrodden, and he tended to excuse them. He observed that most "blue collar" crimes were committed by persons who had deprived, abusive, or traumatic childhoods. Because they were "ill" by what he considered to be psychiatric standards, Bazelon felt these persons should be treated instead of punished.[39] He equated social incompetence with illness. Dershowitz described Bazelon as "a remarkably innovative judge."[40] Years later, in a reversal, Dershowitz found disturbing the implications of race- or gender-specific excuses because they create generalizations about entire groups of people.[41]

Bazelon stated that the purpose of the Durham rule was to get good and complete psychiatric testimony. He sought to remove the shackles of *M'Naghten*. Bazelon thought he was helping not only offenders but psychiatry as well. He wrote: "I really cannot say it too strongly, psychiatrists have a great opportunity under a liberal rule like *Durham*, an opportunity to help reform the criminal law and also to humanize their own work and increase its relevance."[42] He advocated penal reform along psychiatric lines. Here is what he had in mind:

> [W]e have been assisted in the District of Columbia by the fact that we have a notable mental hospital, Saint Elizabeths, directed by Dr. Overholser, a leading figure in forensic psychiatry. Persons acquitted by reason of insanity are committed to that institution until recovered or until it is safe to return them to the community. The existence of such an institution, and of an automatic commitment procedure, has done a great deal to make the public feel more secure.[43]

In the euphoria that surrounded the decision, Menninger described it as "more revolutionary in its total effect than the Supreme Court decision regarding desegregation." Forensic psychiatrists Lawrence Z. Freedman, Manfred Guttmacher, and Winfred Overholser together published a statement recommending its wide adoption, saying, "The *Durham* decision permits free communication of psychiatric information." Dr. Gregory Zilboorg called it "a step toward enlightened justice." The American Psychiatric Association awarded Judge Bazelon a certificate of commendation proclaiming that "he has removed massive barriers between the psychiatric and legal professions and opened pathways wherein together they may search for better ways of reconciling human values with social society."

As it turned out, Bazelon rued the day that he had handed down his ruling. Instead of serving as a bridge between law and psychiatry, it resulted in confusion, a plethora of appeals, and scholarly debates about the complexities of the defense. In subsequent years, Menninger was embarrassed by his statement on its effect and did not like to be reminded of it.[44]

Bazelon's opinion attracted enormous attention, but had virtually no followers. The *Durham* test failed, Bazelon conceded, because it allowed the psychiatric profession to have too much say in determining how responsible a defendant is. Instead, in 1973, in *United States v. Alexander & Murdock*,[45] Bazelon argued in a dissent that the law should eliminate any requirement of mental disease or defect and instruct juries to acquit whenever the defendant's behavioral controls were so impaired "that he cannot justly be held responsible." Under such a test, a jury could conclude that the defendant's "rotten social background" rendered his actions inevitable and, therefore, not responsible. For "it is simply unjust to place people in dehumanizing social conditions, to do nothing about those conditions, and then to command those who suffer, 'Behave or else!'"

Judge Carl McGowan, writing the majority opinion in the case, said that Bazelon's radical position would result in abandoning responsibility. He wrote: "As courts, we administer a system of justice that is limited in its reach. We deal only with those formally accused under laws, which define criminal accountability narrowly. [The jury is to be reminded] that the issue before them for decision is not one of the shortcomings of society generally, but rather that of appellant Murdock's criminal responsibility for the illegal acts [which he had committed]."[46]

Bazelon retired as chief judge of the United States Court of Appeals for the District of Columbia in 1986, after 35 years on the court (he died in 1993, at the age of 83). For his decisions, particularly in the realm of insanity and criminal responsibility, he was lionized by mental health professionals. Among many honors by various mental health organizations, he was elected president of the American Orthopsychiatric Association.

A month after his death, at a gala affair in Washington, D.C., the Mental Health Law Project, the preeminent national legal advocate for children and adults with mental disabilities, celebrated its renaming as the Judge David L. Bazelon Center for Mental Health Law. Dr. Melvin Sabshin, medical director of the American Psychiatric Association, was on the celebration committee along with a number of other psychiatrists.

For psychiatrists to celebrate Bazelon is masochism, as forensic psychiatrist Emanuel Tanay aptly put it.[47] Although by all accounts Warren Burger was one of the least successful chief justices in the modern era, the honors for decisions on insanity and criminal responsibility go to him, not Bazelon. Burger had served with Bazelon on the D.C. Court of Appeals before his appointment to the Supreme Court. Between them there was spirited but bitter antagonism. Burger was not on the list of the more than 200 members of the celebration committee. He debunked Bazelon's decisions in the realm for which he was honored.[48] In the 1960s, on the D.C. Court of Appeals, one of the bitterest Bazelon–Burger feuds was waged over the application of psychiatry to criminal law. In memos and in published opinions, with Burger usually in dissent, the two judges battled over the handling of insanity pleas in criminal cases.

As Judge Frank would recommend, Bazelon was for years on the couch in psychoanalysis (which he acknowledged), and he studied (and misapplied) psychiatric literature. That was especially evident in Bazelon's opinion in *Miller v. United States*,[49] where he abandoned the common assumption about flight from the scene of a crime as being indicative of a consciousness of guilt. Instead he took the contrary position, and he said, the jury should be advised that flight does *not* indicate consciousness of guilt. Among other references from the psychiatric literature, he quoted from Freud's article "Psychoanalysis and the Ascertainment of Truth in Courts of Law":

> You may be led astray ... by a neurotic who reacts as though he were guilty even though he is innocent—because a lurking sense of guilt already in him assimilates the accusation made against him on this particular occasion. You must not regard this possibility as an idle one; you have only to think of the nursery, where you can often observe it. It sometimes happens that a child who has been accused of a misdeed denies the accusation, but at the same time weeps like a sinner who has been caught. You might think that the child lies, even while it asserts its innocence; but this need not be so. The child is really not guilty of the specific misdeed of which he is being accused, but he is guilty of a similar misdemeanor of which you know nothing and of which you do not accuse him. He, therefore, quite truly denies his guilt in the one case, but in doing so betrays his sense of guilt with regard to the other. The adult neurotic behaves in this way and in many other ways just as

the child does. People of this kind are often to be met, and it is indeed a question whether your technique will succeed in distinguishing such self-accused persons from those who are really guilty.[50]

Bazelon then went on to conclude:

When evidence of flight has been introduced into a case, in my opinion, the trial court should, if requested, explain to the jury, in appropriate language, that flight does not necessarily reflect feelings of guilt, and that feelings of guilt, which are present in many innocent people, do not necessarily reflect actual guilt. This explanation may help the jury to understand and follow the instruction which should then be given, that they are not to presume guilt from flight; that they may, but need not, consider flight as one circumstance tending to show feelings of guilt; and that they may, but need not, consider feelings of guilt as evidence tending to show actual guilt.[51]

Once again Burger took issue with Bazelon. While recognizing that flight is relevant evidence, he disagreed with giving the instruction fashioned by Bazelon and, indeed, of giving any instruction. He worried that it would only confuse the jury. In a dissenting opinion, he wrote:

Fact issues and the reasonable inferences from accepted fact are for juries—not judges—in criminal trials, and if we trust the jury system we do not need to attempt to guide every detail of jury deliberations. Left alone with a minimum of basic instructions juries can infuse the law with a sense of reality and can temper judicial technicality with the leaven of the common experience and community conscience. We should not attempt to limit the scope of jury deliberations by telling jurors to ignore their own experience and common sense, and in a case like the one before us, denigrate other evidence in the case, which plainly suggests that flight was indeed indicative of guilt.[52]

With the passage of time, Bazelon conceded his blunder in *Durham*, but he blamed psychiatric testimony. In a number of writings, he castigated psychiatrists for letting him down. In an oft-quoted statement, he said, "Psychiatry, I suppose, is the ultimate wizardry. My experience has shown that in no case is it more difficult to elicit productive and reliable expert testimony than in cases that call on the knowledge and practice of psychiatry ... . Unfortunately, in my experience, they try to limit their testimony to conclusory statements couched in psychiatric terminology."[53]

In another what may be regarded as a pie-in-the-sky opinion, *Lake v. Cameron*,[54] Bazelon, in a majority opinion, talked about "least restrictive alternative" (LRA) and ordered community placement rather than hospitalization of 60-year-old Mrs. Lake, who carried her worldly possessions around with her in a shopping bag, appearing disoriented and wandering about in the downtown crime-ridden district of the nation's capital. In a vigorous dissent, Burger quarreled with placing an investigatory burden on the trial court. He suggested that the burden of making an investigation of alternatives—if there are any—should be reserved for social agencies because the court is not equipped to carry out such specific inquiry or to resolve the social and economic issues involved. Burger also said, "This city [the nation's capital] is hardly a safe place for able-bodied men, to say nothing of an infirm, senile, and disoriented woman to wander about with no protection except an identity tag advising police where to take her." The LRA doctrine, enunciated by Bazelon, played an important role in the deinstitutionalization of the mentally ill. The end result is well known: The mentally ill are on the streets or in jail.

Depending on one's point of view, the Mental Health Law Project gets kudos or brickbats. During the tumultuous 1960s and 1970s, it was at the forefront in litigation to close mental hospitals. In the book *Madness in the Streets* (1990),[55] in a chapter titled "The Law Becomes Deranged," Rael Jean Isaac and Virginia C. Armat describe how the young lawyers in the project became enamored of antipsychiatry doctrine. Bruce Ennis, the "father of the mental health bar," called mental patients "prisoners of psychiatry." He and his followers were engaged in a "mental patient liberation movement."

In Burger's view, one of Bazelon's worst opinions was in 1966, in *Rouse v. Cameron*.[56] In that case Bazelon became the first appellate judge to say that civilly committed mental patients had a right to treatment, that the government, when holding people involuntarily, had an obligation to provide psychiatric care. Burger thought this was judicial activism at its worst. While psychiatrists would endorse a "right to treatment" (it is high-sounding), Burger could not find it in the Constitution or in legislation. Hospital staffs not enjoying immunity would have been opened up for lawsuits, or hospitals would be closed.

That is what happened in 1971 when in *Wyatt v. Stickney*,[57] a federal district court judge in Alabama ruled that involuntarily committed patients "unquestionably have a constitutional right to receive such individual treatment as will give each of them a realistic opportunity to be cured or to improve his or her mental condition." As the State of Alabama could not comply with that order, the end result was abandonment of civil commitment and the closure of hospitals. And that was actually the aim of the Mental Health Law Project. As Ennis wrote in *Prisoners of Psychiatry*,[58] "The goal should be nothing less than the abolition of involuntary hospitalization, and with it, the larger public mental hospitals." Most mental health professionals were unaware of the Project's aim in pursuing a "right to treatment."

In 1979, in a case that came before the Supreme Court, *Addington v. Texas*,[59] the Mental Health Law Project sought to introduce the "proof beyond a reasonable doubt" standard of criminal justice into the civil commitment process. With an appreciation of the consequences, then Chief Justice Burger, writing the opinion of the Court, said that the criminal law "beyond a reasonable doubt" standard was inappropriate because "given the lack of certainty and the fallibility of psychiatric diagnosis, there is a serious question as to whether a state could ever prove beyond a reasonable doubt that an individual is both mentally ill and likely to be dangerous."

As Chief Justice, Burger rendered another important decision in 1979 regarding civil commitment of minors. In *Parham v. J.R.*,[60] the question was presented as to what process is constitutionally due a minor whose parents or guardian seek state-administered institutional mental health care for the minor, and specifically whether an adversary proceeding is required prior to or after the commitment. The petitioner in the case challenged the traditional presumption of parental beneficence along with the role of the admitting physician as a neutral fact finder as being insufficient to protect minors. Burger, writing for the majority, turned back the challenge. He wrote, "Due process has never been thought to require that the neutral and detached trier of fact be law-trained or a judicial or administrative hearing officer ... . Surely, this is the case as to medical decisions, for neither judges nor administrative officers are better qualified than psychiatrists to render psychiatric judgments." And he noted: "One factor that must be considered is the utilization of the time of psychiatrists, psychologists, and other behavioral specialists in preparing for and participating in hearings rather than performing the task for which their special training has fitted them." The decision has been criticized by advocates for children's rights who point to abuses in the treatment of minors,[61] but a barrier to hospitalization is not a panacea for those abuses.

In one of the most important decisions of the last century—the school desegregation case of *Brown v. Board of Education* and consolidated cases—psychiatrists and social scientists testified at trial as to the harmful effects of state-imposed segregation on black children. On appeal, a statement to that effect was filed by 32 sociologists, anthropologists, psychologists, and psychiatrists who worked in the area of American race relations. To the question: "Does segregation of children in public schools solely on the basis of race, even though the physical facilities and other 'tangible' factors may be equal, deprive the children of the minority group of equal educational opportunities?" a unanimous Supreme Court responded: "We believe that it does." Chief Justice Earl Warren, writing for the Court, declared, "Separate educational facilities are inherently unequal." In a celebrated footnote, the Court cited the writings of Kenneth B. Clark, Max Deutscher, Simon Frazier, and Gunnar Myrdal. It is widely considered that the references were simply window dressing.[62]

To return to Freud's lecture to the law class in Vienna (the law has much to learn from psychiatry and psychoanalysis), but there must be caution in their application in a particular case. Ascertaining unconscious motivation or even conscious motivation is fraught with uncertainty. Thus, when sexual-psychopath legislation was enacted in the mid 20th century in various states (the predecessor to the current sex-predator laws), it was suggested that the concept of sex crime be made broad enough to include "any criminal act in which some type of sexual satisfaction is the motivating force of the crime." It is true that some persons with sex problems may obtain sexual stimulation and pleasure by committing arson or by plunging a knife into a woman's back, but there the victim has not been sexually offended, and it could only be inferred that the act might have some sexual significance. If the courts operated on the basis of such an inference, then practically anything under the sun could be labeled sexual. So interpreted, sexual psychopath legislation might encompass all criminal activity, not simply behavior traditionally outlawed as a crime such as rape.[63]

In psychoanalysis, where the analysand lies on a couch and free associates, dreams are said to be the royal road to the unconscious, but, as Theodore Reik argued, that may not be helpful in evaluating outer reality. In contrast to the observation of Justice Clark claiming that "psychiatry is beyond a doubt wedded to the effective administration of justice," others have not been so sanguine. Frederic Wertham, testifying on behalf of the defendant at a 1934 murder trial, said he believed that the accused had been temporarily insane, acting in a psychotic frenzy, but while he was on the stand, he took the opportunity to interject that he also believed that virtually all psychiatric testimony in criminal trials was specious. He made the statement at the risk of undermining his own testimony and the case of the defendant he had been called upon to help. The *New York Times* on the next day reported, "Alientists' Testimony Is Usually 'Bunk.'"[64] Wertham headed the psychiatric clinic connected to the New York Court of General Sessions, where he conducted evaluations of convicted felons (he also headed the movement to ban comic books that featured crime and violence).[65]

In a case in the 1950s that occasioned academic commentary, Marmion Pollard, for several years a member of the Detroit Police Department, robbed banks in an inept way. What motivated the robberies? His conscious need for money? His unconscious guilt feelings? An irresistible impulse? Psychiatrists testified for the defense that an unconscious desire to be apprehended and punished prompted his behavior.[66]

Judges unless they have been psychoanalyzed tend not to be receptive to psychoanalytic explanations, jurors even less so. In the case involving Marmion Pollard, the trial judge asked one of the psychiatrists to explain an apparent inconsistency with his attempts to escape and to deny his acts. The psychiatrist responded that although the defendant had an unconscious desire to be apprehended and punished, the more dominating desire for self-preservation asserted itself when the possibility of apprehension became direct and immediate. Then too, we may recall, kleptomaniacs have a compulsion to steal yet usually try to escape detection. Though Pollard was tried under the ALI test of criminal responsibility, which asks about volitional impairment as well as cognitive impairment, he was convicted (his sentence is not known).[67] However, in all states, be it under *M'Naghten* or ALI, severely abnormal compulsions may be taken into account in sentencing.

Formulating legislation on the basis of knowledge of human behavior must be distinguished from the resolution of a particular case. Any attempts in a particular case to base a decision on speculation or "expert testimony" about unconscious motives would put the reputation of the law at risk. The unconscious cannot be responsibly accessed in a legal proceeding. There are a number of factors in the legal setting that make it difficult, sometimes even impossible, to obtain a reliable psychiatric evaluation, inasmuch as a competent psychiatric evaluation rests on complete trust. In therapy the psychiatrist is totally on the patient's side, will not reveal information the patient has confided, and is primarily concerned with the patient's welfare rather than with that of society in general. Those are not the circumstances when an individual charged with a crime is being evaluated by a forensic expert.

At the turn of the 20th century and for nearly three-quarters of the century psychoanalytic theory was the mainstay of psychiatry, and psychoanalysis was regarded as the gold treatment for all kinds of disorders and also as a means for self-knowledge. For better or worse, during that time Bazelon was regarded by his colleagues and others as the spokesman of psychiatry or psychoanalysis on the judiciary.[68] Though the couch remains the symbol of psychiatry, the reality has changed in the 21st century. In 2001, the American Academy of Psychoanalysis changed its name to the American Academy of Psychoanalysis and Dynamic Psychiatry, as few of its members practiced psychoanalysis even part time. More and more, a psychodynamic interpretation of behavior is giving way to a diagnosis of "chemical imbalance" in the brain.

It may be recalled that Albert Einstein was not impressed by psychoanalysis. "It may not always be helpful to delve into the subconscious," he once said. "Our legs are controlled by a hundred different muscles. Do you think it would help us to walk if we analyzed our legs and knew the exact purpose of each muscle and the order in which they work?" Einstein never expressed any interest in undergoing psychoanalysis. "I should like very much to remain in the darkness of not having been analyzed," he declared. "I think Freud placed too much emphasis on dream theories. After all, a junk closet does not bring everything forth … . On the other hand, Freud was very interesting to read and he was also very witty. I certainly do not mean to be overly critical." Freud wrote to his colleague Sandor Ferenczi in 1927, "Einstein understands as much about psychology as I do about physics."[69]

Be that as it may, Freud and Einstein engaged in a public exchange of letters on psychology and the need for world government. The only method of containing aggression, they argued, was a world organization that had the power to police member nations. At the initiative of President Franklin Roosevelt, Freud and Einstein published the booklet "Why War?" Freud said to Einstein, "Why do we, you and I and many another, protest so vehemently against war, instead of just accepting it as another of life's odious importunities? For it seems a natural enough thing, biologically sound and practically unavoidable"?[70] In *Civilization and Its Discontents*, Freud cited *Homo homini lupus* (man is a wolf to man).[71] Religions persist in proclaiming the Apocalypse and the Day of Judgment.

Just as Judge Frank called on judges to undergo psychoanalysis, there have been calls for political leaders to do the same. In 1977, Egyptian president Anwar el-Sadat issued an invitation to mental health professionals to work side by side with diplomats. Query: Would it be designed to manipulate the public?[72]

Endnotes

1. T.C. Clark, "Introduction." M. Binder (Ed.), *Psychiatry in the Everyday Practice of Law.* (Eagan, MN: West, 2003), p. xiii.
2. As Freud would have it, psychoanalysis would become a substitute for religion. He rejected religious belief as a disguised infantile longing for a father's protection, and interpreted religious observances as ritual ways of defending the self against the incursion of unacceptable instinctive forces. In Freud's view, religion was no more than a universal obsessional neurosis. Marx called religion a narcotic. Psychoanalysis as the new religion is described in A. Storr, *Feet of Clay.* (New York: Free Press,1996), pp. 190–225.

3. New York: Hawthorn Books, 1973; reviewed in R. Slovenko, *Psychiatry and Criminal Culpability* (New York: Wiley, 1995), pp. 275–287. "Sin" came up in discussion by presidential hopefuls on the CNN program, "Faith and Politics" (June 4, 2007). John Edwards was asked whether he would be willing to discuss the "biggest sin you've ever committed." He paused, then said that the list is too long, and he added, "We all fall short, which is why we have to ask for forgiveness from the Lord." All of the candidates expressed belief in God and that they prayed. See P. Healy & M. Luo, "Edwards, Clinton and Obama Describe Journeys of Faith," *New York Times*, June 5, 2007, p. 20.

4. A. Chekhov, "Ward No. 6 (1892)", in D. Plante (Ed.), *Ward No. 6 and Other Stories* (New York: Barnes and Noble, 2003), p. 190. The Pew Forum on Religion and Public Life in 2008 reported (based on 35,000 interviews) that some 60% of Americans say religion is "very important" to them, compared with 12% for the French and 25% for the Italians, but 44% of American adults have switched religious affiliations at some point. People who leave one denomination for another may be more concerned with fulfilling their boutique church-going desires than with meeting the moral obligations of a religious group or the demands of a doctrine. Editorial, "God's country," *Wall Street Journal*, March 1–2, 2008, p. 8. Karl Marx famously called religion "the opium for the masses." Recent debunking of religion include R. Dawkins, *The God Delusion* (New York: Houghton Mifflin, 2006); S. Harris, *The End of Faith* (New York: W.W. Norton, 2004); C. Hitchens, *"god is not Great/How Religion Poisons Everything"* (New York: Twelve, 2007). Response: D. Aikman, *The Delusion of Disbelief* (Nashville, TN: Salt River, 2008); C. Hedges, *I Don't Believe in Atheists* (New York: Free Press, 2008).

5. See R.M. Restak, "Psychiatry in America," *Wilson Quarterly*, Autumn 1983, p. 95.

6. P. Rieff, *The Triumph of the Therapeutic/Uses of Faith After Freud* (New York: Harper & Row, 1996). See also J.D. Hunter, "When Psychotherapy Replaces Religion," *Public Interest*, Spring 2000, p. 5, excerpted from *The Death of Character* (New York: Basic Books, 2000).

7. (1906), in *Collected Papers* (London: Hogarth Press, 1955), vol. 2, pp. 13–24. Earlier Freud wrote, "He that has eyes to see and ears to hear may convince himself that no mortal can keep a secret. If his lips are silent, he chatters with his fingertips; betrayal oozes out of him at every pore." S. Freud, "Fragment of an Analysis of a Case of Hysteria" (1901), in *Collected Papers* (London: Hogarth Press, 1955), vol. 7, pp. 77–78.

8. It is widely believed that psychiatrists or psychoanalysts are omniscient and can straightaway know one's inner thoughts—they supposedly can "read minds" even in a brief encounter in whatever situation. For that reason, even in a social gathering, anxiety is aroused by their presence.

9. Letter dated June 29, 1924. See E. Jones, *The Life and Work of Sigmund Freud* (New York: Basic Books, 1957), vol. 3, p. 103. An excellent discussion of the Leopold and Loeb case and its background appears in S. Baatz, *For the Thrill of It* (New York: HarperCollins, 2008); excerpted in "Criminal Minds," *Smithsonian*, August 2008, pp. 70–79.

10. A.R. Heinze, *Jews and the American Soul* (Princeton, NJ: Princeton University Press, 2004), pp. 93, 367. See also H. Higdon, *Leopold and Loeb and the Crime of the Century* (Chicago: University of Illinois Press, 1999). It is now believed that Nathan Leopold is likely to have suffered from Asperger's Disorder and that Richard Loeb likely was an antisocial personality. See B.G. Haskins & J.A. Silva, "Asperger's Disorder and Criminal Behavior: Forensic-Psychiatric Considerations," *J. Am. Acad. Psychiat. & Law*, 34 (2006): 374.

11. T. Reik, *The Unknown Murderer*, reprinted in *The Compulsion to Confess* (New York: Farrar, Straus & Cudahy, 1959).

12. In his book *On the Witness Stand* (New York: Clark Boardman, 1923) and in a series of magazine articles, Hugo Munsterberg demonstrated how eyewitness testimony—even confessions—could be mistaken, how false memories could be planted by police interrogation, and how difficult it was for students to recall staged crimes accurately. In 1970, Munsterberg got a chance to try these truth-testing techniques in the most prominent trial of the time. Prosecutors in Idaho asked him to assess the honesty of Harry Orchard, a political assassin whose confession to the murder of the state's governor had implicated labor leaders. After testing, he assured prosecutors that he had "not the slightest doubt" Orchard was telling the truth. But he moderated his view after a labor leader "Big Bill" Haywood was acquitted. The press thereupon referred to Munsterberg as "Monsterwork." In any event, it was not long before other scientists echoed his hope that "truth-compelling machines" would soon be adopted by the courts. An article in the *New York Times* (September 11, 1907) predicted a time when judicial questions would be decided by impartial machinery. It wrote: "There will be no jury, no horde of detectives and witnesses, no charges and countercharges, and no attorney for the defense. These impediments of our courts will be unnecessary. The state will merely submit all suspects in a case to the tests of scientific instruments, and as these instruments cannot be made to make mistakes nor

tell lies, their evidence would be conclusive of guilt or innocence, and the court will deliver sentence accordingly." Quoted in K. Adler, *The Lie Detectors/The History of an American Obsession* (New York: Free Press, 2007), p. 47.

13. J.H. Wigmore, "Professor Munsterberg and the Psychology of Testimony," *Ill. L. Rev.* 3(1909): 999. Functional imaging as a substitute for polygraph tests has recently become a highly debated topic in academic, commercial, government, and legal communities. Recent brain imaging studies using functional magnetic resonance imaging (MRI) maintain distinct neural circuitry is engaged during false versus true responses. It is highly unlikely that it will meet the standards at trial for scientific evidence, demonstrate its probative value and lack of prejudicial effect, and not intrude into the province of the fact-finder. See D.D. Langleben *et al.*, "Telling Truth From Lie in Individual Subjects With Fast Event-Related fMRI, *Human Brain Mapping,* 26 (2005): 262.

14. J.H. Wigmore, *A Treatise on the Anglo-American System of Evidence in Trials at Common Law,* (Boston: Little, Brown, 2nd ed., 1923), vol. 1, p. 544.

15. *United States v. Hiss,* 88 F. Supp. 559 (S.D. N.Y. 1950). To this day the courts are divided on the admissibility of psychiatric opinion on the credibility of a witness. See Chapter 6 on credibility of witnesses.

16. M.A. Zeligs, *Friendship and Fratricide/An Analysis of Whittaker Chambers and Alger Hiss* (New York: Viking Press, 1967).

17. A summary of some of the books appears in M.K. Beran, "To Be as Gods," *Claremont Review of Books,* Fall 2004, p. 36; see also T.P. Gorman, "Spies, and a Witness to Analyze," *Litigation* 30 (2004): 53–60.

18. J. Frank, *Courts on Trial* (Princeton, NJ: Princeton University Press, 1949), p. 250.

19. J. Frank, *Law and the Modern Mind* (New York: Tudor, 1936), pp. 8–21.

20. Obituary by A. McCulloch, *New York Times,* Oct., 2004, p. C-12.

21. J. Katz, J. Goldstein, & A.M. Dershowitz (Eds.), *Psychoanalysis, Psychiatry and Law* (New York: Free Press, 1967).

22. A.S. Watson, *Psychiatry for Lawyers* (New York: International Universities Press, 1968).

23. See P.R. McHugh, "Psychiatric Misadventures," *American Scholar,* Autumn 1992, pp. 497–510; reprinted in P.R. McHugh, *The Mind Has Mountains* (Baltimore, MD: Johns Hopkins University Press, 2006), pp. 3–17; see also pp. 129–143. See also S. Jacoby, *The Age of American Unreason* (New York: Pantheon Books, 2008), pp. 224–225.

24. J. Goldstein, A. Freud, & A.J. Solnit, *Beyond the Best Interest of the Child* (New York: Free Press, 1973).

25. F.G. Alexander & A.J. Selesnick, *The History of Psychiatry* (New York: Harper & Row, 1966), p. 432.

26. S. Freud, "Criminality from a Sense of Guilt: Some Character Types I Have Met in Psychoanalytic Work," in *Collected Papers,* (London: Hogarth Press, 1955) vol. 4, pp. 342–344.

27. New York: Free Press, 1929.

28. K.A. Menninger, *Man Against Himself* (New York: Harcourt, Brace & World, 1938), p. vii.

29. New York: Viking Press, 1963.

30. New York: Viking Press, 1968.

31. *Ibid.,* 138.

32. Kansas Stat. Ann. 76-24ao3.

33. Kansas Stat. Ann. 62-2239.

34. J. Rogers *et al.,* "Insanity Defenses: Contested or Conceded?" *Am. J. Psychiatry,* 141 (1984): 885.

35. L.B. Erlich, *Textbook of Forensic Addiction Medicine and Psychiatry* (Springfield, IL: Thomas, 2001); Symposium, "Specialty Courts," *Int. J. Law & Psychiat.* 26 (2003): 1–110; A.J. Grudzinskas & J.C. Clayfield, "Mental Health Courts and the Lesson Learned in Juvenile Court," *J. Am. Acad. Psychiat. & Law* 32 (2004): 223; D.P. Lay, "Rehab Justice," *New York Times,* Nov. 18, 2004, p. 29.

36. Durham v. United States, 214 F.2d 862 (D.C. Cir. 1954).

37. D.L. Bazelon, *Questioning Authority/Justice and Criminal Law* (New York: Knopf, 1988).

38. A.M. Dershowitz, *Chutzpah* (New York: Simon & Schuster, 1991), p. 58.

39. Personal communication (April 5, 1993) from Dr. Norman Q. Brill, one of Bazelon's friends, to Ralph Slovenko.

40. A.M. Dershowitz, *op. cit. supra* note 38.

41. A.M. Dershowitz, *The Abuse Excuse* (Boston: Little, Brown, 1994).

42. D.L. Bazelon, "Equal Justice for the Unequal," (Isaac Ray Award Lecture, 1961), reprinted in D.L. Bazelon, *Questioning Authority/Justice and Criminal Law* (New York: Knopf, 1988).

43. *Ibid.*

44. Personal communication to Ralph Slovenko.

45. 471 F.2d 923 (D.C. Cir. 1973).

46. 471 F.2d at 965, 968.
47. Personal communication to Ralph Slovenko.
48. R. Slovenko, "Should Psychiatrists Honor Bazelon or Burger?" *J. Psychiat. & Law* 20 (1992): 635.
49. 320 F.2d 767 (D.C. Cir. 1963).
50. 320 F.2d at 772.
51. 320 F.2d at 773.
52. 320 F.2d at 775.
53. Rollerson v. United States, 343 F.2d 269, at 271 (D.C. Cir. 1964).
54. 364 F.2d 656 (D.C. Cir. 1966).
55. New York: Free Press, 1990.
56. 373 F.2d 451 (D.C. Cir.).
57. 344 F. Supp. 387 (M.D. Ala.).
58. New York: Harcourt, Brace & Jovanovich, 1974.
59. 441 U.S. 418 (1979).
60. 442 U.S. 584 (1979).
61. J. Sharkey, *Bedlam* (New York: St. Martin's Press, 1994).
62. 347 U.S. 483 11 (1954). Psychiatrist Fredric Wertham, famous for his crusade against the depiction of crime in comic books, claiming that they led to juvenile delinquency, carried out a study on the psychological effects of segregation on African Americans that was used by the Supreme Court in the *Brown* decision. See L. Menand, "The Horror," *New Yorker*, March 31, 2008, p. 124.
63. Since 1990, 16 states (Arizona, California, Florida, Illinois, Iowa, Kansas, Massachusetts, Minnesota, Missouri, New Jersey, North Dakota, South Carolina, Texas, Virginia, Washington, and Wisconsin) have enacted new laws called "sexual predator laws" to confine mentally abnormal and dangerous sex offenders in secure mental health facilities until it is safe to release them. The states have also passed community notification laws that allow or require law enforcement agencies to disclose the names and addresses of registered sex offenders to potential victims in the community.
64. *New York Times*, March 21, 1934. See Chapter 16 on sex offender legislation.
65. See D. Hajdu, *The Ten-Cent Plague* (New York: Farrar, Straus & Giroux, 2008). Dr. Karl A. Menninger, renowned as dean of American psychiatry, also was of the same opinion, but believed that psychiatric testimony should be used in posttrial proceedings. Two members of the staff of the Menninger Foundation, however—Dr. Herbert Modlin and Dr. Joseph Satten—testified frequently at trial. See K.A. Menninger, *The Crime of Punishment* (New York: Viking, 1968).
66. United States v. Pollard, 171 F. Supp. 474 (E.D. Mich. 1959). Near the end of his life, with his country in ruins largely because of his arrogant misrule, Benito Mussolini said: "I did not create fascism; I drew it from the Italians' unconscious minds. If that had not been so, they would not all have followed me for 20 years. I repeat, all of them, because a tiny, really microscopic minority can have no weight." R.J.B. Bosworth, *Mussolini's Italy: Life Under the Dictatorship, 1915–1945* (New York: Penguin Press, 2003).
67. Pollard entered a plea of NGRI. Three psychiatrists testified that at the time he committed the criminal acts, he knew the difference between right and wrong and knew that the acts he committed were wrong, but that he was suffering from a "traumatic neurosis" or "dissociative reaction," characterized by moods of depression and severe feelings of guilt. They further stated that he had an unconscious desire to be punished by society to expiate these guilt feelings, and that the governing power of his mind was so destroyed or impaired that he was unable to resist the commission of the criminal acts. The ALI test of criminal responsibility, under which Pollard was tried in Michigan, asks about volitional impairment as well as cognitive impairment as a result of mental illness. Mich. Comp. Laws § 768.21a (1).
68. Comment by Judge J. Skelly Wright, Bazelon's colleague on the D.C. Court of Appeals, in a personal communication to Ralph Slovenko. The author served as a commissioner for Judge Wright when he was a federal district court judge.
69. Quotes from W. Isaacson, *Einstein/His Life and Universe* (New York: Simon & Schuster, 2007) pp. 209, 366, 615.
70. Paris: Internationale Institute of Intellectual Co-operation, League of Nations (1933).
71. Quoted in C. Trueheart, "Organized Violence," *American Scholar*, Winter 2007, p. 141. The conditions that turn people into killers are well known: extreme coercion, obedience to authority, dehumanization of the victim, social bonding, hatred, indoctrination, revenge, survival. Alcohol or drugs can also help produce an "altered state" conducive to violence. Bloodletting can itself be intoxicating, even erotic. American soldiers in Vietnam are quoted as saying that killing was like "getting screwed for the first time," producing "an ache as profound as the ache of an orgasm." H. Slim, *Killing Civilians:*

Method, Madness and Morality in War (New York: Columbia University Press, 2008). See also J. Hillman, *A Terrible Love of War* (New York: Penguin, 2004). In an essay written during World War I, "Thoughts for the Times on War and Death," Freud argued that war signified the reassertion of primitive instincts that society had previously repressed. "When the frenzied conflict of this war shall have been decided," he wrote, "every one of the victorious warriors will joyfully return to his home, his wife and his children, undelayed and undisturbed by any thought of the enemy he has slain … . If we are to be judged by the wishes in our unconscious, we are, like primitive man, simply a gang of murderers … . Our unconscious is just as … murderously minded towards the stranger, as divided or ambivalent towards the loved, as was man in earliest antiquity … War … strips us of the later accretions of civilization and lays bare the primal man in each of us." Quoted in N. Ferguson, *The Pity of War* (New York: Basic Books, 1999), p. 357. See also N. Ferguson, *The War of the World* (New York: Penguin, 2007); J. Hillman, *A Terrible Love of War* (New York: Penguin, 2004).

72. See V. Volkan, *Blood Lines* (New York: Farrar, Straus & Giroux, 1997).

PSYCHIATRY IN LAW

PART I
Expert Testimony

1
Experts in the Adversary System

The adversary system is the distinguishing characteristic of Anglo-American justice, along with the importance attached to formal rules of evidence. The continental legal procedure, on the other hand, is without the formalism found in the Anglo-American system. Objections, such as "inadmissible evidence," "hearsay," "opinion," or "leading question," customary in an Anglo-American trial, are unknown in a continental trial. In Anglo-American law, the key to a fair trial is not only the presentation of evidence according to formal rules of evidence, but also the opportunity to use cross-examination, rebuttal evidence, and argument to meet adverse evidence. A cross-examining procedure, guaranteed by the confrontation clause of the Sixth Amendment to the U.S. Constitution, is at the very heart of the adversary system.

The adversary proceeding, in an impartial and public forum, provides a mechanism by which differences can be settled in a decision-making process that people generally trust. It provides a means of making even big government and big business accountable. The ability to assert a legal right in a proceeding where an individual has reasonable equality with his opponent buttresses self-image and sense of worth. It is the modern-day scene where David may defeat Goliath. To be sure, there are critics, particularly among losers. Charlie Chaplin in his autobiography said of the paternity suit that ruled against him, "Listening to the legal abracadabra of both attorneys, it seemed to me a game they were playing and that I had little to do with it."

Under the adversary system, the judge acts as arbiter to assure conformity to the rules of fair play that have evolved over time. The jury then decides the issues on the basis of those facts which the judge as a gatekeeper permits them to hear. Simply put, the adversary system is a process of contention in which the role of the lawyer is to initiate suit following the dispute, raise the issues, and propel the controversy. The judge does not venture forth like a Don Quixote seeking justice as he does under the inquisitorial system, which prevails in most countries. The inquisitorial judge has the responsibility to arrive at the truth by his own exertions in conjunction with those of the official prosecutor. Experimental studies lend support to the claim that an adversary form of presentation, in contrast to an inquisitorial presentation, counteracts bias in decision makers.

The physical setting of the courtroom reflects the system of justice. Under the adversary system, in civil and criminal cases, the chairs of the parties in the courtroom are situated on the same level, without benefit of elevation above the floor, and are equidistant from the judge. The parallel location of the parties is designed to indicate to judge and jury that the word of one counsel—prosecutor (plaintiff in civil cases) or defense counsel—carries no more weight than that of the other. The scales of justice are thus held evenly. In countries employing the inquisitorial system, the prosecutor has a place well above that of the defense counsel, and he carries, by virtue of that location, a certain majesty, hardly distinguishable from that of the judge. In all systems, a judge sits elevated, a position communicating dominance or superiority, representative of his symbolic authority and the finality of judgment under law.

In the Anglo-American adversary proceeding, the rules governing the action are as formal and ritualistic as those of an ancient tournament or a game of chess. Each side is charged with presenting the strongest possible case on its own behalf and expects to be countered with the strongest possible case by the adversary, creating conditions like those of an ancient tournament.

The adversary proceeding requires that the lawyers, like gladiators, carry out their task in a fair or sporting manner.

The adversary system is based on the theory that truth (or viewpoints) emerges best out of the open combat of ideas. While physicians are trained to discover medical truth, lawyers are trained to represent any point of view. The theory of the adversary system, as Professor Edmund Morgan once put it, is that "each litigant is most interested and will be most effective in seeking, discovering, and presenting the materials that will reveal the strength of his own case and the weakness of his adversary's case, so that the truth will emerge to the impartial tribunal that makes the decision."[1] Richard A. Posner, the venerable chief judge of the U.S. Court of Appeals for the Seventh Circuit, views the adversary system as relatively efficient—not ideal by any means, but better for Americans than feasible alternatives. In general, Judge Posner likes its competitiveness and the incentives it provides, and he supports the lay jury.[2]

The adversary system is also employed in nonlaw forums. The American Psychiatric Association at its annual meetings uses an adversary system to debate topics such as whether "depressive personality is a useful construct that should be included in *DSM-IV* (*Diagnostic and Statistical Manual of Mental Disorders*, 4th edition)." In the Roman Catholic Church, a postulator (a priest assigned to investigate the possibility that someone is a saint) goes before a church tribunal to argue the case for sainthood against another priest whose job is popularly known as "the devil's advocate."

The Widening Use of Expert Testimony

The potential use of expert testimony expands with wider knowledge of the world and as the world becomes more complicated. In the film *Bananas*, Woody Allen is a products tester trying out electrically heated toilet seats and coffins with piped-in music. As the modern age continues to become more complex, it is not surprising that modern litigation requires more expert opinion evidence than ever before. Not only is reliance on expert witnesses increasing, but new types of experts are developing.

At a time when trial by jury was not much developed, only two modes of using expert knowledge existed: first, to select as jurymen such persons as were especially fitted by experience to know the class of facts that were before them and, second, to call to the aid of the court skilled persons whose opinions it might adopt. The existence of the judge's power to call witnesses generally included the power to call expert witnesses who were regarded originally as *amici curiae* (friends of the court).

Technological advances along with the liberalization of the rules of evidence have prompted the use of a wider range of experts. In complex and technical cases, the expert is often crucial because the evidence is beyond the ken of the jury, but even in a single slip-and-fall case an expert may be used to establish the way premises are usually maintained. As recent as 30 years ago, nearly all tort cases were very simple. There was virtually no medical malpractice and mass injury, which today constitutes 40% of cases. New technologies have created "high stakes" litigation calling for expert testimony. As a consequence, the use of expert witnesses in recent years has been growing rapidly, but their use in courts is far from new. A 17th century treatise numbered as experts only five: locksmiths, cutlers, peruke makers, washerwomen, and rope makers.[3] Earlier courts called on physicians to help determine whether a defendant was "bewitched."

The concept of "expert" in litigation, however, does not necessarily mean being at the top in one's field. It includes anyone whose knowledge of a subject extends beyond that of the average juror. By legal definition, an "expert" is almost anybody who can reasonably be expected to know more about a given subject than the average person. As Rule 702 of the Federal Rules of Evidence puts it, anyone with "knowledge, skill, experience, training, or education" who can assist the trier of fact may qualify as an expert. Sometimes the choice of an expert may seem bizarre— a narcotics user has testified as an expert to the identification of a drug;[4] an "expert burglar" has qualified as an expert witness.[5] The court's ruling on the competency of the expert falls within its broad discretion and is reviewed under the abuse of discretion standard. The court's ruling is not reversed absent a showing of a clear abuse of discretion. The more complicated the expertise, the more likely the court is to be demanding about qualifications.

Along with the growing complexity of life, the liberalization of expert testimony rules in the last decade has had a prolific effect on the use of experts. Unlike an ordinary witness, an expert may now not only testify in the form of an opinion or otherwise, about the past or the future, but, in forming an opinion, rely on inadmissible evidence, such as hearsay, if "reasonably relied upon by experts in the particular field" (subject to the amendment in 2000 to Rule 703 as discussed in Chapter 2).[6] Evidence though relevant may be excluded, however, if it is likely to be confusing or misleading. The test, under Rule 403, is whether the probative value of the evidence is substantially outweighed by the danger of "confusion of the issues or misleading the jury."

A number of critics have charged that psychiatrists (and psychologists) have no useful place in the courtroom. These critics say that psychiatrists cannot answer forensic questions with reasonable accuracy, and they cannot help the fact-finder reach more accurate conclusions than would otherwise be available. In fact, they claim, the involvement of psychiatrists as expert witnesses is not only not helpful, but actually harmful as they mislead by testimony that has little scientific underpinning.[7]

In criminal trials, where so much controversy surrounds psychiatric testimony, we must recall that a trial is very much a morality play. A trial without a psychiatrist is usually dull—indeed, without psychiatric testimony, jurors tend to go to sleep. Psychiatric testimony makes headlines. The public wants some understanding of why the accused acted as he did. Without psychiatric testimony trials are not very interesting or satisfying. Indeed, the press even insists on obtaining and printing off-the-cuff comments by psychiatrists on any and all facets of life and behavior.

The "battle of the experts," as it is called, heightens tension, prompting the trier of fact to pay attention. It stimulates thought; it enhances the deliberations. The evidence can serve as a guideline that the jurors can integrate with their own moral, social, philosophical, and religious backgrounds to arrive at an appropriate decision.[8]

Psychiatric testimony, whether or not accepted, opens options to judge and jury. It brings flexibility and an element of humanity into the law. The jury, following their conviction of Jean Harris for the killing of the Scarsdale diet doctor, Dr. Herman Tarnower, wondered why no psychiatric testimony was presented. The jury wanted some excusing evidence, though it may have been conflicting, but got none. Whether in a given case judge or jury accepts or declines evidence is for them to decide, but without some testimony they may not be able to rationalize a decision they would like to return. The scale is the symbol of justice, but measurement alone would subvert the nature of a trial as a morality play. A trial, of course, has more to do with justice than show business, but a trial (especially a criminal trial) is, in large measure, a morality play.

The Doctrine of Judicial Notice

While the parties, and not the court, are responsible under the adversary system for gathering and presenting facts, there are many facts that need to be supplemented or cannot be established by formal proof. The doctrine of judicial notice recognizes the right or the necessity of the judge to notice evidence outside the record which is "a matter of general knowledge." The judicial notice apparatus, however, does not work well unless it is fed with information. Judge Frank of the Second Circuit once observed that judicial notice often amounts to nothing more than "cocktail hour knowledge." He suggested that "competently to inform ourselves, we should have a staff of investigators like those supplied to administrative agencies."[9]

Almost any case can be used to illustrate the need for, and the propriety of, supplying the court with information. The usual method of establishing adjudicative facts—the facts of the particular case—is through the introduction of evidence, ordinarily consisting of the testimony of witnesses, whereas judicial notice is the usual method of finding those facts having relevance to legal reasoning and the lawmaking process.

In judicial lawmaking a prominent illustration is *Durham v. United States*,[10] a decision subsequently cast aside, where Judge Bazelon, without support in the evidence developed at the trial, declared: "Medicolegal writers in large numbers … present convincing evidence that the right-and-wrong test is 'based on an entirely obsolete and misleading conception of the nature of insanity.'" The court had no hesitation in using this "convincing evidence" even though it was not in the record. In the landmark case of *Wolf v. Colorado*,[11] Supreme Court Justice Murphy wrote to district attorneys of various cities to learn of police practices there and obtained from their replies information that he used to confront the issue of illegally obtained evidence at trial. In the historic case in 1954 of *Brown v. Board of Education of Topeka*,[12] the Court cited Kenneth B. Clark and Gunnar Myrdal on the adverse effect of school racial segregation on personality development. Sociological and psychological theories also controlled the Court's separate-but-equal decision in *Plessy v. Ferguson*, decided in 1896, even though these theories were neither formally presented to the Court nor given formal recognition. In *Powell v. Texas*,[13] the Supreme Court resorted to various extra-record facts to determine the prevailing view of the medical profession concerning whether alcoholism is a disease.

Participation as *Amicus Curiae*

The role of the professional expert as *amicus curiae* is an important function in providing the court with information. Apart from testifying, professionals in a pertinent field can offer invaluable suggestions to an attorney preparing an *amicus curiae* brief on a point of law or of fact for the information of the judge. In recent decades, the role of the *amicus curiae* brief has expanded, and it is quite common now to see an organizational presentation of a brief. It constitutes a modification of the adversary system that provides a form of information gathering that is the judicial counterpart of lobbying and congressional hearing in the legislative process. Fairly speaking, it is often a "political statement" or "lobbying before the court."[14]

Should it be allowed? Permission to participate as a friend of the court is and has always been a matter of grace rather than of right. The theory of trial by duel between two contestants precludes an unlimited right of third persons to intervene or file a brief. "The fundamental principle underlying legal procedure," one court observed, "is that parties to a controversy shall have the right to litigate the same, free from the interference of strangers." The late Chief Justice Burger as well as many other judges was of the view that the role of the court is not to decide broad social issues, but rather to decide a contest between two litigants, and "friends" should remain outside the courtroom.

On the other hand, access to the judicial process on the part of third-party individuals or organizations is an extension of the view that the law is a process of social choice and policy making. The outcome of litigation indirectly affects interests other than those formally represented. Groups organized to promote altruistic goals are likely, as *amici*, to represent important widespread public interests. Organizational participation in the judicial process focuses public attention on the judge's decision, and as a consequence, he is particularly cautious and deliberate in these cases. The National Association for the Advancement of Colored People (NAACP), almost from its inception, has participated as *amicus curiae* in litigation. The American Civil Liberties Union (ACLU) also found early on that the *amicus curiae* brief is a useful instrument in drawing widespread attention to its causes. The American Jewish Congress over the past years is one of the most active filers of *amicus curiae* briefs.

The American Medical Association, American Psychiatric Association, American Psychological Association, and American Orthopsychiatric Association (Ortho) at one time or another have participated as *amici* on various mental health issues. These associations, however, have no rational scheme for submitting *amici* briefs or instituting suit, but do so when attention is called by their attorneys, staffs, or interested members to a particular case judged directly relevant to their field, and if there are sufficient time and money. One or another of these associations—in a happenstance, often fortuitous manner—has submitted briefs on issues of criminal responsibility, competency to stand trial, admissibility of expert testimony by psychologists, psychological test validity in assessing employment placement, privileged confidential communication, services to the mentally retarded, adequacy of treatment in mental hospitals and mental retardation institutions, peonage in mental institutions, psychosurgery, capital punishment, unusual punishment in solitary confinement, denial of admission of a candidate to medical school because of a prior mental hospital stay, imprisonment for possession of marijuana, and abortion. In addition, these associations on occasion have offered sundry proposals for model legislation.

The Supreme Court's rulings on competency to stand trial in *Jackson v. Indiana* and *Beze v. Rees* and the death penalty in *Furman v. Georgia* drew heavily on the issues formulated and researched in the *amicus* briefs. In fact, most of the issues discussed by the Court in *Jackson* were not touched on by attorneys for the state or for the defendant, but were raised only in Ortho's *amicus* brief. The brief called the Court's attention to the broad implications of the procedure used in commitment for incompetency to stand trial, and the Court, although it did not permit filing of the brief, responded by addressing itself to these issues.

While it may encumber the judicial process, many courts are grateful for the participation of *amicus curiae*. A court's opinion often incorporates verbatim the *amicus* brief, which has come to represent the intersection of scholarship and advocacy. An *amicus* may enter at the trial or appellate level although rarely is afforded the opportunity to participate at the trial level, as it did in *Wyatt v. Stickney*, the right-to-treatment case, where *amici* were actively engaged in the proceeding presenting numerous witnesses on all aspects of the case. In helping to formulate minimum medical and constitutional standards in hospital treatment, the court expressed gratitude for exemplary service to Ortho, ACLU, American Psychological Association, and American Association on Mental Deficiency.

Today, individuals look to their organizations to represent and further their professional interests and concerns. As individuals, they have neither the time nor the inclination to pursue a matter that does not directly and immediately impact their pocketbooks, and they have come to expect organizational representation in the courts on general professional matters. While there has been much criticism of the role of mental health professionals as expert witnesses in the adversary system, it is at the same time recognized that in some way their viewpoint should enter the judicial process.[15]

As an avenue of publicity, *amici* briefs are often published in the *Congressional Record*—any congressman can put anything in the *Record*, and on request he will usually do so. The *Record* makes it possible to publish at a low printing price (the cost is absorbed by the public). Each day, within 13 hours of the close of debate, congressional presses turn out 49,000 copies of another thick edition of the *Record*. While production may be impressive, content unfortunately is not. In effect, the *Record* is a subsidiary copying service for congressmen, producing by the thousands whatever items they choose. Nader's Study Group, which calls the *Record* a big charade, says that shrewd doctors soon will learn to stock their waiting rooms with copies of the *Record*. In any event, the *Record* is a means to heighten visibility and citizen consciousness of an issue, which is also the goal of much litigation.

Mass Litigation (Class Actions)

Organizational activity in the legal process has found a broad new field with the recent development of mass litigation (class actions), which allows representation of all those in a similar position.[16] For over a decade, mass litigation has become increasingly common in the areas of personal injury, product liability, and workplace discrimination. In the area of law and psychiatry, class action suits have notably been brought in regard to the right to treatment and the right to refuse treatment.[17]

Mass litigation is sometimes called "public interest" litigation. Today, entire industries—cigarette producers, gunmakers, lead paint manufacturers, and health maintenance organizations (HMOs)—are struggling to protect their profits, or even their survival, in the face of new, outsized forms of litigation. The courts are increasingly being called upon to make public policy in areas vacated by politicians (such as gun violence, smoking, and HMO reform). In the lawsuits against gunmakers, the tobacco industry, and healthcare industries, contentious economic, social, or political matter has been transformed into an ostensibly "legal" issue. The lawsuits were prompted by the general feeling of the public that legislative policies were hamstrung and that these industries needed to be curbed. Of course, at the same time, there are outbursts against over-zealous lawyers, silly lawsuits, and outrageous fees. Turning difficult political choices into legal issues (disputes that can be litigated) usually involves a narrowing process that excludes important social considerations. In any event, the pace of legal change has suddenly accelerated as the third branch of government, the judiciary, assumes responsibilities from the other two branches, resulting in judicial regulation of whole segments of the country's industry.

The growth of mass litigation, and especially the newest kind of big lawsuit—civil suits brought by government to fight social problems, such as smoking and gun violence—raises vexing questions about the role of law in U.S. society: Can mass justice be done without jeopardizing individual rights? Does the sheer size of these lawsuits exert undue pressure on defendants to settle? Are these lawsuits good for society—or just good for lawyers? In mass cases, the lawyers do not maintain meaningful one-to-one contact with their clients, nor can they represent these people as individuals, each with his or her own needs and interests.

Up to a point, litigation has been "good for America," as Professor Alan Dershowitz put it. It provided something of a social safety net, in a country without a national health scheme and with only limited disability insurance. It helped to level the playing field between private citizens and large corporations. But, is all the vast litigation still worth the price? Judge Jack Weinstein, of the U.S. District Court in New York, concedes the costs, but stresses the benefits: "It has defects, and it has undoubtedly, to some extent, discouraged innovation and put economic pressure on some industries, perhaps unnecessarily. But, in general, it has fulfilled an equalizing function. This is a justice system open to everybody."[18]

Participation as Partisan Expert

While the *amicus* role is significant, partisan experts called by the contesting parties remain the familiar source of expert testimony. The appointment of experts by the court is expressly allowed under the rules of evidence, but it is rare in the United States because it is viewed as an undesirable departure from the dueling nature of the adversary system. As such, in the United States, experts are usually called by the parties. This is contrary to most countries where the court itself appoints expert witnesses allegedly to ensure scientific objectivity. The advocates of party selection of expert witnesses maintain that the impartial witness is a myth and empowering the parties to choose the witnesses in judicial proceedings gives them some effective control over the proceedings and thereby vindicates democratic values.[19] To most observers of court proceedings, the concept of an "impartial expert" echoes hollowly.[20]

In procuring the assistance of an expert, the attorney typically talks in terms of "if" ("if you take the stand"), reviewing the topics and the facts of the case. Once the expert agrees to serve, the attorney expects the expert to take on the role, in effect, of an advocate. That is, to make the best case he can for the lawyer's client. The expert is expected to carry out an evaluation and then if he feels he can be helpful, testify for the party and do all that is possible for the party without fabrication. The witnesses and immediate parties to a legal action are adversaries; they are labeled as witnesses *for* the plaintiff or *for* the defendant.

The adversarial process might be likened to a multilane highway with several lanes going in one direction and several lanes in the opposite direction. The witness, like the traveler, must go one way or the other. To use another metaphor, the witness cannot be like a Roman candle, shooting sparks in every direction without aim.

Because each side is allowed to present its best version of the contested issue, the adversarial system ensures that both sides will be aired. Yet, to make out their cases, lawyers crudely say, quite often, that they "buy" experts. They call them "hired guns." In a sense, they are right, but it is not unethical so long as they do not ask the expert to fabricate or falsify his or her opinion. Who can say that the opinion of the so-called impartial expert, the expert called by the court, is less biased or more truthful and objective than that of the adversary witness? The partiality of the impartial expert is masked as impartiality, more or less deceiving the fact finder. The traditional adversary system of calling witnesses for each side and then examining witnesses by direct and cross-examination has evolved specifically for the purpose of exposing shortcomings and biases, of probing the accuracy and veracity of the opposition witness's testimony.[21]

Experience reveals that there is almost no subject that cannot be viewed in at least two ways. The adversary system, the battle of the experts that it entails, and the frequent reversals on appeal may all reflect the natural working of the human mind. In the very nature of things, every event has different versions. The famous Japanese film *Rashomon* is a dramatization of the classic enigma of truth, a metaphor of life reminding us that there is no one truth, that there are many truths, some valid for one, some for another. Events are seen in different ways. Sigmund Freud has shown that ambivalence is the normal manner of human thought. The "adversary rumination" keeps the law in correspondence with human nature. Erik Erikson observed, "The conflicting evidence which parades past the paternal (or parental) judge, the fraternal jury, and the chorus of the public, matches the unceasing inner rumination with which we watch ourselves."[22]

To be sure, there are at least two sides to every story. Life is Janus-faced. In every war there have been virtuous and reasonable men earnestly fighting on both sides. Socrates would allow an adversary to pick any side of an argument. In the same spirit, Ralph Waldo Emerson would give a lecture on one side of a subject, then on the other side.[23]

Types of Expert Testimony

The role of the expert may be to reconstruct the past, analyze the present, or predict the future. In doing this, the expert may offer testimony of two general kinds: testimony as to facts and opinion testimony. The admissibility of each rests upon different theories. Expert testimony as to facts is admissible because special skill and experience are needed for the understanding of certain matters. For example, any person of ordinary understanding can testify as to whether a man had a cut or to the color of stains that may have appeared on his clothes. It requires special experience and knowledge, however, to say what arteries, nerves, or bones were injured and to determine whether the stains, if yellow, were due to urine or semen, or if brown, were human blood. Because the ordinary witness is not capable of making the determination, an expert is needed.

Unlike expert witnesses, lay witnesses are not allowed to give opinion testimony. Hence, the lay witness may not give a retrospective judgment or make a prediction. The lay witness is restricted to a presentation of facts with the judge or jury drawing the inferences or conclusions from such facts. In an amendment in 2000 to the Federal Rules of Evidence, a lay witness may not give testimony in the form of opinions or inferences based on scientific, technical, or other specialized knowledge.[24] The amendment is designed to eliminate the risk that the reliability requirements for expert testimony would be evaded through the simple expedient of proffering an expert in lay witness clothing (but it also results in the added cost of expert fees). Under the amendment, a witness's testimony must be scrutinized under the rules regulating expert opinion to the extent that the witness is providing testimony based on scientific, technical, or other specialized knowledge. The amendment does not distinguish between expert and lay *witnesses*, but rather between expert and lay *testimony*. Certainly it is possible for the same witness to provide both lay and expert testimony in a single case, as, for example, a law enforcement agent could testify that the defendant was acting suspiciously, without being qualified as an expert, but the rules on experts would be applicable where the agent testified on the basis of extensive experience that the defendant was using code words to refer to drug quantities and prices.[25] Similarly, a therapist testifying about his patient may be providing both expert and lay testimony.

In many instances, the court, judge or jury, is not able to reach an intelligent decision because of the difficulty of the question involved, and the opinion of those skilled in the particular subject at issue may be obtained for assistance. Here the function of the expert's testimony is advising the jury by giving an opinion rather than proving facts. For example, the jury would be incapable of determining whether death resulted from a particular cut, even though it had before it a description of the wound; hence, the opinion of a medical person is of assistance to the jury. However, when experts disagree, as they do more often than not, one may wonder how a jury composed of lay persons can fairly render a decision. For example, how can a jury decide whether an individual suffered from "repressed memory syndrome" if even the professional organizations point out that it is very difficult for an expert to determine this?[26] The answer may be in credibility. Simply, some experts are more convincing than others. Jurors may also decide on the basis of their own personal view of things.[27]

The problem of expert testimony, particularly that of a psychiatric character, whether as to facts or opinion, is somewhat different in criminal than in civil cases because of certain constitutional privileges of the accused. Because of the accused's privilege against self-incrimination, the expert witness for the state in a criminal prosecution is much more restricted when the accused's mental, rather than physical, condition is an issue. The accused may be compelled to submit to a physical examination by the medical witness for the prosecution because this does not involve testimonial compulsion.[28] The accused cannot be compelled to answer any questions asked by the expert in a mental examination, however, because this would violate his privilege against self-incrimination.[29] A proviso: An accused who pleads insanity must submit to a psychiatric examination and, if he refuses, he forfeits the right to present psychiatric testimony. The psychiatrist may testify only on the issue of mental status and may not reveal any statement made to him as to the commission of the offense.

"Helpfulness" as the Touchstone of Expert Testimony

The touchstone on the role of the forensic expert is "helpfulness." It is on this basis, for pretrial or trial purposes, that a lawyer engages an expert. The expert may be engaged to serve as a consultant or as a witness at trial, or both. Even before filing a complaint, the lawyer might use an expert in order to develop knowledge about a technical area and to help him frame the complaint and understand relevant issues. The lawyer's familiarity about the subject matter will determine the need of assistance. Once the complaint is filed, the expert can be of assistance with discovery or identifying documents. The expert can also be helpful in preparing for depositions, whether of lay or expert witnesses, or in identifying licensing agencies and, sometimes, specific persons within agencies with whom the lawyer may find communication helpful.[30]

Experts often play a pivotal role in the settlement of a case, thereby avoiding a trial. More than 95% of tort cases are resolved without a trial. The expert's deposition or report is most important in the determination of whether to go to trial or in determining the settlement amount. Insurance companies can be persuaded by the expert's report or by the reputation of the expert.

At trial, the use of expert testimony poses two interrelated but separate questions: (1) whether the subject matter of the litigation is such that the trier of fact (judge or jury) may appropriately receive assistance in the form of specialized knowledge, and (2) whether the witness at hand is qualified to render the assistance. In resolving the first question, the test, under Rule 702 of the Federal Rules of Evidence and its state counterparts, is whether the testimony of the expert "will assist the trier of fact to understand the evidence or to determine a fact in issue." The helpfulness requirement means that experts may testify not only on subjects beyond the ken of lay juries (as common law courts often held), but also to aid the jury to understand even familiar matters, by virtue of experience or training that provides a more thorough or refined understanding than ordinary experience provides.[31]

Once at trial, the first step is to qualify the witness as an expert, not only to satisfy fundamental evidentiary and procedural rules, but also to inform the jury about the expert's credentials. The better the credentials, the greater the witness's credibility, and the more weight the jury will give the testimony. It is apparently best that an expert be neither virgin nor prostitute—an expert who has never testified may have difficulty in getting qualified while one who testifies often is discredited as a hired gun.[32]

Endnotes

1. See J. Frank, *Courts on Trial* (Princeton: Princeton University Press, 1949).
2. R.A. Posner, "An Economic Approach to the Law of Evidence," *Stanford L. Rev.* 51 (1999): 1477. On the other hand, in the book *The Argument Culture* (New York: Random House, 1998), Deborah Tannen criticizes the adversarial system. Polarized arguments, she contends, leave us without the facts we need to make up our minds. To avoid needless squabbling, Tannen recommends mediation or adoption of the French system, in which cases are decided not by a jury, but by the *conviction intime de juge*—the judge's private belief. What Tannen is missing is the drama of conflict and the importance of a trial as a morality play.
3. *Causes Celebres* 3:309, quoted in J. Bentham, *Rationale of Judicial Evidence* (London: Hunt & Clarke, 1827), pp. 37–38.
4. United States v. Johnson, 575 F.2d 1347 (5th Cir. 1978); People v. Boyd, 65 Mich. App. 11, 236 N.W.2d 744 (1975); Anno., 95 A.L.R.3d 978 (1979).
5. State v. Briner, 198 Neb. 766, 255 N.W.2d 422 (1977).
6. Federal Rules of Evidence, Rule 701. For commentary on the subjective nature of expert testimony, see M. Angell, *Science on Trial* (New York: Norton, 1996); C.A.G. Jones, *Expert Witnesses* (New York: Oxford University Press, 1994). An excellent historical survey of expert testimony appears in S. Landsman, "Of Witches, Madmen, and Products Liability: An Historical Survey of the Use of Expert Testimony," *Behav. Sci. & Law* 13 (1995): 131.
7. See, e.g., B.J. Ennis & T.R. Litwack, "Psychiatry and the Presumption of Expertise: Flipping Coins in the Courtroom," *Cal. L. Rev.* 62 (1974): 693; D. Faust & J. Ziskin, "The Expert Witness in Psychology and Psychiatry," *Science*, July 1, 1988, p. 31; discussed in D. Goleman, "Psychologists' Expert Testimony Called Unscientific," *New York Times*, Oct. 11, 1988, p. 19.
8. James McElhaney, professor of trial advocacy, writes: "Within the limits of relevance and the constraints of ethics, the lawyer as playwright decides whether and how the trial will be a fascinating experience that will keep the judge and the jury on the edge of their seats, or a turgid, stultifying affair that will leave everyone in a stupor." J. McElhaney, "Creating Tension," *A.B.A.J.*, June 1, 1988, p. 84.
9. Triangle Publication v. Rohrlich, 167 F.2d 969 (2d Cir. 1945).
10. 214 F.2d 862 (D.C. Cir. 1954).
11. 338 U.S. 25 (1949).
12. 347 U.S. 483 (1954).

13. 392 U.S. 514 (1968).
14. E.R. Beckwith & R. Soberheim, "*Amicus curiae*—Minister of Justice," *Fordham L. Rev.* 17 (1946): 38; F.V. Harper & E.D. Etherington, "Lobbyists Before the Court," *U. Pa. L. Rev.* 101 (1953): 1172; S. Krislov, "The *Amicus Curiae* Brief: From Friendship to Advocacy," *Yale L. J.* 72 (1963): 694.
15. With the exception of governmental units, which can file *amicus* briefs as a matter of right, an individual or group desiring to file must obtain the consent of all parties or file a motion describing their interest in the case and showing that the brief will cover matter not presented, or inadequately presented by the parties. 28 U.S.C. §1706. Under the regulations of the Internal Revenue Service, § 1.501(c)(3), the status of contributions as gifts and the charitable classification of an association would not be jeopardized by involvement in court proceedings, either on its own behalf or as *amicus curiae*. There are, though, other limitations placed upon an organization as a nonprofit, tax-exempt organization that should be noted. It may not use any "substantial portion of its resources" in attempting to influence the legislative process. It may produce educational and informational materials, but it may not lead crusades or propaganda campaigns. It may respond to requests to testify before legislative hearings, and members of the staff may voluntarily appear, but only as individuals and not representing the organization. If these restrictions are too confining, an organization could establish a coordinate activity organization, which would not be tax-exempt and, thus, could become involved in political, propaganda, or legislative campaigns. Thus, the ACLU and the NAACP are, respectively, the activist organizations of the ACLU Foundation and the NAACP Legal Defense Fund.
16. The "class action" is a device by which one or more representatives of a group of people affected by a particular defendant's actions can file suit and press claims on behalf of the entire group of similarly situated individuals. Class actions are often used when individual actions would be impractical because of the low value of the claims involved, such as in an action by consumers against a drug company for overcharges on medicine. On occasion the class action device is resorted to in mass tort cases involving personal injuries to a number of people, but in most such cases personal injury plaintiffs prefer to assert their claims as individuals. To certify a class, the judge must find that the named or representative plaintiff will adequately represent the interests of the class of persons on whose behalf a suit is brought. Notice must generally be provided when money damages are sought to allow class members to "opt out" of the class and file their own suit if they choose. All settlements must be approved by the judge after notice to the class at a "fairness hearing." See H.B. Newberg, *Newberg on Class Actions: A Manual for Group Litigation at Federal and State Levels* (New York: McGraw Hill, 1977); Jenkins v. Raymark Industries, 782 F.2d 468 (5th Cir. 1986).
17. Class action lawsuits over Ritalin were filed against the American Psychiatric Association and various pharmaceutical companies alleging that they conspired to create the diagnosis of attention-deficit disorder and attention-deficit hyperactivity disorder as a way to reap pharmacologic profits. D. Fulton, "Class Action Suits Over Ritalin Filed Against APA," *Clinical Psychiatry News*, Oct. 2000, p. 1; K.P. O'Meara, "Writing May Be on Wall for Ritalin," *Insight*, Oct. 16, 2000, p. 16.
18. J.B. Weinstein, *Individual Justice in Mass Tort Litigation* (Evanston, IL: Northwestern University Press, 1995). See also P.M. Barrett, "Why Americans Look to the Courts to Cure the Nation's Social Ills," *Wall Street Journal*, Jan. 4, 2000, p. 1; P. Waldmeir, "Legal Eagles Rule the Roost," *Financial Times*, Dec. 11–12, 1999, p. 1.
19. See Federal Rules of Evidence, Rule 706; E.J. Imwinkelried, "The Court Appointment of Expert Witnesses in the United States: A Failed Experiment," *Med. & Law* 8 (1989): 601.
20. Dr. Bernard Diamond debunked the idea of an "impartial expert" in a classic article, "The Fallacy of the Impartial Expert," *Arch. Crim. Psychodynam.* 3 (1959): 221, and together with Professor David W. Louisell in another article, "The Psychiatrist as an Expert Witness: Some Ruminations and Speculations," *Mich L. Rev.* 63 (1965): 1335. See also N. Miltenberg, "Myths About 'Neutral' Scientific Experts," *Trial*, Jan. 2000, p. 62.
21. R.L. Goldstein, "Psychiatrists in the Hot Seat: Discrediting Doctors by Impeachment of Their Credibility," *Bull. Am. Acad. Psychiat. & Law* 16 (1988): 225. In a Louisiana case, the expert had just expressed his opinion that the claimant was not suffering from posttraumatic neurosis, but was, instead, a malingerer. The attorney asked: "Is that your conclusion that this man is a malingerer?" To which the expert replied, "I wouldn't be testifying if I didn't think so, unless I was on the other side, then it would be a posttraumatic condition." Ladner v. Higgins, 71 So.2d 242, 244 (La. App. 1954).

22. E. Erikson, "The Ontogeny of Ritualization," presented in June 1965 to the Royal Society as a contribution to a symposium on Ritualization in Animals and in Man. In a well-known joke about a couple who come to a rabbi, the husband gives his side of the story, and the rabbi says, "You're right." Then the wife gives her side of the story, and the rabbi says, "You're right." Then the husband says, "But, rabbi, how can we both be right? She's right, and I'm right?" The rabbi says, "You're right."

23. Apparently every proverb—that pithy summary of popular wisdom—can be matched by another that contradicts it flatly, as, for instance, "a rolling stone gathers no moss," against "the traveling bee gets the honey"; or "look before you leap," against "he who hesitates is lost"; "The Lord loveth a cheerful giver," but "fools and their money are soon parted"; "absence makes the heart grow fonder," but "out of sight, out of mind." R. Slovenko, "Mixed Messages in Proverbs," *J. Psychiat. & Law* 21 (1993): 405.

24. Federal Rules of Evidence, Rule 701.

25. See United States v. Figueroa-Lopez, 125 F.3d 1241 (9th Cir. 1997). The amendment incorporates the distinctions set forth in State v. Brown, 836 S.W.2d 530 (Tenn. 1992), where the court noted that a lay witness would have to qualify as an expert before he could testify that bruising around the eyes is indicative of skull trauma.

26. In Bertram v. Poole, 597 N.W.2d 309 (Minn. App. 1999), the experts disagreed whether there is any scientific basis for repressed memory, or whether the individuals involved in the case suffered from repressed memory syndrome.

27. "Where expert witnesses offer conflicting opinions, it is for the jury, as the ultimate trier of fact, to consider their qualifications and determine the weight to be given their opinions." McKay's Family Dodge v. Hardrives, 480 N.W.2d 141, 146 (Minn. App. 1992).

28. In the leading case of Schmerber v. California, 384 U.S. 757 (1966), the defendant was compelled to give a blood test against his will in a drunk-driving prosecution. Tracing the development of the law, the Supreme Court held that this did not violate the defendant's constitutional rights, noting that "the distinction which has emerged, often expressed in different ways, is that the privilege [against self-incrimination] is a bar against compelling 'communications' or 'testimony,' but that compulsion, which makes a suspect or an accused the source of 'real or physical evidence' does not violate it." Thus, the privilege is no bar to compelling the defendant to submit to such tests as fingerprinting, photographing, urine analysis. State v. Tarrance, 252 La. 396, 211 So.2d 304 (1968) (defendant compelled to give a handwriting sample).

29. People v. Stevens, 386 Mich. 579, 194 N.W.2d 370 (1972). The U.S. Supreme Court in its controversial decision in *Miranda* in 1966 ruled that persons suspected of a crime must be advised of their rights before interrogation or their confessions may not be used in court. See H.A. Davidson, Psychiatric examination and civil rights, in R. Slovenko (ed.), *Crime, Law and Corrections* (Springfield, Ill.: Thomas, 1966), p. 459; Comment, "Pretrial Psychiatric Examination and the Privilege against Self-Incrimination," *J. Ill. L. For.* 1971: 232.

30. R.E. Brooks, "Expert Witness, Used Properly, Can Expedite Fact-Finding Process," *Natl. Law J.*, Sept. 5, 1988, p. 20.

31. *In re* Japanese Elect. Prods. Antitrust Litig., 723 F.2d 238 (3d Cir. 1983); Garbincius v. Boston Edison Co., 621 F.2d 1171 (1st Cir. 1980).

32. I owe this observation to Dr. Emanuel Tanay.

2

Obligations and Responsibilities
of Lawyers and Experts

Questions arise regarding the obligations and responsibilities of lawyers in their interaction with forensic experts. This chapter discusses the necessity at trial of expert testimony, selection of the expert, the underlying data of the expert opinion, fabrication and the providing and withholding of data, sequestering witnesses, compelling expert testimony, depositions, discovery of expert opinions and reports, instructions to the jury, and the fee arrangement.

Necessity of Expert Testimony

The underlying theory of the adversary system is that each side presents its best version of the case, without perjury or manufactured evidence, subject to cross-examination and rebuttal by the adversary.[1] The lawyer is not free, as he might like to be, in the representation of a client.[2] In many cases expert testimony is helpful and would be permitted as proof, but at other times it is absolutely essential and required as a matter of law. In these cases, the court will not entertain the litigation without expert testimony. The testimony of lay witnesses in these cases would be insufficient as a matter of law. As a consequence, the lawyer is at the mercy of experts—he *must* find and engage one.

That is the situation in a professional negligence (malpractice) case where "the standard of care is that degree of skill and learning which is ordinarily possessed and exercised by members of the profession in good standing." The plaintiff must, as a matter of law, produce an expert to establish that standard and that there was a deviation from it (unless the negligence is sufficiently obvious as to lie within common knowledge, as where a foreign object, such as a sponge or needle, is left within the body of the patient).[3] In rendering professional services, a practitioner is held, with few exceptions, to a provider-defined standard of care. To put it differently, the law allows the profession to establish its own liability standards. On the other hand, in the ordinary negligence action (e.g., a collision case), "the standard of care to which the defendant must conform is that degree of care which, in the jury's view, a reasonable person of ordinary prudence would have exercised in the defendant's place in the same or similar circumstances."[4]

In a medical malpractice case based on negligent nondisclosure, expert testimony is necessary to establish that a risk of the procedure exists, that it is accepted medical practice to know that risk, and that it is more probable than not that the undisclosed risk materialized in harm. (Informed consent is the theoretical construct, but, needless to say, both physician and patient are beholden to the auditor and policy maker.) Nationwide, as a rule, the action for failure to disclose risks is deemed one of malpractice, requiring expert testimony.[5]

Is expert testimony necessary when the propriety of seclusion or restraint is the question? In *Reifschneider v. Nebraska Methodist Hospital,*[6] it was argued unsuccessfully that the question of restraint is custodial or nonmedical and within the grasp or knowledge of ordinary laymen, and, therefore, no expert testimony as to the defendant's duty to restrain is necessary. In line with other decisions, the Nebraska Supreme Court required expert testimony to establish a duty of the defendant to restrain a patient. The court said that assessing the status of a patient and determining whether restraints are needed are matters calling for expert testimony.[7]

One small but important and much publicized area of the law of medical malpractice involves duties or standard of care mandated by the legislature or the courts. One illustration is the Washington Supreme Court's requirement of glaucoma tests not apparently required by the medical profession (or by legislation) as a matter of routine for patients under 40 years of age.[8] Another illustration is the decision that outraged nearly all psychiatrists—the *Tarasoff* case in California,[9] and progeny in other states, calling upon psychotherapists to protect potential victims from the acts of a patient. The court in *Tarasoff* characterized the case as one of professional negligence, calling for expert testimony. The question whether a patient poses a serious danger of violence to others is measured, the court said, by whether the "therapist does in fact determine, or under applicable professional standards reasonably should have determined," the danger.[10] The court, while imposing the duty, at the same time deferred to the profession in assessing the danger, though, in fact, the profession has no standards on the prediction of dangerousness.

On the other hand, expert testimony was not mandated on the propriety of the course of behavior taken in view of the danger. The court in *Tarasoff* said that "the adequacy of the therapist's conduct must be measured against the traditional negligence standard of the rendition of reasonable care under the circumstances."[11] The court pointed out, "The discharge of this duty may require the therapist to take one or more of various steps, depending upon the nature of the case. Thus, it may call for him to warn the intended victim or others likely to apprise the victim of the danger, to notify the police, or to take whatever other steps are reasonably necessary under the circumstances."[12] Placing an advertisement in the newspaper would likely not be found reasonable. It would be a jury question not necessarily aided by expert testimony.[13]

In criminal cases, failure to engage an expert may constitute ineffective assistance of counsel warranting reversal of a conviction. That is the implication of *Ake v. Oklahoma*,[14] a murder case, where no psychiatrist was called to testify, though the only issue was insanity. In this case, the U.S. Supreme Court overturned the conviction on the ground that the defendant, an indigent, should have access to psychiatric assistance in preparing an insanity defense.[15]

In some cases, the courts want psychiatric testimony as window dressing. Decisions on civil commitment, child custody, and also criminal responsibility are difficult and uncomfortable to make. Such decisions, however, have to be made and the courts, mindful of public opinion, often abdicate their decision-making responsibility to psychiatrists or want to decorate their decision with psychiatric testimony. It is passing the buck, so to speak. It may give the impression of undue power of experts in the judicial process, but that is more appearance than reality. Taking it at face value, however, Dr. Jonas Robitscher in *The Powers of Psychiatry* concluded that "the psychiatrist is the most important nongovernmental decision maker in modern life."[16]

In still other cases, an attorney may engage an expert in order to have a report that will provide leverage in bargaining, rather than to assist in the quest for truth. In many cases, civil or criminal, the report may lead to a settlement without having been tested by cross-examination. Insurance companies, in settling a case, place great reliance, by and large, on the expert's report. Of course, the expert is subject to the time-honored crucible of cross-examination at trial—provided the case goes to trial. Most divorce cases (including those involving distribution of assets) are not tried; they are settled after the experts' reports are received. In domestic litigation, it may well be that, as time goes on, the role of the parties or lay witnesses may be relatively minor compared with that of the experts.

Selecting the Expert

Under the rules of evidence, the lawyer has wide discretion in selecting an expert. The task of qualifying a witness as an expert is not a major obstacle though it is becoming more difficult as the result of widespread complaints about "junk science" in the courtroom. The door to Plato's Academy in Athens bore the forbidding inscription, "Let no one enter who is not a mathematician." Webster's dictionary defines an expert as "a person who is very skillful, or highly trained and informed in some special field." The temple of justice, however, is not nearly so exacting. The expert need not have "special" or "complete" knowledge of his field of expertise[17]—the testimony, as we have noted, need be merely "helpful" to the court.[18] To be helpful, the expert must have knowledge of the matter in issue, but also as a practical matter, the expert must be skillful in presenting his testimony. What the lawyer wants in an expert medical witness is the knowledge of Michael DeBakey, the looks of George Clooney, and the presence of Ronald Reagan, but alas, not many doctors fill that prescription.[19] Those attributes may help overcome the widespread bias against experts.

The selection of several experts on an issue may not be advantageous. Having several experts on an issue can create problems as any difference of opinion among them can be exploited. Multiple experts can create contradictions. In the trial of John E. DuPont, the defense called twelve mental health professionals. In the trial of John W. Hinckley, Jr., who shot and wounded President Ronald Reagan, the various defense experts did not agree on his diagnosis. Many trial judges limit one expert to an issue.

Sometimes in serving as an expert, the expert may have unfavorable information about a colleague on the other side of the case. There is divided opinion whether the expert should relate that information to the attorney retaining him. Is it within the proper scope of the expert's role in the case? Dr. Paul Appelbaum is of the opinion (not widely held) that it is not the role of the expert to help the attorney who has hired him to win the case, but rather to provide honest and accurate testimony about the person who has been evaluated. He suggests that one goes beyond that role when one provides not generally known information regarding an expert. By and large, experts are of the opinion that if it is a matter of public record, such as the board of medicine having censured the expert for alcoholism or for being dishonest in court, it should be pointed out to the attorney as it may be useful in cross-examination or qualification as an expert.[20]

An orthopedic surgeon wrote to Randy Cohen, who writes a column on ethics in the *New York Times*, saying that he treated a woman who was obviously crippled by a surgeon, and as she was unaware of her right to sue for malpractice, he asked whether he was obligated to inform her, particularly when he knew that she would need the money for continuing care. Randy Cohen responded:

> [Y]ou must give your patient a true understanding of her present condition, and that conversation may reasonably address the past treatment that brought it about. If you were discussing the case with a colleague, surely you'd opine that the patient was ill served by her last doctor. Your patient herself is entitled to the same candor.
>
> Her legal options, too, are germane. Physicians often consider a patient's economic circumstances. (Is a patient insured? Can she afford her medication?) As you note, the economic relief she might gain through the courts can have a significant effect on her medical care and thus is within your purview. You may not offer legal advice, but you should encourage her to seek it.
>
> I understand your reluctance to disparage a colleague or embroil another doctor in a malpractice suit. But your primary obligation is to your patient's health, not to your colleague's reputation. If you do not give her this meaningful information, how is she to get it?
>
> UPDATE: The physician not only discussed his patient's previous treatment, but also referred her to an attorney specializing in medical malpractice. He told this attorney that he could not testify in any proceeding, lest his receiving payment as an expert witness suggest a conflict of interest.[21]

Of special concern in the administration of justice are the conflicts arising out of the need to present expert testimony and the willingness of experts to say whatever is needed to prevail in a case. Unquestionably, there are experts who have no business being in a courtroom much less in their profession. Lawyers say, "Some experts are willing, upon request, to find a muscle spasm in a statue."[22] Lawyers too, it must be noted, are often willing to say anything to advance their cause. The prominent attorney F. Lee Bailey is also known as F. Lie Bailey.

The courts traditionally deferred to the profession to set out the standard of care in malpractice cases and, in doing so, they adopted a "school" method for qualifying expert witnesses, but in recent years, at the behest of medical societies, various states have required that the testifying expert not simply be familiar with the practice of the defendant, but that they be of the same specialty.[23]

In a suit in California against a church and its pastors for wrongful death, arising out of a suicide, an order was initially entered forbidding testimony of a psychiatrist.[24] The order was subsequently withdrawn because the court said that the action was not one of malpractice (professional negligence), which calls for expert testimony, but one of intentional infliction of mental distress, which requires no expert testimony.[25] The court thus avoided the issue whether a psychiatrist may testify in a clergy malpractice case. "We need not decide," the court said, "whether [the pastor] had a duty to refer [the individual] to a psychiatrist or other mental health professional or whether [the pastor] or the church had a duty to adequately train the pastors in methods of psychological counseling."[26]

In psychiatric malpractice cases, the plethora of therapeutic techniques and the eclectic nature of much psychiatric practice inevitably results in a blurring of "school" boundaries. This fact, together with the dogmatism of many practitioners, makes it likely that experts, though familiar with a "school," will disagree as to the standard of care for that school. Indeed, the principal controversy in mental health care is over the development of standards of treatment.[27] Frederic Worden, a noted psychoanalyst and brain researcher, once observed that, unlike violinists, who all play violins and know what one looks like, psychiatrists "are not all playing the same instrument"; indeed, he said, "Some are playing instruments that others disapprove of or disbelieve in or even, in some cases, instruments whose very existence is unknown to others in the group."[28] Following Illinois, a New York court ruled that psychologists are not qualified to testify as expert witnesses in malpractice suits against psychiatrists or the hospitals with which the psychiatrists are affiliated.[29]

The "locality rule" at one time was generally followed along with the "school" rule in regard to the medical profession, but usually not in regard to other professions. The rule further constricted the pool of professionals qualified to testify as to the relevant standard of care. The expert testifying in a medical malpractice case had to be one who could testify as to the standard of knowledge and skill in terms of the practitioner in good standing in the community in which he practices or a similar one. The definition of "community" was a narrow one. Under the rule, to show what is the standard of learning or the customary practice in a small town, the only expert is a doctor who knows about this (or a similar) small town. Conjoined with the protective, provider-defined standard of care, the rule served to insulate the medical profession from liability. Current efforts to hold expert testimony by physicians as the practice of medicine is another attempt to curtail experts coming from a different state.

The locality rule arose in the days when medical education was not standardized and there was a wide variance in the knowledge and skill of doctors in different parts and areas of the country. As this situation has changed, the courts have held that there is a minimum national standard especially for specialists. As a consequence, experts may come from places other than the locality of the practitioner on trial, subject to the "schools" rule. This is evident in legal journals that are now replete with advertisements of experts offering their services nationwide. The use of experts has become so common that thriving businesses have been formed to serve as clearinghouses for witnesses. The lawyer looking for a medical expert, or other expert, can also search by computer for an expert by state or specialty. Trial attorney associations (plaintiffs' or defendants') maintain a regularly updated index of experts ranging from accidentalist to zoologist. In short, the lawyer, for a fee, now has a cornucopia of available services. Most law firms maintain a list, or "stable," of experts whom they call upon as needed.[30] However, in child custody litigation, some experts lose credibility the more they appear as a witness for a given lawyer, as these cases are tried before judges alone and they get to know the credibility of the witness.

In criminal cases, in order to avoid reversible error, trial judges tend to be more liberal in accepting the qualifications of a witness when tendered by the defense as an expert and in admitting the evidence as probative (thus the trial court allowed the defense to introduce as evidence the CAT scans of the slightly shrunken brain of John Hinckley, Jr.).

The Underlying Data of the Expert Opinion Under the Federal Rules of Evidence

Questions are presented: Given that the polygraph or hypnosis itself is deemed so untrustworthy that it may not be admitted in evidence, may an expert rely on the results of the polygraph or hypnosis in forming an opinion? May an expert rely on inadmissible hearsay? On a criminal record in assessing a party? Rule 703 of the Federal Rules of Evidence, adopted in 1975, allows experts to rely on sources of information that are not admissible in their own right. Hence, the lawyer, by using an expert, would have passage around the exclusionary rules of evidence, and that may prompt the use of an expert. Rule 703 provides that an expert may base an opinion on facts or data "if of a type reasonably relied upon by experts in the particular field … the facts or data need not be admissible in evidence." The focus of the rule is not on the admissibility of the underlying data of the expert's opinion, but on its validity and reliability as measured by the practice of experts when not in court. Thus, under it, a doctor as an expert witness may relate hearsay statements of other doctors or investigators in explaining the basis for his opinion.[31] The expert, however, may not be a mere "conduit" for the opinions of other doctors or investigators.[32]

An amendment in 2000 to Rule 703 provides that when experts reasonably rely on inadmissible information to form opinions or inferences, they may not disclose the underlying data on direct examination merely because their opinions or inferences are admitted, unless the court determines that the prejudicial effect of the date is substantially outweighed by its value in assisting the jury's evaluation of the expert's opinion. Nothing in the amendment, of course, limits the right of the adverse party upon cross-examination to bring out details of inadmissible data relied upon by the expert, typically for the purpose of impeaching the witness by questioning the reliability or completeness of the data upon which the expert relied. Various states in their rules of evidence provide that the trial court may require that underlying facts or data essential to an opinion be in evidence.[33]

The degree to which the trial judge allows experts to rely upon hearsay evidence for their testimony depends on a finding that it was reasonable for the expert to rely on the hearsay evidence in forming the opinion. Take the case of *United States v. Madrid*[34] as an example of expert testimony based, in part, on the criminal record of the accused. Ordinarily, testimony as to past crimes, standing alone, is excludable as impermissible character evidence.[35] However, in *Madrid*, involving a defense of insanity, the state's psychiatrist was allowed to testify that the defendant was sane, an opinion based, in part, on the fact that the accused "had committed armed robberies of stores prior to the offense in question in order to support a heroin addiction."[36]

Indeed, under the Federal Rules of Evidence, the lawyer in offering an expert need not even present the data underlying an opinion, unless the court requires otherwise. Under the Rules, it is left to the cross-examiner to attack the opinion and to ferret out its basis, if any. As a matter of trial tactics, however, the expert on direct presents the data for the opinion, otherwise it would not be persuasive. The examination of the expert may begin thus:

"Doctor, do you have an opinion whether stress had a bearing on the defendant's conduct?"

"Yes."

"What is that opinion?"

"It caused the defendant to act involuntarily."

"Doctor, would you tell the court the basis for your opinion?"

[The doctor thereupon provided the basis for his opinion.]

Fabrication and the Providing and Withholding of Data

In a cartoon: "Just remember that lying can get you into a lot of trouble if not done properly," says a lawyer to a witness, but many would say it is true to life.[37] Professional regulations define the duties of the lawyer to the court, to the client, to the profession, and to the public. It is the duty of the lawyer "to employ, for the purpose of maintaining the causes confided to them, such means only as are consistent with truth and never to seek to mislead the judge or juries by any artifice or false statement of the law."[38] To put it simply, the lawyer is ethically bound not to fabricate evidence. Preparation of a witness is good lawyering, but coaching of a witness is grounds for reversal.

In the situation involving client-intended perjury, it may be noted, the well-defined duty to preserve client confidences conflicts with the lawyer's duty of candor and honesty toward the court. Disciplinary standards prohibit a lawyer in the course of representation from (1) knowingly using perjured testimony or false evidence, (2) participating in the creation or preservation of evidence when he knows or it is obvious that the evidence is false, or (3) counseling or assisting his client in conduct that the lawyer knows to be illegal or fraudulent. The Supreme Court imposed an additional, judicially created duty on lawyers when it held in 1986 that "it is the special duty of an attorney to prevent and disclose fraud upon the court."[39]

As an expert may also express an opinion, for this reason as well, lawyers engage an expert. An opinion, unlike a statement of fact, is not subject to perjury. "That's my opinion," says the expert. In *United States v. Roark*,[40] a psychologist was permitted to testify that the defendant's confession was voluntary. And, in many cases, the opinion, as we shall discuss, may go to the "ultimate issue." Thus, in *People v. Whitfield*,[41] a physician was allowed to give an opinion as to whether the victim's injuries were caused by sexual assault.

An expert may base an opinion on facts about which the expert has personal or firsthand knowledge—doctors usually base their opinions in part on conditions and symptoms they personally observed during an examination of the patient—or the expert may rely on reports from third parties (as long as it is customary practice in the specialty to consider that kind of data). The expert may also express an opinion in response to a hypothetical question. In the hypothetical, the lawyer specifies the facts that the expert is to assume. Dr. Jonas Rappeport enters a criticism: "Often such [hypothetical] questions do not actually contain the full information necessary to enable a professional opinion to be reached. This is a serious defect with hypothetical questions and arises unless the expert helps prepare or actually prepares the question."[42] In all cases, whether or not based on a hypothetical question, the expert must be willing to testify that he has formed his opinion to a reasonable medical or scientific certainty or probability.[43]

The rules of evidence entitle the adversary to inspect any notes that a witness uses to refresh recollection at trial or prior to testifying.[44] The adversary has a right to use them on cross-examination. The witness is obliged to bring to court any notes that were viewed in preparation for trial. However, any list of questions prepared by the witness and given to the lawyer engaging him as an aid in asking questions is considered work product, protected from inspection by the adversary, if not reviewed by the witness to refresh recollection and intended solely as a trial aid for the attorney.

Lawyers vary in their ability, of course, in using expert witnesses (as in other matters). Some lawyers although famous and successful (among them F. Lee Bailey and Melvin Belli) did not use experts well (say the experts). These lawyers wanted to be center stage, taking the limelight away from the expert. One may recall the song, "Oh Lord, it's hard to be humble." Still, others use too many experts. Too many experts on a side tend to dilute the transference (to use psychiatric language) with the jury, and differences get exaggerated. Court rules generally limit the number of experts on an issue unless special circumstances can be shown. Within a time period as set out in the court rules, the attorneys must exchange lists of all witnesses to be called at trial. No witness, lay or expert, may be called at trial of the case unless listed, except by leave granted upon a showing of good cause.[45]

To maintain relevancy, the lawyer in preparing a case with an expert will quite frequently discuss the report that the expert is planning to write or will go over a draft of the report and edit it. Litigation manuals instruct the lawyer: "An expert should never write a report until he has first discussed his conclusions with you orally."[46] Properly done, the lawyer provides useful guidance so that the report will focus on the key issues in the case. The process becomes improper, however, when misleading or manufactured statements are put into the report. At trial, the lawyer who withholds potentially damaging information from the expert may find, on cross-examination, that doing so has proven counter productive. In many cases, experts have been forced to change their conclusion when, on cross-examination, they are confronted with additional or different data. This occurs, for example, when an expert is provided with only parts of hospital records or an incomplete history.

Experienced forensic experts usually advise the lawyer that they want to see everything that is available and they caution that withholding information will likely boomerang at trial. The forensic expert would want all the information that is available in order to base his opinion on the best possible information, rather than on a limited amount. There are times, however, when lawyers tell the expert that they are not going to provide everything because they choose not to (as, for example, when they have information that they do not wish to make available to the opposing attorney) and that the expert should form his opinion on the information given and not to worry about the rest.

Generally speaking, experts are provided all the information that is available and relevant, but is it unethical for a lawyer to withhold information from an expert? The ethics of the attorney are to provide the best possible defense for a client, which may include not showing certain materials to the expert at the risk of having that backfire in court. That is a legal judgment call, the lawyer's prerogative as part of his decision making or strategy. When an expert is on the witness stand, it is left to the lawyer to bring out what he wants and to deal with what he may not like in his own way.[47] That is his job under the adversary system; the job of the expert is to present his findings or opinion as clearly and honestly as the system will allow.

Sequestering Witnesses

The trial judge's power to control a witness has traditionally included a broad power to sequester witnesses before, during, and after their testimony. The U.S. Supreme Court has pointed out that the aim of imposing "the rule of witnesses," as the practice of sequestering witnesses is sometimes called, is twofold: (1) it exercises a restraint on witnesses "tailoring" their testimony to that of earlier witnesses, and (2) it aids in detecting testimony that is less than candid.[48] Rule 615 of the Federal Rules of Evidence provides that at the request of a party the court "shall" order witnesses excluded so that they cannot hear the testimony of other witnesses. In view of the use of the word *shall*, the Rule makes exclusion of witnesses mandatory at the request of a party.

Rule 615 contains exceptions. One exception, most frequently invoked in the case of expert witnesses, exempts a person whose presence is shown by a party to be essential to the presentation of his cause.[49] It has been held that where a party seeks to except an expert witness from exclusion under the Rule on the basis that he needs to hear firsthand the testimony of the other witnesses, the decision whether to permit him to remain is within the trial judge's discretion. On the other hand, where a fair showing has been made that the expert witness is required for the management of the case, the trial court must accept any reasonable representation to this effect by counsel.[50]

To form an opinion, the expert may wish to hear the testimony of the witnesses at trial. An expert opinion may be based on testimony heard during the trial. Questions arise: Did the expert hear all of the evidence? On what witnesses did the expert rely? On demeanor? In the much-publicized trial of Alger Hiss, accused by Whittaker Chambers of passing secrets to Communists, Dr. Carl Binger testified that Chambers was a "psychopath with a tendency toward making false accusations." Binger testified that his opinion was based, in part, on personal observation of Chambers at trial.[51] The cross-examination of Dr. Binger is widely regarded as the single most devastating cross-examination of an expert ever conducted.[52]

Prosecutors have generally been permitted to have an investigative agent or expert at counsel table throughout the trial eventhough the agent or expert may be a witness. The investigative agent's or expert's presence may be extremely important to counsel, especially when the case is complex or involves some specialized subject matter. The agent, too, having lived with the case for a long time, may be able to assist in meeting trial surprises where the best-prepared counsel would otherwise have difficulty.[53] Most of the cases have involved allowing a police officer who has been in charge of an investigation to remain in court despite the fact that he will be a witness.[54] In Canada, the parties are not concerned about the costs of the experts, as the Crown pays them, and both sides tend to agree to allowing their experts to sit throughout the trial.

Rule 615 does not resolve the debate over whether sequestration includes limitations on conduct outside of trial, e.g., limitations on counsel in informing witnesses of other testimony, on witnesses reading transcripts, and on presence at depositions. In doubt, counsel requests the court to acknowledge that the sequestering order prohibits counsel informing sequestered witnesses as to what happened in court before the witnesses testify. In holding that providing a witness daily transcript copy constitutes a violation of Rule 615, one court stated: "The opportunity to shape testimony is as great with a witness who reads trial testimony as with one who hears the testimony in open court. The harm may be even more pronounced with a witness who reads trial transcript than with one who hears the testimony in open court because the former need not rely on his memory of the testimony, but can thoroughly review and study the transcript in formulating his own testimony."[55] As a sanction, the court may hold the witness in contempt or exclude him from testifying.[56]

Compelling Expert Testimony

May an expert be compelled to give testimony at trial (or in pretrial discovery)? A lawyer looks for a willing expert because one willing is more likely to be helpful than one who is not, but there are times when a willing expert is unavailable and compelling an unwilling expert may be the only way to establish a case. As we have noted, there are areas of the law where it is absolutely essential to have expert testimony. In compelling testimony, the lawyer is not asking the expert to make any special preparation. It is agreed that an expert cannot be compelled to prepare for his testimony because this would be in the nature of involuntary servitude. However, when a lawyer is convinced that a particular expert's testimony will be of benefit, the testimony will be sought regardless of the expert's willingness to testify or familiarity with the particular facts of the case. The lawyer may feel the expert will be helpful by virtue of a publication, lecture, or testimony in a prior trial of a related matter, or simply because the expert's knowledge derived from his training and experience would make his testimony helpful.[57]

In many cases of medical malpractice, the lawyer is often faced with summoning a treating physician who is reluctant to testify against a doctor, the defendant, who previously treated and allegedly harmed the patient. The treating physician, should he testify, would make a more convincing witness against the defendant doctor than one called in merely as an examiner, but more often than not, he will not testify willingly. He could be called as a fact witness, if not as an expert witness.

Is an expert who is called upon to answer a hypothetical question or to set out a standard of care being required to do merely that which every good citizen is required to do on behalf of public order? The answer is apparently "yes," but abuse of the expert must somehow be curtailed. Would a famous surgeon, for example, be compellable to testify in every malpractice case involving a unique operating procedure? The danger is that he might end up spending more time in the courtroom than in the operating room. Society would hardly benefit. In this age of litigation, involving sundry matters, unwilling experts could be made subject to the beck and call of attorneys. In a democracy, should not the expert be allowed the freedom to choose the best use of his time and who is to receive his labor and service? Compensating the expert is not an adequate remedy.

Is there a rational basis for applying different rules to witnesses furnishing "scientific" as opposed to "observed" facts? Certainly, one is the product of the witness's learning and experience, the other of direct perception, but, if the purpose of witness evidence is to assist the trier of fact, what is the functional difference? The arguments raised by experts as to why they should not be compelled to testify can be made as well by the nonexpert. Reliance on whether the proposed evidence is "fact" or "opinion" is not realistic, as these terms themselves escape workable definition. Further difficulty results when the litigants seeking to compel expert testimony must show that other "qualified" witnesses are unavailable. Who is qualified and what makes a witness unavailable? Is an expert "available" if he lives in another part of the country?

Is there not inequity in forcing an expert to go to the expense of hiring a lawyer to vindicate his position? How much in advance of trial must the judge decide whether to require the expert to appear? Must the judge determine how much time the expert will spend in the courtroom? Should the judge require a statement by counsel of what testimony he seeks to elicit from the expert before allowing such a subpoena to be deemed properly issued? Can the matter be decided on paper rather than on oral testimony? Must such a subpoena be served sufficiently in advance of trial to permit its resolution before trial begins?[58]

In contrast to factual witnesses who possess knowledge that is unique and often irreplaceable, expert testimony is not based on any singular personal knowledge of the disputed events. Rather it depends on specialized training or other acquired knowledge that allows the expert to draw conclusions or to set out a standard of practice. In most areas of expertise, because many individuals possess the necessary qualifications to render expert opinions, this kind of testimony is not unique and a litigant will not usually be deprived of critical evidence if he cannot have the expert of his choice.

The courts in the United States are not in agreement as to when experts can be compelled to testify. The cases concerning the compulsion of expert testimony vary greatly depending on the factual situations and legal approach taken.[59] The commentators in law journals are also in disagreement.[60] The only reference in the Federal Rules of Evidence to the need of consent by an expert is in Rule 706(a), dealing with court-appointed experts. This provides in part that "an expert witness shall not be appointed by the court unless he consents to act."[61] The situation of the court-appointed expert who is expected to explore the problem and arrive at an informed and unbiased opinion differs markedly, however, from that of an expert called by a party to state the facts as he knows them and what opinion he may have formed on the basis without being asked to make any further investigation. If any inference is to be drawn from the Federal Rules of Evidence, it is against the claim of privilege by an expert, not for it.

In a noted case, *Kaufman v. Edelstein*,[62] the U.S. Court of Appeals for the Second Circuit held that the trial court did not abuse its discretion in allowing the government in its antitrust action against IBM to compel testimony from two individuals with considerable expertise in the computer industry. Specifically, the government wanted these witnesses "to explain the nature of their duties as computer systems consultants and especially to recount advice they gave to various users and potential users of computer systems." Significantly, the government was not asking for an expert evaluation of their evidence in the IBM case, but instead stated that the witness's testimony would be confined to events that occurred between 1960 and 1972. In a concurring opinion, Judge Gurfein noted that these experts differed from the ordinary expert who has no personal relationship with the subject matter of the litigation. Indeed, they were intimately involved as observers of and participants in the growth and development of the electronic data processing market. The author of the majority opinion, Judge Friendly, indicated that these particular experts could only give a substantial part of the testimony sought by the government. They possessed unique information unavailable from any other source, though most of the testimony sought in the *Kaufman* case was factual rather than opinion.

In a case less known, *Wright v. Jeep Corp.*,[63] the defendant in a personal injury action, Jeep Corporation, sought discovery of a crash vehicle researcher who had published an adverse report on the safety of certain vehicles manufactured by the defendant. The information desired by Jeep concerned all research data and memoranda pertaining to a study of highway safety in which the researcher had participated and out of which grew the adverse report. Jeep was interested in the factual basis underlying the researcher's conclusion because it felt the study might be used against it at trial. Although the researcher objected to discovery, on the basis that, among other things, he was an expert and could not be compelled to testify, the court held otherwise. In its ruling, the court noted that the researcher was not being required to assist in explaining technical matters, but rather was simply being required to disclose the underlying factual basis for his conclusions so that the parties and the court could judge their validity. As in *Kaufman*, the particular information sought from the experts was not readily available from other sources. Moreover, while the factual observation sought in discovery may have involved some of the expertise and experience of the expert, neither the court nor the litigant in *Wright* was seeking an expert opinion per se from the researcher. Thus, although both *Wright* and *Kaufman* affirm the general principle that an unwilling expert is not immune from compulsory process merely because he is an expert, they do not support the contention that the party has an unlimited right to compel the expert of his choice to provide opinion testimony. The decisions in these cases were based, in large part, on the peculiar need of the compelling party for the information sought and its unavailability from other sources.

Can we adhere to a rule that an expert may not be compelled to give testimony? Were this the rule, it would lie within the discretion of the expert to prevent some cases from being tried and the lawyer or court would be powerless to provide the jury with any sort of basis for a decision. It would be, in a manner of speaking, an obstruction of justice. In *Kaufman*, the question was whether IBM had monopoly power. The experts on the subject were so uncommon that, were they to decline to testify, the court would be without crucial evidence.[64] In professional malpractice cases, as noted, the plaintiff is obliged to produce an expert to establish the proper standard and that there was a deviation from it. The use of learned treatises is not a happy substitute. As the law defers to the profession on standard of care, it behooves the profession to provide testimony on that standard of care. According to a number of reports, however, experts in the medical field are threatened by their insurers with a loss of insurance coverage or increase in premium rates should they testify in a malpractice case.

Wigmore, the leading authority on evidence, once wrote: "The giving of … testimony may be a sacrifice of time and labor, and, thus of ease, of profits, of livelihood. This contribution is not to be regarded as a gratuity or a courtesy or an ill-required favor. It is a duty not to be grudged or evaded. Whoever is impelled to evade or to resent it should retire from society of organized and civilized communities, and become a hermit. He who will live by society must let society live by him, when it requires to." And he added, "All privileges of exemption from his duty (of giving testimony) are exceptional, and are, therefore, to be discountenanced. There must be good reason, plainly shown, for their existence."[65]

Depositions

Depositions are taken in order to preserve testimony, to make discovery, or for cross-examination (to impeach the credibility of the witness). Originally, depositions were done solely and only for the purpose of preserving testimony for trial. A relic of this historic root is that depositions for preservation of testimony were once required to be specifically noticed as *de bene esse* (of well being) depositions. Today, in contrast, any deposition not specifically limited (as for example, for discovery only) may be used for preservation of testimony for use at trial. Of course, if a witness dies or is, for some reason, unavailable at trial, what the lawyer thought originally was not to be a deposition seeking to preserve testimony may turn out to function as the trial testimony of the deponent. As there is the opportunity to cross-examine at the time of the taking of the deposition, it is admissible at trial (where it may be read by anyone of the attorney's choice). In a discovery deposition, designed to gather information prior to trial, almost all the questions are asked by opposing counsel. Depositions take place in an office with attorneys for both sides and a court reporter present. Despite the informal setting, the deponent is under oath, and what is said can be brought up at trial, notably in cross-examination, and it can be the basis for a charge of perjury if deliberately inaccurate.

It is generally required that oral testimony from live witnesses be presented in any trial proceeding.[66] Exceptions permit the use of depositions for witnesses who are dead, at an inconvenient distance from the forum, the elderly, sick, insane, infirm, and the imprisoned who are not subject to subpoena. Such "unavailability" is required before a lay witness's deposition may be admitted. The deposition of an expert witness, however, may be used by any party for any purpose.

Experts' depositions are often *de bene esse* depositions, usually taken by videotape. At any time before trial a party may depose a witness expected to be called as an expert at trial.[67] In some instances, a witness will make a better appearance on videotape and will be more believable than if presented to a jury in person. The deposition is usually taken in the expert's office or where the demonstrative evidence of his profession (diplomas, etc.) can be seen as this lends authority and credibility to his testimony. The deposition of a physician or physical therapist demonstrating an injured plaintiff's physical limitations often is better than an in-court demonstration, which can sometimes be distasteful to a jury.

In preparing the expert for a deposition, the attorney will use some or all of the techniques that he uses in preparing a client for a deposition, except that he will adapt them to the expert and take some special precautions. The expert is expected to review the materials that he has been furnished. The expert should understand that his file, minus any privileged materials, is open to the opposing lawyer. Usually that would be the entire file except for those materials giving the attorney's thoughts and impressions of the case, which are privileged under the attorney–client work product rule. The attorney should learn beforehand, where possible, what the expert may have testified to in similar cases. The attorney should obtain, beforehand, through discovery other information the expert believes is necessary to formulate an opinion in the case, and (if he knows) he should familiarize the expert with such terms as *cause, reasonable degree of medical certainty*, and other key phrases as they are defined in law and which may be important to the case. A legitimate technique of preparation of a witness, particularly a client or an expert witness, is to practice with that witness; however, the danger is that the witness may later try to remember the "right" answers to questions, or will relax too much or give testimony at trial that sounds stale.

Most cases are settled without trial; the depositions play an important role in this settlement. Throughout the preparation for a deposition, the lawyer keeps in mind its context in the case, i.e., its relationship to settlement negotiation, its use for preparation of mediation summaries, and its potential use at trial. Before the deposition, the lawyer considers what facts can be developed in the deposition that will assist him in presenting his theory of the case to the other lawyer, to the mediators, to the judge, and to the jury. Some lawyers will try to talk to the opponent's expert, particularly in cases such as medical malpractice cases, where they believe they can influence the expert. The expert ought to be advised not to talk to anyone concerning the case prior to the deposition. When the expert is deposed by the adversary, the fee is owed by that party (and it is a good idea to be paid in advance). The high cost of litigation is due, in large measure, to the taking of depositions and other discovery.

Discovery of Expert Opinions and Reports

Rules on discovery are designed to avoid unfair surprise at trial and, at the same time, to protect the work product of the lawyer. The expert consulted is, in effect, an extension of the attorney's law firm and is bound by the obligation of confidentiality covering all of the lawyer's staff, including secretaries, investigators, and accountants, whether employees or independent contractors. The expert, for whatever reason, may not switch over to the side of the adversary.

Experts may be classified into three categories, with varying limits on discovery of their opinions and reports.[68]

These three categories of experts include:

1. *Experts expected to be used at trial.* The opponent may learn by interrogatories the names of these trial witnesses and the substance of their testimony, but further discovery concerning them can be had only on motion and court order. By local rule or the practice of individual judges, a date is set in advance of trial for the declaration of experts. Failure to declare will preclude using the expert at trial.

2. *Experts retained or specially employed in anticipation of litigation or preparation for trial, but not expected to be used at trial.* Except in the case of an examining physician, the facts and opinions of experts in this category can be discovered only on a showing of "exceptional circumstances" that make it impractical for the party seeking discovery to obtain the information by other means. The party seeking disclosure "carries a heavy burden."[70] Invoking the attorney work-product privilege to shield a consulting expert is an election not to use that expert at trial.[71]

3. *Experts informally consulted in preparation for trial, but not retained for service in the litigation.* In the majority of jurisdictions, no discovery may be had of the names or views of these experts.[72] Problems arise in drawing a line between informally consulted experts and experts retained in anticipation of litigation. The determination is made on an ad hoc basis, depending on the manner in which the consultation was initiated; the nature, type, and extent of information or material provided to, or determined by the expert in connection with his review; the duration and intensity of the consultative relationship; and the terms of consultation, if any.

The lawyer must make an early decision when consulting an expert whether to use him as a trial witness. Consulting opinions and reports are placed at the risk of discovery when the expert crosses over the line and becomes a trial witness.

Discovery about nontestifying experts is treated very differently from discovery about persons who are expected to be called at trial. Within the category of nontestifying experts, a distinction is made about the discovery of information about nontestifying experts who were specially employed or retained and those who were merely informally consulted. Learning the identity of the former category of experts, facts known or opinions held by them, and the ability to depose them may occur only "upon a showing of exceptional circumstances under which it is impracticable for the party seeking discovery to obtain facts or opinions on the same subject by other means."[69] Nothing about informally consulted experts is discoverable.

What is the basis for treating these experts differently? Routine discovery of any nontestifying expert would deter thorough preparation by the attorney. The attorney is to feel free to discuss strategies and trial preparation with nontestifying experts without worrying about eventual disclosure of that information.

Instruction to Jury

Out of concern that the expert will be unduly persuasive or will usurp the province of the jury, the adversary may request the judge to instruct the jury on the expert's testimony. The jury is told that it is not bound to accept it. On this, a typical instruction provides the following:

> Certain witnesses have been called who testified as expert witnesses. You are not required to take the opinions of experts as binding upon you, but they are to be used to aid you in coming to a proper conclusion. Their testimony is received as that of persons who are learned by reason of special investigation, study, or experience along lines not of general knowledge, and the conclusion of such persons may be of value. You may adopt, or not, their conclusions, according to your own best judgment, giving in each instance such weight as you think should be given under all the facts and circumstances of the case.
>
> In determining the weight to be given such testimony you should consider, among other things:
>
> 1. The education, training, experience and knowledge of the expert with respect to the matters about which he testified.
> 2. The reasons given for his opinion.
> 3. The sources of his information.[73]

There is little, however, to warrant the concern over usurpation of the jury by expert testimony. Actually, studies tend to show that in the majority of cases juries develop a strong leaning or make up their minds on the basis of the opening statements and closing arguments of the lawyer (though technically not evidence) and the demeanor of the parties (the court may specifically instruct the jury that demeanor is evidence). In the Hinckley trial, the jury looked at the accused during the course of the trial, saw his bizarre behavior, and concluded that he was not guilty by reason of insanity. The conflicting testimony tends to wash out, as lawyers say.

The Fee Arrangement

The expert may be a "hired gun," but, quite often, he may need a gun to get paid. Who has the obligation to pay? Who has the ability to pay? The alternative arrangements for compensation of an expert include litigant-paid fees, attorney-advanced or promised fees, and fees taxed as costs or paid out of public funds as in the case of a court-appointed expert. The litigant may be unable or undisposed to pay the fee, especially when the outcome of the case is unfavorable. In cases handled by the lawyer on a contingency fee basis, the fee of the expert is taken as one of his expenses. He may, or may not, pay. In a number of situations, experts have turned to litigation to collect their fee. Hence, payment "up front" is the recommended advice commonly given to those who would serve as experts. Failing that, the expert is advised to serve only on the condition that the attorney assume full responsibility for payment of all services in connection with the case. Court approval must be obtained for the payment of expert witness fees.[74] Attorneys paid on a contingency basis are more likely to advance expert fees.

The contingency fee—either a percentage or fixed amount conditioned on recovery of a judgment or settlement—is an option not available to an expert witness. This is based on the theory that it would unduly intensify the expert's interest in the outcome of the case and would undermine the credibility of his testimony. That it would degrade testimonial reliability beyond present practices may be exaggerated, however.[75] Still others argue that the ban on expert contingency fees deprives litigants in many cases of the services of an expert.[76] Legislation enacted in Michigan in 1986 makes testifying on a contingency fee basis a misdemeanor.[77] An expert retained on a contingency basis violates ethical guidelines, and so any member of the profession learning of it has an obligation to report it to the Board of Medicine.

The compensation available for an examination often determines the length of time that the expert spends on the case. In many criminal cases where the defendant pleads "not guilty by reason of insanity," the forensic experts spend hundreds of hours interviewing the defendant and witnesses, when in actuality the evaluation could have been done in a few hours, especially when the defendant is patently delusional. The late Dr. Robert Myers, prominent forensic psychiatrist in Australia, was dismayed by the number of hours spent by forensic experts in the United States. He would carry out an evaluation in two or three hours.

The adversary has the right to challenge all credentials, including fee arrangements. On cross-examination, the expert is likely asked, "How much are you being *paid* for your testimony?" (The reply ought to be, "I am not being paid for my testimony. I am being paid for my time, like the other professional people in the courtroom.")[78] Fees for forensic services are usually higher than fees for treatment. The California Law Revision Commission of its rules of evidence states in a comment: "The jury can better appraise the extent to which bias may have influenced an expert's opinion if it is informed of the amount of his fee—and, hence, the extent of his possible feeling of obligation to the party calling him."[79] A lawyer strategy of portraying a witness as a "professional expert" whose testimony has been purchased may be deemed so prejudicial as to require a new trial. In one case, the Michigan Supreme Court said, "We do not view … remarks concerning plaintiffs' experts as being merely 'breaches of good manners'; we perceive a studied purpose to prejudice the jury and divert the jurors' attention from the merits of the case … . [w]e cannot believe that plaintiffs had a fair trial where defendants' counsel succeeded in characterizing plaintiffs' witnesses as 'professional experts' who made their living traveling around the country as a trio providing 'bought' testimony."[80]

In another malpractice case, the Michigan Supreme Court said, "Fairness to physicians requires the rule requiring expert testimony, but fairness to injured persons requires the plaintiff's expert witnesses not be impugned simply because they have testified for plaintiffs in other cases … . To allow the defendant to challenge a plaintiff's expert witness simply because he testifies for plaintiffs with some frequency is to permit the defendant to exploit unfairly the rule requiring, for defendant's protection, expert testimony, and the reluctance of physicians to testify against another member of their profession."[81] In a criminal case, the Michigan Supreme Court, reversing a conviction, found that the prosecutor argued matters not in evidence in saying (in closing argument) that the defense expert on insanity had testified in the manner he did only because he was paid to do so.[82]

A Final Comment

Invariably, in what may be described as a Catch-22, the witness proffered as an expert, who is a "virgin" in testifying, is attacked as unqualified to testify while, on the other hand, the witness, who testifies frequently as an expert, is disparaged as a "whore."[83] One judge said to an expert witness, "Aren't you ashamed to be seen here in court so often?" To which the expert replied, "Why no, Your Honor, I always thought it was a very respectable place."[84]

To enhance one's credibility as an expert witness, psychologist Stanley Brodsky recommends measuring devices suggested by Edward Colbach: a "contrary quotient" (CQ) and perhaps also a "validity quotient" (VQ). The CQ could calculate how many times the expert's opinion was or was not that desired by retaining counsel, and that, of course, he was called only when his opinion fitted with the case of the retaining attorney. The VQ would calculate the number of court decisions that were in accord with the expert's opinion, but this quotient is based on the assumption that the validity of the expert opinion is affirmed by legal standards as demonstrated by the court decisions. Time and again, it has been shown that experience, by itself, is unrelated to the accuracy of clinical assessments.[85]

Endnotes

1. The proposition—that the task of each side under the adversary system is to put forward its best case—is not without criticism. Judge Harry T. Edwards of the U.S. Court of Appeals for the District of Columbia says, "As a judge, I see far too many examples of abusive litigation tactics, such as the withholding of critical information from the court." H.T. Edwards, "Do Lawyers Still Make a Difference?" *Wayne L. Rev.* 32 (1986): 201 at 206. Putting one's best foot forward, keeping silent on the negative, is not unique to the adversary system, of course. In one of Luigi Pirandello's short stories, "Moon Sickness," a husband tells his bride shortly after their marriage that he becomes like a werewolf at a full moon. "Why didn't you tell me before our marriage?" she asks.
2. While the use of "he" as universal reverberates with a not-so-subtle glorification of the male and a dismissal of the female, I want to assure that is not intended. Writing "he or she" is cumbersome, so in this book I simply use "he." David Gelernter, professor of computer science at Yale, ponders whether the damage to the English language can be undone in "Feminism and the English Language," *Weekly Standard*, March 3, 2008, p. 25.
3. See Koeller v. Reynolds, 344 N.W.2d 556 (Iowa App. 1983) (attorney malpractice); Annot., "Necessity of Expert Testimony to Show Malpractice of Architect," 3 A.L.R.4th 1023 (1981). In medical malpractice actions, a plaintiff must establish through expert medical opinion (1) the standard of care in the locality where treatment occurred, (2) that defendant breached that standard of care, and (3) that the breach of the standard of care was the proximate cause of injury. Gibson v. D'Amico, 97 A.D.2d 905, 470 N.Y.S.2d 739 (3d Dept. 1983); Bivins v. Detroit Osteopathic Hospital, 258 N.W.2d 527 (Mich. App. 1977).
4. W. Prosser & W.P. Keeton, *The Law of Torts* (St. Paul, MN: West, 5th ed. 1984). Expert testimony is sometimes required in breach-of-contract cases just as in malpractice cases. See, e.g., Steinmetz v. Lowry, 17 Ohio App.3d 116, 477 N.E.2d 671 (1984). In Blatz v. Allina Health System, 622 N.W.2d. 376 (Minn. 2001), the court held that the appropriate standard of care for paramedics in attempting to locate the home of a patient was that of an ordinary person and, therefore, expert testimony was not required to establish standard of care.
5. See Chapter 31 on informed consent.
6. 387 N.W.2d 486 (Neb. 1986).
7. 387 N.W.2d at 489.
8. Helling v. Carey, 83 Wash.2d 514, 519 P.2d 981 (1974).
9. Tarasoff v. Regents of the University of California, 13 Cal.3d 177, 529 P.2d 553, 118 Cal. Rptr. 129 (1974), *vacated*, 17 Cal.3d 425, 551 P.2d 334, 131 Cal. Rptr. 14 (1976).
10. 551 P.2d at 345, 131 Cal. Rptr. at 25. In Louisiana, a *Tarasoff*-type case is called one of ordinary negligence, not malpractice, as the plaintiff is not a patient but a third party. The holding amends the restrictions on a malpractice suit. As a result, the therapist is exposed to personal liability (unless he has liability insurance). Hutchinson v. Patel, 637 So.2d 415 (La. 1994). See the Chapter 36 on duty to third parties.
11. 551 P.2d at 345, 131 Cal. Rptr. at 25.
12. 551 P.2d at 340.
13. See J.C. Beck, "Violent Patients and the *Tarasoff* Duty in Private Psychiatric Cases," *J. Psychiat. & Law* 13 (1985): 361.
14. 105 S. Ct. 1087 (1985).

15. 105 S. Ct. at 1092.
16. J. Robitscher, *The Powers of Psychiatry* (Boston: Houghton Mifflin, 1980).
17. Rule 702 of the Federal Rules of Evidence in an earlier version called for "special" knowledge, but the qualification was omitted in the final version.
18. Rule 701, Federal Rules of Evidence.
19. For psychiatric testimony, Terence F. MacCarthy, the Federal Public Defender in Chicago, said he would "get someone with a foreign accent and Freud as his middle name." Quoted in S. Taylor, "Hinckley Trial: $2 Million So Far in Case Where Experts Plus Time Equal Money," *New York Times*, June 14, 1982, p. 16.
20. See McDonnell v. Commission on Medical Discipline, 301 Md. 426, 483 A.2d 76 (1984); discussed in Chapter 4 on holding the expert accountable.
21. R. Cohen, "The Ethicist," *New York Times Magazine*, May 27, 3007, p. 20.
22. Comment by Sheldon Miller, well-known Detroit trial lawyer, in an address at Wayne State University School of Law. While the law may require expert testimony in a particular case, experts—one and all—must overcome the impression that because they are "paid witnesses," their credibility is impugned, and, in particular, psychiatric experts must overcome the impression that their testimony is fanciful. Parodies of psychological testimony abound. The psychologist, as distinguished from the psychiatrist, was, for a long time, not allowed to testify as an expert on insanity and competency. The leading case on allowing testimony by a psychologist is Jenkins v. United States, 307 F.2d 637 (D.C. 1962). See the cases collected in 78 A.L.R.2d 919. Today, generally speaking, the testimony of a psychologist is often preferred over that of the psychiatrist because it is based on testing. Depending on the type of testimony sought to be elicited, the courts have been inconsistent in the degree to which they insist on professional qualifications when an expert proffers psychological opinions. See A.A. Moenssens, D.C. Henderson, & S.G. Portwood, *Scientific Evidence in Civil and Criminal Cases* (New York: Foundation Press, 5th ed., 2007), pp. 1302–1306.
23. See Mich. H.B. 5154; P.A. 178 of 1986, § 2192 (d) (e); *Tate v. Detroit Receiving Hosp.*, 249 Mich. App. 212, 642 N.W.2d 346 (2002); Dolan v. Galluzzo, 77 Ill.2d 279, 396 N.E.2d 13 (1979). See Chapter 27 on establishing malpractice liability.
24. Nally v. Grace Community Church of the Valley, Civ. No. 67200 (not published, but available through West Law or Lexis database services).
25. Nally v. Grace Community Church of the Valley, 157 Cal. App. 3d 912, 204 Cal. Rptr. 303 (Cal. App. 1984). Following several years of coverage in newspapers and magazines (e.g., *National Law Journal*, July 16, 1984, p. 6), the case was featured on NBC's *20/20* April 6, 1986. See E. Barker, "Clergy Malpractice," *Trial*, July 1986, p. 58.
26. 204 Cal. Rptr. at 309.
27. See S. Brownlee, *Overtreated* (New York: Bloomsbury, 2007); R.O. Pasnau, "Response to the Presidential Address; Health Care Crisis: A Campaign for Action, *Am. J. Psychiat.* 143 (1986): 955.
28. Quoted in R.M. Restak, "Psychiatry in America," *Wilson Q.* 7 (1983): 95.
29. McDonnell v. County of Nassau, 492 N.Y.S.2d 699 (Sup. 1985). In Taormina v. Goodman, 63 A.D.2d 1018, 406 N.Y.S.2d 350 (2d Dept. 1978), a medical doctor was not allowed to testify to the alleged malpractice of a chiropractor.
30. In a bit of satire, humorist Art Buchwald has a lawyer saying, "We have lists of shrinks who believe anyone who commits a major crime is crazy, just as the government has lists of doctors who are willing to testify that anyone involved in one was sane. We don't use their lists and they don't use ours." Syndicated column, May 11, 1982. The epithet "whores of the court" is widely used to denigrate expert witnesses. See, e.g., M.A. Hagen, *Whores of the Court* (New York: Harper Collins, 1997); S. Moss, "Opinion for Sale/Confessions of an Expert Witness," *Legal Affairs*, March/April 2003, p. 52. Dr. Douglas Mossman cites cases where the psychiatric or psychological witness is described as a hired gun, whore, or prostitute, and he responds to the experts. See D. Mossman, "'Hired Guns,' 'Whores,' and 'Prostitutes': Case Law References to Clinicians of Ill Repute," *J. Am. Acad. Psychiat. & Law* 27 (1999): 414; see also B. Bursten, *Psychiatry on Trial* (Jefferson, NC: McFarland, 2001). In his writings, Judge Richard Posner excoriates judges who in their opinions denounce experts by name, and experts cannot respond to judges because they have immunity from suit for defamation or from anything else they say. See L. Mac Farquhar, "The Bench Burner," *New Yorker*, Dec. 10, 2001, p. 78.

By the way, if the experts are "whores," then who are the pimps? Who is blameworthy: the buyer or seller, or both? In the case of controlled substances (narcotics) both buyer and seller are condemned, while in prostitution only the seller. The prominent advocate C.P. Harvey, one of her Majesty's counsel, said that to practice law, one must have "flexible morality." See C.P. Harvey, *The Advocate's Devil*

(London: Stevens & Sons, 1958), p. 92. Michael Brock, a forensic mental health professional in Michigan, responds, "Attorneys with whom I have worked as a forensic mental health expert sometimes like to needle me about being a whore. Of course, they say it with a good-natured smile, but we both know they mean it. Sometimes I let it go, but sometimes I smile good naturedly and say, 'Well, it may be true that all the whores in our business are mental health experts, but all the pimps are lawyers.' They laugh, but of course, they know that I mean it, too." M.G. Brock, "A look at the judiciary," *Detroit Legal News*, March 21, 2007, p. 3. In a Gallup poll rating the "ethical standards" of various professionals, 38% of respondents would trust psychiatrists, 18% of respondents would trust lawyers, and only 7% would trust car salesmen. E. Bender, "Public Has Trust Issues with Psychiatrists, Survey Finds," *Psychiatric News*, March 2, 2007.

31. O'Gee v. Dobbs Houses, 570 F.2d 1084 (2d Cir. 1978): Hernandez v. Faker, 137 Ariz. 449, 671 P.2d 427 (1983); Ballenger v. Burris Industries, 311 S.E.2d 881 (N.C. App. 1984). See D.W. Shuman, *Psychiatric and Psychological Evidence* (Colorado Springs: Shepard's/McGraw-Hill, 1986).

32. Thus, in Linn v. Fossum, 2006 WL 3093186 (Fla. 2006), the Florida Supreme Court held that an expert witness's trial testimony on direct examination stating she consulted with colleagues and others when formulating her opinion about the conduct of a physician named in a malpractice suit was inadmissible. In this case, the expert testified on direct examination that although she might have taken a different approach to the patient's treatment, after conferring with other physicians and experts she thought the defendant physician had met the standard of care. The Florida Supreme Court noted that under state law, experts can rely on "facts or data" not admissible in forming their opinions, but, the court said that where an expert solicits the opinions of other experts who lack firsthand knowledge of the case at hand, this information constitutes not facts or data, but unverifiable hearsay opinions. The court added that an expert's testimony must not be used merely as a conduit for the introduction of otherwise inadmissible evidence, as the opposing party would not be able to cross-examine the nontestifying experts.

33. See, e.g., Michigan Rules of Evidence, Rule 703.

34. 673 F.2d 1114 (10th Cir. 1982).

35. See Federal Rules of Evidence, Rules 403 and 404(b).

36. 673 F.2d at 1122.

37. "Pepper and Salt," *Wall Street Journal*, Sept. 4, 1986, p. 23.

38. Ga. O.C.G.A. 15-19-14.

39. Nix v. Whiteside, 106 S. Ct. 988, 995 (1986).

40. 753 F.2d 991 (11th Cir. 1985).

41. 388 N.W.2d 206 (Mich. 1986).

42. J.R. Rappeport, "Ethical Issues in Forensic Psychiatry," in A. Carmi, S. Schneider, & A. Hefez (Eds.), *Psychiatry—Law and Ethics* (New York: Springer-Verlag, 1986), p. 308. A typical instruction to the jury on expert opinion based upon a hypothetical question is as follows: "An expert witness answering a hypothetical question assumes as true every material act stated in the question. The value of his opinion is dependent upon, and is no stronger than, the material facts upon which it is based. Therefore, the opinion of the expert should be disregarded by you, unless you find the material facts stated in the question are true." Nebraska Jury Instruction 1.43. This instruction is based on the general principle that "the premise being false, the conclusion based thereon cannot be accepted as true." Williams v. Watson Bros. Transp. Co., 145 Neb. 466, 16 N.W.2d 199 (1945).

43. J.R. Rappeport, "Reasonable Medical Certainty," *Bull. Amer. Acad. Psychiat. & Law* 13 (1985): 5.

44. Congress amended the Rules of Evidence to provide that a writing used to refresh the memory of a witness *before* he testifies needs to be produced only if the court in its discretion determines it is necessary in the interest of justice. A writing used *while* testifying must be shown to the adversary on request. Federal Rules of Evidence, Rule 612.

45. Thus, in Davis v. Lhim, 124 Mich. App. 291 (1983), involving a psychiatrist's duty to protect a third person endangered by a patient, defense counsel was not allowed to present expert witnesses as they were not timely listed. Thus, it is essential that the attorney determine at the outset whether this case is one of malpractice or ordinary negligence, which does not require expert testimony. (see Chapter 26). Query: Should Dr. Lhim, found liable, have sued his lawyer for legal malpractice? As a state hospital employee, he was represented by the state attorney, who enjoys immunity.

46. Under Federal Rule of Civil Procedure 26, the expert is obliged to prepare a report that sets out all opinions and their bases, qualifications, publication list for the past 10 years, and testimony at trials and depositions. Various states do not require a report, but if a report is prepared, testimony at

trial may not go beyond the report. Hence, reports in these states are not prepared except when it is considered that they may aid in settlement. See P.I. Ostroff, "Experts: A Few Fundamentals," in *The Litigation Manual/A Primer for Trial Lawyers* (Chicago: American Bar Association, 1983), p. 84.

47. Humorist Art Buchwald has written (syndicated column, May 11, 1982):
    "I asked a defense attorney ... suppose you hire a psychiatrist to examine your client and he decides the person was sane at the time he committed the crime."
    "I'd fire him ... . I've had cases where five shrinks have examined my client before I could get one to say he was crazy."
    "And that was the one you called to the stand?"
    "If I called the other four, I could have been sued for malpractice."

48. Geders v. United States, 425 U.S. 80 (1976). And as the court in Miller v. Universal City Studios, 650 F.2d 1365 (5th Cir. 1981), put it: "The purpose of the sequestration rule is to prevent the shaping of testimony by one witness to match that of another, and to discourage fabrication and collusion."

49. Federal Rules of Evidence, Rule 615(3).

50. Morvant v. Construction Aggregates Corp., 570 F.2d 626 (6th Cir. 1978), *cert. denied,* 439 U.S. 801 (1978). In Morvant, the court stated that it could "perceive little, if any, reason for sequestering a witness who is to testify in an expert capacity only and not to the facts of the case" 570 F.2d at 629. The court in Morvant further held, however, that Rule 703, providing wide bases of opinion testimony, does not furnish an automatic ground for exempting an expert from sequestration under Rule 615, 570 F.2d at 630.

51. United States v. Hiss, 88 F. Supp. 559 (S.D. N.Y. 1950). See the discussion in Chapter 6 on witnesses and the credibility of testimony.

52. The transcript of the cross-examination by prosecutor Thomas Murphy of Dr. Binger is used in trial tactics courses as illustrative of effective cross-examination. Transcripts are available from Professional Education Group in Hopkins, Minnesota.

53. Report of Senate Committee on the Judiciary on Rule 615, Federal Rules of Evidence.

54. United States v. Alvarez, 755 F.2d 830 (11th Cir. 1985).

55. Miller v. Universal City Studios, 650 F.2d 1365, at 1373 (5th Cir. 1981).

56. The remedy for sequestration violation is discretionary with the trial judge. United States v. Oropeza, 564 F.2d 316 (9th Cir. 1977), *cert. denied,* 434 U.S. 1080 (1978).

57. D.W. Shuman, "Testimonial Compulsion: The Involuntary Medical Expert Witness," *J. Legal Med.* 4 (1983): 419.

58. In Karp v. Cooley, 493 F.2d 408, 424-25 (5th Cir. 1984), Dr. Michael DeBakey refused to answer whether it was bad medical practice in 1969 to put a mechanical heart in a human being. Vindicating his position was no easy task.

59. In People v. Barnes, 11 Cal. App. 605, 295 Pac. 1045 (1931), a handwriting expert was asked for an impromptu opinion on the stand as to the possibly identical authorship of several specimens of handwriting, some of which he had never seen. It was held he did not have to express an opinion. See also Mason v. Robinson, 340 N.W.2d 236 (Iowa 1983); Commonwealth of Mass. v. Vitello, 367 Mass. 224, 327 N.E.2d 819 (1975).

60. See P.L. Porterfield, "The Right to Subpoena Expert Testimony and the Fees Required to Be Paid Therefore, *Hastings L.J.* 5 (1953): 50; Comment: "Requiring Experts to Testify in Maine," *U. Me. L.Rev.* 20 (1968): 297; Comment: "Compelling Experts to Testify: A Proposal," *U. Chi. L. Rev.* 44 (1977): 851.

61. This language is taken verbatim from former Federal Rules of Criminal Procedure, Rule 28.

62. 539 F.2d 811 (2d Cir. 1976).

63. 547 F. Supp. 871 (E.D. Mich. 1982).

64. I. Younger, "On Technology and the Law of Evidence," *U. Colo. L. Rev.* 49 (1977): 1.

65. J. Wigmore, *Evidence* (McNaughton Rev. 1961), vol. 8, §1292.

66. Fed. Civ. P. 32(A); Mich. Court Rules 2.308.

67. Mich. Court Rules 2.302(B)(4)(d).

68. For a detailed discussion, see C.A. Wright & A.R. Miller, *Federal Practices and Procedure* (St. Paul, MN: West, 1970 and supp.), vol. 8, sec. 2029.

69. Federal Rule 26(b) (4) (B).

70. Ager v. Stormont Hospital & Training School for Nurses, 622 F.2d 496, 503 (10th Cir. 1980).

71. Garrett v. Coast Federal Savings & Loan Assn., 136 Cal. App.3d 266, 186 Cal. Rptr. 178 (1982).

72. Annot., "Pretrial Discovery of Facts Known and Opinions Held by Opponents' Expert Under Rule 26(b)(4) of Federal Rules of Civil Procedure," 33 A.L.R. Fed. 403 (1977).

73. Nebraska Jury Instruction 1.42.

74. See, e.g., M.C.L.A. (Mich.) 600.2164 (expert witness fee statute); Spearman v. Barron, 351 So.2d 856 (La. App. 1977).

75. Note: "Contingent Fees for Expert Witnesses in Civil Litigation," *Yale L. J.* 86 (1977): 1680.

76. Argued in Person v. Assn. of Bar of City of New York, 554 F.2d 534 (2d Cir. 1977).

77. Mich. P.A. 178 of 1986.

78. P.J. Resnick, "The Psychiatrist in Court," in J.O. Cavenar (ed.), *Psychiatry* (Philadelphia: Lippincott, 1986), vol. 3, chap. 37, p. 8.

79. *Cal. L. Rev. Comm. Reports* 7 (1965): 1. See also J.H. Friedenthal, "Discovery and Use of an Adverse Party's Expert Information," *Stan. L. Rev.* 14 (1962): 455.

80. Kern v. St. Luke's Hospital Ass'n. of Saginaw, 404 Mich. 339, 273 N.W.2d 75 (1978). The conduct of defense counsel was perceived as "a studied purpose to prejudice the jury."

81. Wilson v. Stilwill, 309 N.W.2d 898 (Mich. 1981).

82. People v. Tyson, 423 Mich. 357, 377 N.W.2d 738 (1985).

83. In one case involving an expert who testified frequently on product safety, it was noted on cross-examination that he had criticized products literally "from A to Z." The cross-examiner began writing items down on a large pad, starting with automatic garage door openers. He did fine up to J: "Jumping on a trampoline." "I think that that should be under T," quipped the other attorney. The cross-examiner kept up through W, with wood preservatives, then petered out altogether, admitting, "I couldn't find X, Y, Z." C. Guyette, "Anatomy of a verdict," *Metro Times* (Detroit), May 17–23, 2000, p. 12.

84. Reported in E. Tanay, "Money and the Expert Witness: An Ethical Dilemma," *J. Foren. Sci.* 21 (1976): 769.

85. S.L. Brodsky, *The Expert Expert Witness* (Washington, DC: American Psychological Association, 1999), pp. 75–79; E.M. Colbach, "Integrity Checks on the Witness Stand," *Bull. Am. Acad. Psychiat. & Law* 9 (1981): 285. See also B.D. Sales & D.W. Shuman, "Reclaiming the Integrity of Science in Expert Witnessing," *Ethics & Behav.* 3 (1993): 223.

3

Restrictions on Expert Testimony

In the 19th and early 20th centuries the courts asked only whether the expert was "qualified" before the expert's testimony could be admitted. Since then, particularly during the last quarter century, various restrictions—real or perceived—have been put on expert testimony. Notably, with the advent of mass torts, companies have been driven into bankruptcy as a result of court decisions involving expert testimony. In the latter part of the 20th century, expert testimony has frequently been derided as "junk science." Time and again, numerous books and articles, as well as editorials in various newspapers, have criticized the role of lawyers and experts in litigation. In 1986, a prominent federal judge said, "It is time to take hold of expert testimony."[1]

In this chapter, the following topics are discussed: (1) the trial judge as gatekeeper, (2) right of confrontation, (3) testimony on ultimate issue, (4) form of testimony— narrative v. question and answer, (5) special rules on qualification of experts in malpractice cases, (6) ethics guidelines, (7) treating therapist as expert, (8) forensic consultation in states in which the expert is not licensed, and (9) suspension or termination of professional license.

The Trial Judge as Gatekeeper

Many commentators mused that junk science in the courtroom was to end under the U.S. Supreme Court's celebrated decision in 1993 in *Daubert v. Merrell Dow Pharmaceuticals*.[2] The case involved expert testimony concerning the teratogenic effect of the antinausea drug Bendectin. Before *Daubert*, for almost three quarters of a century, the *Frye* test, from the brief (two-page) 1923 decision in *Frye v. United States*,[3] reigned as the standard governing admissibility of scientific testimony. In *Frye*, the D.C. Circuit Court wrote,

> Just when a scientific principle or discovery crosses the line between experimental and demonstrable stages is difficult to define. Somewhere in this twilight zone the evidential force of the principle must be recognized, and while the courts will go a long way in admitting expert testimony deduced from a well-recognized scientific principle or discovery, the thing from which the deduction is made must be sufficiently established to have general acceptance in the particular field in which it belongs.[4]

In *Frye*, the defendant sought to use the testimony of an expert who would opine, on the basis of blood pressure readings, that the defendant was telling the truth when he denied having committed the alleged offense. The D.C. Court of Appeals rejected the evidence on the ground that it was the product of a scientific theory that was not yet generally accepted within the relevant professional community.

The *Frye* test presents numerous difficulties in application. Who must have accepted the principle in question? What is the field to which the principle must belong? What is meant by "general acceptance"? What degree of dissent will render the evidence inadmissible? To what subjects is the *Frye* test applicable? To all scientific matters or only to "novel" scientific matters? To "scientific" matters but not to nonscientific matters?

Under *Daubert*, in implementing Rule 702 of the Federal Rules of Evidence (FRE; adopted in 1975) that allows "scientific, technical, or other specialized knowledge [that] will assist the trier of fact to understand the evidence or to determine a fact," the Supreme Court called upon trial judges to be active gatekeepers to ensure that "any and all scientific testimony or evidence admitted is not only relevant but reliable." In less than a decade there were thousands of appeals based on *Daubert*; hundreds of these appeals related to the testimony of mental health experts.

At a hearing (which has come to be known as a "Daubert hearing"), the parties make their claims about the validity of the evidence. The effective application of *Daubert* requires the trial judge to learn about the scientific notion or technique in question. The judge is not bound by a scientific "party line," as required under *Frye*, and allows researchers using new techniques in the vanguard of scientific knowledge to bring their knowledge to court. Novel scientific evidence, not admissible under *Frye*, may be admissible under *Daubert* (*novel* means that which is not generally accepted in the particular field).[5]

The *Frye* decision focused exclusively on "novel" scientific techniques. The Court in *Daubert* said that the requirements of FRE 702 do not apply specially or exclusively to unconventional evidence. Of course, well-established propositions are less likely to be challenged than those that are novel, and they are more handily defended. Indeed, theories that are so firmly established as to have attained the status of scientific law, such as the laws of thermodynamics, properly are subject to judicial notice.

Under *Daubert*, "general acceptance" within the relevant field of science is but one consideration in ascertaining reliability or validity. *Daubert* did not eliminate the "general acceptance" test, but incorporated it as one of the indicia to be considered in determining whether to admit scientific evidence. To the extent that *Daubert* retains the *Frye* test as one factor to be considered, all of the questions presented under *Frye* remain. As often noted, the judge under *Daubert* is to consider the following: Is the theory or technique testable, and has it been tested? Has the theory or technique been subjected to peer review and publication? What is the known or potential error rate for the technique? Is the expert's field a "well-accepted body of learning" with reasonably well-defined standards?

With expert testimony ranging from alloys to zygotes, the competency of a judge to evaluate under the *Daubert* criteria is questionable. In *Daubert*, on remand, Judge Alex Kozinski of the U.S. Court of Appeals for the Ninth Circuit in 1995 noted that while judges are largely untrained in science and no match for any of the witnesses whose testimony they are reviewing, "it is our responsibility [under the Supreme Court's decision] to determine whether those experts' proposed testimony amounts to 'scientific knowledge,' constitutes 'good science,' and was 'derived by the scientific method.'"[6] He went on to raise the question:

> How do we figure out whether scientists have derived their findings through the scientific method or whether their testimony is based on scientifically valid principles? ... One very significant fact to be considered is whether the experts are proposing to testify about matters growing naturally and directly out of research they have conducted independent of the litigation, or whether they have developed their opinions expressly for purposes of testifying. That an expert testifies for money does not necessarily cast doubt on the reliability of his testimony, as few experts appear in court merely as an eleemosynary gesture. But in determining whether proposed expert testimony amounts to good science, we may not ignore the fact that a scientist's normal workplace is the lab or the field, not the courtroom or the lawyer's office.[7]

In *Daubert*, the Supreme Court said, "[A] pertinent consideration [in determining whether a theory or technique is scientific knowledge that will assist the trier of fact] is whether the theory or technique has been subjected to peer review and publication." "Peer review" refers to the evaluation of submitted manuscripts to determine what work is published in a professional journal. It may be asked whether "peer review" is a rubber stamp and whether publications produced by professional organizations are manufactured in order to defend against lawsuits. Then too, pharmaceutical companies are known to distort the results of clinical trials and, thereby, mislead the merits of their products. In ruling on *Daubert* on remand from the Supreme Court, Judge Kozinski acknowledged that a peer-reviewed publication is no guarantee that testimony is trustworthy, but, nevertheless, he said that the fact "[t]hat the research is accepted for publication in a reputable scientific journal … is a significant indication that … it meets at least the minimal criteria of good science." Hence, since "[n]one of the plaintiffs' experts has published his work on Benedectin in a scientific journal," the court affirmed the lower court's summary judgment once again.

In one way or another, the lower federal courts have resisted a literal application of *Daubert*. By and large, judges are unable or do not want to be thrust into the role of scientific arbiter. In 1995, in *McCullock v. H.B. Fuller Co.*,[8] Federal Court of Appeals Judge Joseph McLaughlin wrote that while trial judges must exercise sound discretion as gatekeepers of expert testimony under *Daubert*, they are not "St. Peter at the gates of heaven, performing a searching inquiry into the depth of an expert witness's soul, separating the saved from [the] damned. Such an inquiry would inexorably lead to evaluating witness credibility and weight of the evidence, the ageless role of the jury."[9]

In *Daubert*, Chief Justice Rehnquist wrote in a dissent, "I defer to no one in my confidence in federal judges, but I am at a loss to know what is meant when it is said that the scientific status of a theory depends on its 'falsifiability,' and I suspect some of them will be, too." He went on to say, "I do not doubt that Rule 702 confides to the judge some gatekeeping responsibility in deciding questions of the admissibility of proffered expert testimony. But I do not think it imposes on them either the obligation or the authority to become amateur scientists in order to perform that role."[10]

From time to time scholars have proposed creating a judicial or quasijudicial "science court" to resolve factual disputes, but the idea has largely been abandoned as unworkable.[11]

Do the *Daubert* criteria apply to any type of science, and do the criteria apply to areas outside of science? Rule 702 speaks about "scientific," "technical," or "other specialized knowledge." The language of Rule 702 makes no distinction between "scientific" knowledge and "technical" or "other specialized" knowledge. It makes clear that any such knowledge may become the subject of expert testimony. As a matter of language, FRE 702 applies its reliability standard to all "scientific," "technical," or "other specialized" matters within its scope. The Court in *Daubert* referred only to "scientific" knowledge because that was the nature of the expertise at issue.

Daubert clearly involved hard science. Indeed, in *Daubert*, the Supreme Court stated that the enumerated criteria do not constitute a checklist—the criteria can be applied as deemed appropriate by the trial judge, not all criteria need be applied, and those that are applied can be given unequal weight. In *Daubert*, Justice Blackmun, author of the Court's opinion, interpreted Rule 702 to require that the content of the expert's testimony be "scientific" in the sense that it be "ground[ed] in the methods and procedures of science." Justice Blackmun understood science to be a method or a procedure rather than simply a body of facts. Upon his death, in a memorial to him, it was stated that his discussion of the factors that make knowledge "scientific"—falsifiability, peer review, error rates, and general acceptance within the relevant scientific community—reflected his "longstanding receptivity to scientific ways in understanding complex events."[12]

What about psychiatry or psychology? They may be categorized as "other specialized knowledge" or "soft science." They are often described as more art than science.[13] (Perhaps the hard sciences could include neuropsychology, given its reliance on quantitative measurement.[14]) Propositions in the soft sciences, by their very nature, cannot be validated in the same manner as in the hard sciences.

For the soft sciences, while there must be a basis for the expert's opinion, the opinions of the courts on the application of *Daubert*, however, have been divided. As we shall illustrate, the majority of courts have held that neither the *Frye* or *Daubert* tests apply, and instead they apply a conventional analysis, i.e., the acceptability of the evidence depends on the experience or training of the expert.[15] In a case involving the child sexual abuse accommodation syndrome, the Michigan Supreme Court in 1990 held that the rules on competency of testimony do not apply to expert witnesses in behavioral sciences. The court said:

> Psychologists, when called as experts, do not talk about things or objects, they talk about people. They do not dehumanize people with whom they deal by treating them as objects composed of interacting biological systems. Rather, they speak of the whole person. Thus, it is difficult to fit the behavioral professions within the application and definition of *Frye*.[16]

In 1995, in *Borawick v. Shay*,[17] involving repressed-memory evidence, the Second Circuit said, "We do not believe that *Daubert* is directly applicable to the issue here because *Daubert* concerns the admissibility of data derived from scientific techniques or expert opinions." Also in 1995, in *United States v. Starzecpyzel*,[18] a federal district court in South Dakota concluded that questioned-document testimony is not scientific knowledge under *Daubert* because there is a lack of systematic empirical validation for many of the assumptions in questioned-document examination. In 1996, in *Compton v. Subaru of America*,[19] the Tenth Circuit emphasized, "[A]pplication of the *Daubert* factors is unwarranted in cases where expert testimony is based solely upon experiences or training." In 1997, in *Jenson v. Eveleth Taconite Co.*,[20] the Eighth Circuit observed, "There is some question as to whether the *Daubert* analysis should be applied at all to 'soft' sciences such as psychology." The assessment of the risk of suicide (danger to oneself) or danger to others is apparently unaffected by *Daubert*.[21] Of course, in all cases, *Daubert* or no *Daubert*, an opinion unsupported by data is excluded as speculation.

On the other hand, a minority of courts have held that *Daubert* does apply to the soft science, but give only lip service to it or the bar is set low.[22] The Texas Court of Criminal Appeals applied *Daubert* to expert testimony using unstructured clinical judgments to predict future dangerousness at capital sentencing, and, lo and behold, it ruled that the testimony meets the *Daubert* test.[23] However, under the majority view, as illustrated by *United States v. Fields*,[24] the Fifth Circuit in 2007 ruled that the *Daubert* factors do not apply in determining the admissibility of expert evidence in death penalty hearings. Moreover, it may be noted, the rules of evidence do not generally apply in sentencing hearings. The Federal Death Penalty Act (FDPA) provides that evidence may be admitted "regardless of its admissibility under the rules governing admission of evidence at criminal trials."[25] FDPA sets a low barrier to the admission of evidence at capital sentencing hearings and by its terms, does not fully implement the Federal Rules of Evidence at the punishment phase. Because the holding in *Daubert* was based on the Federal Rules of Evidence, it is not directly applicable.

Given that *Daubert* allows testimony not generally accepted in the particular field, some courts have used *Daubert* to broaden rather than narrow admissibility of expert opinion in the soft sciences. The traditional rule has been that the opinion of a psychiatrist or psychologist of whether a witness is lying or telling the truth is ordinarily inadmissible because the opinion exceeds the scope of the expert's specialized knowledge. Traditionally, credibility is deemed to be a matter that a jury can decide without the aid of expert testimony. This rule, however, has been bent in the post-*Daubert* era to allow that kind of testimony. In 1995, in *United States v. Shay*,[26] the First Circuit reversed the trial court's exclusion of psychiatric testimony that the defendant's inculpatory statements were caused by *pseudologia fantastica*, a mental disorder rendering the person a pathological liar, one who makes false statements without regard to their consequences. The First Circuit said that the evidence goes to character (or competency) and that under the rules of evidence, truthful or untruthful character (or competency) may be proven by expert testimony.[27] Citing *Daubert*, the court assumed the reliability of the expert testimony.

Similarly, in *United States v. Hall*,[28] the Seventh Circuit in 1996 ruled that the trial court erred when it excluded testimony on false confessions. In denying the use of proffered expert testimony to that effect, the trial judge had said that the jury needed no help in assessing the suggestiveness of the interrogator's techniques. Reversing, the Seventh Circuit noted that the trial judge had failed to comply with, or even mention *Daubert*, and found that the conclusions were based on a misunderstanding of the helpfulness required of expert testimony. The Seventh Circuit noted that the Supreme Court in *Daubert* disclaimed any intention of creating a rigid or exclusive list for admission of expert testimony. It noted that under the Supreme Court's rulings, a trial court has broad discretion to admit or exclude expert testimony, and its decision is reviewed only for an abuse of discretion.[29]

On the other hand, just as prior to *Daubert*, a number of federal courts excluded certain psychological expert testimony, but used *Daubert* as the rationale. In these cases the testimony would have been excluded even before *Daubert*. That is to say, *Daubert* made no difference as to its exclusion.[30] Profile evidence is an example. Likewise, as before *Daubert,* but relying on *Daubert*, the Fourth Circuit in 1995 in *United States v. Powers* excluded the use of the penile plethysmograph as a method to measure sexual arousal (the individual can look away when shown the stimulus or think of something else).[31] The court said, "The government proffered evidence that the scientific literature addressing penile plethysmography does not regard the test as a valid diagnostic tool because, although useful for treatment of sex offenders, it has no accepted standards in the scientific community."[32] Moreover, it "shocks the conscience," as was said in 2006 in a Ninth Circuit case, *United States v. Weber*.[33] Senior Judge John Noonan wrote, "A prisoner should not be compelled to stimulate himself sexually in order for the government to get a sense of his current proclivities … . There is a line at which the government must stop. Penile plethysmography testing crosses that line."

Also, the Abel Assessment for Sexual Interest (AASI), which seeks to provide information about current sexual interests and impulses using computer images and a statistical measurement, did not overcome a *Daubert* challenge.[34]

In 1995, in *United States v. Brien*,[35] the testimony of an eyewitness expert was proffered on memory, image retention, and retrieval. Again, as in most cases prior to *Daubert*, but now relying on *Daubert*, the First Circuit ruled that the failure of the defense to provide adequate data or literature underlying the expert's assumptions and conclusions failed to satisfy *Daubert*. Then too, in 1994, in *United States v. Rincon*,[36] the Ninth Circuit, citing *Daubert*, excluded expert testimony on the fallibility of eyewitness identification, saying as did the trial court that (1) it does not assist the trier of fact, (2) no showing was made that the testimony relates to an area that is recognized as a science, and (3) the testimony was likely to confuse the jury. As other courts say, the courtroom is not a classroom—it deals with individual cases.

What about "technical knowledge"? In a sequella to its 1993 decision in *Daubert*, the U.S. Supreme Court in 1999, six years later, in *Kumho Tire Co. v. Carmichael*,[37] ruled that trial judges are to play the same gatekeeping role when it comes to "technical" or "other specialized knowledge" as for "scientific" knowledge. Technical knowledge (about a tire) was involved in *Kumho*. Nineteen *amicus curiae* briefs were filed. Writing for a unanimous Court, Justice Stephen Breyer said, "There is no clear line that divides ["scientific" knowledge from "technical" or "other specialized knowledge"]. Disciplines such as engineering rest upon scientific knowledge." Justice Breyer also wrote, "[I]t would prove difficult, if not impossible, for judges to administer evidentiary rules under which a gatekeeping obligation depended upon a distinction between 'scientific' knowledge and 'technical' or 'other specialized' knowledge." At the same time, Justice Breyer said that in fulfilling their gatekeeping obligation, judges should take a flexible approach tailored to the potential witness's experience and field of expertise, be it engineering, economics, handwriting analysis, or any of numerous other subjects. Justice Breyer wrote:

> The conclusion, in our view, is that we can neither rule out, nor rule in, for all cases and for all time the applicability of the factors mentioned in *Daubert*, nor can we now do so for subsets of cases categorized by category of expert or by kind of evidence. Too much depends upon the particular circumstances of the particular case at issue.[38]

"The Supreme Court, wisely, waffled," that is the apt evaluation by Professor James Starrs, who publishes *Scientific Sleuthing Review,* about this decision.[39] On the one hand, the Court said that the testimony of nonscientific experts must satisfy the reliability requirements of *Daubert,* but, on the other hand, it said that the four factors described in *Daubert* as guidelines are advisory only, rather than mandatory, with the trial court at liberty to apply one or more, or none, under "the particular circumstances of the particular case at issue."

Together with its decision two years earlier, in 1997 in *General Electric Co. v. Joiner,*[40] the *Kumho* decision means less chance of reversal of a trial court's ruling on appeal. In *Joiner,* the Supreme Court affirmed that on appellate review of a trial court's decision to admit or to exclude expert testimony, it would not do a complete reevaluation of the factual basis for the trial court's decision. Instead, appellate courts were adjured to give great deference to a trial court's admissibility decision unless it was provably an abuse of discretion. That is to say, the judge may be quite arbitrary in making a decision.

In *Kumho,* Justice Breyer's oft-repeated refrain was that admissibility questions in the case of the many and diverse fields of expert testimony must be resolved through the application of "flexible" standards, in the best judgment of trial judges. Thus, in some instances, all of the four *Daubert* factors may be employed, while in others a lesser number, or even different factors, may be called into action by a trial judge. This approach makes the admissibility of expert testimony a very case-specific matter, which is problematic.[41]

Whatever the competency of the testimony under *Frye* or *Daubert,* there are other reasons why the testimony may be excluded, such as relevancy or if its probative value is substantially outweighed by the danger of unfair prejudice, confusion of the issues, or misleading the jury, or by considerations of undue delay, waste of time, or needless presentation of cumulative evidence. More often than not, psychiatric testimony is excluded on one of these grounds, and not whether the evidence meets the *Daubert* criteria. In any event, a *Daubert* hearing adds to the cost and time of a hearing, adding nothing in the case of the soft sciences.

It is to be emphasized that *Daubert* is based on an interpretation of a federal statute, the Federal Rules of Evidence, not the Constitution. Hence, *Daubert,* being a statutory rather than a constitutional case, is not binding on the states, even in the 40 jurisdictions with evidence codes modeled on the Federal Rules of Evidence. Thus, in declining to follow *Daubert,* the Arizona Supreme Court in 1993 noted that it was "not bound by the United States Supreme Court's nonconstitutional construction of the Federal Rules of Evidence when we construe the Arizona Rules of Evidence."[42]

On a count taken in 2007, opinions in 28 states follow *Daubert* or very similar standards. Opinions in 17 other states pointedly decline to follow *Daubert,* preferring something close to a *Frye* standard. Other states continue to defer any decision about *Daubert.* It is problematical whether *Daubert* would make any difference in regard to the soft sciences if it were adopted, as its reception in the federal courts would attest.

Right of Confrontation

In 2004, by a vote of 7–2, the U.S. Supreme Court changed the law on the use of out-of-court statements by a declarant who is not available to testify at trial. Previously, the Court had ruled that such statements were admissible against a criminal defendant under accepted hearsay exceptions.[43] But in *Crawford v. Washington*,[44] the Court held that under the confrontation clause of the Sixth Amendment, statements that are "testimonial" in nature cannot be used against a criminal defendant. In *Crawford*, the Court, in an opinion by Justice Scalia, held that "[W]here testimonial evidence is at issue, the Sixth Amendment demands what the common law required: unavailability and a prior opportunity for cross-examination." Justice Scalia excluded from "testimonial" some hearsay exceptions, such as business records, official records, and statements in furtherance of a conspiracy. They are "nontestimonial." The out-of-court statements of the defendant are not excluded because the defendant may not complain that he was not subject to cross-examination at the time of making the statement. Out-of-court statements that are not "testimonial" may be admitted against the defendant when they fall within a recognized hearsay exception. The decision has no effect on civil cases, in which the confrontation clause does not apply.

The facts of the *Crawford* case are simple. The defendant, Michael Crawford, was charged with attempted murder and assault for stabbing a man who allegedly tried to rape Crawford's wife. The police interviewed the wife, who witnessed the stabbing, and recorded their conversation. She contradicted her husband's claim that he had acted in self-defense. At trial, the prosecution could not call the wife as a witness because the state law precludes a person from testifying against his or her spouse without the spouse's consent. Instead, the prosecution sought to introduce her recorded statements on the grounds that she was unavailable as a witness and that her statements to the police were trustworthy.

The wife's statement to the police was clearly "testimonial," said Justice Scalia, and, hence, inadmissible. "[W]hatever else the term covers," he wrote, "It applies at a minimum to prior testimony at a preliminary hearing, before a grand jury, or at a former trial; and to police interrogation." The ruling expressly left open the question of whether a "dying declaration" could be used: "[M]any dying declarations may not be testimonial." Likewise, the majority opinion left unclear when "spontaneous declarations" could be used as evidence against a criminal defendant.

Immediately following the *Crawford* decision, trial courts were faced with the question whether a 911 call is testimonial.[45] Because complainants in domestic violence cases often do not appear for trial, prosecutors were left with proving their cases by offering out-of-court statements by the victim. Prior to *Crawford*, a call for help to 911 would ordinarily be admitted into evidence as an "excited utterance." The issue went to the Supreme Court. In 2006, in *Davis v. Washington*,[46] the Court held that statements made during emergencies to law enforcement personnel that describe ongoing events are not testimonial, but those made when there is no emergency and that describe past occurrences are testimonial and cannot be used. The Court summarized its overall holding this way:

> Without attempting to produce an exhaustive classification of all conceivable statements—or even all conceivable statements in response to police interrogation—as either testimonial or nontestimonial, it suffices to decide the present cases to hold as follows: Statements are nontestimonial when made in the course of police interrogation under circumstances objectively indicating that the primary purpose of the interrogation is to enable police assistance to meet an ongoing emergency. They are testimonial when the circumstances objectively indicate that there is no such ongoing emergency, and that the primary purpose of the interrogation is to establish or prove past events potentially relevant to later criminal prosecution.[47]

In *People v. Goldstein*, the New York Court of Appeals, the highest court in the state, in 2005 held that statements solicited by a mental health professional during a forensic evaluation and relied on at trial by the state are testimonial under *Crawford*. The case involved Andrew Goldstein, who pushed Kendra Webdale into the path of an approaching subway train. He was charged with murder in the second degree and his principal defense was insanity. His first trial ended in a hung jury. In the second trial, the two main witnesses were forensic psychiatrists, one called by the defense and one by the prosecution. Both agreed the defendant was mentally ill. The prosecution's expert, Dr. Angela Hegarty, relied on facts obtained from interviews of third parties. They included a former landlady, a girlfriend of a man who previously shared an apartment with the defendant, a current roommate, and a security guard who had restrained the defendant during a previous assault on a woman. On the stand, the psychiatrist distinguished forensic psychiatry from traditional clinical psychiatry by noting that the latter largely confines itself to what the client says and to the clinical record. She testified that the purpose of forensic psychiatry is "to get to the truth" and that she believed interviews of people with firsthand knowledge are an important way of accomplishing this goal.

The jury in the second trial rejected the insanity defense and found the defendant guilty. Because the third-parties interviewed by the prosecution's forensic psychiatrist were not called as witnesses and made available for cross-examination, the defense appealed the conviction. The New York Court of Appeals noted that cases prior to *Crawford* had established that a psychiatrist's opinion may be received in evidence even though some of the information on which it is based is inadmissible hearsay if the out-of-court information "is of a kind accepted in the profession as reliable in forming a professional opinion."

The New York court held that under *Crawford* the admission of these statements violated the defendant's constitutional right to confront the witnesses against him. The court rejected the prosecution's assertion that these statements were admitted not to establish the truth of what was said, but only to help the jury in evaluating the forensic psychiatrist's opinion—a distinction that is legal fiction. The court also concluded that this was "testimonial" hearsay because it could be inferred that the third parties knew that they were responding to questions from an agent of the state engaged in trial preparation, were not making "a casual remark to an acquaintance," and reasonably expected their statements to be used by the prosecution.[48] Hence, forensic experts testifying for the government in a criminal case must either (1) ensure that the third party testifies, (2) show that the third party is unavailable and that the defendant had an opportunity to cross-examine him at some earlier proceeding, or (3) obtain a waiver of confrontation rights.[49]

In the wake of the decision, law schools held full-day conferences that attracted large audiences of lawyers and prosecutors. They pondered the meaning of *testimonial*. Apparently every evidence law professor has written about *Daubert*, and now they are writing about *Crawford* (Professor Richard Friedman of the University of Michigan Law School even has a Web site on the case).[50] In *Crawford*, in a dissent, Chief Justice Rehnquist wrote: "I believe that the Court's adoption of a new interpretation of the Confrontation Clause is not backed by sufficiently persuasive reasoning to overrule long-established precedent. Its decision casts a mantle of uncertainty over future criminal trials in both federal and state courts, and is by no means necessary to decide the present case."[51] The Chief Justice reviewed historical material supporting his view that "[t]he Court's distinction between testimonial and nontestimonial states, contrary to its claim, is no better rooted in history than our current doctrine." He expressed approval of prior decisions holding that hearsay falling under firmly rooted exceptions passed muster under the Confrontation Clause. He concluded:

> The Court grandly declares that "[w]e leave for another day any effort to spell out a comprehensive definition of 'testimonial.'" But the thousands of federal prosecutors and the tens of thousands of state prosecutors need answers as to what beyond the specific kinds of "testimony" the Court lists, is covered by the new rule. They need them now, not months

or years from now. Rules of criminal evidence are applied every day in courts throughout the country, and parties should not be left in the dark in this manner.[52]

Testimony on Ultimate Issue

In cases of criminal responsibility, the forensic expert in offering testimony on the impact of mental illness on *mens rea* or *actus reus* is restricted by the parameters of the test of criminal responsibility (the M'Naghten or other test),[53] and also by the restriction on testimony on the ultimate issue. The Federal Rules of Evidence, when adopted in 1975, and their state law counterparts, expressly allowed expert testimony to embrace an ultimate issue of fact, so long as it is helpful to the trier of fact. Rule 704, as then adopted and before the addition of subsection (b) in 1984, abolished the common law "ultimate issue rule." According to the Advisory Committee's notes, the common law rule forbidding that type of testimony "was unduly restrictive, difficult of application, and generally served only to deprive the trier of fact of useful information. ... [Efforts to avoid the prohibition] led to odd verbal circumlocutions, which were said not to violate the rule. Thus, a witness could express his estimate of the criminal responsibility of an accused in terms of sanity or insanity, but not in the terms of ability to tell right from wrong or another more modern standard."[54]

However, in 1984, following the Hinckley trial, a subsection (b) was added to Rule 704 to provide that the expert may testify only as to the defendant's mental disease or defect and the characteristics of such a condition, and may not tender a conclusion as to whether that condition rendered the defendant unable to appreciate the nature and quality or the wrongfulness of his act. The provision bars "an opinion or inference as to whether the defendant did or did not have the mental state or condition constituting an element of the crime charged or of a defense thereto." Under the amended rule (adopted also in most states), the latter is an "ultimate issue" to be determined solely by the jury on the basis of the evidence presented.[55] The expert may inform the court that the defendant is suffering from a mental illness, but that is only part of the equation of "insanity" or criminal responsibility. One may suffer from schizophrenia, but rob a store for purely financial reasons.

Much faith is put in the jury system to resolve disputes, but at the same time, the rules of evidence screen the information that the jury hears and opinion testimony is precluded that would "invade" the province of the jury (though it is not obliged to accept the testimony of any witness). The adoption of Rule 704 (b) is a step back in the trend in the last half of the 20th century to permit expert testimony on the "ultimate issue" (however that may be defined).

Apparently the first appellate decision to allow an expert to give an opinion on the ultimate issue was in 1942 by the Iowa Supreme Court.[56] That ruling was adopted in the Federal Rules in 1975 in Rule 704, which provided simply: "Testimony in the form of an opinion or inference otherwise admissible is not objectionable because it embraces an ultimate issue to be decided by the trier of fact." The restrictions adopted in 1984 have been applied inconsistently. The courts in some cases have interpreted 704(b) narrowly while in others they have given it a broad scope.

In 1990, in *United States v. Kristiansen*,[57] the defendant failed to report to the halfway house where he was confined. He claimed that his addiction to cocaine prevented him from forming the requisite willful intent to escape and called an expert witness to testify to that effect. The trial court would not let the defense ask questions pertaining to the ultimate issue in the case, which was whether the defendant appreciated the wrongfulness of his acts. A jury found that the defendant did intend to escape, and he appealed his conviction. The trial court had barred the question: "Would this severe mental disease or defect, which you've testified that Mr. Kristiansen has, if an individual has that, affect the individual's ability to appreciate the nature and quality of the wrongfulness of his acts?" The trial court sustained the prosecution's objection to the question because it felt that the word *would* asked for an answer that reached the ultimate issue. Writing for the Eighth Circuit Court of Appeals, Senior Circuit Judge Gerald Heaney found that the question was proper under 704(b) "because it relates to the symptoms and qualities of the disease itself and does not call for an answer that describes Kristiansen's culpability at the time of the crime." Rule 704(b), Judge Heaney said, "was not meant to prohibit testimony that describes the qualities of a mental disease."[58]

The rule is that expert testimony concerning the nature of a defendant's mental disease or defect and its *typical* effect on a person's mental state is admissible. In *United States v. Davis*,[59] the defendant, who attempted to establish an insanity defense based on a multiple personality disorder, objected to the testimony of a government expert that such a disorder does not in itself indicate that a person does not understand what he is doing. The Eleventh Circuit in 1988 upheld the admission of this testimony because it "did not include an opinion as to Davis' capacity to conform his conduct to the law at the time of the robbery."[60]

Similarly, in 1993, again before the Eleventh Circuit, in *United States v. Thigpen*,[61] the testimony elicited by the government concerned the *general effect* of a schizophrenic disorder on a person's ability to appreciate the nature or wrongfulness of his actions and was allowed. In this case, the defendant was charged with making false statements concerning his criminal background when purchasing pistols and with illegally possessing these weapons. His sole defense was insanity.

However, in 1990, in a decision also by the Eleventh Circuit, *United States v. Manley*,[62] the court upheld the exclusion of opinion testimony by a defense expert where counsel inquired as to the mental capacity of a hypothetical person with each of the pertinent characteristics of the defendant. The court said that while Rule 704(b) does not bar an explanation of the disease and its typical effect on a person's mental state, "a thinly veiled hypothetical" may not be used to circumvent the rule.

In an opinion rendered in 1982 involving the well-known prosecution of Captain Jeffrey MacDonald, a physician, for the alleged murder of his wife and children, expert testimony was offered to support the defense theory that another person committed the crime.[63] The proffered testimony that the defendant had a "personality configuration inconsistent with the outrageous and senseless murders of [his] family" was excluded, under Rule 403, as confusing and misleading, but Rule 704(b) apparently would not bar this kind of evidence. Testimony about a "personality configuration" is character evidence, well removed from intent or lack of it. A psychiatrist would not appear to violate 704(b) if he testified that the defendant was capable of "loving" or "caring" for people, which presumably would make it less likely that he committed a heinous crime.

Rule 704(b) is interpreted to prohibit only opinions that track the precise statutory language of the insanity defense. In 1987, in *United States v. Edwards*,[64] the Eleventh Circuit observed:

> In resolving the complex issue of criminal responsibility, it is of critical importance that the defendant's entire relevant symptomatology be brought before the jury and explained" [quoting a Fifth Circuit opinion in 1971] … . Congress did not enact Rule 704(b) so as to limit the flow of diagnostic and clinical information. Every actual fact concerning the defendant's mental condition is still as admissible after the enactment of Rule 704(b) as it was before … . Rather, the Rule "changes the style of question and answer that can be used to establish both the offense and the defense thereto." … The prohibition is directed at a narrowly and precisely defined evil … . Rule 704(b) forbids only "conclusions as to the ultimate legal issue to be found by the trier of fact."[65]

In this case, the government expert testified, over objection, that people who are not insane can nevertheless become frantic over a financial crisis. The prosecution put the expert on the stand to dispute the defense psychiatrist's diagnosis. The government's expert explained why the defendant's behavior—his frantic efforts to pay bills, his manifestations of energy, his lack of sleep, and his feelings of depression—did not necessarily indicate an active manic state. The court concluded, "We think that the doctor played exactly the kind of role that Congress contemplated for the expert witness."

It is now widely recognized that Rule 704(b) is an unnecessary addition to the rules of evidence. Judges can rely on other evidentiary rules to minimize jury confusion and ensure that expert testimony assists the trier of fact. As with other types of evidence, the judge has the discretion to exclude expert testimony if it is found that its probative value is substantially outweighed by its prejudicial effect, or that its admission would confuse the issues or create needless delay or waste of judicial resources. In actual fact, just as with the common law "ultimate issue rule," 704(b) obscures a clear summation of the psychiatric viewpoint and promotes form of expression over substance. Ultimately, the rule simply ignores the principle that the touchstone in the law of expert evidence is helpfulness. Rudolph Giuliani, then U.S. Attorney of Manhattan, in a statement in the hearings about the adoption of Rule 704 (b) predicted, "It would be all gobbledygook without the psychiatrist drawing a conclusion as to what he's saying."[66] Guliani can now say, "I told you so."'

Form of Testimony—Narrative v. Question and Answer

The examination of witnesses is conducted predominantly by means of dialogic Q&A sequences. The lawyer may prefer testimony in the form of a narrative because juries would believe the witness is speaking freely, even though in reality the testimony is rehearsed prior to trial. Testimony in narrative form, however, is usually blocked by the adversary. A question phrased in a way that calls for a narrative is objectionable because it eliminates the opportunity for a timely objection. An example is, "Tell the jury what you know about the accident." In the trial of Patty Hearst, the judge admonished F. Lee Bailey, the defense attorney, and Dr. Louis Jolyn West, the expert witness, that testimony was to be given in the form of questions and answers rather than lengthy narratives.[67]

Narration is severely restricted by the cross-examination. On cross-examination, the lawyer is concerned with retaining tight control over the content of the evidence. Questions are put to the witness so as to restrict the testimony of the witness to a "yes" or "no" answer.

Special Rules on Qualification of Experts in Malpractice Cases

Special rules govern the qualification of experts in malpractice cases. Long ago, the courts adopted the "school" method for qualifying expert witnesses. This method of qualifying limited the expert to one who either practices in or is familiar with the particular school of medicine of the practitioner on trial. Subsequently, as we discuss in Chapter 2, various states require that a witness proffered as an expert not only be familiar with, but also practice in the very school to which he seeks to testify.[68] Thus, psychologists are not permitted to testify on the standard of care required of psychiatrists, even though they may be familiar with the practice of psychiatry. In particular, decisions of the Michigan Supreme Court (and increasingly in other states) make it difficult, if not impossible in some cases, to determine who is of the same specialty to qualify as an expert witness.[69] The late Stanley Schwartz, a well-known trial lawyer, wrote: "In recent years, there has accreted around the expert witness statute a body of Court of Appeals decisions, most of them unpublished *per curiams*, which have been barren of essential facts, badly reasoned, at odds with other panel decisions, or all of the above. The muddle makes selection of an unchallengeable expert witness much like a lottery, even for the most experienced and diligent malpractice attorney."[70] Additionally, a number of states by legislation require that a certain percent of an expert's professional time be spent in "clinical practice," that is, nonforensic work, in order to testify about the standard of care for healthcare providers.

Ethics Guidelines

Professional associations set out ethics guidelines that its members are expected to follow. The American Medical Association has Principles of Medical Ethics, the American Psychiatric Association has added "annotations," and the American Academy of Psychiatry and the Law also has additional guidelines that address the special situations found in forensic practice. These ethics guidelines are binding only on members of the organization that sets them. The penalty for serious ethical breach is expulsion from the organization. This does not in itself affect one's medical license, but the courts, legislature, licensing board, or employer may have adopted the organization's ethics guidelines and the result could be suspension or termination of a license to practice. In some measure, the ethics guidelines have been adopted by these bodies and vice versa.[71] The AMA at one time asserted that its statement of ethical standards should not be enforced as law, but in some areas, for example, in regard to the question of sexual misconduct by physicians, the courts have used the AMA standards as evidence of the standard of care despite the AMA's assertion. For example, because treatment to achieve competency to be executed is unethical, it is claimed to not be "medically appropriate" and, therefore, constitutionally impermissible.[72]

Most difficult issues in healthcare that have raised ethical dilemmas have been addressed by law. Indeed, discussions of medical ethics in treatises or lectures sound like an exposition of the law, e.g., the Emergency Medical Treatment and Labor Act (EMTALA) on "patient dumping," the Health Insurance Portability and Accountability Act (HIPAA) on maintaining patient confidentiality, the right of informed consent, and the duty to protect third parties against a danger posed by a patient.[73] The AMA's ethical guidelines call on physicians to "safeguard patient confidence and privacy within the constraints of the law."

The Treating Therapist as Expert

Numerous professional guidelines explicitly state that forensic and clinical roles should be filled by two different individuals.[74] The Ethical Guidelines for the Practice of Forensic Psychiatry point to the problems related to a treating therapist's serving as an expert witness. The relevant guideline states: "Treating psychiatrists should generally avoid agreeing to be an expert witness or to perform evaluations of their patients for legal purposes because a forensic evaluation usually requires that other people be interviewed and testimony may adversely affect the therapeutic and forensic relationship."[75]

The primary role of the forensic expert is to collect the facts of the case, it is said, whereas, in therapy, the emphasis is on "helping" as opposed to getting the facts. Engaging in conflicting therapeutic and forensic relationships exacerbates the risk that experts will be more concerned with case outcome than the accuracy of their testimony. Moreover, it is often claimed that testifying as an expert on behalf of the patient jeopardizes the therapeutic relationship, but apparently there is no empirical evidence to support the claim. Be that as it may, attorneys and juries tend to give more credibility to the testimony of a therapist than to a forensic expert. The therapist spends much more time with the patient, prior to the litigation, and he is not paid for his services as a witness.

In a case in Michigan for breach of an insurance contract, where the jury awarded over a million dollars to the patient, the attorney who represented the patient said the key to winning the case was *not* hiring expert witnesses to explain the plaintiff's condition. Rather, he relied exclusively on the testimony of the plaintiff's treating doctors. Moreover, he indicated, "We never hire an expert psychiatrist. We rely exclusively on the treaters. If you've got good treaters and they are credible, that goes a long way with a jury as opposed to what any expert might say."[76]

For social security disability benefits, regulations provide that administrative law judges are to give more weight to opinions from treating sources than from other examinations, such as consultative examinations. The regulations note that the treating physician is "most able to provide a detailed, longitudinal picture" of the mental impairment.[77]

Then too, as noted, in any type of case, the courts may consider whether an expert's assertions were prepared in the course of litigation when determining whether the testimony is reliable. In *Johnson v. Manitowoc Boom Trucks*,[78] the case cited above, the federal trial court granted the defendant's motion to exclude the expert's testimony on behalf of the plaintiff, holding that it was unreliable because, among other reasons, the expert's opinions were prepared solely for the litigation. The court then granted the defendant a summary judgment based on a lack of expert testimony. Affirming, the Sixth Circuit in 2007 noted that the *Daubert* decision, which delineated several factors to consider in determining expert testimony reliability, did not mention independent research. The court said, however, that it has long recognized that work prepared in the course of litigation is to be viewed with caution because the paid expert may not be an unbiased scientist. Thus, the court said, the trial court did not err in applying a prepared-solely-for-litigation factor in addition to the basic *Daubert* factors.

In any event, the *Crawford* decision restricts the information that a forensic expert may use in testifying for the government in a criminal case.

Forensic Consultation in States in Which the Expert Is Not Licensed

In recent years, at the behest of medical societies, a number of states by legislation have required licensure in the jurisdiction of the forensic examination or testimony. As a consequence, experts may be cited for practicing without a license with associated civil or criminal penalties as well as noncoverage of malpractice insurance.[79] In 1998, the AMA adopted a policy that expert witness testimony by physicians be considered the practice of medicine subject to peer review.[80] It is a position that ignores the clinical, legal, and ethical differences between the practice of clinical medicine and forensic examination and testimony. Prominent Philadelphia lawyer Clifford Haines in a comment to the audience at a recent annual meeting of the American College of Forensic Psychiatry said that he would represent, without fee, any expert so penalized—he would challenge the law. An Alabama appellate court ruled that a psychologist, who was licensed in another state, could not be prohibited from testifying as an expert witness solely on the ground of nonlicensure in Alabama. The court commented, "[T]estifying is [not] a function of practicing psychology."[81]

In one way or another, professional organizations have sought to curtail expert witnesses. It is a Catch-22 situation: On the one hand, the law, deferring to the profession, requires expert testimony in a malpractice case, but, on the other hand, it has been increasingly difficult to obtain competent expert testimony. The American Association of Neurosurgeons has attacked neurosurgeons who are willing to testify for plaintiffs in malpractice cases. In peer reviewing medical testimony, the organization has not found a single case of bad testimony in favor of a defendant physician, but many in favor of the plaintiff. The American Medical Association has endorsed such programs.

Suspension or Termination of Professional License

An expert's professional license could depend on what he says on the witness stand. As a consequence, an expert may wish not to testify. In a first-of-its-kind ruling in 2001, the U.S. Seventh Circuit Court of Appeals, with the prominent Judge Richard Posner writing the opinion, ruled that a professional society might discipline a member on account of testimony presented at trial that is deemed not up to standard. In *Austin v. American Association of Neurological Surgeons*,[82] the court said: "Although [the expert witness] did not treat the malpractice plaintiff for whom he testified, his testimony at her trial was a type of medical service, and if the quality of his testimony reflected the quality of his medical judgment, he is probably a poor physician. His discipline by the Association, therefore, served an important public policy exemplified by the federal Health Care Quality Improvement Act."[83]

To implement the ruling in *Daubert*, Judge Posner said that judges need the help of professional associations. Medical boards are the classic expert agency and, in fact, could be viewed as expert judicial panels or juries. In the *Austin* case, Judge Posner wrote the following:

> By becoming a member of the prestigious American Association of Neurological Surgeons, a fact he did not neglect to mention in his testimony in the malpractice suit against [the defendant doctor], Austin boosted his credibility as an expert witness. The Association had an interest—the community at large had an interest—in Austin's not being able to use his membership to dazzle judges and juries and deflect the close and skeptical scrutiny that shoddy testimony deserves. It is no answer that judges can be trusted to keep out such testimony. Judges are not experts in any field except law. Much escapes us, especially in a highly technical field, such as neurosurgery. When a member of a prestigious professional association makes representations not on their face absurd, such as that a majority of neurosurgeons believe that a particular type of mishap is invariably the result of surgical negligence, the judge may have no basis for questioning the belief, even if the defendant's expert testifies to the contrary.[84]

In a medical case in North Carolina in 2006, the defendant doctor complained to the state medical board about the testimony of neurosurgeon Gary Lustgarten. The board investigated and charged Lustgarten with engaging in unprofessional conduct, saying he had misrepresented the standard of care and had claimed, without evidence, that the defendant had falsified a medical record. The board revoked Lustgarten's license. Lustgarten appealed the decision to a trial court. The court reversed in part, noting that he could not be disciplined for his testimony regarding the standard of care, but found that he had engaged in unprofessional conduct in his statements about the allegedly falsified notes. The court remanded the case, and the board suspended his license for a year. The appeals court reversed, citing parts of Lustgarten's deposition and cross-examination in determining that "the substantial record evidence does not permit an inference that Dr. Lustgarten made an entirely unfounded statement concerning [the] notes." Instead, the court said, Lustgarten merely "stated under oath that he had 'difficulty believing' [the defendant's] notations." The appeals court ordered the lower court to dismiss the disciplinary charges against Lustgarten.[85]

The attorney representing Lustgarten commented, "The doctor who got mad at Lustgarten was going through the back door. He couldn't file a defamation suit against him or a malpractice suit, so he just went to the medical board to get his license revoked, which is the worst sanction because it's not just money, it's his livelihood." He added, "The risk of professional sanction could discourage many medical experts from testifying."[86]

Anyone—even a stranger to the litigation—can file a complaint with a licensing board. Its sweep is broad. Not all experts are members of a professional organization (subject to its peer review), but they may be licensed practitioners subject to the licensing board. The disciplinary action of a licensing board could be the most powerful way to control expert testimony. Yet there is potential for abuse. Disciplinary actions are not covered by insurance. The boards apparently have immunity from suit.[87]

An Ohio pediatrician complained to the Kentucky Medical Licensure Board that Governor Ernie Fletcher, a physician, violated medical ethics by ordering the execution of Thomas Bowling when he signed a death warrant. The Board unanimously held that Fletcher acted as governor and not as a physician and, therefore, did not violate medical ethics. One may query Dr. Josef

Mengele's role at Auschwitz in deciding which concentration camp inmates went to the gas chamber and which to the labor camp. Was he acting as a physician? Dr. A. L. Halpern, an outspoken opponent of the death penalty, says:

> The Kentucky committee chose not to recognize that Dr. Fletcher was a physician when he ordered the execution in clear violation of the ethics code by engaging in an action that could automatically cause an execution to be carried out on a condemned prisoner. The code speaks of no exception to this prohibited action. If the committee's decision was widely accepted, we would be facing a slippery slope, running the risk of emasculating the prohibition against direct physician participation in executions by allowing physicians to claim that they were acting, not as physicians, but in some other role.[88]

Conclusion

The American Academy of Psychiatry and the Law, as its title indicates, is about psychiatry and law, but one member in a presidential address at an annual meeting complained that its meetings and its journal focus more on the law than on psychiatry. Perhaps it should be that way, as a forensic report that is not mindful of the law may be misdirected or even an exercise in futility. The legislature (often at the behest of medical societies), as well as the courts and medical boards, restricts or dissuades the testimony of experts. The codes of ethics of professionals set out standards, but when they are at variance with the law, they are trumped.

On some occasions, the forensic expert believes that there is a restriction when there is none, as under the *Daubert* ruling, or when it is said that the treating psychiatrist is incompetent to testify as an expert. At other times, the expert does not recognize a restriction when there is one, as under the *Crawford* decision. For this reason, and for good reason, expositions of ethics in forensic psychiatry often sound like expositions of the law.

Endnotes

1. Judge Patrick Higginbotham in *In re* Air Crash Disaster at New Orleans, Louisiana, 795 F.2d 1230 at 1234 (5th Cir. 1986). See J. Fisher, *Forensics Under Fire/Are Bad Sciences and Dueling Experts Corrupting Criminal Justice?* (New Brunswick: Rutgers University Press, 2008); M.A. Hagen, *Whores of the Court* (New York: HarperCollins, 1997).
2. 509 U.S. 579 (1993).
3. 293 Fed. 1013 (D.C. Cir. 1923).
4. 293 Fed. at 1014.
5. In *In re* Detention of Robinson, 146 P.3d 451 (Wash. App. 2006), the Washington Court of Appeals in affirming an individual's commitment as a sexually violent predator (SVP) held that the Screening Scale for Pedophilic Interests (SSPI) is an actuarial instrument, rather than a novel scientific theory or principle and, thus, not excludable for that reason under *Frye*. The justification for restricting the test on admissibility to novel scientific evidence under *Frye* are partly historical and partly practical. *Frye* itself concerned a novel technique. The practical justification for restricting admissibility decisions to novel evidence is that it would be a waste of judicial time to relitigate the question with respect to well-settled techniques and methods. See, e.g., Hulse v. Dept. of Justice, Motor Vehicle Div., 289 Mont. 1, 961 P.2d 75 (1998). In jurisdictions that do not distinguish between novel and nonnovel scientific evidence, successful challenges are theoretically possible. See Hartman v. State, 946 S.W.2d 60 (Tex. Crim. App. 1997). As a practical matter, some scientific theories are so well accepted that they are entitled to judicial notice of their admissibility. Trial courts that apply their admissibility test to all evidence are rarely embroiled in determining the admissibility of scientific theories and techniques that have already been well established. See Report of the 2006 Forum for State Appellate Court Judges, *The Whole Truth? Experts, Evidence, and the Blindfolding of the Jury* (Washington, DC: Forum for State Court Judges, 2007), p. 10.
6. Daubert v. Merrell Dow Pharmaceuticals, 43 F.3d 1311 (9th Cir. 1995).

7. 43 F.3d at 1316–1317. The courts may consider whether an expert's assertions were prepared in the course of litigation when determining whether the testimony is reliable. Johnson v. Manitowoc Boom Trucks, 484 F.3d 426 (6th Cir. 2007). Pharmaceutical companies routinely hire writers to prepare "research papers" touting their products for publication in prestigious medical journals, and some physicians are happy to sign their names to them—for a fee. The practice raises serious questions about the integrity of medical literature. J.P. Kassirer, "Ghostwriters and Ghostbusters," *Trial*, Sept. 2007, p. 38. In 2006, the editor of the journal *Neuropsychopharmacology* resigned following a flap over the medical journal's failure to disclose that the authors of a paper reviewing a new treatment for depression had financial ties to the treatment's developer. At the 2007 annual meeting of the American Psychiatric Association, held in San Diego, various speakers pointed out the ways pharmaceutical companies distort the results of clinical trials.
8. 61 F.3d 1038 (2d Cir. 1995).
9. 61 F.3d at 1045.
10. 509 U.S. at 600–601.
11. S. Jasanoff, *Science at the Bar* (Cambridge, MA: Harvard University Press, 1997).
12. Resolution in the U.S. Supreme Court in tribute to Justice Harry A. Blackmun, Oct. 27, 1999. See L. Greenhouse, *Becoming Justice Blackmun* (New York: Henry Holt, 2005).
13. The meetings of the Topeka Psychoanalytic Institute invariably began with the greeting: "Welcome to the scientific meeting," but psychoanalysis is not "science" as the term is commonly understood.
14. See T.W. Campbell, *Assessing Sex Offenders* (Springfield, IL: Thomas, 2nd ed., 2007); E.S. Janus & R.A. Prentky, "The Forensic Use of Actuarial Risk Assessment with Sex Offenders: Accuracy, Admissibility and Accountability," *Am. Crim. L. Rev.* 40 (2003): 1443.
15. In Moore v. Ashland Chemical Inc., 126 F.3d 679 (5th Cir. 1997), the Fifth Circuit said that the four *Daubert* factors—(1) empirical testing, peer review, and publication; (2) known or potential rate of error; (3) the existence and maintenance of operational standards; and (4) acceptance within a relevant scientific community—are relevant only to hard science. Consequently, they "generally are not appropriate for assessing the evidentiary reliability of a proffer of expert clinical medical testimony." In a study of hearings involving "battered woman syndrome" and "rape trauma syndrome" defenses, expert testimony was admitted in 51 of the cases and rejected in 17, largely on the basis of the credentials of the expert. In none did the judges refer to any scientific analysis. The issue that was examined by the judge was the relevance of the expert testimony to the case. Reported in S.L. Brodsky, *The Expert Witness* (Washington, DC: American Psychological Association, 1999), p. 34. See "Symposium, *Daubert's* Meanings for the Admissibility of Behavioral and Social Science Evidence," *Psychol., Public Policy & Law* 5 (1999): 1–242; D.L. Faigman, "The Evidentiary Status of Social Science Under *Daubert*: Is It 'Scientific,' 'Technical,' or 'Other' Knowledge?" *Psychol., Public Policy & Law* 1 (1995): 960–979; H.F. Fradella, A. Fogarty, & L. O'Neill, "The Impact of *Daubert* on the Admissibility of Behavioral Science Testimony," *Pepperdine L. Rev.* 30 (2003): 403; T.G. Gutheil & M.D. Stein, "*Daubert*-Based Gatekeeping and Psychiatric/Psychological Testimony in Court: Review and Proposal," *J. Psychiat. & Law* 28 (2000): 235.
16. People v. Beckley, 434 Mich. 691, 456 N.W.2d 391 (1990).
17. 68 F.3d 597 (2d Cir. 1995).
18. 880 F. Supp. 1027 (S.D. 1995).
19. 82 F.3d 1513 (10th Cir. 1996).
20. 130 F.3d 1287 (8th Cir. 1997).
21. Whether medication prompted a suicide is another question. In Miller v. Pfizer, 196 F. Supp.2d 1062 (D. Kan. 2002), *aff'd*, D.C. No. 99-CV-2326-KHV (10th Cir. 2004), the parents of a teenager, 13-year-old Matthew Miller, who had hanged himself just after taking Zoloft, sued Pfizer, the pharmaceutical firm that produced the medication. The plaintiffs offered Dr. David Healy, an expert on serotonin, depression, and the brain as an expert witness. Pfizer filed a motion to exclude Healy's testimony under *Daubert*. To help evaluate Healy's research, U.S. District Judge Kathryn Vratil appointed two independent experts, Yale epidemiologist John Concato and University of Illinois psychiatrist John Davis. In their report, they called Healy an "accomplished investigator," but they also said that his methodology "has not been accepted in the relevant scientific community" and that Healy holds a "minority view" about SSRIs (selective serotonin reuptake inhibitors) and suicidality. With that, Judge Vratil rejected Healy's testimony, and dismissed the lawsuit. She wrote, "Dr. Healy is an accomplished researcher and his credentials are not in dispute," but his belief in the SSRI–suicide link is a "distinctly minority view," and she added that the flaws in his methodology "are glaring, overwhelming, and unexplained." See B. Yeoman, "Putting Science in the Dock," *The Nation*, March 26, 2007, p. 22. See also D. Healy, *Let*

Them Eat Prozac (New York: New York University Press, 2004). Since then, the FDA has ordered all antidepressants—SSRIs and others—to carry a "black box warning" alerting parents to dangers the medications pose to their children.

22. An illustration of the minority view is Elcock v. K-Mart Corp., 233 F.3d 734 (3d Cir. 2000), where the appellate court held that the district court was required to hold a *Daubert* hearing to determine the reliability of the testimony of a psychologist who sought to testify as a vocational rehabilitation expert in a slip-and-fall action.

23. Nenno v. State, 970 S.W.2d 549 (Tex. Crim. App. 1998). In Barefoot v. Estelle, 463 U.S. 880 (1983), the Supreme Court declined to exclude future dangerousness testimony because the defense could not show that "psychiatrists are always wrong with respect to future dangerousness, only most of the time." 463 U.S. at 900.

24. 483 F.3d 313 (5th Cir. 2007).

25. 18 U.S.C. § 3593 (c).

26. 57 F.3d 126 (1st Cir. 1995).

27. Federal Rules of Evidence, Rule 405(a) and 608(a).

28. 93 F.3d 1337 (7th Cir. 1996).

29. 93 F.3d at 1341. In State v. Shuck, 953 S.W.2d 662 (Tenn. 1997), the Tennessee Supreme Court in reaching a similar result ruled admissible a neuropsychologist's testimony concerning a defendant's acute susceptibility to inducement in support of an entrapment defense.

30. In Gier v. Educational Service Unit No. 16, 66 F.3d 940 (8th Cir. 1995), the Eighth Circuit held that the use of psychological evaluations of alleged child abuse must conform to the standards set forth in *Daubert*. The evaluations in question consisted of (1) reviewing a child behavior checklist completed by parents, (2) clinical interviews involving role playing with anatomically correct dolls, and (3) interviewing the plaintiff's parents. The court distinguished between a methodology reliable enough to determine a course of therapy and a methodology reliable enough to support factual or investigative conclusions in a legal proceeding. The court held, as it would have under *Frye*, that the *Daubert* standard of reliability was not met.

31. United States v. Powers, 59 F.3d 1460 (4th Cir. 1995).

32. 59 F.3d at 1471.

33. 451 F.3d 552 (9th Cir. 2006).

34. *In re* Ready, 63 Mass. App. 171, 824 N.E.2d 474 (2005); United States v. White House, 177 F. Supp.2d 973 (D.S.D. 2001).

35. 59 F.3d 274 (1st Cir. 1995).

36. 28 F.3d 921 (9th Cir. 1994).

37. 526 U.S. 137 (1999).

38. 526 U.S. at 150.

39. J.E. Starrs, "The Admissibility Factor," *Sci. Sleuthing*, 23 (Fall 1999):14. See also P. Giannelli & E. Imwinkelried, "Scientific Evidence: The Fallout From Supreme Court's Decision in *Kumho Tire*," *Crim. Just.* 14 (Winter 2000): 12.

40. 522 U.S. 136 (1997).

41. In the wake of *Kumho Tire*, and citing it, the Tenth Circuit in United States v. Charley, 176 F.3d 1265(10th Cir. 1999), excluded an expert's testimony that a child's symptoms were more consistent with the symptoms of children who have been sexually abused than with the symptoms of children who witness physical abuse of their mother. The court found that no sufficient foundation was laid for this kind of expert analysis, and no reliability inquiry was undertaken. 176 F.3d at 1278.

42. State v. Bible, 858 P.2d 1152, 1183 (Ariz. 1993). In a later Arizona case, Logerquist v. McVey, 1 P.3d 113 (Ariz. 2000), the plaintiff alleged that she had been sexually abused by the defendant, her pediatrician, and that she had repressed these recollections for almost 20 years until her memory was triggered by a television commercial featuring a pediatrician. She sought to introduce expert testimony at trial to support her contention that such memories can be repressed for years, but can be recalled with accuracy once triggered by some external event. Applying the traditional approach articulated in *Frye*, the trial judge determined that the theories advanced by the plaintiff's experts were not generally accepted among trauma memory researchers. Both parties urged the state supreme court to adopt the standard set out by the U.S. Supreme Court in *Daubert*.

In response, the state supreme court said that *Daubert* and its progeny force the trial judge to cross the line between the legal task of ruling on the foundation and relevance of evidence—which is a judge's traditional role—and the jury's task of determining whom to believe and why and whose testimony to accept and on what basis. The court added that it would not adopt the *Daubert* approach even

if it could be shown that trial judges do a better job than juries of weeding out unreliable expert witnesses. It noted that the state constitution preserves each litigant's right to have the jury pass on questions of fact by determining the credibility of witnesses and the weight of conflicting evidence. In fact,
the court said, judges are prohibited from even commenting on the credibility of the evidence, which
would seem to preclude granting them the broader power of excluding proffered relevant evidence
entirely. Returning to the plaintiff's claim the court held that the expert testimony she had sought to
introduce was not sufficiently novel to require application of the *Frye* standard and directed that the
plaintiff's expert witnesses be permitted to testify.

43. Ohio v. Roberts, 448 U.S. 56 (1980).

44. 541 U.S. 36 (2004).

45. See, e.g., People v. Moscat, 777 N.Y.S.2d 875, 2004 N.Y. Misc. 231 (2004); State v. Jensen, 2007 WI 26,
727 N.W.2d 518 (2007); see also M.J. Polelle, "The Death of Dying Declarations in a Post–Crawford
World," *Mo. L. Rev.* 2006: 285.

46. 126 S. Ct. 2266 (2006).

47. 126 S. Ct. at 2273–74. In the absence of a definitive explanation of *testimonial*, the Minnesota Supreme
Court listed the following considerations: (1) whether the declarant was a victim or an observer, (2)
the declarant's purpose in speaking with the officer, (3) whether it was the police or the declarant
who initiated the conversation, (4) the location where the statements were made, (5) the declarant's
emotional state, (6) the level of formality and structure of the conversation, (7) the officer's purpose in
speaking with the declarant, and (8) if and how the statements were recorded. See State v. Krasky, 736
N.W.2d 636 (Minn. 2007). In State v. Bobadilla, 709 N.W.2d 243 (Minn. 2006), the court concluded
that statements by a child sexual abuse victim to a child protection worker were not testimonial by
reference to what it concluded was the "main purpose" of the interview: "assessing and responding to
imminent risks to the child's health and welfare." In State v. Scacchetti, 711 N.W.2d 508 (Minn. 2006),
the court concluded that the child's statements were not testimonial because they were made to a
pediatric nurse practitioner whose purpose in interviewing and examining the child was to assess her
medical condition; no government actor initiated, participated, or was involved in any way. In State v.
Jensen, 727 N.W.2d 518 (Wis. 2007), the Wisconsin Supreme Court allowed the admission of a victim's
statements to a neighbor indicating that she thought the defendant was trying to kill her, but statements in the victim's letter in which she told the neighbor to give to police if anything happened to her
were testimonial and inadmissible under *Crawford v. Washington*. In People v. Cage, Calif. S. Ct., No.
S127344 (April 9, 2007), the California Supreme Court held that a domestic violence victim's statements to a deputy in the emergency room and later at the sheriff's station were inadmissible under
Crawford. They were made in response to focused police questioning whose primary purpose, objectively considered, was not to deal with an ongoing emergency, but to investigate the circumstances of
a crime. In contrast, the court ruled that the victim's statements to the physician who treated him at
the hospital was properly admitted at trial. "In order to help diagnose the nature of the victim's slash
wound, and to determine the appropriate treatment," the court said, "the physician asked the victim
a single question—'what happened?'" The primary purpose of this inquiry "was not to obtain proof
of a past criminal act, or the identity of the perpetrator, for possible use in court, but to deal with a
contemporaneous medical condition about what had caused the victim's wound."

The U.S. Supreme Court was recently called upon to decide whether prosecutors can use crime
lab reports as evidence without having the forensic analyst who prepared them testify at trial. State
and lower federal courts have come to different conclusions about whether the decision in *Crawford
v. Washington* extends to lab reports that are used in many drug and other cases. Defendants argue
that they should be allowed to question the person who prepared the report about testing methods,
how the evidence was preserved, and a host of other issues; Melendez-Diaz v. Massachusetts, 07-591
(March 24, 2008). The application of *Crawford* to mental health testimony, as well as laboratory reports
and medical examiner testimony and reports, is discussed in S. Yermish, "Crawford v. Washington and
Expert Testimony: Limiting the Use of Testimonial Hearsay," *Champion*, Nov. 2006, p. 12. Professor
Gerald Uelman writes, "Since [lab reports] are prepared by police personnel for the purpose of subsequent criminal investigation, there is a very persuasive argument that they come within *Crawford*, and
even those states that recognize a hearsay exception to admit them must now exclude them to protect
the defendant's Sixth Amendment rights." G. Uelman, "Motions FYI: Admissibility of Lab Reports
After Crawford v. Washington," *Champion*, Sept./Oct. 2005, p. 67.

The Justices declined a separate case from Iowa, raising a similar question about the use of video-
taped interviews in child sex abuse cases. The decision leaves in place an Iowa Supreme Court ruling
that bars prosecutors from using the interview of a child against her alleged molester. State and federal

courts have been split on the issue, with some ruling that interviews given to counselors and other nonpolice professionals may be admitted in court even without cross-examination. The topic is of great importance to prosecutors, and 26 states joined Iowa in asking for Supreme Court review. Iowa v. Bently, 07-833 (March 24, 2008).

48. People v. Goldstein, 6 N.Y.3d 119, 843 N.E.2d 727 (2005).

49. C. Slobogin, *Proving the Unprovable* (New York: Oxford University Press, 2007), p. 73.

50. See R.D. Friedman, "Grappling With the Meaning of 'Testimonial,'" *Brooklyn L. Rev.* 71 (2005): 241; T. Lininger, "Prosecuting Batterers After *Crawford*," *Va. L. Rev.* 91 (2005): 747; R.A. Oliver, "Testimonial Hearsay as the Basis for Expert Testimony: The Intersection of the Confrontation Clause and Federal Rule of Evidence 703 after *Crawford v. Washington*," *Hastings L. J.*, 55 (2004): 1539; M.A. Mendez, "*Crawford v. Washington*: A Critique," *Stanford L. Rev.* 57 (2005): 569; R.P. Mosteller, "*Crawford v. Washington*: Encouraging and Ensuring the Confrontation of Witnesses," *U. Richmond L. Rev.* 39 (2005): 511.

51. 541 U.S. at 69.

52. 541 U.S. at 75.

53. Clark v. Arizona, 126 S. Ct. 2709 (2006). See Chapter 11 on criminal responsibility.

54. Advisory Committee's Note to Fed. R. Evid. 704.

55. The legislative history explained the reason for the adoption of Rule 704 (b): "The purpose of this amendment is to eliminate the confusing spectacle of competing expert witnesses testifying to directly contradictory conclusions as to the ultimate legal issue to be found by the trier of fact. Under this proposal, expert psychiatric testimony would be limited to presenting and explaining their diagnoses, such as whether the defendant had a severe mental disease or defect and what the characteristics of such a disease or defect, if any, may have been." S. Rep. No. 225, 98th Cong., 1st Sess. 230 (1983).

56. In Grismore v. Consolidated Products Company, 232 Iowa 328, 5 N.W.2d 646 (1942), a turkey raiser wanted to make his turkeys grow faster and he yielded to the sales talk of the salesman of a food products company. The magic food was called "E Emulsion" and the turkey raiser contracted for quantities of it that he fed to great numbers of healthy poultry. Although assisted by the salesman so as to feed it properly, the turkeys died in great numbers long before their normal execution date. In the lawsuit that followed, the sole issue for the jury to decide was what caused the deaths of the turkeys. The trial court permitted counsel for the turkey raiser to ask of an expert on turkey raising, in substance, what, in his opinion, caused the deaths of the turkeys? To this question, vigorous objections were urged. The court thought the jury ought to know what the expert did think about it, overruled the objections, and permitted the answer. The expert then placed the entire blame on "E Emulsion." On appeal, in an opinion of 34 pages, the state supreme court ruled that the trial court was right to admit the testimony. Six leading cases of the jurisdiction were overruled by name and an endless number of decisions were overruled by implication.

57. 901 F.2d 1463 (8th Cir. 1990).

58. 901 F.2d at 1466.

59. 835 F.2d 274 (11th Cir. 1988).

60. 835 F.2d at 276.

61. 4 F.3d 1573 (11th Cir. 1993).

62. 893 F.2d 1221 (11th Cir. 1990).

63. United States v. MacDonald, 688 F.2d 224 (4th Cir. 1982).

64. 819 F.2d 262 (11th Cir. 1987).

65. 819 F.2d at 265.

66. National Mental Health Association, "Myths & Realities," Hearing Transcript of the National Commission on the Insanity Defense (1983), at p. 30.

67. United States v. Patricia Hearst, trial transcript, reproduced in *The Trial of Patty Hearst* (San Francisco: Great Fidelity Press, 1976), p. 257.

68. Michigan legislation provides that the expert must share the same specialty as the defendant physician. Mich. Comp. Laws Ann. 600.2169(1)(a)(2000). In Woodard v. Custer, 476 Mich. 545, 719 N.W.2d 842 (2006), the Michigan Supreme Court set out a detailed analysis of the requirements for medical experts. The court, interpreting the statute, held that the plaintiff's expert witness must match the one most relevant standard of practice or care, i.e., the specialty engaged in by the defendant physician during the course of the alleged malpractice, and, if the defendant is board certified in that specialty, the plaintiff's expert must also be board certified in that specialty; the statute requires the matching of a singular specialty, not multiple specialties, and does not require the witness to specialize in specialties and possess board certificates that are not relevant to the standard of medical practice or care

about which the witness is to testify. Moreover, if a defendant physician specializes in a subspecialty, the plaintiff's expert witness must have specialized in the same subspecialty as the defendant physician at the time of the occurrence that is the basis for the action. 476 Mich. at 562, 719 N.W.3d at 851. See also Halloran v. Bhan, 470 Mich. 572, 683 N.W.2d 129 (2004). In Reeves v. Carson City Hosp., 274 Mich. App. 622, 736 N.W.2d 284 (2007), the court held that because the defendant physician was a specialist in emergency medicine, the patient's expert needed to be a specialist in emergency medicine. Among other states, California by legislation sets out the same restriction.

Until the 20th century, most physicians were general practitioners. The few that specialized were mainly surgeons. The advances in medical science during the past 40 years have resulted in specialization. In the United State (and Canada), medicine is now divided into 28 recognized specialties, each with its own rule-making and certifying bodies. All of these specialties include various subspecialties (that also have specific educational and training requirements). A license to practice medicine, however, allows the physician to practice in any specialty even though not board certified in that specialty.

69. As noted, the expert testifying for the plaintiff must be of the same specialty (or subspecialty) as the defendant physician (a specialist is one who can become board certified). See Woodard v. Custer, 476 Mich. 545, 719 N.W.2d 842 (2006).

70. S.S. Schwartz, "Where's Dr. Waldo? Finding the Right Medical Malpractice Expert Witness, *Mich. Neglig. Law Sec. Q.*, Spring, 2004, p. 3.

71. See, e.g., Kansas Statutes Annotated 60-3412.

72. Task Force on Mental Disability and the Death Penalty, "Recommendations and Report on the Death Penalty and Persons with Mental Disabilities," *Ment. & Phys. Disabil. Law Rep.* 30 (2006): 668–677.

73. See M. Hall, "Law, Medicine, and Trust," *Stanford L. Rev.* 55 (2002): 463; C. Scott, "Why Law Pervades Medicine: An Essay on Ethics in Health Care," *Notre Dame J. L. Ethics & Public Policy* 14 (2000): 245.

74. For example, American Academy of Child and Adolescent Psychiatry, The American Psychological Association's "Guidelines for Child Custody Evaluations in Divorce Proceedings," American Professional Society on the Abuse of Children.

75. See S. West & S.H. Friedman, "To Be or Not to Be: Treating Psychiatrist and Expert Witness," *Psychiatric Times*, May 2007, p. 50.

76. Joseph Bird, attorney, quoted in *Michigan Lawyers Weekly*, Sept. 10, 2001, p. 1362. In United States v. Villegas, No. Dist. of N.Y., No. 87-CR-151, the testimony of the treating physician along with the testimony of the forensic expert, Dr. A.L. Halpern, were able to establish that the defendant was competent to stand trial. Ltr. of David Homer, assistant U.S. attorney, to Dr. Halpern (Feb. 1, 1989), on file.

77. See 20 C.F.R. § 404.1527 (d) (2). Moreover, in workers' compensation cases, there is a rebuttable presumption in favor of the treating physician's opinion. See Conaghan v. Riverfield Country Day Sch., 163 P.3d 557 (Okla. 2007).

78. 484 F.3d 426 (6th Cir. 2007), cited in Note 7.

79. See R.K. Bailey, V.R. Scarano, & S.R. Varma, "The Practice of Forensic Psychiatry: Is It the Practice of Medicine?" *Am. J. Foren. Psychiat.* 25 (2004): 1; R.I. Simon & T.G. Gutheil, "The Forensic Expert on the Road: New Hazards Along the Way," *Psychiat. Ann.* 33 (2003): 302.

80. Policy H-265, 993 (1998). Dr. Larry Faulkner, dean of the School of Medicine at the University of South Carolina, urged in his presidential address at the 1999 annual meeting of the American Academy of Psychiatry and Law that forensic psychiatry be considered a medical specialty. L.R. Faulkner, "Ensuring That Forensic Psychiatry Thrives as a Medical Specialty in the 21st Century," *J. Am. Acad. Psychiat. & Law* 28 (2000): 14. Dr. Faulkner added (personal communication, Oct. 19, 1999):

> I do believe that forensic psychiatry is indeed medical practice, and I have no problem with licensing boards placing practical and reasonable "restrictions" on conducting "examinations on the road." We can't have it both ways. If we do not consider forensic psychiatry to be medical practice, then we have to also accept the proposition that anybody can do it. I would rather put up with the inconvenience of responding to the "restrictions" of licensing boards.

Approximately 11 states now require local licensing, and 7 states require local licensing unless the out-of-state psychiatrist is a consultant for a state-licensed one. One state allows out-of-state psychiatrists to provide testimony a limited number of times without a local license. J. Arehart-Treichel, "Crossing State Lines May Put Expert Witnesses in Jeopardy," *Psychiatric News*, Dec. 1, 2000, p. 10. The same licensing or certification issue arises in regard "examinations on the road" by psychologists. See E.Y. Drogin, "Prophets in Another Land: Utilizing Psychological Expertise From Foreign

Jurisdictions," *MPDLR* 23 (Sept./Oct. 1999): 767. See also R.I. Simon & D.W. Shuman, "Conducting Forensic Examinations on the Road: Are You Practicing Your Profession Without a License?" *J. Am. Acad. Psychiat. & Law* 27 (1999): 75. Actually, the Attorney General is not likely to proceed against the forensic expert on the grounds that he is practicing medicine without a license, but a disgruntled litigant may create problems for the expert with the medical board. Indeed, should a forensic examination, as suggested, be considered the practice of medicine? In an oft-quoted statement, Dr. Seymour Pollack described the field of psychiatry and law as one in which "psychiatric theories, concepts, principles, and practice are applied or related to any and all legal matters." The current definition of forensic psychiatry, adopted by the American Board of Forensic Psychiatry and the American Academy of Psychiatry and the Law states, "Forensic psychiatry is a subspecialty of psychiatry, in which scientific and clinical expertise is applied to legal issues in legal contexts, embracing civil, criminal, correctional, or legislative matters; forensic psychiatry should be practiced in accordance with the guidelines and ethical principles enunciated by the profession of psychiatry."

The forensic expert usually serves as an agent of the attorney, and the expert in making an assessment is not in a physician–patient relationship with the examinee. Indeed, the forensic expert makes a point of advising the examinee that the examination is not for the purpose of treatment.

81. Mitchell v. Mitchell, 830 So.2d 755 (Ala. App. 2002).
82. 253 F.3d 967 (7th Cir. 2001).
83. 253 F.3d at 975. Austin argued that "the Association acted in bad faith because it never disciplines members who testify on behalf of malpractice defendants." 253 F.3d at 969. Organizations such as the American Psychological Association do not have an obvious partisan position in the sense that they are equally likely to sanction a plaintiff or a defense expert. However, organizations such as the American Association of Neurological Surgeons or other medical associations are more likely to sanction plaintiff experts than defense experts. T. Carter, "M.D. With a Mission: A Physician Battles Against Colleagues He Considers Rogue Expert Witnesses," *A.B.A.J.* 90 (Aug. 2004): 41.
84. 253 F.3d at 975.
85. *In re* Gary James Lustgarten, 629 S.E.2d 886 (N.C. App. 2006).
86. Quoted in *Trial*, Sept. 2006, p. 20. See also H.W. Tesoriero, "Doctor Roils Colleagues in Debate on Fetal Monitors," *Wall Street Journal*, Oct. 26, 2007, p. 1.
87. In Fullerton v. Florida Medical Ass'n, 938 So.2d 587 (Fla. App. 2006), an expert sued the state medical association (of which he was not a member) and a number of physicians who had filed a complaint with the association alleging his testimony fell below reasonable professional standards and that he specifically "presented false testimony and false theories about stroke in the hope to prove negligent medical care." Fullerton alleged in his complaint that the Expert Witness Committee "was organized for the purpose of intimidating, hindering, and deterring persons … from appearing as expert witnesses on behalf of plaintiffs in cases involving medical malpractice." The appellate court reversed a trial court dismissal of the action and held that the Florida peer review immunity statute did not govern this situation. The court, however, expressed no opinion on whether the complaint stated a cause of action. In Deatherage v. Examining Board of Psychology, 948 P.2d 828 (Wash. 1997), the court held that the state's absolute witness immunity rule did not extend to professional disciplinary proceedings. In Huhta v. State Board of Medicine, 706 A.2d 1275 (Pa. 1998), the court similarly held that judicial immunity did not shield a physician from disciplinary proceeding before the state board of medicine—the witness's transgression was the disclosure of confidential patient records. In Budwin v. American Psychological Ass'n, 29 Cal. Rptr.2d 453 (Cal. App. 1994), the American Psychological Association censured the plaintiff after finding that he testified falsely. See J. Sanders, "Expert Witness Ethics," *Fordham L. Rev.* 76 (2007): 1563.
88. Personal communication (Dec. 1, 2006).

4

Holding the Expert Accountable

In many types of cases (for example, malpractice), the law obliges the litigant to present an expert, otherwise the case will be dismissed. The litigant *must*—not simply *may*—present an expert. The testimony of lay witnesses in these cases is insufficient as a matter of law (although, in reality the expert testimony may not be clarifying). As a consequence, the lawyer is at the mercy of experts—an expert must be found and engaged, often at considerable cost.

The Federal Rules of Evidence adopted in 1975 and the various state counterparts widened the use of experts by relaxing the rules on qualification of experts, the basis of their opinion, and testimony on ultimate issues.[1] Rule 702 provides that expert testimony may be used whenever it "may assist the jury."[2] Under that provision, experts have been used in criminal and even civil cases that rest entirely on simple facts. The result has been a battle of experts that confuses rather than assists the jury. Now there is a backtracking on expert testimony.

Various solutions have been offered to curb expert abuses. They include capping expert witness fees, prescreening experts, using only court-appointed experts, adherence to a strict code of ethics, peer review, and a science court.[3] With increasing frequency, the issue is raised: What about expert witness malpractice? The incompetence, negligence, or intentional misconduct of experts prompts a search for ways to hold the expert responsible in tort. Under what circumstances (if any) may an expert be held responsible for his findings made in a report or for his testimony in a deposition or at trial? To what extent does the expert enjoy immunity? Is the expert or other witness subject to a tort of perjury? May there be a claim of defamation? May the adversary party claim infliction of mental distress? May the client or attorney retaining the expert make a claim against him? Does it make a difference whether the expert is hired by a party or is court-appointed? May a licensing board impose sanctions?

Witness Immunity as a General Principle

English common law cases are generally cited as the seminal cases establishing the doctrine of witness immunity (or privilege). These cases reveal that the immunity originated within the limited context of defamation law.[4] In most states, it was later expanded to bar other actions.[5] The purpose of the rule is said to preserve the integrity of the judicial process by encouraging full and frank testimony. In the words of one 19th century court, "[C]laims [against a witness] must yield to the dictates of public policy, which requires that the paths that lead to the ascertainment of truth should be left as free and unobstructed as possible."[6]

A witness's apprehension of subsequent liability might induce two forms of self-censorship. First, witnesses might be reluctant to come forward to testify. Second, once a witness is on the stand, his testimony might be distorted by the fear of subsequent liability. A witness who knows that he might be forced to defend a subsequent lawsuit, and perhaps to pay damages, might be inclined to shade his testimony in favor of the potential plaintiff, to magnify uncertainties, and thus to deprive the finder of fact of candid, objective, and undistorted evidence.[7]

Various states by statute provide in relevant part that: "A privileged publication or broadcast is one made: … In any (1) legislative or (2) judicial proceeding."[8] In response to abuses, several courts modified the absoluteness of the privilege by adopting an "interest of justice" exception.[9]

The California Supreme Court in 1990 overruled a number of lower court decisions in the state that applied the exception.[10] It said that "the evils inherent in permitting derivative tort actions based on communications during the trial of a previous action are … far more destructive to the administration of justice than an occasional 'unfair' result."

In Illinois, in *Renzi v. Morrison*,[11] the immunity or privilege was held not to be absolute. In this case, a psychiatrist discussed test results with a patient's husband who was planning to petition to dissolve the marriage and assume custody of their child. The psychiatrist also appeared at the custody hearing and gave crucial testimony for the husband. The patient was informed that the psychiatrist had discussed the results of her psychological tests with her husband in relation to the dissolution and custody proceedings. The patient contacted the psychiatrist and stated her intention to exercise her right under the state's Mental Health and Developmental Disabilities Confidentiality Act to prevent disclosure of any confidential information. The psychiatrist voluntarily appeared at the custody hearing and offered to testify for the husband. The patient objected, citing confidentiality. The trial court permitted the testimony, and temporary custody of the child was awarded to the husband. The patient thereupon filed an action against the psychiatrist for violation of the Mental Health Act. The psychiatrist argued the common law doctrine of immunity protected a witness who disclosed confidential communications under the Mental Health Act in a judicial proceeding. The appellate court noted that the act provided for disclosure of confidential communication when the interests of substantial justice superseded patient privilege, but that was not the case here. The court noted that the psychiatrist was neither testifying under subpoena nor appointed by the court to testify, hence the patient was entitled to seek damages.

The focus of the privilege is on the proceeding in which the communication takes place. It has its boundaries. Thus, in *Susan A. v. County of Sonoma*,[12] the court held that the privilege did not apply because of the venue of the communication. In this case, a forensic psychologist interviewed a juvenile murder suspect at the request of a public defender, and with the permission of the public defender and the consent of the juvenile, he spoke with the press. The suspect's parents sued for "breach of confidence, invasion of privacy, public disclosure of private facts, false light, defamation, intentional infliction of emotional distress, and negligence." The trial judge granted summary judgment to the defendant, but the court of appeals reversed on the ground that the immunity of the litigation privilege does not apply because the psychologist's statements to the press do not satisfy the requirement that the communication be made in judicial or quasijudicial proceedings. The court rejected the psychologist's argument that the privilege applied because his remarks to the press were designed to obtain a litigation advantage for the juvenile.[13]

Perjury

Immunity from a civil suit is granted a witness, lay or expert, for perjury as well as for defamation. There is no "perjury tort action,"[14] but perjury is subject to criminal prosecution; it is rarely charged because it is difficult to prove. Perjury is defined as the willful giving of false testimony in a judicial proceeding, made under oath, on a point material to the issue or inquiry. (The court has the inherent power to vacate a judgment procured by fraud). In an article quoted in a report by the American Medical Association, Drs. David L. Chadwick and Henry F. Krous give several examples wherein physicians misquoted standard journals and texts, made false statements, and deliberately omitted important facts and knowledge as it pertained to the expert opinion offered.[15] The expert's fraudulent presentation of his qualifications or fabrication of facts may give rise to a charge of perjury, but not for his opinion.[16] An opinion does not have a true or false dimension, just as you cannot say your dream is right and mine is wrong.

Accountability to the Adversary

Does an attorney or expert hired by the attorney owe a duty of care to the adversary to conduct a reasonable investigation prior to filing a lawsuit? A few years ago, physicians who were sued for malpractice were urged by their colleagues to countersue as a way to discourage malpractice claims. The movement got nowhere, as the following cases illustrate.

In an action before a federal district court in Michigan, *Kahn v. Burman*,[17] Dr. Roger Kahn, a defendant in a malpractice suit, brought an action against Dr. Sheldon Burman, consultant and potential expert witness, asserting claims of negligence, fraudulent and innocent misrepresentation, defamation, and intentional infliction of emotional distress. The claims were based exclusively on the expert's reports and deposition testimony in the malpractice case. The court held that Dr. Burman, the expert, owed no legal duty to Dr. Kahn.[18]

The court also noted that while the expert's reports were not statements made under oath in the course of litigation, they may well satisfy the witness immunity prerequisite of relevancy to the judicial proceedings. The court said, "Physicians' reports are so inextricably intertwined with medical malpractice actions that it would be illogical to hold that such reports are not 'relevant' to the underlying judicial proceedings. ... To hold otherwise would defeat the purpose of witness immunity, which is to ensure that the judicial process functions 'unimpeded by fear on the part of its participants that they will be sued for damages for their part in the proceedings.'"[19]

In holding that no duty is owing the adversary, the court referred to the readily analogous case of *Friedman v. Dozorc*,[20] where the Michigan Supreme Court was faced with the issue of whether an attorney who files a malpractice suit against a physician owes any legal duty to him. The physician, upon the dismissal of the suit against him, brought suit against the plaintiff's attorney for negligence, abuse of process, and malicious prosecution. (The title of "malicious prosecution" is often expanded to cover not only criminal prosecutions, but also frivolous or unwarranted civil actions.) The Michigan Supreme Court ruled that the defendant did not owe a duty to investigate before bringing the action. To hold that attorneys owed a duty to adverse parties would unduly inhibit attorneys' prime duty to their clients, the court said. The attorney's duty of care is to his client and to the court, not to the adversary.[21]

Responsibility of Prosecutor in Presenting Incompetent Evidence

On its face, the Civil Rights Act (§ 1983) makes liable every person who deprives another of civil rights in the name of state law. The U.S. Supreme Court, however, has held that the section preserves at least some of the immunities traditionally extended to public officers at common law. State law usually immunizes governmental agencies and their employees against civil damages unless it can be shown that the employees acted with reckless disregard for the individual's welfare or constitutional rights. A prosecutor has absolute immunity for eliciting false statements, but he has only qualified immunity for giving legal advice to police officers or experts. In *Burns v. Reed*,[22] with the approval of the prosecutor, experts obtained a confession based on hypnosis, but it was not revealed to the court that that method was used. On the basis of the misleading presentation, the judge issued a search warrant. The resulting detention was held to be a violation of civil rights.

In the trial of Clay Shaw (alleged to be a participant in the assassination of President Kennedy), District Attorney Jim Garrison would have the medical examiner hypnotize the principal witness in the case, Perry Russo, every morning before the testimony. This was unknown to the defense. The purpose allegedly was not to tamper with the witness, not to have the witness say something different, but to have the witness appear in a confident way, and everybody knows that juries give more credibility to a witness who testifies with confidence. Notwithstanding,

Clay Shaw was acquitted, and thereupon he filed a malicious prosecution suit against Garrison and the medical examiner. Shortly thereafter, however, Shaw died, and that brought an end to the matter.

In the much publicized case involving the Duke lacrosse players, Durham District Attorney Mike Nifong brought patently false charges in an effort to court the black vote in his election race. He has been disbarred, obliged to resign from office in disgrace, and sentenced to jail for a day for lying to the court. Going along with the district attorney, the Duke administration and many of the faculty, led by the university president, condemned the players. They have apologized. The debacle cost the players and their families a year of disgrace and millions of dollars in legal bills.[23]

Prolonged Examination

What about when an expert on behalf of the prosecution carries out a prolonged or rigorous examination of the accused? Is it not expected? (There may be a complaint about the bill.) The expert is on the horns of a dilemma. The expert invariably is asked on cross-examination, "How much time did you spend in carrying out the examination?" Yet, if the examination is grueling, extending over a period of time, the individual may complain and may bring suit for intentional infliction of mental distress (which is likely to be dismissed, but defending it takes time as well as expense). It has happened on a number of occasions. Interrogating a witness, should it resemble an assault, may be tortuous, just as when anyone attacks another wherever it occurs. The fact that an attorney hires an expert does not entitle the expert to physically or mentally harm another.

Testifying in the Presence of the Subject

The practice of giving clinical testimony about the psychological or psychiatric assessment in the presence of the subject at trial raises ethical concerns. Would it inflict trauma on the subject? Should the subject hear about, say, his sexual impulses or his psychological test scores? The code of ethics of the American Psychiatric Association says to "respect integrity and protect the welfare of the person." In law, however, the accused has a right to be present at his trial; however, to avoid psychic harm, his attorney may ask him to leave the courtroom.[24]

Civil Commitment Proceedings

What about responsibility, be it by a therapist or examiner, in regard to participation in a civil commitment proceeding? When a therapist in the course of diagnosis or treatment has determined that the patient is in need of hospitalization, an exception in the law on psychotherapist–patient privilege protecting confidentiality allows the therapist to testify in regard to the need for hospitalization. Others, too, may have immunity in seeking hospitalization of an individual, even a stranger. Texas law provides: "*All persons* acting in good faith, reasonably, and without negligence in connection with examination, certification, apprehension, custody, transportation, detention, treatment, or discharge of any person, or in the performance of any other act required or authorized by [the Mental Health Code], shall be free from all liability, civil or criminal, by reason of such action" (emphasis added).[25] Yet, there is a caveat in regard to a negligent diagnosis in Texas as well as elsewhere.[26] In the Texas case of *James v. Brown*,[27] damages were sought against three psychiatrists arising out of an involuntary hospitalization. The plaintiff alleged libel, negligent misdiagnosis/medical malpractice, false imprisonment, and malicious prosecution. The Texas Supreme Court rejected a blanket immunity from all civil liability for mental health professionals testifying in commitment proceedings. The court did not allow a defamation claim for the testimony at trial, but it did allow a claim for negligent misdiagnosis, which occurred prior to the hearing. The court noted that "[the plaintiff] is not prevented from recovering from the doctors for negligent misdiagnosis–medical malpractice merely because their diagnoses were later communicated to a court in the due course of judicial proceedings."[28]

What about failure to seek a patient's involuntary hospitalization? There is a so-called best judgment rule that shields a physician from liability "for mere errors of judgment provided he does what he thinks best after careful examination."[29] In the context of psychiatry, the rule has most commonly been applied to exculpate psychiatrists for their decision not to seek a patient's involuntary hospitalization. Under the psychotherapist judgment rule, the court would not impose liability on therapists for simple errors in judgment. Instead, the court would examine the good faith, independence, and thoroughness of a psychotherapist's decision not to commit a patient. The factors in reviewing such good faith include the competence and training of the reviewing psychotherapists; whether the relevant documents and evidence were adequately, promptly, and independently reviewed; whether the advice or opinion of another therapist was obtained; whether the evaluation was made in light of the proper legal standards for commitment; and whether other evidence of good faith exists.[30]

Autopsies

Medical examiners or coroners, as well as psychiatrists and others whom they hire, are protected by governmental immunity to the extent that the jurisdiction provides governmental immunity. "Body of Evidence," the cover story of an issue of the *ABA Journal*, looks at what happens when medical examiners or coroners fail to distinguish accidents from murders or suicides. A botched autopsy can impede a fair trial or may be the start of a civil suit. Case in point: When the bloody and partially clothed body of Susan Negersmith was found in an alley in Wildwood, New Jersey, her death was ruled an accident, caused by a lethal combination of alcohol poisoning and hypothermia. Some 3 years later, police reclassified the death as a homicide. The reason for this was that an outside expert hired to review the original autopsy findings concluded that she had been raped and strangled. "What happened in New Jersey happens all over the place, all the time," said Dr. Claus Speth, a consulting forensic pathologist in Woodbury, New Jersey.[31]

It is estimated that up to 70% of the nation is poorly served by its system for investigating deaths, and given governmental immunity, there is no recourse. There is no uniform method for certifying deaths in the United States, and no two states do it exactly alike. Approximately half of the nation's population comes under the jurisdiction of medical examiners, usually physicians appointed based on merit. The rest of the population falls under the jurisdiction of coroners, and only four states require a coroner to be a physician. South Carolina requires only a high school diploma.

Reporting of Sexual Abuse in the Course of a Child Custody Proceeding

Under the law providing for reports of suspected child abuse, immunity protects the act of reporting, but a diagnosis of sexual abuse is fraught with hazard. In the treatment or evaluation of a child, the courts have held that a duty of care is owed not only to the child, but also to the parents. Thus, in the case of revival of memory in therapy of sexual abuse, a duty of care is said to be owing the parent, though the parent is not the patient, and as a consequence the parent as well as the child may bring an action against the therapist or examiner.[32]

Consider a case that occurred in Colorado. A mother, after dissolution of the marriage, took her 4-year-old daughter to a counselor who reportedly observed the child for two sessions and administered no psychological tests, but came to suspect the father of sexually abusing his daughter. When questioned, the counselor described her diagnostic method as "the technique of the nonverbal," which involved analyzing the child's body language. Based on this method of analysis, she concluded that the father was sexually abusing the daughter. The counselor reported this to the appropriate authorities and also advised the mother to restrict the father's visitation. When the father learned of this allegation, he asked for a session with the counselor and she refused. The counselor referred the child to another psychologist who raised the question about the validity of the sex abuse charge. The counselor characterized this input as irrelevant and not helpful. Finally, after several court proceedings, the court appointed a third psychologist, agreed upon by both parties, who observed the family's interactions, separately and as a group, and administered psychological tests. The psychologist concluded that there were serious doubts about the child's veracity. The counselor, however, persisted and when she was called as an expert witness stated that there was no doubt in her mind that the father had sexually abused the child. In an affidavit, the third psychologist expressed concerns that the counselor had no support in the literature to validate her procedures and conclusions, had not conducted psychological testing, had not adequately investigated inconsistent statements made by the child to other parties, had diagnosed the father as a sex abuser without having seen him, and had not taken steps to be aware of and to control the effects of her personal prejudices on the opinion she had formed. The trial court dismissed the father's complaint against the counselor on technical grounds and he appealed.

The Colorado Court of Appeals held that the counselor had a duty to the father to use due care in formulating any opinion, which might reasonably have an adverse effect on him. The counselor sought the refuge of statutory immunity whereby individuals reporting suspected sexual abuse are protected from being sued, but the court found that the counselor's acts went beyond the protection of the law when the counselor recommended that the mother restrict the father's visitation. The father also alleged that the counselor acted in wanton and reckless disregard for his rights and feelings. As a consequence, the father could pursue a tort claim against the counselor for outrageous conduct and intentional infliction of emotional harm. Tort liability for intentional acts and punitive damages falls outside the scope of many malpractice insurance policies, which cover only negligence. The appellate court also found it an error to dismiss the father's complaint against the supervising psychologist who may have negligently supervised the counselor.[33]

Accountability to Retaining Client

What of accountability of the expert to the retaining client? There is immunity for testimony, but what about negligence in investigation or evaluation? Does immunity protect prior preparatory activity leading to the witness's testimony? Would accountability for negligence in preparatory activity in effect undercut witness immunity? Is immunity limited to protecting the expert from an adverse party?

Apparently only a couple of appellate decisions have granted expert witnesses full immunity for preparation as well as testimony at trial. In *Bruce v. Byrne-Stevens & Associates Engineers*,[34] in a plurality opinion of four justices with one justice concurring, and four justices dissenting, the Washington Supreme Court barred any suit against an expert for his testimony or pretrial preparation.[35] In *Bruce*, the plaintiffs sued an engineering group for negligently underestimating the amount of damage sustained when the plaintiff's neighbor performed excavation work and, as a consequence, did not recover the actual amount needed for the repair. The court held that immunity covers not only an expert's negligence on the stand, but also negligence in preparing an opinion before courtroom testimony. The court said, "There is no way to distinguish the testimony from the acts and communications [with the litigant] on which it is based."

The decision was based on several policy assumptions. The basis for the majority's extension of the rule of immunity was the claimed desire to promote "full and frank testimony," but such a rule provides no such impetus. Second, the court contended that "imposing civil liability on expert witnesses would discourage anyone who is not a full-time professional expert witness from testifying." The court reasoned that no one-time expert could carry the needed insurance to testify.

The court, being unable to separate the act of preparing the estimate from the actual testimony about the estimate, broadly defined witness immunity. So, the court said that the "whole integral enterprise [of preparing and testifying] falls within the scope of immunity." The court held that "absolute immunity extends to acts and statements of experts that arise in the course of or preliminary to judicial proceedings." The court rejected the plaintiff's argument that they were suing for negligent engineering, rather than negligent testifying.[36]

In a federal court case in Louisiana, *Marrogi v. Howard*,[37] the defendants, experts in medical billing, were retained by a physician to assist in his lawsuit against a former employer. The physician claimed he was underpaid and he retained the defendants to analyze a year's billing records and testify on his behalf. When the physician's lawsuit against the employer was dismissed, he blamed the experts, alleging that the dismissal was caused by their substandard expert performance. In dismissing the physician's lawsuit against the experts (affirmed on appeal to the Fifth Circuit), the federal district court judge cited "a line of Louisiana cases that uniformly recognize absolute immunity to witnesses in judicial or quasijudicial proceedings."

The vast majority of appellate decisions, however, are holding an expert liable to the retaining client for negligence in the preparation of an opinion.[38] In a Missouri case, *Murphy v. Mathews*,[39] as in *Bruce*, the Washington case, the plaintiff complained his expert was negligent in preparing and documenting the damage claim. In a unanimous opinion, 7–0, the Missouri Supreme Court ruled that witness immunity did not protect the engineers. It ruled that the immunity generally protected only in-court testimony, not pretrial litigation, and that it generally protected only against defamation suits.[40] In the course of its opinion, the court noted that an opposing litigant could not sue an expert because the expert owed no duty to that litigant.

In another case involving experts hired to help a plaintiff prove its damages in litigation, the California Court of Appeals held that immunity does not protect an expert hired by a litigant against a malpractice suit by the expert's own client.[41] In this case, Mattco Forge, a maker of airplane parts, obtained Arthur Young to calculate the profits it lost when General Motors stopped awarding contracts to them. It accused Arthur Young, the manager and his supervisor, of misrepresenting their qualifications and of engaging in a cover-up. In ruling that the suit was not barred by immunity, the court said, "Applying the privilege in this circumstance does not encourage witnesses to testify truthfully; indeed, by shielding a negligent expert witness from liability, it has the opposite effect."

In a Connecticut case, *Pollock v. Panjabi*,[42] the court denied a motion to dismiss a lawsuit against Manohar Panjabi, a Yale University biomechanics expert. He had been retained by the plaintiff, a quadriplegic, in a Canadian police brutality suit, to help determine the cause of the plaintiff's paralysis. The expert concluded that an officer's wresting hold on the plaintiff caused the injury, but the Canadian trial court barred him from testifying, finding that the expert had based his conclusion, in part, on improperly conducted analyses. The plaintiff nevertheless obtained a $783,000 judgment against the police. Notwithstanding, he filed a breach-of-contract lawsuit, alleging that the expert improperly conducted the tests he had been hired to perform. In allowing the lawsuit to go forward, the court ruled that the point of contention was not the expert's testimony, but his failure to meet his obligation to provide scientifically supportable conclusions.

Crucial elements of any tort, be it malpractice or other tort, involve causation and damages as well as fault. Tort liability requires proof that the defendant caused the injury to the plaintiff, and that as a result of the fault of the defendant, the plaintiff suffered harm. It is not always apparent that the expert's testimony was the proximate cause of the failure to obtain a favorable verdict. Causation may be difficult to prove. In the event that causation is established, it then behooves the party to establish damages. What is the monetary damage done by false conviction of an innocent person? For liability, does it matter whether the expert presented his evaluation at trial?

Actually, testifying at trial is a rare event; more than 95 percent of cases, civil or criminal, are settled before trial, but in any event, there may be liability for negligent preparation, as in any situation where one relies on an expert opinion. Research or investigation makes up most of an expert's work, culminating in an oral or written report that evaluates the merits of a claim. Sometimes, in litigation, an expert witness will take part in a deposition, through which the opposing attorney gauges the strength of the other side's case.

Time and again, an employee may lose employment as a result of a negligent evaluation by a company physician of his condition, and the employee sues the examiner.[43] Should the time of the evaluation, or whether the matter ends up in litigation, make a difference as to the examiner's responsibility? Obviously not. These cases are distinguishable from those where an expert on behalf of an attorney evaluates an adversary. In those instances, no duty of care is owed the adversary, as we have noted.

In addition to a claim based on negligence, a cause of action may be asserted for breach of contract. A contract claim evades traditional negligence defenses, such as the short statute of limitation, or contributory or comparative negligence. Malpractice insurance does not cover contract claims. A claim in contract depends on the agreement of the parties as to the scope of the expert's engagement.

Moreover, there may be a claim based on various consumer protection–type statutes that are frequently resorted to in professional negligence situations. The claim may be based either in an alleged violation of professional standards or in alleged misrepresentation by the expert as to his qualifications.

Attacking One's Witness on Account of Unexpected and Contrary Testimony

Under the Anglo-American adversary system, each side presents its witnesses and vouches for them. A party was not allowed to present a witness and then when the witness testified in a contrary way, ask the court *not* to believe the witness; that is to say, a prior contradictory statement could not be used to attack the witness (or impeach, in lawyer vernacular) unless the party was surprised by the testimony. In the event the witness informed the party prior to trial that he would testify differently than previously stated, there would be no surprise and, hence, he could not be impeached.

With the mounting number of turn-tail witnesses, especially in criminal cases where the witness may have been intimidated, the Federal Rules of Evidence adopted in 1975 and the various state counterparts provide that the credibility of a witness may be attacked by any party, including the party calling the witness.[44] The prior statement, however, cannot be used as proof in the case (unless it was made under oath and subject to cross-examination). By virtue of the prior statement, the jury may not give credibility to any of the witness's testimony. And, if the witness is an expert, the attorney will not likely engage him again. Perjury charges are rarely invoked due to inconsistent testimony.

May an expert be held liable to the party calling him when the expert changes his testimony on the stand without having previously notified counsel who called the expert?[45] In *Panitz v. Behrend*,[46] an expert medical witness hired by a law firm brought action to recover the balance of monies the firm had agreed to pay, and the firm counterclaimed for damages resulting from an unfavorable verdict allegedly caused by gross negligence and misrepresentation regarding the substance of the expert's testimony at trial. The witness previously had agreed to testify about a causal connection involving cigarette smokers, but, at trial during cross-examination, she stated that she could not identify a causal connection. After trial, she explained that "she had come to realize prior to trial that the reasoning upon which she had relied in earlier depositions was inaccurate." The court held that she was immune from liability. The court said,

> To allow a party to litigation to contract with an expert witness and thereby obligate the witness to testify only in a manner favorable to the party, on threat of civil liability, would be contrary to public policy. … Fundamentally, no witness can be required to testify, and no witness should be expected to testify, to anything other than the truth as he [or she] sees it and according to what he [or she] believes it to be. The same is expected of expert witnesses. … An expert witness will not be subjected to civil liability because he or she, in the face of conflicting evidence or during vigorous cross-examination, is persuaded that some or all of his or her opinion testimony has been inaccurate.[47]

Attacking the Credibility of a Witness by the Adverse Party

There are several traditional and well-recognized methods by which an adversary can impeach a witness, lay or expert.[48] *Impeach* is lawyer language meaning an attack on the credibility of the witness. The witness is qualified or competent to testify, but the probative value of the testimony is impugned by the impeachment. One way of doing so is showing that the witness has made a prior inconsistent statement (usually in a deposition). A second way involves showing that the witness is affected by some bias or motivation that may tempt him to falsify or shade his testimony. This may involve reference to the fee or to ideology (the expert invariably testifies for the prosecution or defense or for the employer or employee).[49] Another way is cross-examining the witness about prior convictions. Yet another way is cross-examination about particular instances of nonconviction misconduct that involves veracity, such as falsifying an employment application. Then, too, statements contained in published treatises and other similar publications may be used to impeach the witness.[50]

A new technique has recently passed muster, at least in Michigan. The question arose: May an expert who testifies on standard of care in a malpractice case be shown on cross-examination that his professional practices have been failures? That issue came before the Michigan Supreme Court in *Wischmeyer v. Schanz*.[51] In this case, Wade Wischmeyer suffered back pain as a result of a fall at work and consulted Dr. George Schanz, who recommended back surgery. Wischmeyer underwent a surgical procedure known as a posterior lumbar interbody fusion (PLIF). After the operation, Wischmeyer continued to experience pain and decreased mobility. He filed a lawsuit claiming that the surgery was negligently performed. At trial, to establish standard of care, the plaintiff presented Dr. Ronald Ignelzi, who testified that the PLIF procedure was improperly performed. He testified that the injury "should not have occurred unless there was some negligence at the time of the procedure." On cross-examination, Dr. Ignelzi admitted that on the six occasions that he personally had performed similar PLIF procedures, all six could be classified as failures. He also was asked about his suspension from hospital privileges and his malpractice litigation history. The trial court jury granted the defendant a no cause of action verdict. The Court of Appeals reversed, saying, "The trial court abused its discretion in allowing defense counsel to cross-examine plaintiff's expert witness, Dr. Ignelzi, regarding prior poor surgical results and prior medical malpractice claims … . This line of questioning was not probative of truthfulness or untruthfulness, and constituted an improper means of impeaching the credibility of Dr. Ignelzi."[52]

Federal Rule of Evidence 608(b), as well as the state counterpart, provides: "Specific instances of the conduct of a witness, for the purpose of attacking or supporting the witness's credibility … may not be proved by extrinsic evidence. They may, however, in the discretion of the court *if probative of truthfulness or untruthfulness*, be inquired into on cross-examination of the witness (1) *concerning the witness's character for truthfulness or untruthfulness* …" (emphasis added).

Hence, under Rule 608(b), a witness may not be impeached by an inquiry into specific past acts unless the court finds that those acts reflect on the witness's character for truthfulness. The allegations of prior surgical mishaps by Dr. Ignelzi had nothing to do with his truthfulness, and so the Court of Appeals held that permitting such questions was improper.

It has been well established that where not relevant to truthfulness, allegations of professional wrongdoing, misconduct, or negligence that is unrelated to the case on trial is not a proper subject of impeachment of an expert medical witness. This rule of law seeks to avoid the substantial risk of distracting and confusing the jury with a "minitrial" on collateral matters. In order for the jury to assess the past acts in weighing the expert's opinion, the jury would have had to have known, at a minimum, the circumstances of the other cases, the nature of the mistakes made in those cases, how they occurred, and what, if anything, about those cases made it more likely that the expert was mistaken in his opinion in the present case.

Be that as it may, the Michigan Supreme Court, in a 4–3 decision, reversed the Court of Appeals, and reinstated the verdict of no cause for action. The majority said, "Where information is relevant and not unduly prejudiced, it would be unwise to apply [Rule] 608 so that the jury is deprived of information that would assist it in its task." The majority ignored the plain meaning of Rule 608(b) and instead relied on the principle of relevancy. It concluded, "We believe that this cross-examination was proper because during direct examination Dr. Ignelzi testified that he had performed hundreds of back surgeries, including PLIFs, in order to establish his competency."

Why did the court shift away from Rule 608? Trial judges are egregious in not disqualifying a witness offered as an expert. So, what should be a matter of qualification in considering competency to testify is used to attack credibility. The Michigan Supreme Court, by 4–3, allowed it. Given the army of experts at the ready to swear an oath for a fee, many attorneys say, "Let's have more of it."[53] If so, should not Rule 608 be amended to allow it?

Accountability of Court-Appointed Experts

At one time (and still today in some quarters) the court appointment of experts has been recommended as the way to improve the quality of expert testimony. During the first half of the 20th century a number of jurisdictions adopted an "Impartial Expert Testimony Plan" in regard medical testimony, but the hopes for an improvement in testimony did not materialize. Again recently, the American Medical Association in its Report on Expert Testimony urges courts to retain nonpartisan experts so as to obtain objective evidence.[54] In federal law and most states, the rules of evidence adopted in the last quarter of the 20th century, allow for court-appointed experts, but the provision is little used, and when used, it is mainly in child custody cases (where the parties are unable to afford experts) or in evaluating competency to stand trial.[55]

The reasons for nonuse of court-appointed experts are several. For one, the belief in an impartial or unbiased expert has been debunked.[56] For another, it is counter to the adversary system, which, the argument runs, results in a fuller factual record for the decision maker. Still another reason is that a court appointment delegate's quasijudicial power and it is inherently more difficult for judges to rule against the advice of an expert whom they have appointed.

The duty of a court-appointed expert is to the court and, as a consequence, the litigants have no cause of action against this kind of expert, be it for negligent investigation or testimony. (A court-ordered examination may or may not be carried out by a court-appointed expert.) The court-appointed expert acts for the benefit of the court, not for the benefit of the either litigant. Thus, the Arizona Court of Appeals held that court-appointed officials, such as psychiatrists and psychologists, are protected by judicial immunity.[57] The New Jersey Supreme Court held that a husband could sue a court-appointed accountant and his firm for negligent valuation of a business asset that was being divided in a divorce proceeding. The court found that the defendants were not "arbitrators" and that, because they were privately paid by the litigants, they should be held to professional standards.[58]

Suspension of a Professional License

A licensing board may withdraw a license where the practitioner is found to have violated an ethical or legal norm. In *McDonnell v. Commission on Medical Discipline*,[59] Dr. Edmond McDonnell, a defendant in a medical malpractice action, expressed concern to his attorney about two physicians who were scheduled to testify for the plaintiff that they lacked the relevant experience. Through intermediaries, he contacted the two physicians and advised them that he intended to have transcripts of their depositions disseminated to their local and national medical societies. He claimed that his purpose in doing so was "to make certain that the testimony of the witnesses would be honest," but he later admitted that his actions were "wrong, improper, and injudicious." The Maryland Commission on Medical Discipline reprimanded him, but the Maryland Court of Appeals held that his actions were not "directly tied to the physician's conduct in the actual performance of the practice of medicine, i.e., in the diagnosis, care, or treatment of patients," and therefore set aside the reprimand.

In a first-of-its-kind ruling, the U.S. Seventh Circuit Court of Appeals ruled that a professional society may discipline a member on account of testimony presented at trial that is deemed not up to standards. As noted in Chapter 3, in *Austin v. American Association of Neurological Surgeons*,[60] the court said, "Although [the expert witness] did not treat the malpractice plaintiff for whom he testified, his testimony at her trial was a type of medical service and if the quality of his testimony reflected the quality of his medical judgment, he is probably a poor physician. His discipline by the Association therefore served an important public policy exemplified by the federal Health Care Quality Improvement Act."[61]

Malpractice lawsuits by a party against its expert does not do much in regard to the quality of testimony at trial. On the other hand, lawsuits by the adversary may work in that direction, but the courts hold that the attorney or the expert owes no duty of care to the adversary. However, either party—or even a stranger to the litigation—can file a complaint with the licensing board.

In Conclusion

Traditionally, witnesses were given immunity in regard to their participation in the judicial process so that they would not be reluctant to testify. In recent years, however, as a result of the criticisms of expert testimony, immunity is being circumvented by lawsuits arising out of the preparation of an opinion or by suspension of a professional license. The threat is apparently beginning to chill expert testimony. According to a number of attorneys, that is not a plus. They say experts who are aware of the development are becoming reluctant to testify.[62]

Endnotes

1. Rules 701–705, Federal Rules of Evidence.
2. The Advisory Committee's Note to Rule 702 states, "Whether the situation is a proper one for the use of expert testimony is to be determined on the basis of assisting the trier."
3. See J. Sanders, "Expert Witness Ethics," *Fordham L. Rev.* 76 (2007): 1563; J.B. Weinstein, "Improving Expert Testimony," *U. Richmond L. Rev.* 20 (1986): 473.
4. Traditionally, the witness immunity rule was limited to defamation cases. The Restatement of Torts defines the parameters of the privilege as follows: "A witness is absolutely privileged to publish defamatory matter concerning another in communications preliminary to a proposed judicial proceeding or as part of a judicial proceeding in which he is testifying. If it has some relation to the privilege." The traditional witness immunity rule does not offer a wholesale immunity for any civil wrong.
5. In Harris v. Riggenbach, 633 N.W.2d 193 (S.D. 2000), a former husband brought action for defamation, negligence, intentional infliction of emotional distress, and negligent infliction of emotional distress against a counselor who submitted an affidavit in a visitation and custody proceeding. The affidavit by

the counselor stated that she believed that the husband had sexually abused his son. The court held that the affidavit was absolutely privileged. South Dakota legislation provides for an absolute privilege; SDCL 20-11-5(2).

6. Calkins v. Sumner, 13 Wis. 193 (1860).
7. The U.S. Supreme Court spelled out these reasons in Briscoe v. LaHue, 460 U.S. 325 (1983).
8. See, e.g., Cal. Code of Procedure, Sec. 47 (b)(2).
9. See P.T. Hayden, "Reconsidering the Litigator's Absolute Privilege to Defame," *Ohio St. L. J.* 54 (1993): 985; S.M. Smith, "Absolute Privilege and California Civil Code Section 47 (2): A Need for Consistency," *Pac. L. J.* 14 (1982): 105.
10. Silberg v. Anderson, 50 Cal. 3d 205, 786 P.2d 365, 266 Cal. Rptr. 638 (1990).
11. 249 Ill. App. 3d 5, 618 N.E.2d 794 (Ill. App. 1993).
12. 2 Cal. App. 4th 88, 3 Cal. Rptr 2d 27 (1991).
13. See also Kennedy v. Cannon, 229 Md. 92, A.2d 54 (1962).
14. A tort remedy for perjury is recommended in D.W. Eagle, "Civil Remedies for Perjury: A Proposal for a Tort Action," *Ariz. L. Rev.* 19 (1977): 349.
15. D.L. Chadwick, & H.F. Krous, "Irresponsible Testimony by Medical Experts in Cases Involving the Physical Abuse and Neglect of Children," *Child Maltreatment* 2(1997): 313; quoted in Report of the Board of Trustees of the American Medical Association, Report 5-A-98.
16. In a New Jersey case, a general practitioner was convicted of perjury in falsifying medical testimony at the murder trials of certain persons known as the "Trenton Six." The basis of the conviction was the differing testimony between the first trial when all six were convicted and the second, three years later, when four of the six were acquitted. The doctor's testimony was a report of an examination made of the prisoners at the request of the state at the time when they were giving confessions. It was used by the state to show their voluntary nature. The doctor's contention was that it is practically impossible to convict a doctor of perjury. Apart from epistemological problems concerning the imperfections of the senses and the consequent relativity of all knowledge, it was argued that the doctor testified only as to medical opinions and beliefs, which, no matter how erroneous, cannot attain to him in the absence of conclusive proof that they were not actually entertained. By a 4–3 vote, the appellate court affirmed the perjury indictment; State v. Sullivan 24 N.J. 18, 130 A2d 610 (1957).

   There have been many instances of expert witnesses presenting false or fraudulent credentials. Attorneys have an obligation to investigate the credentials of expert witnesses (Model Rules of Professional Conduct Rule 3.3), but they rarely do more than look at their current position. It occurs in all arenas—business, medicine, academia, and even sports. See J.W. Fountain & E. Wong, "Notre Dame Coach Resigns After 5 Days and a Few Lies," *New York Times*, Dec. 15, 2001, p. 1.
17. 673 F.Supp. 210 (E.D. Mich. 1987).
18. Nationwide, courts that have faced the question of a witness's duty to an opposing litigant have concluded that the legal concept of duty does not extend to such bounds. Writing for the Arizona Court of Appeals, Judge Sandra Day O'Connor found that the only duty that a witness owes is to the court, rather than to an adverse party. Filling out this logic, Judge O'Connor reasoned that the witness's breach of the duty owed to the court cannot give rise to a cause of action in tort by the adverse party; Lewis v. Swenson, 126 Ariz. 562, 617 P.2d 69 (Ariz. App. 1980).
19. 673 F. Supp. at 212, citing Collins v. Walden, 613 F. Supp. 1306 (N.D. Ga. 1985).
20. 412 Mich. 1, 312 N.W.2d 585 (1981).
21. The standard for determining whether an attorney had probable cause to initiate and continue a lawsuit was articulated in Tool Research & Engineering Corp. v. Henigson, 45 Cal. App. 3d 675, 120 Cal Rptr. 291 (1975): "The attorney is not an insurer to his client's adversary that his client will win in litigation. Rather, he has a duty "to represent his client zealously [seeking] any lawful objective through legally permissible means [and presenting] for adjudication any lawful claim, issue, or defense (ABA Code of Professional Responsibility, EC 7-1, DR 7-101[A][1])."
22. 500 U.S. 478 (1991).
23. See Taylor & K.C. Johnson, *Until Proven Innocent* (New York: Thomas Dunner, 2007); reviewed in C. Allen, "Durham Bull," *Weekly Standard*, Sept. 24, 2007, p. 40.
24. See L.S. Berger, "Expert Clinical Testimony and Professional Ethics," *J. Psychiat. & Law* 7 (1979): 347.
25. Tex. Rev. Civ. Stat. Ann. Art. 5547-18.
26. In O'Rourke v. O'Rourke, 50 So.2d 832 (La. App. 1951), the plaintiff sued the medical officer who had issued a certificate of commitment without making an examination as required by law. The court held that the medical officer, by so issuing a certificate, was liable for resulting damages. Anyone who maliciously and without probable cause initiates commitment proceedings may be liable. See also

Strahan v. Fussell, 218 La. 682, 50 So.2d 805 (1951); Dauphine v. Herbert, 37 So.2d 829 (La. App. 1948); Pickles v. Anton, 49 N.D. 47, 189 N.W. 684 (1922); and Lindsay v. Woods, 27 S.W.2d 263 (Tex. Civ. App. 1930). Furthermore, a physician who makes a negligent examination as well as one who makes no examination, which causes a competent person to be committed to an institution, may be liable; Bacon v. Bacon, 76 Miss. 458, 24 So. 968 (1899); Ayres v. Russell, 50 Hun. 282, 3 N.Y.S. 338 (1888). But see Williams v. LeBar, 141 Pa. 149, 21 Atl. 525 (1891); herein was a mere error in judgment. Hospital authorities who interfere with the efforts of a committed person to obtain a writ of habeas corpus may be held liable for damages; Hoff v. State, 279 N.Y. 490, 18 N.E.2d 671 (1939).

In Maben v. Rankin, 55 Cal.2d 139, 10 Cal. Rptr. 353, 358 P.2d 681 (1961), a husband requested a psychiatrist to hospitalize his wife and provide treatment. On grounds of the patient's symptoms and the husband's story, the psychiatrist administered a sedative and admitted the wife to a sanitarium of which he was part owner. Subsequently, suing the psychiatrist and hospital, she alleged that she was not mentally ill, but had been upset only because of her husband's questionable conduct in marital matters. The court awarded her damages for false imprisonment and assault and battery.

A similar holding awarding damages is Stolwers v. Ardmore Acres Hospital, 19 Mich. App. 115, 172 N.W.2d 497 (1969), aff'd, 386 Mich. 119, 191 N.W.2d 355 (1971), where the court said that the husband's consent is irrelevant, for he cannot force medical care upon his wife. The Michigan Supreme Court in the course of its decision said: "Psychiatry is a relatively new professional discipline and, as with all disciplines, there is a great deal of controversy within the profession as to precisely what methods of treatment should be used. Psychiatrists have a great deal of power over their patients. In the case of a person confined to an institution, this power is virtually unlimited. All professions (including the legal profession) contain unscrupulous individuals who use their position to injure others. The law must provide protection against the torts committed by these individuals"; 191 N.W.2d at 363. See A. McCoid, "A Reappraisal of Liability for Unauthorized Medical Treatment," Minn. L. Rev. 41 (1957): 381; W. Kelly, "The Physician, the Patient, and the Consent," Kan. L. Rev. 8 (1960): 405.

27. 637 S.W.2d 914 (Tex. 1982).

28. 637 S.W.2d at 917.

29. Littleton v. Good Samaritan Hosp., 39 Ohio St. 3d 86, 529 N.E.2d 449 (1988). It is to be noted that the professional judgment rule applies only where the decision taken has been preceded by a "careful examination"; 529 N.E.2d at 457.

30. 529 N.E.2d at 458.

31. M. Hansen, "Body of Evidence," ABAJ, June 1995, pp. 60–67.

32. See R. Slovenko, "The Duty of Therapists to Third Parties," J. Psychiat. & Law 23 (1995): 383.

33. Montoya v. Bebensee & Smith, 761 P.2d 285 (Colo. App. 1988), noted in C.R. Barback, "Beyond the Guessed Interests of the Child: The Role of the Expert Witness in Child Custody Cases," Carrier Foundation Med. Ed. Ltr., May 1991, no. 161.

34. 776 P.2d 666 (Wash. 1989).

35. The decision is criticized in E.G. Jensen, "When 'Hired Guns' Backfire: The Witness Immunity Doctrine and the Negligent Expert Witness," UMKC L. Rev. 62 (1993): 185. See also C.H. Garcia, "Expert Witness Malpractice: A Solution to the Problem of the Negligent Expert Witness," Miss. College L. Rev. 12 (1991): 39; D. Pahl, Absolute Immunity for the Negligent Expert Witness: Bruce v. Byrne-Stevens," Willamette L. Rev. 26 (1990): 1051; D.J. DeBenedictis, "Off-Target Opinions," ABAJ (Nov. 1994): 76; T.E. Peisch & C.M. Licursi, "Suing Friendly Experts," For the Defense (March 2008): 44.

36. See 776 P.2d at 672.

37. 2000 U.S. Dist. Lexis 8525; on appeal, 248 F.3d 382(5th Cir. 2001); referred to Louisiana Supreme Court, 794 So.2d 778 (La. 2001).

38. "Expert witness malpractice causes of action are gaining momentum," reported in A.A. Moensens, C.E. Henderson & S.G. Portwood, Scientific Evidence in Civil and Criminal Cases (New York: Foundation Press, 5th ed. 2007), p. 105. "The law has been moving in the direction of holding friendly experts liable for their professional errors for the past 10 or 15 years." M. Hansen, "Experts Are Liable, Too: Client Suits Against 'Friendly Experts' Multiplying, Succeeding," ABAJ 86 (Nov. 2000): 17. See also G. McAbee, "Improper Expert Medical Testimony," J. Legal Med. 19 (1998): 257.

39. 841 S.W.2d 671 (Mo. 1992).

40. 841 S.W.2d at 677. Actually, various courts have held that the immunity extends beyond defamation suits. In Brisco v. LaHue, 460 U.S. 325 (1983), the U.S. Supreme Court on the ground of immunity barred a civil rights action by criminal defendants against police officers who had committed perjury.

41. Mattco Forge Inc. v. Arthur Young & Co., 5 Cal. App. 4th 392, 6 Cal. Rptr. 2d 781 (1992).

42. 47 Conn. Supp. 179, 781 A.2d 518 (Conn. 2000).

43. In Mangrum v. Roy, Wayne County Circuit (Michigan), No. 82-217856-NO, the plaintiff, an injured workman, sued an examining insurance company physician, the compensation insurance carrier, and the employer for the tort of intentional infliction of emotional distress. The gravamen of the case concerned two medical reports by Dr. Roy, one of the defendants, a well-known defendant's orthopedic expert. The conclusion in the first report was that the plaintiff could not return to work. Less than four months later, without any new findings or changes in his condition, opined that he could now carry out unrestricted work. On the basis of the second report, workers' compensation proceedings were stopped. The patient was awarded compensation.

44. Federal Rules of Evidence, Rule 607. Still a party may not call a witness primarily to impeach. The courts have imposed a requirement comparable to "surprise" ("good faith"). See, e.g., United States v. Gomez-Gallardo, 915 F.2d 553 (9th Cir. 1990); United States v. Hogan, 763 F.2d 697 (5th Cir. 1985); United States v. Webster, 734 F.2d 1191 (7th Cir. 1984); United States v. DeLillo, 620 F.2d 939 (2d Cir. 1980); Whithurst v. Wright, 592 F.2d 834 (5th Cir. 1979).

45. In his book, The Defense Never Rests (New York: Stein & Day, 1971), defense attorney F. Lee Bailey describes an encounter with Dr. Ames Robey in regard the trial of Albert DeSalvo. Bailey writes (p. 184): "Robey was something, all right. I asked him about the conversation we'd had on Friday, and he admitted it in substance. But he said he'd thought about it over the weekend and decided that DeSalvo had 'conned' him very badly. In view of that, he didn't think DeSalvo was insane under any test [of criminal responsibility]." Bailey and lead attorney Johnnie Cochran used prominent experts to beguile the jury in the O. J. Simpson case. The Family of Ron Goldman, His Name is Ron: Our Search for Justice (New York: Wm. Morrow, 1997).

46. 429 Pa. Super. 273, 632 A.2d 562 (1993).

47. 632 A.2d at 565–566.

48. See Federal Rules of Evidence, Rules 607–610, and counterpart in various states' rules of evidence.

49. The rules of evidence do not expressly set out bias as a way of impeachment, but it is an "established basis of impeachment"; United States vs. Abel, 569 U.S. 45 (1984).

50. Under the Federal Rules of Evidence, Rule 803(18), statements in published treatises and other similar publications may be used either as impeachment or as substantive evidence. The states vary in the permissible use. Under the Federal Rules it is not necessary to show that the expert has relied on the treatise, nor must the expert acknowledge the publication as authoritative, so long as other expert testimony establishes the authority of the work. Once the treatise has been established as reliable, the expert can be impeached in one of two ways: (1) a passage from the work can be read into evidence without questioning the expert on it, or (2) after reading a particular passage, the witness can be asked whether he agrees with it. Even if the expert disagrees, it can later be argued that he failed to recognize established authority.

51. 449 Mich. 469, 536 N.W.2d 760 (1995).

52. 203 Mich. App. 361, 512 N.W.2d 82 (1994).

53. Personal communication.

54. Board of Trustees Report 5-A-98.

55. Rule 706 of the Federal Rules of Evidence adopted in 1975 provides for the court-appointment of experts. The Advisory Committee Note accompanying the rule seems to mandate that federal judges appoint court experts more frequently than they did at common law, but that has not occurred in this case. The various states, too, have been lukewarm to the concept. While the majority of states have adopted rules similar to that of the Federal Rules of Evidence, one notable exception is Rule 706. Only a few states adopted Rule 706 verbatim, a number of states declined to adopt any version of Rule 706, while others amended the language of the rule. One state deleted subsection (c) of Rule 706 authorizing the judge to inform the jury of the expert's court appointment, and another state expressly precluded the judge from informing the jury of the witness's court appointment. In Wisconsin, the Judicial Council Committee added an explanatory note that "[r]outine utilization of the power to appoint experts is an abuse of discretion." G.P. Joseph & S.A. Saltzburg, Evidence in America: The Federal Rules in the States (Charlottesville, VA: Michie, 1987), vol. 2, p. 706.

56. See, e.g., B. Diamond, "The Fallacy of the Impartial Expert," Arch. Crim. Psychodynam. 3 (1959): 221.

57. Lavit v. Superior Court, 839 P.2d 1141 (Ariz. App. 1992).

58. Levine v. Wiss & Co. 478 A.2d 397, 400 (N.J. 1984).

59. 301 Md. 426, 483 A.2d 76 (1984).

60. 253 F.3d 967 (7th Cir. 2001).

61. 253 F.3d at 975. See also Mississippi State Board of Psychological Examiners v. Hosford, 508 So.2d 1049 (Miss. 1987) (withdrawal of license for breach of confidentiality). It has been ruled that a medical board oversteps its authority by threatening to punish physicians for participating in the carrying out of the death penalty. News report, "Execution Policy Rejected," *New York Times*, Sept. 22, 2007, p. 12; see Chapter 14 on the death penalty.
62. Personal communication.

PART II
Evidentiary Issues

5
Testimonial Privilege

At common law (*common law* is a phrase for court precedent rather than statutory law), the physician had no legal right or privilege to remain silent when called as a witness. The only two relationships given a testimonial privilege at common law were the attorney–client and husband–wife relationships. In the United States, the medical privilege was a statutory innovation originating in New York in 1828, a time when a person sedulously wanted to conceal from the community the fact that he was the victim of some "dreadful" disease that was rampant at the time. In the years following, legislatures of most other states enacted some form of medical privilege, protecting "communications" revealed by permitted examination or by word of mouth.

From the viewpoint of litigation, the medical privilege was of comparatively little importance when most of these statutes were enacted. At the turn of the 20th century, however, the development of life and accident insurance, workers' compensation, and liability of common carriers rapidly expanded the role of the medical privilege. Personal injury litigation came to represent approximately 90% of all litigated cases, and the medical privilege penetrated these cases.

As a consequence, insurance interests came into conflict with the privilege, or shield law, as otherwise known. Furthermore, strong antipathetic comment on the part of authorities in the law of evidence contributed to the privilege's unpopularity at law. Numerous exceptions were made by the courts to the privilege, to the extent that little remained of it. Surveys of decisions of appellate courts revealed that, for one reason or another, the privilege was held not to shield the physician–patient communication.[1] The Iowa Supreme Court in 1942 put it thus: "[There has been] considerable criticism of physician–patient privilege statutes in recent years, on the ground that such statutes [have] but little justification for their existence and that they [are] often prejudicial to the cause of justice by the suppression of useful truth, the disclosure of which ordinarily [can] harm no one."[2]

Litigants claiming personal injury while trying to conceal their medical history brought disrepute to the medical privilege. Charles McCormick, a leading authority in evidence, wrote in 1954: "More than a century of experience with the [medical privilege] statutes has demonstrated that the privilege in the main operates not as a shield of privacy but as the protection of fraud. Consequently the abandonment of the privilege seems the best solution."[3] Earlier, in 1938, the American Bar Association's Committee on Improvements in the Law of Evidence made a recommendation that was conciliatory in nature. It stated the following:

> The amount of truth that has been suppressed by this statutory rule must be extensive. We believe that the time has come to consider the situation. We do not here recommend the abolition of the privilege, but we do make the following recommendation: the North Carolina statute allows a wholesome flexibility. Its concluding paragraph reads: "Provided that the presiding judge of a superior court may compel such a disclosure if in his opinion the same is necessary to the proper administration of justice." This statute has needed but rare interpretation. It enables the privilege to be suspended when suppression of a fraud might otherwise be aided.[4]

The National Conference of Commissioners on Uniform State Laws, which seeks to promote uniform legislation throughout the country, voted in 1950 that the physician–patient privilege should not be recognized. However, in 1953, the conference reversed its previous action and by a close vote decided to recommend the privilege as optional. The recommendation contained so many exceptions that it would be difficult to imagine a case in which it might be applied.

The medical privilege over the years has been invoked most often in three areas, to wit: contested will cases where the testamentary capacity of the patient is under inquiry, actions for bodily injuries where the plaintiff's prior physical condition is at issue, and actions on life and accident insurance policies where misrepresentations of the insured as to state of personal health are at issue. In all of these situations, in one way or another, the privilege was circumvented by an exception or waiver.

In many jurisdictions, death of the patient terminated the privilege, so a legatee to a will in testamentary actions or a beneficiary of life insurance policy could not claim the privilege of the deceased patient (except perhaps when it may be regarded in the interest of the patient).

In suits for personal injuries, the privilege was considered waived by the patient by instituting litigation. In an oft-quoted expression, the patient cannot make the medical statute both a sword and a shield. A good-faith claimant suing for personal injuries presumably would not object to the testimony of any physician who examined or treated him, but rather would want the physician to testify. The defendant is entitled to learn whether the injury complained about predated the alleged incident. Individuals who file a lawsuit and resist the release of their medical record can forget about their case—it would be presumed that the evidence is unfavorable or it would have been produced.

In actions on life and accident insurance policies wherein the truth of the insured's representations as to his health are vital, the insurer may desire to introduce testimony of the insured's physician to show fraud on the part of the insured in making his application. The medical privilege may be circumvented quite easily by the insurer by inserting a provision in the application whereby the insured waives the right to the privilege, both for himself and his beneficiary. The same procedure is often followed in employment applications, and also for disability benefits, pensions, and compensation claims. Such a waiver by contract is generally upheld. For large life insurance policies, the insured is required to undergo a medical examination by the company's physician. As a result, most undesirable risks are eliminated and the problem of the medical privilege is diminished in importance.

Psychiatrists came to find that the medical privilege enacted in the various states was so riddled with exceptions that they sought a special psychiatrist–patient privilege. The Group for the Advancement of Psychiatry (GAP), an organization of some 200 psychiatrists, in 1960 urged enactment of legislation granting a privilege to psychiatrist-patient communication that would parallel the attorney–client privilege. It issued a 24-page report on the need of privilege to protect confidentiality in the practice of psychiatry.

Shortly thereafter, at the suggestion of Law Professor Joseph Goldstein and Dr. Jay Katz of Yale University, GAP revised its proposal, realizing that privilege by analogy would be unworkable, and it urged the enactment of a psychotherapist–patient privilege similar to that enacted in 1961 in Connecticut (Goldstein and Katz were members of the committee that prepared the Connecticut bill).[5] The Connecticut law was the model of the statute subsequently adopted by the various states and proposed for the Federal Rules of Evidence (FRE) of 1975. All 50 states have now adopted varying forms of the psychotherapist–patient privilege. Following is a typical statute:

(a) *Definitions*
  (1) A "patient" is a person who consults or is examined or interviewed by a psychotherapist.
  (2) A "psychotherapist" is

      (A) A person authorized to practice medicine in any state or nation, or rea-
          sonably believed by the patient so to be, while engaged in the diagnosis or
          treatment of a mental or emotional condition, including drug addiction.

      (B) A person licensed or certified as a psychologist under the laws of any state
          or nation, while similarly engaged.

  (3) A communication is "confidential'" if not intended to be disclosed to third persons
     other than those present to further the interest of the patient in the consultation,
     examination, or interview, or persons reasonably necessary for the transmission of
     the communication, or persons who are participating in the diagnosis and treat-
     ment under the direction of the psychotherapist, including members of the patient's
     family.

(b) *General rule of privilege.* A patient has a privilege to refuse to disclose and to prevent
    any other person from disclosing confidential communications, made for the purposes
    of diagnosis or treatment of his mental or emotional condition, including drug addic-
    tion, among himself, his psychotherapist, or persons who are participating in the diag-
    nosis or treatment under the direction of the psychotherapist, including members of
    the patient's family.

(c) *Who may claim the privilege.* The privilege may be claimed by the patient, by his guard-
    ian or conservator, or by the personal representative of a deceased patient. The person
    who was the psychotherapist may claim the privilege, but only on behalf of the patient.
    His authority to do so is presumed in the absence of evidence to the contrary.

(d) *Exceptions*

  (1) *Proceedings for hospitalization.* There is no privilege under this rule for communi-
     cations relevant to an issue in proceedings to hospitalize the patient for mental ill-
     ness, if the psychotherapist in the course of diagnosis or treatment has determined
     that the patient is in need of hospitalization.

  (2) *Examination by order of judge.* If the judge orders an examination of the mental or
     emotional condition of the patient, communications made in the course thereof are
     not privileged under this rule with respect to the particular purpose for which the
     examination is ordered unless the judge orders otherwise.

  (3) *Condition an element of claim or defense.* There is no privilege under this rule as to
     communications relevant to an issue of the mental or emotional condition of the
     patient in any proceeding in which he relies upon the condition as an element of his
     claim or defense, or after the patient's death, in any proceeding in which any party
     relies upon the condition as an element of his claim or defense.

History has a way of repeating itself. The psychotherapist–patient privilege, like the medical
privilege, is a form of zero-sum game. What it gives with one hand it takes away with the other.
Virtually nothing of relevance in litigation is shielded by the shield. In every jurisdiction, the
exceptions make it difficult to imagine a case in which the privilege applies.

First of all, as the term *testimonial privilege* would indicate, it concerns a privilege not to
provide "testimony." Of course, outside the judicial process, society has a strong interest in protecting confidentiality, but that is protected not by privilege, but possibly by a tort action for
infliction of mental distress, invasion of privacy, defamation, a breach of the fiduciary duty of
confidentiality, or a disciplinary sanction. Whether testimony may be barred in a judicial (or
administrative) proceeding as a consequence of a privilege does not control the issue of liability
for unauthorized extrajudicial disclosures. In *State v. Beatty*,[6] an impoverished mental patient
confided to her psychiatrist that she committed a robbery to pay for food for herself and a sick
friend. The psychiatrist called Crime Stoppers and provided enough information to allow the

police to obtain a search warrant that was challenged as "a gross violation of defendant's rights under the doctor–client privilege and use of that information, and its subsequent use in the search warrant, was a violation of defendant's constitutional rights." As ought to be expected, the Missouri Court of Appeals held that the testimonial privilege was not involved because the telephone call did not constitute "testimony." As generally understood, the court explained that the only prohibition dictated by a privilege statute is to bar testifying in a court proceeding. The court left for another day the question of whether the revelation of the type made by the psychiatrist was an ethical violation or whether there is a cause of action in tort law for the breach of confidentiality. That question was not before the court.

Then, too, testimonial privileges are narrowly interpreted because they work against a fair trial. Evidence is the basis of justice—the very essence of a fair trial. Having all the facts helps to make better judgments. When a privilege keeps out relevant evidence, the goal of a fair trial is less attainable. Testimonial privileges are usually the result of political lobbying. The word *privilege* stems from the Latin *privata lex*, a prerogative given to a person or to a class of persons; the word is a composite derived from the words *privus* and *lex*. Because a privilege is contrary to general law, it is strictly construed. Of course, as one might expect, the attorney–client privilege fares best of all. The determination of whether an individual or communication in a particular case falls under an enacted privilege depends on its scope, as interpreted by the court. The traditional judicial preference is for the "truth" (i.e., determining historical facts accurately) rather than the protection of confidentiality of a given relationship, but other goals may also be claimed: protecting the sanctity of the individual (e.g., the Fifth Amendment) or providing disincentives for governmental abuses (e.g., Fourth Amendment exclusionary rule). The sporting theory of justice may call for the exclusion of probative as well as nonprobative or prejudicial evidence.

It is to be noted, however, that when an attorney refers a client to a physician for examination, the attorney–client privilege protects a report made by the physician to the attorney. This is especially important in jurisdictions where there is no medical privilege. In cases of referral for examination, the physician acts as the agent of the attorney. In this situation, the physician is serving as an examining physician, rather than as a treating physician, and is performing the examination on behalf of the attorney in the preparation of a case. The physician, as an agent of the attorney, comes under the umbrella of the attorney–client privilege.[7] The attorney will call upon the physician to testify if the physician's opinion is favorable to the attorney's theory of the case, but if the opinion is unfavorable, the attorney will discharge him and seek another expert or will drop the case.[8]

The essence of any testimonial privilege is that it may be waived or terminated by the person who enjoys it. The confidential communication is protected from disclosure at the option of the person who owns the privilege (or one acting on his behalf). The medical or psychotherapy privilege belongs to the patient, not to the physician, just as the attorney–client privilege belongs to the client. The privilege is for the benefit of the patient or client. Thus, patients have the option to require either silence or testimony from their physician (under ordinary process of summoning witnesses) on any communication made on the basis of the professional relationship that existed between them.

Because the privilege is the patient's, the physician or psychiatrist can be compelled to testify when the patient or ex-patient so desires. The patient is given legal control over his destiny, irrespective of other factors. The patient may believe, quite unrealistically, that testimony by his therapist may aid his legal position. A patient's waiver of the privilege may conceivably be a self-destructive technique; it may be an expression of hostility toward the therapist; or it may be an attempted repetition of an early power struggle. Even an attempt to clarify to a patient why it would be inadvisable to call upon the therapist to testify can be markedly prejudicial to effective therapy, especially when it comes at an inappropriate stage in treatment.

It has been argued that privilege in the psychiatrist–patient relationship should belong to the psychiatrist as well as, or rather than to the patient. When an individual waives a privilege such as the attorney–client privilege, or the privilege against self-incrimination, the decision is made with awareness of what will be disclosed. However, in psychotherapy, it may be detrimental for patients to see, for example, the report of projective tests, which they have taken. When patients waive the psychotherapy privilege, they do not know what they are waiving. It may be harmful to reveal to patients that they have been labeled schizophrenic (whatever that might mean). Should the law allow an individual to make an irrational or irresponsible decision? Should the privilege be waivable? Privacy of the unconscious or of one's fantasy life is a requisite of man's dignity; no one, it is said, can remain dignified when the contents of his unconscious are disclosed.

Dr. Joseph Lifschutz of California, among others, has argued for a right of privacy separate from that of any individual patient, a right derived from what he sees as a duty not to a particular patient alone, but to all patients. He argued that the disclosure of one patient's confidential communications causes damage to all the therapist's other patients.[9] That argument is echoed in the book *The New Informants* by Christopher Bollas and David Sundelson.[10] It is to be noted that a priest must keep absolutely secret anything told to him in a confession, even when the penitent (confessor) requests that the priest divulge what was communicated. The Episcopal Church's *Reconciliation* states: "The secrecy of a confession is morally absolute for the confessor, and must under no circumstances be broken."[11] Be that as it may, the professional's urging of confidentiality allegedly on behalf of patients is often a facade to serve self-interest. The privilege is designed to protect the privacy of the patient, not that of the therapist; it is not to serve as a fig leaf to cover up incompetency or wrongdoing.[12]

Tort Cases

As in the case of the medical privilege, the most common form of waiver of the psychotherapist–patient privilege is the one when the patient injects his condition in tort litigation, as when his condition is an element of claim or defense. In this vein, no-fault automobile insurance legislation expressly and completely eliminates the statutory physician–patient privilege.

California's psychotherapist–patient privilege, a copy of the Connecticut statute and a model for the proposed Rule 504 of the Federal Rules of Evidence, was tested shortly after its enactment in 1965 in the much-publicized case involving Dr. Joseph Lifschutz.[13] The case was featured in national news weeklies and was reported at numerous meetings of psychiatric societies and in psychiatric and psychoanalytic bulletins and newsletters. The Northern California Psychiatric Society made a nationwide appeal to psychiatrists for contributions to cover legal expenses. The American Psychoanalytic Association and the National Association for Mental Health filed *amicus curiae* briefs. Although great effort was exerted on behalf of privilege, the case illustrates the irrelevancy of privilege law (as well as the irrelevancy of much psychiatric testimony at trial).

Joseph Housek, a high school teacher, brought a damage suit against John Arabian, a student, alleging an assault that caused "physical injuries, pain, suffering, and severe mental and emotional distress." During a deposition taken by defense counsel, Housek stated that he had received psychiatric treatment 10 years earlier from Dr. Lifschutz over a six-month period. The defendant then sought Housek's psychiatric records from Dr. Lifschutz. He refused to produce any of his records, assuming there were any, and also declined to disclose whether or not Housek had consulted him or had been his patient. Thereupon defendant Arabian sought a court order to compel Dr. Lifschutz to answer questions on deposition and to produce the subpoenaed records. The court determined that the plaintiff had put his mental and emotional condition in issue by instituting the pending litigation, so privilege was waived. To no avail, Dr. Lifschutz argued a right of privacy separate from that of any individual patient, a right derived from what he saw as a duty not to Housek alone but to all his patients. He argued that compelling him to testify unconstitutionally impairs the practice of his profession. The court was unpersuaded. It said: "[W]e cannot blind ourselves to the fact that the practice of psychotherapy has grown, indeed flourished, in an environment of a nonabsolute privilege."[14]

Because the privilege is intended as a shield and not a sword, it is considered waived by the patient when he makes a legal issue of his physical or mental condition. Thus, when plaintiff Housek claimed that he had suffered "emotional distress" as a result of the injuries he had suffered, the privileged status of his communications with his psychiatrist was waived, said the trial court. However, on appeal, the California Supreme Court doubted that "the 10-year-old therapeutic treatment sought to be discovered from Dr. Lifschutz would be sufficiently relevant to a typical claim of 'mental distress' to bring it within the exception."

Thus, the real test in protecting patient confidentiality is one of relevancy or materiality (which arises regarding all evidence in every trial), so it must be asked: What are the material issues, and what is relevant or competent to establish them? In other words, does the item of evidence tend to prove that precise contention or fact, which is sought to be proved? In every case where the testimony or records of a physician or psychotherapist have been required by a court, it was because the evidence was deemed relevant or material to an issue in the case. As a consequence, in the last analysis, the confidentiality of a physician–patient or psychotherapist–patient communication is protected from disclosure in a courtroom only by a showing that the communication could have no relevance or materiality to the issues in the case.

A motion to quash a subpoena is in order when other evidence more relevant and material is available or would be less intrusive to obtain. Such a procedure might even protect a patient from having to state in discovery processes whether he ever saw a psychiatrist. Quite often, mental health professionals and others automatically give up records simply because a subpoena has arrived in the mail, without realizing that a subpoena is not a court order, or they believe that it would be futile to challenge a subpoena, but the attorney who is representing the patient can be called upon to seek a quashing of the subpoena.

It is often contended that a forensic examiner can ascertain whether an injury predated the alleged complaint just as well as the patient's therapist, if not more accurately, but that may not always be the case. In his book *The New Psychiatry*,[15] Dr. Jack Gorman of Columbia University gives a vivid example from his practice of a case that justifies discovery of records:

> Once I received a request from a patient's attorney to produce my office notes about [a patient]. She was apparently suing a driver following an automobile accident in which she claimed she had injured her back. The problem was that when I first saw the patient she had told me that she had suffered from back trouble for many years preceding the car accident. I had written that down. My records would obviously reveal that the patient was lying about the car accident; in fact, it hadn't hurt her back at all. When I told her what was in my records she was forced to amend her lawsuit.[16]

Privilege is also waived in a wrongful death action in which a party relies on the deceased's condition as an element of his claim or defense. In this type of action, the patient is not a party litigant, but rather the subject of the litigation. The defendant is entitled to discover evidence, including the testimony of a treating psychiatrist, to establish that the patient died, not as a result of any wrongful act on the part of the defendant but, on the contrary, as a suicide.[17]

It is held that the patient–litigant exception applies whenever either party, plaintiff or defendant, relies on the condition of a patient as part of that party's claim or defense, even when the patient does not personally place the condition at issue. Such a case is one in Texas, a personal injury action brought against a parent by a stepdaughter for allegedly sexually assaulting her, and also against a counselor for negligence in counseling.[18] The Texas Court of Appeals held that the counselor was not entitled to exercise the psychotherapist–patient privilege to protect treatment records. The court's order to turn over the mental health records was based on the exception to privilege for disclosure of records when "relevant to an issue of the physical, mental, or emotional condition of a patient in any proceeding in which any party relies upon the condition as a part of the party's claim or defense." The court also rejected the defendant's argument that his right against self-incrimination precluded discovery of the records (on the ground that he would not lose any privilege against self-incrimination because the disclosure would not be voluntary.)[19]

What about privilege in lawsuits where the patient is not a litigant, but where a third-party sues the therapist? Unlike when a patient sues a therapist, a third party suing a therapist on account of harm inflicted by the patient faces obstacles in obtaining information as to what occurred in therapy. There may have been a duty to warn or protect and in that event the dangerous patient exception to the therapist–patient privilege would come into play. The privilege is not applicable when the therapist has reasonable cause to believe that the patient was dangerous. A duty to report a patient who poses a danger to others, whether or not a report is made, may undercut any privilege, obliging the therapist to testify or provide information, as in the trial of the Menendez brothers.[20]

Certainly, a therapist's duty to third parties would have little meaning if third-party plaintiffs were not able to procure the information needed to vindicate their claims. In the usual case when a third party (family members) sues a therapist such as in the case of "revival of memory of childhood sexual abuse," the patient has retracted the allegation and joins the parents in a lawsuit against the therapist, or when the patient sues her parents, the parents implead the therapist. In these situations, by filing a lawsuit, the patient waives the privilege. In any event, privilege can be overcome by joining the patient along with the therapist as a party defendant.[21]

In a variation of the theme in which the record of a patient may be relevant to a resolution of a lawsuit, yet is not a party to the litigation, are cases where third parties file a lawsuit against a pharmaceutical company claiming that its product had a disinhibiting effect on the patient and resulted in injury or death to third parties. In a much-publicized case, Joseph Wesbecker at the Standard Gravure printing plant in Louisville killed or wounded 20 people with an AK-47 assault rifle, then turned the gun on himself. He had been on disability leave from Standard Gravure for a year, reeling from setbacks in his personal life and on the job. Suffering from severe depression, he was given Prozac, the popular antidepressant. The survivors and victims' families sued its maker, Eli Lily and Company. Both sides to the litigation had an interest in disclosing Wesbecker's psychiatric history, so no objection to disclosure of records was made. In the defense of Prozac, it was argued, "Joseph Wesbecker's attack on Standard Gravure on September 14, 1989, was not the act of a man suddenly turned mad by Prozac … . It was the final chapter in a very complex life, filled with hostility, fueled by job stress. It grew out of a life twisted by insidious mental illness. It was generated out of a lifetime of estrangements and isolation, and hostile withdrawals from spouses, parents, children, friends, co-workers, and bosses." In any event, Wesbecker's family brought a wrongful death action against his psychiatrist, Dr. Lee Coleman, and, as a consequence, privilege was waived.[22]

The question has arisen as to a waiver of the privilege shielding the health records of the plaintiff's family in a lawsuit involving a condition that is arguably genetic. Because the privilege belongs to the patient and is waivable only by the patient, as by filing a lawsuit, the privilege is not waived as to the records of other members of the family. Upholding the privilege as to other members of the plaintiff's family may make it impossible for the defendant to explore the cause of the condition. The issue thus becomes under what circumstances, if any, the defendant may gain access to the medical records of the plaintiff's family members in order to show genetic causation.[23]

Criminal Cases

Criminal cases, as other cases, may involve a treating or examining psychiatrist. The shield law is applicable, at best, only to a treating psychiatrist and not to an examining one. In the examining situation, the relationship is likely to be one entered into at arm's length (the person examined is called an examinee or evaluee, not a patient). In criminal cases, however, even in the treating situation, there is in many jurisdictions no medical or psychotherapist privilege whatsoever.[24] In all states, by statute or case law, the medical privilege or the psychotherapist–patient privilege is inoperative when a defendant raises an insanity defense or a mental disability defense.[25] By and large, the courts hold that raising the insanity defense does not, by itself, waive the attorney–client privilege for retained, nontestifying experts.[26]

In the case of a defendant who asserts a defense of insanity (or other diminished capacity defense), the prevailing law is that he cannot claim possible self-incrimination with respect to psychiatric evidence, be it by a treating or examining psychiatrist. If the defendant does not cooperate with the court's or prosecutor's psychiatrist, he is deemed to have waived his insanity defense, or is denied the right to present expert testimony on his behalf. By pleading and offering evidence of insanity, the accused puts his mental state in issue and thus waives any psychotherapist–patient privilege; his medical or psychiatric history is open to the prosecution, as occurred, for example, in the trial of John Hinckley Jr., the would-be assassin of President Reagan.[27] The very nature of an insanity defense is premised on a broad inquiry into every aspect of the defendant's life. As a matter of practice, the fact of treatment is often brought up by defense counsel in plea bargaining to demonstrate an interest in rehabilitation.

The Illinois psychiatrist–patient privilege expressly states that it does not apply in criminal proceedings in which the mental condition of the defendant is introduced by him as an element of defense.[28] Indiana and Wisconsin have similar statutory provisions.[29] Nebraska states that "[t]here is no privilege ... in any judicial proceedings ... regarding injuries to children, incompetents, or disabled persons or in any criminal prosecution involving injury to any such person or the willful failure to report any such injuries."[30] New Jersey's privilege does not cover cases of driving while under the influence of alcohol.[31] And, as a general rule, the privilege is inapplicable when the "services of the therapist were sought, obtained, or used to enable or aid anyone to commit or plan a crime or fraud or to escape detection or apprehension after the commission of a crime or fraud.[32]

The privilege, moreover, does not cover communications involving fraud in receiving Social Security benefits.[33] Various states exclude the privilege in any judicial proceeding involving narcotics or to communications made to procure narcotics unlawfully.[34] And therapists have a duty to reveal information about the contemplation of a crime or harmful act.[35]

The various rules that have been developed to restrict the role of an examining psychiatrist in criminal cases are rooted in constitutional principles against self-incrimination and coerced confession, not the shield law. It is well established that a psychiatric examination does not violate the constitutional rights of the accused. As one court put it, "Even a cat can look at a queen."[36] However, the psychiatrist may testify only as to his evaluation of the defendant (although in reaching this evaluation inferences are made from the facts of the crime or other crimes). Under the law of the various states, he may not reveal admissions made to him by the defendant in the instant proceeding or in another proceeding.[37]

In the case of a defendant in a criminal case who seeks discovery regarding the alleged victim, there comes into play the right under the Constitution to summon witnesses and to obtain evidence to establish innocence. The U.S. Supreme Court has recognized on a number of occasions that a state's interests as expressed in its evidentiary laws are secondary to the constitutional considerations of fully confronting witnesses who testify against the defendant and of fairness to a defendant seeking to defend against criminal charges.[38] It is prevailing law that a criminal defendant is entitled to review the psychiatric records of a prosecuting witness, but only after a judge has determined there is good cause for disclosure and that the material will in some way be relevant to the defense.[39]

This principle applies when an accused seeks evidence from a victim treatment or rape crisis center. A woman who claims to have been raped, for example, and identifies the defendant as the rapist, may confess in therapy that she had, in fact, consented to the sexual activity. This behavior ought to be regarded as criminal as crimes committed by a patient in the course of therapy. The psychiatrist's response should give precedential concern to the protection of society. The victim treatment center or rape crisis center may or may not have evidence that would be important in a criminal proceeding.[40] Alan Dershowitz posed the legal and ethical issues in his novel *The Advocate's Devil*.[41]

In an Alaska case, a young woman whose records in a rape counseling center were sought by defense protested strenuously, "[The defense] thinks there's something big in the records, but there's not. That's the funny thing. There's stuff in there I haven't even told my parents. There's stuff in there I don't want to review. There's stuff I just wanted to get off my chest and never think about again … [T]here written down [are] all my humiliating moments, my happy moments, and my sad moments. They might as well strip me naked and make me walk in front of everybody naked. I'll tell you, it would be easier."[42]

In dealing with any privilege, the courts have recognized that before a judge can determine whether communications are to be protected, the judge should conduct an *in camera* inspection in order to determine whether the requirements of the privilege are met.[43] Accordingly, when a psychotherapist–patient or sexual assault counselor–victim privilege is asserted, the trial judge under proper circumstances should conduct an *in camera* inspection. The court must determine whether there are statements of the victim that may relate to important issues, such as identity of the assailant or consent. Due process and confrontation does not require disclosure of all the victim's statements, only those that are relevant to the preparation and presentation of the defense.[44]

A refusal by the alleged victim to release her psychological records for *in camera* review will result in the exclusion of her testimony at trial. An *in camera* review is not granted based solely on a defendant's request. There must be a threshold showing by the defendant that the records may reasonably be expected to provide information material to the defense. A general assertion that inspection of the records is needed for a possible attack on the victim's credibility is insufficient to meet this threshold showing.[45]

To avoid involvement in the criminal justice system, counseling centers over the years have announced that they do not keep records, and make no evaluation or diagnosis. Failure to keep records, however, has generally lost its immunizing value. The fact that most psychiatrists or other therapists give reports to third parties for various purposes tends to cast doubt on not keeping records. In the current malpractice climate, the best defenses are records that detail the clinical factors that determine the judgment of the therapist to hospitalize or not to hospitalize in situations where hospitalization might be considered, or not to report behavior patterns that might be questioned in the future, where an infinite number of ambivalent situations requiring hairline judgments might be made. And, of course, third-party payers nowadays require the keeping of records and without them, therapists will not be compensated for their services. Certainly, one must be circumspect about what is included in a record because the current vogue of easily getting search warrants is a threat to every record.

Military

Until recently, no privilege whatever was recognized in military law for the physician–patient or psychotherapist–patient relationship, regardless of whether the physician or therapist is military or civilian. The basis for not extending privilege to the relationship is that the harm done to the relationship by disclosure is considered of less seriousness than the harm done by nondisclosure to the securing of military order and justice. Then, in late 1999, President Clinton signed an executive order extending a psychotherapist–patient privilege to court-martial proceedings. The definition of a psychotherapist in the amended Military Code of Justice encompasses psychiatrists, clinical psychologists, clinical social workers, and assistants to a psychotherapist (assistants are people who the psychotherapist assigns to provide professional service to a patient).

This addition to the Uniform Code of Military Justice, known as Rule 513, does not extend the shield to any aspects of military life other than court-martials. In disciplinary or administrative proceedings that do not come to trial, such as those involving dismissal of service members because they are gay, psychiatrists and other mental health professionals may still be subject to orders to provide information on a soldier's sexuality. The privilege, moreover, does not hold when the patient is dead, even if his family wants the confidentiality maintained. Military personnel also lose the privilege when any communication with their therapist contains evidence of spouse or child abuse or when federal, state, or military law specifically exempts such abuse allegations from confidentiality protection. Additional exclusions allowed under the new rule occur in cases in which a therapist believes that a patient's mental status makes him a danger to self or others, when the patient communicates intent to commit "fraud or crime," and when the information is "necessary to ensure the safety and security of military personnel, military dependents, military property, classified information, or the accomplishment of a military mission." The specific interpretation of the limits of these exclusions is left to the discretion of military judges who can thus choose to view them broadly or narrowly on a case-by-case basis. In sum and substance, the exceptions viscerate the privilege.

Proceedings to Hospitalize

In proceedings to involuntarily hospitalize a patient, there is no privilege for communications relevant to the issue when the doctor has determined, during the course of diagnosis or treatment, that the patient is in need of such care. The Advisory Committee to the Federal Rules of Evidence commented, "The interests of both patient and public call for a departure from confidentiality in commitment proceedings. Since disclosure is authorized only when the psychotherapist determines that hospitalization is needed, control over disclosure is placed largely in the hands of a person in whom the patient has already manifested confidence. Hence damage to the relationship is unlikely."[46] And as one court put it, "The evidence is not used against the individual, but to aid the court in evaluating alternate treatment plans. Involuntary commitment proceedings are not penal in nature, but humanitarian."[47]

The hospitalization exception does not mention guardianship but the justification for the exception would seem to apply as well to guardianship. Under the law, there are provisions for appointment of a guardian of one's person (e.g., with authority over health care decisions) and a guardian of one's estate (e.g., with authority over the making of contracts to sell one's property). In some jurisdictions, a guardian might be appointed for the specific purpose of consent to psychiatric hospitalization.[48] In a number of states, guardianship and civil commitment of a "gravely disabled person" take place through a conservatorship proceeding (a guardian of one's estate is often called a "conservator" or "committee").[49] In most cases where a psychiatrist is involved in giving testimony in a guardianship proceeding, it is as an examining rather than as a treating psychiatrist.

The intent of the hospitalization exception in the typical psychotherapist–patient privilege is for the treating psychiatrist to play a key role in commitment proceedings (and presumably in guardianship proceedings). In nearly all jurisdictions, as a matter of law, no warning as to privilege against self-incrimination or right to silence need be given prior to examination or treatment.[50] Michigan is apparently an exception. Michigan's Mental Health Code (applicable to the public sector and agencies or clinics under contract with the state to provide services) sets out a requirement of notice. It states that privileged communications shall be disclosed "[w]hen the privileged communication is relevant to a matter under consideration in a proceeding to determine the legal competence of the patient or the patient's need for a guardian, but only if the patient was informed that any communications made could be used in such a proceeding."[51]

A patient opposed to hospitalization, however, may be angered by the breach of confidentiality. The issue of whether disclosures by a therapist to a court-appointed examiner are reasonably necessary to protect the interests of the patient or others is one for the jury, said the Michigan Court of Appeals; hence, the therapist is not entitled to summary disposition.[52] This ruling came out of a case where the patient's estranged wife (later divorced) petitioned for the patient's commitment. The patient and his wife quarreled over finances and he contended that she wanted to "put him away." The psychiatrist who was appointed to undertake an examination consulted with the treating psychiatrist. In a lawsuit called unprecedented, the patient sued the treating psychiatrist for breach of confidentiality. The trial court held that the defendant was entitled to judgment on motion for summary disposition, but the Michigan Court of Appeals held that the issue of whether the disclosures were reasonably necessary to protect the interests of the patient or others was one for the jury because the facts of the case were such that reasonable minds could differ. The appellate court rendered that decision though the psychiatrist was in private practice and, hence, not governed by the Michigan Mental Health Code, which provides that a patient must be informed that communication may be used in a hospitalization (or guardianship) proceeding.[53] In Australia, among other countries, the treating psychiatrist must have the consent of the patient as a requisite for discussions with an examiner.

Child Custody

In a dispute between parents over the custody of a child, the "best interest of the child" sets the standard for decision making. It opens the door to a wide range of evidence pertaining not only to the fitness of the parents, but also to the environment in which the child will be raised. As a general principle, the "best interest" standard overrides any psychotherapist–patient privilege, thereby allowing access to therapy records and to compelling the testimony of the therapist. The statutory law mandates that the court consider, among other factors, the mental and physical health of the parties.[54]

In contentious proceedings, attorneys search for data that will support their case. The case law reveals that the privilege provides some, but uncertain, protection of confidentiality. The majority of courts say, under the mandate of the statutory law, or otherwise, that the privilege yields automatically in child custody or related matters.[55] Other courts order disclosure only when health is in issue or when the circumstances indicate abuse or neglect. According to these decisions, the question is whether there is a compelling need to have past psychiatric records to evaluate the capacity of the parent with respect to current parenting abilities.[56] Various legislation provides that there is no privilege concerning matters of adoption, adult abuse, child abuse, child neglect, or other matters pertaining to the welfare of children or any dependent person, or from seeking collaboration or consultation with professional colleagues or administrative supervisors on behalf of the client.[57]

"In every custody proceeding and in every proceeding for the modification of a custody decree," as one court put it, "the mental and physical health of not only the parents but of the child is of great concern and importance to the court." The court went on to say, "Whenever custody of infants is in dispute, the parties seeking custodial authority subject themselves to extensive and acute investigation of all factors relevant to the permanent and, hopefully, proper award of custody. Of major importance is the mental and physical health of all of the parties and whether the child is in an environment likely to endanger his physical, mental, moral or emotional health." As another court put it, "The paramount consideration in a child custody matter is the child's best interest … . A court cannot determine the best interests of the child without considering whether [the parent] is physically, financially, or mentally able to care for the child."[58]

Quite often, the testimony, as well as the records of the treating therapist, are demanded. To quote an attorney, who has been involved in considerable child custody litigation, in an address to a law group: "The more I know about a parent the better. I would depose the treating doctor. The record standing alone is not sufficient."[59] Moreover, as a matter of routine, court-appointed or lawyer-appointed evaluators ask for the psychiatric records of the parents or child, and they usually get them. An evaluator would be remiss in not obtaining these records, for on cross-examination, the evaluator would likely be asked about matters revealed there, and legitimately so. Typical questions might include: "Didn't you know that she (or he) was diagnosed as schizophrenic?" "Didn't you know that she (or he) threatened the life of the child?" Even if the expert may not need the records to carry out an evaluation, the expert will want them to defuse a cross-examination, and also to confirm the evaluation, thereby enhancing the probative value of the report. This is all the more true where a party resists production of the records. When a party refuses a request, suspicion arises that the party is hiding something, and the records gain even more importance. Moreover, refusing to disclose psychiatric records is usually an expensive and time-consuming exercise in futility as the trial judge will likely order disclosure, but disclosure without court order may result in liability for breach of confidentiality.

There may be circumstances when the confidentiality of reports will be protected, particularly if it can be shown that the "best interest of the child" is advanced by confidentiality rather than disclosure. In some cases, disclosure of statements of the parents or the child could harm the parent–child relationship. In the process of evaluation, children may make statements that may result in a vendetta against the child. The evaluator is in a dilemma: How to inform the court and at the same time protect the child? A youngster says, "I hate my father." The data, put in a report in raw form, will expose the child negatively. In this type of situation, the trial judge might very well shield these communications. Disclosure may then be limited to communications relevant to fitness, or to the interaction and interrelationship of the child with the parent.[60]

It is argued that the "best interest of the child" is enhanced by confidentiality of parental psychotherapy records, by encouraging parents to obtain treatment that might otherwise not be sought. Discouraging people from consulting a psychotherapist, out of fear that confidences will be used against them in later court appearances, does not inure to the welfare of the child. The protection of confidentiality, with its attendant encouragement to seek help, may better serve the child. As one Florida Court of Appeal observed, successful therapy can be dependent upon the psychiatrist's ability to assure confidentiality.[61]

Records of treatment of a parent or child occurring years ago might be protected on relevancy grounds. A Michigan Court of Appeals said:

> [W]e do not find relevant to a party's present condition the testimony of a physician who has not treated the party for years … . Moreover, the … court was able, with the [party's]

participation, to gather information with regard to her mental condition … . We also reject as meritless defendant's argument that by virtue of submitting to a court-appointed psychological examination and introduction of the psychologist's testimony, plaintiff waived her medical privilege.[62]

Privilege claims aside, judges must decide the relevancy of all proffered evidence and must also consider whether there is less intrusive, but equally probative, evidence available. In any kind of case, when the psychotherapist–patient privilege is raised, the guideline on the admissibility of evidence is relevancy, not privilege.

Group Therapy

With the increasing number of psychotherapy groups, questions have frequently arisen (mainly in nonlegal circles) regarding privileged communication in that type of therapy. While there has been some litigation involving confidentiality of joint marital counseling and family therapy, there is little involving group therapy, notwithstanding its wide use. Is, then, the prevailing concern warranted?

Various medical and psychiatric societies have sought to organize therapy or support groups for members who are facing malpractice lawsuits. During this time, while these individuals may have the support of an attorney, they feel under stress and isolated during the years awaiting the outcome of the litigation. In general, lawyers advise their clients not to talk to anyone about the litigation and this increases their sense of isolation. Many hesitate to enter a therapy or support group, it is said, out of concerns about confidentiality.

More commonly than medical or psychiatric societies, bar associations in various states have sponsored therapy groups for their members who have a problem with alcoholism. While their competency to practice law may be questionable, they usually are not facing a malpractice suit as are the members of medical and psychiatric societies who have been sued and enter a therapy group. Anyway, "if criminals can be rehabilitated, then why not lawyers?" said a Michigan lawyer about a proposal to permanently disbar lawyers for misconduct.[63]

Nationwide, group therapists express different views about the concern of group members concerning confidentiality. In an article in the *American Journal of Psychiatry*,[64] Dr. Howard Roback and colleagues surveyed 51 therapists who led psychotherapy for physicians recovering from substance abuse and they reported that concern about confidentiality was a significant factor in the group members' willingness to share secrets. Of those group therapists surveyed, 49% rated physician group members as exhibiting a moderate amount or a great deal of concern over potential confidentiality infractions. Moreover, they report, 27% of group therapists who treat impaired physicians have been subpoenaed at some time in the past to testify about physician members. Some states require physicians to report impairment of other physicians. They suggest that group therapy would provide a safer milieu for patients to share highly personal information if the members themselves could be held liable for violating confidentiality. They recommend legislation making group members liable for violating confidentiality.

To survey the concern, if any, of group members about confidentiality, I interviewed several group therapists and members of a group. In my survey, I discovered that therapists are far more concerned about confidentiality than are members of the group. Some group therapists say that a person involved in litigation should not be in group therapy for his or her own protection. I am told by group therapists, novice and veteran alike, that while they have many times discussed the problem of confidentiality with colleagues and students, they know of no actual instance where there has been any serious problem in connection with lack of confidentiality. For example, Dr. Joseph J. Geller, who had been doing group therapy for many years, said:

Over all the years, with many people becoming privy to a wealth of personal details about others, there seems to have been very little harmful use of the material. This is true of my own practice as well as the experiences of others. Each of us, having this rather uneventful experience, assumed it was unusual, but without comparing notes with others, we learned that it is fairly generally true.[65]

The executive director of the National Commission on Confidentiality of Health Records advised that no incidents of group therapy breaches of confidentiality have been reported to the Commission.[66] In any event, as a shield against a demand for disclosure in legal proceedings, the enactment of a legal privilege that would excuse testimony from a group member or therapist has often been suggested. The American Group Psychotherapy Association, desiring greater protection for group therapy, recommended the enactment of a specific privilege to cover group therapy. The history of privilege, however, reveals that it has not been very much of a shield. When push has come to shove, the privilege had ended up not shielding very much, if anything. It is like the warranty where the bold print giveth and the fine print taketh away.

A rule of privilege law, which is of particular significance in group therapy is that a communication loses any privileged status it may have had if it takes place in the presence of a "third party." The privileges are formulated with the dyadic relationship in mind (attorney–client, physician–patient, accountant–client), and the presence of a third party is said to "pollute" confidentiality. The law equates disclosure to a third person with a general publication to the world. The rationale is, "The world knows about it, why not the court?" Will group members (and the insurance company) be considered a third party, polluting privilege, or will they be considered as agents taking part in the therapy process.[67] It may be noted that following adoption of the medical privilege in the early 19th century, a number of courts ruled that a nurse does not come under its umbrella and, because of this, later statutes on the medical privilege specifically include nurses and other attendants within the scope of the privilege (for whatever the privilege may be worth).

The prominent legal commentator Charles McCormick discussed the issue of whether the presence of third parties renders a statement to a physician nonprivileged, and he argued that the court should analyze the problem in terms of whether the third persons were necessary and customary participants in the consultation or treatment and whether the communications were confidential for the purpose of aiding in diagnosis and treatment.[68] In a Minnesota case,[69] where the defendant was charged with criminal sexual conduct, the prosecutor sought the records of group psychotherapy sessions in which the defendant participated. The Minnesota Supreme Court applied McCormick's approach and upheld privilege:

> Under [McCormick's] approach, we conclude that the medical privilege must be construed to encompass statements made in group psychotherapy. The participants in group psychotherapy sessions are not casual third persons who are strangers to the psychiatrist/psychologist/nurse–patient relationship. Rather, every participant has such a relationship with the attending professional, and, in the group therapy setting, the participants actually become part of the diagnostic and therapeutic process for co-participants.[70]

Likewise, in a California case, an appellate court held that disclosing information in the presence of members of a therapy group does not defeat the privilege.[71] The court said the following:

> Communications made by patients to persons who are present to further the interests of the patient comes within the privilege. "Group therapy" is designed to provide comfort and revelation to the patient who shares similar experiences and/or difficulties with other like persons within the group. The presence of each person is for the benefit of the

others, including the witness/patient, and is designed to facilitate the patient's treatment. Communications such as these, when made in confidence, should not operate to destroy the privilege.[72]

In a Connecticut case,[73] the Connecticut Court of Appeals remanded for a determination of whether a murder suspect's alcohol treatment facility records were protected by the psychiatrist–patient privilege. In this case, Michael Skakel, the scion of Greenwich wealth, completed a required alcohol treatment program at Elan, a licensed treatment facility, after he was convicted of driving while intoxicated. Pursuant to a murder investigation, the state moved to compel the person who owned the facility to testify and produce records regarding Skakel's treatment. Skakel applied for an injunction on the grounds that the information was privileged under the psychiatrist–patient privilege. The trial denied the motion because Skakel failed to (1) establish that Elan was a "mental health facility" within the meaning of the statute and (2) demonstrate that the communications and records related to the diagnosis or treatment of a "medical condition" within the meaning of the statute. The appellate court said that interpreting "mental condition" in the statute to include alcohol-related disorders would effectuate the legislature's objective by providing individuals who have such disorders with an incentive to seek treatment and make a full disclosure to a psychiatrist. Because the trial court did not determine whether any of the communications and records sought by the state were related "to diagnosis or treatment" of the plaintiff's alcohol-related condition, the appeals court remanded.[74]

By and large, it appears that group therapists are more concerned than members of the group about confidentiality issues and testimonial privilege. In or out of court, group members assume confidentiality, though increasingly the assumption is being made explicit, sometimes in a contractual agreement. Be that as it may, therapists fear that one celebrated case, should it arise, would create a great deal of anxiety about group therapy. In fact though, the likelihood of assault by subpoena is slight, but should it come, there are circumstances that tilt toward the maintenance of confidentiality.

Identity of Patient

Whether the identity of a patient is discoverable is problematical. In its formulation, a testimonial privilege covers only the content of communications and not the fact of a relationship. For a person to seek to invoke the privilege, there must be an initial showing, by affidavit or otherwise, that the person is one covered by the privilege. It is necessary to set out the existence of a therapist–patient relationship—the privilege does not cover communications between social guests.

While sometimes acknowledging that the identity of a psychiatric patient must be protected to maintain the purpose of the privilege, many courts nonetheless adhere to the formula and hold that the identity of patients, the dates on which they were treated, and the length of treatment on each date do not fall within the scope of the privilege.[75] Other courts, however, say that when disclosure of the fact of consultation also of necessity discloses the nature of the condition for which the patient sought treatment, then the fact of disclosure also becomes privileged.[76]

Given the context, disclosure of even a name may reveal much about the person. A story tells about a young man who goes to confession: "Forgive me, Father," he murmurs, "for I have sinned. I have sinned the cardinal sin with one of the female members of the congregation." "Who was it?" asks the priest. "Oh, I cannot betray that confidence," the young man says, but the priest is persistent. "Was it, by any chance, the lovely Mrs. Callahan?" The young man says no. "Was it, then, the vivacious Miss O'Malley?" He says no again. "Well, was it Michael's beautiful daughter?" He still says no. On leaving the church, he meets a friend outside. "Did the priest give you absolution?" "No," says the sinner. "But he did give me three good leads."

"Clearly," it is argued by commentators, "the idea of confidential communication must encompass the identity of the patient as well."[77] Illinois expressly includes the fact of psychotherapeutic treatment within the privilege.[78] Federal law prohibits the use or disclosure of "patient identifying information" concerning anyone diagnosed or treated for substance abuse at facilities receiving federal funds.[79] The principles of ethics of the profession declare that "the identification of a person as a patient must be protected with extreme care."[80]

In a discovery proceeding, individuals are asked whether they have ever been in treatment and, if so, where, when, and by whom. In a *Tarasoff*-type case, should the therapist have given a warning about the patient? In an assault case, the fact of psychiatric care might suggest that the patient was the aggressor in the fray. However, there is no justification in asking the question unless there is some basis in fact that would raise a legitimate question concerning the individual's condition.

In a malpractice action, a plaintiff may attempt to discover the names and addresses and, sometimes, the case histories of other people who have been treated by the defendant's physician. The attorney for the complainant wants the opportunity to talk to other patients of the physician in order to establish a pattern that would give credence to the complaint.[81] For example, a claim that the physician sexually exploited the plaintiff is more credible when supported by testimony of similar incidents with other patients. As a rule, discovery is disallowed on the ground of privilege or relevancy.[82]

In an article in *Trial*,[83] Linda Jorgenson, Pamela Sutherland, and Steven Bisbing cite research suggesting that "up to 80% of therapists who have had sexual contact with one patient, had sexual contact with other patients" (a debatable statistic), and they recommend the admission of evidence of these other acts to prove a case against an alleged abusing therapist. But how is evidence of these other acts to be obtained? Newspaper publicity of a lawsuit against a therapist for undue familiarity may bring forth other patients who have been violated, as occurred in *Roy v. Hartogs*.[84] But in lieu of that, is an attorney to be allowed to discover the names of all the therapist's patients, and then is the attorney to be allowed to contact the patients and ask them whether they have been sexually involved with their therapist? What will these patients think of the invasion of their privacy? What will they think of their therapist? What will it do to the therapeutic relationship with their therapist?

Demands for patient identification abound. A physician or a hospital who is a defendant in a malpractice action urges that a discovery order for information about patients not privy to the lawsuit be set aside on the ground that it violates the physician–patient privilege. The physician or hospital may claim the privilege on behalf of a patient not privy to the action. In a California case,[85] the plaintiff sought to recover damages from a physician and hospital for injuries allegedly arising out of various tests performed on him. The plaintiff sought disclosure of the names and addresses of other patients to whom the defendants had given the same (angiographic) tests. The purpose of this information was to enable investigators to seek out and interrogate these patients and attempt to persuade them to discuss their experiences regarding the tests. The California Court of Appeals barred discovery. It concluded that disclosure of identity of patients receiving such tests would necessarily be revealing confidential information.[86]

In a Michigan case, *Dorris v. Detroit Osteopathic Hosp.*,[87] the plaintiff, Deborah Dorris, claimed that she was given the medication Compazine intravenously even though she tried to refuse that medication and asked for another. The medication allegedly triggered an abrupt drop in her blood pressure. The doctor who treated her denied giving her the medication against her wishes, but she insisted a patient who shared her room heard the dispute and she sought a court order requiring the hospital to disclose the patient's name. Reluctantly, the Michigan Court of Appeals declined to order disclosure of the patient's name, feeling bound by the precedent of a 32-year-old ruling of the Michigan Supreme Court in *Schechet v. Kesten*,[88] where it was held that the privilege "prohibits the physician from disclosing, in the course of any action wherein his patient or patients are not involved and do not consent, even the names of such noninvolved patients." The Michigan Supreme Court in *Schechet* held that the identity of noninvolved patients was privileged. However, a few years before *Dorris*, in *Porter v. Michigan Osteopathic Hosp. Assn.*,[89] the Michigan Court of Appeals, over a strong dissent, allowed discovery, in a case where the plaintiff was allegedly raped in a hospital, of the names and addresses and the room assignments of any and all suspected assailants and also the name of a patient who may or may not have overheard a conversation between the plaintiff and medical personnel. Distinguishing *Porter*, the Michigan Court of Appeals in *Dorris* said that *Porter* presented stronger policy reasons than *Dorris* for disclosure. The Michigan Supreme Court affirmed *Dorris* (that had disallowed discovery) and it overruled *Porter* (that had allowed discovery).[90] The Michigan Legislature also amended the psychiatrist–patient privilege by including an identity privilege.

In a case featured in the American Psychiatric Association's *Psychiatric News*, someone scratched graffiti on a bathroom wall in a building housing the offices of Maryland psychiatrist David Irwin. The police looked upon it as a hate crime because of its messages and ordered the psychiatrist to turn over the names, addresses, phone numbers, and appointment history of patients he had seen the day of the crime. The police suspected, with no supporting evidence, that one of his patients might have been responsible for the crime. The psychiatrist refused to comply with the police order and soon was served with a subpoena ordering him to appear in court to explain why he was not complying. None of the other professionals with offices on the same floor, including a dentist and two chiropractors, were ordered to turn over patient lists. The court ruled that the data the police wanted were not protected by psychiatrist–patient privilege or by the state's medical record confidentiality law and ordered the psychiatrist to provide the police with the information they sought. He appealed, and the appeals court affirmed that psychiatrist–patient privilege does not apply, but disagreed with the lower court's order that the state confidential law mandates that patient records are subject to release in a situation such as this. That law states that law enforcement and prosecution agencies must have written procedures in place describing how they will protect the confidentiality of the medical records they obtain during a criminal investigation. The appeals court said because the record of the case provided no indication that such written procedures do exist, the lower court, on account of this technicality, erred in ordering the psychiatrist to turn over the patient data to the police.[91]

Parents in Mississippi brought a negligence action against a hospital that mistakenly placed their infant with an unidentified female patient, who breast-fed the infant. Subsequently, the infant's health deteriorated. In response to the parents' request for discovery of the patient's identity, the hospital asserted the patient's privilege of confidentiality. Reasoning that the patient was a potential witness to the alleged negligence, the Mississippi Supreme Court ordered disclosure of her identity. The court said that the privilege "must give way where it conflicts with the sensible administration of the law and policy."[92]

Death of Patient

It is not uncommon for therapists to receive requests for disclosure of confidential information after the death of a patient. Such requests may be by relatives contesting the patient's will, police or life insurance companies investigating the cause of death, or bereaved family members attempting to deal with their own guilt or emotional distress.[93] The therapist is bound, both ethically and legally, to maintain confidentiality to the same extent after death of the patient as before, unless the law otherwise authorizes disclosure. The great weight of authority is that the right to waive the privilege extends to the patient's legal representatives after the patient's death.[94] (The writing of articles or books about a deceased patient occurs in an extrajudicial context and, therefore, raises issues of confidentiality, not privilege.)

In will contest cases, where the testamentary capacity of the testator is often under inquiry, there may be an attempt to overthrow a will through proof of the mental capacity of the testator at the time of the making of the will.[95] As a general rule, the courts say that those who stand in the place of the patient (the owner of the privilege) may waive the privilege. This is generally held to include the heirs of the deceased as well as the executor or administrator of the estate. The reason given is that the heir or personal representative will be as concerned with the preservation of the decedent's reputation and estate as was the decedent.

The majority of courts hold that a person having the right of waiver may exercise it as either a proponent or contestant of the will. The purpose of contesting the will is to determine whether the purported testament is, in fact, that of the decedent, or whether it is void as a result of the decedent's mental incapacity at the time of its making. Thus, in a Minnesota case, the court decided that the beneficiary of an insurance policy, the husband of the deceased, could waive the privilege, and implied that any personal representative or heir claiming an interest would be allowed to do the same.[96] A New York statute limits the right of waiver of the deceased patient's representative to those communications that are not confidential and do not tend to disgrace the memory of the decedent. In a case that generated considerable critical comment in the law reviews, the physician was not allowed to answer questions concerning the effect of arteriosclerosis on the individual's mental capacity in writing a will.[97] The heir's waiver of the privilege permitted the doctor to testify only as to matters a layman could notice and describe, namely, that the patient had arteriosclerosis. The physician could not testify, however, as to information derived by reason of treating the patient.

There is, however, no restriction in most other states in a waiver provision excluding confidential communications. A few courts suggest that disclosures that would tend to disgrace the decedent's memory should be barred. The Connecticut statute on the psychiatrist–patient privilege provides that when a deceased patient's mental condition is introduced by any party claiming or defending through or as a beneficiary of the patient, there is no privilege if the judge finds "that it is more important to the interests of justice that the communication be disclosed than that the relationship between patient and psychiatrist be protected."[98]

The Self-Defense Exception

Any professional who is bound by confidentiality has the right of "self-defense." The self-defense exception is justified on the well-established theory that a patient or client impliedly "waives" the privilege by making allegations against the professional. As the Advisory Committee to the Federal Rules of Evidence puts it: "The exception is required by considerations of fairness and policy when questions arise out of dealings between attorney and client, as in cases of controversy over attorney's fees, claims of inadequacy of representation, or charges of professional misconduct." John Wigmore in his classic treatise on evidence likewise stated, "When the client alleges a breach of duty to him by the attorney, the privilege is waived as to all communications relevant to that issue."[99] This applies to other professionals as well as attorneys; hence, a therapist may disclose privileged information to defend against malpractice action.[100]

For waiver, it is not necessary for the client or patient to bring formal charges or proceedings against the professional. In the attorney–client context, the self-defense exception arises most frequently in a convicted defendant's posttrial assertions that put in issue the legitimacy of advice provided by the attorney, the effectiveness of the attorney's representation, or the attorney's competence.

Thus, as one court said, "It is well established that if a client assails his attorney's conduct of the case, or if a patient attacks his physician's treatment, the privilege as to confidential communications is waived, since the attorney or physician has a right to defend himself under the circumstances."[101] And in another case, the court said, "While the rule with respect to privileged communication between attorney and client should be zealously guarded, yet this privilege may be destroyed by the acts of the client in attacking the attorney on a charge of dereliction of duty.[102]

James Earl Ray, the assassin of Rev. Martin Luther King, Jr., claimed that he was "coerced" by his attorney, Percy Foreman, to enter a plea of guilty so as to avoid a trial that might have implicated high-level accomplices. In response, Foreman said that he never recommended that Ray plead guilty to the murder of King, but advised Ray that "there is a little more than a 99% chance of your receiving a death penalty" if the case went to trial. Foreman displayed a letter he wrote to Ray. Foreman also disclosed that interviews with Ray convinced him that Ray alone assassinated King in the hope of becoming a white hero.[103]

The media, in the early 1990s, carried numerous articles describing the alleged misconduct of Harvard psychiatrist Margaret Bean-Bayog, whose patient, Paul Lozano, a medical student at Harvard, had committed suicide after being treated by her. These accounts were based on 3,000 pages of documents filed in court by the lawyer for the deceased patient's family. They included allegations that the psychiatrist had fallen in love with her patient, had seduced him into a sexual relationship, and had regressed him to a stage where he believed she was his mother. Lozano killed himself about a year after Bean-Bayog stopped treating him.

The patient's family settled out of court for $1 million, but with the stipulation that the settlement contain no admission of liability on the part of the psychiatrist. Bean-Bayog also resigned her license rather than face a televised hearing before the Massachusetts Board of Registration in Medicine, which alleged that she provided substandard care causing harm to her patient. Then came a report from the Committee on Therapy of the Group for the Advancement of Psychiatry (GAP) that said:

> An immediate consequence that emerges from the Bean-Bayog case is that because a practitioner must adhere to the rules of confidentiality he or she cannot respond, without risk of a lawsuit, against charges of a patient or patient's family, regardless of how unfounded those charges may be. If a celebrity, such as Michael Jackson or Woody Allen, is accused of misconduct, he or she is free to call a press conference and openly refute the charges, revealing any information to strengthen his or her defense. This is not the case for physicians or other mental health therapists, who are required to keep the details of their patients' treatment confidential.[104]

In a press interview, Bean-Bayog stated, "It is important for a psychiatric audience to understand that if anything like this ever happened to them, they will not be able to say anything because of patient–therapist confidentiality." "As the law now stands," the GAP committee said, "any accused therapist must bear all such accusations in silence."

Not so. While the privilege of confidentiality belongs to the patient (or the representatives of the patient in the event of the death of the patient), it is waived when the patient charges the practitioner with misconduct or malpractice.

Federal Law on Privilege

What about psychotherapist–patient testimonial privilege in federal courts? The Federal Rules of Evidence, when adopted in 1975, omitted a medical privilege, given the numerous exceptions that had been made to it. Its Advisory Committee, however, recommended a psychotherapist–patient privilege, modeled on the Connecticut law, but the proposal, along with several others, evoked considerable criticism. Two committees of the American Bar Association recommended to the ABA House of Delegates "the complete abolition of any and all privilege in the physician–patient area including the proposed 'psychotherapist–patient privilege.'" The Committee on the Judiciary of the House of Representatives, after extensive hearings, recommended and the House approved the scrapping of all the proposed rules on privileges and left federal law of privileges unchanged, to wit, that the federal courts are to apply the state's privilege law in actions founded upon a state-created right or defense, while in other civil cases and in criminal cases, according to Rule 501 of the Federal Rules of Evidence, the principles of the common law, as interpreted by the federal courts in "the light of reason and experience," would be applied. In subsequent years, the federal courts in the "the light of reason and experience" adopted only an attorney–client privilege and a marital privilege, though by legislation all 50 states and the District of Columbia adopted some form of psychotherapist privilege. For a long time, privileges were said to arise only by statute, not common law, but Rule 501 provides that the law of privileges in the federal courts shall be determined by principles of federal common law, as developed in light of "reason and experience."

After the adoption of Rule 501, the U.S. Second, Sixth, and Seventh Circuit Courts of Appeals have held in recent years that "reason and experience" compel the recognition of the psychotherapist–patient privilege in both civil and criminal cases. In contrast, the Fifth, Ninth, and Eleventh Circuits rejected the privilege. Given the conflict among the circuits, the U.S. Supreme Court granted *certiorari* in *Jaffee v. Redmond*.[105] In this civil rights case, coming out of the Seventh Circuit, surviving family members of a man who was shot and killed by a police officer sought the therapy records of the officer. Dr. Joseph Lifschutz, who was involved earlier in seeking to protect testimonial privilege, filed an *amicus curiae* brief.

Mary Lu Redmond, a police officer in an Illinois town, fatally shot Ricky Allen after responding to a report of a disturbance at an apartment complex. She said she shot Allen because he was holding a butcher knife and was about to stab another man, but Allen's mother and other relatives alleged that he was unarmed. Redmond had undergone counseling with a licensed clinical social worker after the shooting, and Allen's relatives sought to have communications between Redmond and the social worker divulged. Both Redmond and the social worker refused, and the trial judge told jurors they could presume the information would be unfavorable to both Redmond and the town. The Seventh Circuit ordered a new trial. It upheld privilege under Rule 501 because "key to successful treatment lies in the ability of patients to communicate freely without fear of public disclosure."

The Seventh Circuit said that the privilege was not absolute and should be determined by balancing the interests protected by shielding the evidence sought with those advanced by disclosure. In this case, the court found in favor of applying the privilege, noting the strong interest in encouraging officers who are frequently forced to experience traumatic events by the nature of their work to seek qualified professional help. At the same time, the court noted that there were many witnesses to the shooting, and the plaintiffs' need for the officer's personal, innermost thoughts about the shooting were cumulative at best, compared with the substantial nature of the officer's privacy interest. So, once again, privilege or no privilege, the outcome depended essentially on relevancy or materiality.

In oral argument before the U.S. Supreme Court, these issues were raised:

1. Do the Federal Rules of Civil Procedure provide trial judges with adequate tools to protect privacy interests involved in confidential communications with a psychotherapist without creation of new evidentiary psychotherapist–patient privilege under the Federal Rules of Evidence?
2. Should any privilege for psychotherapist–patient communications be extended to social workers, rather than being limited to psychiatrists and clinical psychologists?
3. Should a psychotherapist–patient privilege be recognized, and, if so, what would be the scope of the privilege?

In the course of oral argument, Justice Scalia asked: "If somebody comes up to me and, let's say, my nephew comes up to me and says, 'You know, Unc, I want to tell you something in strictest confidence,' and I say, 'Yes, you tell me that; I promise you I won't tell this to anybody.' Is that enough that I've undertaken a duty of confidentiality to justify the creation of a privilege?" And Justice Breyer asked, "Why in logic or policy distinguish between physicians who treat physical problems and psychotherapists? Is there any reason in logic or policy; is there any reason, other than what the courts have held? I'm not interested, for this question, what courts have held in the past. I'm interested in whether there is a reason in logic or policy for drawing the line that I just referred to."

In its decision the Supreme Court declared the privilege to be absolute, or so it said, concluding that anything else would be worthless. "Making the promise of confidentiality contingent upon a trial judge's later evaluation of the relative importance of the patient's interest in privacy and the evidentiary need for disclosure would eviscerate the effectiveness of the privilege," Justice Stevens wrote for the majority. The decision went farther than the appellate decision that it affirmed. The Seventh Circuit had created not an absolute privilege, but a qualified one, to be balanced in appropriate cases by the "evidentiary need for disclosure."[106]

Although the ruling applies generally to federal litigation, the Court found the law enforcement context of the case to be particularly persuasive. "The entire community may suffer if police officers are not able to receive effective counseling and treatment after traumatic incidents," Justice Stevens said, "either because trained officers leave the profession prematurely or because those in need of treatment remain on the job." Two law enforcement organizations, the International Union of Police Associations and the National Association of Police Organizations, joined numerous organizations of mental health professionals in urging the Court to adopt the privilege. Given that all of the states and several circuits had adopted the privilege, it was justified in federal law, Justice Stevens wrote, in "the light of reason and experience."

Under the ambit of the privilege, the Supreme Court included social workers who provide counseling. The Court noted that when Americans turn to psychotherapy, it is often provided by social workers who generally are less expensive than psychiatrists or psychologists. "Their clients often include the poor and those of modest means who could not afford the assistance of a psychiatrist or psychologist," Justice Stevens wrote.[107]

Justice Scalia wrote one of his fiery dissents, suggesting that people would be better advised to seek advice from their mothers than from psychiatrists, yet there is no mother–child privilege. Justice Scalia wrote:

> When is it, one must wonder, that the psychotherapist came to play such an indispensable role in the maintenance of the citizenry's mental health? For most of history, men and women have worked out their difficulties by talking to, *inter alios*, parents, siblings, best friends and bartenders—none of whom was awarded a privilege against testifying in court. Ask the average citizen: Would your mental health be more significantly impaired by preventing you from seeing a psychotherapist, or by preventing you from getting advice from your mom? I have little doubt what the answer would be. Yet there is no mother–child privilege.[108]

Justice Scalia's suggestion that people would be better advised to seek advice from their mothers rather than from psychiatrists prompted a comment in a letter to the *New York Times*: "Apparently he has never heard the old story of the mother who boasted about the devotion of her son: 'Not only did he buy me a condo, a Cadillac and a mink coat, but he also pays a psychiatrist $250 for a visit every week and all he talks about is me.'"[109]

Justice Scalia in his dissent argued that the privilege would interfere with the truth-finding function of the courts and cause the courts "to become themselves the instruments of wrong." He wrote:

Even where it is certain, that absence of the psychotherapist privilege will inhibit disclosure of the information, it is not clear to me that that is an unacceptable state of affairs. Let us assume the very worst in the circumstances of the present case: That to be trustful about what was troubling her, the police officer who sought counseling would have to confess that she shot without reason, and wounded an innocent man. If (again to assume the worst) such an act constituted the crime of negligent wounding under Illinois law, the officer would, of course, have the absolute right not to admit that she shot without reason in criminal court. But, I see no reason why she should be enabled *both* not to admit it in criminal court (as a good citizen should) *and* to get the benefits of psychotherapy by admitting it to a therapist who cannot tell anyone else. And even less reason why she should be enabled to *deny* her guilt in the criminal trial—or in a civil trial for negligence—while yet obtaining the benefits of psychotherapy by confessing fault to a social worker who cannot testify. It seems to me entirely fair to say that if she wishes the benefits of telling the truth she must also accept the adverse consequences. To be sure, in most cases the statements to the psychotherapist will be only marginally relevant, and one of the purposes of the privilege (though not one relied upon by the Court) may be simply to spare patients needless intrusion upon their privacy, and to spare psychotherapists needless expenditure of their time in deposition and trial. But, surely this can be achieved by means short of excluding even evidence that is of the most direct and conclusive effect.[110]

What about Common Sense?

An individual who shoots and kill another, as in *Jaffee,* may feel guilty about it whether or not it was done in lawful self-defense or defense of others. Expressing such feelings in the course of therapy, however, may appear as a confession of wrongdoing when it is used in a legal proceeding. But, absolute confidentiality is not acceptable to common sense, as illustrated by a Michigan case involving the murder of Dr. Deborah Iverson, an ophthalmologist.

In this case, as in all cases, trust meshed with common sense—not absolute confidentiality—has to be the measure of confidentiality. Every Thursday morning for several years, Dr. Iverson would drive to see her psychiatrist, Dr. Lionel Finkelstein, and would park in an adjoining area. One Thursday morning, she disappeared after leaving his office and was found strangled a distance away the next day in the backseat of her car. As the media reported, law-enforcement officials questioned Dr. Finkelstein for possible clues. Was the patient threatened? Did she fear someone? Apparently unsatisfied with their interview, the law-enforcement officials obtained a search warrant and seized the patient's file. It will be recalled that privilege is no bar to a search warrant.

Confidentiality cannot be turned into a holy grail without concern for good judgment in these matters. From the file on Dr. Iverson, the law-enforcement officials learned that she was having problems with hospital co-workers and also "troubles or conflicts" with some relatives. Using that information, detectives focused much of their probe on relatives and co-workers, but it shed no light on the killing. Assuredly, the patient or the patient's family would want law enforcement to be informed about any fear that the patient may have had of an attack.[111] It turned out that Dr. Iverson was killed by a young couple who stole her car.

Exceptions to the Federal Privilege

In a footnote to the majority opinion in *Jaffee,* Justice Stevens, while calling the privilege absolute, wrote, "Although it would be premature to speculate about most future developments in the federal psychotherapist privilege, we do not doubt that there are situations in which the privilege must give way, for example, if a serious threat of harm to the patient or to others can be averted only by means of a disclosure by the therapist." Justice Stevens also said, "Because this is the first case in which we have recognized a psychotherapist privilege, it is neither necessary nor feasible to delineate its full contours in a way that would govern all conceivable future questions in this area." The court did not base its decision on some notion of privacy grounded in the Constitution; rather, the decision was an interpretation of the Federal Rules of Evidence that apply in federal cases.[112]

In the wake of *Jaffee*, no time was lost in the setting out of exceptions. Does the privilege cover unlicensed therapists? In *United States v. Schwensow*,[113] the defendant claimed the psychotherapist privilege recognized in *Jaffee* protected statements made to Alcoholics Anonymous volunteers. The government argued the volunteers were not licensed counselors nor was the relationship justifying confidentiality present. The district court noted that the Supreme Court failed to designate who was considered a "psychotherapist" for purposes of the privilege. It then stated that lower courts would determine such details on a case-by-case basis. Ultimately, the district court held the two volunteers were not "psychotherapists."[114] In *United States v. Lowe*,[115] the district court stated, "*Jaffee* does not control a determination of whether the federal privilege extends to communications with a rape crisis center employee or volunteer who is not a licensed social worker or psychotherapist." The court concluded that the policies of *Jaffee* call for some form of the psychotherapist privilege to be applied to communications with a rape crisis counselor.[116]

The First Circuit in 1999 held that the nascent psychotherapist–patient federal privilege encompasses a crime-fraud exemption similar to that of the established attorney–client privilege.[117] The decision arose out of subpoenas issued to two psychiatrists in the course of a grand jury investigation. It was alleged that the accused trumped up an array of disabilities, which he communicated to selected healthcare providers, who in turn provided the information to insurance carriers that had underwritten credit disability policies, thus fraudulently inducing payments. As with the attorney–client privilege, the exception applies even when the psychiatrist is an unknowing pawn of the patient.

Inevitably other exceptions will follow (and have followed), as in the case of the state-adopted privilege.[118] As we have noted, when push comes to shove, the principle of relevancy or materiality rather than privilege provides the protection of confidentiality. And, as we would emphasize, because these are elastic terms given to interpretation, the therapist should withhold information until the patient consents or the court orders disclosure (and, of course, a subpoena is not a court order). The courts tend to find communications in therapy irrelevant, immaterial, or prejudicial, and do not call for their production.

In any event, psychotherapists have been enthused by the news of the Supreme Court's decision in *Jaffee*; at least it did not deflate the myth in the public mind and in the mind of therapists that the privilege is a solid shield.[119] Given the extensive publicity to decisions of the Supreme Court, a decision against privilege would have punctured the myth of privilege, though in practice, privilege or no privilege, the outcome is usually the same.[120]

Endnotes

1. See United States *ex rel.* Edney v. Smith, 425 F. Supp. 1038 (E.D. N.Y. 1976); C. DeWitt, *Privileged Communications Between Physician and Patient* (Springfield, IL: Thomas, 1958).
2. Boyles v. Cora, 232 Iowa 822, 6 N.W. 2d 401, 414 (1942).
3. C. McCormick, *Handbook of the Law of Evidence* (St. Paul, MN: West, 1954), p. 224.
4. American Law Institute, *Model Code of Evidence*, Rules 220–223 (1942).
5. J. Goldstein & J. Katz, "Psychiatrist–Patient Privilege: The GAP Proposal and the Connecticut Statute," *Conn. B. J.* 36 (1962): 175.
6. 770 S.W.2d 387 (Mo. 1989).

7. It is to be noted that an attorney may, but is not obliged to, report a client who poses a danger, unlike a therapist who is obliged to report under the *Tarasoff* doctrine. A psychiatrist examining a litigant at the request of an attorney would fall under the attorney–client privilege and, thus, would not be obliged to report under *Tarasoff*. See United States v. Glass, 133 F.3d 1356 (10th Cir. 1998); Antrade v. Superior Court of Los Angeles County, 54 Cal. Rptr. 2d 504 (Cal. App. 1996); see S. Saltzburg, "Privileges and Professionals: Lawyers and Psychiatrists," *Va. L. Rev.* 66 (1980): 597; Comment, "Function Overlap Between the Lawyer and Other Professionals: Its Implications for the Privileged Communication Doctrine," *Yale L. J.* 71 (1962): 1266. It has occasionally been held, however, that the interests of public safety may outweigh the attorney–client privilege calling for divulgence of the intention of a client to commit crimes in the future. Smith v. Jones, Vancouver Reg. C8876491 (Dec. 18, 1997), discussed in R.J. O'Shaughnessy, G.D. Glancy, & J.M. Bradford, "Canadian Landmark Case, Smith v. Jones, Supreme Court of Canada: Confidentiality and Privilege Suffer Another Blow," *J. Am. Acad. Psychiat. & Law* 27 (1999): 614.

8. In United States v. Talley, 790 F.2d 1468 (9th Cir. 1986), the court held that the government should not have been allowed to call as a rebuttal witness a psychiatrist, appointed for the defendant's benefit, but who was not called as a witness by the defendant. In White v. State, 1999 W.L. 124310 (Okla. Crim. App.), the prosecutor called as a witness a psychiatrist appointed by the trial court to aid the defense in presenting an insanity defense. The defense had elected not to call the psychiatrist as a witness in its behalf because, in reporting to the court, the psychiatrist had apparently found the defendant not to have been insane at the time of the commission of the crime. The prosecution summoned the psychiatrist, the defense expert, to give testimony to rebut the claim of insanity. The Oklahoma Court of Criminal Appeals ruled that the attorney–client privilege protected the findings of the psychiatrist from disclosure to or use by the prosecution. The defense's raising the issue of insanity was not considered a waiver of the protection of the privilege. See T.G. Gutheil & R.I. Simon, "Attorneys' Pressures on the Expert Witness: Early Warning Signs of Endangered Honesty, Objectivity, and Fair Compensation," *J. Am. Acad. Psychiat. & Law* 27 (1999): 546.

9. Matter of Lifschutz, 2 Cal.3d 415, 85 Cal. Rptr. 829, 467 P.2d 557 (1970). As pointed out in the case, a large segment of the psychiatric profession concurs in Dr. Lifschutz's strongly held belief that an absolute privilege of confidentiality is essential to the effective practice of psychotherapy; cf. Annotation, 20 A.L.R.3d 1109, 1112. An oft-cited study found in a survey of a group of lay people that "93% of those surveyed 'would have sought help for serious emotional problems' without the privilege and 74% 'did not know whether there was a privilege statute or guessed incorrectly that there was no privilege statute.'" D. Shuman & M. Weiner, "The Privilege Study: An Empirical Examination of the Psychotherapist–Patient Privilege," *No. Car. L. Rev.* 60 (1982): 893; expanded version, *The Psychotherapist–Patient Privilege* (Springfield, IL: Thomas, 1987).

10. Northvale, NJ: Jason Aronson, 1995; reviewed in D.J. Kevles, "The Suspect on the Couch," *New York Times Book Review*, Dec. 31, 1995, p. 9.

11. *Reconciliation*, p. 446.

12. In the course of investigating a psychiatrist for fraudulent billing of his patients' insurance companies, a grand jury may subpoena his records identifying his patients' names, the period of treatment, and their billings. The psychiatrist may not successfully assert privilege to avoid compliance. *In re* Zuniga, 714 F.2d 632 (6th Cir. 1983).

13. Matter of Lifschutz, supra note 9.

14. 2 Cal.3d at 426.

15. New York: St. Martin's Press, 1996.

16. P. 353.

17. Annot., 25 A.L.R.3d 1401.

18. In this case, a mother alleged that a counselor was negligent in his diagnosis of the stepfather and in representing to her that his condition was no threat to their daughter. The mother claimed that, during their marriage, the stepfather sexually assaulted the daughter. The mother, on behalf of the daughter, a minor, brought suit against the stepfather for assault and against the counselor for negligence in diagnosis. The court noted that the condition of the stepfather would necessarily have to be determined in order to decide if the counselor was negligent. Easter v. McDonald, 903 S.W.2d 887 (Tex. App. 1995).

19. The court noted that Texas Rule of Evidence Rule 510 provides for exceptions to nondisclosure, including those communications and records "relevant to an issue of the physical, mental, or emotional condition of a patient in any proceeding in which any party relies upon the condition as a part of the party's claim or defense." The court noted that the exception "represents a significant departure from the historical scope of the patient–litigant exception." The court noted, "The exception now terminates

the confidentiality privilege whenever any party relies on the condition of a patient as part of that party's claim or defense, even when the patient does not personally place the condition at issue or is not a party." 903 S.W.2d at 890. However, in Reaves v. Bergsrud, 982 P.2d 497 (N.M. App. 1999), the New Mexico Court of Appeals in a malpractice action declined to allow the plaintiff to discover the physician's history of mental health treatment on the basis of the psychotherapist–patient privilege. Actually, the information would be irrelevant as it was not alleged that the physician's mental health was the cause of the plaintiff's postoperative problems. See the discussion in Chapter 31 on informed consent. See also Jaffee v. Redmond, 518 U.S. 1 (1996), discussed hereinafter.

20. People v. Hopkins, 119 Cal. Rptr. 61 (Cal. App. 1975). See also San Diego Trolley v. Superior Court of San Diego Cty, 105 Cal. Rptr.2d 476 (Calif. App. 2001); United States v. Glass, 133 F. 3d 1356 (10th Cir. 1998). In contrast, in a 2–1 ruling, in United States v. Hayes, 227 F.3d 578 (6th Cir. 2000), the U.S. Court of Appeals, Sixth Circuit, ruled that issuing a *Tarasoff* warning does not abrogate the testimonial privilege. The court stated that such an exception would negatively affect the "atmosphere of confidence and trust" in the psychotherapist–patient relationship. Second, the court stated that although allowing a psychotherapist to testify against his patient in a criminal prosecution about statements made for treatment purposes may serve a public end, this end does not justify the means. And third, the court stated that the absence of the state's adoption of a dangerous patient exception supported rejecting such an exception. In writing the opinion for the majority, Judge James Ryan reasoned that issuing a warning would not disrupt therapy as would testifying against the patient. In *Tarasoff*, however, the patient quit therapy when his therapist reported him to the police, then he killed Tatiana Tarasoff. Judge Ryan commented, "There is no question that the issue addressed in the *Hayes* case is difficult and that the resolution the court reached is subject to disagreement among reasonable people. We did what we thought was right and we recognized that the rule laid down in the case would not appeal to everyone." Personal communication (Dec. 19, 2000). Law Professor Vincent Johnson writes: "Students may be interested to learn that not all patients would be upset by learning that their therapists intend to divulge their threats to the intended victims. Indeed, [I have] a friend who works at the Counseling Service of Addison County. That doctor (who, needless to say, was greatly distressed by the decision in *Peck*) routinely tells any patient who makes a threat that the doctor intends to relay the threat to the intended victim. The doctor says that most patients are pleased to learn that the threat will be communicated because it gives them a sense of power." V.R. Johnson & A. Gunn, *Teaching Torts/A Teacher's Guide* (Durham, NC: Carolina Academic Press, 1995), p. 167.

   A decision in New York also ruled that issuing a warning does not result in having to testify at trial. State of New York v. Bierenbaum, No. 8295/99, discussed in "*Tarasoff* Warning Does Not Waive Psychotherapy Privilege, Judge Rules," *Psychiatric News*, Oct. 20, 2000, p. 2. In this case, Robert Bierenbaum, a plastic surgeon, discussed his serious marital problems with a psychiatrist who was alarmed by threats of violence he made against his wife. He carried out his *Tarasoff* duty by alerting Bierenbaum's wife, an action to which Bierenbaum assented. Two years later, the wife disappeared; her body was never found. Some 15 years later, Bierenbaum was convicted of killing his wife. He was suspected of dismembering her and dumping her into the ocean. P. Rogers et al., "Judgment Day," *People*, Nov. 6, 2000, p. 15.

21. See also Easter v. McDonald, 903 S.W.2d 887 (Tex. App. 1995), discussed supra notes 18–19. In Johnson v. Rogers Memorial Hosp., 238 Wis.2d 227, 616 N.W.2d 903 (2000), the Wisconsin Supreme Court stated that lack of therapy records is not sufficient to dismiss a third-party case. In other cases, if the parents did not have access to therapy records, the case did not go forward.

22. Fentress v. Shea Communications, Jefferson Circuit Court, Louisville, KY, case no. 90-CI-06033; see P.R. Breggin, *Brain-Disabling Treatments in Psychiatry: Drugs, Electroshock, and the Role of the FDA* (New York: Springer, 1997); id., *Medication Madness* (New York: St. Martin's Press, 2008); J. Cornwall, *The Power to Harm* (New York: Viking, 1996); M.L. Harris, "Problems with Prozac: Defective Product Responsible for Criminal Behavior?" *J. Contemp. Legal Issues* 10 (1999): 359; "Colorado Psychiatrists Fight Propaganda About Psychiatric Meds," *Psychiatric News*, Feb. 4, 2000, p. 8. See also M.J. Grinfeld, "Litigation Raises New Questions About Safety and Effectiveness of Depression Treatment," *Psychiatric Times*, Aug. 2001, p. 18.

23. In Palay v. Superior Court, 22 Cal. Rptr.2d 839 (Cal. App. 1993), the California Court of Appeals held that a mother's records relating to her prenatal care were discoverable and not protected by physician–patient privilege in a medical malpractice case she brought on behalf of her 16-month-old son. In Jones v. Superior Court, 119 Cal. App.3d 534, 174 Cal. Rptr. 148 (1981), an adult plaintiff instituted a product liability action for injuries allegedly sustained due to her mother's ingestion of a drug while pregnant with the plaintiff. The defendants sought to secure records of the mother's ingestion of the

drug and of her physical condition during her pregnancy. The court held that although the mother may still have had the right to assert the privilege to protect that information after the plaintiff instituted the action, she waived the right by her subsequent deposition disclosures, which revealed the circumstances of her drug ingestion and the related communications with her physician. See L.O. Gostin, "Genetic Privacy," *J. Law, Med. & Ethics* 23 (1995): 320; L.B. Wright, "Genetic Causation and the Physician–Patient Privilege in Michigan: Shield or Sword?" *Wayne L. Rev.* 36 (1989): 189.

In Baker v. Oakwood Hosp. Corp., 239 Mich. App. 461, 608 N.W.2d 833 (2000), the plaintiff, a research nurse coordinator for a doctor, was allegedly fired after confronting the doctor about reportedly illegal and unethical conduct on his part. She subsequently filed suit against the doctor and hospital, alleging, among other claims, wrongful discharge. During discovery, the plaintiff requested patient records related to the research she worked on during her employment. Because none of the patients whose records were sought by the plaintiff had waived the physician–patient privilege, the Michigan Court of Appeals concluded that the records were protected from disclosure, even though patients' names would be redacted from the records.

24. The statutes are set out in R. Slovenko, *Psychotherapy and Confidentiality* (Springfield, IL: Thomas, 1998), pp. 150–185. In the District of Columbia, there is no medical privilege in criminal cases where "the accused is charged with causing the death of, or causing injuries upon, a human being, and the disclosure is required in the interests of public justice;" D.C. Code Ann. § 14–307. In jurisdictions where a psychotherapy or medical privilege applies in criminal cases, the question arises whether it is applicable in the emergency treatment of an unconscious patient. In People v. Childs, 243 Mich. App. 360, 622 N.W.2d 90 (2000), the defendant was charged with having started a fire while intoxicated. The defendant was unconscious when taken to the hospital, where blood was drawn and tested for alcohol content. The Michigan Court of Appeals affirmed the trial court's decision precluding the admission of the blood test results under the state's physician–patient privilege. It rejected the prosecutor's argument that the privilege should not apply to an unconscious patient on the ground that the privilege was designed only to protect and encourage communication between a patient and a physician. The court held that the plain language of the state's privilege statute provides that the privilege applies to "information" acquired in attending to a patient if the information is necessary to treat the patient. Thus, the court held that the statute applies to any "information" acquired, including blood test results, and is not limited to information acquired through communication with the patient.

25. Mark David Chapman, who shot and killed John Lennon, a former member of the Beatles, pleaded guilty to the crime, but if he had asked for a trial and raised an insanity defense, his prior visits to a psychotherapist would have been subject to discovery by the prosecution because his claim of insanity created an implied waiver of the psychotherapist–patient privilege. See, e.g., Ariz. Rev. Stat. Ann. § 13-3933.

26. See, e.g., Smith v. McCormick, 914 F.2d 1153 (9th Cir. 1990); Miller v. District Court, 737 P.2d 834 (Colo. 1987); People v. Hilliker, 185 N.W.2d 831 (Mich. App. 1971). *But see* Lange v. Young, 869 F.2d 1008 (7th Cir. 1989); Haynes v. State, 739 P.2d 497 (Nev. 1987).

27. United States v. Hinckley, 525 F. Supp. 1342 (D.C. 1981).

28. Ill. Stat. Ch. 740, § 110/10.

29. Ind. Code Ann. § 25-33-1-17; Wis. Stat. Ann. § 905.04(4)(d).

30. Neb. Rev. Stat. § 27-504.

31. State v. Schreiber, 122 N.J. 579, 585 A.2d 945 (1991).

32. See, e.g., Alaska R. Evid. 504(d)(2). In *In re* Grand Jury Proceedings of Violette, 183 F. 3d 71 (1st Cir. 1999), Gregory Violette was under a grand jury investigation for allegedly making false statements to financial institutions for the purpose of obtaining loans and credit disability insurance and fabricating disabilities in his communications to his healthcare providers. He was alleged to have prompted the communications of these falsehoods to the companies that underwrote the credit disability policies. The United States subpoenaed two psychiatrists who had seen Violette to appear before the grand jury. The crime-fraud exception to privilege allowed the inquiry.

33. D.C. Code Ann. 4-307(b)(4).

34. See, e.g., Neb. Rev. Stat. § 27-504.

35. See, e.g., Ill. Stat. Ann. Ch. 740 § 110/10.

36. McDonough v. Director of Patuxent Institution, 183 A.2d 368 (Md. 1962).

37. See People v. Stevens, 386 Mich. 579, 194 N.W.2d 370 (1972).

38. The U.S. Supreme Court addressed the issue in State of Pennsylvania v. Ritchie, 480 U.S. 39 (1987). In this case the accused was charged with the sexual assault of his daughter, a minor, whereupon the matter was referred to the Pennsylvania Children and Youth Services Agency for investigation and treatment. The accused sought production and disclosure of the agency's confidential records on the

basis of the Sixth Amendment of the Constitution. The Court held that if information "material" to the defense of the accused had been disclosed to the defense—evidence is "material" if there is a reasonable probability that had the evidence been disclosed to the defendant, the result of the proceeding would have been different. A "reasonable probability" is a probability sufficient to undermine confidence in the outcome. 480 U.S. at 57.

The threshold test is not construed too strictly so as to avoid placing the accused in a Catch-22 situation. It is designed to prevent speculative or frivolous applications only. In Commonwealth of Massachusetts v. Bishop, 617 N.E.2d 990 (Mass. 1993), the defendant was accused of sexually assaulting members of his Boy Scout Troop. After the alleged incidents, two victims were treated by a psychologist. The accused sought pretrial production of the psychologist's records pursuant to his right to a fair trial. The court held that confidential documents were to be produced to the court where the accused demonstrated "a likelihood that the records contain[ed] relevant evidence." The accused was not required to demonstrate the actual existence of relevant evidence, only some factual basis indicating how the impugned records were likely to be relevant. A low threshold was preferred because the court did not want to leave the accused in the Catch-22 situation or interfere with his right to present a full answer and defense. The court expressed the opinion that the stated threshold was sufficient to prevent the accused from merely grasping at straws; 617 N.E.2d at 1000.

39. Shartzer v. Israels, 51 Cal. App. 4th 641, 59 Cal. Rptr.2d 296 (1996).
40. A. Meisel, "Confidentiality and Rape Counseling," *Hastings Center Report* 11 (1981): 5.
41. New York: Warner Books, 1994. The Canadian Supreme Court upheld the constitutionality of a law that prevents psychiatric records from being disclosed routinely in sexual assault cases. In a 7–2 ruling, the court upheld a 1997 law that requires trial judges to decide whether a request to examine psychiatric records is relevant to the case. R. v. Mills, (1999) 3 S.C.R. 668.
42. Quoted in E.J. Pollock, "Mother Fights to Keep Daughter's Records in Rape Case Secret," *Wall Street Journal*, Aug. 22, 1996, p. 1.
43. See United States v. Nixon, 418 U.S. 683 (1974).
44. West Virginia v. Roy, 460 S.E.2d 277 (W. Va. 1995).
45. State v. Cisneros, 535 N.W.2d 703 (Neb. 1995). In a prosecution in California for forcible sex offenses, Farrell L. v. Superior Court, 203 Cal. App.3d 521, 250 Cal. Rptr. 25 (1988), the defendant sought to cross-examine the victim, his minor daughter, regarding persons in her therapy group at a state hospital to whom she had revealed details of the offenses allegedly perpetrated against her. The victim declined to provide the names of the persons in her therapy group on the ground of confidentiality. After a hearing in chambers in which the victim's counselor at the state hospital testified, the trial court refused to allow defense counsel such line of cross-examination on the basis that it fell within the psychotherapist–patient privilege. The California Court of Appeals denied the petition. It held that the identification of persons in the victim's group counseling could only have been relevant in a subsequent attempt to impeach her testimony at trial and that the exclusion of the cross-examination did not deny the defendant a fair hearing; 203 Cal. App.3d at 528.
46. Federal Rules of Evidence, Rule 504 (as proposed).
47. Matter of Winstead, 67 Ohio App.2d 111, 425 N.E.2d 943 (1980).
48. Some 20 states have statutory provisions that allow commitment by guardians. See D.M. English, "The Authority of a Guardian to Commit an Adult Ward," *Mental & Phys. Disabil. L. Rept.* 20 (1996): 584.
49. Cal. Welf. Inst. Code §§ 5350–5371.
50. Matter of Farrow, 41 N.C. App. 680, 255 S.E.2d 777 (1979).
51. Michigan Compiled Laws (MCL) 330.1750.
52. Saur v. Probes, 190 Mich. App. 636 (1991).
53. MCL 330.1750.
54. See, e.g., Ala. Code 26-18-7(a) (2).
55. See, e.g., Matter of A.J.S., 630 P.2d 217 (Mont. 1981). See also United States v. Burtrum, 17 F. 3d 1299 (10th Cir. 1994) (criminal child sexual abuse context).
56. Laznovsky v. Laznovsky, 745 A. 2d 1054 (Md. 2000). See C.P. Malmquist, "Psychiatric Confidentiality in Child Custody Disputes," *J. Am. Acad. Child Adolesc. Psychiat.* 33 (1994): 158.
57. Mo. Rev. Stat. 17:337.639.
58. Matter of von Goyt, 461 So.2d 821, at 823 (Ala. Civ. App. 1984).
59. Address by Marianne Battani on April 30, 1991, at Michigan's Institute of Continuing Legal Education.
60. Critchlow v. Critchlow, 347 So.2d 453 (Fla. App. 3d Dist. 1977).

61. Roper v. Roper, 336 So.2d 654, at 656 (Fla. App. 4th Dist. 1976). In a bitterly contested divorce and custody battle, the father, an attorney, complained to the Maryland State Board of Physicians that Dr. Harold I. Eist overmedicated his wife and two of the children. In keeping with its policy, the board automatically demanded the entire charts on all three patients. Acting in accordance with medical ethics, Dr. Eist contacted the patients to obtain permission, which was refused by the patients and their attorneys. However, when Dr. Eist notified the board, he was told, "For your information, receipt of those medical records is not contingent upon the consent of the patients." Dr. Eist was charged with failure to cooperate with a lawful investigation. In more than five years of costly litigation, an administrative law judge (twice), two separate Maryland circuit judges, and an appellate court consisting of three judges ruled in a 56-page opinion that the prosecution of Dr. Eist was unfounded. The court stated that if a patient or physician challenges a request for medical records, the burden rests with the board to prove that its need to invade privacy outweighs the patient's right to privacy. The court said that the application of the balancing test would have failed to result in a subpoena for the patient records. J.G. Chester & R.L. Pyles, "Absolute Power: The Eist Case," *Clinical. Psychiatry News*, Nov. 2007, p. 13.
62. Navarre v. Navarre, 191 Mich. App. 395, 479 N.W.2d 357 (1991).
63. Comment by East Lansing attorney Steven A. Mitchell, quoted in Editorial, *Detroit News*, Jan. 22, 2000, p. C7.
64. H.B. Roback, R.F. Moore, G.J. Waterhouse, & P.R. Martin, "Confidentiality Dilemmas in Group Psychotherapy with Substance-Dependent Physicians," *Am. J. Psychiat.* 153 (1996): 10.
65. Personal communication.
66. Personal communication.
67. In Blue Cross v. Superior Court & Blair, Super. Ct. No. 32612 (Sept. 10, 1976), it being agreed that the patient's name and ailments were disclosed to Blue Cross for the purpose of paying the doctor's fees, the court held that confidentiality was not lost and the privilege was not waived.
68. McCormick's *Handbook of the Law of Evidence* (St. Paul, MN: West, 5th ed., 1999). This point is more fully developed in W. Cross, "Privileged Communications Between Participants in Group Psychotherapy," *L. & Soc. Order* 1970: 191.
69. State v. Andring, 342 N.W.2d 128 (Minn. 1984); see P.S. Appelbaum & A. Greer, "Confidentiality in Group Therapy," *Hosp. & Comm. Psych.* 44 (1993): 311.
70. 342 N.W.2d at 133.
71. Farrell L. v. Superior Court, 203 Cal. App.3d 521, 250 Cal. Rptr. 25 (1988); discussed supra note 45.
72. 203 Cal. App.3d at 527.
73. Skakel v. Benedict, 738 A.2d 170 (Conn. App. 1999).
74. See T. Scheffey, "Beyond Rich Man's Justice," *Conn. Law Tribune*, Aug. 16, 1999, p.1. In a New York case, Paul Cox, who broke into his boyhood home in Larchmont and fatally stabbed the husband and wife doctors who lived there, was arrested four years later, when seven AA members told the police about the killings. He was then linked to the crime by fingerprints at the victims' house. The defense contended that Cox was drunk and temporarily insane and thought he was killing his parents. He was convicted of manslaughter rather than murder under the theory that he suffered from extreme emotional disturbance. AP news release, "Lawyer says AA testimony should have been barred in Cox case," June 18, 1999. An attempt to apply a psychotherapist-type privilege to "confidential" communications among Alcoholics Anonymous members failed in Cox v. Miller, 296 F.3d 98 (2d Cir. 2002); State v. Boobar, 637 A.2d 1162 (Me. 1994); see T.J. Reed, "The Futile Fifth Step: Compulsory Disclosure of Confidential Communications Among Alcoholics Anonymous Members," *St. John's L. Rev.* 70 (1996): 693.
75. *In re* Zuniga, 714 F.2d 632 (6th Cir. 1983); Ley v. Dall, 150 Vt. 383, 553 A.3d 562 (1988).
76. City of Alhambra v. Superior Court, 110 Cal. App.3d 513, 168 Cal. Rptr. 49 (1980).
77. D. Louisell & C. Mueller, *Federal Evidence* (Rochester, NY: Lawyer's Cooperative, rev. ed., 1985), vol. 2, § 216, p. 857. See also E.S. Soffin, "The Case for a Federal Psychotherapist–Patient Privilege That Protects Patient Identity," *Duke L. J.* 1985: 1217. Some state statutes specifically protect the identity of a patient. For example, Rule 510 of the Texas Rules of Evidence provides that records of the identity, diagnosis, evaluation, or treatment of a patient shall not be disclosed (subject to the exceptions to nondisclosure).
78. 740 Ill. Comp. Stat. Ann. 110/2 (Supp. 1995).
79. 42 C.F.R. §§ 2.11, 2.12.
80. "The Principles of Medical Ethics With Annotations Especially Applicable to Psychiatry" (1995 ed.); P.B. Gruenberg, "Some Thoughts on Confidentiality," *So. Calif. Psychiat. Newsl.*, Sept. 1996, p. 4.

81. Annot., Discovery in Medical Malpractice Action, of Names of Other Patients to Whom Defendant Has Given Treatment Similar to That Allegedly Injuring Plaintiff, 74 A.L.R.3d 1055. In N.O. v. Callahan, 110 F.R.D. 637 (D. Mass. 1986), an action by inmates at a state mental health facility alleging systematic failures to provide adequate medical care, the plaintiffs sought medical records of nonparty patients. Although the court found that such records are privileged under state law, it held that a strong showing of need had been made and that the records could be discovered. The court required deletion of the names of the patients and limited disclosure of the records to counsel, clerical assistants, and experts.

82. *Ex parte* Abell, 613 S.W.2d 255 (Tex. 1981); see also Ltrs., "Ethics of Contacting Past Patients of Alleged Molester," *Clinical Psychiatry News*, Feb. 1989, p. 9.

83. "Evidence of Multiple Victims in Therapist Sexual Misconduct Cases," *Trial*, May 1995, p. 30.

84. 381 N.Y.S.2d 587 (1976).

85. Marcus v. Superior Court of Los Angeles County, 18 Cal. App.3d 22, 95 Cal. Rptr. 535 (1971).

86. In a commentary, Law Professors Jon R. Waltz and Roger C. Park say, "One would think that the information was much more important to the plaintiff than it would be to the patient enquired about, and that in justice, the plaintiff should get the information. Certainly the physician defendant has no interest in keeping the information confidential except insofar as it shields him from liability for malpractice. It would seem that it should be privileged if this were a test for a sexually transmitted disease or various other things in which the other patients of the physician had a real privacy interest. Here it is hard to think that the third party interest is very strong. One is tempted to hold that a patient's angiogram is not a communication, but the problem is that it is clear that the patient would have had to make certain communications before the doctor would do an angiogram upon her, so the privilege is not nonexistent on that account." J.R. Waltz & R.C. Park, *Evidence* (New York: Foundation Press, 9th ed., 1999), p. 607. See also Smith v. Superior Court, 118 Cal. App.3d 136, 173 Cal. Rptr. 145 (1981; income of psychiatrist in action for spousal support could be learned in other ways); Costa v. Regents of the University of California, 116 Cal. App.2d 445, 254 P.2d 85 (1953); Boddy v. Parker, 45 App. Div.2d 1000, 358 N.Y.S. 218 (1974).

87. 220 Mich. App. 248, 559 N.W.2d 76 (1996).

88. 372 Mich. 346, 126 N.W.2d 718 (1964).

89. 170 Mich. App. 619, 428 N.W.2d 719 (1988).

90. Dorris v. Detroit Osteopathic Hosp., 460 Mich. 26, 594 N.W.2d 455 (1999). In Falco v. Institute of Living, 757 A.2d 571 (Conn. 2000), the court held that the psychiatrist–patient privilege prevents disclosure of the identity of a patient who attacked the plaintiff in a psychiatric hospital. On the other hand, in Baptist Memorial Hospital–Union County v. Johnson, 754 So.2d 1165 (Miss. 2000), the court ruled that the hospital must disclose the identity of a patient who mistakenly breast-fed another patient's baby. See annot., 66 A.L.R. 5th 591 (1999).

91. Shady Grove Psychiatric Group v. State of Maryland, 128 Md. App. 163, 736 A.2d 1168 (1999); "Psychiatrist Wins Refusal to Release Patient Names," *Psychiatric News*, Nov. 5, 1999, p. 2. See, in general, W. Winslade, "Confidentiality of Medical Records," *J. Legal Med.* 3 (1982): 497; see also J.B. Sloan & B. Hall, "Confidentiality of Psychotherapeutic Records, *J. Legal Med.* 5 (1984): 435.

92. As for the production of medical records, the court noted both the parents' need for the medical history information from the unidentified patient to protect their infant's health and the unidentified patient's privacy interest in nondisclosure of her identity and medical records. The court ruled that the woman's medical records would have to be produced *in camera* for review to determine whether the infant's health was at risk; Baptist Memorial Hosp.–Union County v. Johnson, 754 So.2d 1165 (Miss. 2000).

93. R.L. Goldstein, "Psychiatric Poetic License? Post-Mortem Disclosure of Confidential Information in the Anne Sexton Case," *Psychiat. Ann.* 22 (1992): 341; J.N. Onek, "Legal Issues in the Orne/Sexton Case," *J. Am Acad. Psychoanal.* 20 (1992): 655.

94. The son of a decedent requested to see his father's hospital records in Emmett v. Eastern Dispensary & Cas. Hosp., 396 F.2d 931 (D.C. Cir. 1967). The court recognized the duty of physicians to protect the interests of their patients under the privilege, but it also said there was a duty to reveal what the patient should know. "This duty of disclosure," the court said, "extends after the patient's death to the next of kin." In Drouillard v. Metropolitan Life Ins. Co., 107 Mich. App. 608, 310 N.W. 2d 15 (1981), it was held that an insurance beneficiary or personal representative may waive a physician–patient privilege that had existed between a physician and the deceased insured. See also Scott v. Henry Ford Hosp., 199 Mich. App. 241, 501 N.W.2d 259 (1993).

95. G.L. Usdin, "The Psychiatrist and Testamentary Capacity," *Tul. L. Rev.* 32 (1957): 89; see generally H. Weihofen, "Guardianship and Other Protective Services for the Mentally Incompetent," *Am. J. Psychiat.* 121 (1965): 970.

96. Olson v. Court of Honor, 100 Minn. 117, 110 N.W. 734 (1907).

97. Matter of Coddington, 307 N.Y. 181, 120 N.E.2d 777 (1954); noted in *Cornell L. Q.* 40 (1954): 148; *Minn. L. Rev.* 39 (1955): 800; *N.Y. U. L. Rev.* 30 (1955): 202; *Syr. L. Rev.* 6 (1954): 213.

98. Conn. Gen. Stat. §17-183; § 17-206d. In Swidler & Berlin v. United States, 118 S. Ct. 2081 (1998), the U.S. Supreme Court held the attorney–client privilege prevents disclosure of confidential communications after a client has died even where the information is relevant to a criminal proceeding. The case involved notes taken by a Washington lawyer whom Vincent Foster, then White House deputy counsel, consulted about a week before his suicide. Independent counsel Kenneth Starr contended he needed the notes as part of his inquiry into whether administration officials lied in order to conceal first lady Hillary Rodham Clinton's alleged role in the 1993 firing of employees in the White House travel office.

99. The courts have also permitted an attorney to disclose client confidences when a third party alleges wrongdoing. The Model Rules of Professional Conduct, Rule 8.3(a), provides: "A lawyer having knowledge that another lawyer has committed a violation of the Rules of Professional Conduct that raises a substantial question as to that lawyer's honesty, trustworthiness, or fitness as a lawyer in other respects, shall inform the appropriate professional authority." To defend against such an allegation, the attorney may disclose client confidences. See Application of Friend, 411 F. Supp. 776 (S.D. N.Y. 1975).

100. Ill. Comp. Stat. Ch 735, § 5/8-802; M. Graham, *Handbook of Illinois Evidence* (St. Paul, MN: West, 6th ed., 1994), pp. 279–280.

101. Pruitt v. Payton, 243 F. Supp. 907, 909 (E.D. Va. 1965).

102. United States v. Butler, 167 F. Supp. 102 (E.D. Va. 1957).

103. AP news release, "Lawyer Denies He Advised Ray to Admit Killing King," *Detroit Free Press*, Nov. 14, 1978, p. D3.

104. For the GAP report, see "Aftermath: Repercussions of the Bean-Bayog Case, *Psychiatric Times*, Feb. 1995, p. 7.

105. The decision in the case, 518 U.S. 1, was rendered in 1996. The oral arguments and decision appear in R. Slovenko, *Psychotherapy and Confidentiality* (Springfield, IL: Thomas, 1998).

106. See E. Inwinkelried, "The Rivalry Between Truth and Privilege: The Weakness of the Supreme Court's Instrumental Reasoning in *Jaffee v. Redmond*," *Hastings L. J.* 49 (1998): 969; C.B. Mueller, "The Federal Psychotherapist–Patient Privilege After *Jaffee*: Truth and Other Values in a Therapeutic Age," *Hastings L. J.* 49 (1998): 999.

107. See M.S. Raeder, "The Social Worker's Privilege, Victim's Rights, and Contextualized Truth," *Hastings L. J.* 49 (1998): 991. In *Henry v. Kernan*, 177 F. 3d 1152 (9th Cir. 1999), the defendant believed that a medical doctor whom he consulted was a psychotherapist and, therefore, his communications should not be discoverable. The court said, "There can be no psychotherapist–patient privilege … if there is no psychotherapist," 177 F. 3d at 1159.

108. 518 U.S. at 22.

109. E. Muravchik (ltr.), *New York Times*, June 19, 1986, p. 14.

110. 518 U.S. at 23.

111. J. Martin, "Slain Doctor Talked of Conflicts," *Detroit Free Press*, June 20, 1996, p. B1.

112. The Ninth Circuit ruled *en banc* that the federal psychotherapist–patient privilege does not contain a "dangerous patient" exception. See United States v. Chase, 340 F.3d 978 (9th Cir. 2003), *cert. denied*, 124 S. Ct.1531 (2004). See also United States v. Hayes, 227 F.3d 578 (6th Cir. 2000). But, see United States v. Glass, 133 E.3d 1356 (10th Cir. 1998). It is asked: What would a dangerous patient exception of the kind referred to in the footnote in *Jaffee* embrace? Only evidence necessary in a proceeding to commit or imprison the patient to prevent him carrying out the danger he exhibited in the therapy session? Or evidence in any kind of case, so long as dangerousness was exhibited in the therapy session and the information was relevant? Would the exception apply in a prosecution or civil suit against the patient for a killing he indicated to the therapist he would commit, but had already committed by the time of the prosecution or civil suit, so disclosure is not necessary for prevention of the killing? See P.F. Rothstein, M.S. Raeder, & D. Crump, *Evidence: Cases, Materials, and Problems* (Newark, NJ: LexisNexis (3d ed., 2006), p. 938.

113. 942 F. Supp. 402 (E.D. Wis. 1996).

114. 942 F. Supp. at 406–408.

115. 948 F. Supp. 97 (D. Mass. 1996).

116. 948 F. Supp. at 98–100.
117. *In re* Grand Jury Proceedings of Violette, 183 F.3d 71 (1st Cir. 1999), discussed at supra note 32. See D. W. Shuman & W. Foote, "*Jaffee v. Redmond's* Impact: Life After the Supreme Court's Recognition of a Psychotherapist–Patient Privilege," *Prof. Psychol. Res. and Pract.* 30 (1999): 479.
118. United States v. Glass, 133 F. 3d 1356 (10th Cir. 1998), the Tenth Circuit held that the privilege does not extend to a criminal case in which the confidential communication constituted the sole basis for the government's prosecution and conviction for threatening the life of the president (the case was remanded to determine whether the threat was serious when it was uttered and whether its disclosure was the only means of averting harm to the president when the disclosure was made).
119. It was headline news on page one of the *New York Times*. L. Greenhouse, "Justices Uphold Psychotherapy Privacy Rights," *New York Times*, June 4, 1996, p. 1. APA President Allan Tasman wrote that the decision provides "additional needed protections for the psychotherapist–patient relationship." A. Tasman, "APA Fighting Hard for Better Medical-Record Privacy Rights," *Psychiatric News*, Dec. 3, 1999, p. 3. In the first-ever mental health report released by a Surgeon General, David Satcher asserted that the decision "leaves little doubt that there is broad legal protection for the principle of confidentiality." The full report, "Mental Health: A Report of the Surgeon General," is available on the Web. "Satcher Focuses National Spotlight on Mental Illness," *Psychiatric News*, Jan. 7, 2000, p. 1.
120. For extended discussion of testimonial privilege, see R. Slovenko, *Psychotherapy and Confidentiality* (Springfield, IL: Thomas, 1998).

6
Witnesses and the Credibility of Testimony

The early method of settling disputes was by fist or club. Gradually, the concept of a trial evolved with its concomitant rules regarding the competency of witnesses and the admissibility of evidence. The early method of deciding disputes, however, has influenced the development of the rules of procedure; within this evolving framework various psychological notions are being used to assess the credibility of testimony.

Historically, litigation is a substitute for trial by ordeal or by battle. During the feudal period, the issue in important cases, such as a disputed claim to land or an accusation of unjustifiable homicide, was generally determined by judicial combat between the principals or their legally appointed champions rather than in a courtroom. In knightly array, the two fought it out and the vanquished, if still alive, suffered whatever penalty the law prescribed.[1]

Around AD 1100, ambitious princes took heed of the political systems of Athens and republican Rome and adopted many of the same concepts in order to support and expand their jurisdiction. The function of the jury at this time was to give support to the king's administrative officials and, later, to his traveling justices in their efforts to extend the jurisdiction of the king's courts throughout England. The strong men of the locality were drawn to the aid of the judges and, as the jury, were not only witnesses, but a determining body. These functions were not split as they are today between our modern jury and witnesses; rather these men had, or were supposed to have had, information regarding the matters in issue.[2] It is interesting to note that the original meaning of the word *juror* is one who took an oath and swore to declare truly what he knew or believed in a given case. There were no rules concerning the way in which the jurors acquired their knowledge.[3] During this period the independent witness was thought of as a meddler and, if he intervened, was in peril of being held guilty of maintenance.

The advent of the modern witness took place in the 16th century, the time of the end of the feudal order. Disputes were no longer provincial matters, and the jury gained in importance, becoming a symbol of political freedom. The Elizabethan Act of 1562, which created the statutory offense of perjury and provided for compulsory attendance of witnesses, initiated a new epoch in the law of evidence. Thereafter, the facts of the case were presented by outside witnesses and not by members of the jury. Previously the jurors were to know everything about the case, now they were to know nothing. The *tabula rasa* dictum, soon to be current in philosophy, found judicial application.

Initially, however, these outside witnesses were received with some circumspection as possible perjurers, and if there was any reason to suspect that a witness might be inclined to lie, he was considered incompetent to testify.[4] The common law borrowed heavily from the canon law in designating certain persons as incompetent to serve as witnesses. In his *History of English Law*, Sir William Holdsworth points out:

> The canon law rejected the testimony of all males under fourteen and females under twelve, of the blind and the deaf and the dumb, of slaves, of infamous persons, and those convicted of crime, of excommunicated persons, of poor persons, and of women in criminal cases, of persons connected with either party by consanguinity and affinity, or belonging to the household of either party, of the enemies of either party, and of Jews, heretics, and pagans.[5]

The grounds of incompetency, as developed through the centuries, may be broadly categorized under five I's:

1. *Interest*: A witness, whether or not a party to the controversy, if pecuniarily interested in the outcome of the cause, was not allowed to testify because of the temptation to falsify.
2. *Insanity*: A person considered insane was thought not to have the mental capacity to testify.
3. *Infancy*: A child was considered incompetent to understand the nature of an oath or to narrate with understanding the facts of what he had seen.
4. *Infidelity*: A person who did not believe in a Supreme Being who was a rewarder of truth and an avenger of falsehood was deemed incapable of taking an oath and, therefore, of testifying.
5. *Infamy*: Part of the punishment for crime in early common law was to render the guilty person infamous and, among other sanctions, he lost the right to testify in a court of law. In addition, a wife was not permitted to testify for or against her husband because in theory husband and wife were one (and that one was the husband).

A number of general basic reforms in trial procedure were accomplished during the 17th century, and major reforms also occurred during the 19th century, in large measure stimulated by the writings of Charles Dickens. Today the rules on competency of witnesses have been replaced with the general principle that any person of "proper understanding" is a competent witness. The rules on competency have been converted into rules of credibility whereby nearly every proposed witness is allowed to testify, but on cross-examination his credibility may be impeached.[6] The question of competency, when raised, is a preliminary matter for the trial judge, whereas, once the witness is allowed to testify, his credibility is a question for the jury.

Cross-examination includes the right, as the courts typically say, "to place the witness in his proper setting and put the weight of his testimony and his credibility to a test, without which the jury cannot fairly appraise them." The credibility of the witness is always relevant in the search for truth. Unquestionably, judges or juries are swayed by the relative attractiveness or unattractiveness of the parties or of the witnesses. As a consequence, cross-examination sometimes ends up being a smearing rather than a discrediting process.

The main lines of attack upon the credibility of a witness are (1) by showing that the witness on a previous occasion has made statements inconsistent with his present testimony; (2) by specific contradiction, proving that some statement of fact made by the witness is, in fact, otherwise; (3) by showing that the witness is biased by reason of such influences as kinship with one party or hostility to another, or motives of pecuniary interest, legitimate or corrupt; (4) by showing a defect of capacity in the witness to observe, remember, or recount the matters testified about; (5) by attacking the character of the witness; and (6) by showing that the witness lacks the religious belief which would give the fullest traditional sanction to his obligation to speak the truth (now obsolete).

Under the rules of evidence, evidence of traits of the character of the witness other than honesty or veracity, or their opposites, is inadmissible to attack or support the credibility of the witness. Other character traits are not deemed sufficiently probative of a witness' honesty or veracity to warrant their consideration on the issue of credibility. Evidence of specific instances of a witness's conduct is inadmissible to prove a trait of character for the purpose of attacking or supporting credibility, with the exception that certain kinds of criminal convictions may be used, and specific instances indicating bias may be shown. Character evidence in support of credibility is admissible only after the witness's character has first been attacked, it being presumed that the witness is credible. The law of evidence on character for credibility of a witness is different from that on propensity of a defendant to commit an act, which is discussed in Chapter 7 on propensity.

The rules of evidence, including the method of challenging credibility, may appear to be an affront to common sense, but, as Chief Justice Vanderbilt once remarked, "The entire history of the law of evidence has been marked by a continuous search for more rational rules, first as to competency of witnesses, and then as to the admissibility of evidence."[7] The courts frequently point out that the rules of evidence are designed to obtain the truth by excluding unreliable testimony, such as hearsay, lay opinion, and biased testimony.

The concept of the Anglo-American system is that truth is best discerned by application of the rules of evidence in an adversarial proceeding, a procedure well suited to the popular American conditioning to games. The witness may feel that he goes through an ordeal just as harrowing as the ancient ordeal by battle. In various ways, the witness is placed under stress as it is believed that this will aid in the ascertainment of truth, whether the witness be shy or bold. The unfamiliar courtroom procedure and legal language are built-in stress factors. At one time, and still in most countries, the witness had to stand (from which derives the term *witness stand*), which increased his anxiety. The witness must swear to tell the truth, and he may be subjected to a vigorous cross-examination,[8] which lawyers say is "one of the principal and most efficacious tests that the law has devised for the discovery of truth."[9]

To be sure, there is need for a better test in the search for truth than the notion expressed by one trial judge: "Wiping hands during testimony is almost always an indication of lying."[10]

The Rules of Evidence on Challenging Credibility and the Role of Psychiatry

Testimony on the credibility or trustworthiness of a witness, vouching testimony as it is sometimes called, is not permitted. Thus, a psychiatrist or other witness may not testify as to the believability of the complainant's or other witness's testimony.[11] To allow it would reconstruct the "oath helpers" of the old common law ("oath helpers" were usually relatives or close friends brought along by the parties to testify to their veracity rather than to the occurrence of facts). The decisions are beyond count that an expert or other witness may not render an opinion as to one's veracity.[12] In no uncertain terms, the Oregon Supreme Court said, "We have said before, and we will say it again, but this time with emphasis—we really mean it—*no psychotherapist may render an opinion on whether a witness is credible in any trial conducted in this state.*"[13] Credibility is an assessment to be made by the jury: "Credibility ... is for the jury—the jury is the lie detector in the courtroom."[14]

To be sure, the words are emphatic, but nationwide, in quite a number of instances (as hereinafter noted), the prohibition on testifying about credibility is circumvented by testifying about the *ability* of a witness to tell the truth. As herein after discussed, the ability to tell the truth and not tell the truth is distinguished from whether the witness is telling the truth.

The late Dr. Henry Davidson, the well-known forensic psychiatrist, observed that the major clinical conditions affecting testimonial capacity are psychosis, mental deficiency, drug addiction, alcoholism, personality disorders, certain organic involvements of the brain, and sometimes certain forms of psychoneurosis. The schizophrenic person, he claimed, can report an event with carbon paper fidelity, but may make an unreliable witness because of defective observation, distorted memory processes, or paranoid ideas. A senile psychotic person is unreliable as a witness because of frequent delusions of infidelity, impairment of memory, and delusions of ingratitude. The hypomanic witness is dangerous because his speech is plausible and positive, but the things he says can be the stuff of which dreams are made. The drug addict may not be a good witness because he may be under the toxic influence of a drug, or his testimony may not be reliable because the issue happens to concern his source of supply. The mental defective may make an adequate witness if the event is one that can be described simply, but, because most events are complex, involving many subtle details, the defective would make a poor witness because of his deficient powers of observation and his inability to paint a vivid verbal picture. The alcoholic is often at the mercy of mixed and unpredictable emotions; the memory defects of chronic alcoholics are well known to psychiatrists. The psychopath will twist his tongue to say anything. Among psychoneurotics, recessional states or obsessional reactions may result in distorted interpretations of events.[15]

A paranoid patient, if not deteriorated, may appear to talk sense, but his testimony may be part of the delusional network. The late psychiatrist Ralph S. Banay, said:

> The problem of the paranoid personality offers an illustrative example of the usefulness of psychiatric testimony, especially in civil cases. Paranoids who have a marked proclivity for getting into legal difficulties, often make a favorable appearance in court when not crossed or agitated, and they may impress the untrained observer as rational and sincere. They could conceivably mislead a judge, an attorney, or a jury into the sincerity of their claim but they would less likely deceive a clinically experienced psychiatrist. Similarly, in many borderline cases or in maladies of obscure manifestation, the root of the trouble may be discernible to the clinician although it is hidden from other observers.[16]

The Hiss Trial

In the spectacular Hiss trial of the early 1950s, the defense offered psychiatric testimony designed to impeach the credibility of the government witness, Whittaker Chambers, who accused Alger Hiss of passing secrets to Communists in the 1930s.[17] In general, more leeway is given to the defense than to the prosecutor on the proffer of evidence. In this spirit, at the outset of his opinion, Judge Henry Goddard ruled the psychiatric testimony admissible, saying:

> It is apparent that the outcome of this trial is dependent, to a great extent upon the testimony of one man: Whittaker Chambers. Mr. Chambers' credibility is one of the major issues upon which the jury must pass. The opinion of the jury—formed upon their evaluation of all the evidence laid before them—is the decisive authority on this question, as on all questions of fact. The existence of insanity or mental derangement is admissible for the purpose of discrediting a witness. Evidence of insanity is not merely for the judge on the preliminary question of competency, but goes to the jury to affect credibility.[18]

Until the end of 1958, Chambers was senior editor of *Time*, but his family had no social or community ties—his grandmother, who went around the house brandishing a carving knife, was put in an asylum; his grandfather was an alcoholic; his father was unfaithful to his mother; his brother committed suicide; and Whittaker himself made an unsuccessful attempt at "self-execution" (his own label) prior to the first Hiss trial. Dr. Carl Binger gave his opinion after listening to a 70-minute hypothetical question that accentuated unpalatable aspects of Mr. Chambers' life.

Binger authored what the Hiss defense called the "theory of unconscious motivation." He claimed that Chambers' accusations were rooted in an obsession with Hiss; he developed feelings of love and admiration for the charming New Dealer, but when Hiss had cut off the friendship, the obsession allegedly metamorphosed into its opposite, an irrational hatred and rage that had set Chambers upon his vengeful course. That theory was also set out by psychoanalyst Meyer A. Zeligs in a 476-page book, *Friendship and Fratricide/An Analysis of Whittaker Chambers and Alger Hiss.*[19]

On cross-examination, Binger's testimony that Chambers was a "psychopathic liar" was discredited. On direct examination, he had pointed out Chambers' untidiness, and on cross-examination he was made to acknowledge that the trait was found in many famous people. He testified that Chambers habitually gazed at the ceiling while testifying and seemed to have no direct relation with his examiner. The prosecutor in a turnabout told him, "We have made a count of the number of times you looked at the ceiling ... . We counted a total of 59 times that you looked at the ceiling in 50 minutes. Now I was wondering whether that was any symptom of a psychopathic personality?" Shifting uneasily, he replied, "Not alone." He had testified that stealing was a psychopathic symptom and the prosecutor asked him, "Did you ever take a hotel towel or Pullman towel?" He replied, "I can't swear whether I did or not, I don't think so." The prosecutor thereupon asked, "And if any member of this jury had stolen a towel, would that be evidence of a psychopathic personality?"[20] The jury believed Whittaker Chambers, and a number of recent studies have vindicated Chambers.[21]

Assessing Credibility by Proof of Character

Historically, the most widely used method of attacking a witness as lacking veracity was by the personal opinion of those acquainted with him. Gradually, evidence of reputation in the community in regard to veracity replaced personal opinion. In judicial opinions, the terms *reputation* and *character* in regard to veracity were (and are) often used interchangeably.[22]

The Federal Rules of Evidence and their counterparts in various states now allow not only reputation evidence, but also opinion evidence as to the character of a witness (including, in regard to truthfulness, an accused who testifies). This rule makes it clear that the belief of a character witness whose conclusion as to a witness's character is based on personal acquaintance rather than on reputation will not be excluded. Rule 608(a) provides the following:

> The credibility of a witness may be attacked or supported by evidence in the form of opinion or reputation, but subject to these limitations: (1) the evidence may refer only to character for truthfulness or untruthfulness, and (2) evidence of truthful character is admissible only after the character of the witness for truthfulness has been attacked by opinion or reputation evidence or otherwise.

With the change allowing opinion evidence, the question was raised: Should evidence in assessing credibility pass from the "crucible of the community" to the "couch of the psychiatrist"?[23] What is "character for truthfulness"? In the *Hiss* case, Dr. Binger looked at the character of Chambers in assessing his credibility. The question today is most frequently raised in sex-offense cases where the credibility of the accused or the prosecuting witness is in question. The victim frequently is a child of such early age that the report often cannot be considered reliable.

Is psychiatry capable of devising a test that can measure character for truthfulness? Test results of so-called lie detectors, truth serum, we may note, are uniformly rejected by the courts.[24] The development of DNA evidence (which may be described as "do not argue") has resulted in overturning a number of convictions or preventing wrongful convictions. What about the psychiatrist as "a walking lie detector"? Davidson asserted that psychiatrists can play a major role in the administration of justice by appraising the credibility of witnesses.[25] There is a strong emotional component in the motivation and memory of witnesses, Davidson said, and, thus, credibility represents an area that should fall within the special field of the psychiatrist. Observation is selective and in large part dependent on the condition of the observer as well as on inner motivations. To give effective and accurate testimony, a witness must observe intelligently, remember clearly, speak coherently, and be free of any emotional drive to distort the truth. According to Davidson, the analysis of these traits should be a job for the psychiatrist.

Impeachment by use of medical records or other evidence indicating treatment for psychiatric problems, however, raises concerns over the personal privacy of the witness. The attack may be demeaning and unfair and would be precluded if the problems did not relate in important ways to capacity to observe or communicate.[26] In any event, suggestions are made that psychiatric diagnosis, whether based on clinical examination or courtroom observation alone, should be admitted whenever it is offered to show the unreliability of a witness. Those who make these suggestions would have the psychiatrist sit with a cross-examining attorney, at the counsel table, and thus "direct the cross-examination, thereby approximating a personal interview with the witness."[27]

In the courtroom, the psychiatrist may observe the witness's mood, pressure of talk, stream of thought, brightness, content of thinking, memory. But, in the courtroom, where nobody believes anybody, the aura of cross-examination, with its concomitant implication of hostility and adversity of interest, provides an emotional climate far different from that of the ideal psychiatric interview. The witness feels attacked and abused, which immediately elicits defense mechanisms that can only shut out or distort pertinent psychiatric material.[28]

In the oft-cited 1921 case, *State v. Driver*, a 12-year-old girl, upon whom an attempted rape was allegedly committed, was called as a witness. The defendant offered to show by the testimony of a psychiatrist that the girl was a moral pervert and not trustworthy. On the basis of courtroom observation, the expert was prepared to testify that he would classify the girl as a lying moron and unworthy of belief. The evidence was designed to be an attack on her truthfulness, aimed at her credibility; and the inference to be drawn from the testimony, if it had been permitted, would have been that she was a habitual and confirmed liar because of her mental defectiveness. The court refused to hear the proffered evidence and said: "It is yet to be demonstrated that psychological and medical tests are practical and will detect a lie on the witness stand."[29]

To vary the facts in *Driver*, consider the case of a woman in her late twenties who had a very poor childhood relationship with her father. Although rather attractive, she dated rarely and never married. She meets a man at a social gathering and, following some pleasant conversation, he offers to take her home. She accepts, but he drives to a secluded spot. She reports that her memory was a "complete blank" from that time until she recalls finding herself in his arms. Let us assume that she regularly sees a psychiatrist and on the day following the alleged incident, she sees him and, still in a very anxious and overwrought condition, she tells him that she was raped. If this event becomes the subject of prosecution, does the psychiatrist have probative evidence to offer unavailable to others? The psychiatrist may know her to be a hysterical woman who regularly mixes fact with fantasy, and he is also aware, we must assume, that hysterical women are not immune from rape.[30]

In the trial of Lewis "Scooter" Libby, aide to Vice President Dick Cheney, the question was whether he was lying or had a lapse of memory in regard to the unmasking of Valerie Plame Wilson, the CIA operative. The Libby defense planned to call Robert A. Bjork, a distinguished member of the faculty at UCLA, to testify about memory. The trial judge barred the testimony, saying that the science of memory is not "science" at all, but common knowledge and common sense. He held that the right of cross-examination was an effective substitute for the right to offer evidence about it. Moreover, he held that the proposed evidence was more likely to confuse the jury than educate it.[31]

According to a number of decisions, testimony may be offered by a mental health professional as to whether the emotional or mental condition of the witness affected his *ability* to accurately perceive, recollect, or communicate information.[32] Testifying on the ability or capacity of a witness is a way to sidestep the rule against testifying on a witness's credibility. This tactic has passed muster in a number of cases.[33] In *United States v. Lindstrom*,[34] a decision that appears in a number of law school casebooks, the Eleventh Circuit observed,

> Although the debate over the proper legal role of mental health professionals continues to rage, even those who would limit the availability of psychiatric evidence acknowledge

that many types of "emotional or mental defect may materially affect the accuracy of testimony; a conservative list of such defects would have to include the psychoses, most or all the neuroses, defects in the structure of the nervous system, mental deficiency, alcoholism, drug addiction and psychopathic personality."[35]

The court, reversing a conviction, said, "The jury was denied any evidence on whether [the] key witness was a schizophrenic, what schizophrenia means, and whether it affects one's perceptions of external reality. The jury was denied any evidence of whether the witness was capable of distinguishing reality from hallucinations."[36]

Then, too, the North Carolina Supreme Court said: "What could be more effective for the purpose than to impeach the mentality or the intellectual grasp of the witness? If his interest, bias, indelicate way of life, insobriety, and general bad reputation in the community may be shown as bearing upon his unworthiness of belief, why not his imbecility, want of understanding, or moronic comprehension, which go more directly to the point?"[37]

Logically, an individual who does not have the ability to tell the truth ought not be allowed to testify. On taking the oath, the rules of evidence provide: "Before testifying, every witness shall be required to declare that he will testify truthfully, by oath or affirmation administered in a form calculated to awaken his conscience and impress his mind with his duty to do so."[38] The witness swears that he will tell "the truth, the whole truth, and nothing but the truth." In early history, the oath was the factor that decided the issue, and it rendered a judicial decision unnecessary. Operating as proof, it was absolute proof. Originally, the oath was not incidental to testimonial evidence; rather the reverse was the case—witnesses supported the oath. Through the centuries, variations in oath formulae record the transition from proof by oath to testimonial proof.[39] Nowadays, just about anyone is competent to take the oath and testify, but the credibility or competency of the testimony is subject to attack.[40]

At trial in *United States v. Shay*,[41] the defense introduced psychiatric evidence to establish that the defendant was not capable of telling the truth. The defendant's confession to aiding and abetting an attempt to blow up his father's car was impugned. Psychiatrist Robert Phillips testified that the defendant was a pathological liar; that is, he suffered from pseudologia fantastica, a condition that caused him "to spin out webs of lies that are ordinarily self-aggrandizing and serve to place him in the center of attention." An ordinary liar has a purpose in mind when telling a lie, whereas a pathological liar obtains gratification by telling lies, not by the fruits of lying. The pathological liar is driven to make up stories (a polygraph test is of no value because the pathological liar has no qualms about lying). The First Circuit ruled that the psychiatric testimony "would be beneficially informative to the jury." The court, after an examination of the law and the psychiatric literature, concluded that factitious disorders are an appropriate topic for expert testimony.[42]

There is argument whether "pseudologia fantastica" or pathological lying should be included in the *Diagnostic and Statistical Manual of Mental Disorders (DSM)*. Proponents contend that pathological lying is an impulse disorder different from confabulation, delusions, and factitious disorder in that individuals who suffer from pseudologica fantastica are not out of touch with reality and do not suffer organic amnesia. Instead, the pathological lying is not only the end in itself, but also it is compulsive and uncontrollable.[43]

The condition is, however, referenced in the *DSM* as a symptom of factitious disorder, such as Munchausen syndrome, where patients induce psychological or physical symptoms in order to assume the sick role. Yet pseudologia fantastica is not induced by a desire to appear sick and seems to more closely resemble the case of the real Baron Munchausen, who told exaggerated stories that were entirely unrelated to medical complaints. Moreover, studies have correlated pseudologia fantastica with neurological disorders. The discussion of compulsive lying as a mental defect has been going on since the early 20th century and continues to this day.[44] Recently, the confession of John Mark Karr that he murdered and sexually assaulted JonBenet Ramsey propelled the phenomenon of false confessions back into the limelight (he was ruled out as a suspect by DNA evidence).

The leading case where an expert was allowed to testify about false confessions is *United States v. Hall*.[45] In this Seventh Circuit case, the defendant was convicted of kidnapping a child for sexual purposes. The district court excluded testimony of a psychologist and a psychiatrist who were to testify about false confessions, that individuals can be coerced into giving a false confession and that certain signs can be seen where a false confession is likely to occur. The court held that the jury could determine on its own whether certain techniques were suggestive or not. On appeal, the Seventh Circuit held that as long as the proffered testimony was found to be scientifically valid, it should have been allowed.

About the time of the decision in *Hall*, the Wyoming Supreme Court rejected the testimony of a psychologist about "false confession syndrome." The court found that the expert did not base his testimony on any documented data, that this so-called syndrome was not accepted in the field of psychology, and that rather than a syndrome, the psychologist's testimony was really just a collection of reasons that a person may make a false confession.[46]

Quite often, as a review of the cases would reveal, the admissibility of the expert's opinion depends on "doublespeak," where one testifies about credibility in a roundabout way, and quite often, the defense is allowed to offer testimony that would be precluded if offered by the prosecution. Some examples may be noted. In an Oregon case, *State v. Gherasim*,[47] it was ruled that the trial court committed reversible error when it excluded a psychiatrist's testimony opining that a sexual assault victim had dissociative amnesia affecting her credibility to recall what took place. In this case, the defendant, charged with attempted rape, asserted that he had not been the attacker, but had tried to help the victim when he found her on the side of the road. At trial, he sought to have a psychiatrist testify that inconsistencies in the victim's descriptions of what took place indicated she had developed dissociative amnesia, a condition that impairs one's ability to remember traumatic experiences.[48] The trial court, in excluding the testimony, said that it was a comment on credibility and that it was so within the common experience of jurors that it would not assist the fact-finding process. The defendant was convicted.

The Oregon Court of Appeals reversed, saying it was not a direct comment on the witness's credibility, and it concluded, "[T]he psychiatrist's testimony was no different from that of an ophthalmologist who testifies that an eyewitness has impaired vision or that of a psychologist who testifies that a witness suffers from dementia.[49] The Oregon Supreme Court (the same court that a decade earlier had exhorted against psychiatric opinion on credibility) affirmed, holding that the psychiatrist's testimony was admissible because it would be helpful to the trier of fact's understanding of the issue. No one witnessed the crime, so the jury could find the defendant guilty only if it considered the victim's version of events more credible than his. The defendant was entitled to present the testimony as evidence that would help the jury assess the victim's credibility, the court ruled, and it added that even though the psychiatrist did not give a detailed explanation of his diagnosis, this did not make it unhelpful to the jury.[50]

In *Westcott v. Crinklaw*,[51] a tort action brought under the civil rights law, it was claimed that the defendant, a police officer, was not justified in shooting the deceased. After the shooting, police officers questioned the defendant about the shooting at which time he said he "didn't know" if he was "in fear" and that he "did not know" if the deceased had a gun in his hand. At trial, to defuse these statements, a psychiatrist testified that the defendant suffered from posttraumatic stress syndrome after the shooting, and that it may cause a person to make inaccurate, unreliable, and incomplete statements. It was permissible for the expert to testify that the defendant suffered posttraumatic stress, but it was an error, the Eighth Circuit ruled, for the expert to testify as to the reliability of the statements, as that was a credibility issue that should have been left in the exclusive province of the jury. The following is the testimony:

Q. Just focus upon the physiological, emotional, and psychological reactions that the officer has afterwards in dealing with [a situation such as a shooting]?

A. Usually the heart is racing, adrenaline is flowing. Many officers report a numbness, an unrealness, difficulty making sense, an immediate attempt to try to reconstruct the events that have happened. Oftentimes incomplete, inaccurate, or in some cases even total memory lapses of what's occurred.

Q. Is there a name applied in the psychological profession for this reaction that you're talking about?

A. Posttraumatic stress.

Q. Could you focus on how posttraumatic stress and these symptoms that you have listed would affect the police officer's ability to write reports and give oral accounts of what had happened?

A. Officers in this type of situation very frequently, in fact as a standard rule, give varying accounts … basically the ability to accurately report immediately following a situation's [sic] seriously impaired.

Q. Was Joseph Crinklaw exhibiting the symptoms of posttraumatic stress syndrome?

A. Yes, he was.[52]

In a similar holding in *Schutz v. State*,[53] which involved a charge against the defendant of aggravated sexual assault of his 6-year-old child, the Texas Court of Appeals noted that the general capacity for truthfulness evidence admissible in a criminal proceeding includes evidence as to whether the person can distinguish between reality and fantasy or whether the person's physical or mental condition adversely affects that person's ability to accurately perceive or relate events, but the expert may not testify that the complainant's allegations "were not the result of fantasy" as that would constitute a direct comment upon the truth of the complainant's allegations. In a concurring opinion, Judge Paul Womack questioned the drawing of the line:

The Court's rule is [that] it is not error to admit testimony of the major premise of a syllogism (children who are fantasizing or being manipulated behave in certain ways) and the minor premise (this child did not behave in those ways), but it is error to admit testimony of the inevitable conclusion (this child was not fantasizing or being manipulated). Could jurors, who have heard the expert's opinion on the major premise and the minor premise, not be aware that the expert must hold the inevitable opinion about the conclusion? The conclusion is ineluctable after the premises have been admitted. It would be more natural and straightforward to admit the expert's opinion on the conclusion.[54]

Confirmation Hearings of Clarence Thomas

At the confirmation hearings of Clarence Thomas for the U.S. Supreme Court, psychiatric language abounded and there was much psychologizing about Thomas and Anita Hill. As everyone knows, Anita Hill accused Thomas of sexually harassing her in the early 1980s when Thomas was her superior at the Education Department and Equal Employment Opportunity Commission. According to the news reports, Sen. John Danforth, who was Thomas's chief sponsor, called on Dr. Park Dietz, a leading forensic psychiatrist, for an opinion. Not having examined the parties, he declined to offer a diagnosis, but provided a description of the disorder known as "erotomania," in which "the delusion is that another person, usually of a higher status, has romantic interest in the subject."

Other psychiatrists were more willing to render a diagnosis without examination of the subject, though it may violate a dubious professional ethic. The Senate offices were inundated with calls, faxes, and letters from psychiatrists offering theories about Thomas and Hill, and both camps had psychiatrists prepared to take the stand.

A number of forensic psychiatrists that year at the annual meeting of the American Academy of Psychiatry and the Law privately expressed the opinion that Hill fits the diagnosis of erotomania. At the meeting, Dietz insisted that he did not pin a diagnosis on Hill, but only provided "general information" about diagnostic categories. Another psychiatrist at the meeting expressed the opinion that Hill was lying because "a woman traumatized as she allegedly was, though 10 years ago, would not testify in her dispassionate manner." Another found it surprising how she seemed to stick to a kind of script, and there was so little variation. To that psychiatrist, Thomas's anguish seemed honest and believable.

However, there surely was no consensus among the psychiatrists offering an opinion in the corridors at the meeting. One psychiatrist, a renowned expert in the detection of deception, concluded that Thomas was lying because an innocent person would have listened to Hill's testimony. Another psychiatrist noted Thomas's slip of the tongue, "I want to say *uncategorically* that I deny every allegation."

The opinions of these psychiatrists were as divided as lay opinion. Richard Starr, deputy managing editor of a now defunct magazine, was not at the meeting, but he wrote, "The profession has reason to be thankful that the struggle to enlist psychiatry in the Hill–Thomas controversy remained mostly behind the scenes. Had the psychiatrists taken the stand for the two sides, the public indeed would have been educated—not about sexual harassment, but about the limits of psychiatric expertise."[55]

Be that as it may, Harvard Law Professor Alan Dershowitz, in a luncheon address at the meeting, wondered about the character of Hill—using Thomas to advance herself over a period of ten years, and then turning on him. Character, after all, goes to credibility; she wanted to torpedo him, in secret no less, like an enemy submarine. Like Munsterberg years earlier, Dershowitz beseeched the psychiatrists to bring to bear their knowledge of human behavior to assist in the ascertainment of truth.

Is a psychiatrist better able to assess credibility when the witness has talked over the matter with him in psychotherapy? Theodor Reik, in his book *The Unknown Murderer*,[56] it will be recalled, claimed that psychoanalysis has no contribution to make to evidence of guilt, as it is concerned with mental (inner) reality rather than material (outer) reality. A therapist does not ordinarily check on material reality. He is ordinarily concerned with the patient's view of the world rather than with what the world actually is. He does not cross-question the patient. Some therapists say that outside information about the patient interferes with their clinical work, and they prefer to close their eyes to it. They know the situation only through the eyes of the patient. Something more, then, is needed to test veracity. By and large, credibility is accorded witnesses who testify with confidence or certainty. The witness who testifies in that way is considered more likely to be accurate than the less positive witness. Intuitively, credibility is related to the confidence of the witness.

Reliability of Eyewitness Identification

The standard jury instruction on eyewitness identification states, in part: "Think about ... how sure the witness was about the identification."[57] It also instructs: "How did the witness look and act while testifying?"[58] Jurors tend to assume that a witness who is nervous is lying. Witnesses who appear anxious tend not to be believed. Wiping one's hands while testifying is taken almost always as an indication of lying.[59]

Experiments, however, show that witnesses who say that they are 100% certain the accused is the culprit are just as likely to be wrong as witnesses who are vague or ambivalent about their identification. Dr. Daniel L. Schacter, chairman of the Psychology Department of Harvard University, writes: "Even though juries believe confident witnesses more than uncertain ones, eyewitness confidence bears at best a tenuous link to eyewitness accuracy: Witnesses who are highly confident are frequently no more accurate than witnesses who express less confidence. To make matters worse, eyewitness confidence can be inflated when a witness is told that another witness identified the same suspect, or when witnesses rehearse their testimony repeatedly during trial preparations. Clearly, eyewitness confidence is not set in stone at the time an event occurs."[60] Psychologists' study of eyewitness identification has a long history, particularly in the United States and England, going back at least to the early influential work of Hugo Munsterberg around the turn of the 20th century.[61]

Can expert testimony be used to show that credibility is not related to the confidence of the witness? Because it is counterintuitive, as a witness who speaks with confidence is taken as trustworthy, expert testimony may be helpful to the jury. Testifying with confidence, albeit inaccurately, may stem out of various considerations. For example, a victim wanting revenge testifies with confidence. Witnesses who feel a social role in seeking justice help out by testifying with confidence. Witnesses who have been hypnotized testify with confidence. The delusional paranoid person has immutable beliefs even though they are contradicted by every shred of physical evidence. Then, too, there is the psychopath, or con artist, who is very convincing.[62]

When the expert testimony is about witnesses generally, however, the courtroom is turned into a classroom. And because the experts would be called in by the defense, they would tend to emphasize those experiments that would undermine any eyewitness's testimony.[63] In a civil case, the burden of proof is a preponderance of the evidence, but in a criminal case the state has the burden of proving the case beyond a reasonable doubt, and, as a consequence, testimony on eyewitness testimony, though of a general nature, can inject a reasonable doubt.

Psychologists, when allowed to offer expert testimony on eyewitness identification, trace the process of eyewitness observation and testimony from the initial acquisition phase (the initial observations of the event) to the retention phase (when these observations are organized and stored in memory) to the retrieval phase (when the eyewitness, on interrogation, reports on the observations as modified and then retrieved from memory). There follows the stage of matching and recognition, during which the images of the persons involved in the crime, retrieved from memory, are matched against a showup, a photo lineup, or a live lineup. Then, there is the formation of opinions and judgment by the eyewitness, and further identification and testimony in the courtroom.[64]

Psychologists claim that the rate of mistaken identification is significantly higher than most people tend to believe. They point out that witnesses have particular difficulty in making an accurate identification in cross-ethnic identification. By and large, the trial courts are left to decide whether they will allow expert testimony on the fallibility of eyewitness testimony (appellate courts usually defer to their judgment). The trial courts mostly rule against admissibility.[65] In a conference dealing with eyewitness testimony, Michigan trial judge Donald Shelton stated that he would be "reluctant to allow expert testimony on the credibility of eyewitnesses generally, but would allow it, of course, about a particular witness" (e.g., to show that the witness had poor eyesight).[66]

While usually deferring to the ruling of the trial court, the appellate court decisions nationwide reveal increasingly divided opinion. In *United States v. Hall*,[67] the Seventh Circuit cites a long line of cases excluding expert testimony on eyewitness identification. In *United States v. Rincon*,[68] the Ninth Circuit suggested educating jurors through cautionary instructions on eyewitness identification rather than by expert testimony. It would be less costly, said the court, and unlike expert testimony, it would not confuse or mislead the jury.[69]

In *United States v. Amaral*,[70] defense counsel sought to introduce the expert testimony of Bertram Raven, a social psychologist, on the effect of stress on perception and, more generally, on the unreliability of eyewitness identification. The trial court considered this a novel question and, in view of the prosecutor's opposition, requested both sides to submit authorities supporting their respective contentions. No appellate or trial court decision was cited by either counsel. The trial court excluded the proffered testimony on the ground that "it would not be appropriate to take from the jury their own determination as to what weight or effect to give to the evidence of the eyewitness and identifying witnesses and to have that determination put before them on the basis of the expert witness testimony as proffered."[71] The Ninth Circuit Court of Appeals, in an opinion of 1973, ruled that the trial court did not err in excluding the testimony. Six years later, a trial judge allowed Dr. Raven's testimony and he, thereafter, similarly testified a number of times, as have several other social psychologists.[72]

In *United States v. Fosher*,[73] the First Circuit in 1979 upheld a trial court's exclusion of such expert testimony on the ground that "the average lay juror, on the basis of his own life experiences and common sense, can make an informed evaluation of eyewitness testimony without the assistance of a psychologist, particularly when the jurors are aided by professional argument and skilled cross-examination."

The Arizona Supreme Court in 1983 took a different position in *State v. Chapple*,[74] the first appellate decision in the United States to rule that a judge abused his discretion in excluding expert testimony concerning eyewitness reliability. In this case, a murder prosecution in which the only issue was accuracy of eyewitness identification, the court held it erred to exclude expert testimony offered by the defendant regarding factors relevant to identification accuracy: the effect of stress on perception, the rate of forgetting, transference—the tendency to believe a person was seen at a certain time and place when the person was actually seen at that place at a different time or at another place, and the tendency of witnesses who have talked together to reinforce one another's identifications. The court said, "Depriving [the] jurors of the benefit of scientific research on eyewitness testimony force[d] them to search for the truth without full knowledge and opportunity to evaluate the strength of the evidence. In short, this deprivation prevent[ed] [the] jurors from having 'the best possible degree' of 'understanding the subject' toward which the law of evidence strives."

A number of federal circuits have joined the ranks of *Chapple*. In *United States v. Downing*,[75] the Third Circuit in 1985 held that excluding expert testimony of the accuracy of eyewitness testimony is inconsistent with the liberal standard of admissibility under the Federal Rules of Evidence adopted in 1975. In this case, the defendant sought to adduce, from an expert in the field of human perception and memory, testimony concerning reliability of eyewitness identifications. The trial court refused to admit the testimony, apparently because it believed such testimony can never meet the "helpfulness" standard under the rules of evidence. The Third Circuit, holding error by the trial court, said that admission of such testimony is conditional, not automatic.[76]

The Fifth Circuit in 1986 concluded, "Expert testimony on eyewitness reliability is not simply a recitation of facts available through common knowledge. Indeed, the conclusions of the psychological studies are largely counterintuitive, and serve to 'explode common myths about an individual's capacity for perception.'"[77]

A number of state appellate courts have also joined the ranks of *Chapple*. In 1984, the California Supreme Court held that when an eyewitness identification "is a key element of the prosecution's case, but is not substantially corroborated by evidence giving it independent reliability, and the defendant offers qualified expert testimony on specific psychological factors shown by the record that could have affected the accuracy of the identification, but are not likely to be fully known to or understood by the jury, it will ordinarily be error to exclude that testimony."[78]

In 1988 in New York, a professor of psychology, an expert in the field of memory and perception, was permitted to testify at trial, on behalf of the defendant, as to the effect of stress on identification, the psychological effect of delay between the criminal event and subsequent identification, and the lack of correlation between a prospective witness's confidence *and* accuracy of recollection.[79] Then, in 2001, New York State's highest court ruled that expert testimony on the reliability of eyewitnesses could be admitted at trial. The court ruled such testimony "is not inadmissible per se" and warned judges not to exclude it solely on the grounds that jurors are already equipped to make an informed judgment.[80]

In 1991, the South Carolina Supreme Court, reversing a conviction, ruled it prejudicial error to exclude a psychologist's testimony on the unreliability of eyewitness identifications by white victims of black defendants.[81] The New Jersey Supreme Court, taking judicial notice of studies on the inaccuracy of cross-racial recognition, ruled in 1999 in a cross-racial rape case that even without expert testimony the jury should be told that cross-racial identifications may be less reliable than same-race ones.[82] The court urged caution:

> [W]e recognize that unrestricted use of cross-racial identification instructions could be counterproductive. Consequently, care must be taken to insulate criminal trials from base appeals to racial prejudice. An appropriate jury instruction should carefully delineate the context in which the jury is permitted to consider racial differences. The simple fact pattern of a white victim of a violent crime at the hands of a black assailant would not automatically give rise to the need for a cross-racial identification charge. More is required.[83]

There's a Russian saying: "He lies like an eyewitness." In sum and substance, expert testimony on eyewitness identification in general invariably puts into question its accuracy. It makes jurors wary of all eyewitness testimony. Therefore, the prevailing view would have it that, as set out by Michigan Judge Donald Shelton, the appropriate role of the expert is to assist the attorney in attacking the credibility of a particular witness, not to discuss as in a classroom the credibility of eyewitnesses generally.

When testifying generally about eyewitness testimony, the expert may have no particular reason to challenge the witness. A cigar may be a cigar, as Freud said; in this case, an accurate witness. Ann Wollner, associate editor of the *Fulton County Daily Report*, writes: "The point is not to blunt the effect of all eyewitness identifications. The point is to inform juries when to be wary of them, when to look harder for corroborating evidence, when to remind themselves that just because the witness is certain doesn't mean the witness is right."[84]

Reliability of Messenger and Message

Who are unreliable as witnesses? Children are not very reliable. Mental defectives are unreliable. People with organic brain disease are unreliable. Psychotics are unreliable. Psychopaths are liars. Obsessive compulsives deny various things and obviously cannot be reliable about these things. The law is replacing the old categories (those involved in the five I's of interest, insanity, infancy, infidelity, and infamy) whereby large groups of people were excluded as incompetent with psychiatric categories. Popular disapproval of drug addiction and chronic alcoholism is so strong that it would be imprudent to introduce an addict as a witness. The courts say: "The habitual use of opium is known to utterly deprave the victim of its use and render him unworthy of belief."[85] "We believe it will be admitted that habitual users of opium, or other like narcotics, become notorious liars. The habit of lying comes doubtless from the fact that these narcotics users pass the greater part of their life in an unreal world, and thus become unable to distinguish between images and facts, between illusion and realities."[86]

A minority of courts take the position that addicts per se are predilected toward untruthfulness and, by so holding, the court takes away the jury's prerogative to assess credibility. In an old parallel, St. Thomas maintained with the authority of St. Chrysostom, *Daemoni, etiam vera dicenti, non est credendum* (the devil is not to be believed, even when he tells the truth). In the absence of other proofs, it was said, one must not proceed against those who are accused by devils. Christ imposed silence on the demons when they spoke the truth.

Obviously, though, no one can judge the reliability of a group of people as a class. It may be expeditious, but a great error, to generalize. For example, it is sometimes said that a person is an alcoholic and then his testimony is excluded on the ground that alcoholics are not reliable witnesses. However, many persons are alcoholics (or have an alcoholic problem) even if they have not drunk any alcohol in a year or more. Many who have an alcoholic problem hold most responsible positions and are reliable when not drinking to excess. If all alcoholics were disqualified as reliable observers, we should disqualify many judges, lawyers, psychiatrists, and clergy. But suppose, instead of deciding on the basis of class, we consider each individual as an individual, try to understand his reactions to various situations, and examine the reliability of his stories under various circumstances. Would that be of any help in resolving disputes?

To estimate one's reliability presumably calls for knowing something of his unconscious motivation. Lawyers are specialists in verbal communication and usually deal with conscious motivation, but psychiatrists, specialized in listening with the third ear, are concerned about unconscious motivation and nonverbal communication. Of course, lawyers such as Perry Mason read between the lines, understanding unconscious motivation though not identifying it as such. Research has found, however, that even those skilled at lie detection, such as Jo-Ellan Dimitrius or police and customs officers, are no better than the general public at successfully detecting deception.[87] The only professional group found by psychologists to be consistently better than the general public at detecting deception were secret service agents selected for bodyguard duty, but their advantage appears to lie in the fact that they do not trust anyone.

On a practical and personal level, we all have known friends who are not alcoholic or addictive or psychopathic, but when they make out their federal income tax return, it becomes very questionable how far they are reliable. There may be times when perhaps no one is reliable. On the other hand, there are individuals who list every conceivable item on their tax return. They are scrupulously honest. We might say that they are reliable honest people. But the psychiatrist looks behind the scene and asks, "Why does this person have to be so honest?" Hamlet, looking behind his mother's pretenses, said: "The lady doth protest too much, me thinks." When somebody is too scrupulously honest, he may be worried about his dishonest tendencies and distrustful of himself. An individual may be very compulsive, a perfectionist, always being sure that he is clean, etc., but when we look carefully at him, we may find that underneath his clean shirt, he has not bathed or wears dirty underwear.

What Is the Relationship of Man to His Message?

Philosophy traditionally has taught that words lead a life independent of the messenger. Under the correspondence theory of truth, the relation studied is strictly that between the statement and the world. Personalizing is ruled out under the well-known *ad hominem* objection. But, we may ask, does the *ad hominem* (or *ad feminam*) objection need reevaluation? What is the relationship between ideas, mentation, and biography? A person gains in understanding his own philosophy and ideas by examination and analysis of his mental processes and motivations, as psychoanalysis may attest. Do we likewise, in examining the philosophy or message of another person, add a dimension to it by understanding his personality? Man's message reveals the man; does man reveal the message?

Freud, although never concealing his background as a Jew, often worried about protecting his new science from a closeness with the personality of its creator. Notwithstanding, psychoanalysis is often called a "Jewish science." David Bakan in his book, *Freud and the Jewish Mystical Tradition*, says that Freudianism is a laic transformation of the Jewish mystique. Bakan shows the decisive importance of Freud's Jewishness in the formulation of his work and the need to be aware of this fact for the best interpretation of his work.

That Immanuel Kant's neighbors set their clocks by his routine is not surprising to one having knowledge of his obsessive behavior. Schopenhauer, too, is known to have been an obsessional neurotic. Jean-Jacques Rousseau's noble savage and state-of-nature philosophy may be linked with his psychosexual infantilism, which expressed itself also in exhibitionism, narcissism, and homosexual trends. Bishop Berkeley's idealism and denial of reality may be tied in with his attitudes regarding excretion. Nietzsche's mother was considered to be hereditarily tainted. Hegel's philosophical system begins where repression is involved, where thesis turns into antithesis. Albert Deutsch in his book, *The Mentally Ill in America*, raises the issue of the credibility of Mrs. E. P. W. Packard, the famous crusader for the enactment of commitment laws, pointing to her psychiatric history.

Is such biography helpful to a study of a message? The roots of psychohistory, as it is called, may go back to Freud's *Leonardo da Vinci: A Study in Psychosexuality*, published in 1916, which analyzed the Renaissance genius on the basis of his work and from available records, and to his work, in 1939, *Moses and Monotheism*, which attempted to discover in Moses' life the origins of Christianity. Historian Robert G. L. Waite in a postscript in *The Mind of Adolf Hitler* praises Dr. Walter Langer's use in his secret wartime report of psychoanalytic principles to investigate Hitler's psyche. The technique, he says, led not only to predictions of uncanny accuracy, but to insights never provided by historians relying on traditional research methods.

It is necessary, it seems, to distinguish the various functions of language—informative, expressive, directive—that is, to transmit information, to express mood, and to promote action. Different criteria are relevant in evaluating each function: truth and falsehood for the informative; sincerity or insincerity, valuable or otherwise, for the expressive; and proper or improper, right or wrong, for the directive. Of all disciplines, there is the fullest exploitation of the genetic dimension in psychoanalysis; psychoanalysis links the present with genesis, but that is for the purpose of treatment. Genesis or biography has little relevance to a person's message if the message is to be evaluated in terms of truth and falsehood. The fact that Kant's neighbors set their clocks by his afternoon walks has no logical bearing on the truth or informative significance of his philosophy. From his character, we may surmise that he would ponder his statements at length, but the psychological origin of a belief, the motive for holding it, and the condition that leads to its acceptance are all irrelevant to its truth or falsehood. Kekule, the chemist who formulated the benzene ring, dreamed the night before of a snake with its tail in its mouth, but the theory of benzene rings is not to be equated with a dream about a snake. Freud's explanation of how belief in God is born need not be inconsistent with that belief. A message is substantiated by the available evidence, not by its genesis.

If the function of a message, however, is expressive and directive as well as informative (and usually all three functions are included) then, because criteria other than truth and falsehood are involved in its evaluation, biography should be not only helpful, but essential to an evaluation and understanding of the message.

The court is essentially concerned with the informative function of a message, and the fact that an individual may be an unreliable witness does not imply that he will be unreliable. No witness is completely unreliable at all times, just as the sky in Texas is not cloudy all the time. The courtroom process is a practical one, however, and when testimony conflicts and the evidence of a witness is crucial, the *ad hominem* approach may be practically, but not theoretically, justified. There are posters in some libraries that say, "If it is the truth, what does it matter who said it?" But in the mundane world, it is not only what a witness says, but how he says it and who he is that is important. This is not epistemology. To look at a man, including his sacroiliac, is justified in terms of convenience and public policy, resulting in a rough sense of justice. It is a question of fair judgment, and it is thought that psychiatry may lend a hand in reaching that judgment. Yet, as pointed out, a number of factors in the legal setting make it difficult, perhaps impossible, to obtain a reliable psychiatric evaluation. A psychiatric evaluation usually rests on the complete trust between the patient and psychiatrist. This trust implies that the psychiatrist is totally on the patient's side, will not reveal information the patient has confided, and will be primarily concerned with the patient's welfare rather than that of society.

Psychiatrist as Detective

Freud in one of his lectures pointed out that a psychiatrist with a patient is different from a lawyer with a witness. A psychiatrist can allow himself to be hoodwinked because if the psychiatrist does not show his belief in the patient, he will not be able to establish a successful relationship with him. The patient does not hurt the psychiatrist in hoodwinking him. Rather he is hurting himself. On the witness stand, however, in an attempt to hoodwink, the witness seeks to protect rather than to hurt himself.

A sharp poker player probably knows better than a psychiatrist whether a person is lying or, as the legal test puts it, whether the emotional or mental condition of the witness may affect his ability to tell the truth. A psychiatrist is a doctor, not a lie detector. A lawyer, too, has his shortcomings as an investigator. Although Perry Mason solves cases on the stand (he also solves cases out of court), skillful interrogation and evaluation can more readily take place in the police station than in the courtroom. Such a procedure, however, is against our tradition of law enforcement. In *Leyra v. Denno*,[88] working in a room that was wired, rather than rendering medical aid that the accused was expecting, the psychiatrist "by subtle and suggestive questions simply continued the police effort" to obtain a confession. The police may use trickery, but not psychiatrists. The Supreme Court invalidated the confession and denounced the admission of statements made to the psychiatrist as "so clearly the product of mental coercion that their use as evidence is inconsistent with due process." Nowadays the role of psychiatrists in interrogating alleged terrorists is controversial. After much discussion, the American Psychiatric Association, in 2006, approved a Position Statement, "Psychiatric Participation in Interrogation of Detainees," declaring that no psychiatrist should participate directly in interrogation of prisoners.

Refusal by a trial court to order a psychiatric examination of a witness has almost always been held not to be an abuse of discretion. When the court does order such examinations, what sanctions does it have available to compel compliance? Rule 35 of the Federal Rules of Civil Procedure and similar state statutes authorize trial courts to order a physical or mental examination of a party when his physical or mental condition is in controversy, that is, to determine injury sustained by a party in a personal injury suit. The rule probably does not include psychiatric examination as to credibility, especially of an ordinary witness, as credibility is not a matter directly in controversy. The power to order a psychiatric examination, although not provided by statute, may be said to be part of inherent or implied judicial power;[89] but even in rape cases some courts have been hesitant to order psychiatric examination of the complainant.[90]

Hypnosis is accepted by the American Medical Association as a valid medical technique. It is accepted by both the American Medical Association and the American Psychological Association as a legitimate psychiatric method of inquiry, but its use in the legal process at the pretrial or trial stage is highly dubious. The use of hypnosis by District Attorney Jim Garrison of his star witness in the alleged investigation of President Kennedy's assassination was a national scandal; the defense was unaware that the witness had been hypnotized prior to this testimony.

Not long before, Dr. Joseph Satten, then of the Menninger Foundation, at the behest of defense counsel, made a videotape of a sodium amytal (truth serum) interview of a person accused of murdering his wife. Its use was allowed at trial, resulting in the exculpation of the accused and was announced in television newscasts as a breakthrough in the search for truth.

An Ohio case is one of the few examples of in-court hypnosis (the subject in this case being the defendant).[91] On examination the hypnotist in the case contended that the subject had very little conscious control and, therefore, would be unable to lie in response to questions asked by the hypnotist. He testified that the statements made by a person under hypnosis would, with "reasonable medical certainty," be truthful and correct. He further stated that, except in the case of certain mental disorders, the use of hypnosis would discover the facts. In this case, the court allowed the hypnotist to ask questions whenever it appeared that the defendant was having difficulty understanding the attorney's questions. The procedure has been criticized as inherently suggestive.

Whether hypnosis is done for forensic or clinical purposes, the individual who has been hypnotized may be precluded from testifying. A number of courts have ruled that witnesses who have undergone hypnosis cannot be allowed to testify because of the possibility of the "pollution" of their testimony or because they cannot be properly subjected to cross-examination. Based on a ruling in 1982 by the California Supreme Court in *People v. Shirley*,[92] and followed by a number of other jurisdictions,[93] even a rape victim would not be allowed to testify about the rape if she had undergone hypnosis for any reason.[94] In so holding, these courts have restricted the use of hypnosis as an investigative device.[95] These rulings, however, do not preclude a defendant from giving testimony even though he has been hypnotized. With four justices dissenting, the U.S. Supreme Court held that a state may not bar the testimony of the accused. The majority opinion was "bottomed" on recognition of an accused's "constitutional right to testify in [his] own defense." It said: "A State's legitimate interest in barring unreliable evidence does not extend to per se exclusions that may be reliable in an individual case. Wholesale inadmissibility of a defendant's testimony is an arbitrary restriction on the right to testify in the absence of clear evidence by the State repudiating the validity of all posthypnosis recollections."[96] In 1989, California joined the many other jurisdictions refusing to apply the exclusionary rule to any witness to testimony about events recalled and recorded prior to the hypnotic session.[97]

Conclusion

To obtain an ideal climate for an effective psychiatric evaluation of a witness, a number of legal reforms would be necessary that might be unwise either from a social or legal point of view. If this is the case, then psychiatrists and jurists should realize the limitations that the legal procedure places on the accuracy and effectiveness of the psychiatric examination and, in turn, on the psychiatric opinion. But is psychiatry here being used more for its prestige value than for its probative value? And who is the reliable witness? Just thou and me, and I am not so sure about thee and thou is not so sure about me.

Endnotes

1. An early and graphic illustration is provided by the "Song of Roland"—the duel between Thierry and Pinabel to decide the fate of Ganelon. See C. Stephenson, *Mediaeval Feudalism* (Ithaca, NY: Cornell University Press, 1942), p. 34.
2. L. Green, "Jury Trial and Mr. Justice Black," *Yale L. J.* 65 (1965): 482.
3. A. Goodhart, "A Changing Approach to the Law of Evidence," *Va. L. Rev.* 51 (1965): 759, 761.
4. S. Rowley, "The Competency of Witnesses," *Iowa L. Rev.* 24 (1939): 482, 491–492.
5. W.S. Holdsworth, *History of English Law*, (London: Methuen, 3d ed., 1927).

6. It is unusual for a proposed witness today to be ruled incompetent and disqualified, except possibly in the case of the very young or the very old. That it does occur occasionally, however, is illustrated by the criminal case of People v. McCaughan, 49 Cal.2d 409, 317 P.2d 974 (1957), which involved the prosecution of a psychiatric aide at a state mental hospital charged with the involuntary manslaughter of one of the patients resulting from use of excessive force in spoon feeding. The patient, a 70-year-old woman, had refused to eat, believing that the food was poisoned. The prosecutor offered, as witnesses against the accused, other patients at the hospital. Perhaps seeking to protect the aide from criminal conviction, the California Supreme Court ruled that the court below had committed error because these witnesses had a history of insane delusions regarding the same matter as did the deceased. The decision is criticized in Note, *So. Cal. L. Rev.* 32 (1957): 65.

   In another criminal case, People v. Lapsley, 26 Mich. App. 424, 182 N.W.2d 601 (1970), patients in a state mental home were allowed to testify against the defendant for torturing another patient, a 14-year-old girl. The witnesses, all minors with mental problems, were examined by the judge prior to their testimony and deemed to be mentally competent for testimonial purposes.

7. Robertson v. Hackensack Trust Co., 11 N.J. 304, 317, 63 A.2d 515, 521 (1949; concurring opinion).

8. The chapter titles in one book on cross-examination include "Break Your Witness," "Step by Step Attack," "Witness on the Run," "The Kill," "Shock Treatment." Chapter titles of another book include "The Deposition Game," "Hold the Eye of the Witness," "Roll with the Punch," "Don't Beat a Dead Horse," "When Should Mud Be Thrown?" "Making Speeches While Objecting," "Endure the Torment," "Indirectly Depreciating the Witness, How about Sarcasm?" "Hot on the Trial," "Stay in Command," "Don't Telegraph Your Punch," "Preserve the Damaging Answer," "You Are Awfully Expensive, Doctor." See J.A. Appleman, *Cross-Examination* (Fairfax, VA: Coiner Publications, 1963).

9. "Psychiatry and drugs may have given us new insights into motivation, but the classic Anglo-Saxon method of cross-examination is still the best means of coping with deception, of dragging the truth out of a reluctant witness, and assuring the triumph of justice over venality." L. Nizer, *My Life in Court* (New York: Doubleday, 1961). On the misbegotten "brain fingerprinting" in lie detection, see P.S. Appelbaum, "The New Lie Detectors: Neuroscience, Deception, and the Courts," *Psychiat. Serv.*, 58 (April 2007): 460.

10. Reversed in Quercia v. United States, 289 U.S. 466, 471-72 (1933). See also NLRB v. Universal Camera Corp., 190 F.2d 429, 430 (2d Cir. 1951).

11. In United States v. Azure, 801 F.2d 336 (8th Cir. 1986), the Eighth Circuit held that the trial court's admission of a pediatrician's testimony that an alleged victim of childhood sexual abuse "was believable" and that he could "see no reason why she would not be telling the truth in this matter" constituted reversible error. The court reasoned that, although some expert testimony may be helpful in child sexual abuse cases, "putting an impressively qualified expert's stamp of truthfulness on a witness's story goes too far"; 801 F.2d at 339–340.

12. "It is well settled that an expert witness may not render an opinion as to a complainant's veracity … . Matters of credibility are to be determined by the trier of fact." People v. Miller, 418 N.W.2d 668 (Mich. App. 1987). In State v. Heath, 341 S.E.2d 565 (N.C. 1986), the North Carolina Supreme Court overruled a lower court decision allowing a psychologist to state concerning a witness that there was "nothing in the record or current behavior to indicate that she has a record of lying." The appellate court held that the expert had gone beyond the scope of her expertise and had testified to the victim's credibility or record for truth or veracity, a matter upon which the jury was as qualified as the witness to decide.

13. State v. Milbradt, 756 P.2d 620, 624 (Ore. 1988; emphasis by court).

14. United States v. Barnard, 490 F.2d 907, 912 (9th Cir. 1973), *cert. denied*, 416 U.S. 959 (1974). See M.A. Berger, "*United States v. Scop*: The Common-Law Approach to an Expert's Opinion About a Witness's Credibility Still Does Not Work," *Brooklyn L. Rev.* 55 (1989): 559. However, the attorney in closing argument quite often says that a witness was not telling the truth, or in cross-examination will ask the witness which of his statements is to be believed, and objection is often not made, or there is no reversal.

15. H. Davidson, "Appraisal of the Witness," *Am. J. Psychiat.* 110 (1954): 481; see also his classic book, *Forensic Psychiatry* (New York: Ronald Press, 1952).

16. R. Banay, "The Psychiatrist in Court," in R. Slovenko (Ed.), *Crime, Law and Corrections* (Springfield, IL: Thomas, 1966), p. 433. Hitler and his propagandists and ideologists carried on a paranoid anti-Semitic account of the world war. The literary scholar Viktor Klemperer wrote in his diary in 1944, "[T]he Jew is in every respect the center of the language of the Third Reich, indeed of its whole view

of the epoch." The art historian E.H. Gombrich wrote that what characterized Nazi propaganda was "the imposition of a paranoic pattern on world events." See J. Herf, *The Jewish Enemy/Nazi Propaganda During World War II and the Holocaust* (Cambridge, MA: Harvard University Press, 2006).

17. United States v. Hiss, 88 F. Supp. 559 (S.D.N.Y. 1950).

18. 88 F. Supp. at 559.

19. New York: Viking, 1967.

20. Fifteen years later, Dr. Binger, reflecting on the Hiss case, had this to say:

> My opinion of Chambers and the Hiss trial was based almost entirely on the seven volumes of sworn testimony, which he deposed in Baltimore before the trial. This was an exposition of a life so irregular and so delinquent that one could only interpret it as the story of a psychopath. Many of my psychiatric friends agreed with me in this decision, but were less willing to expose themselves to ridicule and contumely than I was. Perhaps they were wiser. But I never regretted my stand nor had I any serious doubts about Hiss's innocence. I did suspect some hidden, unconscious relationship with Chambers, of which I believe Hiss was unaware, and that this led him into an involvement which might well have looked like a conspiracy. He certainly never gave signed state documents to Chambers … . The prosecutor, Mr. Murphy, who looked like a dumb cop, turned out to be highly astute and tricky. He resorted to all kinds of subterfuges to trip me up. He tried to turn words around in my mouth and forced me to answer "yes" and "no" to questions framed in such a manner that the answers did not convey the meaning that I wished to present. I know that this is all part of the game, but it seemed to me shocking and preposterous. I had only one wish and that was to tell the truth and not lose my temper. I think I did both. Mr. Murphy, on the other hand, was determined to try to have me lose my temper and to distort the truth.

Correspondence of November 23, 1965, to Ralph Slovenko from Dr. Carl Binger, quoted with permission. See W.P. Hill, "The Use and Abuse of Cross-Examination in Relation to Expert Testimony: The Second Alger Hiss Trial," *Ohio St. L. J.* 15 (1954): 458.

21. S. Tanenhaus, *Whittaker Chambers: A Biography* (New York: Random House, 1997); A. Weinstein, *Perjury: The Hiss-Chambers Case* (New York: Random House, 1978); see M. Ladd, "Techniques and Theory of Character Testimony," *Iowa L. Rev.* 24 (1939): 498. Still, there are studies maintaining that Hiss was not a Soviet spy, the most recent being K. Bird & S. Shervonnaya, "The Mystery of Ales," *Am. Schol.* 76 (Summer 2007): 20.

22. See, e.g., Knode v. Williamson, 17 Wall. 586 (U.S. 1873).

23. This phrase is used in the state's Supplemental Memorandum to People v. Jones, 42 Cal.2d 219, 266 P.2d 38 (1954), a pioneering case in which the court said that if the crime on charge involved a trait indicating a tendency toward sexual perversion, the accused may adduce expert psychiatric testimony that he is not a sexual deviate. The case is critically examined in J.F. Falknor & D.T. Steffen, "Evidence of Character: From the 'Crucible of the Community' to the 'Couch of the Psychiatrist,'" *U. Pa. L. Rev.* 102 (1954): 980; but it is viewed with favor in W. Curran, "Expert Psychiatric Evidence of Personality Traits," *U. Pa. L. Rev.* 10 3(1955): 999. In Hopkins v. State, 480 S.W.2d 212 (Tex. Crim. App. 1972), the court said that the divergence of psychiatric opinion and its frequent inexactness render its value minimal in enabling the jury to decide the issue of credibility. In fact, the court said, the jury after being subjected to several conflicting, equivocating, and highly technical psychiatric opinions may actually be more confused than before. Another court failed to perceive the benefit to be gained from "an amateur's voyage on the fog-enshrouded sea of psychiatry." See Note, *St. Mary's L. Rev.* 4 (1972): 460.

24. See, e.g., Barrel of Fun v. State Farm Fire & Cas. Co., 739 F.2d 1028 (5th Cir. 1984); D.T. Lykken, *A Tremor in the Blood: Uses and Abuses of the Lie Detector* (New York: Plenum, 1998). Yet polygraph use is now at the highest level in two decades. Government agencies from local police departments to the CIA are increasingly using the technology for job interviews. In courts lately, judges have expended the instances in which polygraph testing is mandated or admitted as evidence. Polygraphy is used increasingly in parole and probation programs that are designed to dissuade sex offenders and other felons from committing more crimes. Polygraph testing is becoming a standard for supervising probationers of all kinds. It is increasingly being used in administrative hearings (such as in medical board hearings). See L.P. Cohen, "The Polygraph Paradox," *Wall Street Journal*, March 22–23, 2008, p. 1.

25. H. Davidson, "Appraisal of the Witness," *Am. J. Psychiat.* 110 (1954): 481. See also H.B. Dearman, "Psychiatric Examination of the Client," *Tenn. L. Rev.* 32 (1965): 592; E.H. Moore, "Elements of Error in Testimony," *Ore. L. Rev.* 28 (1949): 293. See, generally, P.H. Hoch & J. Zubin, (Eds.), *Psychopathology of Perception* (New York: Grune & Stratton, 1965); A.A. Smirnov, *Problems of the Psychology of Memory* (New York: Plenum Press, 1973).

26. In United States v. Butler, 481 F.2d 531 (D.C. App. 1973), the court said, "The question of when a trial judge should order a physical and psychiatric examination of a prosecution witness was directly considered by this court in United States v. Benn & Hunt … . We, therefore, explained that such an examination 'may seriously impinge on a witness's right to privacy; … the examination itself could serve as a tool of harassment'; and the likelihood of an examination could deter witnesses from coming forward … . The resultant presumption against ordering an examination must be overcome by a showing of need." Quoting United States v. Benn & Hunt, 476 F.2d 1127 (D.C. App. 1973).

   In People v. Carter, 128 Mich. App. 541, 341 N.W.2d 128 (1983), rev'd on other grounds, 42 Mich. 941, 369 N.W.2d 842 (1985), the Michigan Court of Appeals held that the trial court did not abuse its discretion on grounds of relevancy in precluding the defense from impeaching the complainant with evidence of her alleged drug use and psychiatric problems. A witness's history of prostitution was excluded in People v. Chaplin, 412 Mich. 219, 313 N.W.2d 899 (1981); the Michigan Supreme Court ruled that prior acts of prostitution have no relation to veracity. See C.B. Mueller & L.C. Kirkpatrick, *Evidence* (New York: Aspen, 2d ed., 1999), p. 541.

27. Comment, "Psychiatric Evaluation of the Mentally Abnormal Witness," *Yale L. J.* 59 (1950): 1324.

28. R. Monroe, "The Psychiatric Examination," in R. Slovenko (Ed.), *Crime, Law and Corrections* (Springfield, IL: Thomas, 1966), p. 439.

29. 88 W. Va. 479, 107 S.E. 189 (1921).

30. In sex cases, less so today than previously, considerable latitude in cross-examination of witnesses is permitted, on the theory that the accusation is easily made and difficult to disprove. The courts have permitted psychiatrists to expose mental defects, hysteria, and pathological lying in sex prosecutrices. See, e.g., People v. Rainford, 58 Ill. App. 2d 312, 208 N.E.2d 314 (1965); see S. Estrich, *Real Rape* (Cambridge, MA: Harvard University Press, 1987); A.E. Taslitz, *Rape and the Culture of the Courtroom* (New York: New York University Press, 1997); M.G. Blinder, "The Hysterical Personality," *Psychiatry* 29 (1966): 227; R. Cavallaro, "A Big Mistake: Eroding the Defense of Mistake of Fact About Consent in Rape," *J. Crim. L. & Criminol.* 86 (1996): 815; S. Estrich, "Rape," *Yale L. J.* 95 (1986): 1087; D.N. Husak & G.C. Thomas, "Date Rape, Social Convention, and Reasonable Mistakes," *Law & Phil.* 11 (1992): 95; C.L. Muehlenhard & L.C. Hollabaugh, "Do Women Sometimes Say No When They Mean Yes? The Prevalence and Correlates of Women's Token Resistance to Sex," *J. Personal. & Soc. Psychol.* 54 (1988): 872.

   Women who make false accusations of rape tend not to be prosecuted. The North Carolina attorney general declined to charge a stripper with making false accusations that several Duke University lacrosse players had sexually assaulted her because of her "mental health history." It was a travesty of justice that lasted 395 days. Google the names of the lacrosse players and up come 1,000 stories that mention "arrest," "charge," "accusations," and "rape," but the name of the accuser is not widely released, as if an obligation remains to protect her (her name and photo are revealed in the *Weekly Standard*, Sept. 24, 2007, p. 40). During the course of the proceedings, protest rallies were held against the Duke players. One of the signs at these rallies read "Take Back the Night," though the woman they were supporting worked nights as an exotic dancer. With its overtones of race, sex, and privilege, the Duke case instantly drew national media attention. See M. Albom, "Where Do They Go to Get Their Names Back?" *Detroit Free Press*, April 13, 2007, p. D1; D. Wilson & D. Barstow, "Duke Prosecutor Throws Out Case Against Players," *New York Times*, April 12, 2007, p. 1.

   In 1987, a 15-year-old girl named Tawana Brawley claimed that six white men had raped her and covered her face in feces while shouting racial slurs. The Rev. Al Sharpton hurried to Duchess County, New York. He accused a local white prosecutor, Steve Pagones, of being one of the rapists. The problem was, Pagones did not do it, and for that matter, nobody did. Brawley made the whole thing up. Pagones eventually sued and, 11 years later, won a defamation verdict with Sharpton owing $65,000 (which was paid by the late Johnnie Cochran and others). See R.T. Ford, *The Race Card* (New York: Farrar, Straus & Giroux, 2008).

31. E.F. Loftus & R.L. Steinberg, "If Memory Serves," *Wall Street Journal*, March 9, 2007, p. 14.

32. Evidence of mental illness is introduced on grounds that it affects the witness's "capacity to perceive, to recollect, or to communicate." United States v. Partin, 493 F.2d 750 (5th Cir. 1974). Impeachment with evidence of mental health problems is subject to the standard considerations of Rule 403, such as prejudice or confusion of the issues; United States v. Lopez, 611 F.2d 44 (4th Cir. 1979). Considerations

of embarrassing the witness are not often mentioned, but undoubtedly are also taken into consideration. Some conditions, such as schizophrenia, have more probative value in showing that the witness's testimony may have been deluded than do others.

33. People v. Francis, 5 Cal.App. 3d 414, 85 Cal. Rptr. 61, 64 (1970).
34. 698 F.2d 1154 (11th Cir. 1983).
35. Quoting M. Juviler, "Psychiatric Opinions as to Credibility of Witnesses: A Suggested Approach," *Cal. L. Rev.* 48 (1960): 648.
36. 698 F.2d at 1168.
37. State v. Armstrong, 232 N.C. 727, 62 S.E.2d 50 (1950). See also People v. Schuemann, 190 Colo. 474, 548 P.2d 911 (1976); Mosley v. Commonwealth, 420 S.W.2d 679 (Ky. 1967). Taking a different view, the Oregon Supreme Court declined to overturn a trial court's refusal to order the prosecutrix in a rape case to submit to psychiatric examination, saying: "It has not been demonstrated that the art of psychiatry has yet developed into a science so exact as to warrant such a basic intrusion into the jury process"; State v. Walgraeve, 243 Ore. 328, 413 P.2d 6095 (1966). See R.J. O'Neale, "Court Ordered Psychiatric Examination of a Rape Victim in a Criminal Rape Prosecution: Or How Many Times Must a Woman Be Raped?" *Santa Clara L. Rev.* 18 (1978): 119.
38. Rule 603, Federal Rules of Evidence.
39. See H. Silving, "The Oath," *Yale L. J.* 68 (1959): 1328.
40. Rule 601, Federal Rules of Evidence.
41. 57 F.3d 126 (1st Cir. 1995).
42. The case is discussed in A.W. Scheflin & D. Brown, "The False Litigant Syndrome: 'Nobody Would Say That Unless It Was the Truth,'" *J. Psychiat. & Law* 27 (1999): 649. See also United States v. Gonzalez-Maldonado, 115 F.3d 9 (1st Cir. 1997).
43. K. Hausman, "Does Pathological Lying Warrant Inclusion in DSM?" *Psychiat. Ann.* 38 (Jan. 3, 2003): 1, 24.
44. C.C. Dike, M. Baranoski, & E.E. H. Griffith, "Pathological Lying Revisited," *J. Am. Acad. Psychiat. & Law* 32 (2005): 342; D. Grubin, "Getting at the Truth About Pathological Lying," *J. Am. Acad. Psychiat. & Law* 33 (2005): 350; R. Sharrock & M. Cresswell, "Pseudologia Fantastica: A Case Study of a Man Charged With Murder," *Med. Sci. Law* 29 (1989): 323; A. Vaughan, "Believe Me—I Cannot Tell the Truth," *Independent*, July 9, 1991, p. 13.
45. 93 F.3d 1337 (7th Cir. 1996).
46. Kolb v. State, 930 P.2d 1238 (Wyo. 1996).
47. 153 Or. App. 313, 956 P.2d 1054 (1998), *aff'd*, 329 Or. 188, 985 P.2d 1267 (1999).
48. It may be noted that statements made by a declarant under hypnosis are not simply attacked for credibility, but are excluded as incompetent evidence, yet statements made by a declarant who is suffering multiple personality disorder or is in a dissociative state are not excluded. See Dorsey v. State, 206 Ga. App. 709, 426 S.E.2d 224 (1992).
49. 956 P.2d at 1058.
50. The psychiatrist's proffered testimony was as follows (985 P.2d at 1269–70):

> Q. Doctor, have you had a chance to review a transcript of the testimony of [the victim] and the police reports in this case?
> A. Yes.
> Q. After reviewing the police reports, do you have an opinion with respect to [the victim], as to whether or not she suffered from any disorders as a result of the incident?
> A. Yes, I do.
> Q. Would you please tell us that opinion.
> A. My opinion, from looking at this material, is that she suffers from a dissociative amnesic disorder.
> Q. Why?
> A. The information would seem to indicate a degree of amnesia or lack of memory of what went on, conflicting kinds of responses to what went on at that incident. She admits in her testimony, on a number of occasions, that she was very nervous, very frightened, that her mind wasn't functioning on what was going on, which is not uncommon after a traumatic incident of this nature, with normal people.
> Q. Under our legal standards, the law does not permit a witness to testify with respect to the credibility or truthfulness of a particular witness. Are you testifying to that effect here?

A. No. I think that the transcript and the written statement of the victim, there is no question as to her, in my opinion, conscious intent at truthfulness. I think that the inconsistencies that appear in the police reports and in her own words, saying "I don't remember," validate my conclusion in terms of the diagnosis. I think she's credible in terms of her efforts to do the best she can. It's not a question of truthfulness. It's a question of her mental ability to perform, having experienced what would appear to be a traumatic encounter.

Q. If a group of individuals had suffered a traumatic encounter, such as being kidnapped and being sexually assaulted, would a person that had been subjected to that kind of an assault have emotional factors that would influence their ability to remember the events with precision?

A. Yes.

Q. And would this hold true with respect to a group of people, as opposed to a particular individual?

A. Yes.

The state's cross-examination included the following:

Q. Would you repeat for me the words of what you called the disorder —

A. Dissociative amnesia.

Q. Is it a condition or a disorder?

A. A condition.

Q. A condition. So, when you say "dissociative amnesia," is that a diagnosis?

A. Yes.

Q. A medical diagnosis?

A. Yes.

Q. Are you making a medical diagnosis in this case?

A. It's a medical opinion.

Q. Can you tell the jury that you are diagnosing [the victim] with dissociative amnesia?

A. I can tell the jury that from the information available to me, it would appear that the condition pertains to the situation.

Q. But you can't tell them that you are diagnosing her as suffering from that?

A. Well, "suffering" is an ongoing term. It is related to this incident and her recall of the incident, it would seem, by virtue of my looking at her written information, the police information, and the transcripts of her testimony.

Q. So you are giving an opinion about her mental ability to perform when she is reporting the crime, her mental ability to—

A. Her recall of the incident.

Q. —to recall.

A. Memory.

Q. So you're saying that she cannot recall the incident?

A. Yes.

Q. And, in your opinion, she's confused about what she's saying?

A. It's my opinion she's confusing the events.

Q. The events? Which events?

A. The activities of the defendant here and the activities wherein she was assaulted.

Q. Well, where do you find the information on the police reports or her transcript that there were two separate events?

A. She describes different information than would apparently pertain to the arrest of the defendant.

Q. I'm sorry. I don't understand what you mean.

A. For instance, she doesn't describe a colored shirt, and defendant was apparently wearing one. She doesn't describe the seat belt in his car. There is quite a bit of questioning about a seat belt situation, and she says that the only type of seat belt she knows is one that goes around your waist. And then it looks like she's sort of led in questioning, one way or another. It would be my opinion that she's combining two incidents—one of a rescue situation, one of an attack situation—in her mind, retrospectively. It seems as though she's confused the two together.

Q. So the bottom line is that you don't believe the story she's telling?

A. I believe she believes what she's saying.

Q. But you believe that's not the truth?

A. I didn't say anything about truth. I believe she's telling the truth as she knows it.

Q. But you believe that it isn't the truth.

A. No. I believe that she has confused a situation because of an amnesic problem.

Q. You believe that there are other facts that she's not talking about?

A. No. I don't think she's doing anything volitionally.

Q. You believe that there are other facts that she is not able to talk about?

A. I think there are other facts that she doesn't remember.

On redirect examination, the defense asked the expert:

Q. Do you believe that [the victim's] conduct, as it relates to having this dissociative amnesia, compares with similarly situated people who have been subjected to violent attacks?

A. Yes.

985 P.2d at 1269-70.

51. 68 F.3d 1073 (8th Cir. 1995).

52. 68 F.3d at 1076.

53. 957 S.W.2d 52 (Tex. Cr. App. 1997).

54. 957 S.W.2d at 78. See Chapter 8 on syndrome evidence.

55. R. Starr, "Psychiatrists Take Note: Sometimes Silence Is Golden," *Insight*, Nov. 18, 1991, p. 40. In his book *My Grandfather's Son* (New York: HarperCollins, 2007), Justice Thomas says he was pilloried during the 1991 confirmation hearings because liberal advocacy groups feared he would vote to overturn abortion rights and they stooped to "the age-old blunt instrument of accusing a black man of sexual misconduct." N.A. Lewis, "In New Book, Justice Thomas Weighs in on Former Accuser," *New York Times*, Sept. 30, 2007, p. 24. Justice Thomas also made those accusations in a rare interview on CBS's *60 Minutes*, Sept. 30, 2007. In response, Anita Hill reiterated her allegation of sexual harassment; letters that were published mainly supported her. A. Hill, "The Smear This Time," *New York Times*, Oct. 2, 2007, p. 25; Ltrs., "Anita Hill vs. Clarence Thomas, Redux," *New York Times*, Oct. 3, 2007, p. 24. During the hearings, the tide began to turn in favor of Thomas when he described the conduct of the Judiciary Committee as tantamount to a "high-tech lynching." He portrayed himself as a defiant black man who was being unfairly imposed upon by a hypocritical, all-white gang of politicians eager to find some reason, any reason, to prevent an African-American male from attaining a coveted position of authority and honor. Thomas thus expertly played the race card. See R.T. Ford, *The Race Card* (New York: Farrar, Straus & Giroux, 2008); R. Kennedy, *Sellout: The Politics of Racial Betrayal* (New York: Pantheon Books, 2008).

56. Reprinted in Theodor Reik's *The Compulsion to Confess* (New York: Farrar, Straus & Cudahy, 1959).

57. Michigan CJI 2d 7.8.

58. Michigan CJI 2d 3.6.

59. See NLRB v. Universal Camera Corp., 190 F.2d 429, 430 (2d Cir. 1951).

60. D.L. Schacter, *The Seven Sins of Memory* (New York: Houghton Mifflin, 2001), p. 116.

61. H. Munsterberg, *On the Witness Stand* (New York: Clark Boardman, 1923).

62. In United States v. Pacelli, 521 F.2d 135 (2d Cir. 1975), *cert. denied*, 424 U.S. 911 (1976), the court refused to permit a psychiatrist to testify that the major prosecution witness was psychopathic and incapable of telling the truth. See G.L. Wells & E. Loftus (Eds.), *Eyewitness Testimony: Psychological Perspectives* (Cambridge, UK: Cambridge University Press, 1984). See also I. Freckleton & T. Henning, "Lies, Personality Disorders and Expert Evidence: New Developments in the Law," *Psychiat., Psychol. & Law* 5 (1998): 271.

63. J.E. Bishop, "Memory on Trial/Witnesses of Crimes Are Being Challenged as Frequently Fallible," *Wall Street Journal*, March 2, 1988, p. 1; see E. Loftus & K. Ketcham, *Witness for the Defense: The Accused, the Eyewitness, and the Expert Who Puts Memory on Trial* (New York: St. Martin's Press, 1991).

64. See G.L. Wells & E.F. Loftus (Eds.), *Eyewitness Testimony: Psychological Perspectives* (Cambridge, UK: Cambridge University Press, 1984); E.F. Loftus, *Eyewitness Testimony* (Cambridge, MA: Harvard University Press, 1979); R. Buckhout, "Eyewitness Testimony," *Sci. Am.* 321 (1974): 23.

65. In United States v. Smith, 122 F.3d 1355 (11th Cir. 1997), the court said, "[W]e have found only one case where a district court was reversed for excluding expert testimony regarding eyewitness reliability," and it cited United States v. Stevens, 935 F.3d 1380 (3d Cir. 1991). In *Stevens*, the trial court had admitted some of the expert's testimony, but the Third Circuit reversed because it had not admitted all of the relevant expert testimony. 935 F.2d at 1400. In *Smith*, a robbery case, an expert in eyewitness identification proposed to testify that eyewitness identification could be unreliable in the circumstances of the case: disguise, cross-racial identification, weapon focus, presentation bias in law enforcement lineup, delay between the event and the time of identification, stress, and eyewitness certainty as a predictor of accurate identification. The trial court excluded the proposed testimony in its entirety, holding that although the proposed testimony was relevant, it would not assist the trier of fact. Alternatively, the trial court held that the probative value of the testimony was outweighed by the

possible danger of misleading or confusing the jury. The Eleventh Circuit affirmed. Some courts have held that such evidence would be admissible under "narrow" or "certain" circumstances; United States v. Harris, 995 F.2d 532, 535 (4th Cir. 1993).

66. Conference, "Dealing With Eyewitness Testimony," on April 3, 1998 at the University of Michigan; reported in B.K. Hutson, "Eyewitness Testimony: Reliable or Misleading?" *Michigan Lawyers Weekly*, May 4, 1998, p.1. In Michigan in 1978, in People v. Hill, 84 Mich. App. 90, 269 N.W.2d 492 (1978), the Michigan Court of Appeals concluded that the trial court had not committed reversible error in excluding expert testimony regarding the process by which people perceive and remember events, and in 1996, in People v. Carson, 217 Mich. App. 801 (1996), the Michigan Court of Appeals reaffirmed its decision in *Hill*.

67. 165 F.3d 1095 (7th Cir. 1999).

68. 28 F.3d 921 (9th Cir. 1994).

69. 28 F.3d at 925.

70. 488 F.2d 1148 (9th Cir. 1973).

71. 488 F.2d at 1153.

72. B.H. Raven, "Social Psychological Factors in Eyewitness Testimony," presentation at the conference on "International Perspectives on Crime, Justice, and the Public Order," in St. Petersburg, Russia, June 21–27, 1992, sponsored by the St. Petersburg University and John Jay College of Criminal Justice.

73. 590 F.2d 381 (1st Cir. 1979).

74. 660 P.2d 1208 (Ariz. 1983).

75. 753 F.2d 1224 (3d Cir. 1985).

76. See also United States v. Smith, 736 F.2d 1103 (6th Cir. 1984).

77. United States v. Moore, 786 F.2d 1308 (5th Cir. 1986).

78. People v. McDonald, 37 Cal.3d 351, 208 Cal. Rptr. 236, 690 P.2d 709 (1984); see C.W. Walters, "Admission of Expert Testimony on Eyewitness Identification," *Cal. L. Rev.* 73 (1985): 1402. In People v. LeGrand, 8 N.Y. 3d 449, 867 N.F. 2d 374 (2007), New York's highest court said: "[W]e hold that where the case turns on the accuracy of eyewitness identifications and there is little or no corroborating evidence connecting the defendant to the crime, it is an abuse of discretion for a trial court to exclude expert testimony on the reliability of eyewitness identifications if that testimony is (1) relevant to the witness's identification of defendant, (2) based on the principles that are generally accepted within the relevant scientific community, (3) proffered by a qualified expert, and (4) on a topic beyond the ken of the average juror."

79. People v. Beckford, 532 N.Y.S.2d 462 (N.Y. Sup. 1988). In another New York case, where it was alleged that the accused was a victim of mistaken identity, Dr. Elizabeth Loftus testified about academic studies on possible weaknesses in the way crime witnesses identify suspects. She reported that many studies show that when a weapon is visible, the eyes of a witness can focus more intently on it than on the criminal's face; that the memory of a witness can be corrupted by seeing files of police photos or new accounts of the crimes; and that witnesses tend to make more mistakes in identifying suspects whose racial identity is different from their own. C. Drew, "Conflicting Testimony on Identifying Assailant in Brick-Attack Trial," *New York Times*, Nov. 25, 2000, p. B15.

80. People v. Lee, 2001 N.Y. Lexis 1061; reported in J.C. McKinley, "Court Opens Door to Data on Eyewitness Fallibility," *New York Times*, May 9, 2001, p. 27.

81. State v. Whaley, 305 S.C. 138, 406 S.E.2d 369 (1991).

82. State v. Cromedy, 158 N.J. 112, 727 A.2d 457 (1999).

83. 727 A.2d at 497.

84. A. Wollner, "Courts Eye the Problems of Eyewitness Identifications," *USA Today*, Sept. 29, 1999, p. 15. See also J. Gibeaut, "Yes, I'm Sure That's Him." *ABAJ*, Oct. 1999, p. 26. The expert testifying skeptically about eyewitness testimony no matter what is really believed by the expert brings to mind Freud's "skeptical" Jewish joke: Two Jews met in a railway station in Galicia. "Where are you going?" asked one. "To Cracow," was the answer. "What a liar you are!" replied the other. "If you say you are going to Cracow, you want me to believe you're going to Lemberg. But I know that in fact you're going to Cracow. So why are you lying to me?"

85. State v. Concannon, 25 Wash. 237, 65 Pac. 534, 537 (1901). In drug cases, the truth is often battered, ignored, or shaded. From the sworn affidavit of police seeking a search warrant to a defendant's court testimony, what is said under oath often falls short of the promise to speak the whole truth and nothing but the truth. Indeed, in all criminal trials, drug cases or otherwise, lying is commonplace. As a

rule, alcoholism or drug addiction are not deemed to be character traits that bear on truthfulness, but courts often admit such proof on the issue of capacity, that is, impairment of sensory and mental faculties. See United States v. Van Meerbeke, 548 F.2d 415 (2d Cir. 1976).

86. State v. Fog Loon, 29 Idaho 248, 158 Pac. 233, 236 (1916). The record in Irwin v. Ashurst, 158 Or. 61, 74 P.2d 1127 (1938), discloses the following questions and answers:

Q. As much as I hate to I am going to have to ask you a personal question. Do you use narcotics?
A. No, sir, not now.
Q. You don't use any at all?
A. I was ill for 10 years and the doctor gave me morphine at the time I had operations.
Q. You don't use them at all any more?
A. No.

During closing argument to the jury, counsel said the following concerning the witness: "Did you watch her? Did you see how she acted? The mind of a dope fiend, she was full of it, she was full of it when she testified; she showed she was an addict; why, she's a lunatic, she's a crazy lunatic; she's a dope fiend; how nervous she was all through her testimony; she's a hop head; her whole testimony is imagination and delusion from taking dope; all through her testimony she showed it; she testified she had taken dope for 10 years, and you may well know that she is still taking it; you know when a person has taken dope for 10 years, they never stop it; she's a dope fiend; she is lower than a rattlesnake; a rattlesnake gives you warning before it strikes, but this woman gives no warning; she is under a delusion from taking narcotics as long as she has; on account of her being an addict, I wouldn't believe a word she said."

87. See J. Dimitrius & M. Mazzarella, *Reading People* (New York: Ballantine, 1999).
88. 347 U.S. 556 (1954).
89. State v. Butler, 27 N.J. 560, 143 A.2d 530 (1958).
90. The Indiana Supreme Court and the California Court of Appeals have ruled that in sex-offender cases, when there is reason to doubt the truth of the accuser's allegations, a psychiatric examination should be made of the accuser to ascertain his or her mental and emotional condition and whether they have bearing on the accuser's credibility. The rulings stressed that the purpose of a psychiatric examination is "not to determine whether the witness is telling the truth, but to determine whether the emotional or mental condition of the witness may affect his or her ability to tell the truth." Easterday v. Indiana, 256 N.E.2d 901 (Ind. 1970); California v. Francis, 5 Cal. App. 3d 414, 85 Cal. Rptr. 61 (1970). See M. Juviler, "Psychiatric Opinions as to Credibility of Witnesses: A Suggested Approach," *Calif. L. Rev.* 48 (1960): 648.
91. State v. Nebb, No. 39540, Ohio C.P., Franklin Co., June 8, 1962; discussed in Note, "Hypnosis in Court: A Memory Aid for Witnesses," *Ga. L. Rev.* 1 (1976): 269.
92. People v. Shirley, 31 Cal.3d 18, 181 Cal. Rptr. 243, 641 P.2d 775, *cert. denied*, 103 S. Ct. 13 (1982). The California Supreme Court was influenced by the testimony of Dr. Bernard Diamond. See B. Diamond, "Inherent Problems in the Use of Pretrial Hypnosis on a Prospective Witness," *Cal. L. Rev.* 68 (1980): 313. See also A.W. Newman & J.W. Thompson, "The Rise and Fall of Forensic Hypnosis in Criminal Investigation, *J. Am. Acad. Psychiat. & Law* 29 (2001): 75.
93. By a 4–3 decision, the Michigan Supreme Court held that the testimony of a hypnotized witness is inadmissible, absent proof by clear and convincing evidence that the testimony being offered was based on facts recalled and related before hypnosis. People v. Lee, 450 N.W.2d 883 (Mich. 1990). See also People v. Gonzales, 310 N.W.2d 306 (Mich. App. 1981). The North Dakota Supreme Court has ruled that a complaining witness whose memory is enhanced through hypnosis is not incompetent to testify, but rather, hypnosis affects the credibility of the testimony. State v. Brown, 337 N.W.2d 138 (N.D. 1983).
94. J. Swickard, "Woman Can't Testify in Sex Case," *Detroit Free Press*, Nov. 9, 1984, p. B-1; see also, "The Trials of Hypnosis," *Newsweek*, Oct. 19, 1981, p. 96. In a prosecution in Cincinnati of Joseph Howard on a sexual battery charge, it was argued that "multiple personality people are notorious for faulty memory and are not credible." AP news release, Oct. 10, 1994. In Dorsey v. State, 206 Ga. App. 709, 425 S.E.2d 224 (1992), the court held that the bar on statements in a hypnotic state does not apply to testimony of a victim in a dissociative state. The court said, "We believe the nonvolitional nature of a dissociative state itself makes statements made while in such a state inherently more reliable than statements made in a hypnotic trance." That view was rejected in Wall v. Fairview Hosp. & Health Care Services, 584 N.W.2d 395 (Minn. 1998). The denial of the right of confrontation is also urged in

cases of dissociative testimony. In Loeblein v. Dormire, 229 F.3d 724 (8th Cir. 2000), where the alleged sexual assault victim had been diagnosed with a multiple personality disorder (MPD), the court held that allowing one personality to testify to the abuse suffered by another did not violate the defendant's right of confrontation, though an expert witness testified that the various personalities of persons with MPD often do not have the same personal knowledge of what happened to the person. The court concluded that none of the victim's testimony indicated that she did not have first-hand knowledge of everything to which she testified; hence, trial counsel was able to conduct a full cross-examination. See M.A. Miller, "The Unreliability of Testimony From a Witness With Multiple Personality Disorder (MPD): Why Courts Must Acknowledge the Connection Between Hypnosis and MPD and Adopt a 'Per Se' Rule of Exclusion for MPD Testimony," *Pepperdine L. Rev.* 27 (2000): 193.

95. K.M. McConkey & P.W. Sheehan, *Hypnosis, Memory, and Behavior in Criminal Investigation* (New York: Guilford, 1995); see A.W. Scheflin & J.L. Shapiro, *Trance on Trial* (New York: Guilford, 1989); A.W. Scheflin, H. Spiegel, & D. Spiegel, "Forensic Uses of Hypnosis," in A.K. Hess & I.B. Weiner (Eds.), *Handbook of Forensic Psychology* (New York: John Wiley & Sons, 2d ed., 1999); M.T. Orne, "The Use and Misuse of Hypnosis in Court," *Intl. J. Clin. Exp. Hypnosis* 27 (1979): 311.

96. Rock v. Arkansas, 483 U.S. 44 (1987).

97. People v. Hayes, 49 Cal.3d 1260, 265 Cal. Rptr. 132, 783 P.2d 719 (1989). If the proponent of a witness who has been hypnotized is permitted to introduce untainted, prehypnotic memories, proof that these memories existed prior to hypnosis should go beyond a subject's posthypnotic recollections of the timing of his memories because such posthypnotic recollections may not be accurate. Contreras v. State, 718 P.2d 129 (Alaska 1986).

7

Propensity and Other Acts of Evidence

The characteristics of people, we know, make them more or less likely to respond in particular ways to events or circumstances. There is usually regularity of behavior and a link between personality and behavior. Thus, an introverted individual is unlikely (unless under the influence of drugs or alcohol) to tell loud jokes and become the center of attention at a gathering, but this behavior would not be unusual for a histrionic extrovert.

The law, however, on the admissibility of character evidence, otherwise known as propensity evidence, is bewildering, even to the most experienced trial lawyer. This confusion results from the conflict between the sporting theory of justice, which calls for its exclusion, and the reality of the probative value of the evidence, which calls for its admissibility. In excluding such evidence, the rule contradicts everyday experience, e.g., employers routinely ask people furnishing references to discuss the applicant's character and prior behavior, but out of a sporting theory of justice, evidence of the accused's character is not admissible to show propensity. However, the option is given to the accused to "open the door" to evidence of his character, and also about the character of the victim.

In any event, either party can offer evidence of *habit* to show propensity or lack thereof, or evidence of other crimes, wrongs, or acts, not to show propensity, but to establish motive, opportunity, intent, preparation, plan, knowledge, identity, or absence of mistake or accident.

All in all, to be sure, this body of law is bewildering. Its meaning is frequently the topic of litigation and of proposals for change. Supreme Court Justice Robert Jackson once described it as a "grotesque structure"—"archaic, paradoxical, and full of compromises and compensations by which an irrational advantage to one side is offset by a poorly reasoned counter-privilege to the other."[1]

Of course, even without the formal introduction of character evidence, the focus on propensity (or credibility) by way of character takes place at the very outset of a trial. In ordinary thinking, character is judged by appearance, so defense attorneys go to great length to make their clients attractive and presentable. In defending the Menendez brothers, who brutally killed their parents, Leslie Abramson called them "my boys" and dressed them in Oxford shirts. Numerous studies have pointed out that attractive individuals are found guilty less often and sentenced less harshly. Similarly, individuals who appear "loving and warm" or show remorse are treated more leniently than those who seem "cold and unapproachable."[2] People are categorized and judged by characteristics, such as social class, race, gender, education, empathy, marriage, parenthood, religion, political ideology, profession, physical stature, or affiliations with various groups. Fairly or unfairly, consciously or unconsciously, people are judged by these characteristics.[3]

Then, too, apart from appearance, an indictment, which is read to the jury, may name the accused by an alias or nickname (such as "Sammy the Bull" or "Jimmy the Weasel"). References to character are made during opening statement or closing argument, which, though not evidence, tends to be persuasive. Time and again, during opening statement or closing argument, the prosecutor resorts to name-calling that implies propensity, such as referring to the accused as an animal, beast, snake, cunning rascal, or filthy pervert, or by referring to the accused by his nickname, such as "Slick Willie."[4] Name-calling may result in reversible error.[5]

The basic principle of law, as a matter of policy, is that evidence of character is irrelevant in judging the merits of a case. In oft-quoted language: "The business of the court is to try the case and not the man, and a very bad man may have a very righteous case."[6] The rationale is that, in the ordinary case, be it civil or criminal, character evidence has a remote bearing as proof regarding whether the act in question has or has not been committed. In a criminal case, the accused is put on trial for a specific deed; he need not defend an entire life history. Character evidence is usually laden with prejudice, distraction, time expenditure, and surprise, although it may have some value as circumstantial evidence.

That having been said, the rule is then swallowed up by exceptions. Lady Justice's blindfold has as many holes as a poor man's stockings. Character evidence is admissible not only when character is "in issue" (as in cases of defamation, a "fit parent" for child custody, or entrustment of a vehicle to an "incompetent driver"), but also, at the option of the accused, for the purpose of suggesting an inference about the commission of the criminal act. An accused claiming mistaken identity may offer evidence of "inconsistent personality," that is, that he is not the type of person who would or could commit the charged crime. In the event the accused initiates the use of character evidence, the prosecutor may then rebut it.

In the penalty phase of a capital case, assessment of dangerousness is a factor in the imposition of the penalty (discussed in Chapter 14 on the death penalty). Psychopathy (also known as sociopathy or antisocial personality) is highly correlated with violence proneness. Some research suggests that the diagnosis has no predictive power independent of that provided by the number and types of past antisocial acts committed by the individual. The evidence is about character "in issue," so other acts may be shown, but in any event, the rules of evidence are not applicable in sentencing.

Except somewhat in the imposition of the death penalty, evidence of social issues (or social conditions) is not presented in a legal proceeding. To be sure, the focus on the character of the offender or victim obscures social issues, such as poverty, poor schools, broken homes, violence in the media, and availability of guns, but that is not considered relevant consideration at trial. The task of courts is to decide specific disputes.

Pertinent Trait of Character

At trial, on character or propensity evidence, the rules of evidence provide the following:

> Evidence of a person's character or a trait of character is not admissible for the purpose of proving action in conformity therewith on a particular occasion, except: … Evidence of a *pertinent trait* of character offered by an accused, or by the prosecution to rebut the same (emphasis added).[7]

What is a *pertinent* character trait depends largely on the nature of the charges. In a battery prosecution, a court would likely exclude evidence that the accused is "honest," but admit proof that he is "peaceable" or "nonviolent." The cases generally hold that "law-abidingness" is a trait of character and is pertinent to any criminal accusation (as distinguished from good character generally).[8]

Joseph Brill, whose colorful style and record of success made him one of New York's eminent criminal lawyers, would—with a straight face—portray his racketeer clients as being "as pure as snow." In the civil wrongful-death trial, O. J. Simpson took the stand and gently nudged along by his attorneys painted a version of himself as a loving husband, father, and all-around good guy who could not have fatally slashed his former wife, Nicole Brown Simpson, and her friend, Ronald Goldman.[9]

How limiting is evidence of "pertinent trait" of character? In *Shelton v. State*,[10] a murder case, the Arkansas Supreme Court set out a summary of the law:

The prevailing view limits pertinent traits to those involved in the offense charged—proof of honesty in a theft charge or peacefulness in a murder charge .... However, it is necessary to allow evidence of defendant's character, as testimony that the general estimate of his character may be so favorable the jury could infer he would not be likely to commit the offense charged .... [In this case,] the defense proffered opinion evidence that Shelton was not a discipline problem and had an aversion to violence. Both of these traits—probative of law-abiding and nonviolent nature—have been traditionally admissible in a murder case and should have been admitted.[11]

Upon a defendant's introduction of character evidence, the question arises whether the defendant is entitled to an instruction to the jury that positive character evidence "standing alone" can be sufficient to create a reasonable doubt. On this score, the courts are in dispute. Some courts have held that such an instruction is never necessary and often, if not always, is improper because it misleads the jury. As the Seventh Circuit put it:

The "standing alone" instruction conveys to the jury the sense that even if it thinks the prosecution's case compelling, even if it thinks that defendant is a liar, if it also concludes that he has a good reputation, this may be the "reasonable doubt" of which other instructions speak. A "standing alone" instruction invites attention to a single bit of evidence and suggests to jurors that they analyze this evidence all by itself. No instruction flags any other evidence for this analysis—not eyewitness evidence, not physical evidence, not even confessions. There is no good reason to consider *any* evidence "standing alone."[12]

Other courts, however, have stated that a "standing alone" instruction is required where the defendant has presented character evidence.[13] Most courts, though, have held that while a defendant is not entitled to a "standing alone" instruction, it ordinarily is not an abuse of discretion to give one.[14]

Following the discussion of evidence of "habit" and evidence of other crimes or wrongdoing, there is a discussion herein of character evidence of "inconsistent personality."

Evidence of Habit

Evidence of the habit of a person is relevant to prove that the conduct of the person on a particular occasion was in conformity with the habit. It is propensity evidence. Unlike evidence of character, which is admissible only at the option of the accused, evidence of habit, under Rule 406 of the Federal Rules of Evidence and its counterpart in state rules, may be offered initially by either the prosecutor or the accused. In this context, habit refers to the type of nonvolitional activity that occurs with invariable regularity. Habit, a consistent method or manner of responding to a particular stimulus, has a reflexive, almost instinctive quality. Michel de Montaigne said, "Habit is second nature." Put another way, habit is a "trait jacket," but it does not have to amount to what is clinically known as a compulsion (an act that unless performed causes anxiety).

The commentary of the advisory committee in the Federal Rules of Evidence, quoting from Charles McCormick's textbook on evidence, contrasts habit with character:

Character and habit are close akin. Character is a generalized description of one's disposition, or of one's disposition in respect to a general trait, such as honesty, temperance, or peacefulness. "Habit," in modern usage, both lay and psychological, is more specific. It describes one's regular response to a repeated specific situation. If we speak of character for care, we think of the person's tendency to act prudently in all the varying situations of life, in handling automobiles and in walking across the street. A habit, on the other hand, is the person's regular practice of meeting a particular kind of situation with a specific type of conduct, such as the habit of going down a particular stairway two stairs at a time, or of giving the hand-signal for a left turn, or of alighting from railway cars while they are moving. The doing of the habitual acts may become semiautomatic.[15]

The courts give contrasting interpretations of habit. The character versus habit categories may lead to controversy because the categorization of the evidence determines its admissibility. A person who wakes up regularly at 6 a.m. can be described as an early riser or the person can be said to have a habit of getting up early. A person may be described as having a "lustful inclination" or as having a habit of sexually molesting children. Specificity provides the key: If specific conduct usually results from specific stimuli, the conduct is called a habit.

Habit is said to deal with the regularity of certain behavior, whereas character is said to deal with "inner nature." In *Perrin v. Anderson*,[16] the U.S. Tenth Circuit Court of Appeals held that five instances of violent encounters with the police are sufficient to establish habit of reacting violently to uniformed police officers. In the matter of informed consent, physicians have established the evidence of "habit" by "routinely and regularly" informing patients of certain risks involved in a therapy.[17] In *Weil v. Seltzer*,[18] however, the U.S. Court of Appeals for the District of Columbia required that the conduct be "nonvolitional" to qualify as habit. In this case, testimony that a doctor had the habit of prescribing steroids to allergy patients was rejected. Likewise, the District of Columbia court held testimony concerning religious practices not admissible because "the very volitional basis of the activity raises serious questions as to its invariable nature and, hence, its probative value." In *Levin v. United States*,[19] the court excluded a rabbi's testimony as to the defendant's habit of being home on the Orthodox Jewish Sabbath; the crime was committed on a Sabbath. In a South Carolina case, evidence that a motorist was involved in numerous collisions during a 3-year period and is "an habitually reckless driver" was held not admissible as habit evidence.[20] A pattern of intemperate drinking is usually inadmissible to prove drunkenness on a specific occasion, but distinctive drinking practices that are routinely followed may qualify as a habit.[21]

Evidence of Other Crimes or Wrongdoing

As a general principle, under Rule 404(b) of the Federal Rules of Evidence and its counterpart in state rules, evidence of other crimes or wrongdoing may not be used to show propensity, but may be used to establish motive, opportunity, intent, preparations, plan, knowledge, identity, or absence of mistake or accident. The defendant has no option in excluding evidence of other crimes or wrongdoing when offered to establish one or another of these purposes, just as the defendant has no option in excluding evidence of habit. Thus, in the case of William K. Smith of the Kennedy family, who was charged with rape, the court excluded the testimony of three women who would testify that Smith sexually attacked them years ago. The other alleged acts would have been to show propensity and did not fall under one of the exceptions in Rule 404(b) for the admission of evidence of other wrongdoing.[22] Likewise, in a medical malpractice case, reference to other acts of malpractice may not be made unless designed to establish one of the exceptions.[23]

In recent years, a preponderance of the courts have sustained the admissibility of testimony as to prior or subsequent similar crimes, wrongs, or acts in cases involving sexual offenses, such as incest and statutory rape. Among the grounds relied on for the admissibility of such evidence is that it is admissible to show motive or to show plan, with various phrases being used by the courts to describe those concepts. Motive may be inferred from previous occurrences having reference to and connection with the commission of the offense. Thus, in *People v. McConnell*,[24] the Michigan Court of Appeals said that when addiction is offered as the motive for robbery, past drug convictions can be used to show that the defendant is an addict. Motive, if established, would tend to rebut a contention that the defendant was at home and knew nothing of the crime charged against him. In *Elliot v. State*,[25] the Wyoming Supreme Court held that one who has committed acts of pedophilia could well be recognized as having a motive to commit such acts as are complained of by a victim.

Given the concern over sexual assault and child molestation, the U.S. Congress in 1994 enacted Rules 413–415 in the Federal Rules of Evidence (FRE), effective 1995, which marked a significant change in the long-established doctrine restricting evidence of other crimes or wrongdoing as propensity evidence against a defendant in a criminal case. Under Rule 413, to show propensity, evidence of the defendant's commission of another offense of sexual assault is now admissible in a criminal case where the defendant is accused of sexual assault. Rule 414 similarly allows evidence of the defendant's commission of a prior offense of child molestation in a case where the defendant is accused of child molestation. Rule 415 provides that such evidence is also admissible in civil cases "for damages or other relief" predicated on a party's commission of an offense of sexual assault or child molestation. To date, only a few states have enacted provisions similar to FRE 413–415.[26] As the Wyoming decision in *Elliot* would indicate, Rule 404(b) already provides an adequate basis for admitting evidence from prior crimes in those cases where it is most needed.[27]

In a justification of the adoption of Rules 413–415, Chief Judge Richard Posner of the Seventh Circuit wrote the following:

> Most people do not have a desire to sexually molest children. Between two suspects, only one of whom has a history of such molestation, the history establishes a motive that enables the two suspects to be distinguished; prior crimes evidence is admissible to prove motive. Unlike a molester, a thief, unless he is a kleptomaniac, does not have an overwhelming desire to steal. Theft is merely instrumental to his desire for money, and there are many substitute instruments. Committing a prior theft does not show that a defendant "likes" theft and so does not furnish a motive for his committing theft with which he is charged.[28]

On another occasion, Judge Posner noted that the principle under discussion is not limited to sex crimes:

> A "firebug"—one who commits arson not for insurance proceeds or revenge or to eliminate a competitor, but for the sheer joy of watching a fire—is, like the sex criminal, a person, whose motive to commit the crime with which he is charged, is revealed by his past commission of the same crime. … No special rule analogous to Rules 413 through 415 is necessary to make the evidence of the earlier crimes admissible because 404(b) expressly allows evidence of prior wrongful acts to establish motive. The greater the overlap between propensity and motive, the more careful the district judge must be about admitting under the rubric of motive evidence that the jury is likely to use instead as a basis for inferring the defendant's propensity, his habitual criminality, even if instructed not to.[29]

The exceptions in the Rules of Evidence allowing evidence of other crimes, wrongs, or acts can, like an accordion, be contracted or expanded. When expanded, the exceptions swallow the rule and, in effect, allow other acts to show propensity. Consider, for example, the decision by the Michigan Court of Appeals in *People v. Hoffman*,[30] on the admissibility of other acts to show motive. To establish that the defendant's actions were motivated by his misogyny (hatred of women), the prosecutor was allowed to present the testimony of two of the defendant's former girlfriends that the defendant had beaten and threatened. One of the witnesses testified that the defendant told her that "women are all sluts and bitches and deserve to die." Writing the opinion, Judge Griffin turned to *Black's Law Dictionary* for a definition of motive: "Cause or reason that moves the will and induces action. An inducement, or that which leads or tempts the mind to indulge a criminal act." Judge Griffin noted that "the distinction between admissible evidence of motive and inadmissible evidence of character of propensity is often subtle." He offered the following hypothetical to clarify the distinction:

> In midafternoon, on the outskirts of a rural Michigan village, an African-American man is savagely assaulted and battered by a white assailant. The assailant neither demands nor takes any money or property. The assailant is a total stranger to the victim. The defendant is later apprehended and charged with the attack. After the arrest, the prosecutor discovers that the defendant had been involved in several other violent episodes in the past, including bar fights, an assault on a police officer, and a violent confrontation with a former neighbor.

Under this scenario, "[a]bsent a proper purpose (such as to prove a common plan, scheme, or other exception), these other acts evidence would be inadmissible on the basis that its only relevance is to establish the defendant's violent character or propensity towards violence," Judge Griffin wrote, and he went on to say:

> However, if we were to add to this scenario that all of the defendant's prior victims were African-American and that the defendant had previously expressed his hatred toward blacks, then the evidence of defendant's prior assaults would be admissible to prove the defendant's motive for his conduct. By establishing that the defendant harbors a strong animus against people of the victim's race, the other acts evidence goes beyond establishing a propensity toward violence and tends to show why the defendant perpetrated a seemingly random and inexplicable attack.

Judge Griffin then turned to a New Jersey decision to support the hypothetical. In *New Jersey v. Crumb*,[31] the defendant was charged with hitting an elderly black man in the head and kicking and stomping him on his face and chest. The defendant allegedly told a friend that he had beaten "an old black bum ... just because he was there." The victim was not robbed. At trial, the prosecutor sought to introduce letters, verse, and drawings found in the defendant's apartment containing language that showed that the defendant was a racist. In overruling the trial court's ruling excluding the evidence, the New Jersey Superior Court said that "some of the written material directly expresses defendant's hostility toward and hatred of black people and his concomitant desire to see them dead. This material is compellingly powerful evidence of a motive, which helps to explain an otherwise inexplicable act of random violence." The New Jersey Court also noted that, without the evidence of the defendant's bigotry, "a jury would not know the context [of the victim's] death and might be resistant to the idea that a young man purposely would inflict deadly harm on an elderly stranger without any apparent reason, such as theft or substantial provocation."

Judge Griffin agreed with the analysis in *Crumb* and "adopt[ed] it as our own." Accordingly, he wrote the following:

> [W]e hold that in the present case the trial court did not abuse its discretion by admitting the other acts evidence for the purpose of establishing defendant's motive. Similar to the evidence of racism in *Crumb*, evidence that the defendant hates women and had previously acted on such hostility establishes more than character or propensity. Here, the other acts evidence was relevant and material to defendant's motive for his unprovoked, cruel, and sexually demeaning attack on his victim. ... Absent the other acts evidence establishing motive, the jurors may have found it difficult to believe the victim's testimony that defendant committed the depraved and otherwise inexplicable actions.

Inconsistent Personality Evidence

What about inconsistent personality evidence? When "opening the door" to character evidence, the accused seeks to establish innocence by evidence of no propensity to commit the crime. His personality, it is argued, is inconsistent with the crime, but just how probative to an issue is inconsistent personality evidence?[32] It is a common mode of thinking.[33]

Not surprisingly, however, the use of expert psychological testimony to establish innocence by evidence of an "inconsistent personality" is controversial. There is considerable but conflicting jurisprudence as to whether an expert may be asked, "Doctor, do you have an opinion with a reasonable degree of psychological certainty whether or not the defendant has personality characteristics that would make it impossible for him to have committed the criminal act?"[34] The evidence is pertinent, as required under the rules of evidence, but is it probative?

The Third Circuit, in a narcotics case where the defense was entrapment, held it error to exclude testimony of a psychologist that the defendant had a unique susceptibility to inducement.[35] In a prosecution for pointing a gun at an officer who had been trying to arrest the defendant, the Seventh Circuit held it error to exclude testimony of a psychiatrist that the defendant was more likely to injure himself than to direct his aggression at others.[36] In a prosecution for statutory rape and contributing to the delinquency of a minor, the Alaska Supreme Court allowed psychiatric testimony that in view of defendant's personality it was improbable that he committed the offenses charged.[37]

The Arizona Supreme Court, in a murder prosecution, held it error to exclude, as bearing on premeditation, the testimony of a psychologist that the defendant had difficulty dealing with stress and that in a stressful situation his reaction would be more reflexive than reflective.[38] The Iowa Supreme Court allowed psychiatric evidence that one of the participants in a murder was a passive-dependent individual who would allow others to assume responsibility.[39] In a Wisconsin case where the defendant was charged with first-degree murder and first-degree sexual assault, the defendant contended that a conviction for a sexual assault requires the victim to have been alive during the alleged intercourse and that there was inadequate evidence to support a finding that the victim was alive if and when the intercourse occurred. Testimony was allowed that an assailant without necrophilic tendencies could have intercourse with his victim without realizing that she was dead.[40]

On the basis of a psychiatric report that the accused was a nonviolent man who found sexual satisfaction in consensual relationships, a Canadian judge was convinced that the accused did not rape his former girlfriend.[41] Then too, many believed that Supreme Court nominee Clarence Thomas was "not capable" of the sexual harassment claimed by Anita Hill.[42] Woody Allen, confronted with an allegation by Mia Farrow that he sexually molested their adopted 7-year-old daughter, Dylan, in the attic of Mia's summer home, said, "I have never been in an attic. I'm a famous claustrophobic; wild horses couldn't get me into an attic."[43]

The common law rule that proof of the defendant's character is allowed only by evidence of reputation in the community, and not by opinion evidence, was first abandoned when the California Supreme Court in 1954, in *People v. Jones*,[44] allowed the defense to submit expert psychiatric opinion evidence of the personality traits of the defendant as bearing on the unlikelihood that he had committed the crime of sexual abuse of a 9-year-old child. This was also one of the first cases in which a psychiatrist was allowed to testify to an opinion based in part on a narcoanalysis interview with the defendant. The evidence submitted by the defendant was a negative diagnosis, that is, that he was *not* a sex deviate or sexual psychopath.[45]

In *People v. Stoll*,[46] a California child sexual abuse case, the trial court excluded a psychologist's opinion that the defendant had a normal personality function, with a low indication of antisocial or aggressive behavior, thus making it unlikely that he would commit the charged acts. The opinion was based on a combination of personality tests, interviews with the defendant, and the psychologist's professional experience. Moreover, the psychologist testified on *voir dire* as to the statistical accuracy of the personality tests used, but noted that the tests were not the sole determinant of his opinion. He pointed out that psychiatrists and psychologists "always" used the Minnesota Multiphasic Personality Inventory (MMPI)—the primary test—to diagnose patients at various stages of clinical treatment. It also is "frequently" given in "employment and reemployment situations in conjunction with a polygraph," and in "promotion studies in the industry," as well as to inmates and job applicants in correctional facilities. The trial court's exclusion of the evidence was appealed to the state supreme court.

On appeal, the prosecutor argued that the testimony should be admitted only if valid empirical evidence supported both the existence of a rapist profile and that the defendant did not fit that profile. In reversing the trial court, the state Supreme Court held that there was no need to subject the testimony to the kinds of tests (*Frye* and *Daubert*) applied to screening scientific or technical evidence. As a rule, empirical or statistical evidence is not a prerequisite or helpful in the determination of the admissibility of expert testimony in the soft sciences. The court said, "No precise legal rules dictate the proper basis for an expert's journey into [an individual's] mind to make judgments about his behavior."[47]

Opposition to Psychiatric Testimony on Inconsistent Personality

In the face of some support for allowing psychiatric testimony on inconsistent personality, there is at the same time substantial opposition to it. An illustration is the New Jersey case, *State v. Cavallo*,[48] where the defendant, charged with rape, sought to introduce expert psychiatric testimony that he did not have psychological traits common to rapists. In rejecting the proposed testimony, the court said: "The danger of prejudice through introduction of unreliable expert testimony is clear. While juries would not always accord excessive weight to unreliable expert testimony, there is substantial danger that they would do so, precisely because the evidence is labeled 'scientific' and 'expert.'" The court noted that the testimony was based on two unproven and unreliable premises: (1) rapists have particular mental characteristics, and (2) psychiatrists can, by examination, determine the presence or absence of these characteristics.[49]

The U.S. Second Circuit excluded expert psychiatric testimony (the defendant suffered from "dependent personality disorder"), which was offered to show that the defendant did not know that certain property was stolen. It was excluded as unhelpful and as an opinion on the ultimate issue of mental state. The court, in a 2–1 decision, said that "the imprimatur of a clinical label was neither necessary nor helpful for the jury to make an assessment of [the defendant's] mind." In a lengthy dissent, the senior judge on the court argued that the proffered expert testimony should have been allowed.[50]

The U.S. First Circuit rejected a defendant's offer of psychological testimony in a fraud case that he was "too naive to know" as not being "character evidence" within the meaning of the rules of evidence.[51] In a prosecution for shooting at a helicopter, the Fifth Circuit held it not an error to exclude testimony of defense witnesses that, based on psychological tests, the defendant was nonviolent and not likely to shoot at a helicopter. "This character trait was as plainly within the 'ken of lay jurors,'... as it was a proper subject for lay testimony."[52] The Tenth Circuit also said that generalized testimony about the influence of personality traits is excludable as within the common knowledge and experience of lay jurors.[53]

In *United States v. MacDonald*,[54] the defendant, Captain Jeffrey MacDonald, a physician, was on trial for the murders of his wife and daughters. The trial judge excluded psychiatric testimony that the defendant's "personality/emotional configuration" was inconsistent with violent crime as confusing and misleading. The defense sought to offer the testimony of leading forensic psychiatrists who contended that MacDonald's personality was inconsistent with the crime. Dr.

Seymour Halleck said at the end of a 24-page report, "On the basis of my clinical experience as a psychiatrist and criminologist and on the basis of my knowledge of theories and research into the area of violence, I would conclude that there is only an extremely remote possibility that a person of his type would commit a crime of this type. Certainly, no one with Dr. MacDonald's personality organization has ever been known to commit such a crime." Dr. Robert Sadoff, who examined Dr. MacDonald in 1970, 1975, and 1979, says he would say again what he said previously: "Dr. MacDonald's personality is not consistent with the type of personality likely to commit this crime. I think that it is very unlikely that he could have done this. I base this statement today, not only upon my previous examination of him, but upon his total actions and behaviors over the 13 years since the murder." A prosecution psychologist, Hirsch Lazaar Silverman, disagreed, "This man is a pathological narcissist. His personality is such that under certain pressures he would revert to violence."[55]

Profiles

"Round up the usual suspects," said the police chief in the film *Casablanca*. The suspects had a profile of criminality. Generally speaking, the term *profile* describes observable behavior patterns as distinguished from physical or psychological characteristics known as "syndrome evidence" that we discuss in Chapter 8. Put briefly, *syndrome* means a group of symptoms or signs typical of an underlying cause or disease.

A profile is a list of characteristics compiled by a law enforcement agency, which have been found, through experience, to be common characteristics of those engaged in a certain type of criminal activity. The most common example is a drug courier profile, but officers also employ other profiles for specific criminal activity.[56] The primary use of profiles is in police investigation, where they are tools for identifying crime suspects.[57] In this time of terrorism, the authorities profile groups of people. The U.S. Immigration and Naturalization Service also uses profiles of "illegal immigrants."[58]

What about the use of profiles to establish guilt or innocence at trial where the rules of evidence apply? Larry King invited experts to discuss whether O. J. Simpson fit the profile of a stalking spousal killer, and Simpson's prosecutors did the same. At times, profiles have been admitted as evidence.

Prosecutors routinely offer drug-courier profile testimony as the basis of expert opinion of law enforcement witnesses to bolster circumstantially substantive proof of guilt at trial. The fact that an individual matched a "drug courier profile" may be admitted as evidence to prove that the individual must have known that he was carrying drugs and, consequently, that he intended to distribute them.[59]

It has been held that use of the results of the Millon Clinical Multiaxial Inventory and the Minnesota Multiphasic Personality Inventory to identify sex offenders is not sufficiently supported by the data, nor could the science be deemed sufficiently valid or reliable, and so, on the basis of this data, an expert cannot testify that the defendant does or does not fit the profile of a typical sex offender.[60]

A number of courts have allowed testimony that the accused does or does not share the characteristics of individuals who typically abuse children.[61]

Therapists have established a "battering parent" profile (a "battering parent" frequently exhibits low empathy, short temper, and lack of self-esteem). In a case where medical testimony regarding the "battering parent profile" as well as the "battered child profile" was admitted at trial, the Minnesota Supreme Court said:

> We hold that the establishment of the existence of a battered child, together with the reasonable inference of a battering parent, is sufficient to convict defendant herein in light of

the other circumstantial evidence presented by the prosecution. It is very difficult in these prosecutions for injuries and death to minor children to establish the guilt of a defendant other than by circumstantial evidence. Normally, as was the case here, there are no eye-witnesses. ... The prosecution properly presented to the jury the psychological framework that constitutes a battering parent. It did not attempt to point the finger of accusation at the defendant as a battering parent by its medical testimony. Rather, it presented sufficient evidence from which the jury could reasonably conclude that the defendant fit one of the psychological patterns of a battering parent.[62]

Three years later, the Minnesota Supreme Court determined that "battering parent" evidence was not an indispensable element of the state's case in a child abuse prosecution, but held it was not reversible error to receive it into evidence.[63] Then, 5 years later, the same court ruled that the prosecution is not permitted to introduce evidence of a "battering parent" profile or to establish the character of the defendant as a "battering parent" unless the defendant first raises that issue.[64] The court stated, "We feel this finding is required until further evidence of the scientific accuracy and reliability of syndrome or profile diagnoses can be established."[65] In sum and substance, we would say the following: Many people fit a profile, but few act accordingly. As evidence, it would be misleading as there would be too many false positives.

In "undue familiarity" cases, the psychiatrist (or other defendant who is sued) may seek to offer evidence that he is not the type of person who would engage in that type of behavior. In his experience of evaluating, treating, and consulting on many cases of physician sexual misconduct, Dr. Glen Gabbard of the Menninger Foundation finds that the vast majority of the physicians involved fall into four psychodynamically based categories: (1) lovesickness, (2) masochistic surrender, (3) predatory psychopathy and paraphilias, and (4) psychotic disorders.[66] There is no way, however, to establish the known or potential rate of error in the classifications used to establish profile evidence, therefore, this evidence would be excluded at trial. Exploiting therapists cover a wide range of people from the very good to the very bad, as Dr. Gabbard's findings indicate; hence, profile evidence does not offer much to the jury in a particular case.[67]

Even assuming scientific reliability of character evidence, in a criminal case the accused may keep the evidence out by not introducing evidence of character (or by not pleading not guilty by reason of insanity). Once the defendant introduces evidence of good character, however, as we have noted, the prosecution then may rebut it with evidence of bad character.[68] The defendant, however, has no option in excluding evidence of "habit" or evidence of other crimes, wrongs, or acts that tend to establish motive, opportunity, intent, preparation, plan, knowledge, identity, or absence of mistake or accident.[69]

Evidence of the Victim's Character

A defendant in a criminal case who alleges a defense that rests upon the conduct of the victim may offer evidence of the victim's character to prove that conduct. Under the rules of evidence, evidence of a pertinent character trait of the victim is admissible when it is offered by the accused to prove that the victim acted in conformity to his or her character.[70] Thus, when a defendant alleges self-defense, evidence of the victim's character trait of violence may be admissible for one of two purposes. First, the evidence may be offered on the issue of who was the aggressor. As John Wigmore, the leading authority on the law of evidence, put it, "One's persuasion will be more or less affected by the character of the deceased; it may throw much light on the probabilities of the deceased's actions." The second purpose is to prove that the accused was apprehensive of the victim and that his defensive measures were reasonable. For the admission of evidence for this purpose, it must first be established that the accused knew of the victim's acts of violence or aggression. In this situation, the evidence is offered to prove apprehension or state of mind rather than to prove that the person actually was the first aggressor.[71]

It is an old trial strategy to blame or taint the victim. Sometimes rightly, sometimes wrongly. Who has not heard it said that women who dress provocatively invite a rape?[72] And, who has not heard the old Western saying that the first thing to do in a murder case is determine whether or not the victim deserved to die? In Texas, there is a saying, "He needed killing." It was that philosophy that led a Wyoming jury to free a law official in a killing. Ed Cantrell, a former public safety director in Wyoming, shot his own undercover agent between the eyes in front of two other policemen. He was found not guilty. The tactic of the defense attorney, the famed Gerry Spence, was to try the agent who was killed. He was made out to be a violent, unstable man who used and dealt in drugs.[73]

Jack Litman became famous as a defense attorney by blaming the victim. He used this tactic on behalf of Yale student Richard Herrin who not only admitted to killing Bonnie Garland (he told police her head "split like a watermelon"), but testified that when he entered her room with a hammer, he intended to kill her. Litman's defense sympathetically portrayed Herrin as a love-struck young man driven temporarily insane by a manipulative and unfaithful girlfriend. Herrin was convicted of manslaughter rather than murder.[74] In another much publicized case, Litman portrayed Jennifer Levin as sexually aggressive when Robert Chambers choked her one night in Central Park. A mistrial resulted, and when Chambers was tried again, he entered a plea and got off with a few years of imprisonment.[75]

In the trial of Lyle and Erik Menendez, attorney Leslie Abramson portrayed the parents who were killed as abusive. With a shotgun, they blasted their parents, who were watching television, as "a preemptive strike in self-defense." In the first of two trials, blaming the victim succeeded as a defense.[76] It was one of many cases where the "abuse excuse" was offered as a defense.[77] In recent years, women who have been prosecuted for killing their partners have sought exculpation by asserting the defense of self-defense. In some of the cases, the "battered woman" killed the victim while he was asleep or during a significant lull in the violence. The "battered woman" introduces evidence of the decedent's violent nature in support of her claim of self-defense.

And then there is the case of *State v. Clark*,[78] involving a defendant who killed his estranged wife and the man she was living with. At the time of the homicide, he had been separated from his wife for less than a week under a domestic violence protective order. He shot them when he found them in their marital home. At trial he sought to introduce in evidence the fact that his wife had a prior criminal record, used drugs during the marriage, had extra-marital affairs, and had a baby by another man during her marriage to him. The court excluded the evidence on the grounds that the character of a victim is relevant only in cases of self-defense, not diminished capacity as was urged in this case. In oral argument, on appeal, one of the judges analogized the defendant's position to that of a battered spouse, but the court nonetheless ruled against the admission of the evidence. To no avail, his attorney argued that the defendant was traumatized by his wife and, thus, suffered diminished capacity. He was convicted of first-degree murder. Quite likely, had he been represented by a Gerry Spence or Jack Litman, the outcome would have been different.[79]

Endnotes

1. Michelson v. United States, 335 U.S. 469, 486 (1948).
2. The emotional display of the defendant associated with his statements affects the character assessment of the defendant and the recommended sentence. A theory, known as "affect control theory," explains sentencing through the relations between emotions, identities, and behaviors. If an offender displays unconcern after an offense, the emotion confirms a negative identity, perhaps typically engaging in negative behaviors. If the offender displays sadness or remorse after the offense, the emotion disconfirms the negative identity. When a victim displays sadness after the offense, the decision maker may

perceive the victim as undeserving of the offense, in other words, a positive identity. When a victim displays unconcern, the decision maker may perceive the victim as perhaps deserving of the offense, thus, a more negative identity. In turn, the victim's identity may influence perceptions of the offender and the offense. See D.R. Heise, "Effects of Emotion Displays on the Assessment of Character," *Soc. Psychol. Q.* 52 (1989): 10; D. Landy & E. Aronson, "The Influence of the Character of the Criminal and His Victim on the Decisions of Simulated Jurors," *J. Exp. Soc. Psychol.* 5 (1969): 141.

In a Florida death penalty case, Judge Edward Cowart wrote in his opinion, "This court has observed the demeanor and the action of the defendant throughout this entire trial and has not observed one scintilla of remorse displayed, indicating full well to this court that the death penalty is the proper selection of the punishment to be imposed in this particular case." State of Florida v. Robert Austin Sullivan, Circuit Court of 11th Judicial Circuit, Dade County, FL, case no. 73-3236A. See R. Slovenko, "Remorse," *J. Psychiat. & Law* 34 (2006): 397; S.E. Sundby, "The Capital Jury Absolution: The Intersection of Trial Strategy, Remorse, and the Death Penalty," *Cornell L. Rev.* 83 (1998): 1557.

3. See S. Deitz & L. Byrnes, "Attribution of Responsibility for Sexual Assaults: The Influence of Observer Empathy and Defendant Occupation and Attractiveness," *J. Psychol.* 108 (1981): 17; M.J. Saks & R. Hastie, *Social Psychology in Court* (New York: Van Nostrand Reinhold, 1978), pp. 156–160. Many people concluded that Ted Bundy, because he was so photogenic and so articulate, could not have committed the crimes for which he had been convicted, but he was sadistic. R.K. Ressler & T. Shachtman, *Whoever Fights Monsters* (New York: St. Martin's Press, 1992), p. 72. Ann Rule, the author of many books about crime, has written: "In my three decades of writing about actual crimes, only once have I been personally involved in a case before I wrote about it. That, of course, was the story of Ted Bundy, who had been my partner at Seattle's Crisis Clinic a few years before he was exposed as a merciless serial killer. During the years I knew him, I had no more knowledge of the man behind the 'mask' than anyone else who interacted with him. Indeed, I had a contract to write a book about an unknown killer—my first book contract—only to find out I would be writing about my friend." A. Rule, *Every Breath You Take* (New York: Simon & Schuster, 2001), p. xviii.

As World War II was reaching a climax, Henry Morgenthau, Jr., Secretary of the Treasury in President Roosevelt's administration, put forward a plan to deindustralize the Ruhr, reassigning parts of Germany to France and Poland, and divide the remainder of Germany into two purely agricultural states. The aim of weakening and "pastoralizing" Germany was to ensure that it could not again become powerful; and as Morgenthau's book, *Germany Is Our Problem* (1945), argued, it was necessary to ensure this by institutional means because the Germans were in his view by nature "militaristic." More extreme was Theodore Kaufman's *Germany Must Perish!*, self-published in 1940, that called for the systematic sterilization of the German people so that once the existing German population died out there would no longer be an aggressive militaristic nation in the world to threaten its peace. In 1944, the well-known lawyer Louis Nizer in *What to Do With Germany* accused the Germans of being psychiatrically ill, suffering from a variety of sexually based disorders, principally sadism, homosexuality, and bestiality. Akin to the idea of "flawed national character" is the premise for Daniel Goldhagen's *Hitler's Willing Executioners: Ordinary Germans and the Holocaust*, published in 1996, which imputes to the entire German people a practically genetic anti-Semitism and, therefore, capacity for genocide, in which any "ordinary German" is by his nature capable of participating in, and for which the character of the German people as a whole is responsible. See A.C. Grayling, *Among the Dead Cities* (New York: Walker & Co., 2006), pp. 159–166. Leon Gustave Dehon, a French priest who founded the priesthood of the Sacred Heart in 1877, in his writings described the Talmud, the Jewish holy text, as the "manual for the bandit, the corrupter, the social destroyer," and recommended that people of the Jewish faith should wear explicit identifiers, such as badges (reported in "No Saint?" *The American Scholar*, 78 (Winter 2006): 15). In the United States, at the present time, men are considered "high risk" and are kept away from children. John Walsh, host of Fox's *America's Most Wanted*, says, "It's all about minimizing risks. What dog is more likely to bite and hurt you? A Doberman, not a poodle. Who's more likely to molest a child? A male." Airlines use similar reasoning when they seat unaccompanied minors only with women. They are trying to decrease the odds of a problem. "You have to make generalizations for the safety of a child," says an expert in aviation disputes. See J. Zaslow, "Are We Teaching Our Kids to Be Fearful of Men? *Wall Street Journal*, August 23, 2007, p. D-1.

4. In the trial of Conrad Black, aka Lord Black, accused of looting his Hollinger International media empire, the prosecutor in the opening statement said to the jury (referring to Lord Black and three associates), "Bank robbers are masked and they use guns. Burglars wear dark clothing and use crowbars. These men dressed in ties and wore a suit." D. Litterick, "Lord Black Is Like a Bank Robber Dressed in Suit and Tie, Court Told," *Weekly Telegraph*, March 28–April 3, 2007, p. 13.

5. In United States v. Williams, 739 F.2d 297 (7th Cir. 1984), a police detective, in the course of his testimony, stated that he knew the defendant by the sobriquet "Fast Eddie." The Court of Appeals found that this testimony constituted reversible error because it was an impermissible reference to the defendant's character. The court rejected the argument that "Fast Eddie" was a neutral name, concluding that it would "suggest to the jury that the defendant had some sort of history or reputation for unsavory activity." The court recognized that other cases had permitted evidence of a defendant's alias or nickname if it "aids in the identification of the defendant or in some other way directly relates to the proof of the acts charged in the indictment." However, in this case, "the detective's testimony about the defendant's nickname was completely unrelated to any of the other proof against the defendant"; 737 F.2d at 300. See A.N. Bishop, "Name Calling: Defendant Nomenclature in Criminal Trials," *Ohio North. U. L. Rev.* 4 (1977): 38.

6. Michelson v. United States, 335 U.S. 469 (1948).

7. Rule 404(a) (1), Federal Rules of Evidence.

8. United States v. Angelini, 678 F.2d 380 (1st Cir. 1982). The government has often argued that "being prone to law-abiding conduct" is not an actual character trait, but is rather a conclusion that must be drawn from other character traits, such as honesty, reliability, and rectitude. However, the courts have generally held that "character traits admissible under Rule 404(a)(1) need not constitute specific traits of character, but may include general traits, such as lawfulness and law-abidingness." Indeed, the defendant in the landmark case, Michelson v. United States, 335 U.S. 469 (1948), was permitted to prove his "law-abiding" character trait, and the Supreme Court held that a defendant may introduce favorable testimony concerning "the general estimate of his character."

This does not mean, however, that the defendant has unlimited freedom to define a character trait. For example, in United States v. Diaz, 961 F.2d 1417 (9th Cir. 1992), the defendant was charged with possession with intent to distribute more than 500 grams of cocaine. Defense counsel sought to ask a defense witness whether the defendant had a "character trait for being prone to large-scale drug dealing." The Ninth Circuit found no error in excluding this testimony because a defendant propensity (or lack thereof) to engage in large-scale drug dealing "is not an admissible character trait." The proposed testimony was not the same as testimony that the defendant was law-abiding because it was in effect too specific. The court reasoned that an inquiry into a propensity to engage in large-scale drug dealing "would be misleading if addressed to a defendant with a record of criminal offenses other than drug dealing: If answered in the negative [as the defendant, of course, anticipated], the impression may be given that the defendant is a law-abiding person although he has a record of other crimes"; 961 F.2d at 1419. See S.A. Saltzburg, M.M. Martin, & D.J. Capra, *Federal Rules of Evidence Manual* (Charlottesville, VA: Michie, 6th ed., 1994), vol. 1, p. 317.

9. B.D. Ayres, "Simpson Testifies, Portraying Himself as a Loving Husband," *New York Times*, Jan. 11, 1997, p. 6. Psychologist Linda N. Edelstein sets out character traits including profiles of human behaviors and personality types in her book *The Writer's Guide to Character Traits* (Cincinnati, OH: Writer's Digest Books, 1999). The physician Cesare Lombroso, a compassionate 19th-century proponent of social justice, nonetheless promoted the view that the condition of teeth, ears, overhanging brows, jutting jaws, and especially tattoos were signs of the born criminal. Phrenology was launched as a science by the Viennese physician Franz Joseph Gall (1758–1828), who believed bumps on the head and the shape of the head held the key to personality. By inkblots, Hermann Rorschach, a Swiss psychiatrist, sought to create "a key to the knowledge of mankind." See A.M. Paul, *The Cult of Personality* (New York: Free Press, 2004).

10. 287 Ark. 322, 699 S.W.2d 728 (1985).

11. 699 S.W.2d at 734.

12. United States v. Burke, 781 F.2d 1234, 1239 (7th Cir. 1985).

13. See, e.g., United States v. Lewis, 482 F.2d 632 (D.C. Cir. 1973).

14. See, e.g., United States v. Pujana-Mena, 949 F.2d 24 (2d Cir. 1991).

15. The quote appears in the commentary to Rule 406 of the Federal Rules of Evidence and in subsequent editions of *McCormick on Evidence*. See J.W. Strong et al., *McCormick on Evidence* (St. Paul, MN: West, 5th ed., 1999), § 195.

16. 784 F.2d 1040 (10th Cir. 1986).

17. See, e.g., Meyer v. United States, 464 F. Supp. 317 (D. Colo. 1979), *aff'd*, 638 F.2d 155 (10th Cir. 1980); Reaves v. Mandell, 209 N.J. Super. 465, 507 A.2d 807 (1986).

18. 873 F.2d 1453 (D.C. Cir. 1989).

19. 338 F.2d 265 (D.C. Cir. 1964).

20. Williams v. Johnson, 244 S.C. 406, 137 S.E.2d 410 (1964).

21. In Loughan v. Firestone Tire & Rubber Co., 749 F.2d (5th Cir. 1979), the court admitted as habit evidence testimony that a certain employee "routinely carried a cooler of beer on his truck," "was in the habit of drinking on the job," and "normally had something to drink in the early morning hours." In Keltner v. Ford Motor Co., 748 F.2d 1265 (8th Cir. 1984), the court admitted evidence of habit of drinking a six-pack of beer four nights a week.

22. D. Margolick, "3 Women's Testimony on Smith Is Barred," *New York Times*, Dec. 3, 1991, p. 9. The writer Dominick Dunne in his book *Justice* (New York: Crown, 2001) expresses outrage that evidence of a defendant's past offenses is kept from the jury. Moreover, in the trial of his daughter's killer, the defendant was "costumed" like a sacristan in a Catholic seminary and carried a Bible, which he read throughout the trial in a pious fashion.

    The law of evidence on character of a person is distinguished from character of a place. Evidence of other wrongdoing is restricted in establishing an individual's propensity, but evidence of other events is admissible to establish character of a place, such as evidence of a number of accidents at an intersection to establish a dangerous intersection. See, e.g., Simon v. Kennebunkport, 417 A.2d 982 (Me. 1980).

23. Thus, in Persichini v. Beaumont Hosp., 238 Mich. App. 626, 607 N.W.3d 100 (1999), a question on cross-examination of the defendant physician with respect to the number of times he was sued for malpractice was deemed improper and highly prejudicial warranting the grant of a mistrial.

24. 124 Mich. App. 672, 335 N.W.2d 226 (1983).

25. 600 P.2d 1044 (Wyo. 1979).

26. L.S. Eads, D.W. Shuman, & J.M. DeLipsey, "Getting It Right: The Trial of Sexual Assault and Child Molestation Cases Under Federal Rules of Evidence 413–415," *Behav. Sci. & Law* 18 (2000): 169.

27. See C.B. Mueller & L.C. Kirkpatrick, *Evidence* (New York: Aspen, 3d ed. 2003). For a criticism of Rules 413–415, see L.M. Natali & R.S. Stigall, "How Sexual Propensity Evidence Violates the Due Process Clause," *Champion*, Sept./Oct. 1997, p. 24.

28. R.A. Posner, "An Economic Approach to the Law of Evidence," *Stanford L. Rev.* 51 (1999): 1477 at 1525–1526.

29. United States v. Cunningham, 103 F.3d 553 (7th Cir. 1996).

30. 1997 WL 476532 (Mich. App. 1997).

31. 277 N.J. Super. 311, 649 A.2d 879 (App. Div. 1994).

32. M.A. Mendez, "The Law of Evidence and the Search for a Stable Personality," *Emory L. J.* 45 (1996): 221.

33. In a blurb on the dust jacket of Tony Hiss's book, *The View from Alger's Window/A Son's Memoir* (New York: Knopf, 1999), Lawrence Weschler (fellow *New Yorker* writer) wrote:

    > Tony Hiss's book about his father, Alger—remarkable on its own terms (warm, loving, nuanced, and revelatory)—is likely to have a profound effect on the ongoing debate over Alger's character and culpability. Hiss's detractors will now have to square their version of the man with the person who comes shining through Tony's narrative, based largely on a never previously published trove of intimate family papers, especially Alger's letters home from prison. How could a man capable of penning such letters ever have behaved in the manner they persist in alleging?

34. See S. Roll & W.E. Foote, "The Inconsistent Personality Defense," in D.J. Muller, D.E. Blackman, & A.J. Chapman, (Eds.), *Psychology and Law* (New York: John Wiley & Sons, 1984), pp. 125–132; R.H. Woody & J.M. Shade, "Psychological Testimony on the Propensity for Sexual Child Abuse," *Mich. Psychol.*, March–April 1989, p. 12.

35. United States v. Hill, 655 F.2d 512 (3d Cir. 1981).

36. United States v. Staggs, 553 F.2d 1073 (7th Cir. 1977).

37. Freeman v. State, 486 P.2d 967 (Alaska 1971).

38. State v. Christensen, 129 Ariz. 32, 628 P.2d 580 (1981).

39. In State v. Wood, 346 N.W.2d 481 (Iowa 1984), the defendant introduced expert testimony evaluating her as a "passive-dependent personality." The expert testified that a "passive-dependent" individual will allow others to assume responsibility and will act in a manner to maintain such a dependent relationship. The defendant was allowed to offer this testimony to negate evidence that she had the requisite intent to kill her husband. The state law required the prosecutor to prove, on a first-degree murder charge, that the defendant "willfully, deliberately, and with premeditation kills another person"; Iowa Code §707.2(1). In substance, she sought to show it was unlikely she would commit such an act.

40. State v. Holt, 382 N.W.2d 679 (Wis. App. 1985).

41. Canadian Press, "Man Gets Day's Probation in Rape of Ex-Girl Friend," *Globe & Mail*, June 21, 1990, p. 1.

42. Ltr., Hill vs. Thomas, *Commentary*, May 1992, p. 10.
43. J. Adler, "Unhappily Ever After," *Newsweek*, Aug. 31, 1992, p. 40.
44. 42 Cal. 2d 219, 266 P.2d 38 (1954).
45. The case is discussed in W.J. Curran, "Expert Psychiatric Evidence of Personality Traits," *U. Pa. L. Rev.* 103 (1955): 999.
46. 265 Cal. Rptr. 111, 783 P.2d 698 (1989).
47. 783 P.2d at 709. The case is criticized in J.E.B. Myers, *Legal Issues in Child Abuse and Neglect* (Newbury Park, CA: Sage, 1992). In People v. Spigno, 156 Cal. App.2d 279, 319 P.2d 458 (1957), the California Court of Appeals held that there was no scientific recognition of a psychologist's ability to determine propensity for child molestation. See A.E. Taslitz, "Myself Alone: Individualizing Justice Through Psychological Character Evidence," *Md. L. Rev.* 52 (1993): 1. See Chapter 3 on restrictions on expert testimony.
48. 88 N.J. 508, 443 A.2d 1020 (1982), noted in 42 ALR4th 919 (1985).
49. Annot., "Admissibility of Expert Testimony as to Criminal Defendant's Propensity Toward Sexual Deviation," 42 ALR4th 937 (1985).
50. United States v. DiDomenico, 985 F.2d 1159 (2d Cir. 1993).
51. United States v. Kepreos, 759 F.2d 961 (1st Cir. 1985).
52. United States v. Webb, 625 F.2d 709 (5th Cir. 1980).
53. United States v. Esch, 832 F.2d 531 (10th Cir. 1987).
54. 485 F. Supp. 1087 (E.D. N.C. 1979), 688 F.2d 224 (4th Cir. 1982), *cert. denied*, 459 U.S. 1103 (1983).
55. Quoted in D.L. Breo, *Extraordinary Care* (Chicago: Chicago Review Press, 1986), pp. 140–141. Joe McGinniss in a best-selling book, *Fatal Vision* (New York: Putnam, 1983), devotes 663 pages to building a case that Captain MacDonald committed the crime.
56. The profile of a "pimp": track suit, Adidas sneakers, gold chain, sleeves short enough to reveal the bulge of his muscles. R. Cohen, "The Oldest Profession Seeks New Market in West Europe," *New York Times*, Sept. 19, 2000, p. 1.
57. The use of drug courier profiles is discussed extensively in United States v. Berry, 670 F.2d 583 (5th Cir. 1982). See also United States v. Malone, 886 F.2d 1162 (9th Cir. 1989) where the defendant is stopped by the police on the basis of a gang member profile. In an Oregon case, a profile of a serial killer was the basis for a search warrant that resulted in discovery of body parts in the suspect's residence. See R. Turco, *Closely Watched Shadows: Profile of the Hunter and the Hunted* (Wilsonville, OR: BookPartners, 1999). Dr. Philip Resnick provided a profile of a person who would kidnap a pregnant woman, perform a C-section, and steal the baby. A. Garrett, "4 Other Babies Stolen by C-Section," *Plain Dealer*, Oct. 4, 2000, p.1.

The practitioner of criminal profiling looks at the specifics of a crime—the scene, the facts about the victim, the evidence, and the act itself—and extrapolates a portrait of the culprit. See J. Douglas & M. Olshaker, *The Cases That Haunt Us* (New York: Scribner, 2000); R.M. Holmes & S.T. Holmes, *Profiling Violent Crimes* (Thousand Oaks, CA: Sage, 3rd ed., 2002); R.K. Kessler & T. Shachtman, *Whoever Fights Monsters* (New York: St. Martin's 1992); G.B. Palermo & R.N. Kocsis, *Offender Profiling* (Springfield, IL: Thomas, 2005); M.F. Abramsky & K. Ross, "Criminal Profiling in Child Sexual Assault Cases," *Am. J. Forens. Psychol.* 24 (2006): 39; M.G. McGrath, "Criminal Profiling: Is There a Role for the Forensic Psychiatrist?" *J. Am. Acad. Psychiat. & Law* 28 (2000): 315. Profiles of various types of offenders are described in B. Danto, *Dangerous and Mentally Disordered Offenders* (Laguna Hills, CA: Eagle Books, 1985). See also P.C. Ellsworth & R. Mauro, "Psychology and Law," in D.T. Gilbert, S.T. Fiske, & G. Lindzey (Eds.), *The Handbook of Social Psychology* (New York: McGraw-Hill, 4th ed., 1998), chap. 32, pp. 684–732; B. Turvey, *Criminal Profiling* (San Diego: Academic Press, 1999); M. Higgins, "Looking the Part," *ABAJ*, Nov. 1997, p. 48.

Profiling has found a role in screening in the employment context as well as in police investigation. Psychiatrist Martin Blinder has constructed a profile "by which management can identify well in advance those employees most likely to engage in lethal acts of revenge." He postulates that there are 18 traits conducive to lethality and that a person exhibiting "any 10 or more" should give rise to concern. M. Blinder, "Profile of a Workplace Killer," *Wall Street Journal*, Feb. 10, 1997, p. 18.

In a cartoon in the *New Yorker*, a CEO notifies his deputy of a downsizing, "We've got to get rid of some people," and he asks the deputy, "Who are the least likely to come back and shoot us?" For a critical view of the utility of profiling in the workplace, see M. Braverman, *Preventing Workplace Violence* (Thousand Oaks, CA: Sage, 1999); R.V. Deneberg & M. Braverman, *The Violence-Prone Workplace* (Ithaca, NY: Cornell University Press, 1999). In a spoof of profiling, a police chief in a German film shows a threatening letter to a psychiatrist and asks for a profile. The psychiatrist looks over the letter and muses, "It could have been written by a man. It could have been written by a woman. It could have been written by a group."

58. S.H. Verhovek, "Besmirched 'Deportland' Wrestles with the I.N.S.," *New York Times*, Aug. 31, 2000, p. 12.

59. See, e.g., United States v. Jackson, 51 F.3d 646 (7th Cir. 1995). See M. Kadish, "The Drug Courier Profile: In Planes, Trains, and Automobiles; and Now in the Jury Box," *Am. U. L. Rev.* 46 (1997): 747. In Iseley v. Capuchin Province, 877 F. Supp. 1055 (E.D. Mich. 1955), testimony that a defendant did not fit a sex offender profile was held inadmissible as a defense against a sexual assault claim. While posttraumatic stress disorder (PTSD) testimony may be offered to show that a victim has symptoms that are consistent with sexual abuse, PTSD testimony is inadmissible to identify the perpetrator of the alleged sexual abuse. See State v. Alberico, 116 N.M. 156, 861 P.2d 192 (1993).

60. State v. Dobek, 2007 WL 257625 (Mich. App. 2007).

61. Reports are not infrequent about mothers who deliberately induce illnesses in their children in order to elicit sympathy or to play the role of heroic caregiver. Dr. Roy Meadow, chairman of pediatrics at the University of Leeds in England, observed parents simulating and producing dramatic illness in their children, and in a 1977 article, he described the syndrome as Munchausen Syndrome by Proxy (MSBP; the term *by proxy* means that instead of inducing illness in oneself, the person with the disorder creates illness in another person, almost exclusively a child). It has also been called Meadow's syndrome. See R. Meadow, "Munchausen Syndrome by Proxy: The Hinterland of Child Abuse," *Lancet* 2 (1977): 343. See also D.B. Allison & M.S. Roberts, *Disordered Mother or Disordered Diagnosis? Munchausen by Proxy Syndrome* (Hillsdale, NJ: Analytic Press, 1998); C.V. Ford, *Lies! Lies!! Lies!!! The Psychology of Deceit* (Washington, DC: American Psychiatric Press, 1996); L. Pankratz, *Patients Who Deceive* (Springfield, IL: Thomas, 1998); M.M. Brady, "Munchausen Syndrome by Proxy: How Should We Weigh Our Options?" *Law & Psychology Rev.* 18 (1994): 361; R.M. Sapolsky, "Nursery Crimes," *The Sciences*, 39, May/June 1999, p. 20; T. Vollaro, "Munchausen Syndrome by Proxy and Its Evidentiary Problems," *Hofstra L. Rev.* 22 (1993): 495; B.C. Yorker & B. Kahan, "The Munchausen Syndrome by Proxy: Variant of Child Abuse in the Family Courts," *Juv. & Fam. Court J.* 42 (1991): 51; B. Kahan & B.C. Yorker, "The Munchausen Syndrome by Proxy: Clinical Review and Legal Issues," *Behavior. Sci. & Law* 9 (1991): 73.

    In People v. Phillips, 122 Cal. App.3d 69, 175 Cal. Rptr. 703 (1981), the defendant was convicted by a jury of murdering one of her two adopted children and willfully endangering the life or health of the other by adding a sodium compound to their food. In order to suggest a motive for the defendant's conduct, the prosecution, over objection, presented evidence by a psychiatrist of MSBP. The appellate court held that because the conduct ascribed to the defendant was incongruous and apparently inexplicable, the psychiatric evidence was relevant to show a possible motive. The court further held that psychiatric evidence was not rendered inadmissible by the defendant's failure to make her mental state an issue. A significant aspect of the case was that the court allowed the use of psychiatric expert testimony to describe the phenomenon of MSBP and to give an opinion that the defendant mother fit the profile of a perpetrator, notwithstanding the rule that character evidence is admissible under Rule 404(b), which allows a series of acts to establish motive.

62. State v. Loss, 295 Minn. 271, 204 N.W.2d 404 (1973).

63. State v. Goblirsch, 309 Minn. 401, 246 N.W.2d 12 (1976).

64. State v. Loebach, 310 N.W.2d 58 (Minn. 1981).

65. 310 N.W.2d at 64. In United States v. Powers, 59 F.3d 1460 (4th Cir. 1995), the court, citing *Daubert*, excluded testimony that the defendant lacked the profile of a pedophile. See D.G. Saunders, "A Typology of Men Who Batter: Three Types Derived from Cluster Analysis," *Am. J. Orthopsychiat.* 62 (1992): 264.

66. G.O. Gabbard, "Psychodynamic Approaches to Physician Sexual Misconduct," in J.D. Bloom, C.C. Nadelson, & M.T. Notman (Eds.), *Physician Sexual Misconduct* (Washington, DC: American Psychiatric Press, 1999); R.I. Simon, *Clinical Psychiatry and the Law* (Washington, DC: American Psychiatric Press, 2nd ed., 1992).

67. See S.B. Bisbing, L.M. Jorgenson, & P.K. Sutherland, *Sexual Abuse by Professionals: A Legal Guide* (Charlottesville, VA: Michie, 1995), p. 263.

68. Federal Rules of Evidence, Rule 404(a).

69. Federal Rules of Evidence, Rules 404(b), 406.

70. Federal Rules of Evidence, Rule 404(a)(2). The prosecutor may not offer character evidence of the victim unless the accused does so first. In the trial of the four police officers who killed Amadou Diallo, the prosecution was criticized for "failing to humanize the victim" (J. Abramson, "A Story the Jury Never Heard," *New York Times*, Feb. 26, 2000 p. 31), but the prosecution is precluded from initiating character evidence about the victim. The state's accusation does not depend on whether the victim is a saint or a sinner. Unless the defendant brings it up, evidence offered by the prosecution of the victim's character is irrelevant. A person is entitled to the protection of the law regardless of his character, but when the defendant raises it, it is to establish self-defense. S. Gillers, "A Weak Case, but a Brave Prosecution," *New York Times*, March 1, 2000, p. 31. Moreover, prosecutorial argument that invites the jurors to put themselves in the shoes of the victim is considered improper. State v. Bashire, 606 N.W.2d 449 (Minn. App. 2000).

71. R. Alsop, "The Dead Are Psychoanalyzed at Murder Trials; Technique Aids Suspects Pleading Self-Defense," *Wall Street Journal*, July 23, 1980, p. 40.

72. Until fairly recently, the character of a victim was admissible on behalf of the defendant in cases of rape as well as in cases alleging self-defense. It was held that where the defendant had alleged consent as a defense, the "consenting character of the victim" could be shown to make consent more likely. In the 1970s, however, a "shield law" was enacted in virtually every jurisdiction to exclude evidence of a victim's "sexual behavior" in "sex offense" cases. Federal Rules of Evidence, Rule 412. See, generally, G.P. Fletcher, "Convicting the Victim," *New York Times*, Feb. 7, 1994, p. 11. The case of several Duke University lacrosse players wrongly accused of sexual assault fueled debate about the policy of excluding evidence of the character of the prosecutrix. Belatedly, the supposed rape victim has been revealed to be, if not a pathological liar, certainly pathological. C. Allen, "Durham Bull," *Weekly Standard*, Sept. 24, 2007, p. 40.

73. M. Ivins, "Wyoming Jury Frees Law Official in Killing," *New York Times*, Dec. 1, 1979, p. 10.

74. W. Gaylin, *The Killing of Bonnie Garland* (New York: Simon & Schuster, 1982). Writing about the trial of John Sweeney for the murder of his daughter Dominique, Dominick Dunne writes: "From the beginning we had been warned that the defense would slander Dominique. It is part of the defense premise that the victim is responsible for the crime. As Dr. Willard Gaylin says in his book *The Killing of Bonnie Garland*, Bonnie Garland's killer, Richard Herrin, murdered Bonnie all over again in the courtroom. It is always the murder victim who is placed on trial. John Sweeney, who claimed to love Dominique, and whose defense was that this was a crime of passion, slandered her in court as viciously and cruelly as he had strangled her. It was agonizing for us to listen to him, led on by [his attorney], besmirch Dominique's name. His violent past remained sacrosanct and inviolate, but her name was allowed to be trampled upon and kicked, with unsubstantiated charges, by the man who killed her." D. Dunne, *Justice* (New York: Crown, 2001), p. 26.

75. K. Johnson, "Private Talks at the Chambers Trial," *New York Times*, Feb. 15, 1988, p. 15.

76. E. Hardwick, "The Menendez Show," *New York Review of Books*, Feb. 17, 1994, p. 14.

77. See A.E. Taslitz, "Abuse Excuses and the Logic and Politics of Expert Relevance," *Hastings L. Rev.* 49 (1998): 1039.

78. 493 S.E.2d 770 (N.C. App. 1997).

79. By amendment to Rule 404(a)(1) of the Federal Rules of Evidence, effective December 1, 2000, it is provided that when the accused attacks the character of an alleged victim, the door is opened to an attack on the same character trait of the accused. Prior to the amendment, the government could not introduce negative character evidence as to the accused unless the accused had introduced evidence of good character. Thus, in United States v. Fountain, 768 F.2d 790 (7th Cir. 1985), where the accused offered proof of self-defense, this permitted proof of the alleged victim's character trait for peacefulness, but it did not permit proof of the accused's character trait for violence. Under the amendment, the accused cannot attack the alleged victim's character and yet remain shielded from the disclosure of equally relevant evidence concerning the same character trait of the accused. The amendment is designed to permit a more balanced presentation of character evidence when an accused chooses to attack the character of the alleged victim.

8

Syndrome Evidence

Syndrome evidence in courts of law is nontraditional. The search for evidence, particularly in child abuse cases, has led to a new species of medical evidence: the "syndrome" diagnosis.[1] Law Professor Christopher Slobogin observes: "Probably the single biggest change in the nature of psychiatric testimony over the past 25 years has been the advent of 'syndrome testimony.' A quarter century ago forensic experts rarely spoke of syndromes in criminal court. Today, this type of testimony abounds."[2]

This type of evidence, designed to establish the cause of a trauma, apparently originated historically in radiology and clinical observation. John Caffey, the father of pediatric radiology, who spent 20 years trying to fit the bony abnormalities seen on childhood x-rays into known syndromes, noted abnormalities that must be associated with child abuse as they were not seen in any known disease.[3] In 1962, Dr. C. Henry Kempe drew the attention of the medical profession to a set of presenting symptoms for which he coined the term *battered child syndrome*.[4]

The term *syndrome* is well known in the medical community as being "a running together," a *sundromos* in the Greek, or, as the *Oxford English Dictionary* puts it, "a concurrence of several symptoms in a disease." Normally a syndrome is regarded as being identifiable when a collection of symptoms occurs together so often that they provide a recognizable clinical entity. There is controversy, however, over the admissibility of syndrome evidence in criminal or tort cases to establish either that a particular traumatic event or stressor actually occurred or to explain the behavior of the victim. In a child abuse case, a psychiatrist or psychologist is presented to testify that the child exhibits the characteristics of a sexually abused child and that, by implication, the child was sexually abused.[5] (Experts use the term *rape trauma syndrome* in the case of a young girl as well as in the case of an adult woman, and they tend to use the term *sexually abused child syndrome* in the case of a child of tender years or when the offender is a family member.[6]) Because the defense in these cases is usually that the abuse did not occur and that the child is making it up, the testimony is designed to bolster the credibility of the child.[7]

Proponents of syndrome evidence argue that it is probative and logical. After all, what could seem more sensible than to look for patterns? Writing about syndrome identification, psychiatrists Randall Marshall, Robert Spitzer, and Michael Liebowitz have this to say:

> Because the etiology of most mental disorders is largely unknown, psychiatric research remains particularly dependent on the principles and process of syndrome identification. Identification of syndrome criteria with acceptable reliability can then facilitate investigation of syndrome validity with methodologies, such as factor and cluster analysis, laboratory study, studies of co-morbidity and distinction from other disorders, followup, family studies, and treatment response. Official recognition of a clinical syndrome can also greatly stimulate scientific interest, as illustrated by the surge of research in posttraumatic stress disorder (PTSD) since its recognition in *DSM-III* [*Diagnostic and Statistical Manual of Mental Disorders*] in 1980. Finally, diagnoses serve the crucial clinical objectives of identifying individuals in need of treatment and guiding treatment selection.[8]

In medical diagnosis, of course, the symptoms of an individual are compared with a pattern and a conclusion is drawn about etiology. As Jimmy Durante once put it, "If something looks like a duck, walks like a duck, and quacks like a duck, it must be a duck." Some courts call it "the duck test." Its application should be cautious, however, when it is based only on symptoms. Dr. Albert Drukteinis puts it thus:

> Medical conditions, generally, can be defined on different levels, depending on structural pathology, etiology, deviation from some physiological norm, observable signs, or symptom presentation. As definitions move from more objective criteria of identifiable and measurable pathology to symptom presentation only, they change from disease to syndrome. Therefore, a syndrome is more likely to include arbitrary or subjective criteria, and to lie in a more gray area of certainty. However, by using the term "syndrome," a word that has its roots in medicine, the symptom pattern described gains medical legitimacy.[9]

Certain assumptions about psychological evidence to ascertain a stressor are particularly questionable. One is the assumption that a certain posttraumatic stress syndrome is the pathway of a particular kind of stressor. In actuality, a wide variety of stressors may result in the trauma. Second is the assumption that victims of a particular stressor react in the same manner. In actuality, the impact of a stressor depends on the interaction between predisposition and environmental influence. One person may break down, another may be stoic. In short, not all victims react with the same characteristics, and many persons with these characteristics have not been abused, but instead may be suffering from something else, or they may be malingering or acting hysterically.[10]

Freud's patients recalled their trauma "with all the feelings that belong to the original experience." In 1895 and 1896, Freud, in listening to his women patients, felt that something dreadful and violent lay in their past. The psychiatrists before Freud who had heard seduction stories believed their patients to be hysterical liars and dismissed their memories as fantasy. Freud believed that his patients were reporting the actuality. However, some 9 years later he publicly retracted his theory about the etiology of hysteria. His patients, he now said in an about face, had been deceiving themselves and him: "I was at last obliged to recognize that these scenes of seduction had never taken place, and that they were only fantasies that my patients had made up."[11] Other therapists, however, find that the incest fantasies of their patients are based on a history of incest.[12] "Revival of memory" therapists link problems of depression, eating disorders, and multiple personality disorders to childhood sexual abuse.[13]

So out of a concern for relevance comes the legal question: Does the victim's clinically observed emotional trauma support the allegation about the stressor? In the usual tort or criminal case, an act is not in dispute, say, an automobile accident, but rather causation and damages are in dispute. In a turnaround, in cases involving syndrome evidence, symptoms are offered as evidence that a certain act occurred, but is the trauma stressor specific? Is there something peculiar about the trauma suffered by a victim of a tort or crime that is different from the trauma suffered as a result of other stressors, such as a hurricane or an automobile accident? Are subcategories of PTSD warranted, such as *sexually abused child syndrome, rape trauma syndrome, battered spouse, battered elderly*, or *incest trauma*?[14] These terms have developed to encompass the recurrent pattern of certain victims. Should they be elevated to the level of diagnostic nomenclature? Should they simply all be called PTSD? They are not listed as separate syndromes in the American Psychiatric Association's *Diagnostic and Statistical Manual of Mental Disorders*, the state-of-the-art, but who knows, perhaps some day they will be.

A number of appellate decisions have been rendered on syndrome evidence. For some purposes, some appellate courts have recognized a number of categories of PTSD and have allowed testimony on them.[15] In rulings followed by many other courts, the California Supreme Court has admitted testimony on the battered child syndrome to prove child abuse, but has excluded the rape trauma syndrome to prove that a rape had occurred. In 1984, in *People v. Bledsoe*,[16] the California Supreme Court made an attempt at explanation, saying that expert testimony concerning the battered child syndrome is admissible because that concept was devised for the purpose of determining whether a child's injuries were intentionally inflicted.

Dr. Kempe's formulation of the syndrome, however, was based on physical evidence. Put another way, the physical injuries sustained by the child do not form any injury pattern normally sustained by children in day-to-day activities. The battered child syndrome indicated that the injuries suffered by the child were not the result of an accident. Following Dr. Kempe's formulation, courts in various jurisdictions allowed an expert medical witness to express an opinion that a child exhibits the battered child syndrome. In these cases, the expert is permitted to give an opinion as to the cause of a particular injury, either on the basis of the expert's deduction from the appearance of the injury itself or from the syndrome.

Sexual child abuse, on the other hand, often leaves no physical injuries on which a diagnosis of battered child syndrome could be based. And what about an alleged rape? Should a rape counselor or other mental health professional be permitted to testify to an individual's postincident emotional trauma—"a constellation of symptoms experienced by the victims of sexual assault" or "rape trauma syndrome"—in order to prove that a rape, in fact, occurred (or a sexual abuse syndrome to prove that molestations occurred)? In a rape case, it is argued that the complainant would not suffer the symptoms if she had consented to the sexual act.[17] (Consent is no defense, of course, in cases of sexual abuse involving children. In these cases, the issue is whether it occurred and whether the accused is the perpetrator.)

In *Bledsoe*, the California Supreme Court noted that the rape trauma syndrome is a fundamentally different concept from the battered child syndrome because "[the rape trauma syndrome] was not devised to determine the truth or accuracy of a particular past event." Rather, the court said, it is "a therapeutic tool" used to treat victims by counselors who consciously "avoid judging the credibility of their clients."[18] That distinction has been widely, but not always, followed.[19] Actually, any of the PTSDs are treatable without regard to the nature of the stressor or even whether a stressor actually occurred. (The rape crisis centers could be crisis centers for all people in emotional distress.)

While courts have more often rejected than accepted rape trauma syndrome in establishing the stressor, they have allowed evidence of a child sexual abuse syndrome to show that the child was sexually abused. As a result of the concern about child abuse, in the trial of accused child molesters, many courts in recent years have allowed mental health professionals to testify that the psychological problems of a child are evidence that abuse has, in fact, occurred.[20] Other courts draw a distinction without a difference, saying that an expert may testify that the particular behavior of the child was characteristic of, or "consistent with," the behavior pattern of child sexual abuse victims generally, but the expert may not testify about whether the victim's allegations are truthful or whether sexual abuse did occur.[21]

In *State v. Kim*,[22] a child psychiatrist was allowed to present, over objection, the following testimony on trauma:

Q: Based upon your experience, Dr. Mann, have you had an opportunity—in the past—to assess the credibility of reported rape cases by children involving family members?

A: Yes.

Q: Approximately how many times have you done this?

A: I would say about 70 times.

Q: And, as a result of your interviews and examinations of these witnesses, have you arrived at conclusions with respect to the truthfulness of these reported rape cases involving family members?

A: Yes.

Q: Upon what do you base your conclusions as to the credibility of such claims?

A: There are several factors. One is the consistency of the account of the alleged sexual abuse. There are some common emotional reactions we frequently find in victims, which consist of a fear about safety, fear of future sexual abuse, feelings of depression or anxiety, embarrassment to have the alleged happenings known to peers or other people around them, a negative view of sex, some doubts that one parent might be strong enough to prevent further sexual abuse.

Q: Now, as a result of your experience and training in this area, did you come to the conclusion as to the truthfulness of the rape case reported by [the complainant]?

A: Yes, I found her account to be believable.

Q: Now, in arriving at that conclusion, what factors did you consider?

A: Many of the factors I listed before. I found [the complainant's] account quite consistent. She was very much preoccupied with a fear about safety, which took on some almost phobic dimensions, telling me that she locked herself in her room and shut the windows when she was alone out of fear that the accused might come back and she might be reabused. She was quite depressed, showed a negative attitude to sex and seemed somewhat naive in sexual matters, which made it very unlikely that she would have fantasized acts in that specific manner. Also a sense of fairness, I think, made it unlikely that she would make up a story just to get back at somebody.

In *Townsend v. State*,[23] the prosecution's expert witness opined that a child had been sexually abused on the basis of PTSD criteria as follows:

Q: As a result of your working with Sheila [the complainant], what was your diagnosis of her?

A: Posttraumatic stress disorder as a result of sexual abuse.

Q: Now, I am sure this jury is like I am, do not understand the posttraumatic stress disorder.

A: Very simply stated, it is a disorder [that] is a function of being exposed to a traumatic or series of traumatic incidents.

Q: What are the characterizations of that disorder that you observed in Sheila?

A: In Sheila, the observation of the anxiety, the fearfulness that was going to be the outcome. She's talked about the fearfulness of other kids hearing about what happened and how they are going to react to her. There are episodes when things—one of the things you see in posttrauma, there could be brushes with violence [that] are precipitated with minimal precipitation. There were also indications of that.

Q: Is this posttrauma stress disorder something that you have observed in other children in the 120 some cases that you worked on, other children that have been sexually assaulted as Sheila had?

A: Yes.

In proving the rape of an adult, however, most courts like the California Supreme Court in *Bledsoe* have concluded that rape trauma syndrome does not meet the standard of general acceptance in the scientific community.[24] The court emphasized, however, that while such testimony is not admissible for the purpose of proving that a rape occurred, it may be admissible for other purposes, such as explaining to the jury certain popular myths concerning rape victims. It may be used to explain a delay in reporting. Likewise, in battered spouse cases, prosecutors call mental health professionals as expert witnesses to explain the individual's failure to make a timely report for fear of reprisal, fear of being blamed, and fear of terminating the relationship.[25]

Quite frequently the prosecutor seeks to introduce evidence to explain behavior unique to victims of sexual assault in order to enhance the credibility of its witnesses. Some child or adult victims of sexual assault, for example, may fear retaliation and may delay reporting the crime for a longer period than the victims of other crimes. Others may delay out of shame, still others may recant their earlier allegations. The *child sexual abuse accommodation syndrome* (developed by Dr. Roland Summit) has as its premise that children do not lie about sexual abuse, but change their stories for other reasons.[26]

Promptness in the report of a crime tends to be taken as evidence of reliability. It is regarded as an indication that the accusation is not a concoction. Indeed, the law of evidence regards spontaneity of a statement as an indicium of trustworthiness and makes an exception for it in the rule against hearsay.[27] How can a prosecutor deal with a delay in reporting, or with a recanting of the story? In *Bledsoe*, the court said: "[I]n such a context, expert testimony on rape trauma syndrome may play a particularly useful role by disabusing the jury of some widely held misconceptions about rape and rape victims, so that it may evaluate the evidence free of the constraints of popular myths."[28] Thus, in another case, in Washington, a worker at a sexual assault center was allowed to testify that, in over 50% of sexual abuse cases involving children, there is a delay in reporting.[29]

Syndromes are multiplying. In the 1970s, there was much publicity about a disorder called the Stockholm Syndrome. The presenting symptom of this affliction affected hostages who showed signs of sympathy for the captors who had terrorized them. This condition was offered as an explanation for Patty Hearst's taking part alongside her former captors in a bank robbery. Not much is heard now about the Stockholm Syndrome, but we hear a lot about many others. London's *Spectator* reported (in 1994) that the Prince and Princess of Wales were both suffering *slighted-spouse syndrome*, the symptoms of which "are a loss of any dignity and a craving to tell the world one's own side of the story."[30] The Montana Supreme Court upheld an award of $240,000 in damages to a Beaverhead County farmer because the state's nearby highway construction was stressful to his pigs. A veterinarian gave expert testimony about *porcine stress syndrome*.[31] After a few days in Jerusalem, the Holy City, apparently normal pilgrims imagine they are biblical figures. The Holy City derangement is labeled *Jerusalem Syndrome*.[32] Then too, turn-of-the-century jubilees caused the premillennium stress syndrome.[33]

In *Werner v. State*,[34] Judge Marvin Teague of the Texas Court of Criminal Appeals described the proliferation in this way: "Today, we have the following labels: The Battered Wife Syndrome, The Battered Child Syndrome, The Battered Husband Syndrome, The Battered Patient Syndrome, The Familial Child Sexual Abuse Syndrome, The Rape Trauma Syndrome, The Battle Fatigue Syndrome, The Vietnam Posttraumatic Stress Syndrome, The Policeman's Syndrome, The Whiplash Syndrome, The Low-Back Syndrome, The Lover's Syndrome, The Love Fear Syndrome, The Organic Delusional Syndrome, and The Holocaust Syndrome. Tomorrow, there will probably be additions to the list, such as The Appellate Court Judge Syndrome."

Werner involved the admissibility of evidence on the Holocaust Syndrome, offered in support of a plea of self-defense (just as evidence of battered spouse is offered to establish a lower threshold for self-defense). The syndrome is one exhibited by children of survivors of the Nazi Holocaust who grew up hearing the stories from their parents of how entire Jewish families perished, without resisting, in the concentration camps during World War II. These children have formed a firm determination that if their lives are ever threatened, they will immediately resist forcibly and not permit injustice to be foisted upon them. This mindset makes them vulnerable to precipitous use of deadly force in what they believe is self-defense when confronted with assaultive behavior.

In this case, a psychiatrist would have testified (if allowed) that the defendant showed "some" of the characteristics of the syndrome associated with children of survivors of Nazi concentration camps. He would also have testified "that one does not need to be thinking of an event for another event in one's life to have an effect, a subconscious effect on him." The State objected to the proffered testimony on the ground of relevancy; that is, if self-defense is urged, the test to be applied is "the standard of an ordinary and prudent person in the defendant's position at the time of the offense." The majority of the Texas Court of Criminal Appeals, sitting *en banc* agreed, but Judge Teague, while mocking the proliferating phenomenon of syndrome evidence, argued in dissent that the Holocaust Syndrome should be given the same deference as the Battered Spouse Syndrome, or other syndrome, that is allowed to explain the effects of abuse on the condition of a defendant's mind.

It remains a controversial issue whether syndrome evidence should be admissible as evidence to establish that a specific stressor in fact has occurred. Because symptoms of a psychological nature are not stressor specific, the "duck test" is of questionable value. These symptoms do not imply etiology. With few exceptions, the American Psychiatric Association's *DSM* does not set out the etiology of the disorders.[35] A wide variety of stressors may give rise to a given symptom, which may also be attributable to normal developmental variations.[36] During a therapy session, the poet Anne Sexton asked, "Do I make up a trauma to go with my symptoms?"

In sum, a number of courts have allowed evidence of PTSD to explain the behavior of the victim in delaying a report or in recanting, while they have been divided on allowing it to establish the nature of a stressor or whether any stressor in fact occurred. To disallow syndrome evidence to directly prove an occurrence, but to allow it to indirectly prove an occurrence by proving the complainant's credibility is to draw a distinction without a difference.[37] In either case, the aim, in the last analysis, is to establish the occurrence of a stressor, either directly or through the truthfulness of the complainant. Explaining the delay in reporting by syndrome evidence is to enhance the credibility of the complaining witness and thereby, in effect, establish the stressor. It is yet another loophole in the bar on credibility testimony.[38]

Endnotes

1. D. McCord, "Syndromes, Profiles and Other Mental Exotica: A New Approach to the Admissibility of Nontraditional Psychological Evidence in Criminal Cases," *Ore. L. Rev.* 66 (1987): 19.
2. C. Slobogin, "Psychiatric Evidence in Criminal Trials: A 25-Year Retrospective," in L.E. Frost & R. J. Bonnie (Eds.), *The Evolution of Mental Health Law* (Washington, DC: American Psychological Association, 2000), p. 246.
3. J. Caffey, "Pediatric X-Ray Diagnosis," *Yearbook* (Chicago: Medical Publishers, 7th ed., 1978), p. 1335; J. Caffey, "The Parent-Infant Traumatic Stress Syndrome," *Am. J. Radiology* 114 (1972): 218.
4. C.H. Kempe, F.N. Silverman, B.F. Steele, W. Droegemueller, & H.J. Silver, "The Battered Child Syndrome," *J. Am. Med. Assn.* 181 (1962): 17.
5. See, e.g., People v. James, 451 N.W.2d 611 (Mich. App. 1990).
6. See, e.g., People v. Bledsoe, 36 Cal. 3d 236, 203 Cal. Rptr. 450, 681 P.2d 291 (1984); State v. McCoy, 400 N.W.2d 807 (Minn. App. 1987).
7. R.J. Roe, "Expert Testimony in Child Sexual Abuse Cases," *U. Miami L. Rev.* 40 (1985): 97.
8. R.D. Marshall, R. Spitzer, & M.R. Liebowitz, "Review and Critique of the New *DSM-IV* Diagnosis of Acute Stress Disorder," *Am. J. Psychiatry* 156 (1999): 1677.
9. A.M. Drukteinis, "Overlapping Somatoform Syndromes in Personal Injury Litigation," presented at the annual meeting of the American College of Forensic Psychiatry in Newport Beach, CA, March 30, 2000.
10. See P.R. McHugh, "How Psychiatry Lost Its Way," *Commentary*, Dec. 1999, p. 32; reprinted in P.R. McHugh, *The Mind Has Mountains* (Baltimore, MD: Johns Hopkins University Press, 2006), pp. 47–59. See also Note, "Unreliability of Expert Testimony on Typical Characteristics of Sexual Abuse Victims," *Georgetown L. J.* 74 (1980): 429.
11. See J.M. Masson, "Freud and the Seduction Theory," *Atlantic*, Feb. 1984, p. 33. See also D.P. Spence, *Narrative Truth and Historical Truth: Meaning and Interpretation in Psychoanalysis* (New York: Norton, 1982).
12. For example, Dr. Bertram Karon of Michigan State University in an address on delusions presented at a meeting of the Detroit Psychoanalytic Society, April 11, 1987, in Ann Arbor.

13. See W.M. Grove & R.C. Barden, "Protecting the Integrity of the Legal System: The Admissibility of Testimony from Mental Health Experts Under *Daubert/Kumho* Analyses," *Psychol., Pub. Pol., and Law* 5 (1999): 224.

14. For a discussion, see D.W. Shuman, "*The Diagnostic and Statistical Manual of Mental Disorders* in the Courts," *Bull. Am. Acad. Psychiat. & Law* 17 (1989): 25.

15. Evidence of rape trauma syndrome was allowed in State v. Marks, 231 Kan. 645, 647 P.2d 1292 (1982), but was rejected in State v. Saldana, 324 N.W.2d 227 (Minn. 1982). See Annot., "Admissibility, at Criminal Prosecution, of Expert Testimony on Rape Trauma Syndrome," 42 ALR4th 879 (1985).

16. 36 Cal.3d 236, 203 Cal. Rptr. 4:50, 681 P.2d 291 (1984).

17. In United States v. Wesson, 779 F.2d 1443 (9th Cir. 1986), the Ninth Circuit allowed a doctor's testimony that the alleged rape victim's injuries were not consistent with consensual intercourse to "aid the jury in determining the credibility of the alleged victim's claim that the intercourse was nonconsensual;" 779 F.2d at 1444. Similarly, in Henson v. State, 535 N.E.2d 1189 (Ind. 1989), the Indiana Supreme Court held that "fundamental fairness" required that the defense be allowed to present rape trauma syndrome evidence to show that the victim's behavior was inconsistent with that of a rape victim. See P.A. Petretic-Jackson & S. Tobin, "The Rape Trauma Syndrome: Symptoms, Stages, and Hidden Victims," in T.L. Jackson (Ed.), *Acquaintance Rape: Assessment, Treatment, and Prevention* (Sarasota, FL: Professional Resource Press, 1996), pp. 93–143.

18. The *Bledsoe* case involved a 28-year-old offender and a 14-year-old victim. People v. Bledsoe, 36 Cal.3d 236, 203 Cal. Rptr. 450, 681 P.2d 291 (1984).

19. Spencer v. General Electric Co., 688 F. Supp. 1072 (E.D. Va.1988); Commonwealth v. Zamarripa, 379 Pa. Super. 20, 549 A.2d 980 (Pa. Super. Ct. 1988). There are decisions to the contrary. See, e.g., State v. Allewalt, 308 Md. 89, 517 A.2d 741 (1986). See T.M. Massaro, "Experts, Psychology, Credibility and Rape: The Rape Trauma Syndrome Issue and Its Implications for Expert Psychological Testimony," *Minn. L. Rev.* 69 (1985): 395; D. McCord, "Syndromes Profiles and Other Mental Exotica: A New Approach to the Admissibility of Nontraditional Psychological Evidence in Criminal Cases," *Ore. L. Rev.* 66 (1987): 19; D. McCord, "The Admissibility of Expert Testimony Regarding Rape Trauma Syndrome in Rape Prosecutions," *Boston College L. Rev.* 26 (1985): 1143.

20. People v. Lukity, 596 N.W. 2d 607 (Mich. 1999); State: v. McCoy, 400 N.W.2d 807 (Minn. App.1987).

21. In Oliver v. State of Texas, 2000 WL 1389677, a Texas appellate court held that an expert may not testify that a person's recitation of events is or is not the product of fantasy or manipulation because such evidence is, in effect, particularized testimony concerning the person's credibility, but the court said, however, that an expert may testify about both the common traits or symptoms of child sexual abuse syndrome and whether the victim exhibits these traits. See also People v. Beckley, 434 Mich. 691, 456 N.W.2d 391 (1990); *In re* Brimer, 191 Mich. App. 401, 478 N.W.2d 689 (1991). The rule applies to child protective proceedings as well as to criminal prosecutions.

22. 64 Hawaii 598, 645 P.2d 1130 (1982).

23. 734 P.2d 705 (Nev. 1987).

24. See Frye v. United States, 293 Fed. 1013 (D.C. Cir. 1923).

25. See Ibn-Tamas v. United States, 407 A.2d 626 (D.C. 1979); Commonwealth v. Craig, 783 S.W.2d 387 (Ky. 1990); State v. Kinney, 762 A.2d 833 (Vt. 2000). For discussion of the " battered woman syndrome," see L. Walker, *The Battered Woman Syndrome* (New York: Springer,1984). The prominent Australian barrister Ian Freckelton argues against the role of syndrome evidence in the legal system and questions whether battered woman syndrome and rape trauma syndrome merit the status that they have been accorded by some courts. I. Freckelton, "Contemporary Comment: When Plight Makes Right—The Forensic Abuse Syndrome," *Criminal L. J.* 18 (1994): 29. See also A.L. Hyams, "Expert Psychiatric Evidence in Sexual Misconduct Cases Before State Medical Boards," *Am. J. Law & Med.* 17 (1992): 171.

26. R.C. Summit, "The Child Sexual Abuse Accommodation Syndrome," *Child Abuse & Neglect* 7 (1983): 177; see S.J. Ceci & H. Hembrooke (Eds.), *Expert Witnesses in Child Abuse Cases* (Washington, DC: American Psychological Association, 1998); see also T.G. Gutheil & P.K. Sutherland, "Forensic Assessment, Witness Credibility and the Search for Truth Through Expert Testimony in the Courtroom," *J. Psychiat. & Law* 27 (1999): 289.

27. Federal Rules of Evidence, Rule 803 (2).

28. 681 P.2d. at 298.

29. State v. Petrich, 101 Wash. 2d 566, 683 P.2d 173 (1984).

30. Oct. 22, 1994, p. 36.

31. State of Montana v. Howery, 204 Mont. 417, 664 P.2d 1387 (1983).

32. D. Sontag, "On Millennium's Heels, One for Jews," *New York Times*, Dec. 31, 1999, p. 3; E. Umansky, "Jerusalem Syndrome and Other 'Narcissistic Delusions,'" *Forward*, June 4, 1999, p. 18.

33. R.D. Rosen, "Millencholy," *New York Times*, Dec. 29, 1999, p. 25.

34. 711 S.W.2d 639 (Tex. Cr. App. 1986).

35. For example, the most common childhood diagnosis—attention deficit/hyperactivity disorder—describes behavior without in any way explaining its origin. The medication Ritalin is commonly given to treat the symptoms. For a critique, see P.R. Breggin, *Reclaiming Our Children* (New York: Perseus Books, 2000); R. DeGrandpre, *Ritalin Nation* (New York: W.W. Norton, 1999); L.H. Hiller, "Running on Ritalin," *Doubletake*, Fall 1998, p.46.

36. In United States v. Charley, 176 F.3d 1265 (10th Cir. 1999), the Tenth Circuit ruled that a mental health counselor's opinion that the child's symptoms were more consistent with symptoms of children who have been sexually abused than with the symptoms of children who witness physical abuse of their mother was erroneously admitted, the court held, citing Kumho Tire Co. v. Carmichael, 119 S. Ct. 1167 (1999), because no sufficient foundation was laid for this kind of expert's analysis, and no reliability inquiry was undertaken; 176 F.3d at 1281.

37. In State v. Hall, 330 N.C. 808, 412 S.E.2d 883 (1991), evidence that a victim's symptoms are consistent with those of the typical sexual or physical abuse victim was held admissible, but only to aid the jury in assessing the complainant's credibility.

38. Hypothetical: In a prosecution for rape, the complainant testifies that on a certain day she was at the Orange Blossom Bar where she met the defendant, a former boyfriend. She alleged that when the bar closed, she went to her automobile in the parking lot, the defendant followed, took out a knife, and forced her to drive to her apartment where he raped her. Some time later, she again visited the Orange Blossom Bar. By way of defense, defense counsel sought to introduce the testimony of an expert that he had "worked with patients who had suffered posttraumatic stress syndrome, including patients with rape in their backgrounds," and that in his opinion a person who had been raped would be unlikely to revisit the place where the incident had occurred. Should the court exclude the testimony? It likely would be allowed. P. Reidenger, "Private Nightmares," *ABAJ*, May 1990, p. 92.

   In Commonwealth v. Rather, 37 Mass. App. Ct. 140, 638 N.E.2d 915 (1994), the Massachusetts Court of Appeals held that it was reversible error for the expert psychologist to testify about the "pattern of disclosure of child sexual abuse victims," saying that, given the circumstances in the case, "the jury could reasonably have concluded that the [expert] witness had implicitly rendered an opinion as to the general truthfulness of the victims." The court cited as support a prior holding that "while the proposed testimony fell short of rendering an opinion on the credibility of the … [victims] before the court, we see little difference in the final result. It would be unrealistic to allow this type of … testimony and then expect the jurors to ignore it when evaluating the credibility of the complaining [witness]"; 37 Mass. App. Ct. at 149. In general, see C. Bleil, "Evidence of Syndromes: No Need for a 'Better Mousetrap,'" *S. Texas L. Rev.* 32 (1990): 37.

9

The Role of Psychiatric Diagnosis in the Law

Does or should psychiatric diagnosis play a role in the legal process? In a cautionary statement in the American Psychiatric Association's *Diagnostic and Statistical Manual of Mental Disorders* (*DSM-IV-TR*), it is set forth:

> The purpose of *DSM-IV* is to provide clear descriptions of diagnostic categories in order to enable clinicians and investigators to diagnose, communicate about, study, and treat people with various mental disorders. It is to be understood that inclusion here, for clinical and research purposes, of a diagnostic category, such as pathological gambling or pedophilia, does not imply that the condition meets legal or other nonmedical criteria for what constitutes mental disease, mental disorder, or mental disability. The clinical and scientific considerations involved in categorization of these conditions as mental disorders may not be wholly relevant to legal judgments, for example, that take into account such issues as individual responsibility, disability determination, and competency.[1]

Notwithstanding, the *DSM* is used frequently in the legal process. It is not surprising, given that it is recognized as state-of-the-art in psychiatry, and psychiatry is intertwined with the law on a number of matters. The *DSM* also states:

> When used appropriately, diagnoses and diagnostic information can assist decision makers in their determinations. For example, when the presence of a mental disorder is the predicate for a subsequent legal determination (e.g., involuntary civil commitment), the use of an established system of diagnosis enhances the value and reliability of the determination. By providing a compendium based on a review of the pertinent clinical and research literature, *DSM-IV* may facilitate the legal decision makers' understanding of the relevant characteristics of mental disorders. The literature related to diagnoses also serves as a check on ungrounded speculation about mental disorders and about the functioning of a particular individual. Finally, diagnostic information regarding a longitudinal course may improve decision making when the legal issue concerns an individual's functioning at a past or future point in time.[2]

In various legal matters, the law uses various terms for mental incompetency. The term *mental illness* is used for the purpose of civil commitment, *insanity* for a criminal defense, *incompetence* for triability or to justify guardianship or conservatorship, and *disability* for government disability assistance and vocational rehabilitation programs or for protection against discrimination.[3] Sometimes the same term is used in various legal matters. For example, *unsound mind* is used in contract law to determine whether a contract is voidable or in testamentary law whether a will is valid; in evidence, it is used to decide whether a witness may testify, and in torts or contracts to suspend the statute of limitations.[4]

The meaning of the term, or the diagnoses that fall under it, depends on the context. Thus, to suspend the statute of limitations, an *unsound mind* means an "inability to manage ordinary daily affairs," whereas to bar a witness from testifying, the same term means "deprived of the ability to perceive the event or of the ability to recollect and communicate with reference thereto." Providing a psychiatric diagnosis may help to explain why the individual is unable to manage ordinary daily affairs or why a witness is not credible, but in these matters a psychiatric diagnosis is not crucial to a determination. The one thing that all of these legal matters have in common is that if a person's mental state is at issue, the attorneys or the courts turn to mental health experts and they usually call upon them for a diagnosis. The examination at trial of the expert is as follows:

> Q. Does the plaintiff (the accused in a criminal case) suffer a mental illness?
> A. Yes.
> Q. What kind of mental illness? What is the diagnosis?
> A. What difference does it make? Why do I have to classify the mental illness?
> Q. Isn't the *DSM* state-of-the-art? We want to show whether the individual truly suffers a mental illness relevant to the case.
> A. Posttraumatic stress disorder.

The consequences of a diagnosis in law depend on the context. Thus, posttraumatic stress disorder as a diagnosis may entitle a veteran to benefits, but it may not serve to support a disability discrimination claim or a defense in a criminal case. Borderline personality is considered a serious, lifelong diagnosis in disability discrimination, civil commitment, and parental termination cases, but it is considered a far less serious condition when offered as a defense in the criminal context.[5]

Insurers limit coverage to only certain diagnoses set out in the *DSM* (to obtain coverage therapists are mindful of the limitations when writing a report or providing a diagnosis).[6] Proposals of mental health parity are met with the criticism that infers that the making of a diagnosis is subjective. Independent groups representing businesses and other insurers express alarm about the financial burden that would result from mental health parity. They contend that mandatory expanded coverage of mental illness would be prohibitively expensive.[7]

Criminal Responsibility

In criminal cases, under a plea of not guilty by reason of insanity (NGRI), evidence of mental illness is required as a threshold. The alleged inability to understand the nature of the act or to appreciate the wrongfulness of the act does not establish mental illness, but must be the consequence of the mental illness. Put another way, evidence of mental illness is necessary, but not sufficient, to establish NGRI. The legislatures or the courts have set parameters on mental illness that qualify for the NGRI plea.

The diagnostic classification is used as a means in criminal cases of explanation or exculpation. By diagnosis, socially unacceptable behavior is classified as the product of a psychiatric condition. When it was proposed that "rapism" be included in the *DSM*, objections were made that it might lead to NGRI verdicts of those who commit rape. In 1976, in the first draft of *DSM-III*, the Task Force on Nomenclature and Statistics of the American Psychiatric Association proposed a diagnostic category: sexual assault disorder. In a conference to review the proposal, Dr. A. L. Halpern, a representative of the American Academy of Psychiatry and Law, pointed out that while at first blush the introduction of the classification of the act of rape as being due to a sexual assault disorder might seem harmless, it could be considered by some as a move on the part of the American Psychiatric Association to foster the decriminalization of rape. In his statement, Dr. Halpern claimed that classifying sexually assaultive behavior under a specific psychiatric diagnosis would have the effect of minimizing the wrongfulness of the perpetrator's conduct and would open the door to even more widespread misuse of psychiatry than existed at that time. Prosecutors, he claimed, would seek to hospitalize offenders when there was insufficient evidence to convict, and defense attorneys would seek to hospitalize offenders when there was overwhelming evidence making conviction otherwise inevitable. Joining Dr. Halpern were women's groups throughout the country. Subsequent drafts of *DSM-III* did not include the proposed diagnosis.[8]

The various tests of criminal responsibility do not define mental illness or mental disease or defect. The M'Naghten test of criminal responsibility simply asks whether on account of mental disease or defect the individual did not "know the nature or quality of the act he was doing" or did not "know what he was doing was wrong." As in other formulations of a test of criminal responsibility, the threshold is that the individual have a mental disease or defect.

In these cases, does it really matter what diagnostic label is placed on the mental illness? Categories are not dimensional. They do not inform about the context or motives for action. They do not indicate how a person acts and relates to others in changing situations. Nor do they indicate the kinds of fantasies that are tied to actions and relationships. Prior to trial, the defense in criminal cases must inform the prosecution that evidence of insanity will be introduced, nothing more, and that is done by entering the special plea of NGRI. In that way the prosecution is given the opportunity to obtain an expert and to obtain his evaluation of the accused. The Federal Rules of Criminal Procedure, which governs introduction of expert testimony relating to a defendant's mental condition, does not require the expert to specify or categorize the mental condition from which the accused is suffering.[9]

What about at trial? Must a diagnosis be given? In 1961 in *Blocker v. United States*,[10] Judge Warren Burger, then sitting on the U.S. Court of Appeals for the District of Columbia, lamented the lack of a concrete definition of "mental disease or defect" in the test of criminal responsibility. He commented, "Not being judicially defined, these terms mean in any given case whatever the expert witnesses say they mean." Because of the vagaries of psychiatric diagnosis, the D.C. Court of Appeals in 1962, in *McDonald v. United States*,[11] suggested a legal definition of mental disease or defect and was unwilling to leave the definition to psychiatry only. The court said:

> Our purpose now is to make it very clear that neither the court nor the jury is bound by ad hoc definitions or conclusions as to what experts state is a disease or defect. What psychiatrists may consider a mental disease or defect for clinical purposes, where their concern is treatment, may or may not be the same as mental disease or defect for the jury's purpose in determining criminal responsibility. Consequently, for that purpose the jury should be told that a mental disease or defect includes any abnormal condition of the mind, which substantially affects mental or emotional processes and substantially impairs behavior controls. Thus, the jury would consider testimony concerning the development, adaptation, and functioning of these processes and controls.[12]

In the *Hinckley* case, the judge instructed the jury as follows:

> You have heard the evidence of psychiatrists and a psychologist who testified as [expert witnesses]. An expert in a particular field, as I indicated, is permitted to give his opinion in evidence, and in this connection you are instructed that you are not bound by medical labels, definitions, or conclusions as to what is or is not a mental disease or defect. What psychiatrists and psychologists may or may not consider a mental disease or defect for clinical purposes where their concern is treatment may or may not be the same as mental disease or defect for the purposes of determining criminal responsibility. Whether the defendant had a mental disease or defect must be determined by you under the explanation of those terms as it was given to you by the Court.[13]

Given a definition by decisional or statutory law, the term becomes a mixed question of law and fact. Rules setting out specific standards or requiring special types of proof narrow the expert's and jury's role. Given a legal definition, the trial judge may exclude evidence on certain mental illness, eliminating it from the concern of the jury. The expert or jury is not then left with unbridled discretion in determining what is mental illness. Thus, for example, under the definition in *McDonald*, evidence of anxiety disorder or personality defect would be excluded because it is not an "abnormal condition of the mind, which substantially affects mental or emotional processes and substantially impairs behavior controls," and the court would frame instructions to the jury on the basis of the definition.

A number of jurisdictions have adopted the *McDonald* formulation. Those jurisdictions that follow the American Law Institute's (ALI) test of criminal responsibility exclude, by definition, the sociopath from mental disease or defect. The ALI test excludes as a disability "an abnormality manifested only by repeated criminal or otherwise antisocial conduct."[14] A number of jurisdictions have considered excluding other personality disorders as well.[15] By legislation, Georgia, Maine, and Oregon exclude personality disorders.[16] Also by legislation, Connecticut excludes pathological or compulsive gambling.[17] Some jurisdictions exclude dissociative identity disorder.[18] When an expert gives a diagnosis, the cross-examiner thereupon challenges the expert on whether the accused fits the category. The law's exclusion of certain categories brings about the need to categorize. The result is "trial by category," or "battle of categories." A legal definition excluding evidence of certain categories of mental illness invariably results in controversy of whether the individual falls within or outside an excluded category. In the Hinckley case, experts gave numerous diagnoses. It may not be sufficient to simply say that the defendant suffers or does not suffer a serious mental disorder.

The categorical system of the *DSM* is inherently dichotomous (i.e., an individual either meets criteria for a disorder or does not), creating artificial boundaries between disorder and nondisorder and between disorders despite a lack of evidence that such boundaries naturally exist. The *DSM* was designed to facilitate research into the etiology and treatment of mental disorders by providing widely accepted and reliable definitions of disorders. However, despite years of intensive investigation, researchers have failed to identify a single neurobiological, phenotypic marker or gene that is useful in making a diagnosis of a major psychiatric disorder or for predicting response to psychopharmacological treatment.[19]

May the expert testify as to the consequences of the diagnosis? In 1984, following the Hinckley trial, the Federal Rules of Evidence and various state counterparts were amended to provide that the expert in a criminal case may testify only as to the defendant's mental disease or defect and the characteristics of such a condition, and (theoretically) may not tender a conclusion as to whether that condition rendered the defendant unable to appreciate the nature and quality or the wrongfulness of his act.

Competency to Stand Trial

A person accused of a crime is put to trial only if he is able to understand the nature of the charge against him and aid counsel in preparing his defense. The rule on triability originated in cases of physical disability (such as a heart attack or appendicitis), and the notion developed subsequently that a person so disoriented or removed from reality that he could not properly participate and aid in a meaningful defense ought not to be put to trial until such time as competency is achieved. Evidence of mental disorder (whatever the diagnosis) gives credibility to an allegation of incompetency.

Generally speaking, when the incompetency is the result of mental disease or defect (unlike physical disability), the accused is denied bail. One is considered a threat to society to be free on bail when unable even to meet the test of triability. As discussed in Chapter 10, deaf-mute is detained the same as one who is mentally disordered.[20]

Sexually Violent Predator (SVP) Laws

The recently enacted Sexually Violent Predator (SVP) statutes provide for commitment of sex offenders following a prison sentence. Under these statutes the offender must suffer from either a mental abnormality or a personality disorder that causes the likelihood of future predatory acts of sexual violence. In using the concept of mental abnormality, the Washington legislature invoked terminology that can cover a large variety of disorders. Some, such as the paraphilias, are covered in the *DSM*, others are not. In upholding the statute, the Washington Supreme Court said:

> The fact that pathologically driven rape, for example, is not yet listed in the *DSM-III-R* does not invalidate such a diagnosis. The *DSM* is, after all, an evolving and imperfect document. Nor is it sacrosanct. Furthermore, it is in some areas a political document whose diagnoses are based, in some cases, on what American Psychiatric Association leaders consider to be practical realities. What is critical for our purposes is that psychiatric and psychological clinicians who testify in good faith as to mental abnormality are able to identify sexual pathologies that are as real and meaningful as other pathologies already listed in the *DSM*.[21]

As noted in Chapter 16 on sex offenders, the court turned the *DSM* disclaimer on its head. The petitioner in the case argued that the term *mental abnormality* found in the statute is not a true mental illness because it is a term coined by the legislature rather than the psychiatric and psychological community. The court said, "Over the years, the law has developed many specialized terms to describe mental health concepts. … The *DSM* explicitly recognizes … that the scientific categorization of a mental disorder may not be 'wholly relevant to legal judgments.'"[22]

Civil Commitment

For civil commitment, the threshold requirement is mental illness. The statutes also require that as a result of the mental illness, the individual is dangerous to self or others, or lacks the capacity to recognize the need for treatment. A typical definition of mental illness in the legislation provides: "Mental illness means a substantial disorder of thought, mood, perception, orientation or memory, any of which grossly impairs judgment, behavior, capacity to recognize reality, or ability to meet the ordinary demands of life, but shall not include mental retardation."[23] Several jurisdictions exclude not only mental retardation, but also epilepsy and conditions resulting from alcohol or substance abuse. Some statutes specifically exclude personality disorders from the definition of mental illness, probably because these disorders are considered less treatable or best handled through the criminal justice system or through special sex legislation. When a certain disorder is excluded as a basis for commitment (e.g., drug addiction), commitment can be achieved by stating that it is secondary to a diagnosis that allows commitment.[24]

Various states prohibit individuals with certain diagnoses, whether or not they have been hospitalized, from having a firearm, but there is no databank, so the law is ineffective.

Tort Law

In tort cases, posttraumatic stress disorder (PTSD) is a favored diagnosis by plaintiffs because it is incident specific. It tends to rule out other factors important to the determination of causation. Thus, a plaintiff can argue that all of his or her psychological problems issue from the alleged traumatic event and not from myriad other sources encountered in life. A diagnosis of depression, on the other hand, opens the issue of causation to many factors other than the stated cause of action.

Whatever the accuracy of the diagnosis, be it schizophrenia or PTSD or something else, the question is what difference in a tort case does a diagnosis make when before-and-after determines the measure of damage? A diagnosis is not necessary to establish what the claimant was able to do before and after the trauma. Lay witnesses can attest to that. Yet the *DSM* is state-of-the-art and the forensic expert is invariably asked to label the claimant's suffering.

In theory, a diagnosis in medicine is supposed to provide information about cause (etiology) and treatment, but a diagnosis in psychiatry does not inform about cause, and treatments vary tremendously. In law, cause is important in allocating fault and prognosis is important in assessing damages. Studies show that diagnoses do not predict rehabilitation outcomes except in the broadest terms, and there are wide variations in outcomes within diagnostic groups.[25]

Child Custody

The issue of child custody involves an evaluation of the psychological status of the parties, not only in determining the best interests of the child, but also in reaching a decision as to whether a parent has the quality of fitness requisite to a granting of custody. A parent with a mental disorder resulting in a propensity to cause harm to others, including his or her children, would be an "unfit" parent.

A psychiatric diagnosis supposedly says something about behavior. At the same time, certain diagnoses tend to stigmatize the individual. Is it then an advantage or disadvantage to ascribe a diagnosis? Outside of trial, a diagnosis may assist an attorney in persuading a client to seek psychiatric treatment or counseling. However, at trial a diagnosis may complicate rather than elucidate the issues under consideration. Nonetheless, a number of experts on their own initiative or at the request of attorneys or the court give a diagnosis though it is not required as under an NGRI plea where categories are excluded from the test of insanity. Sometimes a party seeks an evaluation or diagnosis of the adversary in order to impugn the adversary.

Does a diagnosis of a parent assist in the determination of what is in the best interests of a child or in determining fitness? Is one diagnosed as schizophrenic a better or worse parent than one diagnosed as an obsessive-compulsive? Is one diagnosed as hysteric a better or worse parent than a psychopath? For years an individual diagnosed as homosexual would be denied custody.

The late Dr. Richard A. Gardner, who testified frequently in child custody cases, advised that there is much to lose, and little if anything to gain, by using diagnostic labels. As in the case of NGRI, it results in a "battle of categories." Gardner put it thus, "Not even the most astute diagnosticians are likely to agree about which diagnostic label best fits a particular person. As a result, no matter what diagnosis the evaluator provides, an opposing attorney is likely to find another serious and competent examiner who will come up with an entirely different diagnosis. Predictably, the lawyers will spin off on this issue in that it provides an ostensibly important reason to lengthen the litigation down this diversionary track."[26]

Others have come forth with a similar caveat. In an article in the *Journal of Psychiatry & Law*,[27] attorney David B. Saxe warned against the use of diagnoses in custody proceedings and discussed how misleading they can be and how they may complicate rather than elucidate the issues. He pointed out how the use of such diagnoses as schizophrenia and psychosis may mislead a court into believing that these disorders are invariably associated with an inability to function as a parent. In an article in the *American Journal of Psychiatry*,[28] Judge David Bazelon of the U.S. D.C. Court of Appeals deplored the psychiatrist's penchant for diagnostic labeling and described how it can narrow options for individuals once they have been put into a particular niche by a diagnosis.

Application for Admission to the Bar

Edward Ronwin was not allowed to take the Arizona bar examination because he could not demonstrate that he was mentally able to practice law. The Arizona Supreme Court indicated he has a paranoid personality, but it said that the phrase "mentally able to engage in active and continuous practice of law" is to be construed to exclude "persons whose longstanding personality traits indicate an obvious inability to get along with authority figures under situations of minor stress and conflict, whether or not these personality deficiencies rise to the level of medically recognized and categorized mental disorders."[29] Many states, for example, California, make "litigiousness" a barrier to admission.

Conclusion

In answer to the question presented at the opening: "Does or should psychiatric diagnosis play a role in the legal process?" The answer is that it plays a role, but it is not always a *sine qua non* in the resolution of a legal matter. It may result in a "battle of categories," diverting from the issue at hand.

Endnotes

1. *DSM-IV-TR* (Washington, DC: American Psychiatric Association, 2000), p. xxxvii.
2. P. xxxiii. *DSM-I* (1952) had 60 categories, *DSM-II* (1968) had 145 categories, *DSM-III* (1980) had 230 categories, and *DSM-IV* (1994) has 382 categories. See P. Conrad, *The Medicalization of Society* (Baltimore, MD: Johns Hopkins University Press, 2007).
3. The Americans with Disabilities Act (ADA) prohibits discrimination in the workplace on the basis of disability. The ADA defines *disability* as a physical or mental impairment that substantially limits one or more major life activities. In Toyota Motor Manufacturing, Kentucky, Inc. v. Williams, 122 S. Ct. 681 (2002), the U.S. Supreme Court clarified the legal principles governing the determination of disability under the statute. The Court ruled that an employee must show that the impairment "prevents or restricts the individual from doing activities that are of central importance to most people's daily lives. The impairment's impact must also be permanent or long-term." The inquiry focuses on the ability of an individual to perform tasks essential to most people's daily lives, rather than tasks associated with the individual's employment.

   The lower courts have recognized certain mental disabilities as falling under the ADA: paranoid schizophrenia, bipolar disorder, depression, anxiety neurosis or disorder, panic disorder, posttraumatic stress disorder, apraxia, agoraphobia, and claustrophobia. They have excluded from the ADA: transvestism, transsexualism, pedophilia, exhibitionism, voyeurism, compulsive gambling, kleptomania, pyromania, and substance abuse disorders. Also out of scope of the law's coverage are chronic lateness syndrome and personality traits, such as violent temper, arrogance, rudeness, and poor judgment. Most courts have held that only conditions that are included in the *DSM* and diagnosed with *DSM* criteria are psychiatric disorders. B. Boughton, "ADA Fitness Exams Need Forensic Psychiatrists," *Clinical Psychiatry News*, Aug. 2002, p. 42. For extensive discussion, see R.J. Bonnie & J. Monahan, *Mental Disorder, Work Disability, and the Law* (Chicago: University of Chicago Press, 1997).
4. Susan Stefan notes the various terms in her book *Unequal Rights* (Washington, DC: American Psychological Association, 2001), p. 40. See also B.J. Winick, "Ambiguities in the Legal Meaning and Significance of Mental Illness," *Psychol., Pub. Policy & L.* 1 (1995): 534.
5. Stefan, at p. 41.
6. See M.J. Schwartz, "Legal Issues in Managed Psychiatric Care: Managed Behavioral Healthcare Issues of Ambiguity and Due Process," *Am. J. Foren. Psychiat.* 28 (2007): 29. The more difficult physicians think it will be for them to obtain approval from an HMO for a medical procedure they think a patient needs, the more likely they are to exaggerate the severity of the patient's condition. R.M. Werner, G.C. Alexander, A. Fagerlin, & P.A. Ubel, "The 'Hassle Factor': What Motivates Physicians to Manipulate Reimbursement Rules?" *Arch. Internal Med.* 162 (May 27, 2002): 1134.
7. See, e.g., K.P. O'Meara, "Money and Madness," *Insight*, June 24, 2002, p. 12.

8. Newsletter, Psychiatric Society of Westchester, May 1986, p. 1. It is also argued that viewing pedophilia (now very much in the news) as an illness, like pneumonia, implies that the individual is not responsible for it and that it is treatable. T. Szasz, "The Psychiatrist as Accomplice," *Washington Times*, April 28, 2002, p. B3.

9. Fed. R. Crim. Proc. 12.2. In meeting the requirement of informing the prosecution of a defense based on mental condition, the court in United States v. Buchbinder, 796 F.2d 910 (7th Cir. 1986), noting that Rule 12.2(b) does not require the defense to specify the "exact mental disease" from which the defendant is suffering, stated that it is sufficient for the defense to notify the prosecution that he "intended to explore the possibility of a psychiatric examination." 796 F.2d at 915.

10. 288 F.2d 853 (D.C. Cir. 1961).

11. 312 F.2d 847 (D.C. Cir. 1962).

12. 312 F.2d at 851.

13. United States v. Hinckley, 525 F. Supp. 1342 (D.D.C.), op. clarified, reconsideration denied, 529 F. Supp. 520 (D.D.C.), *aff'd*, 672 F.2d 115.

14. ALI Model Penal Code § 4.01.

15. S.M. Reichlin, J.D. Bloom, & M.H. Williams, "Excluding Personality Disorders from the Insanity Defense: A Follow-Up Study," *Bull. Am. Acad. Psychiat. & Law* 21 (1993): 91.

16. Georgia's legislation states: "'Mentally ill' means having a disorder of thought or mood which significantly impairs judgment, behavior, capacity to recognize reality, or ability to cope with the ordinary demands of life, or having a state of significantly subaverage general intellectual functioning existing concurrently with defects of adaptive behavior which originates in the developmental period. The term 'mentally ill' shall not include a mental state manifested only by repeated unlawful or antisocial conduct." Ga. Crim. Proc. Law 27-1503. See Me. Rev. Stat. Ann. ch. 149, § 39-A (Supp. 1961); see also S. Rachlin, A.L. Halpern, & S.L. Portnow, "The Volitional Rule, Personality Disorders and the Insanity Defense," *Psychiat. Ann.* 14 (1984): 139; S.E. Reynolds, "Battle of the Experts Revisited: 1983 Oregon Legislation on the Insanity Defense," *Willamette L. Rev.* 20 (1984): 303; A. Van Leeuwen, "Personality Disorders and Criminal Responsibility," *Med. & Law* 9 (1990): 1250.

17. Conn. Pub. Acts 83-486 (1983); see R.J. Bonnie, "Compulsive Gambling and the Insanity Defense," *Newsl. Am. Acad. Psychiat. & Law* 9 (1984): 5.

18. State v. Greene, 139 Wash.2d 64, 984 P.2d 1024 (1999).

19. See R.L. Spitzer, J. Endicott & E. Robins, "Research Diagnostic Criteria: Rationale and Reliability," *Arch. Gen. Psychiat.* 35 (1978): 773.

20. See Jackson v. Indiana, 406 U.S. 715 (1972); see also E. Tidyman, *Dummy* (Boston: Little, Brown, 1974).

21. *In re* Petition of Andre Young, 122 Wash. 2d 1, 857 P.2d 989 (1993).

22. 857 P.2d at 1001, citing *DSM-III-R*, at xxix. See R.F. Schopp & B.J. Sturgis, "Sexual Predators and Legal Mental Illness for Civil Commitment," *Behav. Sci. & Law* 13 (1995): 437.

23. Vt. Stat. Ann. Tit. 18, § 7101(17).

24. For a historical discussion of commitment for substance abuse, see K.T. Hall & P.S. Appelbaum, "The Origin of Commitment for Substance Abuse in the United States," *J. Am. Acad. Psychiat. & Law* 30 (2002): 33.

25. C.J. Wallace, Draft Report, "Psychiatric Rehabilitation: Summary for NIMH," (1993); see also G. Mellsop & S. Kumar, "Classification and Diagnosis in Psychiatry: The Emperor's Clothes Provide Illusory Court Comfort," *Psychiat., Psychol. & Law* 14 (2007): 95.

26. *Testifying in Court* (Cresskill, NJ: Creative Therapeutics), pp. 78–79.

27. "Some Reflections on the Interface of Law and Psychiatry in Child Custody Cases," *J. Psychiat. & Law* 3 (1975): 501.

28. "The Perils of Wizardry," *Am. J. Psychiatry* 131 (1974): 1317.

29. Application of Edward Ronwin to be admitted as a member of the bar of Arizona, 113 Ariz. 357, 555 P.2d 315 (1976).

PART III
Criminal Cases

10

Competency to Stand Trial and Other Competencies

For the validity of the criminal process, a defendant must be competent at every stage of the proceeding, including competency to be executed. In this chapter, following the discussion on competency to stand trial, competency to plead and competency to confess are discussed. The question whether the defendant was competent to confess is likely to be raised prior to trial, at a suppression hearing.

The issue of an accused's competency to stand trial, otherwise known as triability, has become one of high visibility, and it has become one of the more controversial issues in criminal law. As a consequence, the use of the plea is subject to greater scrutiny than ever before. While it has not received the publicity of the insanity plea, at least a hundred defendants are determined to be incompetent to stand trial for each defendant found not guilty by reason of insanity.[1] An estimated 25,000 triability evaluations are carried out annually, with about one fourth to one half of the evaluees (according to various estimates) found incompetent to stand trial and hospitalized in a forensic setting.[2]

The standard for determining triability is often confused with, but is distinct from, the insanity defense. The issue of triability focuses on competency for trial (it is forward-looking) while, in contrast, the insanity defense focuses on the defendant's mental condition at the time of the offense (backward-looking). Incompetency to stand trial abates the action and is procedural in effect, while insanity is substantive and renders the defendant not guilty. In law, unlike psychiatry or medicine, a term is context-defined—it depends on the legal issue. Thus, the term *insanity* or *competency* is variously defined according to the context, for example, competency to commit a crime, to stand trial, or to make a will.

The rule on competency to stand trial originated in cases of physical disability. Thus, the trial of an accused who had a heart attack or appendicitis would be postponed until such time as he would be physically able to be present. Subsequently, the notion developed that a person so disoriented or removed from reality that he could not properly participate and aid in a meaningful defense ought not to be put to trial. Simply put, the rule says, "A case is to be put off until the accused is able to stand trial," that is to say, a continuance of the trial. The rule is designed (1) to safeguard the accuracy of the adjudication, (2) to allow the defendant to protect himself in the proceeding in order to have a fair trial, and (3) to preserve the dignity and integrity of the legal process. As frequently happens, however, rules take on new purpose in the process of application.

Triability has been used for legal maneuvering by both sides in criminal trials. The plea brings "flexibility" to the administration of the criminal law. The defense may use it to delay a trial or to lay a foundation for the introduction of mitigating circumstances or to avoid the difficult and usually unsuccessful trial based on a claim of insanity. The prosecution might raise the question of triability to preclude pretrial release or to obtain a lengthy commitment of the accused, especially when the case is weak on the merits or is controversial.[3]

In either event, the demonstrated effect of raising the plea has been to delay or interrupt the trial process. Although indefinite or prolonged delay is theoretically no longer permissible, the plea continues to be used for that purpose, and increasingly as a device to procure an otherwise unobtainable psychiatric examination for consideration in plea bargaining or sentencing. Thus, psychiatric evaluation remains a part of the process and, sometimes, the very reason for the triability plea. The vast majority of insanity cases are "walkthroughs"; that is, most cases involving competency to stand trial determinations never reach the contested trial stage. They are plea bargained.

Since the mid-17th century, the common law rule has been that one cannot be required to plead to an indictment or stand trial when one is so disordered as to be incapable of putting forth a "rational" defense. For triability, it requires presence of mind as well as presence of body. The accused must have the ability to cooperate with counsel in his own defense (a communicative ability) and the ability to understand the proceedings against him (a cognitive ability). Much depends on the complexity of the case. The issue can be raised at any time.

The Test of Triability

Virtually every court opinion nowadays on competency to stand trial quotes the standard of competency set forth in the 1960 U. S. Supreme Court two-paragraph *per curiam* opinion in *Dusky v. United States*,[4] which established the test of whether or not the defendant "has sufficient present ability to consult with his lawyer with a reasonable degree of rational understanding— and whether he has a rational as well as factual understanding of the proceedings against him." The Court said that it is not enough (as was the case previously) for the trial judge to find simply that the defendant is oriented to time and place and has some recollection of events. To apply the *Dusky* standard adequately, "the court must thoroughly acquaint itself with the defendant's mental condition."[5] In this seminal case, the Court did not state that the requirements are based on the Constitution, but in subsequent cases it has been said that the criminal trial of an incompetent person violates the right to substantive due process.

The test is generally considered to represent a constitutional principle binding on the various states. In any event, state rules regarding competency are generally consistent with the *Dusky* test. It appears to be widely recognized that *Dusky* establishes a minimal constitutional standard on competency. In 1975, in *Drope v. Missouri*,[6] the Supreme Court stated that it is a violation of due process to require a person to stand trial while incompetent, but the Court once again declined to spell out the precise meaning of "incompetent." The logical inference is that, although the test of incompetency is vague, the states may not abolish the rule of incompetency to stand trial, even though such action has been recommended by yours truly and others.[7]

Some jurisdictions have attempted, with varying success, to spell out with more particularity the test for triability. Extensive criteria, for example, have been adopted by statute in New Jersey.[8] These specific criteria include the following:

> (1) That the defendant has the mental capacity to appreciate his presence in relation to time, place, and things; (2) that his elementary mental processes are such that he comprehends: (a) that he is in a court of justice charged with a criminal offense; (b) that there is a judge on the bench; (c) that there is a prosecutor present who will try to convict him of a criminal charge; (d) that he has a lawyer who will undertake to defend him against that charge; (e) that he will be expected to tell to the best of his mental ability the facts surrounding him at the time and place when the alleged violation was committed if he chooses to testify and that he understands the right not to testify; (f) that there is or may be a jury present to pass upon evidence adduced as to guilt or innocence of such charge or, that if he should choose to enter into a plea negotiation or to plead guilty, that he comprehends the consequences of a guilty plea, and that he be able knowingly, intelligently, and voluntarily to waive those rights that are waived upon such entry of a guilty plea and (g) that he has the ability to participate in an adequate presentation of his defense.

Florida adopted, slightly paraphrased, a list of 13 "qualifiable clinical criteria" for assessing competence that were formulated by the Laboratory of Community Psychiatry at Harvard

University.[9] Still another list of 20 similar, yet somewhat different, criteria was proposed in Nebraska.[10] Arizona has directed examining experts to file with the court reports addressing seven specific matters.[11]

Insofar as the compilation of numerous specific findings may lead to an overall picture of the defendant's mental state, such criteria can significantly aid the expert and the court in reaching a determination of competence, but insofar as each separate finding is mandated to support a finding of competence, the list becomes counterproductive, substituting particularized judgments on superficial aspects of the defendant's mental state for the more important ultimate conclusion of competence. The Supreme Court in *Dusky* and in *Drope* established a minimum standard, understandably and necessarily imprecise, in order to permit individual judges to evaluate each case in the light of the individual defendant's level of functioning in relation to the complexity of that case.

Prosecutors have often raised the issue of competency, but in many cases, the prosecutor and defendant have a joint commitment to the success of the motion. When initiated by the prosecutor, the process is often labeled "preventive detention." When raised by the defense, it is called "medical immunity" from trial. The prosecutor is allowed to raise the motion on the ground that the state has a responsibility to seek justice and to protect society. A defendant may not block an inquiry into competence. In a number of well-known cases in England in the latter part of the 19th century, the prosecutor was allowed to raise the issue of fitness to proceed, a practice subsequently confirmed in the United States by the Supreme Court.[12] As a result, it is argued, the defendant is denied the right to a speedy trial.

Indeed, incompetency, however defined, may not be waived, even with the consent of the court. The trial court itself is obliged to raise the issue and to convene a hearing on the question at any time during proceedings when the evidence before the court raises a bona fide doubt as to the defendant's competence. In the leading case of *Pate v. Robinson*,[13] setting the precedent firmly, the undisputed facts were that the defendant, Robinson, had committed shocking acts of violence. He killed his wife and infant son. He also attempted suicide. Given "the uncontradicted testimony of Robinson's history of pronounced irrational behavior," the Supreme Court said that the trial court could not dispense with a hearing on competency, even though the defendant appeared alert and rational at trial.

Time Limit on Confinement

In 1972, in a much discussed case, *Jackson v. Indiana*,[14] the U.S. Supreme Court set a time limit on confinement for pretrial commitment for incompetency to stand trial, though it did not specify an exact period. Prior to this decision, the pretrial commitment procedure was widely used as a method for final disposition of a defendant's case. Commitment for incompetency was tantamount to confinement for life, especially when the accused was permanently retarded.

In this case, Theon Jackson, a 27-year-old mentally defective deaf-mute who could not read, write, or communicate intelligently, had been charged in 1968 with robbery. The testimony at the competency hearing indicated that Jackson's condition precluded his comprehension of the nature of the charges against him or his effective participation in his own defense. The prognosis was "dim" that he would ever develop the necessary communicative skills. Nevertheless, following the usual practice, the state court, finding Jackson incompetent, ordered him committed until such time as he could be certified by the health department as sane and possessing "comprehension sufficient to understand the proceedings and make his defense."

The Supreme Court ruled that such prolonged commitment violates the due process clause of the 14th Amendment. It stated that a person committed on account of incapacity to proceed to trial cannot be held more than the "reasonable period of time necessary to determine whether there is a substantial probability that he will attain that capacity in the foreseeable future." The Court further stated:

> If it is determined that this is not the case, then the State must either institute the custom-ary civil commitment proceeding that would be required to commit indefinitely any other citizen or release the defendant. Furthermore, even if it is determined that the defendant probably soon will be able to stand trial, his continued commitment must be justified by progress toward that goal.[15]

In oft-quoted language, the Court said, "At the least, due process requires that the nature and duration of commitment bear some reasonable relation to the purpose for which the individual is committed." Inasmuch as Jackson was committed because he was incompetent to stand trial, the Court concluded that the purpose of such commitment must be to make the defendant com-petent. The Court in *Jackson* did not address the issue of the disposition of the criminal charge in the case of one for whom restoration of competency was not a foreseeable possibility. It stated only that if such a defendant was to be further confined, the confinement would have to be based on the criteria for civil commitment applicable in that jurisdiction.[16]

Following *Jackson*, various states either by judicial decision or legislation have limited the term of commitment to either a "reasonable period" or a term of 12, 15, or 18 months or not to exceed a maximum sentence for the offense charged. Some say that having a maximum period encourages malingering. It is to be noted, however, that the *Jackson* limitation on confinement is not faithfully followed in all places. Approximately half of the states have not implemented *Jackson*. Who is there to seek out the inmate and represent him? (Quite frequently, there is an issue of transportation: the forensic unit advises the court that the individual is now competent to stand trial, but there is no response from the court, and the forensic unit does not have the authority to return the individual.) Not infrequently, no one wants the inmate out on the streets. Unlike the case of physical disability, the mentally disabled defendant is not, as a matter of pre-vailing practice, released on bail or on recognizance while awaiting trial, on the ground that the mentally ill are dangerous or a nuisance.[17] A number of states now provide for release on bail or on recognizance during the period of examination.[18]

Hearing and speech defects or illiteracy do not constitute mental illness and, thus, are not grounds for commitment under civil commitment statutes. Moreover, in a civil commitment, the hospital has control over discharge; the courts are concerned about the discharge of certain individuals and do not want to leave disposition to the hospital. The triability issue is a way for the court to retain control over the discharge of committed individuals. Before it became one of high visibility, the test of triability was not taken literally. The court, when calling on a psychiatrist for an opinion, did not really want to know whether the accused was capable of standing trial. The court itself could decide that by a few simple questions. What the court really wanted to know was whether the accused was likely to be dangerous or unduly bothersome in the community. In other words, labeling a person "incompetent to stand trial" signified that he was either dangerous or a nuisance and should be confined. That was then, and remains to some extent today, the hidden agenda.[19]

Before triability became an issue of high visibility, courts quite often failed to respond to communications from the hospital that the accused was able to stand trial. The hospital on its own initiative does not have the authority to return the accused to the local jailhouse whence he came or to discharge the accused. Saying one thing but meaning another was clearly demon-strated by the difficulties encountered by the hospital superintendent who certified to the court that a defendant was "competent to stand trial" under a literal interpretation of the test, but still maintained on medication. Just as an athlete may not use drugs to improve performance, an accused had to come to trial *au naturel*. Refusal to accept a defendant wanting to go to trial who was only "synthetically competent" strikingly indicated that the judge was concerned not with the defendant's capacity to undergo trial, but with his ability to get along in the community without medication. In these cases, the judge was concerned that the accused, an individual who has already shown himself—albeit allegedly—to be troublesome to the community, may not continue pharmacological treatment in the event of release and may again become a threat to society.

Modern advances in medication, science, and technology might be expected to affect the status of persons otherwise deemed incompetent. The competency rulings based on the use of psychotropic medication have been inconsistent, and they have also been one-sided. When the issue of competency was raised by the prosecutor or judge, it was usually held that a defendant had to be in a natural state, but, on the other hand, a plea raised by the defendant that he should not be put to trial when on medication has been rarely successful.

Trying Minors as Adults

The trend nowadays in trying minors as adults poses a triability issue, but trying minors as adults is not as new as it might appear. Before juvenile courts were established, minors were tried—and often sentenced—as adults. The courts applied common law guidelines on criminal capacity. Those rules defined the age of adulthood for purposes of criminal responsibility as being 7 years of age; the period between 7 and 14 was a zone of presumptive incapacity. The juvenile court system, which came into being at the turn of the 20th century, had the aim of treating, rehabilitating, and protecting the young from exposure to the adult criminal system, but with the increase in violent crime committed by minors, approximately 45 states have now passed laws to make it easier to prosecute minors as adults. In many cases, the court is finding the juvenile incompetent to stand trial as an adult.

Stress of Trial

A problem is presented when the accused, though able to cooperate with counsel and understand the proceedings, alleges that the stress of trial (or nowadays the televising of the trial) will cause a physical or mental breakdown. In common law, the issue of incompetency could be raised as a bar not only to arraignment, but also to trial, judgment, or execution. It is to be recalled that centuries ago there were many capital offenses, some 170 in number. The incompetency plea is allowed at any stage of the proceedings to undercut the penalty.

In various ways a witness or the accused who chooses to testify at trial is placed under stress; it is believed that stress aids in the ascertainment of truth. The idea that a witness "breaks" under heavy pressure or skillful cross-examination and finally tells the truth is depicted in countless tales. At one time in the United States, and still the practice in most other countries, the accused or witness had to stand while testifying (hence, the term *witness stand*). The occasional physical strain of prolonged standing increased the anxiety. And, of course, he may be subjected to a vigorous cross-examination, which is regarded as one of the principal and most efficacious tests that the law has devised for the discovery of truth. The chapter titles in a book by John Allen Appleman on cross-examination are illustrative of the practice: "Break Your Witness," "Step by Step Attack," "Witness on the Run," "The Kill," "Shock Treatment."[20]

What is the measure of competency to undergo the stress of trial? In a way, it is the type of question faced by many parents in deciding whether to push their child another step or to wait. At the wrong time, the ordeal will upset one's equilibrium. Given a particular stress, of whatever kind, anyone can break down. Can a given person's stress threshold be measured? Are stress and its effect predictable? Are the parameters known and fixed? In the case of the criminal defendant, is it the accusation, the pretrial wait, the trial, the decision, the sentence, or the lawyer's fee that will prove overwhelming? Will it make a difference whether the accused will take the stand to testify on his own behalf?

The televangelist Jim Bakker, accused of siphoning millions from his Praise the Lord ministry, crumpled to the floor of his lawyer's office and hid his head under a couch. He rolled into a fetal position and began to weep. The court suspended the trial and ordered Bakker to the Federal Correctional Institution in Butner, NC, for psychiatric evaluation, where it was reported that he was suffering from a Goyaesque hallucination in which "suddenly people took the form of frightening animals, which he felt were intent on destroying him, attacking him, and hurting him." Sometime later he was declared competent for trial, and the trial was resumed.[21]

Right to Refuse Medication

Medication may alleviate anxiety, as we all know, but in a number of cases the defendant has urged a right not to be tried under medication. A defendant may claim that medication will make him appear glassy-eyed or drugged and that appearance would prejudice him in the eyes of the jury. Some defendants have argued that they have an absolute right not to be tried while under medication. In certain cases, tranquilizing drugs may be necessary to control a defendant's disruptive behavior during trial.

Some defendants seeking trial immunity have argued for a "right to appear in court with mental faculties unfettered." In allowing a defendant under medication to be tried, the New Mexico Supreme Court justified its decision in this way:

> There is no evidence that [tranquilizing drugs, such as Thorazine] affected defendant's thought processes or the contents of defendant's thoughts; the affirmative evidence is that Thorazine allows the cognitive part of the brain to come back into play. The expert witnesses declined to call Thorazine a mind-altering drug. Rather, Thorazine allows the mind to operate as it might were there not some organic or other type of illness affecting the mind.[22]

Another claim is that courtroom demeanor may be relevant to the theory of defense (insanity at the time of the crime) and demeanor is affected by medication. In *United States v. Charters*,[23] the Fourth Circuit observed, "The sanity of the defendant at the time he committed the crime is usually the primary issue in the trial of an 'incompetent' defendant made 'competent' through the administration of drugs. However, if the defendant is heavily medicated during the trial, the jury may get a false impression of the defendant's mental state at the time of the crime." The court in *Charters* also rejected the state's argument that forcible medication should be permitted on *parens patriae* grounds. Likewise, in a death penalty case in Washington, the defendant was given tranquilizers and at trial he appeared calm, collected, and somewhat lackadaisical as he related the details of the murder for which he was charged. The Washington Supreme Court reversed his conviction on the ground that there was reasonable possibility that his attitude and demeanor as observed by the jury had substantially influenced their judgment.[24]

This view has wide support, especially among members of the legal profession, who by and large have a skewed impression of the effects of medication.[25] B. J. George, a prominent law professor and one-time law school dean, argued that in these cases medication should be barred as a matter of procedural due process. He wrote: "Due process can be denied by producing such a calming effect on a defendant that he or she cannot, through conduct or mode of testifying, demonstrate to a jury the irrationality or lack of control under pressure important to establish the insanity defense."[26] The courts hold that the defendant's demeanor, coupled with the content of his testimony, is sufficient to make the issue of his sanity a jury question even though he was the sole defense witness.[27]

In a case that reached the U.S. Supreme Court, David Riggins while awaiting trial in a jail in Nevada on murder and robbery charges complained about hearing voices and having trouble sleeping. After advising the prison psychiatrist that he had been successfully treated with the antipsychotic drug Mellaril in the past, the psychiatrist prescribed it for him. At the same time, through his lawyer, he asked for a determination of his competency to stand trial. Several months before his trial was to begin, he asked for a termination of his medication until the end of trial. He contended that continued medication would deny him due process because of the adverse effect the drugs would have on his demeanor and mental state during the trial, and violate his right to show the jury his "true mental state" as part of the insanity defense he planned to raise.

The trial court denied the motion and he continued to receive medication each day through the completion of his trial. At trial, he testified on his own behalf in support of his insanity defense. The jury found him guilty and sentenced him to death. He appealed to the Nevada Supreme Court, claiming that the forced medication had interfered with his ability to assist in his defense and prejudicially affected his attitude, appearance, and demeanor at trial. The Nevada Supreme Court affirmed the conviction, holding that the denial of his request to terminate medication was not an abuse of discretion.[28] A dissent argued that forced antipsychotic medication should never be permitted solely to allow a defendant to be prosecuted.[29] In a decision in 1992, the U.S. Supreme Court reversed, finding that the trial court had failed to make findings sufficient to justify the administration of medication. The Supreme Court said that as a condition for forced medication, the state must show both an overriding justification and medical appropriateness. In this case, the Court said, the state failed to justify the "need" for the medication.[30] Arguably, however, the need for medication for therapeutic purposes is co-extensive with the need for medication to render the individual competent to stand trial. Electroconvulsive therapy is apparently not used to achieve triability (it may cause memory loss in those treated).

In a Michigan case involving the shooting death of Dr. John Kemink, an otolaryngologist at the University of Michigan, it was undisputed that Chester Lee Posby, the defendant, shot and killed the doctor. The sole issue at trial was the defendant's sanity at the time of shooting. At the time of trial the defendant was on antipsychotic medication. Defense counsel requested discontinuance of the medication so that the jury could observe the defendant in a nonmedicated state. Without the medication, defense counsel urged, the jury would get a truer picture of the defendant's mental condition. In other words, defense counsel wanted the jury to observe the defendant "as he was during the time of the shooting, in an nonmedicated state." The psychiatrist who prescribed the medication testified that if the defendant were taken off it, he would in a matter of days again become delusional and disorganized and would not be competent to stand trial.

The trial court found an overriding state interest in maintaining the competency of the defendant that outweighs any right that he may have to be absent medication during the pendency of the trial. The state has a right, as does the defendant, the trial court said, to a speedy trial and to grant the motion would be to restrict that right. The Court of Appeals overruled the trial court, saying that the request to be taken off antipsychotic medication implicates the defendant's right to present a defense. Citing the Supreme Court's decision in Riggins, the court noted that there was no evidence, and the trial court made no findings with regard to whether the medication was essential for the sake of the defendant's own safety or the safety of others.

Taken off medication for a few days, the defendant could testify in a nonmedicated state, and that, the court found, did not implicate the question of competency during trial. The defendant had already assisted in his defense and there would not have been any further adjournments needed, the court said, because the defendant would then be administered the medication immediately after testifying.[31]

Andrew Goldstein, a schizophrenic who pushed a young woman in front of a subway train, was advised by his lawyers to go off his drugs in an effort to demonstrate to the jury the debilitating effects of his mental illness, but experts described the move as desperate and unethical.[32] In civil commitment proceedings, a few days before a scheduled hearing, psychiatrists often take the individual off medication to demonstrate to the judge his psychotic condition and, thereby, convince the judge of the need of hospitalization. Taking the individual off medication for the hearing is considered preferable to having the person on the streets where he will go off medication.

In lieu of taking the person off medication, what about allowing expert testimony to describe the effect of medication on demeanor? On this there is divided opinion. The Washington Court of Appeals said: "The ability to present expert testimony describing the effect of medication on the defendant is not an adequate substitute. At best, such testimony would serve only to mitigate the unfair prejudice that may accrue to the defendant as a consequence of his controlled outward appearance. It cannot compensate for the positive value to the defendant's case of his own demeanor in a [non]medicated condition."[33] On the other hand, the New Mexico Supreme Court said: "The defense can introduce any prior unusual behavior of the defendant as evidence at the trial and, in addition, can introduce at trial as evidence the fact that he [is] using [antipsychotic medication] and the effect that the drug medication has on the defendant by expert testimony, unless the Court is persuaded to rule otherwise during trial proceedings."[34] The ABA Criminal Justice Mental Health Standards recommend allowing "either party … to introduce evidence regarding the treatment or habilitation and its effects" and "to require the court to give appropriate instructions."[35]

A practical alternative may lie in allowing the defendant to present a video tape deposition of testimony given by him prior to trial in a medication-free state. In this way, the defendant could present probative evidence of his insanity through his manner and demeanor on the witness stand, thereby preserving his right to be tried while mentally competent and, at the same time, recognizing the state's interest in courtroom safety and order.

Would the defendant's demeanor on the witness stand while in a nonmedicated state have approximated his mental state at the time of the shooting? The passage of time and circumstances and the treatment that he had received in the intervening time would attenuate its probative value. Actually, in the substantial time that elapses between offense and trial, no one, to a greater or lesser degree, is the same. One is not in the same emotional state—one integrates or disintegrates, and, if nothing else, one is older. In the murder trial of Nathaniel Abraham, the 13-year-old boy who was tried as an adult for a killing he had committed, the trial attorney sought to have the case dismissed arguing that "the young person in front of the court today is not the same person as 2 years ago, and the jury will not be able to see what he was like then."[36]

The first rule of medicine is "do no harm." Is there a similar rule in the practice of law? Taking the individual off medication would have been antitherapeutic—relapses cause brain damage— and to what end? Suppose the defendant testifies in an nonmedicated state. What would be the likely outcome? Put aside the empirical evidence that juries rarely return a verdict of not guilty by reason of insanity, the odds of an NGRI verdict are even less when the defendant at trial appears crazy. Ironically, the crazier a person appears to a jury, the more likely they would not return a verdict of NGRI. They would not want him out on the streets, an outcome generally believed to follow an NGRI verdict.

The issue of forced medication to render an individual competent to stand trial again came before the U.S. Supreme Court in the case of Charles Sell, a St. Louis dentist.[37] He was indicted on counts of mail fraud, Medicaid fraud, and money laundering. As the trial approached, he became too delusional to understand the charges against him or to participate in his defense, and he declined to take antipsychotic medication. The Court set a high standard for forced medication: medical appropriateness, ensuring that side effects do not interfere with trial fairness, employment of less intrusive measures, and proof of governmental necessity. The Court said that these criteria need not be met if the purpose of the forced medication is related to the defendant's dangerousness or to "the individual's own interests where refusal to take drugs puts his health gravely at risk." Because the lower court had found him not dangerous to himself or to others, the Court assumed that he was not dangerous. The court remanded the case for further proceedings to determine the fairness of a trial given the likely effects of specific drugs.[38] Incompetent mentally ill defendants (including defendants who are actually innocent of the crime charged against them), who do not meet the criteria for forced medication, will languish untreated in a psychiatric hospital, most likely, a maximum security forensic hospital.[39]

Amnesia

A claim made by a defendant of general inability to reconstruct the events of the period in question (when the claim is opposed by the state) has generally been held insufficient to establish denial of due process. As the Louisiana Supreme Court put it, amnesia does not make the defendant incapable of understanding the proceedings against him or of assisting in his defense, even if brain injury or emotional state impairs his recollection of the crime.[40] A general claim of being unable to remember events for the period in question is insufficient, the courts say, because if such a claim had to be accepted, almost every defendant could successfully assert such a defense.[41] The Third Circuit has held that a defendant's feigning mental illness in his trial competency evaluation is an appropriate basis for a sentencing enhancement for obstruction of justice under the U.S. Sentencing Guidelines.[42]

Were amnesia a basis for nontriability, how much amnesia would be required? How many of the accused remember everything? Other reasons militate against a ruling of nontriability. Amnesia is not a mental illness, therefore commitment would not be possible. Then, too, defense lawyers do not want the accused to tell them about their complicity in the commission of a crime, as that would ethically preclude or inhibit their presentation of evidence. The Arizona Supreme Court said that it is a reproach to justice to try a person suffering from amnesia of an uncertain type and extent when it appears that reasonable continuance of the trial may provide the time needed to effectuate a limited or full recovery from the amnesic state. The court emphasized that each case must be considered on its own merits and that no absolutes may be justified without investigation.[43]

Generally, courts give little weight to amnesia in support of an incompetency plea. In *Wilson v. United States*,[44] the D.C. Circuit outlined in some detail the mechanism of *post facto* review of fairness. The court suggested that the trial judge should, before imposing sentence, make detailed findings, after taking any additional evidence deemed necessary concerning the effect of the amnesia on the fairness of the trial. The practical objection to the procedure outlined in *Wilson* is based on the possibility that a lengthy trial, carried to a verdict, would be a nullity.[45]

Multiple Personality Disorder and Hypnosis

The individual diagnosed as having a multiple personality disorder has posed perplexing problems. Multiples are often self-destructive and tend to emerge during periods of stress; a trial is a stressful event. A key dimension of the multiple personality disorder is amnesia, but as noted, the courts usually hold that amnesia alone is not sufficient grounds for a finding of incompetence to stand trial. But, how can an attorney talk with a personality who comes and goes? Forensic experts muse: Which personality does one examine for competency? Does one examine all as they appear? And, if so, which one was involved in the offense?[46]

Because hypnosis is the primary tool utilized in the diagnosis of multiple personality, one must be concerned about the court rulings that witnesses who have undergone hypnosis cannot be allowed to testify due to the impact of hypnosis on their testimony.[47] Most states hold that the testimony of a hypnotized witness is inadmissible, absent proof of clear and convincing evidence that the testimony being offered was based on facts recalled and related before hypnosis. In a Michigan case,[48] the prosecutor argued that hypnotically refreshed testimony of a complaining witness in a rape case should be admitted because the hypnosis was therapeutic in nature and not forensic or investigative. The purpose of the hypnosis was not specifically to refresh the victim's memory and, therefore, it was argued, was less suggestive. The Michigan Court of Appeals rejected this limitation, stating that the dangers associated with hypnotically induced testimony still existed. However, in the case of a defendant in a criminal case, the U.S. Supreme Court has ruled that the state may not bar his testimony, hypnotically enhanced or not. The defendant in a criminal case has a constitutional right to testify.[49]

Hearing Procedures

Some states (e.g., Texas) provide for a jury hearing on the issue of triability, but it is not required on the theory that the question is procedural, that is, it is not a substantive one that involves guilt or innocence. Apart from the statutory requirement in a few states, no duty rests upon the court to impanel a jury on the issue, but the court must consider and determine it in a judicial manner.

In 1992, in *Medina v. California*,[50] the U.S. Supreme Court upheld a state statute, which (1) put the burden of proving incompetency on the party asserting it, and (2) established a presumption of competency. In 1996, in *Cooper v. Oklahoma*,[51] the Court held unconstitutional a statute, which placed the burden on the defendant to show incompetency by clear and convincing evidence. The Court held that under the constitutional guarantee of due process, a "preponderance of the evidence," the lowest evidentiary standard available, is all that can be required of a defendant to demonstrate incompetence. Under that relaxed test, a defendant must show only that he is more likely than not to be incompetent. The court rejected a state argument that the higher burden of proof served the state's interest in efficiency and made it harder for malingerers to pretend to be mentally ill.

Who should assess the competency? Who is in the best position to assess it? The rules of evidence allow expert testimony when it will "assist" the court.[52] Does the court need help in assessing triability? If so, can expert psychological testimony provide this help? Might the assessment be left to defense counsel? After all, the defense attorney is not only in close and continuing communication with a client, but also knows the extent to which defenses may turn on the client's ability to understand them and assist counsel in advancing them. The D.C. Court of Appeals once observed that because of this proximity to client and case, "counsel's first-hand evaluation of a defendant's ability to consult on his case and to understand the charges against him may be as valuable as expert psychiatric opinion on his competency."[53]

But, can the defense attorney be entrusted to make a trustworthy evaluation? That aside, important as counsel data may be bearing on client competency, they cannot be offered or demanded by a court if they rest on or are derived from confidential communications under the protective umbrella of the attorney–client privilege. Moreover, the attorney becoming a witness may strain the attorney–client relationship if a defendant observes defense counsel apparently testifying against the client's best interests as the client perceives them.[54]

Then, why not leave the assessment to the judge or to another attorney? Why call for the assistance of mental health practitioners? The idea of assistance by mental health practitioners in this regard seems strange, but their evaluations are sought in an estimated 2 to 8% of all felony cases.[55]

As we have noted, prosecutors, having the power to inject the issue of triability, have viewed the process as a mechanism to remove from society defendants against whom they might have a weak case or as a means of curbing anticipated violent behavior. In this respect, *nontriable* was a code word for dangerous. What the court really wanted to know from the mental health professional was whether the accused was dangerous or an incorrigible nuisance. To say "incompetent" was another way of saying, "We should put him away." The process entailed automatic commitment, without right to pretrial release on bail (which was allowed a defendant suffering a physical disability, such as a heart condition). It achieved preventive detention.

Since 1972, when the Supreme Court in *Jackson* set out a durational limit for the length of commitment, that reason for engaging mental health professionals has disappeared, so what is the justification now for engaging the mental health professional? To ascertain whether the accused is suffering amnesia? That ascertainment is unnecessary as courts give little or no weight to amnesia in support of an incompetency plea. To ascertain whether the accused is malingering? In general, the best way to detect malingering is by police investigation or surveillance of the accused. Psychiatric experts are surely not needed.

The original intent of the test of triability in mental cases was to excuse only flagrantly psychotic and defective individuals. An unsophisticated layman or the custodial officer is able to apply the test; a commonsense point of view is all that is needed for a literal application of the test. Surely, in a literal application of the test, there would be no need for a diagnosis in depth, or for Rorschach protocols. Assuredly, the sort of evaluation needed for measuring triability is not the same as that needed for treatment. Anything more subtle than what a custodial officer can detect ought not to be a basis to stay a trial and, indeed, results in injustice and perversion of the criminal process. Moreover, the custodial officer, who has a great deal of experience with the criminal element and is able to observe the accused around the clock, is especially adept at detecting malingering.

It is not the suggestion here that the custodial officer or other jail attendants should serve as the "experts" on an accused's fitness to stand trial. The point is that fitness to stand trial can be and ought to be measured by an ordinary view. Psychiatric examination does not further the inquiry. For a literal application of the test, the judge can by himself make as valid a decision as anyone on the basis of a few ordinary and simple questions put to the defendant.

It is often said that a key issue in the determination of triability is whether the person is incompetent because of mental illness. For example, Joseph T. Deters, prosecuting attorney in Cincinnati, has this to say:

> In order for there to be an issue of triability, the defendant must first, as a threshold issue, demonstrate a mental condition, which affects his ability to understand the proceedings or aid in his defense. I am not sure whether the determination of whether a person has a mental condition is one which could be made without the aid of an expert. Once that prong is established, however, I agree that courts could rely on their own inquiry to determine the nature of the defendant's understanding. Having relied on the expert for the primary determination and not being fluent in the nature of mental conditions, however, it is no wonder that courts look to the expert to make their recommendation as to triability. Psychobabble is as confusing to the jurist as to any other laymen in the field of psychiatry.[56]

But, is diagnosis really relevant as to triability? If a defendant is capable of meeting the articulated requirements for competence, the presence or absence of mental illness would seem to be irrelevant. Indeed, a deaf-mute, though not mentally ill, may nonetheless be incompetent to stand trial. Legal criteria, not medical or psychological diagnostic categories, govern competency. Diagnosis is relevant only as to the question of potential restorability of competency with treatment. The possibility of restorability will be different in the case of psychotic depression than in that of dementia. Restorability is the question to be properly put to the mental health professional, not triability. Triability may be accomplished by education (particularly in the case of the low I.Q. defendant), anxiety management, or medication for depression or psychosis.[57]

Onsite Examination

Studies indicate that a majority of mentally disordered defendants, who are unfit, can, with active treatment, attain fitness within a relatively short period of time, often less than 90 days. As a consequence, onsite examination is increasingly required, and this procedure prevents stowing the accused in some remote facility. Onsite examination is also recommended as a less expensive procedure. Statutory changes in a number of states have made provisions for onsite examinations by a mental health team. Some states employ the principle of "least restrictive alternative" to the extent it is consistent with the defendant's pretrial release status. Like the defendant with a physical disability, the defendant with a mental disability may be placed in any appropriate public or private facility that agrees to accept him or with the Department of Mental Health on a "no decline" basis.

A Reevaluation of Triability

Should it really matter *why* the accused is unable to cooperate with counsel or to understand the proceedings against him or to endure the stress of trial? Is psychiatric diagnosis necessary? What difference does it make whether the cause of the disability is organic or functional? In the case of a physical disorder, such as a heart condition, the accused may be able to assist counsel or understand the proceedings against him, but be unable to withstand the stress of trial. On the other hand, in the case of mental disorder, whether organic or functional, the accused may not have the necessary communicative and cognitive ability to plead or go to trial. With it no longer being possible to use the triability issue to detain mentally disordered offenders indefinitely, the trend is away from the issue of the accused's mental condition.

A purely operational procedure would ask simply whether the person understands the charges and can assist counsel, or whether he can undergo trial or punishment. A clinical evaluation, however, follows from a "mental illness" interpretation of competency to stand trial. A number of courts in various states have ruled that evidence regarding triability may consist of lay observations as well as expert clinical testimony. The duty of the court to acquaint itself thoroughly with the defendant's mental condition may be satisfied by lay or clinical witnesses.[58]

The commentators who have urged abolition of the incompetency-to-stand-trial plea (a theoretical proposal in view of the Supreme Court's decisions) question whether we are prisoners of the past, adhering to old rules in the face of wholly changed circumstances. Without the assistance of counsel, as was the case in early law, the defendant's physical and mental presence is essential if he is to use the right to cross-question witnesses and make a defense; but today, given the assistance of counsel, the defendant's presence would seem to be less important. (Actually, from a practical point of view, the crucial question is not the competency of the accused, but rather the competency of the attorney.) Apart from medication, the so-called "restoration of competency" of the defendant is high comedy. One might think that the defendant is being trained to be a lawyer.

While a defendant may not waive the right to be present at trial (physically or mentally), he may forfeit it, as by misbehavior in the courtroom. In Russia, the defendant is in a cage in the courtroom. In the course of upholding the trial court for excluding the defendant from the courtroom when his behavior was contumacious, Justice Hugo Black wrote in 1970 in *Illinois v. Allen*:[59]

> Although mindful that courts must indulge every reasonable presumption against the loss of constitutional rights … we explicitly hold today that a defendant can lose his right to be present at trial if, after he has been warned by the judge that he will be removed if he continues his disruptive behavior, he nevertheless insists on conducting himself in a manner

so disorderly, disruptive, and disrespectful of the court that his trial cannot be carried on with him in the courtroom.[60]

Is an exception to the prohibition against trials *in absentia* to be made only when the defendant has apparent control over his behavior? In factitious incompetency, it may be said that if the defendant wants to be present, he has an easy choice, he can decide to behave, but such an option is not available to the person who is mentally "out of it." The Supreme Court in *Allen* ruled as it did in spite of the questionable mental competence of the defendant. In condoning trial *in absentia*, the Court may have implied that there are no longer any substantial societal interests underlying the defendant's ancient right to be present and that exceptions to the general prohibition against trials *in absentia* might be developed or expanded.

In support of the argument to abolish the triability plea, it is to be noted that the ability of the accused to consult with his lawyer as required by the test of triability is hardly important in actual practice. Defense lawyers do not want the accused to make any admission of guilt because ethical rules bar lawyers from knowingly offering false testimony. Then too, a claim made by a defendant of amnesia or a general inability to reconstruct the events of the period in question has generally been held insufficient for nontriability. Then, too, in every case, defense counsel enters a plea of not guilty, perhaps a plea of not guilty by reason of insanity; the defendant says nothing and need not say anything, and later there is bargaining on sentencing. Moreover, increasingly these days, accused persons are channeled through mental health or drug courts where treatment is mandated as an alternative to incarceration.

Competency to Plead

Should a distinction be drawn between competency to stand trial and competency to plead? The practical question is really not whether the accused is able to undergo trial, but rather whether he is fit to plead. In the vast majority of criminal cases (roughly 90 percent), there is no trial. The criminal convictions are entered by a guilty plea after plea bargaining. A trial, on the other hand, is open and public, and the state is put to its proof beyond a reasonable doubt. Theoretically, in plea bargaining or in the acceptance of a guilty plea, the plea must be entered voluntarily, with an understanding of the charge and consequences of the plea, and the judge must satisfy himself that a factual basis exists for the plea. But because the proceeding is clandestine, it might be suggested that only incompetency to plead not be waivable. The Court of Appeals for the Ninth Circuit, like a number of other courts, held that the competency of a defendant to waive counsel or plead guilty must be determined by a higher standard than for assessing competency for trial,[61] but the Supreme Court reversed this line of decisions.[62] Holding a defendant incompetent to plead, but competent to stand trial, would result in forcing the defendant into a trial that the defendant would rather avoid to obtain a more favorable negotiated sentence.[63]

In the past, serious difficulties arose when, on arraignment, the accused did not plead at all, or, in the ancient legal phrase, "remained mute." As joinder of issue (*litis contestatio*) was essential, it made possible a legal maneuver by which the defendant would attempt to block the proceeding by not pleading. Prior to the 19th century this difficulty was harder to overcome because, at that time, the accused was not entitled to legal representation in court if the charge was treason or felony. There was then no one to act on his behalf, and the court had no method of proceeding. When the court came to the conclusion that the accused remained obstinately mute, or "mute of malice," he was subjected to a form of judicial torture to compel him to plead. Increasingly heavier weights were placed on his chest—he was literally "pressed for his answer."

This *peine forte et dure* was abolished in England in 1772, and by an act of 1827, a plea of not guilty was entered wherever an accused person remained mute of malice. Prior to the beginning of the 19th century, it was not for the court to decide whether an accused who stood mute was mute of malice or mute by visitation of God. In this period, a jury was impaneled to try the issue. In such proceedings, witnesses were called to give evidence of the defendant's condition. If the accused was found unfit to plead, the judge would have no alternative but to order his detention.

Competency to Proceed *pro se*

The trials of Jack Kevorkian of "assisted suicide" fame and Colin Ferguson, who was charged with carrying out a massacre on the Long Island Railroad, were highly publicized cases where the defendant represented himself. They had "a fool for a client," as it is said whenever an individual represents himself. As they were deemed competent to stand trial, it followed, it was said, that they had a right to represent themselves. Illogically, precedents of the Supreme Court proclaimed that the standards for competence to stand trial and competence to represent oneself are one and the same (the Court revisited the issue in 2008 in State of Indiana v. Edwards and ruled that competency is not a unitary, all-or-nothing concept). Kevorkian no longer had the services of Geoffrey Feiger, who had defended him over the years, and he wanted no other attorney. Ferguson wanted no part of the "black rage" defense being prepared for him by his lawyers—basically a contention that he had been driven to murder by the effects of white racism. He insisted instead that he simply was not the killer. The trial was a spectacle (as was that of Kevorkian). "Obviously," said his one-time defense lawyer, "we should not allow an insane man to represent himself."[64] And, the Supreme Court now agrees.

Competency to Confess

What about a confession made to the police during an investigation? For the validity of a confession, must a suspect be "competent to confess"? What if the suspect is tricked by the police into confessing? The mentally incompetent are especially vulnerable to trickery. The Supreme Court has held that the concept of "ordered liberty" (or "the sporting theory of justice") is fundamentally at odds with the use of overt coercion, such as physical torture and extreme psychological pressure, to extract a confession, but the Court has given wide leeway to police trickery. Lying meant to effectuate a search or seizure or fabrication in the interrogation context is routine practice. To induce a confession, the police may show fake sympathy for the suspect, or they might mislead the suspect into believing that only written statements are admissible. They might also tell the suspect that "whatever you say may be used *for* or against you in a court of law," though they are not likely to testify on behalf of the defendant in any subsequent prosecution.[65]

A confession is deemed admissible despite the fact that it was a product of "command hallucinations" caused by the defendant's mental illness. In *Colorado v. Connelly*,[66] the majority of the U.S. Supreme Court concluded that to consider such a confession "involuntary" as a constitutional matter, without some form of coercive police conduct, would unduly infringe upon the evidence laws of the states. In this case, the defendant told a psychiatrist that God's voice had told him to confess. There was internal, but not external coercion. "Absent police conduct causally related to the confession," the majority said that a confession is "voluntary" under the due process clause.[67]

For there to be a constitutional violation, there must be not simply police "causation" but police "coercion." A subjective standard of voluntariness, taking into account all the defendant's weaknesses and infirmities, would make it exceedingly difficult to procure admissible confessions.[68] The standards of the ABA recommend, however, the use of expert testimony not on the admissibility (whether or not it was voluntary), but on the reliability or credibility of a mentally disabled defendant's statements.[69]

To what extent, if any, may the manner of response, or silence, of an arrested person to a Miranda warning be used against him in a criminal prosecution? Recall that *Miranda* provides that when an individual is advised of his rights to an attorney and to remain silent, anything he says can be used against him. No less than the bar on the use of silence as an impeachment device, the use of silence as an admission by the defendant in the prosecutor's case-in-chief is prohibited. Under the Supreme Court's ruling in *Wainwright v. Greenfield*,[70] an expert or other witnesses for the state cannot testify about the way the accused reacted to the Miranda warning. To make it explicit, the Miranda warning might be revised to read as follows: "You have the right to remain silent, and anything you say can be used against you. If you choose to plead insanity, your silence or the way you behave will not be used against you." In this case, a psychiatrist on behalf of the state expressed an opinion on the accused's sanity based in part on his post-Miranda warning behavior. It was deemed in error.

Yet when a defendant elects to present an insanity defense, the critical question is the criminal responsibility of the accused at the time he committed the offense, and, therefore, one might suggest, in determining sanity or lack thereof, the trier of fact should have access to all evidence reasonably bearing on the behavior of the accused at or near the time of the offense. However, under the Supreme Court's ruling, the trier of fact may not be apprised of the defendant's post-Miranda warning behavior.

Conclusion

The question still remains: What is to be done with the troublesome and possibly dangerous person who is unfit to stand trial? One should first ask whether he is indeed troublesome or dangerous and whether he would be responsive to treatment in a hospital setting. Moreover, how can he be kept under the control of the court? As a general principle of Anglo-American procedure, it is deemed irrelevant prior to determination of guilt for the court to inquire about what kind of person is before the bench. Apart from youthful offender laws that have a built-in provision for psychiatric evaluation, the only other way that the criminal law provides a means of getting this type of evaluation is when the accused pleads insanity at the time of offense. The presentence report that is possible following conviction often comes too late; the options open to the court at that time are more limited.

In contrast, courts in other countries allow great leeway in the testimony admitted as evidence. In these systems, the court seeks to find out as much as possible about the circumstances behind the acts that brought the accusation. For that, courts in the United States often turn to the incompetency issue. Under the guise of obtaining a triability evaluation, the court is able to obtain a psychiatric evaluation of the offender, and it wants the evaluation of the offender to be related to the need for institutionalization. Many defense attorneys, too, want a psychiatric report that they might use in litigation or as material for defense, and so they resort to the incompetency plea.

Now that the use of the incompetency plea by the prosecution to confine an individual is restricted, new questions have been posed. Should there be a moratorium on special buildings for the criminally insane? What shall be done with the troublesome and possibly dangerous person? What shall be done with the untried accused whose trial is impeded, or with the defendant who is found NGRI? Given that triability is constitutionally required, and cannot be abolished, should it apply only to the flagrantly psychotic?

Endnotes

1. D.L. Bacon, "Incompetency to Stand Trial: Commitment to an Inclusive Test," *So. Cal. L. Rev.* 42 (1969): 444.
2. B. Winick, "Restructuring Competency to Stand Trial," *UCLA L. Rev.* 32 (1985): 921.
3. Poet Ezra Pound, who spent World War II broadcasting for Mussolini, was found mentally unfit to face treason charges and he spent 13 years in the criminal ward of St. Elizabeths Hospital in Washington, D.C. Had he been tried, he would have insisted on testifying that America's entry into the war was a conspiracy between Roosevelt and the Jews. His long detention aroused the ire of the literary world

here and abroad and he was released in 1958. On his release, he returned to Italy ("America is a lunatic asylum," he said). During his confinement, he wrote his masterful *Pisan Cantos*. On the abuse of the triability plea, see T.S. Szasz, *Psychiatric Justice* (New York: Macmillan, 1965); C. Foote, "A Comment on Pre-Trial Commitment of Criminal Defendants," *U. Pa. L. Rev.* 108 (1960): 832.

4. 362 U.S. 402 (1960).
5. United States v. Makris, 535 F.2d 899, at 907 (5th Cir. 1976). For a comprehensive overview, see the *AAPL Practice Guideline for the Forensic Psychiatric Evaluation of Competence to Stand Trial*, supplement to the *J. Am. Acad. Psychiat. & Law* 35 (2007): S1–S72.
6. 420 U.S. 170 (1975).
7. R.A. Burt & N. Morris, "A Proposal for the Abolition of the Incompetency Plea," *U. Chi. L. Rev.* 40 (1972): 66; A.L. Halpern, "Use and Misuse of Psychiatry in Competency Examination of Criminal Defendants," *Psychiat. Ann.* 3–4 (1975): 123.
8. N.J.S. 2C:4-4.
9. *Florida Review Criminal Proceedings* 3 (1980): 211.
10. State v. Guatney, 207 Neb. 501, 299 N.W.2d 538 (1980).
11. D. Wexler et al., "The Administration of Psychiatric Justice: Theory and Practice in Arizona," *Ariz. L. Rev.* 13 (1971): 1–259. It has been held that the assessing professional must know what would normally go into the defense of the case. See United States v. Duhon, 104 F. Supp.2d 663 at 669 (W.D. La. 2000), citing M.N. Burt & J.T. Philipsborn, "Assessment of Client Competence: A Suggested Approach," *Champion* 22 (June 1998): 18.
12. Pate v. Robinson, 383 U.S. 375 (1966).
13. 383 U.S. 375 (1966).
14. 406 U.S. 715 (1972).
15. 406 U.S. at 738.
16. The case of Donald Lang in Illinois paralleled that of Theon Jackson in Indiana. See D. Paull, *Fitness to Stand Trial* (Springfield, IL: Thomas, 1993); E. Tidyman, *Dummy* (Boston: Little, Brown, 1974).
17. See G. Morris & J.R. Meloy, "Out of Mind? Out of Sight: The Uncivil Commitment of Permanently Incompetent Criminal Defendants," *U.C. Davis L. Rev.* 27 (1993): 1.
18. Conn. Public Act No. 76-353 (1976). Professor Bruce Winick reports the "staggering costs" of competency evaluations. B. Winick, "Restructuring Competency to Stand Trial," *U.C.L.A. L. Rev.* 32 (1985): 921.
19. For a readable account of cases, see D. Woychuk, *Attorney for the Damned* (New York: Free Press, 1996).
20. In 1965, David O. Selznick, the Hollywood studio mogul, who had produced *Gone With the Wind* and other major films, died while being questioned in a deposition for a case involving film distribution payments. Two years later, his son, L. Jeffrey Selznick, during a deposition in a case involving royalties from *Gone With the Wind*, said, "This is terrible," turned to his lawyer and collapsed into his arms and died shortly thereafter.
21. M. Brower, "Unholy Roller Coaster," *People*, Sept. 18, 1989, p. 98.
22. State v. Jojola, 553 P.2d 1296, 1299 (N.M. 1976).
23. 829 F.2d 479 (1987), *rev'd*, 863 F.2d 302 (4th Cir. 1988).
24. State v. Murphy, 56 Wash.2d 761, 355 P.2d 323 (1960).
25. See, e.g., L.C. Fentiman, "Whose Right Is It Anyway? Rethinking Competency to Stand Trial in Light of the Synthetically Sane Insanity Defendant," *U. Miami L. Rev.* 40 (1986): 1109; S. Tomashefsky, "Antipsychotic Drugs and Fitness to Stand Trial: The Right of the Unfit Accused to Refuse Treatment," *U. Chi. L. Rev.* 52 (1985): 773.
26. B.J. George, "Emerging Constitutional Rights of the Mentally Ill," *Natl J. Criminal Defense* 2 (1976): 35.
27. People v. VanDiver, 140 Mich. App. 484, 364 N.W.2d 357 (1985).
28. Riggins v. State, 808 P.2d 535 (Nev. 1991).
29. 808 P.2d at 541-543 (J. Springer, dissenting).
30. Riggins v. Nevada, 112 S. Ct. 2752 (1992).
31. People v. Posby, 574 N.W.2d 398 (Mich. App. 1997).
32. D. Rohde, "For Retrial, Subway Defendant Stops Taking His Medication," *New York Times*, Feb. 23, 2000, p. 21.
33. State v. Maryott, 6 Wash. App. 96, 492 P.2d 239 (1971).
34. State v. Jojola, 553 P.2d 1296 (N.M. 1976).
35. Standard 7-4.14(b).
36. B. Ballou, "Feiger Takes Over Murder Defense," *Detroit Free Press*, Oct. 20, 1999, p.1.
37. See Sell v. United States, 539 U.S. 166 (2003).

38. In United States v. Ghane, 392 F.3d 317 (8th Cir. 2004), the Eighth Circuit, citing *Sell v. United States*, pointed out that the government bears the burden of showing each of the following factors: "(1) important government interests are at stake; (2) involuntary medication is substantially likely to render the defendant competent to stand trial, and substantially unlikely to have side effects that will interfere significantly with the defendant's ability to assist counsel at trial; (3) involuntary medication is necessary to further the government's interests, and less intrusive means are unlikely to achieve substantially the same results; and (4) the administration of the drugs is medically appropriate"; 392 F.3d at 319. An important government interest exists when one is accused of a "serious" crime and "special circumstances" do not undermine the government's interest in trying the defendant for that crime. The seriousness of a crime is measured by its maximum statutory penalty. A statutory maximum term of 10 years imprisonment is a "serious" crime. United States v. Evans, F.3d 227 (4th Cir. 2005). In United States v. Dallas, 461 F.Supp.2d 1093 (D. Neb. 2006), the court concluded that (1) the government did not meet its burden of proving the second prong of the *Sell* test, i.e., that the administration of a drug or drugs would be substantially likely to render [the defendant] competent to stand trial, but substantially unlikely to cause side effects that will interfere significantly with his ability to assist counsel in conducting a trial defense, and (2) the government did not meet its burden of proving the fourth prong of the *Sell* test, i.e., that the administration of the specific kinds of drugs at issue is medically appropriate. Therefore, the matter was remanded for further evidentiary hearing.
39. See G.J. Annas, "Forcible Medication for Courtroom Competence: The Case of Charles Sell," *N. Engl. J. Med.* 350 (May 27, 2004): 2297; S. Satel, "Insanity Goes Back on Trial," *New York Times*, March 3, 2003, p. 23.
40. State v. Pellerin, 286 So.2d 639 (La. 1973).
41. United States v. Atkins, 487 F.2d 257 (8th cir. 1973).
42. United States v. Batista, 483 F.3d 193 (3d Cir. 2007).
43. State v. McClendon, 103 Ariz. 105, 437 P.2d 421 (1968); Comment, "Amnesia: A Case Study in the Limits of Particular Justice," *Yale L.J.* 71 (1961): 109.
44. 391 F.2d 460 (D.C. Cir. 1968).
45. In United States v. Andrews, 469 F.3d 1113 (7th Cir. 2006), the Seventh Circuit set out five nonexclusive factors to guide the trial court in assessing an amnesiac defendant's competency: (1) whether the defendant has any ability to participate in his defense, (2) whether the amnesia is temporary or permanent, (3) whether the crime and the defendant's whereabouts at the time of the crime can be reconstructed without the defendant's testimony, (4) whether access to government files would aid in preparing the defense, and (5) the strength of the government's case against the defendant. In contrast to *Wilson*, the court ruled that the trial court is not required to make a formal finding at the conclusion of trial regarding the amnesiac defendant's competency.
46. R. Slovenko, "The Multiple Personality: A Challenge to Legal Concepts," *J. Psychiat. & Law* 17 (1989): 681.
47. B. Diamond, "Inherent Problems in the Use of Pretrial Hypnosis on a Prospective Witness," *Calif. L. Rev.* 68 (1980): 313.
48. People v. Reese, 149 Mich. App. 53 (1986).
49. Rock v. Arkansas, 483 U.S. 44 (1987).
50. 505 U.S. 437 (1992).
51. 517 U.S. 348 (1996). In *Cooper*, the Court commented that an erroneous determination for competence "threatens a 'fundamental component of our criminal justice system'—the basic fairness of the trial itself"; 517 U.S. at 364.
52. Federal Rules of Evidence 702.
53. United States v. Davis, 511 F.2d 355, 360 (D.C. Cir. 1975).
54. American Bar Association Criminal Justice Mental Health Standards 7-4.8
55. R.J. Bonnie, "The Competence of Criminal Defendants: A Theoretical Formulation," *Behav. Sci. & Law* 10 (1992): 291.
56. Personal communication.
57. See R. Roesch & S.L. Golding, "Treatment and Disposition of Defendants Found Incompetent to Stand Trial: A Review and a Proposal," *Intl. J. Law & Psychiatry* 2 (1979): 349.
58. United States v. Makris, 535 F.2d 899 (5th Cir. 1976).
59. 307 U.S. 337 (1970).
60. 307 U.S. at 343 (1970).
61. Moran v. Warden, 972 F.2d 263 (9th Cir. 1992).
62. Godinez v. Moran, 113 S. Ct. 2680 (1993).
63. 113 S. Ct. at 2686.

64. J. Scott, "A Murder Trial: Through the Looking Glass," *New York Times*, Feb. 4, 1995, p.1. Scott Panetti, a mentally ill killer from Texas who was judged competent to stand trial and allowed to represent himself, was convicted and sentenced to death after arguing that only an insane person could prove the insanity defense. He dressed in cowboy clothing and submitted an initial witness list that included Jesus Christ and John F. Kennedy. The Supreme Court blocked his execution in June 2007, in a ruling that did not address his role in his own defense. Panetti v. Quarterman, 127 S. Ct. 2842 (2007); discussed in Chapter 14 on the death penalty.

   In State of Indiana v. Edwards, 128 S. Ct. 2379 (2008), the Supreme Court considered whether the defendant, Ahmad Edwards, found competent to stand trial, could be found incompetent to represent himself. He was charged with attempted murder. The Indiana Surpeme Court held that his competency to stand trial meant that he was competent to represent himself. On the other hand, the trial court had concluded that he should not be permitted to represent himself. One motion to dismiss that he filed included this sentence, "Defendant prays Psalm 15.5 for innocent of court property to be dismissed wherefore, so shall it be done." The U.S. Supreme Court, in a 7–2 decision, ruled that a defendant can be judged competent to stand trial, yet incapable of acting as his own lawyer. Justice Stephen Breyer, writing the opinion of the Court, cited arguments made by the American Psychiatric Association and the American Academy of Psychiatry and the Law in an *amicus* brief, to wit, that "[d]is-organized thinking, deficits in sustaining attention and concentration, impaired expressive abilities, anxiety, and other common symptoms of severe mental illnesses can impair the defendant's ability to play the significantly expanded role required for self-representation, even if he can play the lesser role of represented defendant." Justice Breyer then observed that even a layperson would recognize "the commen sense of this general conclusion." 126 S. Ct. at 2387. The Court distinguished *Godinez* on two grounds: (1) *Godinez* concerned the competence of a defendant who wanted to plead guilty, not, as in this case, a defendant who wanted to go to trial; and (2) *Godinez* held only that a state may permit a mentally ill defendant to plead guilty, but did not decide the converse, that is, whether a state may deny a mentally ill defendant the right to represent himself. In the dissent, Justices Scalia and Thomas expressed the view that "the Constitution does not permit a state to substitute its own perception of fairness for the defendant's right to make his own case before the jury." 128 S. Ct. at 2389. A holding that competency to stand trial includes a right to proceed *pro se* would require that a defendant be educated to be something of a lawyer, and it would impede the expeditious disposition of cases.

65. See Symposium, "Citizen Ignorance, Police Deception, and the Constitution," *Texas Tech. L. Rev.* 39 (2007): 1077–1435; see also C. Slobogin, "Deceit, Pretext and Trickery: Investigative Lies by the Police," *Ore. L. Rev.* 76 (1997): 775; C. Slobogin, "Lying and Confessing," *Texas Tech. L. Rev.* 39 (2007): 1275.

66. 479 U.S. 157 (1986).

67. The American Psychological Association submitted an *amicus curiae* brief, which stated: "Behavioral science does not use or rely upon the concepts of 'volition' or 'free will.' Accordingly, Dr. Metzner was not testifying as a scientist when he testified that respondent's command hallucinations impaired his 'volitional capacity.' Furthermore, even if Dr. Metzner only meant to testify that command hallucinations are, in a statistical sense, coercive, his testimony finds no support in the professional literature, and is contrary to clinical experience."

68. See J.D. Grano, *Confessions, Truth, and the Law* (Ann Arbor: University of Michigan Press, 1993).

69. Mental illness may contribute to confessions for a variety of reasons. Depression can promote abnormal feelings of guilt and remorse. Depression with psychotic features can produce a confession to a crime not committed. A condition of mania tends to result in poor judgment and feelings of grandiosity or invulnerability that would taint the individual's ability to appreciate the threat of self-incrimination or the risk in declining counsel. Delusions or hallucinations may compel someone to make a false confession. Subnormal intelligence/mental retardation by itself or in combination with mental illness may lead to confessions that are not fully voluntary, knowing, or intelligent. The acquiescent/compliance response is yet another reason that an individual might confess to a crime. The acquiescence response is a psychological term for the tendency to respond to any question in the affirmative regardless of context. An individual might desire to please authorities with the belief that confessing will end questioning, which may be viewed as an ordeal or may result in their release. Then, too, conditions such as intoxication or withdrawal can affect both judgment and comprehension. See K.J. Weiss, "Confessions and Expert Testimony," *J. Am. Acad. Psychiat. & Law* 31 (2003): 451; see also T. Reik, *The Compulsion to Confess* (New York: Grove Press, 1959).

70. 106 S. Ct. 634 (1986).

11

Criminal Responsibility

Criminal responsibility is based on two elements: *actus reus*, a wrongful act, and *mens rea*, a criminal intent.[1] The state has the burden of establishing these elements by proof beyond a reasonable doubt. The accused is not obliged to present any evidence (the accused may be a spectator at his trial), but in the usual case the accused will try to negate evidence of *actus reus* or *mens rea*, or in the situation where the evidence by the prosecution satisfies these elements of the crime charged, the accused may claim an affirmative defense.

Affirmative Defenses

"Justification" and "excuse" are affirmative defenses; the terms are commonly used synonymously as they both have the same effect: acquittal of the accused. For an affirmative defense, the accused has the burden of persuasion, but only by a preponderance of the evidence.

Justified conduct, strictly speaking, is conduct that is "a good thing, or the right or sensible thing, or a permissible thing to do." On the other hand, an accused in asserting an excuse says, in essence, "I admit that I did something I should not have done, but I should not be held criminally accountable for my actions." Justification negates the social harm of an offense, whereas an excuse negates the moral blameworthiness of the actor for causing the harm.

Self-defense may justify killing provided the reasonable person under the circumstances would have also responded with deadly force. Defendants who claim to have killed in self-defense must demonstrate that they believed the dangers they faced were lethal and imminent and that a "reasonable person" would have acted similarly. Provocation is a partial excuse, provided the accused's loss of control was reasonable. Provocation is what distinguishes intentional killings that are murder from those treated as the much less serious crime of manslaughter.[2]

In claims of self-defense, duress, or provocation, the law examines these matters by a "reasonable person" standard, i.e., what the reasonable person would have done under similar circumstances. In principle in these cases, there is often no need for expert testimony because judges and jurors are able to assess reasonableness, justification, provocation, and such.[3] However, there may be situations, such as that of the battered spouse, in which the trier of fact would find it of assistance to have a psychodynamic explanation to assess reasonableness or provocation.[4]

Over the centuries, the concepts of self-defense and justification have been tainted by absurd claims—the more absurd, it seems, the more widely they are believed. Throughout Christendom, Jews were often accused of murdering Christian infants for their blood to add flavor to their matzos. The Nazi destruction of Jews was based on the paranoid fantasy about an all-powerful international Jewry bent on destroying Germany. President Mahmoud Ahmadinejad of Iran says that the global economic system is a Jewish–Crusader conspiracy to keep Muslim nations in a position of weakness and dependency. On and on it goes. With the proliferation of lethal weapons combined with fanaticism, our species is given no better than a 50% chance of surviving this century.[5]

The Elements of a Crime

Actus reus and *mens rea*, we have noted, are the two elements of a crime, which the state must establish by proof beyond a reasonable doubt. Under the concept of *actus reus*, within the meaning of the criminal law, *act* is "voluntary action."[6] Thus, the convulsive movement of an epileptic is not an act, nor is the reflex movement of a person suddenly stung by a bee.[7]

The American Law Institute's Model Penal Code sets out the voluntary act requirement for criminal responsibility, and it gives examples of involuntary acts. The examples are illustrative, not exhaustive, leaving to the court a case-by-case development of the voluntary act requirement. It states:

1. A person is not guilty of an offense unless his liability is based on conduct that includes a voluntary act or the omission to perform an act of which he is physically capable.
2. The following are not voluntary acts within the meaning of this section:

   a. A reflex or convulsion.
   b. A bodily movement during unconsciousness or sleep.
   c. Conduct during hypnosis or resulting from hypnotic suggestion.
   d. A bodily movement that otherwise is not a product of the effort or determination of the actor, either conscious or habitual.[8]

In ordinary affairs, a child who vomits on another is not punished for it because the vomiting was an involuntary act; otherwise stated, not his fault. This sense of justice pervades the law. Therefore, one who urinates on the street violating an ordinance may get, to negate evidence of an unlawful offense, a doctor's note that he has bladder trouble. In common parlance, the formula is, "I couldn't help it" or "I didn't know what I was doing."

It may be said that one can always find—or not find—a voluntary act (or premeditation) on which to predicate criminal responsibility depending on how narrowly or broadly one frames the time period during which one looks. Thus, falling asleep at the wheel may be considered involuntary, but not if it is considered that the person earlier could have avoided driving at the time. On an occasion at the theatre, the man seated next to me belched so often and so loud that I could not hear the performance. He apologized, and said he could not help it. Before coming to the theatre he said he had eaten pickles and that was causing the belching. His eating the pickles was voluntary, but not the belching.[9]

What about self-induced incapacity? By not taking medication, does not an offender create the conditions of his defense?[10] In many cases, the symptoms of mental disorder present at the time of an offense are often the direct consequence of the offender's failure to take medication. Is it feasible, however, for a jury to evaluate the accused's behavior at a past time (when he caused the defense condition) with respect to the then-future ultimate offense? Moreover, it may be argued, the failure or refusal to have treatment is part and parcel of a pathological process. Those who suffer paranoid psychosis more often than not refuse treatment. They do not recognize their fears, which they perceive with extraordinary intensity, to be to the result of a pathological process, but believe them to be based in fact.

The legal significance of noncompliance with treatment has been broached in a number of cases. In *State v. McCleary*,[11] the accused had a history of chronic paranoid schizophrenia that predated the criminal conduct by more than a decade. He had been taking antipsychotic medication continuously since his first episode of illness, until 3 or 4 days prior to going to a park where he disrobed and wrestled a handgun from a park ranger. He was charged with robbery and pleaded not guilty by reason of insanity (NGRI). The court reviewed the psychiatric status of the defendant at the time of the offense, which supported his contention that he was insane at that time. The trial court ruled that he was not entitled to an insanity defense and convicted him, stating unequivocally that "there is a distinction between insanity and insanity that can be controlled." The appellate court, however, reversed on the ground that the accused by a preponderance of evidence had established insanity. As to the trial court's conclusion that noncompliance with medication should give rise to responsibility, the appellate court concluded that, in spite of demonstrating a cause for the accused's illness, it did not rebut the existence of his mental disorder at the time of the offense.

The result in *McCleary* is similar to that in a number of other cases. These cases reflect the view that conduct may be excused under a plea of NGRI as long as a "true" mental illness resulted in a substantial impairment of the individual's cognitive and volitional capacities at the time of the offense, whatever the cause of the mental illness or failure to take medication.[12]

Cases involving automatism or "unconsciousness" from sleepwalking or similar dissociative states are sometimes regarded as involving no action (no *actus reus*) and at other times they are characterized as instances of no intent (no *mens rea*), or at other times as predicated on a mental disorder (NGRI), resulting in postacquittal requirements (i.e., civil commitment) found with an insanity acquittal. Types of automatism are delineated as sleep automatism, epileptoid automatism, alcohol and drug automatism, hypoglycemic automatism, and psychogenic automatism.[13] In practice, a claim of automatism has typically required providing a cause for it.[14]

At times, it is claimed that an act was involuntary on account of a command hallucination. Forensic psychologist J. Reid Meloy opines, "Most individuals with auditory hallucinations will resist those that command activity, but hallucinations of a persecutory nature may precipitate such autonomic arousal and be perceived as so imminently threatening that affective violence results."[15]

Some may hear a command from God or Satan. Sometimes it is argued that a command hallucination negates wrongful intent as well as voluntariness. Obeying Satan is one thing, it is said, but obeying God is quite another. No biblical narrative is more dramatic than God's command to Abraham that he sacrifice his son Isaac. (Command hallucinations apparently are always to kill, not love.) Should obeying God make a difference in the halls of justice? Michael Abrahm, who broke into the home of George Harrison, the former Beatle, and stabbed him 10 times, was found NGRI because he believed himself to be St. Michael the Archangel, instructed by God to kill the "alien from Hell." He was convinced that Harrison was one of the phantom menaces predicted by Nostradamus. Needless to say, Harrison was outraged by the insanity verdict.[16]

In the prosecution of Andrea Yates for the drowning of her five children, Dr. Park Dietz testifying for the prosecution claimed that the fact that she attributed her actions to Satan was an indication that she knew her actions were wrong. For the defense, Dr. Philip Resnick testified, in effect, that even though she knew killing her children was legally wrong, she believed it was morally right because of her religious delusions. She was convicted (the verdict was overturned on account of misstatements by Dietz that she copied a television show).[17]

The leading case on a command from God dates from 1915, *People v. Schmidt*.[18] The defendant Hans Schmidt was accused of killing and dismembering a woman and throwing her remains into the Hudson River. Claiming that God had commanded the killing "as a sacrifice and atonement," he pleaded insanity. Judge Benjamin Cardozo, one of the country's most renowned judges, wrote the opinion of the court. He wrote: "[T]here are times and circumstances in which the word 'wrong' ... ought not to be limited to a legal wrong." In particular, if a person has "an insane delusion that God has appeared to [the accused] and ordained the commission of a crime, we think it cannot be said of the offender that he knows that act to be wrong."[19] The Model Penal Code comments on this situation: "A madman [who believes that God has commanded him] is plainly beyond reach of the restraining influence of law; he needs restraint, but condemnation is entirely meaningless and ineffective."[20]

During the mid-19th century and earlier, American asylum superintendents frequently made the diagnosis of "religious insanity." Benjamin Rush in 1812 noted that 10 percent of individuals came to mental hospitals because of religious feelings causing unbearable guilt. Religious melancholy frequently resulted in suicide or homicide. Not long ago, in Uganda, 5,000 people were killed in the "movement for the restoration of the Ten Commandments." Religious insanity is an ideologically distinct mental illness, but it is always debatable whether an individual is mentally ill or exuberantly religious.[21]

Judge Cardozo's language in *Schmidt* may appear to warrant an insanity acquittal of a mentally ill person who, though knowing his act was legally wrong, felt "morally justified" in committing it. He expressed caution:

> It is not enough that he has views of right and wrong at variance with those that find expression in the law. The variance must have its origin in some disease of the mind. The anarchist is not at liberty to break the law because he reasons that all government is wrong. The devotee of a religious cult that enjoins polygamy or human sacrifice as a duty is not thereby relieved from responsibility before the law.[22]

According to the Washington Supreme Court, "If wrong meant moral wrong judged by the individual's own conscience, this would seriously undermine the criminal law, for it would allow one who violated the law to be excused from criminal responsibility solely because, in his own conscience, his act was not morally wrong."[23] However, the court also created a "deific decree" exception to the general rule that wrong means legal wrong, thus allowing a defense like that in *Schmidt*. The court, nonetheless, upheld the homicide conviction of a person who had been hospitalized on several occasions with a diagnosis of paranoia. He contended that he followed the Moscovite faith and that Moscovites believe it is their duty to kill an unfaithful wife. The court said that "[t]his is not the same as acting under a deific command." Citing *Schmidt*, the court said, "It is akin to the devotee of a religious cult that enjoins human sacrifice as a duty and is not thereby relieved from responsibility before the law. [The accused's] personal 'Moscovite' beliefs are not equivalent to a deific decree and do not relieve him from responsibility for his acts."[24]

Just about every psychiatrist who examines an accused who claims a command from God or the Devil makes a diagnosis of some kind of delusional disorder. Should that make a difference in regard criminal responsibility? A few years ago, the deeply religious Judge John Noonan of the Ninth Circuit spoke at the University of Detroit College of Law on the primacy of freedom of religion as set out in the Constitution. He stated that an individual's religious belief ought to be respected at law. Following his address, I asked him how he would rule in cases when an individual commits a socially harmful act, but claims to have acted out of a spiritual dictate. He said he would want more facts, and he walked away. What facts?, I wondered.

The claim that "the devil made me do it" (comic Flip Wilson's repeated alibi) or a variation of it is frequently urged as a defense to criminal liability. A new twist was the defense raised in the trial in 2003 in Virginia of sniper Lee Boyd Malvo. Here the plea was not "not guilty" (on a theory that the act of shooting was involuntary), but rather it was NGRI. Defense counsel in collaboration with expert witnesses argued that 17-year-old Malvo was so brainwashed by John Muhammad, age 42, that he could not distinguish right from wrong and could not resist Muhammad's commands to commit crimes. Forensic experts called by the defense contended that Malvo's self-identification was so deteriorated under Muhammad's sway that he was little more than a puppet of the older man. They compared Malvo's relationship with Muhammad to that of a cult member with a charismatic leader or a child soldier with a warlord. They contended that as a result, he lost all sense of morality, all sense of identity, and became little more than an extension of Muhammad's ego.

According to the forensic experts, Muhammad exploited Malvo's hunger for a father figure and "trained" him to be a soldier "in his war against America." According to their testimony, Muhammad used an array of techniques to indoctrinate him, including isolating him, controlling his diet and sleep, forcing him to watch violent videos, training him to use guns, and teaching him a violent brand of Islam and black separatism. The indoctrination, they said, desensitized him to violence, broke down his already shaky sense of self, and made him unable to resist Muhammad's commands. In psychiatric terms, they said, he suffered from dissociative disorder, a loss of his sense of identity.

In the defense of Patty Hearst, the well-known criminal defense attorney F. Lee Bailey for the first time raised brainwashing as a defense to a crime, specifically the armed robbery in 1974 of a bank. The plea was "not guilty" (her behavior was claimed to have been involuntary); brainwashing was urged as an extension of the defense of duress. Some observers felt it was simply a ploy to gain sympathy for Patty Hearst by connecting her with prisoners of war (POWs) in the minds of the jurors, while others feared that brainwashing as a defense might be recognized and warned that the very foundations of a criminal law system based on free will and responsibility were threatened.[25]

The jury in the Hearst case was faced with the question of where coerced behavior ends and truly voluntary action begins for persons who appear to have changed their loyalties and values while in captivity. The ordeal described by Patty Hearst during the first weeks of her capture by a radical group known as the Symbionese Liberation Army allegedly resembled POW brainwashing conditions: isolation, sensory deprivation, torture, threats of death, arousal of suppressed guilt and hostility, and so on. The allegations were to no avail. The jury dismissed brainwashing as a defense. The media opinion of the testimony was critical, even derisive.

In the Malvo case, the defense did not claim that his actions were involuntary as was claimed in the Hearst case, but rather that they were the result of mental illness. That was claimed because under prevailing law, psychiatric and other background testimony is admissible on criminal responsibility only when a plea of NGRI is entered. That kind of testimony would not have been admissible under a not guilty plea. Under an insanity defense, the traditional rules of evidence go by the wayside.

The tactic was disingenuous. Though the insanity defense failed at trial, as expected, it allowed the defense to expose the jury to many of the same arguments it would make during the sentencing phase of the trial. During the trial, Malvo's estranged father, Leslie, testified that he taught his son, when he was about 5 years old, to ride a bicycle and play catch, and bought him ice cream almost every night. Then, too, Malvo's teacher in Jamaica described him as "a sad boy searching for love."

To no avail, the prosecutors complained frequently during the trial that the insanity defense was simply a tactic designed to present sympathetic testimony that would usually not be allowed in the guilt phase of a trial. Speculation has it that the trial judge, as is often the case, wanted to give the defendant every benefit of the doubt, and to avoid claims of racism if the evidence had been excluded.

There was no evidence that Malvo was psychotic. Any change of beliefs caused by brainwashing has not been found to constitute a mental disease or defect as required under the insanity defense.[26] Moreover, to establish a defense on the ground of insanity, it must be clearly proved that, as a consequence of the mental disease or defect, the party accused did not know the nature and quality of the act he was doing, or, if he did know it, that he did not know what he was doing was wrong. In all of the POW cases and in the Hearst case, the defendants were aware of what they were doing, so was Malvo.

Malvo was sentenced to life without parole. It was a victory for the defense—the death penalty was avoided, and that was what the case was all about (the jurors who wanted the death penalty gave in to those who did not want it). A month earlier, another jury in Virginia sentenced Muhammad to death. (Malvo and Muhammad have been linked to 20 shootings, including 13 deaths in Virginia, Maryland, Georgia, Alabama, Louisiana, and Washington, DC)

Jeffrey Toobin, the CNN senior legal analyst, said that the defense of Malvo was a "terrifically presented defense," i.e., a manipulation of law and fact.[27] In a posttrial interview, Craig Cooley, the defense counsel, let the cat out of the bag when he described Malvo as very immature.[28]

Immature he was, but immaturity is not mental disease or defect. He did not lose his identity as a result of brainwashing, as the experts contended, but like Woody Allen's *Zelig*, he had no identity of his own, but fitted himself according to the circumstances.

The legitimacy of the insanity defense, already held in low regard, was degraded even more by the tactics in this case, but disingenuousness in the defense of a client does not violate legal ethics. Moreover, in a capital case, failure to present expert testimony would be regarded as ineffective assistance of counsel. The forensic experts supported the disingenuous theory of the defense.

What about duress or necessity (as well as self-defense) constituting not an affirmative defense, but going to the presence of an essential element of a crime, that is, *actus reus*, whether the act was voluntary? An accused is permitted a defense of duress if, due to human threats, he acts in an unlawful way; an accused is permitted a defense of necessity if, due to natural events, he has no alternative but to act in an unlawful way. Both defenses are similar to self-defense, which is the necessary use of reasonable force to protect oneself, as measured by a reasonable person standard; except that in self-defense, the accused uses force against the source of the threat, whereas in duress and necessity, harms are usually inflicted on nonthreatening and innocent persons.[29]

At common law, we may note, if a wife committed a crime in the presence of her husband, the law presumed that he coerced her misbehavior and the crime was attributed to him (and so the husband had the right to chastise his wife). A new excuse from criminal responsibility, an excuse that in practice essentially applies to only women, is self-defense based on the so-called "battered woman syndrome" that is invoked when a woman kills her abusive male partner. The syndrome posits that the battered woman is too dysfunctional to leave the abusive male long before resorting to homicide. The acceptability of the evidence is due to the surge in consciousness about spousal abuse, irrespective of the law's definition of exculpatory or excusing conditions (the law of self-defense traditionally requires imminence, necessity, and proportionality). In the majority of states, evidence of battered woman syndrome is allowed in support of self-defense, or in other states, in support of an insanity defense.[30]

Recent genetic research indicates that some persons are endowed with a gene for impulsivity and aggression. Then, too, tests have shown that in the brains of people diagnosed as schizophrenic there is less activity in the prefrontal cortex, the part of the brain that governs thought and higher mental function. Psychiatrists say that individuals in the throes of an acute episode of schizophrenia often have associated with it impulsivity and aggression. Should defense attorneys ask for routine genetic or neurological testing of their clients?[31]

Though biological, sociological, and psychological determinism have had an influence on the criminal justice system, they have not made an appreciable inroad in its method of assessing responsibility. Genetic factors may be considered in mitigation after guilt has been assessed, but there is considerable evidence to suggest that individuals with genetic liability factors are less likely to learn from experience and more likely to commit further crimes.[32] Of course, to answer the question: "What made Hitler"? and seeing his baby pictures, the epitome of wide-eyed innocence, it would be fanciful to attribute his implacable hatred of the Jews to genes.[33] An article in the *New York Times Magazine* begins with the discussion of how neuroscience is transforming the legal system, but then concludes with quotes from Professor Stephen Morse that the claims are overblown. Morse says,

There's nothing new about the neuroscience ideas of responsibility; it's just another material, causal explanation of human behavior. How is this different than the University of Chicago School of Sociology, which tried to explain human behavior in terms of environment and social structure? How is it different from genetic explanations or psychological explanations? The only thing different about neuroscience is that we have prettier pictures and it appears more scientific. … Some people are angry because they had bad mommies and daddies and others because their amygdalas are mucked up. The question is: When should anger be an excusing condition?[34]

The perception that people are subject to forces beyond the individual's control would swallow any rule of responsibility. The test of criminal responsibility is delimiting. Most criminal offenders have poor control over their impulses or think poorly, so if that were an excuse, prisons would be empty. Over the years, however, a number of "sympathy defenses" have been raised, sometimes successful, such as the "adopted child syndrome," where the defense claims that the trauma of adoption, a fear of abandonment, and feelings of powerlessness and rejection produced a psychotic, insane rage that caused sufferers to strike out, often at the adoptive parents.[35]

Impact of Mental Disorder on *Mens Rea* or *Actus Reus*

Mental disorder may prevent the formation of a required *mens rea* or *actus reus*, the elements of a crime that the state must establish by proof beyond a reasonable doubt, or it may establish a complete or partial excusing condition. A mental disorder defense is raised when it is obvious that the accused committed the crime. It is called a *desperation defense*.

The controversy in criminal law on responsibility involving mental disorder reduces to this: Under what banner will evidence of mental disorder be presented, if at all, and what will be the consequences? Under a plea of not guilty (rather than a plea of NGRI), will an expert be allowed to testify that the defendant did not intend the consequences of his act or did not voluntarily act?

The courts and sometimes legislature provide that evidence of mental disease or defect is inadmissible where the defendant proceeds to trial on a plea of not guilty and does not place his sanity at the time of the offense at issue through a formal plea.[36] The U.S. Congress in the Insanity Defense Reform Act of 1984 stated that mental disease or defect constitutes a defense only under the insanity defense.[37]

The insanity plea, given its adoption in the United States and some other countries, is thus the route when evidence of mental illness affecting criminal responsibility is to be offered at trial. It is designed to give notice to the prosecutor that evidence of mental illness will be forthcoming, it channels the psychiatric evidence, and it provides commitment consequences. The late Professor Norval Morris, leading authority on criminal law, said that the insanity defense is not some kind of novel defense, but rather a refinement in proving *mens rea* or *actus reus*.[38]

The courts have held that due process is not offended by a rule that without pleading NGRI, a defendant cannot rebut evidence of intent by presentation of psychiatric testimony.[39] In this line of cases, in *United States v. Esch*,[40] the Tenth Circuit held that, in the absence of any claim of mental disease or defect, the trial judge may exclude expert opinion as to the accused's capacity to form the requisite intent. Following this line of cases, in *Clark v. Arizona*,[41] the U.S. Supreme Court in a lengthy opinion even upheld Arizona's restriction of psychiatric testimony in a truncated M'Naghten test.[42]

To put it another way, experts may speak on abnormality, but not on normality. The reason generally adduced for this is that the testimony is not helpful, or that the role of the judge and jury must not be usurped by experts unnecessarily testifying on matters within ordinary knowledge. The English Court of Appeal has said:

> We all know that both men and women who are deeply in love can, and sometimes do, have outbursts of blind rage when discovering unexpected wantonness on the part of their loved ones: the wife taken in adultery is the classical example of the application of the defense of "provocation"; and when death or serious injury results, profound grief usually follows. Jurors do not need psychiatrists to tell them how ordinary folk who are not suffering from any mental illness are likely to react to the stresses and strains of life.[43]

Thus, under this view, psychiatric evidence that an individual is not violent, but is susceptible to provocation in the "ordinary way" is not admissible. An expert witness may not be an expert on the "ordinary man"—this is the exclusive province of the jury. The jury is held not to be in need of assistance from expert testimony on the accused's ability to form the intent to commit the crime so long as the accused does not fall into the abnormal category. The law has the presumption that, absent evidence of insanity, we are all alike. Unless one pleads insanity, he is to be judged on the assumption that he has the same capacity as everyone else to judge whether an action is right or wrong, reasonable or unreasonable.

Definition of Mental Disease or Defect

The insanity tests do not identify the mental disorders that constitute mental disease or defect. They identify only the specific effects that must result as a consequence of the disorder. Judge Charles Doe of the New Hampshire Supreme Court in correspondence with Dr. Isaac Ray, the most influential American writer on forensic psychiatry in the 19th century, noted that the law never wanted to restrict the insanity defense to particular forms of illness.[44] On the bench, Judge Doe refused to grant judicial sanction to controversial medicolegal tests and definitions of mental illness or legal insanity. Instead, he would tell the jury that mental illness defies definition and that no test is applicable to every case. The jury, he said, must decide the case on its individual merits. If they believed from the lay and expert testimony that the act in question was the result of mental illness, the verdict must be "not guilty by reason of insanity." In 1869, in State v. Pike,[45] Judge Doe told the jury that there was no single rigid test of mental disease, rather "all symptoms and all tests of mental disease are purely matters of fact," grist for the jury's mill.[46]

Judge Warren Burger, when on the U.S. Court of Appeals for the District of Columbia, lamented the lack of definition of *mental disease or defect*. In a concurring opinion in 1961, he noted that the critical threshold issue is whether the defendant has a mental disease or defect and he said, "Not being judicially defined, these terms mean in any given case whatever the expert witnesses say they mean."[47]

A definition of mental disease or defect in the test of criminal responsibility that differs from that in the law on commitment of the insanity acquittee may result in no confinement of the defendant, and, as a result, the public safety may be put at risk. Take, for example, the prosecution in Illinois of Jearl Wood. Expert testimony at trial was that the offense grew out of his traumatic Vietnam experience. He had severely wounded a foreman at the plant where he was working. The jury found him not guilty by reason of insanity, and in a separate commitment hearing after the trial, a psychiatrist for the Illinois Department of Mental Health confirmed the posttraumatic stress disorder (PTSD) diagnosis, but it did not warrant commitment in the mental health system. He "slipped through the cracks" of the two systems, as it was put.[48] Sometimes the defendant is found NGRI on one count (to provide hospitalization) and guilty on another count (that would result in imprisonment following hospitalization).[49]

For the diagnosis of psychological disorders, as is well known, use is made of the American Psychiatric Association's compendium of mental disorders, the *Diagnostic and Statistical Manual of Mental Disorders* (DSM). As the history of the *DSMs* would reveal, defining mental disorders has been not only conceptually difficult, but also politically controversial. There has been debate about whether the definition of mental disorder has been used systematically to decide what is pathological and belongs in the compendium. In any event, none of the various psychiatric diagnoses set out in the *DSM* of necessity entails impairment of cognition or control, although it is sometimes argued at trial. In the *Hinckley* case, the trial judge instructed the jury as follows about the diagnostic labeling:

You have heard the evidence of psychiatrists and a psychologist who testified as [expert witnesses]. An expert in a particular field, as I indicated, is permitted to give his opinion in evidence, and in this connection you are instructed that you are not bound by medical labels, definitions, or conclusions as to what is or is not a mental disease or defect. What psychiatrists and psychologists may or may not consider a mental disease or defect for clinical purposes where their concern is treatment may or may not be the same as mental disease or defect for the purposes of determining criminal responsibility. Whether the defendant had a mental disease or defect must be determined by you under the explanation of those terms as it was given to you by the court.[50]

Given a legal definition, by decisional or statutory law, the term becomes a mixed question of law and fact. Rules setting out specific standards or requiring special types of proof narrow the expert's and jury's roles. Given a legal definition, the trial judge may exclude evidence on certain mental illness, eliminating it from the concern of the jury. The expert or jury is not then left with unbridled discretion in determining what is mental illness.

A number of jurisdictions have adopted a legal test of mental illness by using the definition of mental illness that is codified in the state's mental health code on civil commitment. Mental illness is there defined as a "substantial disorder of thought or mood that significantly impairs judgment, behavior, capacity to recognize reality, or ability to cope with the ordinary demands of life." Though using the definition in the mental health code, Michigan courts, however, have held that the definition of mental illness in the test of criminal responsibility is not limited to psychosis.[51] A jurisdiction providing a definition of mental illness that is of the level allowing civil commitment is Georgia.[52]

Those jurisdictions that follow the ALI (American Law Institute) test of criminal responsibility exclude, by definition, the psychopath (also called sociopath or antisocial personality) from mental disease or defect. In a caveat paragraph, the ALI test excludes as a disability "an abnormality manifested only by repeated criminal or otherwise antisocial conduct."[53] That exclusion followed what came to be known as the "weekend flip-flop case." A St. Elizabeths' psychiatrist on Friday afternoon testified that the defendant, diagnosed as a psychopath, was not suffering from a mental disease, but on the following Monday morning the St. Elizabeths staff decided to classify psychopathic personality as a mental disease. Returning to the stand on Monday, the psychiatrist changed his testimony and declared that the defendant was suffering from a mental disease.[54] The ALI thereupon excluded psychopathy from the definition of mental disease or defect.

A number of jurisdictions have considered excluding other personality disorders as well as excluding psychopathy or repeated antisocial acts. Oregon legislation excludes from the insanity defense persons suffering "solely a personality disorder." California excludes personality disorders, adjustment disorder, and seizure disorder. Connecticut excludes pathological or compulsive gambling. Florida excludes mental retardation or autism. Arizona excludes character defects, psychosexual disorders, and impulse control disorders. Arizona also excludes momentary temporary conditions arising from the pressure of circumstances; moral decadence, depravity or passion growing out of anger, jealousy, revenge, or hatred; or other motive of a person who does not suffer from a mental disease, defect, or abnormality that has manifested itself only by criminal conduct.

All jurisdictions exclude voluntary intoxication in their definition of mental disease or defect; a few jurisdictions (e.g., Oklahoma) expressly exclude it by statute. In all jurisdictions, however, involuntary intoxication is defined in essentially the same terms as insanity.[55] Involuntary intoxication as an insanity defense has arisen from the use of prescribed medications such as Prozac® or Halcion®. In a number of cases, it has been claimed that the medication had a disinhibiting effect resulting in an explosion of aggression.[56] Sleeping pills may cause disorientation.

Impact of Intoxication on Criminal Responsibility

What is the consequence of intoxication or illicit drug use on criminal responsibility? There is the notion that a person's true nature is revealed when controls are loosened by alcohol or drugs. When James K. Logan was dean at the University of Kansas Law School (he was later on the Tenth Circuit Court of Appeals), a candidate being interviewed for a faculty appointment would be urged to drink at an evening gathering so that his true nature could be revealed.

That notion about a person's true nature finds expression as well in court opinions. In the appellate opinion in *Heideman v. United States*,[57] the trial judge is quoted:

> Many people get drunk, but when honest people get drunk, they do not go out and commit crimes. In other words, you could say if a person committed a crime while drunk he must have a criminal instinct in him because they say, as you probably know, that in a state of intoxication a person exhibits his true desires.[58]

It is not uncommon for individuals to commit criminal acts while high on alcohol or illicit drugs. Keeping in mind that alcoholism or drug addiction is not a basis in most jurisdictions for civil commitment (unless secondary to a mental disorder), exculpation in the criminal law would remove the law of any control in these cases.[59] In the early part of the 19th century, a number of judges asked whether a sufficient degree of intoxication might not preclude any *mens rea* and, thus, any punishment for the offense in question. In England, in a number of instances, the accused were acquitted on precisely these grounds, but on policy grounds some means were sought to hold them responsible for their acts.[60]

Various jurisdictions in the United States to resolve the dilemma have taken the position that intoxication or a drugged condition can negate the *mens rea* of a "specific intent" crime, but does not negate the *mens rea* of a "general intent" crime or lesser-included offenses (such as manslaughter). Thus, a voluntarily intoxicated killer is not punished as a murderer, but neither is he given a complete defense.[61] In 1969, the California Supreme Court addressed the question of whether to designate a mental state as general intent, so as to prohibit consideration of voluntary intoxication, or as specific intent, so as to permit such consideration.[62] In the face of argument that intoxication should not be the basis for acquittal or diminished responsibility, the court stated:

> The distinction between specific and general intent crimes evolved as a judicial response to the problem of the intoxicated offender. That problem is to reconcile two competing theories of what is just in the treatment of those who commit crimes while intoxicated. On the one hand, the moral culpability of a drunken criminal is frequently less than that of a sober person effecting a like injury. On the other hand, it is commonly felt that a person who voluntarily gets drunk and while in that state commits a crime should not escape the consequences.

Before the 19th century, the common law refused to give any effect to the fact that an accused committed a crime while intoxicated. The judges were apparently troubled by this rigid traditional rule, however, for there were a number of attempts during the early part of the 19th century to arrive at a more humane, yet workable doctrine. The theory that these judges explored was that "evidence of intoxication could be considered to negate intent, whenever intent was an element of the crime charged. ... [S]uch an exculpatory doctrine could eventually have undermined the traditional rule entirely, since some form of *mens rea* is a requisite of all but strict liability offenses." To limit the operation of the doctrine and achieve a compromise between the conflicting feelings of sympathy and reprobation for the intoxicated offender, later courts both in England and this country drew a distinction between so-called specific intent and general intent crimes.[63]

Just what *general* and *specific intent* mean in a particular setting has been the subject of considerable controversy. Rape is a general-intent crime and, therefore, an individual will not be entitled to claim that as a result of voluntary intoxication his mind was so clouded that he did not or could not form the intent to have sexual intercourse with the victim. However, paradoxically, if he is arrested during the assault and charged with the specific-intent crime of assault with intent to rape, the individual is entitled to introduce evidence regarding his intoxication in order to prove that because of his condition he lacked the specific intent to rape the victim, either because he was too intoxicated to know what he was doing or because he mistakenly believed that the victim was consenting. The charge "assault with intent to rape" is a specific-intent crime because it refers to an intent to do a further act or achieve a future consequence.[64]

Modern penal codes in the definition of offenses expressly set out the *mens rea* terms. It is what it is because the statute says so. Bank robbery, for example, is a general-intent crime because Congress says so. In sum and substance, it is rather arbitrary whether a crime is a general-intent or specific-intent crime. As the Michigan Court of Appeals stated, "Neither common experience nor psychology knows of any such phenomenon as 'general intent' distinguishable from 'specific intent,'" and in either case the individual is equally dangerous.[65]

What Is the Insanity Defense?

Actually, what is the insanity defense? It is, we maintain, just another way of saying that an essential element of the offense is lacking. In terms of substantive criminal law, the insanity defense is not an affirmative defense, or excuse, as some commentators would have us believe, but rather failure of proof of one of the two fundamental elements of criminal responsibility. As an evidentiary matter, testimony on mental illness goes to the credibility of a defendant's claim that the consequences of his act were not intentional or that the act was not voluntary. A textbook illustration is the man who strangles his wife believing that he is merely squeezing a lemon; his defense is that he lacked the intent to kill another human being. Evidence of mental illness gives credibility to his defense. Likewise, a defense of uncontrollable or involuntary behavior is substantiated by evidence of insanity.

Evidence of insanity is actually a form of character evidence, though it is not formally considered as such in the law of evidence. The Federal Rules of Evidence and state codes only deal with the use of character evidence where the identity of the offender is in doubt. The accused is allowed to introduce evidence relating to a pertinent character trait that would suggest that he is not the type of person who would commit the type of crime charged, but character evidence might create a reasonable doubt not only as to identity, but also as to *actus reus* and *mens rea*, and courts have long allowed its use for those purposes as well.

Though the insanity defense is a negation of an essential element of the crime alleged, cases and procedural law have progressed over the years in a way as to make the insanity defense appear to be a separate defense, as some theorists maintain. At one time, the legal system called upon the accused to plead either "guilty" or "not guilty" at his arraignment and under a "not guilty" plea he could present any evidence at trial, including that of insanity to negate *actus reus* and *mens rea*. Trials in criminal law were trials by surprise because of the absence of pretrial discovery. When the defense offered lay or expert witnesses on insanity at trial, the prosecutor would have to ask for a continuance of the trial to get expert testimony in rebuttal, in order to carry its burden of proving *actus reus* and *mens rea*.

Development as a Practical Matter of the Insanity Defense

To elaborate on what has been noted, the plea of not guilty by reason of insanity (NGRI), or the insanity defense as it is commonly known, serves three purposes:

1. It informs the prosecutor that psychiatric testimony will be forthcoming at trial. It provides an opportunity for the prosecutor to obtain an evaluation of the accused prior to trial, thereby avoiding a continuance at trial to obtain the evaluation. Efficiency dictated that the use of insanity evidence be pleaded before trial.[66] Accordingly, as a rule, psychiatric testimony on *actus reus* or *mens rea* is not allowed unless NGRI was entered as a plea at arraignment.
2. It channels the psychiatric testimony according to the terms of the test of criminal responsibility.
3. Most importantly, it results in a commitment rather than an acquittal under a not guilty plea that discharges the defendant. While theoretically an acquittal, a NGRI verdict results in a commitment.

What would happen in regard to these three purposes with the abolition of the insanity defense? First, it would make trials *less*, not more, streamlined and bring back the "surprise" trial system. Second, it would provide less control over psychiatric evidence and would exacerbate the jury's problem of deciding about mental illness. Ironically, it likely would increase the importance of the psychiatrist's role in that determination. Third, the commitment of the individual would be achieved in other ways. The several states that have abolished the insanity defense have turned more to detaining the accused as incompetent to stand trial.[67] As often happens, when the law is reformed in one area, it is deformed in another. Nearly all countries in the world do not have a special plea of not guilty by reason of insanity; they allow psychiatric testimony under a not guilty plea for challenging *mens rea* or *actus reus*.

The Conceptual Center of Law and Psychiatry

The interplay of law and psychiatry has found most expression in the area of criminal responsibility. The consequence of this focus has been to make it the conceptual center of law and psychiatry. The annual Isaac Ray award lectures, begun in 1952 under the auspices of the American Psychiatric Association, have dealt mainly with criminal responsibility. The trials of John Hinckley, Jr., the would-be assassin of President Reagan, and Jeffrey Dahmer, the Milwaukee anthropophagite, have in recent years again spotlighted the function and significance of the NGRI plea, which at times has made the psychiatrist himself and his theories seem frivolous.

For centuries, it has been considered unjust to label a person as criminal or blameworthy unless his unlawful act was performed with a guilty mind (*mens rea*). Professor Alan Dershowitz has written:

> No matter how the law reads, it is a deeply entrenched human feeling that those who are grossly disturbed, whether they are called "madmen," "lunatics," "insane," or "mentally ill," should not be punished like ordinary criminals. This feeling, which is as old as recorded history, is unlikely to be rooted out by new legislation.[68]

In the place of an eye for an eye, a tooth for a tooth, the Greeks allowed an excuse, the first time, in the case of Orestes, who was "driven" to kill his mother in order to avenge his father. Reduced states of competency vary in terms of their power to excuse. The law on criminal intent, as Justice Holmes once said, takes account of incapacities only when the weakness is marked, such as infancy and madness. Otherwise expressed, one is held accountable in criminal law only when one is competent to commit crime. The formulation of the rule theoretically determines the function of the court, the function of the jury, the instructions of the judge to the jury, and the scope of the evidence. Various tests have been formulated to determine when a person is sufficiently demented or defective as not to be held accountable for his acts.

In 1256, the English judge Henry de Bracton formulated what came to be known as the "wild beast" test. He asserted that an insane person should not be held morally accountable because he was not far removed from a "beast." He wrote, "Such (mad)-men are not greatly removed from beasts for they lack of reasoning." It was approved as a test during the next 5 centuries to be finally dogmatized by Judge Tracy in 1724 at the trial of Edward Arnold. Thirty-six years later the "wild beast" test was abandoned in favor of the defendant's capacity to distinguish between "right and wrong," the precursor of the M'Naghten test.[69]

The *M'Naghten* Test

Today, criminal responsibility is determined in England and in many jurisdictions in the United States according to the rule formulated in 1843 following the trial in England of a Scotsman by the name of Daniel M'Naghten. In this well-known case, M'Naghten (a paranoid schizophrenic, if labeled today) felt persecuted by the Tories, who were then in power. He decided to take action against them by killing Sir Robert Peel, the prime minister. He kept a watch on Peel's house, and when he saw a man come out, he shot Edward Drummond in the mistaken belief that he was shooting Peel. A defense of self-defense would be unavailing as the perceived threat was not imminent and the perception of the threat was not that of a reasonable person. Instead, the jury, as instructed, found the defendant not guilty on the ground of insanity. He premeditated, but the premises of his thinking were bizarre. The acquittal was the beginning rather than the end of this celebrated case.

Although acquitted of crime, M'Naghten was certified as being of unsound mind and detained in a lunatic asylum, where he spent his remaining 22 years. The verdict of not guilty on the ground of insanity, however, created a furor, and within a few days after the trial, the case was debated in the House of Lords. It was speculated that M'Naghten, a Scotsman, was a political assassin. The times were turbulent. Shortly before, Queen Victoria had been the target of an attempted assassination by an assailant who was also found not guilty by reason of insanity. On learning of the M'Naghten acquittal, she summoned the House of Lords to an extraordinary session. They were instructed to clarify and tighten the concept of criminal responsibility. They came forth with the so-called *M'Naghten* rules. These rules are extensive, but the pronouncement of greatest import provides:

> The jurors ought to be told in all cases that every man is presumed to be sane and to possess a sufficient degree of reason to be responsible for his crimes, until the contrary can be proved to their satisfaction, and that, to establish a defense on the ground of insanity, it must be clearly proved, that, at the time of the committing of the act, the party accused was labouring under such a defect of reason, from disease of the mind, as not to know the nature and quality of the act he was doing or, if he did know it, that he did not know he was doing what was wrong.[70]

M'Naghten himself probably would not have been exculpated under the legal definition of insanity laid down in the test that bears his name. In a literal application of the *M'Naghten* rule, two (and probably only two) classes of lawbreakers would be exempted from punishment. For example, in the case of homicide: (1) the person thought that the gun with which he shot somebody was not a deadly weapon, but a water pistol and, therefore, was unaware of the fact that it would kill (he did not "know the nature and quality of the act he was doing"), or (2) a person labored under the delusion that he was physically attacked and acted in legitimate self-defense ("he did not know he was doing what was wrong"). The question to be asked under the *M'Naghten* rule is not whether the lawbreaker knew the difference between right and wrong in general. Rather, the question is whether in the particular matter he "knew he was doing what was wrong," that is, whether he was under such a delusion that he thought he acted in legitimate self-defense.[71]

The *M'Naghten* rule has been criticized mainly because it concerns itself with cognition or intellectual understanding and makes no reference to emotion or control. A person, although not laboring under a defect of reason, may be incapable of controlling his behavior. The judges formulating the *M'Naghten* rule were aware that crime, like all human conduct, has multiple etiology, but they decided upon a narrow exculpatory provision. Under the *M'Naghten* rule as formulated, a person is not exempted from criminal responsibility because his capacity for self-control is affected by pathology. He is exempted when, laboring under a defect of reason from disease of the mind, he lacks moral judgment.

For years, the *M'Naghten* rule has been given lip service. Psychiatric testimony has been freely admitted in establishing "disease of the mind" and in interpreting the word *know* in the phrase: "know he was doing what was wrong." *To know* includes more than simply knowledge that something is wrong; it includes, the courts say, a reasonably adequate grasp of the implications of the act. The interpretation of "premeditation" like that of "voluntary action" depends on how narrowly or broadly one frames the time period—some courts look at the few minutes before the commission of the act, others a longer period.[72]

The *Durham* Test

Notwithstanding the broad scope being given the *M'Naghten* rule, Judge David Bazelon of the Court of Appeals for the District of Columbia in 1954 in *Durham v. United States* ruled that the trial had not been adequate because the expert witness had not been permitted to present his full testimony. In the place of the *M'Naghten* rule, Judge Bazelon, looking at the New Hampshire law, formulated a "disease defect product" test, which provides that "An accused is not criminally responsible if his unlawful act was the product of mental disease or mental defect."[73] Unlike the *M'Naghten* rule, the *Durham* rule does not inquire about the impact of mental disease or defect on cognition.

In *Durham*, Judge Bazelon expressly stated that the purpose of the rule is to open the inquiry to the widest possible scope of medical or psychiatric testimony. He sought to remove the shackles, although theoretical, of the M'Naghten rule. In formulating his opinion, he relied heavily on the advice of leading forensic psychiatrists. The decision was widely heralded. Dr. Karl Menninger at the time described it as "more revolutionary in its total effect than the Supreme Court decision regarding segregation." Forensic psychiatrists Lawrence Z. Freedman, Manfred Guttmacher, and Winfred Overholser together published a statement recommending its wide adoption, saying, "The Durham decision permits free communication of psychiatric information."[74] Dr. Gregory Zilboorg called it "a step toward enlightened justice." The American Psychiatric Association awarded Judge Bazelon a certificate of commendation proclaiming that "he has removed massive barriers between the psychiatric and legal professions and opened pathways wherein together they may search for better ways of reconciling human values with social safety."

As it turned out, however, the *Durham* rule resulted in confusion and a plethora of appeals. In cases where the rule was employed, judges and jurors alike were mired in confusion over the terms *disease*, *defect*, and *product*. With the exception of Maine, and a modification of it in New Mexico, the rule did not spread beyond the District of Columbia.

The sweeping use of the terms *mental disease* or *defect* was only part of the problem. The product test brought in all the controversies of psychic determinism versus free will. What does *product* mean? Is every criminal act related to mental disorder? Is anyone accountable for his acts? Judge Holtzoff, district judge in the District of Columbia, observed: "It is not inconceivable that perhaps the so-called *Durham* formula would not have been adopted if it had been foreseen at the time that it would lead to the exculpation of sociopaths or psychopaths from criminal liability."[75] Judge Bazelon, too, became disillusioned. In 1964, he said, "The frequent failure to adequately explain and support expert psychiatric opinion threatens the administration of the insanity defense in the District of Columbia."[76] In 1967, in an apparent act of desperation, Judge Bazelon took the unusual step of writing a set of instructions to accompany all orders requiring mental examinations, advising psychiatric witnesses as to how they should function.[77] Dr. Menninger, having once expressed great optimism about the possibilities of the Durham decision, did not want to be reminded of it and recanted in his 1968 book, *The Crime of Punishment*.[78]

The ALI Test

The American Law Institute's (ALI) Model Penal Code, prepared during the years 1952 to 1962, recommended a combination of the right–wrong test and an updated version of "irresistible impulse":

1. A person is not responsible for criminal conduct if at the time of such conduct as a result of mental disease or defect he lacks substantial capacity either to appreciate the criminality (wrongfulness) of his conduct or to conform his conduct to the requirements of the law.
2. As used in this article, the terms "mental disease or defect" do not include an abnormality manifested only by repeated criminal or otherwise antisocial conduct.

Subsection 1 of the ALI test has two prongs that may be affected by mental disease or defect: cognition and control. Of the cognition prong, whereas *M'Naghten* spoke in terms of whether the defendant did or did not know, the ALI test refers to a lack of "substantial capacity" to "appreciate." The use of the word *appreciate* is designed to allow testimony about the defendant's emotional and affective attitude about the crime. The second prong excuses those whose mental disease or defect causes a loss of control over their actions at the time of the offense. A number of states that operate under the *M'Naghten* rule have extended the ground of the insanity plea through an addition known as irresistible impulse, popularly characterized as "the policeman at the elbow" test, under which an offender will be found insane only if he would have committed the offense in the presence of an officer. The defendant may have known what he was doing and known that it was wrong, but nevertheless may have been unable to resist an overwhelming impulse to commit the crime. This test is included as the second prong in subsection 1 of the ALI standard. The "irresistible impulse" test when originally formulated in 1897 read: "Though conscious of [the nature of the act he is committing] and able to distinguish between right and wrong and know that the act is wrong, yet his will, [i.e.,] the governing power of his mind, has been otherwise so completely destroyed that his actions are not subject to it, but are beyond his control."

The formulation in subsection 2 of the ALI standard is designed specifically to include persons diagnosed as psychopath or antisocial personality within the scope of criminal responsibility. In a cartoon, the artist Honoré Daumier depicted an arrested man slouched despondently against the wall of his prison cell. "What really bothers me," he says, "is that I've been accused of twelve robberies." His lawyer is nonplused and replies, "So much the better. I will plead monomania." The cartoon was drawn at a time when a disease entity of "monomania" was identified by a French physician who treated the insane.[79] The ALI rejects as an abnormality that which is manifested only by repeated criminal or otherwise antisocial conduct.

Rejection of *Durham*

Then, in 1972, some 18 years after its adoption of the *Durham* rule, the U.S. Court of Appeals for the District of Columbia took the occasion to discard it in *United States v. Brawner*.[80] In this case, the American Psychiatric Association, American Psychological Association, American Civil Liberties Union, National District Attorneys Association, National Legal Aid and Defender Association, and the Georgetown Legal Intern Project filed briefs as *amici curiae* on such issues as the adoption of the ALI test for criminal responsibility and the possibility of the complete abolition of the insanity defense. The case was argued twice. In its *amicus* brief, the American Psychiatric Association suggested the rejection of the *Durham* test and endorsed instead the ALI standard. The *amicus* brief further suggested that if the court were to reject the ALI test, then the abolition of the insanity defense would be an alternative acceptable to the psychiatric profession. It stated that it would favor, with appropriate safeguards, abolishing the insanity defense, but it recognized that the abolition of the defense would have to be accomplished by constitutional amendment. The court, all nine members sitting *en banc*, including Judge Bazelon, unanimously decided in a 143-page opinion to throw out its *Durham* rule and adopt in its place the ALI standard.

In a year of deliberation of the case, the court considered and rejected the alternatives of abolishing the insanity defense entirely or of adopting a standard allowing the jury to decide sanity based simply on the question of whether the accused "can justly be held responsible." The court said that it rejected the abolition of the insanity defense because such an action should come from the legislative branch of government, not the judicial. (The Supreme Court on a number of occasions has indicated that where an insanity defense is raised, the failure to afford a defendant a fair and impartial hearing on the question is a denial of due process of law.) It rejected allowing juries to decide sanity based on their own judgment because such a procedure "would place too heavy a burden on the jury." In general, the court reasoned that the *Durham* rule did not work because of the latitude it gives expert witnesses to make value judgments in front of the jury. The value judgments referred to come in the form of medical or psychiatric testimony.

Acceptance of the ALI Test

The ALI test of criminal responsibility rapidly became accepted throughout the country. Over the next 2 decades, a majority of the states adopted the first paragraph, and many of these also adopted the second.[81] Of the 11 federal jurisdictions, all but one (the First Circuit, which has jurisdiction over federal cases in Maine, Massachusetts, and New Hampshire) used it. Volitional impairment or the "irresistible impulse" concept, however, raised the difficult question: How can an impulse that was truly irresistible be differentiated from one that simply was not resisted? The psychiatric expert would invariably be asked the policeman-at-the-elbow question on cross-examination. "Would the defendant have committed this act if a policeman were standing next to him at the time?" An effective answer may be, "Your guess is as good as mine." Jack Ruby fatally shot Lee Harvey Oswald before a television audience right inside Dallas police headquarters. There is less likelihood that a defense of irresistible impulse will stand up when there is evidence of premeditation and planning as they tend to demonstrate well-reasoned behavior or reasoned intent.

The Impact of the Hinckley Trial

In 1982, a District of Columbia jury shocked the nation by finding the would-be assassin of President Ronald Reagan, John W. Hinckley Jr., not guilty by reason of insanity.[82] The news ignited swift reactions from coast to coast. The verdict engendered countless editorials calling on lawmakers to abandon or modify the law. Television and radio call-in shows were swamped. The jurors were occasionally ridiculed in the media, and they were actually summoned before Congress to explain their decision, ostensibly to obtain information on any needed changes in the law. More or less, it dampened NGRI verdicts.[83]

In the aftermath of the trial, President Reagan submitted a bill to Congress to limit the scope of the insanity plea, which was followed by another bill submitted by Senator Strom Thurmond.[84] When submitting his bill, Senator Thurmond said, "We in the Senate would be shirking our duty to protect law-abiding citizens if we fail to take the time of this Congress to reform the insanity defense." More than 40 bills were introduced in Congress to abolish or reform the defense.[85] Responding to the outcry, the American Bar Association and the American Psychiatric Association (APA) issued statements calling for a change in the law.[86]

The APA urged that insanity acquittals be granted only for impaired cognition (not for impaired control) resulting from mental disorders of the severity (if not always of the quality) of psychoses, and not for personality disorders or antisocial personalities. The APA's suggested standard was that the defendant be "unable to appreciate the wrongfulness of his conduct" because of "severely abnormal mental conditions that grossly and demonstrably impair a person's perception or understanding of reality." Likewise, the ABA recommended that insanity acquittals be granted only for impaired cognition (not for impaired control) as a result of a substantial process of functional or organic impairment, a recommendation adopted in federal law and the law of a number of states. Professor Stephen Morse, prominent scholar in law and psychology, proposed a "craziness" test:

> A defendant is not guilty by reason of insanity if, at the time of the offense, the defendant was so extremely crazy and the craziness so substantially affected the criminal behavior that the defendant does not deserve to be punished.[87]

Shortly after the Hinckley trial, Congress enacted legislation that substantially changed the insanity defense in federal courts, and various states did the same. It put the burden to prove insanity on the defendant, it tightened the definition of insanity, and it restricted the scope of expert testimony. Since then, there have been few successful insanity defenses, particularly in federal courts.

The insanity defense has always been controversial, but, in the past, the controversy was mainly concerned with the formulation of the test to determine criminal insanity. Now there was intense controversy whether there should be any insanity defense at all. The *Hinckley* case quickened the debate in the United States, but the defense, for one reason or another, has been under attack for a long time. There was, for example, a great uproar following the *M'Naghten* verdict in 1843 in England and Queen Victoria sought a tightening of the defense. Professor Henry Weihofen began his book published in 1933, *Insanity as a Defense in Criminal Law*, with the statement: "Probably no branch of the criminal law has been the subject of so much criticism and controversy as the defense of insanity."[88]

During the late 1970s, before the *Hinckley* verdict, 24 states passed laws tightening the test for determining insanity, and a few states enacted a "guilty but mentally ill" (GBMI) verdict.[89] President Nixon, like President Reagan, also attempted to abolish the insanity defense for federal crimes.[90] Advocates of reformation or abolition of the insanity defense argue that reform will bring many benefits including streamlined trials, heightened law and order, and a return to jury decisions on the culpability of criminals without a battle of expert witnesses.[91]

To determine criminal responsibility, the issue is not simply whether the accused did or did not cause injury or harm, but whether he acted voluntarily and intended to cause the harm as well, knowing it was wrong. Most criminal trials focus on what and who (what crime was committed and who committed it?), but the insanity defense focuses on the more difficult issue of why the crime was committed. In the *Hinckley* case, the shootings took place in full view of television cameras, so there was no question of who did the shootings.

On the importance of knowing who, Professor Herbert Wechsler, an esteemed authority on criminal law, addressed an audience with the following example: "Suppose your elderly father, in an advanced arteriosclerotic state, is taken to the hospital and while there experiences a tantrum or delusion and knocks over a lamp, resulting in the death of an attendant. Would you be satisfied with a legal system in which he could be indicted and convicted of a homicidal crime? We would not."[92] Justice Holmes put it this way: "[A] law which punished conduct that would not be blameworthy in the average member of the community would be too severe for the community to bear. ... Even a dog distinguishes between being stumbled over and being kicked."[93] Thus, long before Freud or the advent of psychiatry, the law has required a determination of blameworthiness in the ordinary moral sense and has acquitted defendants who acted without moral culpability.[94]

Who Pleads Insanity?

As the defendant by pleading insanity admits causing the injury, attention is focused not on whether he committed the offense, but on the history of the defendant to ascertain the intent or controllability of his conduct.[95] The accused is allowed to paint a more complete picture of his character and the interaction between his character and his conduct. According to John Wigmore, the leading authority on the law of evidence, when insanity is in issue, "any and all conduct of the person is admissible in evidence."[96] Thus, once the defendant has raised the insanity defense, evidence of prior arrests, conviction, and antisocial conduct is admissible, a result not ordinarily permitted because it could unfairly prejudice the jury as to whether the defendant is guilty in a specific instance. As a consequence, in the majority of cases, a defendant with a criminal history does not raise the defense out of concern that his background will be brought to the attention of the jury and will tend to guarantee conviction, rather than acquittal.[97]

Usually, the defense is urged on behalf of those who have committed one episodic act of violence; the accused is a theretofore law-abiding citizen who explodes, often in a domestic dispute.[98] He may call the police and confess to committing the act, and he may call his lawyer who is more likely to be a specialist in negligence, workers' compensation, or real estate than in criminal law. The criticism that the defense is used extensively by dangerous criminals, who thereby escape punishment, has no basis in fact.

Nevertheless, in quite a number of cases, the prosecutor charges the one-time psychotic with murder, and then declines to plea bargain. He is mindful of public opinion, particularly when soon up for reelection, and prefers to let judge or jury make the appropriate response to the charge. The evidence against the accused causing the harm is usually overwhelming, but his state of mind warrants a charge of manslaughter rather than first-degree murder.[99] A plea of insanity may prompt a lesser, more appropriate verdict. Studies report that 89% of insanity acquittees are schizophrenic, and as a group are less likely to recidivate than felons as a group, or that the two groups are about the same in the rate of recidivism.[100]

By classifying a person as either mad *or* bad, as the law would have it, the insanity defense tries to sort out the respective roles of the penal and hospital systems. It provides a way to determine, with the flexibility necessary in judging human minds, the difference between troubled and troublesome individuals and their dispositions. In many cases, as psychiatrists would say, an individual may be mad *and* bad, but in any event, criminal condemnation or imprisonment of a mentally ill person would be considered an affront to the moral sense of the community. In the judgment of many, for example, a mother suffering from a psychosis, who kills her infant, belongs not in prison, but in a hospital. Our collective conscience, it is often said, does not allow punishment when the individual is not morally culpable.[101]

Frequency of the NGRI Plea

While the literature on criminal insanity is vast, the defense comes up only infrequently in trials (but more often in plea bargaining). In a lifetime of practice in forensic psychiatry, the practitioner may be involved in only a few trials involving a plea of insanity. In cases that go to trial, the insanity plea is a last-ditch defense. At best, it is estimated, insanity is raised in only 1 or 2% of the cases that go to trial (95% of criminal cases are plea bargained), though at least 30% of the prison population have psychiatric problems (at the time of the crime as well as during imprisonment) sufficient to justify psychiatric intervention. Of that 1 or 2% of cases that go to trial, only about 10% end in an NGRI verdict, mostly involving crimes against property.[102] An NGRI verdict is far more likely when the case is tried by a judge without a jury, but when the case is high profile (as Andrea Yates), it is put to a jury, especially when the prosecutor is up for reelection in the near future (as in the Andrea Yates case). Cases such as *Yates* or *Hinckley* go to trial because the victim, the offender, or the nature of the crime is extraordinary. The trials become media showcases because the individuals are well-known or the crimes so bizarre or atrocious as to make for "good copy." And they invariably involve the presentation of conflicting psychiatric evidence.

The statistic that the insanity plea is involved in only 1 or 2% of cases that go to trial is misleading as to the varied uses of the plea. While evidence of insanity may not result in a verdict of NGRI, it may result in a conviction of a crime less than that charged, and in that sense, it is a victory for the defense. In nonserious cases, the prosecutor will often stipulate to an NGRI plea, and there is no trial.[103]

In some parts of the country, where civil commitment standards are stringent, individuals are charged with a minor offense (vagrancy or disturbing the peace) and under an NGRI plea are institutionalized, at least for a short period of time. Ironically, while now used frequently in misdemeanor cases, the plea in former times was mainly used in capital cases to avoid the death penalty. Every felony, of which there were many, carried the death penalty.

As a result of the California legislation enacted in 1994, known as the Three-Strikes and You're Out Law, there occurred a resurgence of the NGRI plea in order to avoid the lengthy penalty under that law. A person convicted of a third felony after two prior serious felonies would under the Three-Strikes law typically receive a sentence of no less than 25 years to life. Prior to Three-Strikes, it was uncommon to see criminal defendants malingering the symptoms of mental illness in any but the most serious of felony cases, typically murder and rape. Subsequent to the adoption of the Three-Strikes law, malingering is seen in individuals charged with anything from murder and rape all the way down to petty theft (typically petty theft with a prior felony), presumably because any new felony conviction of a person with two prior strikes against him will result in a 25-year to life sentence. Quite often, the prosecutor and defendant enter into a NGRI plea bargain.[104]

There is an old saying that statistics are like a bikini—what they reveal is interesting, but what they conceal is vital. And that is the way it is with the statistics on the insanity defense. Most of the research reports acquittal data, not plea data, and approximately 95% of cases are plea bargained. Plea data are difficult to obtain. As a consequence, it is problematic how often the defense is utilized and how it fares in various jurisdictions.[105]

Burden of Proof

A factor almost as controversial and problematic as the test used to legally define insanity is the assignment of the burden of proof.[106] The allocation of the burden of proof on insanity is important because psychiatric evidence is usually not sufficiently clear-cut to prove or disprove insanity beyond a reasonable doubt. The burden of proof may be understood as composed of three parts: (1) the burden of pleading, (2) the burden of production or going forward with the evidence, and (3) the burden of persuasion.[107] The burden of production only requires that evidence be introduced to place a fact at issue in a trial, while the burden of persuasion requires that enough evidence be introduced to persuade the judge or jury of the actual existence of the fact.

In a criminal trial, the prosecution has the burden of proving the essential elements of the crime charged. The prosecution's burden of proof does not extend to proving the sanity of every defendant; instead the law presumes that defendants are sane at the time the alleged offenses are committed. It would be too time-consuming to offer evidence of sanity in every case. However, defendants may challenge this presumption of sanity by pleading NGRI. The *M'Naghten* rule states that jurors are to be told in all cases that every man is to be presumed to be sane and to possess a sufficient degree of reason to be responsible for his crimes until the contrary is proved to their satisfaction.

Once the defendant's mental condition becomes an issue, the burden of persuasion becomes important. By virtue of the presumption of sanity, the onus is placed on the accused to come forward with evidence of insanity. Under any test of criminal responsibility, it is usually sufficient to have "some evidence" of insanity in order to put the matter into controversy. There is, as noted, a distinction between "going forward with the evidence" (which may shift during the course of the trial) and "burden of persuasion." It is problematic whether the prosecutor or the court has the authority or duty to impose an insanity defense on an apparently mentally disabled defendant.[108]

Two views are extant as to who must carry the burden of persuasion. About half of the state jurisdictions place the burden of persuasion on the prosecutor to disprove the elements of the defendant's insanity defense beyond a reasonable doubt. The other states, the federal courts, and the District of Columbia label insanity an affirmative defense, on which the defendant has the burden of persuasion by "clear and convincing evidence."[109] Following Hinckley's trial, the law was changed for the federal courts and within a number of states to place the burden of persuasion on the defendant, making it more difficult for the defendant to achieve an NGRI verdict. (Some states place the burden of persuasion on the defendant by a "preponderance of the evidence.")

The courts and legislatures have based their allocation of the burden of proof of sanity or insanity on their perceptions of the relationship between sanity and *actus reus* or *mens rea*. Those courts that place the burden of persuasion on the prosecution view sanity as necessary to the formulation of the requisite culpable mental state or voluntariness of the conduct and, hence, as an essential element of the crime. Those that place the burden on the defendant do not perceive a necessary relationship between sanity and *actus reus* or *mens rea*, or they simply want to make it harder for a defendant to be found NGRI.

After the *Hinckley* trial, the American Bar Association (ABA) recommended that the prosecution bear the burden of disproving the defendant's claim of insanity beyond a reasonable doubt in jurisdictions utilizing any test for insanity that focused solely on whether the defendant, as a result of mental disease or defect, was unable to know, understand, or appreciate the wrongfulness of his conduct. The ABA recommended that, in jurisdictions utilizing the ALI Model Penal Code test for insanity, the defendant bear the burden of proving a claim of insanity by a preponderance of the evidence.

The control prong of the insanity test raised the difficult question, according to a post-*Hinckley* statement of the American Psychiatric Association, of how can the psychiatrist differentiate between an impulse that was truly irresistible and one that simply was not resisted?[110] There is less likelihood that a defense of irresistible impulse will stand up when there is evidence of premeditation and planning, which tend to demonstrate well-reasoned behavior or reasoned intent. The serial killer claims an urge that he could not resist.

No matter which test of criminal responsibility is applied, the psychiatrist's testimony must describe the offender's state of mind at the time of the commission of the offense. It is necessary to project back from the time of examination to the time of the offense. The validity of an opinion on the defendant's mental condition at some given moment in the past—weeks or months prior to the examination—is invariably challenged on cross-examination. Information obtained from acquaintances and those who had custody of the defendant (jailers) following the crime is helpful.

In arriving at his opinion, the expert is often expected to have or have had carried out the full battery of psychological tests (Rorschach, Thematic Apperception Test, Bender Gestalt, Minnesota Multiphasic Personality Inventory) and physiological tests (x-ray examination, physical examination, electroencephalogram, and neurological examination). Failure to apprise oneself of certain facts or test results or failure to use available examination techniques makes the expert vulnerable for the question, "Would that change your opinion, doctor?" Another attack on adequacy of examination involves questioning the amount of time that the expert spent with the accused.[111]

Post-Act Behavior

Flight from the scene, attempts to avoid detection, and the circumstances of the apprehension of the accused are all relevant to the psychiatric examination. If the defendant after the crime said that he was sorry that he did it or showed regret or remorse, the prosecutor may argue that this is an indication that he knew he had committed a wrongful act. In one case, the prosecutor proceeded this way in cross-examining the defense psychiatrist:[112]

> Q. So I ask you, sir, in your opinion ... was he or did he indicate in any way that he was sorry that he killed this girl?
> A. He did not say he was sorry he had killed this girl and he was expecting the electric chair.
> Q. Doctor, can't you answer that question Yes or No?
> A. I can only answer it on the basis of what I observed. I observed that ...
> Q. What is your opinion, doctor? Was he or was he not sorry that he killed the girl?
> A. My opinion was that he regretted killing the girl, but somehow felt it was in the cards, that something like this was going to happen in his life and that he had no control over it, and this is the way it was going to be, he was going to get the chair and here it comes.
> Q. So your answer is, doctor, that in your opinion from your examination of him, he was sorry that he killed the girl. That is true, isn't it?
> A. I would say he was sorry, but felt there was nothing he could do about it.
> Q. Doctor, are you trying to hedge on the answer?
> A. I am trying to give you an accurate answer as to what I felt was going on in this man's mind.

Ironically, remorse and lack of remorse have both been used to indicate culpability or the lack thereof. In *United States v. McRae*,[113] the accused killed his wife by shooting her through the head with his deer rifle at point-blank range. That he did so was admitted; his defense was that the shooting was not intentional, but accidental. His testimony at trial dwelt on his grief and his intense devotion to his wife, all in an attempt to cast his wife's death as accidental. He was allowed to introduce medical testimony of his hospitalization during a 2-week period following the killing for "grief syndrome."

In the trial of O. J. Simpson, the prosecution sought to prove guilt (apart from other evidence) by the fact that he did not ask how Nicole Simpson was killed. In Albert Camus' novel *The Stranger*, the prosecution "proved" that the accused killed a stranger because he did not show proper grief at his own mother's funeral. The prosecutor found the reaction of the accused to be relevant and concluded with the statement, "I accuse the prisoner of behaving at his mother's funeral in a way that showed he was already a criminal at heart."[114]

Jury Decision Making

How do juries actually decide whether the accused is legally insane? Do the various formulations of criminal responsibility make a difference? To answer this question, Rita James Simon reported on a controlled experiment, introducing three variations into the record. The first variation was designed to test whether it makes any difference which criteria of mental incapacity—*M'Naghten*,

Durham, or neither—a court directs the jury to apply. It was found that a jury instructed under the *M'Naghten* test is more likely to convict than is a jury instructed under *Durham*; whereas an uninstructed jury is likely to return the same verdict as a *Durham* jury.

The second variation in the record was designed to test the effect were the jury to hear a considerably more elaborate evaluation of the accused's illness than is ordinarily given by psychiatrists in a case involving mental incapacity. No difference in the verdicts was found. The third variation was designed to determine whether verdicts would vary when there was an instruction that a verdict of not guilty on grounds of mental incapacity would necessarily result in commitment of the accused to a psychiatric hospital. Again, the variation was found to result in no difference.[115] Ironically, in the operation of the law, the crazier the accused, the more likely the jury will return a verdict of guilty, rather than NGRI. They want the crazy locked up. Their decision very much depends on the nature of the crime. The court's vacating a guilty verdict and entering NGRI is rarely done, but it does happen at times.[116]

Consequences of NGRI Verdict

Judges in many states, at the request of the defendant, instruct the jury on the consequences of an NGRI verdict. Otherwise, thinking that an insanity acquittee goes free, jurors would not likely return an NGRI verdict.[117] If and when an accused is found insane, he is exculpated, but nonetheless his freedom is curtailed. He has been shown to be either a person who does not know what he is doing or one who cannot control his conduct, which has resulted in serious harm to another. In the same manner as did the House of Lords following the *M'Naghten* decision, Congress and the various states have enacted legislation providing for commitment of any person who is acquitted on grounds of insanity. Commitment is made to a unit for the criminally insane, subject to release only upon a judicial finding that he "has recovered his sanity and will not in the reasonable future be dangerous to himself or others." Regarding the entire procedure, Menninger aptly said: "Millions of dollars are spent annually to determine who has [responsibility] or who doesn't have it. If one is found to have it, he is locked up; if he is found not to have it, he is also locked up."[118]

In a turgid essay, penned about 1870, Mark Twain ridiculed the insanity defense, saying that rank criminal offenders were resorting to its use to escape the reach of the law, and he called for a law against the practice. The essay is titled, "A New Crime: Legislation Needed," the new crime being the use of the insanity defense. Mark Twain was perhaps unaware that the procedure at the time was a device to temper the use of the death penalty, and he also presumed that these offenders were released. He apparently was not mindful of the fact that offenders acquitted on the plea of insanity are confined in a criminally insane unit of a mental hospital or penal institution. They do not walk out of the courthouse free men.

As the insanity acquittee is not a free man, the prosecution urged the jury in the trial in England of James Hadfield in 1800 to return what was, at that time, a novel verdict, and it did: "We find the prisoner is Not Guilty; he being under the influence of insanity at the time the act was committed." He was detained for the rest of his 40 years. Under the Insanity Bill of 1800, the court was empowered to order persons acquitted on account of insanity to be kept in strict custody, "in such place and such manner as the court may decide, during the King's pleasure."

It is preferable to be sent to the criminal unit of a mental hospital (with the possibility of release) than to be executed; however, when the choice is between prison and a criminally insane unit, the option is for prison. The prison is less stigmatizing and is a more comfortable facility than the criminally insane unit, and the term of confinement is fixed, usually for a shorter period of time, but in recent years the law on disposition of an NGRI acquittee has changed, as we shall discuss.

When facts of the commission of the offense are undeniable (consider, for example, Jack Ruby's slaying of Lee Harvey Oswald or Arthur Bremer's shooting of Governor George Wallace), the defense of insanity, a subjective element, is the only tactic that a defense attorney has available to furnish judge or jury with a reason to acquit, or to return a verdict of a crime less than that charged. Hence, a defense attorney is obliged to argue the apparently fanciful, as was argued in the *Bremer* case, "This kid is pure schizophrenic … the kid's old lady is to blame for his mental disorders."[119]

Disposition of NGRI Acquittee

Without commitment as a consequence of an NGRI acquittal, the insanity defense would likely be considered unnecessary in the administration of the criminal law. The problem today is really not with the insanity defense per se, but with hospital release of the defendant. Until recently, an NGRI verdict was almost always followed by automatic commitment to a mental hospital for a long period, often for life. However, beginning in the 1970s, a number of jurisdictions in the United States began to require that the person be released if found either no longer mentally ill or dangerous or in need of care or treatment, just as in the case of civil commitment.[120] As a result of this change in the law, the American public began to look askance at a system that regarded people who have already committed dangerous acts as largely equivalent to people who have not.

The issue, then, is whether NGRI and civil commitment proceedings on admission and discharge must be identical. An acquittal by reason of insanity is an explicit finding that the defendant suffered from a mental disability at the time of the offense, but it is not dispositive of the question of the defendant's mental condition at the time of acquittal. The verdict refers to the time of the act, but it is reasonable to presume that the mental illness continues up to the time of commitment. Automatic commitment of insanity acquittees for evaluation satisfies due process because it represents "a judicious weighing of the public's right to be protected from possibly dangerous mentally ill persons against the individual defendant's right to be protected against unjustified commitment."[121]

The controversial issue, however, is not so much over initial commitment, but over discharge. Drug therapy may (quickly) remove the symptoms of mental illness without necessarily assuring that the individual is not dangerous. As far as the hospital is concerned, there is nothing more to treat, if ever there was anything to treat, and it feels justified in discharging the individual. The situation also occurs where the individual is mentally ill, but not treatable. Questions arise: Should the hospital be used as a place of confinement? May the acquittee be transferred to a nonhospital facility? Who should have control over discharge? What, if any, conditions on release may be imposed? An individual who has been found NGRI in the case of a violent crime and is quickly discharged stirs up anxiety in the community.[122]

Taking NGRI acquittees as a fair and proper category, the burden of proof and the criteria for their commitment and discharge may be different from that in the case of the civilly committed patient.[123] The hospital and its staff generally prefer not to have control over discharge of the insanity acquittee, as they do over the civilly committed patient, as they do not enjoy immunity from suit. They prefer that control over discharge of the insanity acquittee be in the hands of the court, but that all too often results in an overcrowded hospital.[124]

In a 5–4 decision in *Jones v. United States*,[125] the Supreme Court in 1983 said that an insanity acquittee should be released only when "he has regained his sanity or is no longer a danger to himself or society." It does not matter, the Court said, how long the maximum jail term would have been if the defendant had been convicted. The *Jones* case involved a man who had been in a mental hospital over seven years. He was charged with trying to shoplift a coat from a department store, a misdemeanor that carries a maximum sentence of one year in jail. He pleaded not guilty by reason of insanity, and was committed to St. Elizabeths. He argued that once the maximum criminal sentence had expired, he was entitled as a matter of constitutional due process either to be released from the mental hospital or to be assigned the relatively more favored legal status of a person who is under an order of civil, rather than criminal, commitment. Writing for the majority, Justice Powell said that imprisonment and commitment to a mental hospital serve two different purposes. The purpose of criminal commitment to a mental hospital, he said, is not punishment, but treatment of a mentally ill person and protection of society "from his potential dangerousness." The continued confinement of such a person, Justice Powell said, "rests on his continuing illness and dangerousness." He added: "There simply is no necessary correlation between severity of the offense and length of time necessary for recovery. The length of the acquittee's hypothetical criminal sentence therefore is irrelevant to the purpose of his commitment."[126]

Guilty but Mentally Ill Verdict

Among the various proposals for change, the most fashionable suggestion has been the verdict of guilty but mentally ill (GBMI). This alternative verdict was adopted in Michigan in 1975 and then in a number of other states.[127] GBMI is not a special plea (like not guilty or NGRI), but a verdict that can be returned whenever a plea of NGRI is entered.[128] Proponents claimed a need for this new kind of verdict because the term *guilty* expresses the objective truth that the defendant committed the crime, while the term *mentally ill* expresses the subjective truth about the defendant, that he is sick. The GBMI verdict gives the jury the opportunity "of agreeing that the defendant is mentally ill, yet holding him criminally responsible."[129] Supposedly, GBMI avoids the either–or approach of guilty or not guilty by providing a middle ground.

Michigan's enactment of the GBMI verdict was a reaction to a decision in 1974 by the Michigan Supreme Court in *People v. McQuillan*.[130] In a decision followed by a number of other states, the Michigan Supreme Court held that after an initial period of 60 days, during which the insanity acquittee was to be evaluated, further confinement had to conform with the procedures and standards of the civil commitment process. The case gave rise to the perception that there were too many NGRIs in the state, and they were not being kept in detention. Within a year of the decision, 64 persons who had been found NGRI were released, and within another year, 2 of the 64 had committed violent crimes—Ronald Manlen raped two women and John McGee killed his wife. Public outrage moved the Michigan legislature to promptly adopt the new verdict of GBMI.[131]

The GBMI verdict was clearly designed as an anti-NGRI verdict. It accomplishes its goal by muddying the water. It appears to be a compromise verdict. In fact, it has exactly the same consequences as a guilty verdict—detention in the penal system or the death penalty. It is a second guilty verdict. The GBMI verdict hoodwinks the jury in the decisional process. Given two guilty verdict options, the odds are increased that a jury will return the GBMI verdict rather than one of not guilty by reason of insanity. Juries think that GBMI is a compromise or middle ground because it sounds exculpatory—guilty but mentally ill. It would sound more condemnatory if it said "guilty and mentally ill." The verdict is not a middle ground, but can be described as a misleading distinction without a difference; it is another guilty verdict. The guilty but mentally ill verdict could just as well be guilty but flat feet. The defendant is found guilty, convicted, and imprisoned. He will get special attention if he needs it, as will any other prisoner.

Nor have trial courts in Michigan allowed defense counsel to offer evidence on the consequences of a GBMI verdict. The jury is not informed of the consequences that follow a GBMI verdict. Moreover, while the state is usually not allowed to invoke a plea of NGRI, the Michigan trial courts have allowed the prosecutor, in final argument, to tell the jury that they should find the defendant guilty but mentally ill where the defendant pleads NGRI and the evidence points to insanity.[132] Thus, the jury may believe they are helping the defendant by finding him GBMI rather than just guilty, unaware that the same consequences await him as any convicted person.

The GBMI verdict is misleading not only at trial, but also in the plea-bargaining process. The plea is illusory because there is a false promise that the jurisdiction can ensure the outcome of what is allegedly the purpose of the GBMI verdict, namely treatment for those individuals who are found guilty and who are mentally ill.[133]

The GBMI verdict has clearly reduced the number of NGRI pleas (as distinguished from NGRI verdicts). Given a GBMI option, defense lawyers tend to prefer entering a not guilty plea rather than a plea of NGRI. With a not guilty plea, there is only one chance of being found guilty (a guilty verdict), but with a NGRI plea, there are two chances of being found guilty (guilty and GBMI). Thus, as the American Psychiatric Association stated, the GBMI verdict amounts to a disguised abolition of NGRI and gives juries an easy way out to avoid grappling with difficult issues of guilt, innocence, and insanity.[134]

Conclusion

The defense of insanity is a defense of last resort—it is not a popular defense with defendants, their counsel, or juries. It is interesting, but very much an academic topic. Insanity is raised in few trials, usually by a person without a criminal record who commits one episodic act of violence. Few of these trials end in acquittal, but evidence produced under the defense may diminish the verdict of guilt for a lesser crime, such as reducing murder to manslaughter.

Contrary to popular belief, the test of criminal responsibility is a constraint on psychiatric evidence regarding *actus reus* or *mens rea*, and a verdict of NGRI provides some control over an acquittee. A not guilty plea, on the other hand, has only the limitation of relevancy. The *Hinckley* trial gave the impetus to "guilty but mentally ill" legislation, which in turn has resulted in not guilty pleas replacing NGRI pleas. In any event, following the uproar over the *Hinckley* verdict, jurors became more reluctant to return an NGRI verdict.

The administration of the law is not a mechanical operation; it needs avenues for the exercise of discretion. The insanity plea is an excuse for behavior, the policy question being the extent to which an excuse will be tolerated. In law school courses on criminal law and procedure, emphasis is on rights of suspects and not on rights of victims. Individuals apparently tend to identify more with the offender than with the offended. It may be said that the law on criminal responsibility stems out of our fear of being accused or held accountable for something we may have done or imagined, even though beyond our reason or control. St. Augustine expressed thanks that he was not responsible for his dreams, which caused him embarrassment.

The insanity defense provides society with a vehicle for debating the meaning of criminal responsibility. As Law Professor George Fletcher put it,

> [T]he issue of insanity requires us to probe our premises for blaming and punishing. In posing the question whether a particular person is responsible for a criminal act, we are forced to resolve our doubts about whether anyone is ever responsible for criminal conduct. And if some are responsible and some are not, how do we distinguish between them? Is it a matter for the experts or is it a question of common sense? If it is for experts, why do they persistently disagree; if it is a matter of common sense, why is the issue so difficult to resolve?[135]

The questions do not lend to simple answers, and that is because NGRI is used for various purposes. For that reason, statistics on the frequency or success of the plea of NGRI are less than satisfying. They do not illuminate the various uses of the plea. The plea is like a crystal ball—turn the sphere a little and it casts a whole new light. At a time when the death penalty was possible in nearly all crimes, NGRI was used to circumvent that penalty. Nowadays, the plea is frequently urged in order to bring about a conviction on a crime less than that charged. In that sense, the plea is successful, though it does not result in an acquittal on the basis of insanity. And, as we have noted, it is frequently used in plea bargaining. Unheard of in past times, the plea is used in cases of minor offenses (disturbing the peace or vagrancy) in order to obtain medical treatment for individuals who otherwise might have been civilly committed, but for the difficulties in obtaining a civil commitment. Then, too, as a recent phenomenon, the plea is used to circumvent heavy criminal penalties under the "Three-Strikes" law. In short, like any excuse, the plea of NGRI provides some flexibility in the administration of the law.[136]

Endnotes

1. In State v. Breakiron, 108 N.J. 591, 532 A.2d 199 (1987), the New Jersey Supreme Court observed: "Twelve centuries of debate have yet to resolve the law's attitude about the criminal mind. At common law proof of an *actus reus* and a *mens rea* sufficed to establish criminal liability. It is easier to translate the Latin than to explain the concepts it capsulizes. In today's parlance, we describe these elements as the requirement of a voluntary act and a culpable state of mind, the minimum conditions for liability. ... At early common law, a defendant was not permitted to present witnesses on his or her own behalf and the defendant's own testimony was regarded as especially suspect. ... The issue of mental state was resolved neatly by maxims. The actor was presumed to intend the natural and probable consequences of his or her own act, thus the question of *mens rea* was collapsed into the concept of *actus reus*."

2. Provoking or inducing a police officer to shoot is often called *suicide by cop* or *suicide by proxy*. The phenomenon is difficult to measure. Often, the police shooting is explained as a "crazy person who came at the officer with a knife or gun." Invariably, the family of the deceased claim an unjustified police use-of-force in a civil action brought under 42 U.S.C. § 1983, an 1871 civil rights law that prohibits violations of citizens' constitutional rights by agents of state governments, including police officers. The police claim it was self-defense. See V.B. Lord (Ed.), *Suicide by Cop* (Flushing, NY: Looseleaf Law Publications, 2004).

3. See A. Buchanan, *Psychiatric Aspect of Justification, Excuse and Mitigation* (Philadelphia: Jessica Kingsley, 2000); G.F. Fletcher, *A Crime of Self-Defense: Bernhard Goetz and the Law on Trial* (New York: Free Press, 1988); J. Dressler, "Justifications and Excuses: A Brief Review of the Concepts and the Literature," *Wayne L. Rev.* 33 (1987): 1155.

   From a psychological or subjective perspective, however, the mechanisms of the ego are all called *defenses*: regression, repression, reaction formation, isolation, undoing, projection, introjection, turning against the self, and reversal. They are the ego's struggle against unpleasant ideas or affects. See the classic work by Sigmund Freud's daughter, Anna Freud, *The Ego and the Mechanisms of Defence* (New York: International Universities Press, 1946). See also A.S. Watson, *Psychiatry for Lawyers* (New York: International Universities Press, 1978). Dr. Karl Menninger, renowned as dean of American psychiatry, maintained that every individual, constantly exchanging with his environment, tries to make the best bargain possible with it, considering its threats, demands, opportunities, and dangers. To end a crisis, from birth trauma to an ingrown toenail, he said, one needs an "anticrisis" in order to achieve that "vital balance." See K.A. Menninger, *The Vital Balance* (New York: Viking, 1963); see also R. Slovenko, *Psychiatry and Criminal Culpability* (New York: John Wiley & Sons, 1995, pp. 275–287). Aleksander Pichushkin, known as the Chessboard Killer because he claimed to have marked off a square on a chessboard for every victim, spoke of killing as if it was both ordinary and required. "For me, a life without murder is like a life without food for you," he said. Killing gave him that "vital balance." Quoted in C.J. Chivers, "Man Accused of Killing 49 Goes on Trial in Moscow," *New York Times*, Sept. 14, 2007, p. 3. For a study of psychodynamics in homicide cases, see C.F. Malmquist, *Homicide: A Psychiatric Perspective* (Washington, DC: American Psychiatric Press, 2nd ed., 2006).

4. See United States v. Brown, 891 F. Supp. 1501 (D. Kan. 1995); K.J. Weiss, "Psychiatric Testimony and the 'Reasonable Person' Standard," *J. Am. Acad. Psychiat. & Law* 27 (1999): 580.

5. See M. Rees, *Our Final Hour* (New York: Basic Books, 2003).

6. See M.S. Moore, *Act and Crime* (Oxford, UK: Clarenton Press, 1993); M. Kelman, "Interpretive Construction in the Substantive Criminal Law," *Stan. L. Rev.* 33 (1981): 591.

7. See P.J.J. van Rensburg, C.A. Gagiano, & T. Verschoor, "Possible Reasons Why Certain Epileptics Commit Unlawful Acts During or Directly After Seizures," *Med. & Law* 13 (1994): 373; J.P. McCutcheon, "Involuntary Conduct and the Criminal Law," *Intl. J. Law & Psychiat.* 21 (1998): 305; S.J. Morse, "Culpability and Control," *U. Pa. L. Rev.* 142 (1994): 1587; K.W. Saunders, "Voluntary Acts and the Criminal Law: Justifying Culpability Based on the Existence of Volition," *U. Pitt. L. Rev.* 49 (1988): 443.

8. Model Penal Code §2.01. See also Cal. Penal Code §26; Ill. Ann. Stat. §4–1; N.J. Stat. Ann. §2C: 2–1.

9. Harvard psycholinguist Steven Pinker writes, "What, exactly, is an event? An event is a stretch of time, and time, according to physicists, is a continuous variable—an inexorable cosmic flow, in Newton's world, or a fourth dimension in a seamless hyperspace, in Einstein's. But the human mind carves this fabric into the discrete swatches we call events." S. Pinker, *The Stuff of Thought* (New York: Viking, 2007), pp. 3–4.

10. Prior to killing her five children, Andrea Yates hid her symptoms from her therapist and avoided taking medication, knowing that when off medication she became irritable with her children and had experienced delusional desires to harm them on at least two previous occasions. See E.W. Mitchell, *Self-Made Madness: Rethinking Illness and Criminal Responsibility* (Burlington, VT: Ashgate, 2003); S.L. Halleck, "Which Patients Are Responsible for Their Illnesses?" *Am. J. Psychotherapy* 42 (1988): 338; E.W. Mitchell, "Madness and Meta-Responsibility: The Culpable Causation of Mental Disorder and the Insanity Defence," *J. For. Psychiatry* 10 (1999): 597; P.H. Robinson, "Causing the Conditions of One's Own Defense: A Study in the Limits of Theory in Criminal Law Doctrine," *Va. L. Rev.* 71 (1985): 1; R. Sherlock, "Compliance and Responsibility: New Issues for the Insanity Defense," *J. Psychiat. & Law* 12 (1984): 483; M.D. Slodov, "Criminal Responsibility and the Noncompliant Psychiatric Offender: Risking Madness," *Case West. Res. L. Rev.* 40 (1989–1990): 271.

11. No. CR 42116 (Ohio Ct. App. 1980), noted in M.D. Slodov, "Criminal Responsibility and the Noncompliant Psychiatric Offender: Risking Madness," *Case West. Res. L. Rev.* 40 (1989–1990): 303.

12. Under the Model Penal Code of the American Law Institute, it is proposed that "a person with a mental disability who is *aware* of a potential for violence when nonmedicated may be liable for reckless or negligent homicide if he fails to remain on medication and then kills [someone]—even if at the time of the crime he would meet the test for not guilty by reason of insanity" (emphasis added). See R. Pies, "Psychiatric Naturalism and the Dimensions of Freedom: Implications for Psychiatry and the Law," *Psychiatric Times*, Oct. 2007, p. 10. The epileptic is held responsible for reckless endangerment when causing harm as a result of not taking antiseizure medication—epilepsy is not a defense where an epileptic disregards a known condition. See, e.g., People v. Decina, 138 N.W.2d 799 (N.Y. 1956), where the court noted that the "defendant knew he was subject to epileptic attacks and seizures that might strike at any time." The operation of the vehicle resulted in the death of several persons. The decision in *Decina* implicates the issue of time framing in a determination of voluntariness. Law Professor Joshua Dressler points out, "If a court constructed an extremely narrow time frame—specifically, the conduct at the instant the car struck the victims—the defendant's] conduct did not include a voluntary act. A broader time frame, however, would include the voluntary acts of entering the car, turning the ignition key, and driving." J. Dressler, *Understanding Criminal Law* (New York: Lexis, 3rd ed., 2001), p. 91. In State v. Welsh, 508 P.2d 1041 (Wash. App. 1973), the court held that a jury should be instructed that unconsciousness is not a complete defense when an epileptic seizer is voluntarily induced by intoxication.

13. Somnambulism, commonly referred to as sleepwalking, has fascinated people throughout history. The ancient Persians believed that the wandering body of a sleepwalker was seeking his spirit, which had detached itself and drifted away during the night. Europeans in medieval times explained it as demonic possession or lycanthropy. See F. McAuley & J.P. McCutheon, *Criminal Liability* (Dublin: Sweet & Maxwell, 2000), pp. 148–176; N. Corrado, "Automatism and the Theory of Action," *Emory L. J.* 9 (1990): 1191; D.W. Denno, "Crime and Consciousness: Science and Involuntary Acts," *Minn. L. Rev.* 87 (2002): 269; D.W. Denno, "A Mind to Blame: New Views on Involuntary Acts," *Behav. Sci. & Law* 21 (2003): 601; P. Fenwick, "Automatism, Medicine, and the Law," *Psychological Medicine Monograph* (1990); S.J. Morse, "Causation, Compulsion, and Involuntariness," *Bull. Am. Acad. Psychiat. & Law* 22 (1994): 159; S.J. Morse, "Craziness and Criminal Responsibility," *Behav. Sci. & Law* 17 (1999): 147; M. Rotter, "The Relationship Between Insight and Control in Obsessive-Compulsive Disorder: Implications for the Insanity Defense," *Bull. Am. Acad. Psychiat. & Law* 21(1993): 245.

People with the rare disorder called *sexsomnia* covering the full gamut of sexual activity, from fondling to intercourse, apparently have no conscious awareness of what they are doing and, when wakened, have no recollection of it. It sounds amusing—and some of the cases have comical aspects. One man had been initiating intercourse on almost a nightly basis, which was apparently fine with his wife, until one night he started snoring. Sexsomnia, or "sleep sex" as it is also known, can lead to both physical and psychological harm. Bed partners have been known to suffer lacerations, as it is not uncommon for male sexsomniacs to exercise much rougher behavior during sleep sex than waking sex. One man masturbated in his sleep with such energy that he suffered "repeated bruising of the penis" and avoided sexual intercourse for more than 8 years. Another man masturbated in his sleep every night, leaving his wife feeling "cheated." M. Mangan, *Sleepsex: Uncovered* (New York: Xlibris, 2001); C.H. Schenck, I. Amulf, & M.W. Mahowald, "Sleep and Sex: What Can Go Wrong?" *Sleep* 30 (2007): 683. A. Underwood, "It's Called 'Sexsomnia,'" *Newsweek*, June 11, 2007, p. 53.

Psychologist E. Michael Coles writes, "The law, operating on the premise that only human beings can commit crimes, logically concludes that, since a crime cannot be committed by a machine, a crime cannot be committed by a person who is functioning like a machine." E.M. Coles, "Scientific Support for the Legal Concept of Automatism," *Psychiat., Psychol. & Law* 7 (2000): 33.

14. See, e.g., State v. Johnson, 156 Ariz. 464, 753 P.2d 154 (1988).
15. J.R. Meloy, *The Psychopathic Mind* (Northvale, NJ: Jason Aronson, 1988), p. 194. See also J. Junginer, "Predicting Compliance with Command Hallucinations," *Am. J. Psyciat.*" 1990/47: 245–247;Command Hallucinations and the Prediction of Dangerousness," *Psychiat. Serv.* 46 (1995): 911; M.E. Kasper, R. Rogers, & P.A. Adams, "Dangerousness and Command Hallucinations: An Investigation of Psychotic Inpatients," *Bull. Am. Acad. Psychiat. & Law* 24 (1996): 219; J.S. Thompson, G.L. Stuart, & C.E. Holden, "Command Hallucinations and Legal Insanity," *Foren. Rep.* 5 (1992): 29; see A.M. Dershowitz, *The Genesis of Justice* (New York: Time Warner, 2000), p. 103.
16. N. Bunyan & D. Bamber, "George Harrison Wins Concession to Victims," *Weekly Telegraph*, Nov. 22–28, 2000, p. 3. In Bass v. Aetna Ins. Co., 370 So.2d 511 (La. 1979), the Louisiana Supreme Court declined to allow application of the "Act of God" defense in a personal injury suit brought by one worshiper against another on allegations that the defendant ran into the plaintiff while the plaintiff was in the aisle of a church praying. The defendant contended that he was "trotting under the Spirit of the Lord" when the accident occurred. The court said, "If [the defendant's] defense is that he was not in control of his actions, it can be compared to voluntary intoxication, which will not exonerate one from delictual responsibility"; 370 So.2d at 513.
17. See C.P. Ewing & J.T. McCann, *Minds on Trial* (New York: Oxford University Press, 2006), pp. 229–240. Returning to the United States from France with her two young children, the writer Judith Warner was shocked to see how difficult motherhood was in the United States as compared to France. She notes that Andrea Yates was overextended, under supported, and, topping it off, she ascribed to a very literal form of the Motherhood Religion. Before she went completely over the edge, Warner writes, she was different not so much in kind as in degree from that of a great number of American women. J. Warner, *Perfect Madness* (New York: Riverhead Books, 2005), p. 130. See also S. O'Malley, *Are You There Alone?* (New York: Simon & Schuster, 2004); D.W. Denno, "Who is Andrea Yates? A Short Story About Insanity," *Duke J. Gender Law & Policy* 10 (2003): 1–60.
18. 216 N.Y. 324, 110 N.E. 945 (1915).
19. 110 N.E. at 949. The State of New York having the *M'Naghten* test, Judge Cardozo was obliged to base the decision on impairment of cognition rather than on control.
20. ALI Model Penal Code §4.01, Comments, 46 (Tent. Draft No. 4, 1955). See A.J. Demko, "Abraham's Deific Defense: Problems with Insanity, Faith, and Knowing Right from Wrong," *Notre Dame L. Rev.* 80 (2005): 1961; C. Hawthorne, "Deific Decree: The Short, Happy Life of Pseudo Doctrine," *Loy. L.A. L. Rev.* 33 (2000): 1, 755. In a New York case, Muthanna Shamma was held NGRI on child sex abuse charges, by virtue of a claim that he committed the abuse because an angel told him to do it, and he was hospitalized. D. Margolick, "Madness as an Excuse: Two Similar Arguments in the Same Court, with Starkly Different Results," *New York Times*, Jan. 28, 1994, p. B11. See also Davis v. State, 595 N.W.2d 520 (Minn. 1999).

LaShuan Harris experienced auditory hallucinations that God instructed her to throw her three children into San Francisco Bay, which she did in 2005. By this act, she believed that her children would be united with God in heaven. At trial, the defense presented evidence indicating that, due to psychotic delusions, she had a very concrete understanding of heaven as a living destination. She wrote letters with the envelope addressed "To Heaven" and she inquired about the health of the children. She did not understand the finality or reality of death. She was found NGRI. The case was discussed at the 2007 annual meeting in Miami of the American Academy of Psychiatry and the Law. See S.H. Friedman, S.M. Horwitz, & P.J. Resnick, "Child Murder by Mothers: A Critical Analysis of the Current State of Knowledge and a Research Agenda," *Am. J. Psychiat.* 162 (2005): 1578.

21. The author Jon Krakauer discusses the case of a woman and her infant daughter who were murdered by two brothers who believed they were ordered to kill by God. J. Krakauer, *Under the Banner of Heaven* (New York: Doubleday, 2003). Brian David Mitchell thought that he was divine and he wandered the streets dressed up like Jesus and spouting biblical prophecies, then kidnapped Elizabeth Smart, then 14, to join a polygamous union. J. Morse, "The Missing Nine Months," *Time*, March 24, 2003, pp. 44–47. See P.S. Appelbaum, P.C. Robbins, & J. Monahan, "Violence and Delusions: Data From the MacArthur Violence Risk Assessment Study, *Am. J. Psychiat.* 157 (2000): 566.

22. 110 N.E. at 950. Years later, in describing the case at the New York Academy of Medicine, Cardozo identified the defendant as a priest who had been sexually intimate with the victim. He mentioned neither of those facts in his opinion, although they were relevant to judging the credibility of the defendant's claim that he had acted under God's command. A.L. Kaufman, *Cardozo* (Cambridge: Harvard University Press, 1998), pp. 383–395.

23. State v. Crenshaw, 98 Wash.2d 789, 659 P.2d 488 (1983).

24. 659 P.2d at 494. In State v. Cameron, 674 P.2d 650 (Wash. 1983), a defendant who believed his act was commanded by God was ruled insane. In McElroy v. State, 242 S.W. 883 (Tenn. 1922), the defendant was ruled sane based on similar facts. Washington has recently revisited the deific decree doctrine, allowing the defense to introduce moral wrongfulness for the jury to consider and to inject a "free will" or volitional argument to prove *M'Naghten* insanity. See G.B. Leong, "Revisiting the Deific-Decree Doctrine in Washington State," *J. Am. Acad. of Psychiat. & Law* 36 (2008): 95.

25. See D.T. Lunde & T.E. Wilson, "Brainwashing as a Defense to Criminal Liability: Patty Hearst Revisited," *Crim. L. Bull.* 13 (1977): 341; see also D.T. Lunde, *Hearst to Hughes: Memoir of a Forensic Psychiatrist* (Bloomington, IN: Author House, 2007), pp. 32–44; C.P. Ewing & J.T. McCann, *Minds on Trial: Great Cases in Law and Psychology* (New York: Oxford University Press, 2006), pp. 31–43.

26. See R. Slovenko, *Psychiatry and Criminal Culpability* (New York: John Wiley & Sons, 1995), pp. 67–117.

27. CNN, Dec. 23, 2003.

28. CNN, Dec. 23, 2003.

29. Daniel Goldhagen, impatient with what he calls "the paradigm of external compulsion," sought to show in his book, *Hitler's Willing Executioners,* that the crimes of the Holocaust were carried out by people obeying their own consciences, not blindly or fearfully obeying orders. D.J. Goldhagen, *Hitler's Willing Executioners: Ordinary Germans and the Holocaust* (New York: Knopf, 1996). Adolf Eichmann, who was convicted of crimes against the Jewish people and crimes against humanity, argued, "I did not want to kill; … my guilt is only in my obedience, my dutiful service in time of war, my loyalty to the oath, to the flag." The judge, in his sentencing statement, responded, "Even if we were to find that the defendant acted out of blind obedience, as he claims, we would still say that a man who participated in crimes of these dimensions, over years, must suffer the greatest punishment known to the law, and no order can mitigate this punishment. But, we have found that the defendant acted out of internal identification with the orders given them, and with a great desire to achieve the criminal object, and it makes no difference, in our opinion, in imposing punishment for such horrifying crimes, how this identification and this desire were born or whether they were the product of ideological education given the defendant by the regime that appointed him, as the defense counsel claims." T. Segev, *The Seventh Million* (New York: Henry Holt, 1991), p. 357.

30. For example, in Marley v. Indiana, 729 N.E.2d 1011 (Ind. App. 2000), the court ruled that a murder defendant could introduce evidence of battered woman's syndrome (BWS) only in support of an insanity defense. Because PTSD is a recognized mental disorder, the court said, evidence of BWS is admissible only under an insanity plea. See also State v. LeCompte, 371 So.2d 239 (La. 1979). BWS was first articulated by psychologist Lenore Walker, who posited a theory of "learned helplessness" to explain why a woman might not leave a battering relationship. The theory analogizes to Martin Seligman's work with laboratory dogs that he subjected to repeated electric shocks over which the dogs had no control. When the dogs were later placed in a position from which they could escape, they failed even to try to flee. Walker argued that battered women similarly learn to believe that they are helpless to flee, even when that belief may later prove to be wrong. Furthermore, the battered woman perceives herself to be trapped in a cycle of violence from which there is no escape. The woman seeks to defend herself at the only time that she thinks possible—before the next, inevitable attack. See A.M. Coughlin, "Excusing Women," *Cal. L. Rev.* 82 (1994): 1; A.E. Taslitz, "What Feminism Has to Offer Evidence Law," *Sw. U. L. Rev.* 28 (1999): 171.

31. It is suggested that persons with a serious personality disorder who show marginal functioning in daily life, under severe stress may at times undergo a personality disintegration with a frank psychotic episode and, therefore, should have the right to enter a plea of temporary insanity. G.B. Palermo, "The Future of Criminology and the Law in the Light of New Research," *Intl J. Offender Ther. & Compar. Criminol.* 43 (1999): 259. The late Dr. Bernard Diamond in an article published in 1962 predicted:

> Within ten years, biochemical and physiological tests will be developed that will demonstrate beyond a reasonable doubt that a substantial number of our worst and most vicious criminal offenders are actually the sickest of all. And that if the concept of mental disease and exculpation from responsibility applies at all, it will apply most appropriately to them. And further, that it will apply equally to the vast horde of minor, habitual, aggressive offenders who form the great bulk of the recidivists. The law and the public, whether they like it or not, will be forced by the stark proof of scientific demonstration to accept the fact that large numbers of persons who now receive the full, untempered blow of social indignation, ostracism, vengeance, and ritualized judicial murder are sick and helpless victims of psychological and physical disease of the mind and brain.

B.L. Diamond, "From *M'Naghten* to *Currens* and Beyond," *Cal. L. Rev.* 5 (1962): 189.

Unusual plasma androgen levels are said to "over influence" sexual offenders. R. Rada, "Plasma Androgens and the Sex Offender," *Bull. Am. Acad. Psychiat. & Law* 8 (1980): 456. It has also been claimed that women, just prior to or during early menstruation, may be prone to uncontrollable impulses resulting in violence. J.M. Abplanalp, "Premenstrual Syndrome," *Behav. Sci. & Law* 3 (1985): 103.

As may be obvious, grossly exaggerated claims are made regarding the impact of genes on behaviors and lifestyles. As S.P. Rose observed, "Genes, it is said, are responsible for such diverse features of human conduct as sexual orientation; poor behavior in school; alcoholism; drug addiction; violence; risk-taking; criminal, antisocial, and impulsive behavior; political antiauthoritarianism; religiosity; tendency to midlife divorce; and even compulsive shopping." S.P. Rose, "Neurogenetic Determinism and the New Euphenics; Clinical Review," *Brit. Med. J.* 317 (1998): 1707. The tendency to focus on genetics as a causal explanation for behaviors at the expense of other factors is called "genetic myopia." For a critique of a simple biological explanation of behavior, see R. Sapolsky, *The Trouble with Testosterone* (New York: Scribner, 1997).

32. S.H. Dinwiddie, "Genetics, Antisocial Personality, and Criminal Responsibility," *Bull. Am. Acad. Psychiat. & Law* 24 (1996): 95.

33. The cover of Ron Rosenbaum's book, *Explaining Hitler: The Search for the Origins of His Evil* (New York: Random House, 2000), features a picture of a cuddly infant Adolf Hitler.

34. J. Rosen, "The Brain on the Stand," *New York Times Magazine*, March 11, 2007, p. 48. Then, too, given the plasticity of the brain, it is quite conceivable that repeated, freely chosen commission of violent acts changes the brain. The idea that the brain changes its own structure and function through thought and activity is deemed to be the most important alternation in the view of the brain since its basic anatomy and workings of its basic component, the neuron, were first sketched out. N. Doidge, *The Brain That Changed Itself* (New York: Viking, 2007). See also S. Pollack (Ltr.), "The Brain on the Stand," *New York Times Magazine,* March 25, 2007, p. 10. "Let's get away from looking for easy answers and bumps on (or inside) the head to explain why we act as we do. The world, and we, are much more complex than that." R. Barsky (ltr.), "The Brain on the Stand," *New York Times Magazine*, April 1, 2007, p. 12.

35. The leading "sympathy defenses" or "abuse excuses" are set out in A.M. Dershowitz, *The Abuse Excuse and Other Cop-Outs, Sob Stories, and Evasions of Responsibility* (Boston: Little, Brown, 1994); S. Estrich, *Getting Away With Murder* (Cambridge, MA: Harvard University Press, 1998). See also P.J. Falk, "Novel Theories of Criminal Defense Based Upon the Toxicity of Social Environment: Urban Psychosis, Television Intoxication, and Black Rage," *N. Car. L. Rev.* 74 (1996): 731; A.E. Taslitz, "Abuse Excuses and the Logic and Politics of Expert Relevance," *Hastings L. J.* 49 (1998): 1039.

36. See Art. 651, Louisiana Code of Criminal Procedure.

37. 100 Stat. 3599, sec. 17.

38. See N. Morris, *Madness and the Criminal Law* (Chicago: University of Chicago Press, 1982).

39. State v. Dalton, 98 Wis.2d 725, 298 N.W.2d 298 (1980); Annot., 16 ALR 4th 654. The doctrine of diminished capacity, where recognized, allows the introduction of psychiatric testimony on mental state without an NGRI plea. See R. Slovenko, *Psychiatry and Criminal Culpability* (New York: John Wiley & Sons, 1995).

40. 832 F.2d 531 (10th Cir. 1987).

41. 126 S. Ct. 2709 (2006).

42. Eric Clark was convicted of first-degree murder under an Arizona statute prohibiting the intentional or knowing killing of a police officer in the line of duty. He was age 17 at the time. Evidence indicated that he had previously stated he wanted to shoot police officers and had lured the victim to the scene to kill him. In defense, evidence was offered that he suffered from paranoid schizophrenia with delusions about "aliens" when he killed the officer. In addition to offering this evidence in support of a defense of insanity, Clark offered it to rebut the prosecution's evidence of *mens rea*, claiming that he could not have acted intentionally or knowingly to kill an officer because his perception of reality was so severely distorted that he did not know his actions were wrong. The court held that psychiatric evidence could be admitted only under an insanity plea for the purpose allowed under the state's test of criminal responsibility. Clark was free to offer nonpsychiatric evidence of the everyday "observation" type to show what was on his mind when he committed the act. The Court noted that expert testimony on mental disease and capacity regarding intent has the potential to confuse jurors. It pointed to disagreement among mental health professionals about diagnoses and the effects of mental disease on capacities. Unlike "observational evidence," the Court reasoned that such "capacity evidence" includes judgments that are "fraught with multiple perils." The majority argued that an expert's judgment addressing the basic categories of capacity requires a leap from the concepts of psychology, which are devised for thinking about treatment, to the concepts of legal sanity, which are devised for thinking about criminal responsibility. See R.J. Allen, "Clark v. Arizona: Much (Confused) Ado About Nothing," *Ohio St. J. Crim. L.* 4 (2006): 135; P. Westen, "The Supreme Court's Bout With Insanity: Clark v. Arizona," *Ohio St. J. Crim. L.* 4 (2006): 143.

43. Regina v. Byrne, (1960) 3 All E. R. 1, 4. In R. v. Turner, [1975] Q.B. 834, C.A., the court again set out the proposition that the loss of self-control that is essential to a successful plea of provocation is something regarded by the law as "falling within the realm of the ordinary juryman's experience." In R. v. Emery, [1993] 14 Cr. App. 394, the application of the rule appeared to have been relaxed so as to permit expert testimony relating to a condition which, although not a mental disorder, "is complex and is not known by the public at large." The court noted that the condition of dependent helplessness to which the evidence related "is complex and is not known by the public at large. Accordingly, we are quite satisfied that it was appropriate for the learned judge to decide that this evidence should be allowed." The court commented further that "the question for the doctors was whether a woman of reasonable firmness with the characteristics of [the defendant], if abused in the manner which she said, would have had her will crushed so that she could not have protected the child." 14 Cr. App. R.(S.) at pp. 397–398. See R.D. Mackay & A.M. Colman, "Equivocal Rulings on Expert Psychological and Psychiatric Evidence: Turning a Muddle Into a Nonsense," *Crim. L. R.* (1996) 88.

44. I. Ray, *A Treatise on the Medical Jurisprudence of Insanity* (Cambridge, MA: Harvard University Press, 1962), p. 15. Original work published in 1838.

45. 49 N.H. 399 (1869).

46. 49 N.H. at 402.

47. Blocker v. United States 288 F.2d 853, 859 (D.C. Cir. 1961).

48. C.P. Erlinger, "Paying the Price for Vietnam: Post-Traumatic Stress Disorder and Criminal Behavior," *B. C. L. Rev.* (1984): 305.

49. Of course, the definition of *mental illness* is only the threshold question—the required consequences (impact on cognition or control) of that mental illness are different in the law on civil commitment or criminal responsibility.

50. United States v. Hinckley, 525 F.Supp. 1342 (D.C.C. 1981), *op. clarified, reconsideration denied*, 529 F. Supp. 520 (D.C.C. 1982), *aff'd*, 672 F.2d 115 (D.C. Cir. 1982).

51. See, e.g., People v. Doan, 141 Mich. App. 209, 366 N.W.2d 593 (1985). The Model Penal Code refrained from defining the content of the phrase "mental disease or defect." Rather, those terms are left open "to accommodate developing medical understanding"; Model Penal Code § 4.01 (1985). In State v. Galloway, 133 N.J. 631, 628 A.2d 735 (1993), the New Jersey Supreme Court said, "[T]he Legislature by its use of the term 'mental disease or defect' did not intend to preclude evidence of a mental condition consisting of a 'disorder' as such. Forms of psychopathology other than clinically defined mental diseases or defects may affect the mental process and diminish cognitive capacity, and, therefore, may be regarded as a mental disease or defect in the statutory or legal sense. ... [T]he determination that a condition constitutes a mental disease or defect is one to be made in each case by the jury after the court has determined that the evidence of the condition in question is relevant and sufficiently accepted within the psychiatric community to be found reliable for courtroom use. ... [T]o resolve, as a matter of law, the ultimate factual dispute over whether a mental condition is a 'disease or defect' would involve weighing the evidence and would thereby intrude into the province of the jury."

52. Ga. Crim. Proc. Law § 27-1503(a)(2).

53. ALI Model Penal Code § 4.01.

54. *In re* Rosenfield, 157 F.Supp. 18 (D.D.C. 1957).

55. See e.g., State v. Plummer, 117 N.H. 320, 374 A.2d 431 (1977).

56. See J. Cornwell, *The Power to Harm* (New York: Viking, 1960). See also M.L. Harris, "Problems with Prozac: A Defective Product Responsible for Criminal Behavior?" *J. Contemp. Legal Issues* 10 (1999): 359; C.M. Vale, "The Rise and Fall of Prozac: Products Liability Cases and 'the Prozac Defense' in Criminal Litigation," *St. Louis U. Pub. L. Rev.* 12 (1993): 525; P.B. Herbert, "Not Guilty by Reason of Prozac," *Newsl. Am. Acad. Psychiat. & Law*, April 2000, p. 16; S.H. Jurand, "Lawsuits Over Antidepressants Claim the Drug is Worse Than the Disease," *Trial*, March 2003, pp. 14–18.

57. 259 F.2d 943 (D.C. Cir. 1958).

58. 259 F.2d at 948 n. 4.

59. A state could make voluntary intoxication itself a crime on the ground that it produces an unreasonable risk of uncontrollable harmful conduct (as has been done in the case of drunk driving). In the United States, alcohol is implicated in 100,000 deaths a year, and figures in 40% of the deaths from injury and more than half the murders. Then, too, it is implicated in wife-beating and unemployment. See P. Cook, *Paying the Tab* (Princeton, NJ: Princeton University Press, 2007).

60. See Reg. v. Gamelin, 1 F & F 90 (1858); Reg. v. Moore, 3 C & K 153 (1852); Reg. v. Doody, 6 Cox C.C. 463(1945).

61. See State v. Hall, 214 N.W.2d 205 (Iowa 1974); see also Comment, "Intoxication as a Criminal Defense," *Colum. L. Rev.* 55 (1955): 1210.

62. People v. Hood, 1 Cal. 3d 444, 82 Cal. Rptr. 618, 462 P.2d 370 (1969).

63. 462 P.2d at 377.

64. See J. Dressler, *Understanding Criminal Law* (New York: Lexis 2001), pp. 324–325.

65. People v. Kelley, 176 N.W.2d 435, 443 (Mich. App. 1970).

66. Michigan law, e.g., provides that a defendant who offers an insanity defense must give notice to the court not less than 30 days before the date for the trial of the case or at such other time as the court directs; M.C.L. §768.20a(1).

67. The several states (Idaho, Kansas, Montana, Nevada, Utah) that have abolished the insanity defense typically allow expert testimony "on the issues of *mens rea* where any state of mind is an element of the offense." See Idaho Code § 46-14-214 (1999); Nev. Rev. Stat. Ann. § 174.035 (1997); Utah Code Ann. § 76-2-305 (1999). In Montana v. Cowan, 861 P.2d 884 (1993), the Montana court upheld such abolition noting that the state law allowed evidence with respect to the defendant's mental state on competency to stand trial, proof of his state of mind, and sentencing. See B.E. Elkins, "Idaho's Repeal of the Insanity Defense: What Are We Trying to Prove?" *Idaho L. Rev.* 31 (1994): 153. Kansas replaced the insanity defense with a *mens rea* definition of criminal responsibility. The legislation provides that it is a defense to prosecution of any criminal offense that "the defendant, as a result of mental illness or defect, lacked the mental state required as an element of the offense charged. Mental disease or defect is not otherwise a defense"; Kan. Stat. Ann. §22-3220 (1995).

68. A. Dershowitz, "Abolishing the Insanity Defense," *Crim. L. Bull.* 9 (1973): 434.

69. A.M. Platt & B.L. Diamond, "The Origins and Development of the 'Wild Beast' Concept of Mental Illness and Its Relation to Theories of Criminal Responsibility," *J. History Behav. Sci.* 1 (1965): 355–367.

70. Daniel M'Naghten's Case, 10 Clark & Fin. 200, 8 Eng. Rep. 718 (1843). The defendant's name is variously spelled M'Naghten, M'Naughton, McNaughtan, McNaughten, McNaughton, and Mhicneachdain. The original report of the trial spelled it M'Naughton. The most common spelling (M'Naghten) is probably the least correct. A photograph of his signature seems to read McNaughtun, which prompted Justice Frankfurter to ask, "To what extent is a lunatic's spelling of his own name to be deemed an authority?" B.L. Diamond, "On the Spelling of Daniel M'Naghten's Name," *Ohio State L. J.* 25 (1964): 84.

71. Delusional misidentification (as when an individual believes his spouse has been replaced by an imposter who threatens to harm him) is often seen in individuals suffering from schizophrenia, schizoaffective disorder, or a psychotic disorder due to a general medical condition. Psychotic thinking plays a substantial if not significant role in the genesis of aggression in those suffering from dementia. Aggression arises from viewing the misidentified person as untrustworthy, evil, or threatening. J.A. Silva, G.B. Leong, R. Weinstock, & M. Ruiz-Sweeney, "Delusional Misidentification and Aggression in Alzheimer's Disease," *J. For. Sci.* 46 (2001): 581.

72. See M.H. Pauley, "Murder by Premeditation," *Am. Crim. L. Rev.* 36 (1999): 145; see also S. Pinker, *The Stuff of Thought* (New York: Viking, 2007).

73. Durham v. United States, 214 F.2d 862 (D.C. Cir. 1954).

74. See L.Z. Freedman (Ed.), *By Reason of Insanity: Essays on Psychiatry and the Law* (Wilmington, DE: Scholarly Resources, 1983).

75. O'Beirne v. Overholser, 193 F. Supp. 652, at 660 (D.C. 1961).

76. Rollerson v. United States, 343 F.2d 269, at 271 (D.C. Cir. 1964).

77. Appendix, Washington v. United States, 390 F.2d 444, at 457 (D.C. Cir. 1967).

78. K.A. Menninger, *The Crime of Punishment* (New York: Viking, 1968). Slovenko assisted in the writing of the book.

79. J. Goldstein, "Professional Knowledge and Professional Self-Interest: The Rise and Fall of Monomania in 19th-Century France," *Int. J. Law & Psychiat.* 21 (1998): 385.

80. 471 F.2d 969 (D.C. Cir. 1972); noted in *N.Y.U. L. Rev.* 47 (1972): 962.

81. For an extensive discussion of the test, see People v. Martin, 386 Mich. 407, 192 N.W.2d 215 (1971).

82. United States v. Hinckley, 525 F. Supp. 1342 (D.D.C.), *op. clarified reconsideration denied*, 529 F. Supp. 520 (D.D.C.), *aff'd*, 672 F.2d 115 (D.C. Cir. 1982); S. Taylor, "Jury Finds Hinckley Not Guilty, Accepting His Defense of Insanity," *New York Times*, June 22, 1982, p.1. See R.J. Bonnie, J.C. Jeffries, & P.W. Low, *A Case Study in the Insanity Defense: The Trial of John W. Hinckley, Jr.* (New York: Foundation Press, 3rd ed., 2008). Hinckley was an obsessed fan of Jodie Foster. He shot President Reagan to impress her, thinking that she would then fall in love with him. Little did he know that she was a lesbian. D. Rader, "'I Have a Longing to Connect,'" *Parade*, March 16, 2008, p. 6.

83. "Hinckley Bombshell End of Insanity Pleas?" *U.S. News & World Rep.*, July 5, 1982, p. 12.

84. S. 2902; S. 2903, 97th Cong., 2nd Sess., 128 Cong Rec. 511392-96; 511404-08 (Sept. 14, 1982).

85. For a summary of the bills introduced in Congress, see *Ment. Disabil. L. Rep.* 6 (1982): 340.

86. "The Insanity Defense: ABA and APA Proposals for Change," *Ment. Disabil. L. Rep.* 7 (1983): 136; "American Psychiatric Association Statement on the Insanity Defense," *Am. J. Psychiat.* 140 (1983): 681.

87. S.J. Morse, "Excusing the Crazy: The Insanity Defense Reconsidered," *S. Cal. L. Rev.* 58 (1985): 777.

88. Professor Weihofen went on to say: "It is charged that the rules of law governing insanity as a defense to crime are vague and confused; that in so far as these rules are clear, they are clearly unsound, in that they are based upon notions of mental disorder discredited by modern science; and that the procedural machinery for trying cases where this defense is raised is inefficient and blundering in its results." H. Weihofen, *Insanity as a Defense in Criminal Law* (New York: Commonwealth Fund, 1933), p. 1. See also H. Weihofen, *Mental Disorder as a Criminal Defense* (Buffalo, NY: Dennis, 1954).

89. The GBMI verdict is discussed hereinafter at note 127.

90. In 1972, President Nixon proposed that the insanity defense be abolished for federal crimes, but Congress never acted on his legislation. See A. Dershowitz, "Abolishing the Insanity Defense," *Crim. L. Bull.* 9 (1973): 434.

91. Dr. Abraham L. Halpern, a president of the American Academy of Psychiatry and Law, has worked continuously over the past 35 years for the abolition of the insanity defense, asserting that it makes a mockery of the criminal justice system, and frequently results in the misuse and abuse of psychiatry. Among his writings on the issue, see "The Insanity Defense: A Juridical Anachronism," *Psychiat. Ann.* 7 (1977): 398; "The Fiction of Legal Insanity and the Misuse of Psychiatry," *J. Leg. Med.* 2 (1980):18; "The Politics of the Insanity Defense," *Am. J. Foren. Psychiat.* 14 (1993): 1. See also J. Goldstein & J. Katz, "Abolish the Insanity Defense—Why Not?" *Yale L. J.* 72 (1963): 853. Professor Christopher Slobogin argues that abolishing the insanity defense has three potential practical benefits: (1) It would improve the public's image of the criminal justice system, (2) it may reduce the stigma associated with mental illness, and (3) it should facilitate treatment of those with mental problems. C. Slobogin, "An End to Insanity: Recasting the Role of Mental Disability in Criminal Cases," *Va. L. Rev.* 86 (2000): 1199.

92. See Panel Discussion, "Insanity as a Defense," 37 F.R.D. 365 (1964). Criminal law does recognize some "acts" of omission as criminal acts, such as a parent's intentionally omitting to feed his child, or an epileptic's intentionally driving without taking medicine to prevent a seizure.

93. See O.W. Holmes, *The Common Law* (Boston: Little Brown, Howe ed., 1963), p. 42.

94. The American Psychiatric Association urged that the insanity defense be retained in some form because it rests upon the fundamental premise of the criminal law, namely, that people should be punished only if they are morally responsible for wrongful deeds. The 27,000 member association was stimulated to take a stand on the defense because of public and legislative outrage over the acquittal of Hinckley. In making the statement, the APA made no judgment as to whether the *Hinckley* verdict was proper or whether other standards and procedures would have resulted in a different verdict. See "Psychiatric Group Urges Stiffer Rules for Insanity Plea," *New York Times*, Jan 20, 1983, p. 18.

95. Shifting the focus of attention from the deed to the biography of the defendant is criticized as a perversion of justice. See, generally, W. Gaylin, *The Killing of Bonnie Garland: A Question of Justice* (New York: Simon & Schuster, 1982); P. Meyer, *The Yale Murder* (New York: Harper & Row, 1982).

96. J. Wigmore, *Evidence* (Boston: Little, Brown, 1940), vol. 2, sec. 228 (emphasis omitted). See also People v. Martin, 386 Mich. 407, 192 N.W.2d 215 (1971).

97. Professor Don Linhorst of the St. Louis University School of Social Service reports that in a dataset of 1,066 Missouri insanity acquittees, 25.7% had a felony conviction prior to the insanity acquittal. The dataset did not contain information on the type of crime or the number of prior felony arrests or convictions. The dataset included only insanity acquittees, not defendants who may have pled insanity, but were unsuccessful. See D.M. Lindorst, "The Unconditional Release of Mentally Ill Offenders From Indefinite Commitment: A Study of Missouri Insanity Acquittees," *J. Am. Acad. Psychiat. & Law* 27 (1999): 563.

98. See E. Tanay, *The Murderers* (Indianapolis: Bobbs-Merrill, 1976).

99. Compare this situation with that of a career criminal. In the latter case, the evidence as to the identity of the offender is often circumstantial. Often plea bargaining occurs because of weak evidence, and the defendant receives a relatively light sentence. Especially in large urban areas, there is trading as to the charge or sentence. Indeed, it may be suggested that evidence of mental illness or defect would not be necessary in many cases if there were more appropriate charging by the district attorney or the grand jury.

100. See S.B. Silver, M.I. Cohen, & M.K. Spodak, "Follow-Up After Release of Insanity Acquittees, Mentally Disordered Offenders, and Convicted Felons," *Bull. Am. Acad. Psychiat. & Law* 17 (1989): 387.

101. Whatever the test, Judge Bazelon observed that juries will continue to make moral judgments under the fundamental precept that "[o]ur collective conscience does not allow punishment where it cannot impose blame"; Durham v. United States, 214 F. 2d 862, 876 (D.C. Cir. 1954).

102. The report (1949–1953) of the Royal Commission on Capital Punishment records a higher number. It noted that of 99,463 persons charged with felony crime in a 5-year period, 19.8% of the 374 charged with murder were acquitted by reason of insanity. London: Her Majesty's Stationery Office. See J. Gunn & P.J. Taylor, *Forensic Psychiatry* (Oxford, UK: Butterworth-Heinemann, 1993); C. Cirincione, H. Steadman, & M. McGreevy, "Rates of Insanity Acquittals and the Factors Associated With Successful Insanity Pleas," *Bull. Am. Acad. Psychiat. & Law* 25 (1995): 399; J. Janofsky, M. Vandewalle, & J. Rappeport, "Defendants Pleading Insanity: An Analysis of Outcome," *Bull. Am. Acad. Psychiat. & Law* 17 (1989): 203; R.A. Pasewark, "Insanity Plea: A Review of the Research Literature, *J. Psychiat. & Law* 9 (1981): 14; H. Steadman et al., "Factors Associated With a Successful Insanity Defense," *Am. J. Psychiat.* 140 (1983): 401. In New York State, there were one or two successful insanity cases per year between 1958 and 1965, and approximately nine cases per year between April 1, 1965, and August 30, 1971. Insanity acquittals rose to an average of 48 cases per year for the period 1971 through 1976, and, after holding steady for the next 4 years, again rose to 124 cases in the year after the Insanity Defense Reform Act of 1980 went into effect. A.L. Halpern, "Elimination of the Exculpatory Insanity Rule," *Psychiat. Clin, N. Am.* 6 (Dec. 1983): 611. See also M.A. McGreevy, H.J. Steadman, & L.A. Callahan, "The Negligible Effects of California's 1982 Reform of the Insanity Defense Test," *Am. J. Psychiat.* 148 (1991): 744, where it is reported that 51% of the 1,300 individuals in a 6-year period who entered an insanity plea were acquitted.

103. Peter Plummer, an Assistant Michigan Attorney General and former Assistant Prosecuting Attorney for Marquette County, Michigan, who has over 30 years of experience prosecuting various criminal offenses, commented, "… of thousands of felony and misdemeanor cases that I had, only three to six of them were actual true trials using the insanity defense. There were a lot of attempts to use the defense, but either the defense counsel or defendant would opt out if my plea offer was good enough." Personal communication.

104. H.B. Terrell, "Malingering Since Three-Strikes in California," *Forensic Examiner*, May/June 1999, p.22. Some states require a mental health hearing before accepting a plea based on insanity; Rennich-Craig v. Russell, 609 N.W.2d 123 (S.D. 2000).

105. A few studies explore the extent to which the insanity defense was used in a jury trial, bench trial, or plea agreement, but they acknowledge the lack of information. See J. Petrila, "The Insanity Defense and Other Mental Health Dispositions in Missouri," *Intl. J. Psychiat. & Law* 5 (1982): 81; C.E. Boehnert, "Characteristics of Successful and Unsuccessful Insanity Pleas," *Law & Hum. Behav.* 13 (1989): 31.

106. In Maine, a criminal defendant charged with murder has the burden of proving by a preponderance of the evidence that he acted in the heat of passion or sudden impulse in order to reduce the charge of homicide to manslaughter. The United States Supreme Court ruled that this burden did not comport with the due process requirement that the prosecution must prove every fact necessary to constitute

the crime charged beyond a reasonable doubt; Mullaney v. Wilbur, 421 U.S. 684 (1975). However, 2 years later the Supreme Court upheld a New York law making "extreme emotional disturbance" reducing a crime from murder to manslaughter an affirmative defense; Patterson v. New York, 421 U.S. 197 (1977). The defense of "extreme emotional disturbance" is but a slightly modified version of the defense of provocation, for which many states had long placed the burden of proof upon the defendant.

107. See E.W. Cleary, "Presuming and Pleading: An Essay on Juristic Immaturity," *Ariz. State L. J.* 1979: 115; J. McNaughton, "Burden of Production of Evidence: A Function of a Burden of Persuasion," *Harv. L. Rev.* 68 (1955): 1382.

108. Theodore Kaczynski, also known as the Unabomber, did not want to be considered mentally ill. See J.S. Newman, "Doctors, Lawyers, and the Unabomber," *Mont. L. Rev.* 60 (1999): 67; A. Chase, "Harvard and the Making of the Unabomber," *Atlantic Monthly*, June 2000, p. 41; W. Glaberson, "Judge Orders Unabomber Suspect to Cooperate in Psychiatric Tests," *New York Times*, Jan. 10, 1998, p.1; G. Witkin, "What Does It Take to Be Crazy?" *U.S. News & World Report*, Jan. 12, 1998, p. 7. The appellate courts are divided on the question of the court's authority or duty to impose an insanity defense on a mentally disabled defendant. The court in Frendak v. United States, 408 A.2d 364 (D.C. App. 1979), took note of conflicting holdings in various jurisdictions. A defendant may prefer confinement in prison rather than in a mental institution, or may wish to avoid the stigma associated with mental disorder. At the same time, the state has a duty to see that justice is served. In Whalen v. United States, 346 F.2d 812 (D. C. Cir. 1965), the D.C. Circuit permitted assertion of the defense over the defendant's objection on the ground that it would be morally repugnant to convict a person who was insane at the time of the offense. Given that a conviction is put in jeopardy by a failure by the defense to raise the insanity defense when warranted would seem to justify interposing it. The state, too, is entitled to a fair trial. See also People v. Redmond, 94 Cal. Rptr. 542 (Calif. App. 1971). In United States v. Marble, 940 F.2d 1543 (D.C. Cir. 1991), the D.C. Circuit overturned *Whalen* on the theory that Congress by the Insanity Defense Reform Act of 1984 made the insanity plea the prerogative of the defense. By recent legislation, Canada allows the insanity plea to be raised only by the defendant.

In Alvord v. Wainwright, 469 U.S. 956 (1984), the U.S. Supreme Court said that counsel has a duty to investigate his client's case and make a minimal effort to persuade him to plead insanity when it is his "only plausible defense." Defense counsel's failure to discover facts supporting a potential insanity defense is deemed to constitute ineffective assistance of counsel and a basis for reversal of a conviction. United States *ex rel.* Rivera v. Franzen, 594 F. Supp. 198 (N.D. Ill. 1984), on appeal, 794 F.2d 314 (7th Cir. 1986). How much weight should be given to the question of whether the defendant's articulated reason to refuse to enter an insanity plea is a "rational" one? Can a trial judge or defense counsel ever say that a defendant's claim of factual innocence or self-defense is "irrational"? In State v. Khan, 417 A.2d 585 (N.J. App. 1980), the defendant claimed that he killed in self-defense, but the psychiatric evidence strongly indicated that he acted under a paranoiac delusion. The insanity defense was interposed, but both issues were submitted to the jury—insanity and self-defense—with instructions that if the jury finds the defendant not insane at the time the homicide was committed, then the trial would proceed on the general issue of defendant's guilt or innocence of the crime charged, including the issue of self-defense. Yale Law Professor Mirjan Damaska writes in his book *Evidence Law Adrift* (New Haven: Yale University Press, 1997):

> If criminal law exempts from punishment legally insane individuals or persons who acted under duress, the facts underlying insanity or duress should be established—whenever their existence appears probable—as part of the court's duty. And the court should proceed to inquire into these facts even against the wishes of the accused: If the individual's interests were controlling, the criminal sanction could be misapplied from the relevant (that is, systemic) point of view.

It is argued that the major reason for permitting the imposition of the insanity defense on unwilling defendants is a policy preference for preserving the dignity of the law over the rights of individual competent defendants. See, e.g., R.D. Miller, J. Olin, D. Johnson, J. Doidge, D. Iverson, & E. Fantone, "Forcing the Insanity Defense on Unwilling Defendants: Best Interests and the Dignity of the Law," *J. Psychiat. & Law* 24 (1996): 487. On the other hand, in the article "The Imposition of the Insanity Defense on an Unwilling Defendant," *Ohio St. L. J.* 41 (1980): 637, Anne Singer argues the unconstitutionality and impracticability of imposing the insanity defense on uncooperative defendants.

109. See Rivera v. Delaware, 429 U.S. 877 (1976); R.I. Allen, "The Restoration of *In re* Winship: A Comment on Burdens of Persuasion in Criminal Cases After *Patterson v. New York*," *Mich. L. Rev.* 76 (1977): 30.

110. People who are caught up in a riot may be regarded as lacking the capacity to control their behavior, for the individual who is lost in the anonymity of a crowd bent on mischief is said to have lost any normal ability to hold his impulses in check. Gang rape is discussed in G. Geis, "Group Sexual Assaults," *Med. Aspects Human Sexual.*, May 1971: 101. Impulse control disorders consist of a group of conditions that are said to share the essential feature of being unable to resist an impulse, drive, or temptation to perform an action potentially harmful to the person or others. In most instances, an individual with an impulse control disorder experiences an increasing sense of tension or arousal before committing the act. Impulse control disorders include kleptomania, pyromania, intermittent explosive disorder, and pathological gambling. In individuals with bipolar disorder, these activities are a component of mania or possibly hypomania. See T. Suppes, J.S. Manning, & P.E. Keck, *Decoding Bipolar Disorder* (Kansas City, MO: Compact Clinicals, 2007), p. 109. General George Patton's commander, General Dwight Eisenhower, did not believe that General Patton lacked self-control, only that he was refusing to practice it. He ordered General Patton to publicly apologize for slapping a soldier and put General Patton on probation. After this, there were no reports that General Patton committed more acts of emotional or physical abuse during two remaining years of World War II. In other words, it is said, General Patton—and just about every other person with a bad temper—could control himself when motivated to do so. See J. Telushkin, *The Ten Commandments of Character* (New York: Bell Tower, 2003), p. 38.

111. For research-based guidelines for interview-based assessments, see R. Rogers & D.W. Shuman, *Conducting Insanity Evaluations* (Washington, DC: American Psychiatric Press, 2nd ed., 2000).

112. McGuire v. Almy, 297 Mass. 323, 8 N.E. 2d 760 (1937).

113. 593 F.2d 700 (5th Cir. 1979).

114. See R. Slovenko, "Remorse," *J. Psychiat. & Law* 34 (2006): 397.

115. Another study using five mock cases and different instructions (the "wild beast" test, M'Naghten, M'Naghten plus irresistible impulse, *Durham*, and the ALI test) found no overall significant differences among the instructions in outcome. N. Finkel et al., "Insanity Defenses: From the Juror's Perspective," *Law & Psychol. Rev.* 9 (1985): 77. The American Bar Association concluded that the difference in outcome in jurisdictions with a test that included a volitional prong and those that did not might be significant. ABA, *Criminal Justice Mental Health Standards*, Commentary to Standard 7-6.1 (1989).

116. See, e.g., Wright v. United States, 250 F.2d 4 (D.C. App. 1957). In another case, Lashauan Harris threw her three young sons to their deaths in San Francisco Bay in 2005, the jury found her guilty of second-degree murder, but she was declared NGRI by the judge. The evidence showed that she was schizophrenic and borderline mentally retarded and that she was convinced she was acting on orders from God. News report, *New York Times*, Jan. 18, 2007, p. 7.

117. See B.R. Schwartz, "Should Juries Be Informed of the Consequences of the Insanity Verdict?" *J. Psychiat. & Law* 8 (1980): 167. In Fulghum v. Ford, 850 F.2d 1529 (11th Cir. 1988), posttrial interviews of jurors revealed that they thought the defendant was insane, but feared that an NGRI verdict would be "less effective" in removing him from society. A verdict cannot be overturned, however, by posttrial jury statements describing even serious errors or misunderstandings on points of law or the proper basis of decision; Rule 606(b), Federal Rules of Evidence.

118. K.A. Menninger, *The Human Mind* (New York: Knopf, 3rd ed., 1961), pp. 7–8.

119. See A.R. Matthews, *Mental Disability and the Criminal Law* (Chicago: American Bar Association, 1970).

120. See G.H. Morris, "Dealing Responsibly With the Criminally Irresponsible," *Ariz. St. L. J.* 1982: 855; A.A. Stone, "Psychiatric Abuse and Legal Reform," *Int. J. Law & Psychiat.* 5 (1982): 9; B. Kirschner, "Constitutional Standards for Release of the Civilly Committed and Not Guilty by Reason of Insanity: A Strict Scrutiny Analysis," *Ariz. L. Rev.* 20 (1978): 233; J.R. German & A.C. Singer, "Punishing the Not Guilty: Hospitalization of Persons Acquitted by Reason of Insanity," *Rutgers L. Rev.* 29 (1976): 1011; Comment, "Commitment Following an Insanity Acquittal," *Harv. L. Rev.* 94 (1981): 605.

121. People v. McQuillan, 392 Mich.511, 221 N.W.2d 569, 576 (1974). See also People v. Chavez, 629 P.2d 1040 (Colo. 1981); *In re* Lewis, 402 A.2d 1115 (Del. 1979); *In re* Jones, 228 Kan. 90, 612 P.2d 1211 (1980); Chase v. Kearns, 278 A.2d 132 (Me. 1971). "A finding of not guilty because of insanity shall be prima facie evidence that the acquitted person is presently dangerous to the person's self or others or property of others." *Kan. Stat. Ann.* Sec. 22-3428 (1) (1981).

122. See J. Gunn, "An English Psychiatrist Looks at Dangerousness," *Bull. Am. Acad. Psychiat. & Law* 10 (1982): 143.

123. The Fifth Circuit ruled that the presumption of continuing insanity that Georgia applied to insanity acquittees, but not to persons civilly committed, amounts to a denial of equal protection of the law, but that the provision requiring judicial approval for release of acquittees charged with crimes evidencing dangerousness was constitutional. See Benham v. Edwards, 678 F.2d 511 (5th Cir. 1982); Bolton v. Harris, 395 F.2d 642, 652 (D.C. Cir. 1968); State v. Simants, 330 N.W.2d 910 (Neb. 1983). See also W.J. Ingber, "Rules for an Exceptional Class: The Commitment and Release of Persons Acquitted of Violent Offenses by Reason of Insanity," *N.Y.U. L. Rev.* 57 (1982): 281. An insanity acquittee may be under enforced medical supervision. *In re* Rosenfield, 157 F. Supp. 18 (D.D.C. 1957).

124. The American Psychiatric Association urged tightened procedures to protect the public against premature release of potentially dangerous individuals. At the same time, the Association said it was "quite skeptical" about procedures in many states requiring periodic psychiatric reassessments of whether an individual is still dangerous. Dr. Loren Roth, chairman of the group that drafted the APA's position paper, explained that psychiatrists "have great difficulty in predicting dangerous behavior" and that the best indicator of future violence is a past record of violence, not a psychiatric diagnosis. The Association urged that decisions on whether to release such persons be made not solely on the basis of psychiatric testimony, but by a broader group, perhaps similar to a parole board. No release should occur, the Association said, unless the individual can be given carefully supervised outpatient treatment to protect himself and the public from harm. In Oregon, a program begun in 1980 under the aegis of a multidisciplinary Psychiatric Security Review Board makes all decisions relating to confinement, release, and reconfinement of the insanity acquittee. See R. Rogers, "1981 Oregon Legislation Relating to the Insanity Defense and the Psychiatric Security Review Board," *Bull. Am. Acad. Psychiat. & Law* 10 (1982): 155; J.L. Bloom & J.D. Bloom, "Disposition of Insanity Defense Cases in Oregon," *Bull. Am. Acad. Psychiat, & Law* 9 (1981): 93. This model did not sweep the country, as the various states are generally reluctant to establish new boards and indeed, in these days of tight budgets, the states are eliminating many of their existing boards. Other states, particularly those with only a handful of insanity acquittees, such as Connecticut, would not make the expenditures necessary for this purpose.

125. 463 U.S. 354 (1983).

126. One recent study found that 85% of insanity acquittees were still under commitment 5 years after acquittal and 76% 10 years after acquittal. D.M. Linhorst, "The Unconditional Release of Mentally Ill Offenders From Indefinite Commitment: A Study of Missouri Insanity Acquittees," *J. Am. Acad. Psychiat. & Law* 27 (1999): 563. Justice Powell said in *Jones* that "important differences" between those under civil commitment for mental illness and those who are committed following an insanity defense justify a refusal to apply the same standard of proof to both categories.

 Patti Davis, President Reagan's daughter, notes the irony in the insanity defense: "Initially, prosecutors claim the defendant isn't insane, he's accountable for his actions and should be punished. The defendant claims his mind is so ravaged by mental illness he can't be held responsible. Then the roles reverse. Once the defendant, now the patient, has been in a mental institution for a while, the claim is: I'm fine; I've been treated; I'm no longer a danger to society. The government then says no, he's too unstable, too ill. Keep him locked up." P. Davis, "Don't Let Hinckley Roam Free," *Time*, April 17, 2000, p. 34.

127. See S.L. Sherman, "Guilty But Mentally Ill: A Retreat From the Insanity Defense," *Am. J. L. & Med.* 7 (1981): 237; C. Slobogin, "The Guilty But Mentally Ill Verdict: An Idea Whose Time Should Not Have Come," *Geo. Wash. L. Rev.* 53 (1985): 494.

128. In Nevada, unlike in other states, GBMI is a special plea.

129. See C. Nesson, "A Needed Verdict: Guilty But Insane," *New York Times* (July 1, 1982): 19, arguing that the "alternative verdict of 'guilty but mentally ill' should be adopted more widely to deal with the John Hinckleys of this world, the partly crazies, who deserve neither to be absolved of responsibility nor to be treated just like ordinary criminals." See also S. Taylor, "Too Much Justice," *Harper's* (Sept. 1982): 56, 65.

130. 392 Mich. 511, 221 N.W. 2d 569 (1974).

131. See Mich. Comp. Laws Ann. § 678.36 (West 1982); Mich. Stat. Ann Sec. 28: 1059 (Callaghan 1978). See also G.A. Smith & J.A. Hall, "Evaluating Michigan's Guilty But Mentally Ill Verdict: An Empirical Study," *U. Mich. J. L. Ref.* 16 (1982): 77; G.D. Mesritz, "Guilty But Mentally Ill: An Historical and Constitutional Analysis," *J. Urb. L.* 53 (1976): 471. According to a study of the effects of the *McQuillan* case in Michigan, out of 223 defendants found not guilty by reason of insanity over a 5-year period, 124 were released, following a 60-day assessment period, as noncommittable according to the civil standards. Almost half of the remaining acquittees had been released within 5 years of acquittal, after an average of 9½ months of postevaluation hospitalization. This represented a substantial decrease in

periods of confinement from the rate during the pre-*McQuillan* years. See M.L. Criss & D.R. Racine, "Impact of Change in Legal Standard for Those Adjudicated Not Guilty by Reason of Insanity," *Bull. Am. Acad. Psychiat. & Law* 8 (1982): 261.

132. See J. Swickard, "New Insanity Verdict on Trial," *Detroit Free Press*, Jan. 31, 1983 p. 3; R. Slovenko, "The Case Against 'Guilty But Ill'," *Detroit News*, Jan 31, 1983, p. 11; J. Swickard, "Gunman Guilty But Mentally Ill in Buhl Attack," *Detroit Free Press*, Feb. 5, 1983, p. 1.

133. C.A. Palmer & M. Hazelrigg, "The Guilty But Mentally Ill Verdict: A Review and Conceptual Analysis of Intent and Impact," *J. Am. Acad. Psychiat. & Law* 28 (2000): 47. Transfers of mentally ill prisoners are rarely accomplished. See, e.g., Maxwell v. McBryde, 12 Ariz. App. 269, 469 P. 2d 835 (1970); see also Special Project, "The Administration of Psychiatric Justice: Theory and Practice in Arizona," *Ariz. L. Rev.* 13 (1972): 1, 174–80; A. Brooks, *Law, Psychiatry and the Mental Health System* (Boston: Little, Brown, 1973), p. 411.

134. The American Bar Association also opposed the enactment of statutes that supplant or supplement the NGRI verdict with an alternative verdict of GBMI. See S.J. Brakel & J.L. Cavanaugh, "Crime, Psychiatry and the Insanity Defense: A Report on Some Recent Reforms in the United States," *Austral. & N. Zealand J. Psychiat.* 30 (1996): 134.

135. G. Fletcher, *Rethinking Criminal Law* (Boston: Little, Brown, 1978), p. 835.

136. See R. Rodgers & D. Shuman, *Conducting Insanity Evaluations* (New York: Guilford, 2nd ed., 2000).

The defense of diminished capacity, in one form or another, has been adopted in about one third of the states, mainly in cases in which the defendant is charged with first-degree murder, although in theory it applies to all crimes involving specific intent as an essential element of the prosecution's proof. Judge or jury could always render a verdict of any cognate lesser offense under the charged crime, but it is perplexing what evidence is admissible or what is convincing to bring about a lesser verdict. In the 1920s, in the trial of Leopold and Loeb, who were accused of kidnapping and murder, Clarence Darrow made then-novel use of psychiatric testimony to avoid the death penalty.

The states that have not adopted the diminished capacity defense hold that evidence of mental capacity to negate criminal intent is all or nothing. These jurisdictions contend that to permit the defense of diminished capacity would, in effect, sneak in the insanity defense without labeling it as such without complying with the requirements or consequences of the insanity defense. As one court put it, "The purpose of requiring notice of intent to claim the defense of insanity is to protect the public and avoid unfair surprise to the prosecution. … [It] is also designed to protect the integrity of the evidence regarding an insanity defense."[1]

Just what is diminished capacity? Nearly every commentary on diminished capacity (or diminished responsibility) begins with a statement that the subject is confusing. Law Professor Stephen Morse aptly described diminished capacity as undiminished confusion.[2] Is diminished capacity simply a negation of an element of a crime—*mens rea* or volition—on which a defendant has a constitutional right to present trustworthy evidence, or is it a unique defense? Is it a defense fully covered by other concepts and, hence, ought to be exorcized for the sake of clarity, as Occam's razor would dictate?

Mental state is the principal device used to measure culpability. Diminished capacity addresses whether there was specific intent at the time of the crime. The insanity defense acts as a complete defense to criminal guilt, whereas diminished capacity acts as a partial defense. It means that the intent necessary for a cognate lesser defense, one that requires only a general intent, was present. The evidence of diminished capacity, though not quite meeting the standard for not guilty by reason of insanity (NGRI), may warrant a verdict of manslaughter instead of murder.[3]

In some jurisdictions, the defense of diminished capacity is available only when the defendant's mental impairment leaves him unable or incapable of forming the specific intent needed to commit the crime. In this vein, psychiatric testimony on *mens rea* must be couched in terms of the defendant's capacity to form a specific intent to commit the crime.[4] In legislation enacted in 1981, California provides that evidence of mental illness "shall not be admitted to show or negate the *capacity* to form any mental state," but is admissible solely on "the issue of whether or not the accused *actually formed* a required specific intent, premeditated, deliberated, or harbored malice aforethought, when a specific intent crime is charged" (emphasis added); it is called *diminished actuality*.[5] It is problematical how a forensic examiner without testifying on capacity can be of assistance to the jury in determining whether the accused actually formed a specific intent. Most formulations of the diminished capacity doctrine allow psychiatric testimony to show that the defendant either was not capable of premeditating or deliberating, or, in fact, did not premeditate or deliberate.[6]

There is another doctrine sometimes called "partial *mens rea*" or "diminished responsibility," which permits the fact finder to consider mitigating evidence of cognitive or volitional impairment that negates neither *mens rea* nor volition under the test of insanity. This variant is also sometimes called "diminished capacity," which causes confusion by giving the term another meaning.[7] In establishing partial *mens rea* or diminished responsibility, as we shall later discuss, the issue is raised whether impulsivity or situational stress may be a consideration.[8] It is often said that diminished responsibility might involve either cognitive or volitional impairment, whereas the diminished capacity doctrine concerns only cognitive impairment.

Following the 1981 legislation, the California Court of Appeals in 1990 said in *People v. Saille:*[9]

The special defense of diminished capacity, allowing the defendant to show he is less responsible for his actions, has been abolished. Our state has returned to the strict *mens rea* approach, only allowing the defendant to show that the requisite mental state was not actually formed due to a mental disorder, thus refuting the prosecution's proof of an element of the offense.[10]

Diminished capacity or diminished responsibility has also been used in sentencing, where individualized justice various factors are taken into consideration.[11] However, federal sentencing guidelines and mandatory minimum sentences adopted in recent years, and their counterparts in the various states, give a lesser role to the concepts of diminished capacity in the posttrial phase of a prosecution. The guidelines focus on the nature of the act, with less attention to the psychological makeup of the actor. The exercise of discretion in considering the actor's mental state or capacity now occurs mainly in the pretrial and trial stages of prosecution. As a result, those matters that used to be considered as factors in sentencing are not introduced in the trial stage in regard the elements of the crime (*mens rea* or *actus reus*).[12]

Years ago, as we have noted, the various states of the United States provided that a defendant wishing to offer evidence of insanity had to enter a special plea: not guilty by reason of insanity (NGRI). No longer would evidence of insanity be admissible under a not guilty plea. The special plea would avoid surprise and the need for a continuance to allow the prosecutor an opportunity to obtain an examination of the defendant. Similar concerns have arisen in diminished capacity cases. Evidence of diminished capacity does not call for a special plea; however, beginning in the 1970s, the courts began to rule that notice of the claim must be given to the prosecutor in advance of trial.[13] As in the case of a NGRI plea, a forensic examination of the accused is obtained, and the medical or psychotherapy testimonial privilege is waived allowing access to records.[14]

Also, as in the case of insanity, diminished capacity opens the door to evidence of the accused's criminal and employment record; in effect, the traditional rules of evidence are abandoned.[15] On the other hand, when a defense of self-defense or provocation is asserted, the door is not open to evidence of the defendant's history as those defenses are based on what is expected of a reasonable person. A claim of diminished capacity, however, does not result in an acquittal, but rather a conviction of a crime lesser than the charged offense, and unlike the case of NGRI, a claim of diminished capacity does not result in automatic commitment to a hospital.

Still different rules apply to a claim of intoxication (or use of drugs) at the time of the offense. In law, intoxication is not mental disorder or diminished capacity, hence, evidence of it (by lay or expert testimony) can be offered to negate specific intent under a not guilty plea without prior notice, and it calls for an instruction to that effect.[16] Therefore, evidence of intoxication, as it is not deemed a mental disorder, does not require a plea of NGRI.[17] Indeed, the California Supreme Court ruled that the legislature by virtue of its repeal in 1981 of the diminished capacity doctrine did not thereby eliminate the viability of a jury instruction regarding the effect of intoxication on the defendant's state of mind at the time of the offense.[18] The California Penal Code, like that of many other states, provides that evidence of voluntary intoxication is admissible "on the issue of whether or not the defendant actually formed a required specific intent, premeditated, deliberated, or harbored malice aforethought, when a specific intent crime is charged."[19] There is a split of authority as to whether intoxication can serve as a defense to rape, with some courts holding that because rape is a general intent crime, no amount of intoxication can negate the crime.[20] Intoxication is listed as a mitigating circumstance in the imposition of the death penalty.[21]

A defendant has a right to present any relevant evidence on *mens rea*, it being an essential or fundamental element of a crime. The question is, what type of evidence will be received, and under what banner (or concept) will the evidence be offered? Should the criminal law allow evidence of mental abnormality that does not establish legal insanity?

In *Fisher v. United States*,[22] the U.S. Supreme Court held that restricting mental disorder evidence to an insanity defense is constitutional. Subsequently, citing *Fisher*, the Seventh Circuit said, "A state is not constitutionally compelled to recognize the doctrine of diminished capacity" and, hence, when the defendant does not plead insanity, "a state may exclude expert testimony offered for the purpose of establishing that a criminal defendant lacked the capacity to form a specific intent."[23] Courts have recognized that some defendants, who are acquitted for lack of *mens rea* based on mental disorder, without pleading NGRI, cannot be released without endangering public safety.[24]

In recent years there has been considerable discussion on the interrelationship between automatism and insanity, with courts distinguishing between "sane" automatism and "insane" automatism. A claim of automatism asserts a loss of conscious control over one's bodily movements. Sane automatism may be deemed a complete or affirmative defense to a criminal charge, separate and apart from the defense of insanity.[25] Should psychiatric testimony on that or other type of mental condition be allowed only in the case of NGRI? Many jurisdictions so hold.[26] Somnambulism (sleepwalking) and epilepsy have been held to constitute mental illness, thus falling under the insanity defense.[27] An automatist defendant may be just as dangerous as an insane one, thus justifying treating certain automatist cases as cases of insanity.

The courts vacillate on what constitutes mental illness or mental defect, which in turn would call for a plea of NGRI in order to introduce evidence of it.[28] As we have noted, under the doctrine of diminished capacity, where recognized, psychiatric testimony relevant to *mens rea* may be admitted into evidence without an insanity plea, and at the same time, in order for a defendant to successfully present a diminished capacity defense, under the prevailing view of that defense, the judge or jury must find that the defendant was mentally ill.[29]

A number of state and lower federal courts have held that the doctrine of diminished capacity is constitutionally mandated, quoting the United States Supreme Court in another context, "[F]ew rights are more fundamental than that of an accused to present witnesses in his own defense."[30] Failure to raise a diminished capacity defense, where recognized, may constitute ineffective assistance of counsel calling for reversal of a conviction.[31] Moreover, under this view, a trial court's exclusion of diminished capacity evidence would be deemed a miscarriage of justice.[32]

In a dissent in *Fisher*, where the Supreme Court held that limiting mental disorder evidence to an insanity defense is constitutional, Justice Frank Murphy said, "There is no absolute or clear cut dichotomous division of the inhabitants of this world into the sane and the insane," and quoting Professor Henry Weihofen, said, "Between the two extremes of 'sanity' and 'insanity' lies every shade of disordered or deficient mental condition, grading imperceptibly one into another …" and he said, "More precisely, there are persons who, while not totally insane, possess such low mental powers as to be incapable of the deliberation and premeditation requisite to statutory first degree murder."[33]

The defense of diminished capacity relates only to the specific intent element of a crime; diminished capacity is not a defense to a general intent crime. Under the common law, courts developed a number of *mens rea* terms to describe various levels of culpability, such as willful and wanton, with a depraved heart, with malice aforethought, and with premeditation and deliberation. These various mental states have been subsumed under the traditional terminology of *specific intent* and *general intent*.[34] The late Dr. Karl Menninger, dean of American psychiatry and student of the criminal law, said that he did not understand any of these terms.[35] But, who does? They are more colorful than defining.

The American Law Institute's Model Penal Code sets out four levels of *mens rea*: purposeful, knowing, reckless, and negligent. It rejects the traditional terminology of *specific intent* and *general intent*. *Specific intent* refers to *purpose* and *knowledge* while *general intent* can be analogized to *recklessness* and *negligence*.[36] *Specific intent* is said to refer to an offender's subjective purpose or belief, while *general intent* is often determined by objective rather than subjective standards.[37]

Be that as it may, the categorization of mental states remains bewildering. The late Dr. Bernard Diamond, leader in forensic psychiatry, wrote, "The difference between general and specific intent can be very confusing and unclear with certain crimes despite the fact that most serious consequences to the defendant hinge upon the distinction."[38] As commonly defined, specific intent refers to a particular state of mind necessary to satisfy an element of an offense. For example, the intent necessary for first degree (premeditated) murder includes "a specific intent to kill." Without specific intent but with general intent, murder is reduced to manslaughter. Sometimes specific intent means an intent to do something beyond that which is done (e.g., assault with intent to commit rape). General intent is usually employed by the courts to explain criminal liability when a defendant did not intend to bring about a particular death. In sum and substance, whether a crime involves specific or general intent depends essentially on the definition of the crime.

Bank robbery, for example, is a general intent crime because Congress said so. Under legislation, Congress chose to distinguish between taking by force and violence (with no specific type of intent other than knowledge) and taking "with intent to steal."[39] In the first case, the manner of taking is that the wrong is being punished, whereas, in the latter example, the wrongful purpose is targeted. Congress apparently intended to cast a broader net for persons wielding guns and threatening people's lives than someone who would break into an ATM machine. On the other hand, there could be situations in which someone takes money by mistake, so it is important to go the extra step of proving the criminal intent with respect to larceny. Commenting on *United States v. Gonyea*,[40] a bank robbery case, Saul Green, then United States Attorney for the Eastern District of Michigan, observed:

> With bank robbery the evil intent is manifest by the act itself—threatening the lives of others. The effect of this in the law of diminished capacity has proven to be important. If someone wishes to put forth a mental defense to a general intent crime, such as bank robbery, they will have to do it by bearing the burden of establishing an insanity defense as required by 18 U.S.C. § 17. Mr. Gonyea unsuccessfully attempted to sidestep this evidentiary burden by using "diminished capacity" as a defense. Essentially the psychiatrist said Mr. Gonyea hated being poor and could not resist attempting to get rich by robbing banks, which apparently had something to do with him serving in Vietnam. In any event, in order to use diminished capacity as a defense it must negate *mens rea* (as distinguished from an insanity defense that excuses the crime). Thus, in the case of a general intent bank robbery, the defendant would have to establish that the act itself was somehow involuntary like a seizure—a virtually impossible burden.[41]

Apart from situations where the statute specifically spells out whether the crime is a specific or general intent crime, the distinction may be problematical. Federal District Court Judge

Avern Cohn says, "Simply put, my criterion for determining whether a crime is a general intent crime as opposed to a specific intent crime is akin to Justice Stewart's criteria for obscenity: 'I know it when I see it.'"[42] By interpreting the crime as one of general intent, the court closes the door on psychiatric testimony. In any event, as a practical matter, categories of intent avoid the all-or-nothing outcome of not guilty or guilty of the charged crime. It makes possible a range of verdicts and, hence, discretion in verdict and sentence. Without this flexibility, for example, the intoxicated individual could readily be absolved of any guilt.

Nowadays, as a result of rulings that a commitment of an insanity acquittee is to be based on the criteria of civil commitment, there is an increasing tendency to have several charges in mental-disordered offender cases, so that acquittal (by NGRI) on one charge and a verdict of guilty of another charge (not requiring specific intent) can result in imprisonment after release from the hospital.[43]

Another move to circumvent an NGRI verdict, or a verdict based on diminished capacity, has been the adoption by a number of states of a guilty but mentally ill verdict. Some call GBMI another form of diminished capacity as it gets away from the all-or-nothing approach of the insanity defense. Some call it a compromise verdict, and juries seem to consider it as such. Theoretically, it is supposed to provide psychiatric care, but, as a practical matter as noted in Chapter 11, the consequence is the same as a guilty verdict.

Diminished Responsibility

Some courts and commentators have expressed the concern that a rule premised on partial *mens rea* or diminished responsibility would open a wide door to unstructured psychiatric or other testimony in a broad array of cases, including situational stress or impulsivity. A parade of pathologies or impulsive behavior passes through the criminal courtrooms on any given day. Some jurisdictions restrict diminished capacity testimony to cognitive impairment as a result of mental illness, just as is done under the *M'Naghten* test of criminal responsibility, and excludes evidence on control, whatever the reason for the impairment.[44] Individuals who are manic are often severely impaired in their capacity to control behavior, while their cognitive impairment is less striking.[45] (Following the *Hinckley* trial, the federal government and a number of states joined those that exclude a volitional prong from the test of criminal responsibility.)

Always testifying for the defense, Dr. Bernard Diamond believed that something could always be said on behalf of the defendant.[46] Indeed, from a psychodynamic point of view, absolutely everything that one does is in the service of reparation, in order to achieve homeostasis. When Thomas McIlvane, a fired letter carrier, exploded with gunfire at the post office in Royal Oak, Michigan, a psychologist said, "I'm not trying to dismiss or discount what he's done, but people don't do things like that because they want to. It's because they don't think they have any other choice."

A person thrown into disequilibrium must do something to reestablish that vital balance or, as it is sometimes expressed, "to stay on one's rocker."[47] In that sense, all thinking and behavior can be explained psychologically as a form of self-defense. Indeed, the adjustive techniques used by the mind are called defense mechanisms.[48] And, so, it is said that the victim is "the cornerstone of the offender's psychic economy."[49] The theme of the film *Juice* is that teenagers on the street can become men and get respect only through committing crime. Thus, the battle of the experts is really a battle over the merit of an excusing condition.[50]

In a memoriam to Dr. Bernard Diamond, Professor Jerome Skolnick of the University of California Law School, had this to say:

> Bernard [Diamond] … perceived the all-or-nothing conceptualization of the insanity defense as central to the difficulties of introducing psychiatric knowledge into the law. At

the same time, he perceived a key to resolving these difficulties in the ancient doctrine of *mens rea*. ... [He] forged the idea of diminished responsibility of the mentally ill—which came in law to be called the doctrine of diminished capacity—out of the implications of a criminal law system that embraces the notion of moral blameworthiness in its determination of guilt. The idea of diminished responsibility can perhaps best be stated as a question: If it is proper to find a psychotic murderer not guilty by reason of insanity, that is, to excuse him entirely from moral blameworthiness because of his mental disorder, isn't it equally appropriate to diminish his criminal liability if he is not psychotic, but nevertheless suffers from a lesser mental disease or defect?

Bernard Diamond would have answered that question with a ringing affirmative. He argued that there were innumerable degrees of *mens rea*. And if there were, an "infinitely graduated" spectrum of legal responsibility was implied—corresponding to our contemporary understanding of the psychological reality of human beings.

[F]or all his accomplishments, he will best be remembered for his work in psychiatry and the law, particularly for his development of the diminished capacity defense. Not only was Bernard the principal architect of the diminished capacity defense, but he was also its chief exponent in the courtroom... .

Largely because of Bernard's courtroom victories and scholarly writings, there was a sharp increase in the use of psychiatric testimony in murder trials in California during the 1960s. Eventually, however, such defenses began to fall out of favor. In part, one can point to a rise in crime from the mid-sixties, which led to increasing punitiveness on the part of the sentencing system. It moved from indeterminate sentencing stressing rehabilitation to a determinate system emphasizing punishment as its goal. Since the practical result of diminished capacity was to reduce the penalty for murder, the public began to look askance at that defense.[51]

The legislation enacted in 1981 in California was designed specifically to nullify the judicial developments advocated by Dr. Diamond.[52] The legislation also enacted, however, a provision permitting evidence of mental disease or defect if it is offered to show the absence of specific intent.[53] Professor Moore won over Dr. Diamond.

Over and over the question continues to arise: Must diminished capacity be linked to a mental disease or defect? Is the mental disease or defect predicate in the insanity context applicable or necessary to diminished capacity? Is a diminished capacity argument foreclosed when there is no mental disease or defect analogous to that required for the insanity defense? Dr. Diamond opened his essay, "Social and Cultural Factors as a Diminished Capacity Defense in Criminal Law," with challenging observations of such questions:

Mental illness, as a defense in criminal law, has traditionally been closely linked to the medical model of psychological deviance. Without exception, every definition of criminal insanity starts with or includes the phrase "mental disease or defect." Although not every degree or kind of mental disease or defect is exculpating, a psychiatric diagnosis of some type is a necessary, if not sufficient, requirement for such a defense in the criminal trial. Social and cultural factors may be relevant evidence, but only insofar as they are material as causation or provocation of the psychiatric condition. The logic of such a restriction is not as clear as formerly when the medical model of mental illness was accepted unquestionably.[54]

Accepting the historical reality of the close association of the insanity defense with the medical model of deviance, should the same hold for the diminished capacity or diminished responsibility defense? The question of whether cultural difference may be taken into account as diminished capacity or diminished responsibility has arisen in a number of cases involving recent immigrants to the United States. One wonders how much the United States will bend its rules to accommodate the new wave of immigrants. In a multicultured society, there is increased demand to explain why people do what they do.[55] To this end, could an anthropologist be used as an expert witness to provide the court with a cultural context for making a determination about the defendant's state of mind?

This issue was raised in *People v. Poddar*.[56] In this case, Prosenjt Poddar, an "untouchable" from India, was charged with the murder of Tanya Tarasoff, who he felt, rejected him. In the much publicized tort case, *Tarasoff v. Regents of the University of California*,[57] Tanya's parents sued the university claiming that the therapist who had treated Poddar was negligent in failing to avert the homicide. In the criminal case, the defense counsel offered the testimony of an anthropologist who had lived more than 20 years in India and who had studied adjustment difficulties of Indian students who had come to American universities. According to the offer of proof, the expert would testify to cultural stresses, which affected the adjustment of the defendant in shifting from the simple culture in which he had lived to the sophisticated milieu of an American university. More particularly, the expert would testify that the cultural strain for Indians becomes acute in relationships between men and women because the normal marriage in India is arranged for the parties. Altogether, the anthropological testimony would give evidence of diminished capacity.

The trial judge ruled that the witness was not qualified to testify on the direct consequences of cultural stresses on the defendant, but the judge offered to allow the witness to testify to facts relevant to cross-cultural difficulties, and then to allow counsel to ask hypothetical questions of psychiatric experts using factual data supplied by the anthropologist. The defense counsel declined, stating that he wished to use the anthropologist as an independent expert witness on the issue of diminished capacity, so that the jury could draw inferences from this testimony itself and not as filtered through the testimony of psychiatrists. The Court of Appeals held that the evidence was properly excluded in the form in which it was offered.[58]

A ruling more restrictive than that in *Poddar* occurred in *Chase v. United States*,[59] where a plea of NGRI was entered. The court completely barred an anthropologist from testifying, on the ground that the proffered testimony was not evidence of insanity (and as to insanity the witness would not likely have qualified as an expert).[60] On the other hand, in a New York case involving Dong Lu Chen, a Chinese man who beat his wife to death with a hammer after she admitted to an affair, a city judge gave him 5 years probation for manslaughter after a cultural anthropologist testified that traditional Chinese values regarding adultery and loss of manhood made him violent.[61]

What should happen, Law Professor Dorian Coleman asks, in a case against a defendant accused of performing a circumcision on a girl by mutilating her genitals, a custom prevalent in some countries, but abhorred by Americans. "Do we want to say that we want to be so sensitive to essentially create a new criminal code?" she said. "Are we treating little girls from Africa differently than we're treating little girls from the United States? We could someday see Balkanization of the criminal justice system, and we really have to ask whether we should go there."[62]

Not only foreign cultures, but subcultures within the United States as well have been said to influence a criminal defendant's state of mind. People are "brainwashed" by the environment in which they live. Quoting Victor Hugo, Martin Luther King, Jr. said, "If a soul is left in darkness, sins will be committed. The guilty one is not he who commits the sin, but he who causes the darkness." The author Phyllis Chesler depicts Aileen Wournos, the killer of seven men in what were known as the I-75 slayings, as a victim of her own life of prostitution and years of abuse.[63]

The subculture of poverty or the ghetto defense has been the prototype for this kind of argument.[64] In these cases, the jury is aware of the cultural or social background of the accused. The issue in the cases is the instruction to the jury. The best known case is the 1972 decision from the

District of Columbia, *United States v. Alexander & Murdock*.[65] In this case, Gordon Alexander and Benjamin Murdock, both black males, in a hamburger restaurant exchanged glares with a group of five white male Marine lieutenants and a woman. Alexander verbally challenged the Marines, one of who responded with a racial epithet. Alexander and Murdock then drew guns and began shooting, killing two Marines and wounding another Marine and the woman. Alexander was found guilty of assault with a dangerous weapon. Murdock raised the insanity defense and was somewhat successful; he was convicted of second-degree murder rather than first-degree murder as charged.

On appeal Murdock claimed that the instructions given by the trial judge unfairly prejudiced his claim to an NGRI verdict. The instructions included the statement: "We are not concerned with a question of whether or not a man had a rotten social background. We are concerned with the question of his criminal responsibility. That is to say, whether he had an abnormal condition of the mind that affected his emotional and behavioral processes at the time of the offense." The appellate court found no error in that ruling, relying primarily on its prior decisions where it had rejected the doctrine of diminished responsibility in seemingly broad terms. The opinion provoked a lengthy dissent by Judge David Bazelon, which has been the subject of extensive commentary.[66]

Were Alexander and Murdock like actors on a stage with their roles set out for them? Should society, the media, or the gun manufacturer share or take the blame? In the never-ending discussion of free will and criminal responsibility, many answer affirmatively. In yet another opinion in the Murdock case, Judge Carl McGowan commented:

> The tragic and senseless events giving rise to these appeals are a recurring by-product of a society, which, unable as yet to eliminate explosive racial tensions, appears equally paralyzed to deny easy access to guns. Cultural infantilism of this kind inevitably exacts a high price, which in this instance was paid by the two young officers who were killed. The ultimate responsibility for their deaths reaches far beyond these appellants.
>
> As courts, however, we administer a system of justice, which is limited in its reach. We deal only with those formally accused under laws, which define criminal accountability narrowly. Our function on these appeals is to determine whether appellants had a fair opportunity to defend themselves, and were tried and sentenced according to law.[67]

On the same day of the decision in *United States v. Alexander & Murdock*,[68] the same court heard arguments in the case of *United States v. Brawner*. In a decision issued some 10 weeks later, Judge Leventhal wrote in the course of a lengthy and scholarly opinion:

> [T]he latitude for salient evidence of, e.g., social and cultural factors pertinent to an abnormal condition of the mind significantly affecting capacity and controls, does not mean that such factors may be taken as establishing a separate defense for persons whose mental condition is such that blame can be imposed. We have rejected a broad "injustice" approach that would have opened the door to expositions of, e.g., cultural deprivation, unrelated to any abnormal condition of the mind. ... Determinists contend that every man's fate is ultimately sealed by his genes and environment, over which he has no control. Our jurisprudence, however, while not oblivious to deterministic components, ultimately rests on a premise of freedom of will. This is not to be viewed as an exercise in philosophic discourse, but as a governmental fusion of ethics and necessity, which takes into account that a system of rewards and punishments is itself part of the environment that influences and shapes human conduct. Our recognition of an insanity defense for those who lack the essential, threshold free will possessed by those in the normal range is not to be twisted, directly or indirectly, into a device for exculpation of those without an abnormal condition of the mind.

Finally, we have not accepted suggestions to adopt a rule that disentangles the insanity defense from a medical model, and announces a standard exculpating anyone whose capacity for control is insubstantial, for whatever cause or reason. There may be logic in these submissions, but we are not sufficiently certain of the nature, range, and implications of the conduct involved to attempt an all-embracing unified field theory. The applicable rule can be discerned as the cases arise in regard to other conditions—somnambulism or other automatisms; blackouts due, e.g., to overdose of insulin; drug addiction. Whether these somatic conditions should be governed by a rule comparable to that herein set forth for mental disease would require, at a minimum, judicial determination, which takes medical opinion into account, finding convincing evidence of an ascertainable condition characterized by "a broad consensus that free will does not exist."[69]

Judge Bazelon, concurring in part and dissenting in part, said: "Perhaps the decision rests on an unstated assumption that change is futile because we lack enough information about human behavior to make possible a meaningful use of the defense, or because we are unwilling or unable to act upon the information that is already at hand."[70] He suggested that a "rotten social background" excuse would spur society to provide effective assistance to the poor. He puts in doubt society's right to punish offenders.

Over a half-century ago, in 1946, a like issue was before the United States Supreme Court in *Fisher v. United States*,[71] where the Court held it constitutional to limit mental disorder evidence to an insanity defense. Fisher, a black janitor in a library in Washington, D.C., killed the librarian, Catherine Reardon, who had complained to supervisors about his care of the premises. According to Fisher's account, one morning when they were alone in the library, Reardon scolded him and called him a "black nigger," whereupon he became angry and struck her. When she ran away screaming, Fisher grabbed a piece of wood, ran after her, struck her on the head with it, then seized her by the throat and choked her until she was silent. A few minutes later, she screamed again and he stuck her in the throat with his pocketknife, killing her.

The defense tried to show that the killing was not deliberate and premeditated, and was, therefore, at worst, only second-degree murder. Although evidence of Fisher's "aggressive psychopathic tendencies, low emotional response and borderline mental deficiency" was introduced, the trial court declined to instruct the jury that they could consider the personality of the defendant in determining whether he was guilty of murder in the first or second degree. Under instructions defining accepted tests of insanity, malice, deliberation, and premeditation, the jury found him guilty of murder with deliberate and premeditated malice. The D.C. Court of Appeals affirmed, saying:

> Modern psychiatry has given us much scientific information which disturbs the former certainty of our judgments of individual responsibility and moral guilt. It has revolutionized the methods of treatment and rehabilitation of prisoners. But the principal place for the application of such a therapeutic point of view where the court exercises discretion in the amount of the sentence and in the treatment of criminals is in our penal institutions. In the determination of guilt age old conceptions of individual moral responsibility cannot be abandoned without creating a laxity of enforcement that undermines the whole administration of criminal law.[72]

The Supreme Court granted *certiorari*. The sole error urged by the petitioner was the trial judge's refusal of an instruction permitting the jury to weigh evidence of mental deficiencies—admittedly short of complete insanity under accepted tests—in determining whether the accused was able to, and did, premeditate and deliberate. In a 5–3 decision, the Supreme Court upheld the trial judge's refusal to give the requested instruction. The Court recognized that "[t]he jury might not have reached the result it did if the theory of partial responsibility for his acts that the petitioner urges had been submitted."[73] But under the case law of the District of Columbia,[74] the Court found that the accused was not entitled to an instruction on this theory, and declined to force the District of Columbia to adopt it.[75]

In *Commonwealth v. Terry*,[76] Benjamin Terry, a prison inmate, killed a prison guard with a baseball bat he had hidden in his trousers, when he was returning to the cellblock from the prison yard and the guard gave him a slight push. This contact allegedly reminded him of a prior altercation with the guard. At trial, the defense argued that Terry should be convicted only of second degree murder, not premeditated, first degree murder. A psychologist testified that Terry suffered from a "dyssocial personality with paranoid hysterical and explosive features and organic syndrome with epileptic seizures." The psychologist also testified:

> It's my opinion that the resentment and rage that he felt brought him to the point where he did make a decision and that decision was that he would protect himself and not let himself be beaten again. So that he decided to protect himself, and if somebody hurt him, he would hurt them.
>
> However, what I believe happened at that moment, then, within that context, is that when the guard grabbed him, he went into a rage; it was immediate, it was reactive, it was based on an emotional response. He didn't stop and deliberate and think and form the intent. He reacted.[77]

The Pennsylvania Supreme Court, upholding Terry's conviction and death sentence, found this testimony irrelevant to the diminished capacity issue because it "directly advances impulsive rage as negating premeditation." According to past case law in Pennsylvania, "only 'mental disorders affecting cognitive functions necessary to form specific intent' are admissible."[78]

Those who put forward a psychosocial portrait have emphasized that extraneous social factors are as much the cause of crime as any evil and harmful desires on the part of the offender.[79] Dr. Ezra Griffith, an African-American psychiatrist at the Yale University Department of Psychiatry and a past president of the American Academy of Psychiatry and Law, says that African-American forensic psychiatrists are likely to be troubled by an ethics framework that ignores the special struggles linked to the matter of race.[80] The existential situation leads to an excuse or rationalization, however, with the result of much crime and little punishment.[81]

In his presidential address to the American Psychiatric Association, Dr. Alan Stone confessed that he has felt so guilty over his testimony in a military trial that he vowed never to testify again; and he asserts that forensic psychiatry has no clear boundaries and that forensic psychiatrists are without any clear guidelines as to what is proper and ethical (he teaches the course in psychiatry and law at Harvard). A black sergeant, facing court-martial for stealing government property, was sent to Stone, then an army psychiatrist, to determine whether his behavior had been driven by kleptomania or any other mental disorder that should excuse him from responsibility, and so testified. A sentence of 5 years at hard labor was imposed. In the course of evaluation, Stone made the discovery that the roots of the sergeant's crime lay not in kleptomania, but in his bitterness over the fate of a black man in a discriminatory society. In Stone's words, "[H]e stole with a sense of entitlement and reparation in protest of the racist world that had deprived him of his hopes." Though testimony about the social origins of the sergeant's actions would not have been exculpatory as a matter of law, Stone is of the opinion that it might have induced leniency in sentencing, and blames himself for omitting it.[82]

The trend away from recognition or acceptance of a diminished capacity defense as suggested by Diamond suggests that the doctrine may be a dying concept. Not quite. In the pretrial stage, the diminished capacity concept (whether or not called that) influences prosecutorial discretion and, thus, plays a role in the charge brought against the defendant. At trial, the defense is infrequently used. It is important more for its symbolism that for its numbers.[83] It is like the insanity defense, always a last ditch argument. It involves evidence of mental disorder, and defense counsel can never be sure whether the evidence will work against or in favor of the accused.

What of the future? Will excuses for behavior have greater or lesser appeal? Will there be an increase in jury nullification (as occurs frequently in the District of Columbia where juries decline to convict in drug-related offenses) or will it decline? The rise in crime prompted the abandonment of Diamond's opening the door to psychiatric testimony. When crime is escalating, there is less interest and less focus on the psychodynamics underlying the behavior of the accused.

Endnotes

1. People v. Wallace, 408 N.W. 2d 87, 89 (Mich. App. 1987).
2. S. Morse, "Undiminished Confusion in Diminished Capacity," *J. Crim. L. & Criminol.* 75 (1984): 1.
3. Experiments have shown the power of situations to influence people's behavior, sometimes even overriding individual personality traits and the dictates of personal conscience. The popular TV show *Survivor* demonstrates the power of circumstances to determine behavior. See E. Goode, "Hey, What if Contestants Give Each Other Shocks?" *New York Times*, August 27, 2000, p. WK3.
4. Once the defendant introduces evidence of diminished capacity, the prosecution must produce evidence that the defendant did not suffer from diminished capacity. People v. Jones, 151 Mich. App. 1, 390 N.W.2d 189 (1986); People v. Denton, 138 Mich. App. 568, 360 N.W.2d 245 (1984); see Michigan Jury Instruction 6.3.
5. For example, in United States v. Bright, 517 F.2d 584 (2d Cir. 1975), the court said that diminished capacity testimony should address *only* the capacity of the defendant to harbor the required mental state, not whether the defendant actually had that mental state.
6. California Penal Code sec. 28(a). See C.R. Clark, "Specific Intent and Diminished Aapacity," in I.B. Weiner & A.K. Hess (Eds.), *Handbook of Forensic Psychology* (New York: John Wiley & Sons, 3rd ed., 2006), pp. 364–391.
7. American Law Institute Model Penal Code § 4.01 (1); see State v. Talbebet, 590 N.W.2d 732 (Iowa App. 1999).
8. See P. Arenella, "The Diminished Capacity and Diminished Responsibility Defenses: Two Children of a Doomed Marriage," *Colum. L. Rev.* 77 (1977): 827. Chief Judge Breitel of the New York Court of Appeals, in People v. Patterson, 39 N.Y.2d 288, 347 N.E.2d 898 (1976), saw as a mark of an advanced criminology "[the enlarging of] the ameliorative defenses based on the nature of the offender and the conditions, which produce some degree of excuse for his conduct."
9. 270 Cal. Rptr. 502, 508, 221 Cal. App.3d 280 (1990).
10. The California Supreme Court affirmed in a much awaited decision, People v. Saille, 54 Cal.3d 1103 (1991). *Saille* was the lead case in a group of cases coming before the California Supreme Court relating to the effect of mental disease, defect, disorder, or voluntary intoxication on the formation of malice aforethought.
11. In England a henpecked husband who battered his wife to death with a hammer was sentenced to only 6 years' imprisonment after a judge told him that the dead woman's behavior "was calculated to impact on your mind." M. Weaver, "Six Years for Man Who Killed Nagging Wife," *Weekly Telegraph*, No. 432 (Nov. 1999), p. 6.
12. P.S. Bamberger (Ed.), *Practice Under the New Federal Sentencing Guidelines* (Englewood Cliffs, NJ: Prentice Hall, 2 vols., 2nd. ed., 1992 supp.). The American Bar Association's Criminal Justice Mental Health Standards recommend that in all cases "[e]vidence of mental illness or mental retardation should be considered as a possible mitigating factor in sentencing a convicted offender." American Bar Association, *Standards for Criminal Justice* 7-9.3 (1984 supp.). In capital cases, the Supreme Court has held that mental condition cannot be excluded from consideration as a mitigating circumstance. Eddings v. Oklahoma, 455 U.S. 104, 116 (1982). However, as a practical matter, evidence of mental illness, while intended to be a mitigating circumstance, is often taken by juries as aggravating.
13. People v. Mangiapane, 85 Mich. App. 379 (1978).
14. M.E. Phelan, "The Pitfalls of Preventing a Diminished Capacity Defense," *Crim. Just.* 5 (1990): 8.
15. "Where insanity is relied upon as a defense, every act of the accused's life, which throws some light on such issues is relevant thereto. ... The issue of insanity gives much latitude, both to the defendant and the State, for the introduction of evidence of defendant's acts, declarations and conduct, prior

and subsequent to the alleged crime, subject to the limitation that the acts, declarations and conduct inquired about must have a tendency to shed light on the accused's state of mind when the act for which he is being tried was committed." Nichols v. State, 276 Ala. 209, 160 So.2d 6619, 621 (1964).

16. In People v. Guillet, 342 Mich. 1, 69 N.W.2d 140 (Mich. 1955), the defendant accompanied a woman to a tavern where they drank, then they went to his house, where they continued to drink. He made indecent advances, which she repulsed, only to be knocked down by the defendant, who continued in the words of the Michigan Supreme Court, "his attempt to commit rape." The jury convicted the defendant of assault with intent to rape. The Michigan Supreme Court reversed the conviction because the judge had failed to tell the jury that intoxication is a defense to a specific intent crime—here, assault *with intent* to rape.

17. In Hope v. Utah, 104 U.S. 631 (1881), the U.S. Supreme Court, after stating the familiar rule that voluntary intoxication is no excuse for crime, said: "[W]hen a statute establishing different degrees of murder requires deliberate premeditation in order to constitute murder in the first degree, the question of whether the accused is in such a condition of mind, by reason of drunkenness or otherwise, as to be capable of deliberate premeditation, necessarily becomes a material subject of consideration by the jury"; 104 U.S. at 634.

18. People v. Ramirez, 50 Cal.3d 1158, 280 Cal. Rptr. 286, 791 P.2d 965 (1990); *In re* Cordero, 46 Cal.3d 161, 259 Cal. Rptr. 342, 756 P.2d 1370 (1988).

19. Calif. Penal Code § 22(b).

20. For example, Walden v. S., 178 Tenn. 71, 156 S.W.2d 385 (1941); but see S. v. Evenson, 237 Iowa 1214, 24 N.W.2d 762 (1946).

21. State v. Reeves, 476 N.W.2d 829 (Neb. 1991).

22. 328 U.S. 463 (1946).

23. Meunch v. Israel, 715 F.2d 1124 at 1144–1145 (7th Cir. 1983. See H.M. Huckabee, "Evidence of Mental Disorder on *Mens Rea*: Constitutionality of Drawing the Line at the Insanity Defense," *Pepperdine L. Rev.* 16 (1989): 573.

24. In State v. Wilcox, 70 Ohio St.2d 182, 436 N.E.2d 523 (1982), the Ohio Supreme Court noted: "The principal effect of the diminished capacity defense is to enable mentally ill offenders to receive shorter and more certain sentences than they would receive if they were adjudged insane. Having satisfied ourselves that Ohio's test for criminal responsibility adequately safeguards the rights of the insane, we are disinclined to adopt an alternative defense that could swallow up the insanity defense and its attendant commitment provisions"; 70 Ohio St.2d at 186.

25. In State v. Cadell, 278 N.C. 266, 215 S.E.2d 348 (1975), Chief Justice Sharp, concurring in result and dissenting in part, wrote, at 215 S.E.2d at 366–367:

> [I]f a person is actually unconscious when he does an act, which would otherwise be criminal, the absence of consciousness not only excludes the existence of any specific mental state, but also excludes the possibility of a voluntary act without which there can be no criminal liability. Unconsciousness, therefore, can never be an affirmative defense, which imposes the burden of proof upon the defendant, because the State has the burden of proving the essential elements of the offense charged, and "a voluntary act is an absolute requirement for criminal liability"; Lafave and Scott, Criminal Law 181 (1972). Although the defense of unconsciousness "is sometimes explained on the ground that such a person could not have the requisite mental state for commission of the crime, the better rationale is that the individual has not engaged in a voluntary act."

In discussing the relationship between the defenses of automatism and insanity, Justice Sharp noted that the defendant acquitted by reason of insanity could be detained in a hospital where he was not a continuing danger to the public, whereas one acquitted on the ground of unconsciousness would be unconditionally released. He noted the judicial tendency to characterize instances in which the condition of unconsciousness is likely to recur as insanity rather than automatism so that the defendant may be committed; 215 S.E.2d at 369. See B. McSherry, "Getting Away With Murder? Dissociative States and Criminal Responsibility," *Intl. J. Law & Psychiat.* 21 (1998): 163.

26. Apparently 14 states and the District of Columbia take this position: Arizona, Delaware, Florida, Georgia, Indiana, Louisiana, Maryland, Minnesota, North Carolina, Ohio, Oklahoma, Virginia, Wisconsin, and Wyoming. In Johnson v. State, 292 Md. 405, 439 A.2d 542 (1982), the Maryland Court of Appeals explained:

[T]he introduction of expert psychiatric testimony concerning the defendant's mental aberrations when the basic sanity of the accused is not at issue conflicts with the governing principle of the criminal law that all legally sane individuals are equally capable of forming and possessing the same types and degrees of intent. Consequently, an individual determined to be "sane" within the traditional constructs of the criminal law is held accountable for his action, regardless of his particular disabilities, weaknesses, poverty, religious beliefs, social deprivation or educational background. The most that it is proper to do with such information is to weigh it during sentencing. ... [B]ecause the legislature, reflecting community morals, has, by its definition of criminal insanity already determined which states of mental disorder ought to relieve one from criminal responsibility, this court is without authority to impose our views in this regard even if they differed.

See H.M. Huckabee, "Avoiding the Insanity Defense Strait Jacket: The *Mens Rea* Route," *Pepperdine L. Rev.* 15 (1987): 1.

27. Tibbs v. C., 128 S.W. 871 (Ky. 1910; somnambulism); P. v. Higgins, 186 N.Y.S.2d 623, 5 N.Y.2d 607, 159 N.E.2d 179 (1959 epilepsy).

28. Query: What about a claim that a sexual advance triggered a violent "homosexual panic"? Provocation may not be claimed as a defense as the behavior is not deemed reasonable. In using provocation as a defense, the personal history of the defendant is not allowed in assessing whether his response was "reasonable." Does homosexual panic constitute "mental illness" calling for a plea of NGRI that would allow evidence of it? Does it constitute diminished capacity? The answer is debatable. See the discussion in Chapter 17 on homosexuality.

Query: What about multiple personality (also known as dissociative identity disorder)? Sidney Sheldon's novel *Tell Me Your Dreams* (New York: Morrow, 1998) is about a multiple personality charged with committing a series of brutal murders. Sheldon claims that 1% of the population suffers from multiple personality disorder and that up to 20% of all patients in psychiatric hospitals have it (p. 15). In State v. Moore, 113 N.J. 239, 550 A.2d 117 (1988), where the defendant was charged with murder and entered a plea of NGRI, the New Jersey Supreme Court ruled that evidence of multiple personality disorder obliged the trial judge to instruct the jury that it may return a verdict of manslaughter. The appellate court ruled failure to charge diminished capacity was reversible error despite the fact that defendant did not request such an instruction. The court said: "In the instant case, where defendant did, in fact, present an insanity defense, the record persuades us that sufficient competent evidence was adduced at trial to support a charge of diminished capacity. As part of her insanity defense, defendant offered evidence that would permit a jury to decide whether she suffered from a condition that diminished her capacity to form the knowing or purposeful mental state required to convict her of murder."

Query: What about "battered spouse"? Originally, in cases of women accused of murdering their spouses or boyfriends who had abused them, the plea was NGRI. The "battered spouse syndrome" was regarded analogous to a posttraumatic stress disorder, but feminists soon regarded NGRI as a stigma and it resulted in commitment, so the defense shifted to self-defense. Expert testimony is allowed to explain the lower threshold of self-defense as a result of the abuse. State v. Kelly, 97 N.J. 1788, 478 A.2d (1984); see A.M. Coughlin, "Excusing Women," *Cal. L. Rev.* 82 (1994): 1; V.M. Mather, "The Skeleton in the Closet: The Battered Woman Syndrome, Self-Defense, and Expert Testimony," *Mercer L. Rev.* 39 (1988): 545: England's Treason Act of 1351 made it a crime of petty treason for a wife to kill her husband because he was her sovereign lord.

See R. Slovenko, *Psychiatry and Criminal Culpability* (New York: John Wiley & Sons, 1995), pp. 67–117.

29. "Mental illness" in diminished capacity may be simply "mental disturbance." See People v. Pickens, 446 Mich. 298, 521 N.W.2d 797 (1994).

30. Hughes v. Mathews, 576 F.2d 1250 (7th Cir. 1978), quoting Chambers v. Mississippi, 410 U.S. 284 (1973). However, in Muench v. Israel, 715 F.2d 1124 (7th Cir. 1983), the Seventh Circuit rejected a *habeas corpus* petition based on similar facts, stating: [I]n Hughes we were not seeking to constitutionalize the law of evidence nor to impose a diminished responsibility doctrine on Wisconsin. ... A theory that the Supreme Court has twice refused to impose upon the state of California, albeit in summary decisions, ... is not one that this lower federal court will impose on the state of Wisconsin as a matter of federal constitutional due process." In Commonwealth v. Walczack, 468 Pa. 210, 360 A.2d 914, 920 (1976), the Pennsylvania Supreme Court held that, under the Pennsylvania constitution, due

process requires the admission of psychiatric testimony that is relevant to *mens rea*. The court stated: "It is inconsistent with fundamental principles of American jurisprudence to preclude an accused from offering relevant and competent evidence to dispute the charge against him."

In Commonwealth v. McCusker, 448 Pa. 382, 292 A.2d 286 (1972), a murder prosecution where the defendant did not plead NGRI, the Pennsylvania Supreme Court in a change of its law allowed psychiatric evidence for the purpose of determining whether the defendant acted in the heat of passion. The court said, "Upon reflection and further consideration, we now conclude that psychiatric evidence, coming as it does from a 'recognized and important branch of modern medicine,' should be admissible at trial for the purpose of determining whether a defendant acted in the heat of passion"; 292 A.2d at 289.

In coming to the same conclusion, the American Law Institute's Model Penal Code, sec. 4.02(1), provides: "Evidence that the defendant suffered from a mental disease or defect is admissible whenever it is relevant to prove that the defendant did not have a state of mind that is an element of the crime." In comments to the provision, the drafters stated: "If state of mind such as deliberation or premeditation [is] accorded legal significance, psychiatric evidence should be admissible when relevant to prove or disprove their existence to the same extent as any other evidence"; Comments to sec. 4.02, 193 (Tent. Draft No. 4, 1955).

More recently, finding that "logical relevance" so requires and "is probably constitutionally required," the American Bar Association has recommended a similar rule. Project of the American Bar Association (1986, 1989), Standard 7-6.2. The commentary states that expert testimony on mental condition "should be admissible on a *mens rea* issue even if a defendant has not pleaded a specific mental nonresponsibility [insanity] defense, as long as it is relevant to a determination of guilt, innocence, or level of culpability." ABA Standard Committee on Association Standards for Criminal Justice, *Criminal Justice Mental Health Standards*, ABA standards for Criminal Justice 2:121 (2nd ed., Ch. 7, supp. 1986).

31. Commonwealth v. Legg, 711 A.2d 430 (Pa. 1998). In this case the defendant, shortly before she killed her husband, had been hospitalized for depression and suicidal and homicidal tendencies. See also People v. Lloyd, 590 N.W.2d 738 (Mich. 1999); State v. Thomas, 590 N.W.2d 755 (Minn. 1999).

32. In People v. Henderson, 60 Cal.2d 432, 35 Cal. Rptr. 77, 386 P.2d (1963), the defendant testified that he had no intention to kill the deceased and that the act was done while he was in a dream-like state. Two psychiatrists testified in corroboration of this explanation of the killing. The California Supreme Court held that the trial court erred in failing to give any instruction that would tell the jury for what purpose they could consider the evidence of that defense.

33. Fisher v. United States, 328 U.S. at 482, quoting H. Weihofen, "Partial Insanity and Criminal Intent," *Ill. L. Rev.* 24 (1930): 505 at 508.

34. The term *malice* in law does not mean evil, enmity, anger, hatred, or the like; it is a term of art. John Hinckley apparently had nothing personally against President Reagan, but would be said to have acted with malice in shooting the President. The California legislation of 1981 provides that malice includes no mental element other than an intent to kill; Calif. Penal Code Sec. 188. Under Maine's statute, malice is implied from "any deliberate, cruel act committed by one person against another suddenly or without a considerable provocation"; Mullaney v. Wilbur, 421 U.S. 684 (1975).

35. Personal communication.

36. See G.B. Melton, J. Petrila, N.G. Poythress, & C. Slobogin, *Psychological Evaluations for the Courts* (New York: Guilford Press, 3rd ed., 2007).

37. Evidence concerning subjective mental state would not be logically relevant in cases involving general intent crimes because culpability will turn not on what a defendant actually perceived, believed, or intended, but on what an ordinary person in the same situation would or should have perceived, believed, or intended. In the great majority of cases, however, evidence concerning a defendant's abnormal mental condition as it relates to *mens rea* will, if believed, reduce the grade of the offense.

38. B.J. Diamond, "Social and Cultural Factors and a Diminished Capacity Defense in Criminal Law," *Bull. Amer. Acad. Psychiat. & Law* 6 (1978): 199.

39. The statutory scheme is set out in 18 U.S.C. § 2113.

40. 140 F.3d 649 (6th Cir. 1998).

41. Personal communication (Sept. 28,1998).

42. Personal communication (March 16, 1999). Justice Stewart's comment appears in Jacobellis v. Ohio, 378 U.S. 184, 197 (1964). See E. Jaeger, "Obscenity and the Reasonable Person: Will He 'Know It When He Sees It?'" *Boston Coll. L. Rev.* 30 (1989): 823.

43. In People v. Massip, 229 Cal. App.3d 1400 (1990), the defendant claimed that she was suffering from depression—commonly known as "baby blues"—that caused her to commit the crime. She claimed that she had heard voices telling her that her child was in pain and to put him out of his misery. She then placed the child under a tire, drove over him and put the body in a trash can. At the trial, she pleaded not guilty by reason of insanity, but a jury found her sane and convicted her of second-degree murder. She then asked for a retrial, but in a ruling that surprised attorneys on both sides, the trial judge reduced the verdict to voluntary manslaughter and also found the defendant not guilty by reason of insanity. See R.D. Miller, J. Olin, E.M. Ball, D.S. Johnson, J.B. Reynolds, & J. Covey, "Dual Commitments to Forensic Hospitals and Prisons: Rational Disposition or Political Compromise?" *J. Psychiat. & Law* 27 (1999): 157.

44. United States v. Pohlot, 827 F.2d 889 (3d Cir. 1987); Commonwealth v. Terry, 513 Pa. 381, 521 A.2d 398 (1987).

45. It has been suggested that the court inquiry apply current scientific knowledge of the nature of impulsive aggression. See D.O. Lewis, *Guilty by Reason of Insanity* (New York: Ballantine, 1998); E.S. Barratt & L. Slaughter, "Defining, Measuring, and Predicting Impulsive Aggression: A Heuristic Model," *Behav. Sci. & Law* 16 (1988): 285; E.S. Barratt, M.S. Stanford, L. Dowdy, M.J. Liebman, & T.A. Kent, "Impulsive and Premeditated Aggression: A Factor Analysis of Self-Reported Acts," *Psychiat. Res.* 86 (1999): 163; E.S. Barratt, M.S. Stanford, T.A. Kent, & A. Felthous, "Neuropsychological and Cognitive Psychological Substrates of Impulsive Aggression," *Biol. Psychiat.* 41 (1997): 1045; M.A. Pauley, "Murder by Premeditation," *Am. Crim. L. Rev.* 36 (1999): 145.

46. Personal communication.

47. The principle of homeostasis can be extended to describe the total biological, psychological, and social behavior of the organism as it seeks to maintain a state of equilibrium. Dr. Karl Menninger states: "Increasing dysfunction, increasing dyscontrol, increasing disorganization can be identified empirically in a series of hierarchical levels, each one reflecting a stage of greater impairment of control and organization." Deviant behaviors or psychiatric symptoms, thus, are looked upon as devices employed by the organism to deal with emergencies, disturbed equilibrium and threatened dyscontrol. K. Menninger, *The Vital Balance* (New York: Viking, 1963). See also S. Halleck, *Psychiatry and the Dilemmas of Crime* (New York: Harper & Row, 1967); M.J. Horowitz (Ed.), *Hysterical Personality* (New York: Aronson, 1977).

48. A. Freud, *The Ego and the Mechanisms of Defense* (New York: International Universities Press, 1946).

49. State v. Herrin, Westchester Cy., N.Y., June 9, 1978; discussed in W. Gaylin, *Killing of Bonnie Garland: A Question of Justice* (New York: Simon & Schuster, 1982); P. Meyer, *The Yale Murder* (New York: Harper & Row, 1982). In People v. Gorshen, 51 Cal. 2d 716, 336 P.2d (1959), Dr. Bernard Diamond testified that Gorshen's rage was a desperate attempt to ward off the imminent and total disintegration of his personality that would occur through regression into a schizophrenic relapse.

50. B.L. Diamond, "Social and Cultural Factors as a Diminished Capacity Defense in Criminal Law," *Bull. Amer. Acad. Psychiat. & Law* 6 (1978): 195.

51. J.H. Skolnick, "Dr. Bernard L. Diamond," *Calif. L. Rev.* 78 (1990): 1433.

52. Cal. Penal Code §§ 188, 189.

53. Cal. Penal Code § 28.

54. *Bull. Amer. Acad. Psychiat. & Law* 6 (1978): 195.

55. "'Die, My Daughter, Die!'" *People,* Jan. 20, 1992, p. 71.

56. 10 Cal.3d 750, 111 Cal. Rptr. 910, 518 P.2d 342 (1974); discussed in W.J. Winslade & J.W. Ross, *The Insanity Defense* (New York: Scribner, 1983).

57. 118 Cal. Rptr. 129, 529 P.2d 553 (1974), vacated, 17 Cal.3d 425, 131 Cal. Rptr. 14, 551 P.2d 334 (1976).

58. The court said:

> Diminished capacity is a mental infirmity. To the extent that it is to be evaluated by experts, the experts should be those qualified in the mental sciences. The effect, therefore, of such matters as cultural stress should be assessed by experts in the fields of psychiatry and psychology, and ultimately by the jury with the assistance of the testimony of such experts. We need not consider whether it would have been proper to exclude the anthropologist's testimony completely because the court was willing … to allow the testimony as furnishing material for the opinions of the psychiatrists. It is desirable to give direction and control to the presentation of expert testimony of such delicate matters as the capacity of a person to deliberate or to entertain malice. To allow independent testimony on sociological, ethnic or like influences, not as reviewed by experts in psycho-

logical sciences, but as directly presented to the jury would be to open the door to a vast amount of argument from various sources, the result of which would often be distraction of the jury and the removing of their deliberation from the essential element of the mental capacity of the accused.

Even without the expert testimony, the jury found Poddar guilty not of first-degree, but of second-degree murder. One might ponder: Would the verdict have been any different—more severe or less severe—if the expert had testified? More often than not, juries are swayed more by the facts of the case than by expert opinions. Defense counsel objected to the exclusion of the expert testimony; as is the practice, to safeguard an appeal, defense counsel raises any and every possible error of the trial court.

59. 468 F.2d 141 (7th Cir. 1972).

60. The case concerned the acts of Frederick Chase and several others, who on May 25, 1969, broke into a Selective Service office, removed draft records, and burned them to protest the Vietnam War. They were tried on charges of destroying government property. Several of the defendants pleaded NGRI, claiming that by reason of mental illness they could not distinguish between right and wrong when they vandalized the Selective Service office. They were convicted. Among the issues on appeal was whether the trial judge had improperly excluded evidence supporting this claim. The Seventh Circuit explained why it did not find the exclusion improper (468 F.2d at 148–149):

> There is virtually nothing in the record to suggest that any of the defendants was suffering from any legally cognizable mental illness on May 24 or May 25, 1969, or that they did not fully under-stand that their conduct was "wrong" as measured by the standards prescribed by society. Their evidence of "insanity" merely tended to prove that their moral judgment as to whether certain conduct—specifically their own deliberate violations of law—was "right" or "wrong" was at odds with the judgment expressed by society at large. Under the standards for determining criminal responsibility ... this defense was manifestly frivolous. ... The trial judge properly excluded certain evidence, which ... would have provided no support for the claim that these defendants could not comprehend the criminal character of their conduct. Thus, an anthropologist was not allowed to testify that the defendants believed their conduct might be considered sane in one culture and insane in another. ... The judge's evidentiary rulings were well within the scope of his discretion. We find absolutely no merit in the contention that these four dedicated intellectuals were not given an adequate opportunity to present their defense of "insanity."

61. Noted in J. Gibeaut, "Troubling Translations," *ABAJ*, Oct. 1999: 93.

62. Ibid. Many countries have laws that reduce or even eliminate sentences for those who kill in defense of family honor. Worldwide, thousands of times each year, a woman is killed by her father or brothers for acts that are seen as besmirching the family's honor, including committing adultery, defying a parental order to marry, being seen in public with a man, or becoming the victim of a rape. Editorial, "Honor Killings," *New York Times*, Nov. 12, 2000, WK14.

63. Quoted in M. Reynolds (Reuters news release), "'Good Girl' to Be Tried in Serial Slaying," *Detroit Free Press*, Jan. 11, 1992, p. 4.

64. As proof that the accused committed the crime, however, evidence of poverty or unemployment is generally not admissible because its probative value is deemed outweighed by unfair prejudice and discrimination. The argument that "poverty causes crime" cannot be used as evidence *against* an accused; People v. Stanton, 296 N.W.2d 70 (Mich. App. 1980).

65. 471 F.2d 923 (D.C. Cir. 1972).

66. Judge Bazelon said (471 F.2d at 926):

> The thrust of Murdock's defense was that the environment in which he was raised—his "rotten social background"—conditioned him to respond to certain stimuli in a manner most of us would consider flagrantly inappropriate. Because of his early conditioning, he argued, he was denied any meaningful choice when the racial insult triggered the explosion in the restaurant. He asked the jury to conclude that his "rotten social background," and the resulting impairment of mental or emotional processes and behavior controls, ruled his violent reaction in the same manner that the behavior of a paranoid schizophrenic may be ruled by his "mental condition." Whether this impair-ment amounted to an "abnormal condition of the mind" is, in my opinion, at best an academic question. But the consequences we predicate on the answer may be very meaningful indeed.

67. 471 F.2d at 965.

68. April 21, 1972.

69. 471 F.2d 969 at 995 (D.C. App. 1972).

70. 471 F.2d at 1012.
71. 328 U.S. 463 (1946).
72. 149 F.2d 28 at 29 (D.C. App. 1945).
73. 328 U.S. at 470.
74. United States v. Lee, 4 Mackey 489 (Sup. Ct. D.C. 1886).
75. The majority stated, "We express no opinion upon whether the theory for which petitioner contends should or should not be made the law of the District of Columbia. Such a radical departure from common law concepts is more properly a subject for the exercise of legislative power or at least for the discretion of the courts of the District"; 328 U.S. at 476. In a dissenting opinion, Justice Frankfurter wrote:

> This case has been much beclouded by laymen's ventures into psychiatry. We are not now called upon to decide whether the antiquated tests set down more than a hundred years ago regarding mental responsibility for crime are still controlling or whether courts should choose from among the conflicting proposals of scientific specialists. This is not the occasion to decide whether the only alternative is between law, which reflects the most advanced scientific tests and law remaining a leaden-footed laggard. The case turns on a much simpler and wholly conventional issue. For the real question, as I see it, is whether in view of the act of Congress defining murder in the first degree for prosecutions in the District and in light of the particular circumstances of this case, the trial court properly sent the case to the jury. That is a very different question from whether the court's charge was unimpeachable as an abstract statement of law. For Fisher is not the name of a theoretical problem. We are not here dealing with an abstract man who killed an abstract woman under abstract circumstances and received an abstract trial on abstract issues. … The preoccupation at the trial, in the treatment of the conviction by the court below and by the arguments at the bar of this Court, was with alluring problems of psychiatry. Throughout this melancholy affair the insistence was on claims of Fisher's mental deficiencies and the law's duty to take into consideration the skeptical views of modern psychiatry regarding the historic legal tests for insanity. I cannot but believe that this has diverted attention from the more obvious and conventional, but controlling inquiry regarding the absence or presence of the requisite premeditation, under the circumstances of this case.
>
> That the charge requested by the defendant and denied did not go to this issue of premeditation unambiguously, but in an awkward and oblique way did not lessen the responsibility of the trial judge to bring this issue—it was the crucial issue—sharply and vividly to the jury's mind. If their minds had been so focused, the jury might well have found that the successive steps that culminated in Miss Reardon's death could not properly be judged in isolation. They might well have found a sequence of events that constituted a single, unbroken response to a provocation in which no forethought, no reflection whatever, entered. A deed may be gruesome and not be premeditated. Concededly there was no motive for the killing prior to the inciting "you black nigger." The tone in which these words were uttered evidently pulled the trigger of Fisher's emotions, and under adequate instructions the jury might have found that what these words conveyed to Fisher's ears unhinged his self-control. While there may well have been murder, deliberate premeditation, for which alone Congress has provided the death sentence, may have been wanting. … I do not believe that the facts warrant a finding of premeditation. But, in any event, the justification for finding first-degree murder premeditation was so tenuous that the jury ought not to have been left to founder and flounder within the dark emptiness of legal jargon. The instructions to the jury on the vital issue of premeditation consisted of threadbare generalities, a jumble of empty abstractions equally suitable for any other charge of murder with none of the elements that are distinctive about this case, mingled with talk about mental disease. What the jury got was devoid of clear guidance and illumination. Inadequate direction to a jury may be as fatal as misdirection.

The case is discussed in H. Weihofen & W. Overholser, "Mental Disorder Affecting the Degree of a Crime," *Yale L. J.* 56 (1947): 959; H.L. Taylor, "Partial Insanity as Affecting the Degree of Crime: A Commentary on *Fisher v. United States*," *Calif. L. Rev.* 34 (1946): 625; Note, *Colum. L. Rev.* 46 (1946): 1005.
76. 513 Pa. 381, 521 A.2d 398 (1987), cited *supra* note 44.
77. 521 A.2d at 405.
78. 521 A.2d at 404.
79. R. Harris, *Murders and Madness* (New York: Clarendon Press, 1989).

80. E.E.H. Griffith, "Ethics in Forensic Psychiatry: A Cultural Response to Stone and Applebaum," *J. Am. Acad. Psychiat. & Law* 26 (1998): 171. In the film *Boesman & Lena* set in South Africa during the days of apartheid, Boesman, a black male, is angry, bitter, and ready for violence at the slightest provocation. Then, too, defense attorneys for Colin Ferguson, who massacred passengers on the Long Island Railroad, wanted to enter a "black rage" defense on his behalf. Paul Harris, an attorney with the Center for Guerrilla Law in San Francisco, pioneered the modern version of the "black rage" defense when in 1971 he successfully defended a young black man charged with armed bank robbery. See P. Harris, *Black Rage Confronts the Law* (New York: New York University Press, 1997); see also A.E. Taslitz, "Abuse Excuse and the Logic and Politics of Expert Relevance," *Hastings L. J.* 49 (1998): 1039. Of course, as we know, juries can return verdict contrary to the law—they do not have to give a reason for their decisions. Returning a verdict contrary to the law is known as jury nullification. See R. Slovenko, "Jury Nullification," *J. Psychiat. & Law* 22 (1993): 545.

81. For a criticism, see S. Estrich, *Getting Away With Murder: How Politics Is Destroying the Criminal Justice System* (Cambridge, MA: Harvard University Press, 1998); J.Q. Wilson, *Moral Judgment: Does the Abuse Excuse Threaten Our Legal System?* (New York: Basic Books, 1997); R. Slovenko, "Crime Revisited," *J. Psychiat. & Law* 18 (1990): 485; L. Weintraub, "Inner-City Post-Traumatic Stress Disorder," *J. Psychiat. & Law* 25 (1997): 249; B. Frank, "Race and Crime: Let's Talk Sense," *New York Times,* Jan. 13, 1992, op-ed, p. 15.

82. A.A. Stone, "Presidential Address: Conceptual Ambiguity and Morality in Modern Psychiatry," *Am. J. Psychiat.* 137 (1980): 887. See also *Ibid.*, "The Ethical Boundaries of Forensic Psychiatry: A View from the Ivory Tower," *J. Am. Acad. Psychiatry & Law* 36 (2008):167. In this article Stone says that what has kept him out of the courtroom is his concern about the ethical boundaries of forensic psychiatry.

83. Steven Kaplan, a prosecuting attorney in Macomb County, Michigan, claims that "diminished capacity is like the Libertarian Party—it's interesting, but it has little role to play." Personal communication.

13
Juvenile Justice

Under ancient biblical codes, the minor and the mental defective were not punished because "their acts are without purpose." In Roman law, a minor under the age of 7 was not responsible (an age that coincides with psychological development). In the early stages of the common law, infancy apparently was not a defense, but children were usually pardoned for their offenses. By the 14th century, it was established that a child under 7 was not criminally responsible, and it was presumed that a child over 7 lacked the capacity to commit a crime. By the 17th century, 14 became the age of full responsibility.[1] Many states enacted statutes specifically directed at youthful behavior, which prohibited, for example, playing ball on public ways or sledding on the Sabbath. Other laws covering children specifically were similar to a Massachusetts statute of 1646:

> If any child[ren] above sixteen years old and of sufficient understanding shall curse or smite their natural father or mother, they shall be put to death, unless it can be sufficiently testified that the parents have been very unchristianly negligent in the education of such children, or so provoked them by extreme and cruel correction that they have been forced thereunto to preserve themselves from death or maiming. ...
>
> If a man have a stubborn or rebellious son of sufficient years of understanding, viz. sixteen, which will not obey the voice of his father or the voice of his mother, and that when they have chastened him will not harken unto them, then shall his father and mother, being his natural parents, lay hold on him and bring him to the magistrates assembled in Court, and testify to them by sufficient evidence that this their son is stubborn and rebellious and will not obey their voice and chastisement, but lives in sundry notorious crimes. Such a son shall be put to death.[2]

A common crime during the 19th century by children was flight from the service of a master to whom they were apprenticed. These offenses were dealt with severely.

Prior to the 1900s, juveniles in violation of the laws were brought to the adult criminal courts. Not only were they tried as adults, but they were sent to adult prisons as well. In 1851, Michigan prison inspectors complained the courts had committed five or six boys to the state prison—one of whom is only 11 years of age. In the late 19th century, according to a history of reform schools in the state, Michigan Governor Andrew Parsons insisted that juveniles be treated "not as men of understanding and hardened in iniquity, but [be trained]."

Starting in the early 19th century, juries began injecting compassion into the law by refusing to convict children, even though the evidence clearly indicated their guilt. Reformers seized on this wave of "jury nullification" and created reform schools, which became homes for children convicted of crimes or found to be "vagrants" or "ungovernable." These schools flourished for several decades until some were revealed to be little more than sweatshops for children.

In 1871, the reform school in Chicago burned in the city's great fire, and many of its charges ended up in the city jails. A year later, three Chicago social leaders, Lucy Flower, Adelaide Groves, and Julia Lathrop, toured the jails and were appalled to find "quite small boys confined in the same quarters with murderers, anarchists, and hardened criminals." These women, who believed that children were innately good and that the state had a moral duty to correct and save wayward youth, began lobbying for a separate "children's court" to handle their cases. Their efforts resulted in the Illinois Legislature enacting a law to establish such a court.[3] On July 3, 1899, Cook County Juvenile Judge Richard Tuthill heard the nation's first juvenile court case, involving an 11-year-old boy who was accused of larceny. The new court system was unique in four ways: (1) it was "rehabilitative" rather than punitive, (2) its records were confidential, (3) it did not place juveniles in adult facilities, and (4) it allowed informal procedures in court, preferring to act "as a wise parent" with a "wayward child," as Judge Julian Mack, one of the original juvenile court jurists put it. By 1935, nearly all states enacted legislation establishing juvenile courts.[4]

Waiver to Criminal Court

In subsequent years, with the increase in juvenile crime, the legislatures of all 50 states passed laws allowing or requiring transfer of juveniles, usually over the age of 14 or 15, to the regular criminal courts. In order to "transfer" or "waive" juvenile court jurisdiction, certain criteria, such as age, nature of the crime, and prior record, had to be met. The waiver was usually for acts that would constitute a felony if committed by an adult.[5]

In 1966, in *Kent v. United States*,[6] the U.S. Supreme Court dealt with the issue of waiver of juvenile court jurisdiction to a court of general criminal jurisdiction. It did not, as was urged, strike down waiver of juveniles to criminal court. In the course of its opinion, Justice Fortas, who wrote the opinion for the Court, commented, "There is much evidence that some juvenile courts lack the personnel, facilities, and techniques to perform adequately as representatives of the state in a *parens patriae* capacity, at least with respect to children charged with law violations." The court was emphatic, however, that the waiver of jurisdiction was a "critically important" action to the juvenile because there are special rights and immunities that accrue from juvenile court handling: he is shielded from publicity, he may be confined, but, with rare exceptions, he may not be jailed along with adults. He may be detained, but only until he is 21 years of age. The child is protected against consequences of adult conviction, such as the loss of civil rights, the use of adjudication against him in subsequent proceedings, and disqualification for public employment.

A felony conviction, on the other hand, whether or not there is imprisonment, is a lifelong handicap, but there is the possibility of expunging at least one conviction from a record. As a consequence, trial as an adult has a number of protections, not available in a juvenile proceeding; in particular, the applicability of the full panoply of the rules of evidence, the defense of not guilty by reason of insanity (NGRI), and the unanimity of a jury of 12. In 1967, in the case of *In re Gault*,[7] the U.S. Supreme Court legalized the juvenile court in considerable measure by establishing that juveniles were owed at least those elements of the due process essential to fundamental fairness (e.g., the right to counsel, written and timely notice of the charges, and the privilege against self-incrimination). In *Gault*, Justice Fortas described juvenile courts as "kangaroo courts" characterized by arbitrariness, ineffectiveness, and the appearance of injustice.[8]

In its 1966 opinion in *Kent*, the U.S. Supreme Court appended eight criteria for waiver, but none specifically called for expert testimony on the prospects for rehabilitation:

1. The seriousness of the alleged offense to the community and whether the protection of the community requires waiver.
2. Whether the alleged offense was committed in an aggressive, violent, premeditated or willful manner.
3. Whether the offense was committed against persons or against property.
4. The prosecutive merit of the complaint, i.e., whether there is evidence upon which a grand jury may be expected to return an indictment.

5. The desirability of trial and disposition of the entire event in one court with the juvenile associates in the alleged offense who will be charged with the crime.
6. The sophistication of the juvenile.
7. The record and previous history of the juvenile in context to the previous findings of the court.
8. The prospects for adequate protection of the public and the likelihood of rehabilitation of the juvenile by use of procedures, services, and facilities currently available to the juvenile court.[9]

The court held that juveniles facing waiver are entitled to representation by counsel, access to social service records, and a written statement of the reasons for waiver. The Fifth Amendment privilege against self-incrimination applies to procedures governing determination as to whether to certify a juvenile for prosecution as an adult.[10]

In a second *Kent* case, the juvenile again appealed the juvenile court's waiver of jurisdiction to criminal court, arguing that he was incompetent to be sent over to the criminal court because he was schizophrenic.[11] Writing the opinion of the U.S. Court of Appeals for the District of Columbia, in 1968, Judge David Bazelon stated that it is implicit in the juvenile court scheme that no criminal punishment is to be the rule, and adult criminal punishment is to be the exception, which must be governed by the particular factors of individual cases. On the facts of the *Kent* case, waiver was deemed inappropriate; allowing insanity to justify waiver, it was said, is not in accord with the prevailing philosophy of the juvenile court. Judge Bazelon wrote: "Since waiver was not necessary for the protection of society and not conducive to [appellant's] rehabilitation, its exercise in this case violated the social welfare philosophy of the Juvenile Court Act. Of course, this philosophy does not forbid all waivers. We only decide here that it does forbid waivers of a seriously ill juvenile."[12] Judge Warren Burger, later Chief Justice of the Supreme Court, vigorously dissented, saying that *Kent*, if waived, would have in the criminal court all the rights in relation to his alleged psychiatric problems that he would have in the juvenile court.[13]

"Waiver hearings" (also known as amenability or transfer hearings) are designed to address these issues: the juvenile offender's "fit" in juvenile court and a determination that rests on the minor's amenability to rehabilitation via those programs, services, and facilities accessible through juvenile court.[14] In 1972, in *Mikulovsky v. State of Wisconsin*,[15] the Wisconsin Supreme Court held that it is not mandatory for a juvenile court to hear expert testimony on a minor's rehabilitative prospects before transferring jurisdiction to adult court. The court apparently followed all of the *Kent* criteria on waiver, the objection being that the court failed to hear certain testimony concerning one aspect, to wit, the psychological and social worker's opinions as to rehabilitation.

All states have established mechanisms whereby some juveniles may be prosecuted within the criminal justice system. These mechanisms, while having different names among the states, fall into three general categories, according to who makes the transfer decision: (1) judicial waiver, (2) statutory exclusion, and (3) concurrent jurisdiction; the decisionmakers are, respectively, the juvenile court judge, the legislature, and the prosecutor. In judicial waivers, a hearing is held in juvenile court, typically in response to the prosecutor's request that the juvenile court judge waives the juvenile court's jurisdiction over the matter and transfers the juvenile to criminal court for trial in the adult system. Most state statutes limit juvenile waiver by age and offense criteria and by "lack of amenability to treatment" criteria. Judicial waiver provisions vary in the degree of flexibility that they allow the court in decision making. Regardless of the degree of flexibility accorded to the court, the waiver process must adhere to certain constitutional principles of fairness, as set out by the Supreme Court in *Kent*.

In a growing number of states, legislatures have statutorily excluded certain young offenders from juvenile court jurisdiction based on age or offense criteria. Some states have defined the upper age of juvenile court jurisdiction as 15 or 16 and, thus, have excluded a large number of youths under age 18 from the juvenile court system. Many states also exclude certain individuals charged with serious offenses from juvenile court jurisdiction.

Under concurrent jurisdiction, state statutes give prosecutors the discretion to file certain cases in either juvenile or criminal court because both courts share original jurisdiction. State concurrent jurisdiction provisions, like other transfer provisions, typically are limited by age and offense criteria. Prosecutorial transfer, unlike judicial waiver, is not subject to judicial review and is not required to meet the due process requirements set out in *Kent*. According to some state appellate courts, prosecutorial transfer is an executive function equivalent to routine charging decisions. Nearly all states rely on a combination of transfer provisions to move juveniles to the criminal system. Moreover, the Sexually Violent Predator laws that have been enacted in some 13 states have been used to commit young men whose sex offenses were as juveniles.

What about the death penalty? In 1988, the U.S. Supreme Court ruled that the states may not execute anyone who was younger than 16 at the time of the crime.[16] The 5–3 decision was followed a year later by a ruling allowing execution of those who were between 16 and 18 at the time of the crime.[17] Then, in 2005, as discussed in Chapter 14, the Supreme Court ruled that those under the age of 18 are too immature to be subject to the death sentence.[18] Presumably, they are sufficiently mature to be transferred to the criminal court.

Responding to the sharp rise in juvenile crimes, at least 44 states since 1992 have adopted new juvenile justice laws that allow more youngsters to be tried as adults. According to the Office of Juvenile Justice, juveniles in 1980 were the offenders in 8% of all homicides in the United States. By 1994, that number had doubled to 16%. Between 1988 and 1994, the arrest rate for males aged 10 to 17 for violent crimes rose 60%. Florida today prosecutes more juveniles as adults than any other state. In recent years, the number of teenagers doing time in adult prisons in the United States has more than doubled. In a number of states—Alabama, California, Florida, Missouri, North Carolina, and Wisconsin—a life sentence may be imposed on juveniles; some 2,400 juveniles in the United States are serving life sentences without parole. The suicide rate of juveniles in prison is appalling.[19]

Transfer research in the 1970s and 1980s found that, contrary to conventional wisdom, transfers (1) were not necessarily violent offenders, (2) did not necessarily receive harsher sanctions in criminal court that they would have received in juvenile court, (3) were not necessarily incarcerated, and (4) if incarcerated, did not necessarily receive longer sentences than their juvenile court counterparts. Research in the 1990s that compared the recidivism outcomes of transfers and of youth retained in the juvenile system found that transfers were more likely to recidivate within 2 years. After a 6-year follow-up period, there was no difference between the groups in the proportion of offenders who recidivated, although the transferred youth who reoffended did so more quickly and more often, on average, than delinquents handled in juvenile court who reoffended.[20]

Juvenile Reform Legislation

The paradigm of developments nationwide was the enactment of juvenile reform legislation in 1996 in Michigan. Under the legislation, the prosecutor is given the discretion to charge a minor of any age as an adult for certain serious crimes. For those under 14, the trial is held not in an adult court (as widely reported), but in family court, and this is significant because the family court has experience with juvenile offenders and rehabilitation services. The most significant aspect of the law is that the sentencing judge has broad sentencing discretion. Upon conviction, the judge may impose a prison sentence not exceeding a similar sentence for an adult. At the other end of the sentencing spectrum, the judge may simply say to the offender, "You are free to go." Most important, the law provides for a "blended sentence" under which the judge can sentence the defendant to a juvenile rehabilitation program with a review every year until age 21. At or before age 21, the judge makes a decision after hearing from professionals, such as psychiatrists and other treatment specialists who have been dealing with the defendant. If the professionals advise the judge that the defendant has not been rehabilitated and poses a significant danger to the public if released, the judge may continue the sentence into the adult prison system.

The law thus gives prosecutors the ability to protect the public from dangerous offenders, while giving judges flexibility to fashion sentences that fit the nature of the crime and the rehabilitative attitude of the juvenile in question. It allows the court to maintain control over the individual at the end of the age of minority, which was not possible under the prior juvenile laws. That is the rationale of the new law—to protect society from an individual who remains dangerous irrespective of the happenstance of reaching age 21. No longer would an individual "age out of the system."

Years ago, Michigan and other states mandated that juveniles 17 or older be tried automatically as adults (many other states and the federal government require that a defendant be at least 18 to be automatically considered an adult). In 1923, the Michigan legislature had provided that a probate court judge, who had jurisdiction at the time over juveniles, could waive jurisdiction of those who had attained the age of 15, charged with a felony, to a court of general criminal jurisdiction,[21] and by an amendment in 1996, the age was lowered to 14.[22] For the 14 to 17 age group, waiver was discretionary. In the law adopted in 1996, Michigan also allowed prosecutors, without court approval, to try any youth as an adult, no matter how young, but those under 14 would be tried in family court. State Senator William van Regenmorter, the key force behind the tougher juvenile offender law in Michigan, said, "I don't think these youngsters are beyond redemption, but whether they are rehabilitable or not is secondary in those rare cases to the incredible danger they pose for all the rest."[23]

In the trial of a minor as an adult, what of competency to confess, competency to stand trial, and criminal responsibility? Would he have understood the Miranda warning.[24] In Michigan, in an appellate opinion in *People v. Givans*,[25] the factors are set forth that a court should consider in deciding whether a statement from a juvenile was properly taken, including a requirement that the offender's parent or guardian be present. That might be called a "Mama Miranda" warning. In *People v. Abraham*,[26] in ruling a minor's confession admissible, the appellate court said,

> We find it a matter of great significance that [the] defendant's mother was present for, and participated in, the entire *Miranda*-waiver process. Parents normally have the duty and authority to act in furtherance of both the physical and legal needs of their minor children. This responsibility includes deciding whether the minor will undergo medical treatment, deciding what school the minor will attend, signing contracts for or on behalf of the minor, and assisting the minor in deciding whether to waive *Miranda* rights.[27]

Of course, a defense attorney always advises a suspect to say nothing to the police, thus cutting off any confession.

What of competency to stand trial?[28] Nationwide, prosecutors seek restoration training of the minor and that involves role playing as well as other training. A number of psychiatrists and psychologists maintain, however, that any minor under the age of 13 is not competent to stand trial, given the minor's undeveloped mental and cognitive skills and decision-making ability.[29] One must view critically, however, the proposition that juveniles under age 13, one and all, do not have the capacity of triability.[30] Apparently out of bias against the criminal prosecution of minors, a number of psychiatrists and psychologists have taken an expanded view of the test of competency to stand trial, almost requiring the accused to have the knowledge of an attorney. In any event, seeing numerous trials on television, youngsters are well versed with the process.

During the time awaiting trial, the youngster grows in size, and in the aforementioned and well-known case involving Nathaniel Abraham, the defense attorney sought to dismiss the case "based on the fact that the young person in front of the court today is not the same person as 2 years ago, and the jury would not be able to see what he was like then."[31] Abraham was at the time of trial less of a sympathy figure. Trials are delayed because of appeals regarding competency to confess and competency to stand trial. The argument is reminiscent of that made in cases of accused persons who plead insanity and are on medication at the time of trial. In those cases, it is claimed that their demeanor is not like that at the time of the offense and would mislead the jury.[32]

What of the criteria for triability set out by the U.S. Supreme Court in *Dusky v. United States*?[33] In numerous studies, psychiatrists and psychologists have done empirical studies on competency in various contexts, but their practical utility at law is problematical. Competency is not independent of the facts of the particular case, and the concept is often used at law as a ploy to reach a desired result. For whatever it may be worth, among the most extensively researched issues in recent decades has been that of competency to stand trial. Psychometric measures of triability have attempted to translate the criteria in *Dusky* that the accused must have a "sufficient present ability to consult with his lawyer with a reasonable degree of rational understanding" and have a "rational as well as factual understanding of the proceedings against him" into psychological and behavioral functions or competency abilities.[34] Not surprisingly, the studies are of no consequence in deciding triability in a particular case.

A trial judge is supposedly obliged to raise the issue of triability *sua sponte* at any time during the proceedings when a bona fide doubt appears as to the defendant's competency.[35] Nationwide, more often than not, when minors aged 14 to 16 are bound over to the criminal court, they are returned to the juvenile court on the ground of incompetency to stand trial.

The tactic of defense lawyers in criminal cases is, more often than not, to put the jury in a fog, as was done in the O. J. Simpson case where the jury was utterly bewildered by the DNA evidence. The defense attorneys and experts blew a lot of smoke. After all, the state has to prove its case beyond a reasonable doubt, and the fog would create a doubt. Invariably, closing arguments by the defense in criminal cases are like those in a dog bite case where defense counsel argued: (1) the defendant's dog didn't bite the plaintiff, (2) the plaintiff provoked the dog into biting him, and (3) the defendant didn't own the dog.

In cases involving minors as criminal defendants, closing arguments are mainly an exhortation for nullification, and that has been the type of argument made by defense counsel. The state, on the other hand, is precluded from making a civic duty argument.[36]

Queries

How should the law handle minors who kill or who are hardened sociopaths? Should juvenile court judges, not prosecutors, decide whether minors charged with serious crimes should be charged as adults or minors? Should there be multiple sentencing of minors; that is, at age 18 or 21, the minor would appear in court for resentencing, at which time the judge would hear evidence about any rehabilitation? Would this rolling sentencing provide an incentive to the minor to improve his life behind bars? Such a system, it is argued, would hold minors responsible for their acts while recognizing that they are minors.

In Conclusion

One who grows up in a dysfunctional family in a dysfunctional environment likely becomes a menace. Children from dysfunctional families usually have some hope when they are exposed to functional adults outside their immediate family, but when these are absent, the situation is bleak. A stable family of two biological parents is the desideratum for molding character, for nurturing, for inculcating values, and for planning a child's future. Then, too, it takes a village to raise a child.

National studies show that an estimated one in five children with mental problems receives treatment, for reasons ranging from lack of services to parental neglect. It is estimated that as few as 5% of children with serious mental problems—or 1 in 20—receive psychiatric help. For the economically disadvantaged, the situation is dire. The number of Medicaid-eligible children needing mental health services who actually receive them varies among the states, depending on the difficulty that psychiatrists have in coping with the state's Medicaid program. They say the technicalities cause so much trouble for them that they cannot hope to accept Medicaid patients and keep their practices solvent. Nationwide, hospital beds for children and adolescents with psychiatric disorders continue to be cut. Some hospitals have discontinued hospital treatment altogether.

Endnotes

1. In the case of State v. Doherty, 2 Overt. Tenn. Rep. 79 (1806), Mary Doherty, a youngster of 12 or 13 years, was prosecuted for the murder of her father. Under the law of Tennessee at the time, if a person under 14 commits an act, such as that charged in the indictment, the presumption of law is that the person cannot discern between right and wrong. Under 7, the individual as a matter of law is deemed incapable of committing a crime. The jury in this case, after deliberation of a few hours, returned a verdict of not guilty. While in jail awaiting trial and during the trial, she spoke only a few monosyllables. A note appended to the original report of the case indicates that on the day after her trial she was observed near the court quite animated and smiling at the judges in a way that indicated her pleasure with what turned out to be deception.
2. III Mass. Records 101.
3. C. Wetzstein, "Kids' Court Centennial," *Insight*, Oct. 4–11, 1999, p. 30.
4. At the turn of the 20th century, Chicago was world famous for crime and it was also world famous for what it was doing to address the causes of crime. Not only was the world's first juvenile court established in Chicago, in 1899, but John Wigmore of Northwestern University Law School in 1910 founded the nation's first criminological research center, the American Institute for Criminal Law and Criminology, and its flagship journal. Then too, Chicago established the nation's first and largest municipal court to deal with tens of thousands of annual quasi-crimes, and a psychopathological laboratory of a eugenic bent to analyze offenders for deviance and feeblemindedness.
5. A collection of 78 appellate decisions in juvenile law that span the range of juvenile opinion in this field during the 20th century appears in J.C. Watkins, *Selected Cases on Juvenile Justice in the Twentieth Century* (Levinston, NY: Mellen Press, 1999). In *The Juvenile Court and The Progressives* (Champaign: University of Illinois Press, 2000), Victoria Getis examines the Cook County Juvenile Court and describes the court's intrinsic flaws and the source of its debilitation in our own time.
6. 383 U.S. 541 (1966).
7. 387 U.S. 1 (1967).
8. 387 U.S. at 18, 19, 26, 28.
9. See R. Borum & D. Verhaagen, *Assessing and Managing Violence Risks in Juveniles* (New York: Guilford, 2006); T. Grisso, G. Vincent, & D. Seagrave (Eds.), *Mental Health Screening and Assessment in Juvenile Justice* (New York: Guilford, 2005); P.H. Witt & F.J. Dyer, "Juvenile Transfer Cases: Risk Assessment and Risk Management," *J. Psychiat. & Law* 25 (1997): 581.
10. In the Matter of the Welfare of S.J.T., 736 N.W.2d 341 (Minn. App. 2007).
11. 401 F.2d 408 (D.C. Cir. 1968).
12. 401 F.2d at 412. Insanity as a defense in a juvenile court proceeding was reviewed in a New Jersey case, which held that a juvenile could be adjudicated a delinquent even though insane. The court noted the distinction between a juvenile case and an indictable offense; the focus in a juvenile proceeding is not upon the commission of the act itself, but upon the consequences of it. In drawing this distinction, the court noted that an adjudication of delinquency brought about the protective and rehabilitative interests of the court; *In re* State of Interest of H.C., 106 N.J. Super. 583, 256 A.2d 322 (1969). A number of states, however, have found the right to assert an insanity defense to be an essential of "due process

and fair treatment" that must be provided to a juvenile charged with delinquency. See Chatman v. Virginia, 518 S.E.2d 847 (Va. App. 1999); State of Louisiana v. Causey, 363 So.2d 472 (La. 1978); *In re* M.G.S., 72 Cal. Rptr. 808 (Cal. App. 1968).

13. 401 F.2d at 414. See T. Grisso, "Juvenile Offenders and Mental Illness," *Psychiat., Psychol. & Law* 6 (1999): 143.

14. B.H. Gross, "The Fitness of Juvenile Court," *J. Foren. Sci.* 44 (1999): 1199; C. Slobogin, "Treating Kids Right: Deconstructing and Reconstructing the Amenability to Treatment Concept," *J. Contemp. Legal Iss.* 10 (1999): 299.

15. 54 Wis.2d 699, 196 N.W.2d 748 (1972).

16. Thompson v. Oklahoma, 487 U.S. 815 (1988).

17. Stanford v. Kentucky, 492 U.S. 361 (1989). A 10-year-old black child was hanged in Louisiana in 1855 and a Cherokee Indian child of the same age was hanged in Arkansas in 1885. See V.L. Streib, "Death Penalty for Children: The American Experience with Capital Punishment for Crimes Committed While Under Age Eighteen," *Okla. L. Rev.* 36 (1983): 613; cited in Thompson v. Oklahoma, 487 U.S. at 828 n. 27.

18. Roper v. Simmons, 125 S. Ct. 1183 (2005); see D.L. Beschle, "Cognitive Dissonance Revisited: *Roper v. Simmons* and the Issue of Adolescent Decision Making," *Wayne L. Rev.* 52 (2006): 1.

19. M. Talbot, "The Maximum Security Adolescent," *New York Times Magazine*, Sept. 10, 2000, p. 41. The Supreme Court declined to review a 30-year prison sentence for a youngster who was 12 when he killed his grandparents; Pittman v. South Carolina, 07-8436 (2008). The case drew wide attention, in part because of the link his lawyers tried to make between the crime and Zoloft®, a widely prescribed antidepressant. In 2004, the FDA ordered Zoloft and other antidepressants to carry "black box" warnings—the government's strongest warning short of a ban—about an increased risk of suicidal behavior in children.

20. Report, *Juvenile Transfers to Criminal Court in the 1990's: Lessons Learned From Four Studies* (Washington, DC: U.S. Department of Justice, 2000). In the book *Cries Unheard* (New York: Henry Holt, 1998), Gitta Sereny reports on the change in the law in England and focuses on the case of Mary Bell who in 1968, at age 11, was tried and convicted of murdering two small boys in Newcastle Upon Tyne. From age 11 to 16, she was confined in a secure unit (a locked educational establishment for a small number of youngsters held for serious offenses), and at age 16, as required under the law, she was sent to a maximum security women's prison, where she remained until she was 23.

21. Mich. Pub. Acts 1923, No. 105 §6, amending Act 325 of Laws of 1907 that had a cut-off age of 17.

22. Mich. Pub. Act 409 (1996).

23. Quoted in L.L. Brasier, "Guilty at 13: What's Ahead for Abraham?" *Detroit Free Press*, Nov. 17, 1999, p. 1. Not all juvenile systems are the same. Missouri's juvenile justice system received accolades for its reorganization of its system. Missouri has established small community-based centers that stress therapy. When possible, young people are kept near their homes so their parents can participate in rehabilitation that includes extensive family therapy. Case managers typically handle 15 to 20 youngsters. In other state systems, the caseloads get much higher. The oversight does not end with the youngster's release. The case managers follow their charges closely for many months and often help with job placement, therapy referrals, school issues, and drug or alcohol treatment. After completing the program, it is reported that only about 10% of their detainees are recommitted to the system by the juvenile courts. Nationwide, on the other hand, the juvenile court system all too often turns nonviolent childhood offenders into hardened criminals. Editorial, "The Right Model for Juvenile Justice," *New York Times*, Oct. 28, 2007, p. WK11.

24. Research in the 1980s said that adolescents did about as well as adults in hypothetical decision-making situations, but that view has changed. Psychologist Thomas Grisso's research on Miranda waivers showed significant differences. While adolescents may reason well cognitively, they also seem to make choices that adults would view as bad choices. So the question arises, do youths arrive at their decisions differently? The hypothetical theory now being studied is that at about the age of 13 to 14, there are no dramatic differences in capacity to understand information and reason between adolescent and adults, but psychosocial factors are more likely to be different. For example, compared with adults, youths do not give as much weight to long-range consequences, they are more accepting of risk, and they are more influenced by peers. T. Grisso & R. G. Schwartz, *Youth on Trial: A Developmental Perspective on Juvenile Justice* (Chicago: University of Chicago Press, 2000); M.N. Norko, "Guttmacher Lecture," *Am. Acad. Psychiat. & Law Newsl.* 25 (Sept. 2000): 1.

25. 227 Mich. App. 113, 575 N.W.2d 84 (1997).

26. 234 Mich. App. 640 (1999).

27. 234 Mich. App. at 651.

28. In *In re* Carey, 615 N.W.2d 742 (Mich. App. 2000), the Michigan Court of Appeals urged the State Supreme Court to promulgate rules of procedure for juvenile competency determinations, or the Legislature to enact any statutory provisions it deems necessary; 615 N.W.2d at 748 n. 4.

29. See T. Grisso, *Forensic Evaluation of Juveniles* (Sarasota, FL: Professional Resource Press, 1998); see also D. Cooper, "Juveniles Understanding of Trial-Related Information: Are They Competent Defendants?" *Behav. Sci. & Law* 15 (1997): 167; V. L. Cowden & G. R. McKee, "Competency to Stand Trial in Juvenile Delinquency Proceedings: Cognitive Maturity and the Attorney–Client Relationship," *J. Family Law* 33 (1994–95): 631; T. Grisso, "Competence of Adolescents as Trial Defendants," *Psych., Pub. Policy & Law.* 3 (1997): 3; E.S. Scott, N.D. Repucci, & J. Woolard, "Evaluating Adolescent Decision Making in a Legal Context," *Law & Hum. Behav.* 19 (1995): 221.

30. Richard III at age 13 was King of England; he read prodigiously. The media frequently interviews minors on worldly affairs. In the Russian magazine *Ogonek* (May 2001, p. 3), six youngsters of ages 7 to 12 are asked the question, "What must be done in order to improve the country?" They gave informed and interesting answers. In Russia's *St. Petersburg Times* (May 22, 2001, p. 15), an 11th grade student wrote an informed op-ed article on trying to make sense of the chaos in the world today. Centuries ago, though minors under the age of 7 were not held responsible under the common law, they were regarded as "miniature adults." In the 10th century, artists were unable to depict a child except as an adult on a smaller scale. See P. Aries, *Centuries of Childhood* (New York: Random House, 1962).

31. Riggins v. Nevada, 112 S. Ct. 2752 (1992); State v. Jojola, 553 P.2d 1296 (N.M. 1976); see B.J. Winick, "Psychotropic Medication in the Criminal Trial Process: The Constitutional and Therapeutic Implications of Riggins vs. Nevada," *N.Y. L. Sch. J. Hum. Rights* 10 (1993): 637.

32. Quoted in L.L. Brasier, *op. cit. supra* note 23.

33. 362 U.S. 402 (1960).

34. On a juvenile's competency to stand trial, see R. Barnum & T. Grisso, "Competence to Stand Trial in Juvenile Court in Massachusetts: Issues of Therapeutic Jurisprudence," *New Eng. J. Crim. & Civil Confine.* 20 (1994): 321; T. Grisso, "Dealing with Juveniles' Competence to Stand Trial: What We Need to Know," *Quinnipac L. Rev.* 18 (1999): 371; G.R. McKee, "Competency to Stand Trial in Preadjudicatory Juveniles and Adults," *J. Am. Acad. Psychiat. & Law* 26 (1998): 88. In 1999 Arkansas enacted legislation that provides that juveniles are to be evaluated according to "age-appropriate" standards, not by the traditional standards used to assess competency of adults; Ark. Code Ann. § 9-27-502 (1999). In Golden v. State, 341 Ark. 963, 21 S.W.3d 801 (2000), the Arkansas Supreme Court held that juveniles have a due process right to have their competency determined prior to adjudication. The Arizona Legislature enacted legislation that provides that developmental immaturity can be used as grounds for finding a juvenile incompetent to participate in juvenile proceedings or to be transferred to criminal court; Ariz. Rev. Stat. Ann. § 8-291 (2000).

35. Pate v. Robinson, 383 U.S. 375 (1966).

36. Such were also the arguments, for example, in the trial of Nathaniel Brazill, a 14-year-old boy who beat a 6-year-old playmate to death. D. Canedy, "Boy Who Killed Teacher Is Found Guilty of Murder," *New York Times*, May 17, 2001, p. 12.

14

Imposing and Carrying Out of the Death Penalty

The psychiatrist may be involved in one or two stages in the death penalty process: (1) imposition of the death penalty, and (2) the carrying out of the death penalty. The criminal law has three concepts of incapacity (insanity), each pertinent to a different stage: the capacity to stand trial, the capacity to commit crime, and the capacity to be executed under a death warrant.

In a recent 10-year period, about 22,000 criminal homicides were recorded annually in the United States. Of these, over the 10-year period, about 4,000 cases were egregious enough to qualify for the death penalty and a total of about 250 actually resulted in a death sentence. However, over the 10-year period only 22 people, on average, were executed annually, a small fraction of the 3,600 who sit on death rows nationwide. Far more death row inmates die of natural causes than are executed. In effect, the process in the United States caters to both proponents of the death penalty (by its imposition) and the abolitionists (by rarely carrying it out). Although juries imposed the death penalty more and more frequently in the 1980s and 1990s, the number of people executed in the United States in any given year has yet to exceed the number killed by lightning.[1]

Imposition of the Death Penalty

On the imposition of the death penalty, the Supreme Court in 1972 rendered highly publicized death penalty opinions in which it ruled, 5–4, that the death penalty in its then form was unconstitutional.[2] While no unifying reason supported the decision, the net result, with each Justice writing his own opinion (243 pages in all), was that the death penalty, as imposed within the discretion of juries, violates the Eighth Amendment, not because it is inherently intolerable, but because it is applied so rarely, "so wantonly and freakishly," that it serves no valid purpose and now constitutes cruel and unusual punishment. Only two justices—Justices Brennan and Marshall—ruled the death penalty unconstitutional *per se*. The dissenting justices felt that the majority had gone beyond judicial jurisdiction and trespassed upon the prerogatives of the legislature.

Thus capital punishment in its then form was rendered "cruel and unusual" by operation of what was intended to be, at the time of its introduction, an ameliorative feature of the criminal justice system—the jury's discretion to impose a lesser sentence than death. The Court, finding no reason to believe that the death sentence was imposed with "informed selectivity," concluded that it was imposed in a way that arbitrarily and capriciously discriminated against minorities and the poor.

Chief Justice Warren Burger then touched on changes that would have to be made to allow the use of the death penalty in compliance with the result of the case. The Court implied that capital punishment would be sanctioned if the penalty is uniformly and consistently applied. It was thought that legislative enactment of mandatory death sentences would seemingly provide an answer.

Following the Supreme Court's decision in 1972 that the death penalty it had under consideration was unconstitutional because of the discriminatory nature in its application, a number of states enacted statutes making the death sentence mandatory for all who committed a designate type of offense. Although their ostensible aim was to avoid discrimination against minority peoples, such statutes did not survive the scrutiny of the Supreme Court. In 1976, in *Woodson v. North Carolina*,[3] the Supreme Court ruled that it is cruel and unusual punishment to mandate the death penalty for all who commit certain crimes.[4] Two years later, in 1978, in *Lockett v. Ohio*,[5] Chief Justice Burger wrote:

> In capital cases, the fundamental respect for humanity underlying the Eighth Amendment requires consideration of the character and record of the individual offender and the circumstances of the particular offense as a constitutionally indispensable part of inflicting the penalty of death.[6]

According to that line of decisions, a death penalty statute is deemed valid if in each case the appropriateness of capital punishment can be ascertained in the light of aggravating or mitigating factors. Under the statutes approved, after a defendant has been found guilty, the court must conduct a hearing and consider, among other things, the mental status of the defendant. Since then, one prime question asked of the expert witness is whether the person is likely to be more violent and dangerous to fellow prisoners and to others than any of the other prisoners who are currently incarcerated.

In *Barefoot v. Estelle*,[7] a case decided in 1983, the Supreme Court was faced with a challenge to the basis of psychiatric opinion in capital sentencing hearings. In the sentencing phase of the bifurcated trial (the defendant had been found guilty of murder of a policeman), the prosecution, in order to establish the aggravating circumstances allowing imposition of the death penalty, introduced the testimony of two psychiatrists who had not examined the defendant (he declined to be interviewed); their testimony was based on information in a lengthy hypothetical question posed to them on the stand by the prosecutor. Nonetheless, they agreed on a diagnosis of the defendant as a sociopath, and agreed "within reasonable medical certainty" that he would commit future acts of violence. One of the psychiatrists claimed that the certainty of this prediction was "one hundred percent and absolute."[8] Errol Morris's documentary film *The Thin Blue Line* ridiculed the psychiatrist, Dr. James Grigson, a.k.a. Dr. Death.[9]

The defendant's challenge to Dr. Grigson's testimony was supported by an *amicus curiae* brief filed by the American Psychiatric Association that argued that psychiatric predictions of future dangerousness ought to be excluded as a matter of law because the empirical data consistently indicate a large margin of error. Justice White, writing for five members of the six-person majority, evidently feared that excluding psychiatric testimony on dangerousness might lead to challenges in a variety of cases (including civil commitment). Thus, he wrote, "The suggestion that no psychiatrist's testimony may be presented with respect to a defendant's future dangerousness is somewhat like asking us to disinvent the wheel." He went on to say, "We are unconvinced ... that the adversary process cannot be trusted to sort out the reliable from the unreliable evidence."[10]

Future dangerousness involves prediction and, hence, is always problematical—a bit of crystal-ball gazing. In a decision handed down in 2000, *Saldano v. Texas*,[11] the Supreme Court vacated a death sentence issued by a Texas court to an Argentine man convicted of a murder committed during a robbery. Under Texas law, the jury deciding on a sentence of death is to consider whether the defendant presents "a continuing threat to society," and in this case, Walter Quijano, a clinical psychologist who testified as the prosecution's expert witness, told the jurors they could take into account the fact that Hispanics were "over represented" in prison compared to their population and might, therefore, be considered dangerous. In statistical terms, ethnicity or gender is correlated—not causative—with dangerousness, but that may not be mentioned by the expert (though ethnicity or gender is apparent to the jury). Ruling that ethnicity had been improperly injected into the sentencing process, the Supreme Court held that the sentencing hearing had violated the defendant's rights to equal protection and due process, and, therefore, vacated the sentence for a new hearing "in which race is not considered."[12] In an earlier case, in 1986, *Skipper v. South Carolina*,[13] a majority of the Supreme Court said that the defendant's behavior in jail between the time of his arrest and trial is indicative of future behavior and, hence, good behavior during that time should be considered as a mitigating factor in the sentencing consideration.[14] In 1992, the Supreme Court ruled that the defendant has a right to inform the jury that because of earlier criminal convictions, he would be ineligible for parole if he were sentenced to life in prison rather than death.[15]

In *Lockett* in 1978, the aforementioned case, the Supreme Court said that in a capital case the accused is entitled under the Eighth and Fourteenth Amendments to present, in all but the rarest kind of capital case, "any aspect of [his] character or records, and any circumstances of the offense that [he] proffers as a basis for a sentence less than death."[16] A statute that restricts mitigating factors is unconstitutional, Chief Justice Burger wrote, because it "creates the risk that the death penalty will be imposed in spite of actions that may call for a less severe penalty." However, Justice Burger noted that "nothing in this opinion limits the traditional authority of a court to exclude, as irrelevant, evidence not bearing on the defendant's character, prior record, or the circumstances of [his] offense."[17] Put another way, for relevancy, the extenuating circumstances must have a causal nexus to the crime. Justice Burger also noted that no opinion is expressed as to whether the need to deter certain kinds of homicide would justify a mandatory death sentence, as, for example, when a prisoner—or escapee—under a life sentence is found guilty of murder.[18]

Commentators have argued that the defendant should be permitted to offer any evidence that might persuade the jury not to impose a death sentence, including evidence calling into question the morality or efficacy of the death penalty or describing the process of execution.[19] The Georgia Supreme Court allowed testimony from the defendant's grandfather that he did not want his grandson executed for killing his parents, though other courts have declined to allow that kind of testimony.[20] Under the Federal Death Penalty Statute and various state statutes, the defendant is allowed to present evidence of any mitigating circumstance. In *Eddings v. Oklahoma*,[21] the U.S. Supreme Court reversed a death sentence because the sentencing court declined to consider that evidence of "a difficult family history and of emotional disturbance" may constitute relevant mitigating evidence. Evidence was presented that the defendant had an antisocial personality.[22]

Various courts do not permit the defendant to testify to his innocence at the penalty phase.[23] In any event, arguing residual doubt may be counter-productive. Studies show that jurors are more likely to sentence to death when a defendant does not show some acknowledgment of the killing and refuses to accept any responsibility.[24] The Model Penal Code provides that "… [i]n the proceeding, evidence may be presented as to any matter the Court deems relevant to sentence, including but not limited to the nature and circumstances of the crime, the defendant's character, background, history, mental and physical condition, and any of the aggravating or mitigating circumstances enumerated in [the Code]."[25]

It is bewildering what is considered as an aggravating or mitigating circumstance. One thing is certain: Defense counsel is obliged to investigate or present evidence relating to the defendant's childhood, educational difficulties, or mental infirmity. That would seem relevant to understanding how the defendant came to be the person that he is, not as to whether he should be sentenced to death. The real consideration ought to be the circumstances of the crime and the characteristics of the offender, not his full life story. The evidence of mitigating circumstances that is offered defies common sense (but the defense attorney is obliged to present it). It is, in essence, a plea for mercy. For example, of Ronell Wilson, who killed two detectives, it was said that he had a miserable childhood, that there were roaches everywhere, he took beatings, and sucked his thumb long past infancy.[26]

Shortly after *Eddings*, the Alabama Supreme Court in a similar case, *Clisby v. State*,[27] stated, "[E]vidence was presented that the defendant had an antisocial personality. Here, the defendant's mental or emotional disturbance must be considered as relevant mitigating evidence." In

State v. Caldwell,[28] the South Carolina Supreme Court held that evidence of antisocial personality that made it difficult for the defendant to obey laws warranted an instruction on the statutory mitigating factor of mental disorder. In this case, a psychiatrist testified for the defense that after his examination of the defendant, his opinion was that he had an "antisocial personality that is synonymous with a psychopathic personality." He described the condition as one in which an individual is not constrained by societal norms. He also stated that if given the opportunity, the defendant could repeat the act and kill again. In reaching his diagnosis, the psychiatrist used a list of criteria suggesting that the disorder begins early in life. The South Carolina Supreme Court concluded, "Because this evidence raised the inference that [the defendant] was suffering from a mental disorder at the time the murder was committed, the trial judge erred in failing to instruct the statutory mitigating circumstances."[29] In other cases, as in *Barefoot v. Estelle*, sociopathy is considered an aggravating circumstance.[30]

The new death penalty laws did not create a new ethical dilemma for psychiatrists, as sometimes alleged. Actually, as fanciful as the courtroom testimony may seem, it is the same type of testimony that is presented in reports and testimony in all types of cases affecting the verdict or sentence, and it has a long history of use in death penalty cases, both in the imposition and in the execution of the penalty. Clarence Darrow decided that the best chance of saving Richard Loeb and Nathan Leopold from execution was to plead them guilty to first-degree murder and then to introduce psychiatric testimony in the form of a plea for mitigation of sentence.

The post-1970s death penalty in the United States bears a striking resemblance to South African law enacted in 1935, which provided that the death penalty may be avoided when there are extenuating circumstances. No definition of extenuating circumstances was given in the law, but they are recognized to be facts associated with a crime that diminish morally, although not legally, the degree of the prisoner's guilt. Among the more important circumstances that were considered in South Africa were mental condition, provocation and other emotional disturbances, intoxication, belief in witchcraft, compulsion, absence of premeditation, youth, political and social and other not ignoble motives, minor degree of participation, repentance and endeavors to assist the victim before *actus reus* is complete, and consent by the victim. Usually, the presence of extenuating circumstances can be determined on the basis of the evidence given before the verdict, but on occasion, it was stated, it may be desirable for the prosecutor and the defense to present evidence and arguments before the sentence is passed because the question arises only after the verdict. The onus of proof of such extenuating circumstances rests on the accused. Likewise, the post-1970s American statutes allow psychiatric testimony to determine whether the death penalty should be imposed. With the demise of apartheid, South Africa abolished the death penalty, as have most other countries.[31]

The typical contemporary capital sentencing statute in the United States sets out a list of both aggravating and mitigating factors, much as did the South African statute. The prosecution must establish, usually by proof beyond a reasonable doubt, of at least one of the aggravating factors. The statutes do not inform the fact finder how to balance the aggravating and mitigating circumstances. These aggravating and mitigating factors call for the participation of psychiatrists or psychologists. Almost without exception, offenders charged with a capital offense have a similar history: they grew up in fractured families marked by drugs, alcohol, violence, and mental illness. Psychiatrist Dorothy Lewis and colleagues studied 14 death row inmates who had committed particularly heinous crimes and found that all but one had a history of severe and sometimes bizarre abuse,[32] but one might wonder, what difference should that make as to the importance of the death penalty?

Supreme Court Justices Blackmun, Scalia, and Thomas have noted that the mandate of unlimited mitigating circumstances has resulted in an arbitrary system. Today's sentencing scheme is also arbitrary because of undefined aggravating factors, unlimited nonstatutory aggravating factors, and victim impact evidence.[33] Phrases such as "relishing of the murder," "gratuitous violence," and "senselessness of the murder" are open to broad interpretation.[34] The courts also have upheld the use of lack of remorse as a nonstatutory aggravating circumstance.[35] Another use of nonstatutory aggravating circumstances is the admission of victim impact statements.[36] The Supreme Court outlawed capital punishment in 1972 because states were arbitrarily imposing it, but the imposition of the death penalty under the new laws is no less arbitrary.

About two-thirds of state capital sentencing statutes expressly incorporate one or more of the mitigating factors listed in the American Law Institute's Model Penal Code, to wit: (1) whether the defendant was suffering from "extreme mental or emotional disturbance" at the time of the offense, (2) whether "the capacity of the defendant to appreciate the criminality of his conduct or to conform his conduct to the requirements of law was impaired as a result of mental disease or defect or intoxication," and (3) whether "the murder was committed under circumstances that the defendant believed to provide a moral justification or extenuation of his conduct."[37]

Two categories of killers (to wit, minors and the mentally retarded) are exempted from the death penalty. In a decision handed down in 2005, *Roper v. Simmons*,[38] the Supreme Court, in a 5–4 decision, barred the imposition of the death penalty for a murder committed by one under 18 years of age. A decade and a half earlier, in 1989, in *Stanford v. Kentucky*,[39] the Court held that the Eighth Amendment prohibition on cruel and unusual punishment does not bar execution of those over age 15 at the time of their crime. In the years following *Stanford*, Justice Kennedy wrote in *Simmons* that a national consensus has emerged that such use of capital punishment is cruel and unusual, but 20 states allowed such executions. (In an appendix to the opinion, the laws in various states dealing with minors are set out.) The heart of Kennedy's opinion, however, was his reliance on international evidence to reach his conclusion. With characteristic asperity, Justice Scalia noted, "To invoke alien law when it agrees with one's own thinking, and ignore it otherwise, is not reasoned decision making, but sophistry."

At the age of 17, when a junior in high school, Christopher Simmons, the defendant in the case, said he wanted to murder someone. In chilling, callous terms he talked about his plans, discussing it for the most part with two younger friends. He proposed to commit burglary and murder by breaking and entering, tying up a victim, and throwing the victim from a bridge. He assured his friends they could "get away with it" because they were minors. Using duct tape to cover the victim's eyes and mouth and bind her hands, they drove to a park and threw the victim from a bridge, drowning her in the water below. An *amicus* brief submitted by the American Psychiatric Association pointed out that the brain of the average 17-year-old is too immature to render the person fully morally accountable.[40] The court did not mention the brief in its opinion, but instead based its decision, 5–4, on the national consensus that had developed against the execution of juvenile offenders. In the majority opinion, Justice Kennedy wrote, "The reality that juveniles still struggle to define their identity means it is less supportable to conclude that even a heinous crime committed by a juvenile is evidence of irretrievable depraved character." He referred, citing the *Diagnostic and Statistical Manual of Mental Disorders* (DSM), to the "rule forbidding psychiatrists from diagnosing any patient under 18 as having antisocial personality disorder."[41]

Three years earlier, in 2002, in *Atkins v. Virginia*,[42] the Court held that the Eighth Amendment barred the execution of a mentally retarded defendant. Daryl Atkins, whose intelligence quotient (IQ) was tested at 59, was convicted in 1996 of killing a truck driver in a carjacking and robbery. The Court set out a presumptive IQ threshold of 70. The Court left undecided whether there are constitutional constraints on the definition of and procedures for determining mental retardation in capital cases. Of course, a declaration that teenagers under age 18 and the retarded must be spared makes irrelevant the issue of proper death penalty jury instructions.[43]

While mental illness is listed as a mitigating factor in sentencing, and mental illness at the time of execution is a basis for a stay of execution, jurors concede (in posttrial interviews) that they consider it an aggravating factor.[44] At trial, jurors are not obliged—indeed, are not permitted—to explain the basis for their verdicts. Studies find a strong correlation between the unsuccessful assertion of an insanity defense and a death sentence. Indeed, a failed insanity defense is one of the most accurate predictors of who will receive the death penalty. Unless the mental illness can be disconnected from dangerousness, defense counsel is best advised not to argue mental illness. Based on interviews with 187 jurors who served on 53 capital cases, Professor Stephen Garvey found that jurors were "more likely to have found the defendant frightening to be near" when the killing was the "work of a madman" or the defendant was "vicious like a mad animal."[45]

In a Georgia case, trial counsel was aware that the defendant, William Lipham, had been institutionalized in mental hospitals, children's homes, and treatment centers and that his records noted several behavioral problems, anxiety disorders, head injuries, and a possible learning disability. The mitigation defense consisted of turning over the 2,500 pages of records to the jury and asking it to look for mitigating evidence itself. The Georgia Supreme Court held that this presentation of mitigating evidence without a mental health expert to evaluate it—along with the expectation that the jury would read all 2,500 pages and understand them without guidance—was unreasonable and constituted ineffective assistance of counsel. This deficiency, the court said, was prejudicial because without it Lipham might not have been sentenced to death.[46]

Proof of an adverse impact on the victim's family (by victim impact testimony) has been held not to relieve the prosecution of its burden to prove beyond a reasonable doubt at least one aggravating circumstance that has been alleged.[47]

An extensive study involving interviews with hundreds of people who have served as jurors in death penalty cases revealed that jurors often misunderstand what will happen to the defendant if they decide not to impose the death penalty, or they believe that their decision is merely advisory, or they misunderstand which factors can and cannot be considered, what level of proof is required, and what degree of concurrence is required for aggravating and mitigating factors.[48]

Professor William Bowers and colleagues found that 48.3% of 864 capital jurors surveyed, drawn from seven states, had predetermined life or death by the conclusion of the guilt phase of the trial, with 28.6% electing death and 19.7% life (51.7% were undecided).[49] Professor Marla Sandys stated that "the data reveal quite dramatically that … the majority of jurors reach their decisions about guilt and punishment at the same time."[50] The finding may not be surprising given that prospective jurors who are opposed to the death penalty are disqualified from serving on the jury. The Supreme Court has held that the Constitution does not prohibit the states from death-qualifying juries in capital cases.[51]

Carrying Out the Death Penalty

Although there may seem to be some novelty in the use of psychiatric testimony to determine whether the death penalty should be imposed, psychiatric testimony has been used for decades to determine the executionability of a person condemned to death. In the first situation, the psychiatrist may be called as a witness to testify whether or not the death penalty ought to be imposed. In the latter situation, the psychiatrist may be called to testify whether it ought to be carried out.

In several ways execution of the death sentence can be avoided. After the trial stage is completed in a capital case, as in other cases, the court machinery continues to operate for some time. The jury's decision is blocked by further litigation and seemingly endless hearings. Legal delays took up 14 years in the case of John Wayne Gacy, who killed 33 young men, though he confessed to the killings and his guilt was never in doubt. He had 523 separate appeals, none of them based on a claim of innocence.

Appeals are made at all levels of the state courts as well as the federal courts. In capital cases, it is said, the courts must be emphatically sure: "No man shall be executed while there is the slightest doubt either as to his guilt or as to the legality of the process by which his guilt was determined." Appellate courts carefully scan the transcript; error is often uncovered and deemed prejudicial, which would have been overlooked in noncapital cases.

Due to the gravity of the sentence, and the obligation of the state to ensure fairness, various jurisdictions impose restrictions on the right of a prisoner to forego appeals (the prisoner must have sufficient rational ability to waive appeals).[52]

The courts are not commended, however, but bitterly criticized for their scrutiny of capital cases. It has been said, "The whole procedure is insane," "the lengthy procedure in capital cases is the enduring shame of American judicial procedure." These criticisms are commonplace because the basis of appeal or writ of *habeas corpus* is recognized as often frivolous. Time and again, a new dodge will appear, a writ will be taken, and years will pass. Any argument is useful. For example, when a black was sentenced to death, the objection of jury discrimination was regularly urged, even when the trial was eminently fair and the black defendant, in fact, would not have wanted blacks sitting on the jury. In one case in California, not especially unusual, there were eight trials, costing the state over $500,000. It is estimated today that a capital case in the United States costs between a half million and a million dollars, draining the treasury and absorbing a great deal of time (other countries having a death penalty do not incur such costs).[53] William Shakespeare said in a different context, "If it were done, when, 'tis done, then 'twere well/it were done quickly."

When court procedures are finally exhausted, when review is no longer pending, the fate of the prisoner passes into the hands of the executive branch of the government, which, under the United States system, is charged with carrying out or executing the orders of the judiciary. It has been generally assumed that the jury's decision imposing the death penalty is carried out—at least following appeals. But what actually has happened at this stage?

In many jurisdictions, the governor has to order the execution, and he often avoids the decision as long as possible. Reprieves have been commonplace. He could, definitively, avoid the execution by pardon or by commutation of the death sentence to a prison term. Governors often hesitated to intervene in this way, however, because they felt they would be usurping the power of the court. Twelve jurors—not the governor—listened at the trial. Interposition often occurred in another way.

The warden (or sheriff) having custody of the prisoner plays a principal role in the implementation of the penalty. The execution of the penalty depends very much on the attitude of the warden toward the penalty and whether he will attest to the incompetency or insanity of the condemned person. The issue of competency to be executed becomes relevant when the date of execution has been set.

In cases tried at common law, execution often followed fairly quickly after trial, so that incompetence at the time of execution was linked as a practical matter with incompetence at the trial itself. No longer. Years may elapse nowadays between the time of trial and time of execution. Gerald Mitchell was age 33 when executed in 2001 for a murder he committed at age 17 in 1984. In *Ford v. Wainwright*,[54] in 1986, the Supreme Court in plurality opinion ruled that the Constitution precludes a state from executing people who have temporarily or permanently become incompetent or insane, but even before 1986. the rule had been well established, either by statute or common law, although the logic behind the rule is vague. In the words of one jurist, "Whatever the reason of the law is, it is plain the law is so." One might argue that, if anyone is to be executed, it should be the criminally insane, but it would go against the sporting theory of justice. One judge, dissenting against the rule, said: "Is it not an inverted humanitarianism that deplores as barbarous the capital punishment of those who have become insane after trial and conviction, but accepts the capital punishment of sane men?" Alvin Ford died a natural death in 1991 while on death row.

In *Ford v. Wainwright*, the plurality did not set forth what standard was applicable in the determination of incompetence or insanity. Justice Powell, the swing vote in the opinion, proposed a standard when he stated in his concurrence that "I would hold that the Eighth Amendment forbids the execution only of those who are unaware of the punishment they are about to suffer and why they are to suffer it." Justice Powell was a voice of one, yet the standard he posited has been embraced by some courts as the constitutional minimum. He discussed in his concurrence the rationale behind the Eighth Amendment prohibition of executing the insane:

> [T]oday as at common law, one of the death penalty's critical justifications, its retributive force, depends on the defendant's awareness of the penalties existence and purpose. Thus, it remains true that executions of the insane both impose a uniquely cruel penalty and are inconsistent with one of the chief purposes of executions generally.[55]

A number of states have more rigorous standards, but none disputes the need to require that those who are executed know the fact of their impending execution and the reason for it.

Justice Powell then addressed the states with more expansive standards in a footnote to his concurring opinion: "States are obviously free to adopt a more expansive view of sanity in this context than the one the Eighth Amendment imposes as a constitutional minimum." This more expansive view is recommended in the American Bar Association Criminal Justice Mental Health Standards. There is a significant common law background for the requirement that a defendant be able to assist in his defense, even after conviction.

Explanations for the exemption rule, as found in the literature, are various. It is said: "If the defendant is sane he might argue some reason not previously considered why the sentence should not be carried out." This theory offers the condemned man a last chance to prove his innocence. Yet the same logic would suffice to postpone, perhaps indefinitely, the execution of a sane man because time for intelligent reflection may disclose new reasons for a stay of execution of the sane as well. To offer another explanation: "Killing an insane person does not have the same moral quality as killing a sane person." The moral basis underlying the forensic responsibility rule at the time of the deed is carried over until the time of execution, although the person was found legally sane and responsible at the time of the deed. A third defense of the rule involves the conception of the self. God would not, on the Great Day, make a person answer for that of which he remembered nothing; he is not the same person. The law likewise says that a man is not subject to execution for a crime when "he is not the same person forensically now which he was then" (but, as Heraclitus long ago explained, "all is flux").[56] Finally, some insist that the rule is based on the lack of retributory satisfaction derived by society in executing an insane person. A related belief is that "a person should not be put to death while insane because in that condition he is unable to make his peace with God." To a modern audience, this argument is hardly convincing, and the condemned man himself often rejects spiritual solace in his final hours and looks instead to a good last meal.

Whatever the underlying reasons, however illogical they may be, the rule has been perpetuated, either by statute or judicial decision, in every state having the death penalty. However, the procedure by which the rule is implemented is slipshod. At common law, the prisoner was brought before a judge who either decided the question of insanity himself or at his discretion impaneled a jury to assist him. But most states in practice, if not in law, entrusted the initial decision to the warden. The condemned person might file a petition for postconviction relief.

The Supreme Court in 1950, in *Solesbee v. Balkom*,[57] said that postponement of execution because of postconviction insanity bears a close affinity not to trial but to reprieves of sentences, which is an executive power, and "seldom, if ever, has this power of executive clemency been subjected to review by the courts." In *Solesbee*, the Court found that Georgia had not violated due process in constituting its governor an "apt and special tribunal" for determining, in *ex parte* proceedings, the sanity of a condemned man at the time of execution. (In federal and military cases, Abraham Lincoln was apparently the first president to intercede in an execution on account of supervening insanity.)

Inquiries have been held entirely behind closed doors without any opportunity for submission of facts on behalf of the person whose sanity is to be determined. It was long recognized that due process does not require that a condemned man who asserts supervening insanity be given a full judicial proceeding to adjudicate his claim. In 1897, in *Nobles v. Georgia*,[58] the Supreme Court said that if such proceedings were required "it would be wholly at the will of a convict to suffer any punishment whatever, for the necessity of his doing so would depend solely upon his fecundity in making suggestion after suggestion of insanity, to be followed by trial upon trial."

In *Solesbee*, the Supreme Court, noting that the governor in deciding on execution had the aid of specifically trained physicians, went on to say:

> It is true that governors and physicians might make errors of judgment. But the search for truth in this field is always beset by difficulties that may beget error. Even judicial determination of sanity might be wrong. … We cannot say that it offends due process to leave the question of a convicted person's sanity to the solemn responsibility of a state's highest executive with authority to invoke the aid of the most skillful class of experts on the crucial questions involved.

The power of the governor was often delegated to agencies, such as pardon and parole boards. In 1958, in *Caritativo v. California*,[59] the Court, extending its decision in *Solesbee*, upheld a procedure whereby the initiation of proceedings to determine the sanity of a condemned man in his custody is made by the warden in his sole judgment. If the warden "has good reason to believe" that a condemned man has become insane, he must so advise the judge or district attorney of the judicial district where the convict was sentenced, and an investigation may be ordered. On some occasions the convicted prisoner is so hated by the correctional officials that they obfuscate evidence of mental disorder.[60]

Justice Harlan in *Caritativo*, said: "Surely it is not inappropriate for [the state] to lodge this grave responsibility in the hands of the warden, the official who beyond all others had had the most intimate relations with, and best opportunity to observe, the prisoner." But Justice Frankfurter, joined by Justices Brennan and Douglas, strongly dissented:

> Now it appears that [the determination of the sanity of a man condemned to death], upon which depends the fearful question of life or death, may … be made on the mere say-so of the warden of a state prison, according to such procedure as he chooses to pursue, and more particularly without any right on the part of a man awaiting death who claims that insanity has supervened to have his case put to the warden. There can hardly be a comparable situation under our constitutional scheme of things in which an interest so great, that an insane man not be executed, is given such flimsy procedural protection and where one asserting a claim is denied the rudimentary right of having his side submitted to the one who sits in judgment.[61]

In its 1986 decision in the aforementioned case of *Ford v. Wainwright*, the Supreme Court found Florida's procedure, which relied on the governor's assessment of clinical reports, as unconstitutional, on three grounds: (1) it provided no opportunity for the condemned individual or his counsel to be heard, (2) it did not permit challenge of the state-employed mental health professionals' findings on the competency issue, and (3) it left the final decision as to competency to the executive, rather than the judicial branch. Although thus ruling Florida's statute unconstitutional, the Court did not explicitly establish a right to counsel at competency proceedings, nor did it require that the condemned individual have a formal opportunity to cross-examine opposing experts or be provided funds for an independent expert.[62] Justice Marshall, who wrote the Court's opinion, suggested that Florida might create a competency procedure similar to that used in the competency-to-stand-trial or civil-commitment contexts, but the majority did not agree on this point, with several members cautioning against requiring, as a constitutional ruling, a full-blown sanity trial.[63]

In a subsequent case involving Thomas Provenzano who was sentenced to death in Florida for murdering a court bailiff, the Florida Supreme Court declared that the state's failure to provide exculpatory information from a mental evaluation did not create reversible error, given the trial counsel's ability to obtain this information from other sources.[64] Six years later, the Florida Supreme Court remanded for a hearing on his competency for execution.[65] A month later, the Florida Supreme Court found that the trial court had abused its discretion for (1) not continuing a hearing so that Provenzano could present psychologist Patricia Fleming, (2) declaring that Fleming was not an expert because she lacked a Ph.D., and (3) refusing to allow Provenzano to cross-examine a state expert.[66] The trial court thereupon held proceedings at which Fleming and other witnesses for both Provenzano and the state gave testimony, and after which defense counsel stated on the record that everything he could offer on Provenzano's behalf had been presented. The trial court determined that Provenzano was competent for execution. The Florida Supreme Court affirmed. Despite his delusions that he was Jesus Christ, Provenzano understood the details of his trial and his conviction, that he is to be executed, and the reasons why. The Florida Supreme Court considered the case troubling, given Provenzano's apparent mental health problems, even though his exaggeration of his symptoms and malingering made determining the exact nature of his condition difficult. However, the Florida Supreme Court, citing the U. S. Supreme Court's decision in *Ford v. Wainwright*, held that the Eighth Amendment requires only that a defendant have an awareness of what penalty he is being given and why he has received it.[67] In 2007, in *Panetti v. Quarterman*,[68] the Supreme Court in a 5–4 decision ruled that the test was too restrictive and does not take into account that the individual may be out of touch with reality on account of delusions.[69]

Challenges to the death penalty stretch the imagination, but leave it to the lawyers and experts to formulate new challenges.

The Trauma of Death Row

A person under a death sentence is sentenced to death; he is not sentenced to prison. He is placed under the custody of the warden. He is not part of the prison population. He is placed in a separate cell.[70] In the United States, where legal maneuvers in capital cases usually take several years, the prisoner during this time sits in isolation on death row. Earlier, during the trial stage, which rarely takes less than a year, he sat in jail, without opportunity for release on bail, and usually without therapy. Following conviction, death even more preys on his mind. In the words of one prisoner: "The days are so long. There is nothing to pass the time. Nothing to keep your mind occupied. I feel like I don't even exist. I'm here and I'm not here. I have headaches. I just want to scream."[71]

Wait long enough and chances are that the prisoner will hallucinate (or he will die a natural death). More likely than not, he will deteriorate. Psychiatrists point out that offenders are usually people who release tension by acting out, by using muscle, and they become very anxious when locked up. Without any activity, they tend to break down and become psychotic. Capital offenders are likely to be unstable anyway, but solitary confinement does much to break down the sanity of the most normal of men, as the experiments of Donald O. Hebb (a Canadian psychologist who was influential in the area of neuropsychology) and others on sensory deprivation have vividly demonstrated. Governor Earl Long once remarked, "Who in hell wouldn't go mad?" (Louisiana at the time of the remark had not carried out an execution in over 10 years.)[72] Tranquilizers are the order of the day.

The condemned man who does not become genuinely psychotic will find it expedient to malinger. He jumps up and down. He seldom does anything correctly. He makes absurd statements. When shown a watch reading 2:30, he may say the time is 6 o'clock. When shown a 50 cent piece, he may call it a dollar bill. Such symptoms are popularly called the nonsense syndrome, and in psychiatry, the Ganser syndrome. The condemned man learns, either through the grapevine or from the subtle advice of his attorney, that under the law insanity precludes execution. As a last-ditch measure, he may act upon this information. The condemned man is entitled to the information, just as a businessman has a right to advice on loopholes in the tax laws.

The following conversation, tape recorded, illustrates the contrivance put on in the prison to affect transfer to the hospital:

> Examiner at Hospital: Tell me what happened at the penitentiary to make them send you to the hospital.
> Patient (formerly prisoner): Nothing.
> Examiner: Huh?
> Patient: My lawyer came and got me.
> Examiner: Your lawyer came and got you? Are you afraid of dying?
> Patient: (No answer.)
> Examiner: Did your lawyer tell you what to do to get out of there?
> Patient: No.
> Examiner: Looks to me like a good lawyer would have told you how to act. He didn't tell you how to act?
> Patient: (Inaudible mumbles.)
> Examiner: I didn't understand you. He told you to act crazy?
> Patient: Uh hum.
> Examiner: What did he say?
> Patient: He kept telling me … (Inaudible).
> Examiner: The last time he came up, what did he do?
> Patient: He asked if I ever had an epileptic fit.
> Examiner: What did you tell him?
> Patient: I told him no.
> Examiner: What did he say then?
> Patient: He said that an epileptic fit was the last straw. [In the lingo, an epileptic fit is the way of a crazy man.]
> Examiner: He told you this?
> Patient: Yes.
> Examiner: Did he tell you how to act?
> Patient: No, he didn't want to incriminate himself.
> Examiner: He told you that he did not want to incriminate himself?
> Patient: That's right.
> Examiner: So, he didn't tell you how to act. But he got his point across to you?
> Patient: (Inaudible.)
> Examiner: Huh? How did you know how to act when he told you about epileptic fits?
> Patient: I just knew.

Sporadic malingering is difficult to prove especially when the motivation to fake is great. In the prison setting, however, as Justice Harlan noted, the individual may be observed on a 24-hour basis; over this period of time, it is difficult to keep up a simulated psychosis. Prison personnel can usually spot an inmate whose bizarre behavior is an act. They know "he's not a real psycho." The problem becomes more difficult when an unstable person begins to fake mental illness, and then, like a man running downhill, finds he cannot stop.

Happily for the condemned man, prison officials in most states have usually closed their eyes to the simulation. Who wants to pull the switch? The condemned man's keepers get to know him, and they develop some feeling for him. As they dislike executing anyone, they have tended to accept feigned craziness as genuine. So, ostensibly for observation or treatment, the condemned man has been referred to a prison psychiatrist or transferred to the security area of a mental hospital (the criminally insane section) where he usually has lived out the rest of his days, often as a trusty (a convict regarded as trustworthy and, thus, granted special privileges).

One easily believes what one wishes to believe. Wardens and psychiatrists, perhaps for different reasons, can readily find a symptom of madness. There is always evidence available, however episodic, to warrant a stay of execution. The Supreme Court has conceded, "The search for truth in this field is always beset by difficulties that may beget error." The law has long recognized that people may have lucid intervals and nonlucid intervals. Psychiatrists use labels such as "dissociative states" and "three-day schizophrenia." We are disoriented when we wake up in the morning and when we are asleep. We "pull ourselves together." We all have "crazy spells." We question at times the judgment of our best friends and colleagues, and at such times we call them crazy. It is not possible to have a touch of pregnancy, but it is possible to have a touch of psychosis; the latter is not an all-or-none condition. Part of one's personality may be affected by a psychotic process, but the remnants of the ego may function properly. Given the type of person who commits a capital crime, mental and emotional aberrations of marked degree are readily in evidence. There is also the syndrome in which the prisoner thinks he is malingering, and the warden or psychiatrist knows the prisoner thinks so, but justifiably considers him crazy nonetheless.

There is a direct corollary between the number and the location of executions. The carrying out of the death penalty has depended to a marked degree on whether the chair is moved around from jailhouse to jailhouse or whether all condemned persons are sent to a centralized place—the state penitentiary—for execution. During the past 20 or 30 years, many states have enacted legislation providing that executions are to be carried out at the state penitentiary rather than at the various county jails. Legislators, possessing the ability to see problems in both ideological and financial terms, realize it is expensive and cumbersome to transport the chair from jail to jail.

When execution of the death penalty is to take place in the local or county jail, it is more likely to be carried out. For one reason, the condemned man, when in the state penitentiary, far removed from the scene of the crime, is more likely to be forgotten by an enraged community than if he remained in close proximity to the scene of the crime. For another, the warden of a penitentiary is in a position very different from that of the sheriff of a local jailhouse. The warden is practically a feudal lord, and his attitude is likely to be every bit as imperious. He feels the inherent power of his position, and he is usually willing to exercise the broad discretion to postpone invested in him by law.

In former times, it was customary for an execution to take place as near as possible to the scene of the crime. A nearby tree was selected or a gallows was erected in a large open space in the town. By the 1930s, with a few exceptions, public executions disappeared from the American scene. Citizens organized to prohibit public executions because, as reports in newspapers of the time disclose, "the crowds often assumed the characteristics of a mob and often indulged in the wildest and most unrestrained orgies." The executions incited widespread agitation, brawling, drunkenness, and crime. Many good citizens got carried away in the heat and violence of the moment and participated in some dreadful acts. So executions were first moved from outdoors to inside the local jailhouse, and then gradually, as noted, from the local jailhouse to the state penitentiary. But what happened there?

The population of the state penitentiary is large, and the atmosphere there is ordinarily tense. It becomes volatile whenever there is an execution. The macabre event provokes brawling and violence among the convicts, as it formerly did on the outside among the citizenry. The warden is motivated to defer the execution not only because he has some feelings for the condemned man, but also because he values his job. All administrators want things to run smoothly. Unpleasant publicity is the bane of officialdom, and riots make ugly headlines.

However, headlines of a different nature may exert influence on the warden in the other direction. The more publicity attending the trial, the more famous or notorious the criminal, the more likely the execution. In such cases, the warden rarely "has good reason to believe" that the prisoner has become insane, and he finds it expedient not to initiate an investigation. Fredric Wertham, psychiatrist and writer, was denied permission to see Ethel Rosenberg when she was at Sing Sing, but in earlier interviews, her attorney reported her as in despair, without lipstick or makeup, her hair uncombed, "not caring how she looked." In Kansas, a young man, Lee Andrews, was sentenced to death for the murder of his parents. He was a university student and spent his time in his cell reading books. He did not act crazy. In addition, prominent citizens intervened asking executive clemency, much to the annoyance of the governor. The case was headlined in the papers. As a result, widespread attention focused on Andrews, and he was executed. California regularly executes its condemned men (following a protracted and expensive judicial process), but even outside California, Caryl Chessman probably would have been executed. The eyes of the world were upon him. Ironically, he protested too much. He made too much noise, and he protested via book writing—the mark of a rational man.

In *Caritativo*, it was held proper for the state to condition a condemned man's right to a sanity investigation upon a preliminary determination by the warden that "good reason exists for the belief that the convict has become insane." More often than not, the various reasons underlying the rule of "competency to be executed" merge or fade away into the simple statement: "You're not supposed to execute someone who doesn't know what's happening." Theoretically, mental illness, of itself, is not sufficient to bring into operation the rule of suspension of execution. Mental illness as a legal concept is not identical with the medical concept of the term. It may be that a person who does not know what is happening is mentally ill, but mental illness alone is not the test. Indeed, a person may be mentally well, but nonetheless may not know what is happening; for example, a person of very low intelligence.

Actually, the test on executionability is void of meaning. In actuality, it would not even exempt the blithering idiot. It is a fiction designed to avoid an execution. In several recent rulings the Supreme Court made no reference to the reasons for the rule, but simply said, in dictum, that it is unlawful to execute a prisoner who has become incompetent or insane after his conviction. Theory notwithstanding, medical status of itself thus serves as a haven from legal action.

Although in *Caritativo*, the Supreme Court specifically stated that wardens are not obliged to obtain a psychiatric examination of the condemned man, they have as a general practice delegated the responsibility to a prison psychiatrist or, with the authorization of the trial court, have transferred him to the security treatment area of a mental hospital for examination and treatment. In this way, the warden guarantees "a responsible and good-faith determination," and he is usually satisfied with the result. The trial court invariably will postpone execution, without a date, when it receives a psychiatric report stating that the condemned man does not realize he is to be executed for the crime he has committed.[73]

To review, the jury (a group so large that individual responsibility is lost) relieves the judge of the death penalty decision at the trial. The judge then transfers the condemned man to the warden who is able to delegate the responsibility to the psychiatrist. Thus, in the end, the decision on execution of the death penalty is essentially left to one individual—the psychiatrist. He is given a nonmedical—and absurd—responsibility. He is asked to report back to the warden when "this man is ready to be electrocuted."

Professor Albert Ehrenzweig of the University of California Law School compared the procedure to a game of ping pong, but this is hardly an apt comparison.[74] The psychiatrist knows that the warden does not want him to make a return play. He rarely reports that his patient, regardless of his mental status, is "ready to be electrocuted," although, as a matter of fact, in this age of tranquilizing drugs, a man could readily be shaped up for execution. The ethical guideline of the American Academy of Psychiatry and the Law calling for "honesty and striving for objectivity" in an evaluation tends to fall by the wayside.

While death may be postponed for the condemned man while in the security treatment unit, his stay there does not always encourage forgetfulness of his sentence. With inadequate facilities, attendants, and security protection, mental hospitals find discipline a stiff problem in these units. Consequently, prisoners transferred from the penitentiary to the hospital are warned that misbehavior will result in their being sent back "to fry." The capital penalty abolitionist may take note that, here, recalcitrant persons already condemned to death can be deterred by the threat of execution. Every now and then, the hospital director, to show he means business, returns an unruly inmate to the penitentiary—and to his death. This accounts for many of the executions in states where, according to statistics, they occur sporadically.

Another punitive practice in the security treatment unit of many hospitals involved the conversion of electroconvulsive treatment (ECT) from a therapy to a threat. In ordinary psychiatric practice, ECT is the somatic therapy of choice in cases of depression. Its potential as a punishment, however, is obvious: a little electricity cures, but it hurts, and too much kills. Furthermore, for a man facing the electric chair, the psychological implications in the threat of being "buzzed" can well be imagined.

None of these unpleasant procedures for controlling the condemned man in the hospital's security area, however, seems half as bizarre on a close look as authority's reason for putting him there. The psychiatrist is asked to treat the prisoner (patient). To what end? Why, so that he may be electrocuted! This goal of therapy is, indeed, a curious footnote to the Hippocratic oath. Little wonder that the psychiatrist, with a prisoner on his hands who has been brought out of his psychotic state by ECT or drugs, fails to report that the man is "ready to be electrocuted." The psychiatrist knows that such a statement from him is tantamount to an endorsement of the death penalty, so he is likely to play it cool and do nothing or use delaying tactics. Ordinarily, he is not in sympathy with the death penalty, but, in any event, he feels that the decision is not for him to make. "Who is fit to be executed?" is a moral, not a scientific inquiry.

Society cannot fairly blame the psychiatrist for taking the law into his own hands. As Dr. Menninger said, "Most psychiatrists dislike very much being called in when somebody wants to know if the accused is well enough so that his head may be chopped off. I don't think the psychiatrist is very interested in acting as assistant to the executioner."[75] Clearly, psychiatrists share the understandable human trait of being reluctant to push a person down the road to death. Moreover, they are doctors whose training and credo aim to preserve life, not to hasten its ending. Their attitude toward the condemned man as patient is readily explained. For many years, Dr. Alfred Freedman and Dr. Abraham Halpern have sought to establish an ethical rule that would prohibit physician participation in legally authorized executions.[76]

The mode of carrying out the death penalty has evolved over the years. The idea of a mechanical form of execution was used in Renaissance Italy and early modern Germany, where it was known as the falling axe or the falling sword. In 1792, Dr. Ignace-Joseph Guillotin, the leading medical authority of the French Revolution, introduced a few minor modifications and the machine he perfected was declared as the sole method of decapitation. The machine removed the status inequalities attached to the variety of pre-Revolutionary capital punishments, in which the nobility were executed with honor and the commonality dispatched with infamy.

In the United States, the Eighth Amendment's prohibition of "cruel and unusual punishments" led to legislative changes in the method of execution. Five different types of execution methods have been used in the United States: hanging, firing squad, electrocution, lethal gas, and lethal injection. As a result of mishaps, hanging came to be regarded as inhumane. Death by firing squad came to be regarded as too bloody and uncontrolled. Electrocution and gas chambers proved no better. For a time, lethal injection appeared to be the sole method of execution accepted by the courts as humane enough to satisfy the requirements of the Eighth Amendment—mainly because it medicalizes the process (Missouri carries out the execution in a prison hospital room).[77] But not only opponents of the death penalty, but also those in the medical field have balked. In 1992, the American Medical Association adopted a provision that specifically forbids any participation in executions, with the exception of prescribing sedation beforehand and later signing the death certificate.[78] Actually, physicians are not needed to carry out an execution. Properly trained personnel can carry it out.

Litigation has raised the question of forcibly medicating a condemned person in order to render him competent to be executed. In *Perry v. Louisiana*,[79] the trial court, after sentencing Perry to death, but finding him incompetent to be executed unless maintained on medication, ordered that he be forcibly medicated to ensure his competence. After exhausting state court remedies, Perry sought relief from the U.S. Supreme Court. It remanded the case for reconsideration in light of its decision in 1990, which allowed forcible medication of penitentiary inmates only when considered medically appropriate.[80] On remand, the Louisiana Supreme Court ruled it impermissible to forcibly medicate individuals to render them competent to be executed.[81] Since then, Louisiana, Maryland, and South Carolina provide for the commutation of a death sentence to life imprisonment without parole when the individual is found incompetent to be executed. They now do not ask psychiatrists to medicate a death row inmate so as to render him rational enough to be put to death.[82]

The question arises whether a physician's decision to treat an ill individual should be dependent on what lies ahead for the individual. Should a physician who is a pacifist decline to treat an ill individual who plans to enter the military service? Should a physician who has a negative view of homosexuality decline to treat an ill individual who will continue to engage in homosexual activity? Should a physician decline to treat an ill individual on death row only when the date of execution has been set? In any event, the odds are against the actual carrying out of the death penalty.[83]

But what about the law—the law of the land—that shall prevail? How do we explain this reluctance, this dalliance and indecision that has marked the course of the law all along the way from death sentence to death row? Although the ultimate punishment issue has evoked national debate for at least a century and a half, it is clear that by a cumbersome and slipshod method, the penalty was, in effect, eliminated long before the Supreme Court's decision in 1972 voiding jury discrimination in sentencing. After the penalty was reinstated in 1976, it took 12 years to carry out 100 executions. Now there are calls to expedite the process. No member of the Court adheres to the view long held by the late Justices Thurgood Marshall and William J. Brennan, Jr., that the death penalty is an affront to a civilized society, let alone the position adopted by Justice Harry A. Blackmun at the end of his career that the "machinery of death," as he called it, was simply not as fair in practice as the Court had deemed it to be in theory by upholding new state death penalty laws in 1976 and permitting the states to resume executions.[84]

Opponents of the death penalty once made broad calls for abolition by arguing that executing people was immoral. Now, while that argument is still made, opponents are focusing their attacks on questions of fairness, racial bias, and guilt or innocence. Skepticism toward and resistance to the death penalty have been building since the late 1990s, after investigations found a number of wrongful convictions.[85] That and the cost of a death penalty case and existing moral objections to it have prompted a number of states to place a moratorium on executions, which have dropped from a yearly high of 98 in 1999 to 53 in 2006. During the 1990s, courts would issue about 300 death sentences annually. Those numbers have plummeted to 128 in 2005 and 102 in 2006.

While the number of death sentences imposed by juries and the number of actual executions are falling, the Supreme Court's interest in capital punishment goes unabated. More than 10% of the cases argued before the Justices from October 2006 to April 2007 involved death row inmates. Chief Justice John Roberts, a dissenter in 6 of the Court's 10 most recent rulings, wrote that contrary to being clear, Supreme Court death penalty law over the years has been a "dog's breakfast," a mess of "divided, conflicted, and ever-changing analyses."[86]

The states are rethinking the death sentence. In 2007, the Nebraska legislature came within one vote of repealing its death penalty law. The new governor of Maryland called for the repeal of the capital penalty, but a legislative committee rejected his plea. New Jersey lawmakers have considered a repeal of that state's death penalty. The governor of Virginia, whose 96 executions since 1976 are exceeded only by Texas, vetoed five bills in 2007 that would have expanded the use of capital punishment. The Montana Senate approved the abolition of the death penalty in 2007, but a House committee defeated the measure. In New Mexico, the House approved a repeal, but a Senate committee said no. Even Texas is wavering.[87]

Be that as it may, opinion polls consistently show support for the death penalty. In years past, and still today, the capacity-to-stand-execution procedure, via the executive department, in many cases achieved the functional abolition of the death penalty. The repugnance felt for the death penalty emerged cloaked as a rational medical decision. Perhaps this was not a chance achievement.

Endnotes

1. D. Frum, "The Justice Americans Demand," *New York Times*, Feb. 4, 2000, p. 27. Most of the death sentences and executions occur in a few states, notably in California, Florida, Texas, and Virginia. A succinct history of the death penalty in the United States appears in C. Crossen, "Use of Death Penalty Over Decades Points to Conflicted Opinion," *Wall Street Journal*, May 7, 2007, p. B1. As of January 2007, the number on death row in California was 660 and the number of executions since 1976 was 13. Texas is special. It now accounts for nearly half of all executions in the United States, of which there have been over 1,000 since 1976. The FBI's crime statistics for 2005 show that the murder rate per 100,000 people in Washington, D.C., which does not have the death penalty, was 35.4, whereas in Texas it was 6.2. See the listing in the various states in "Capital Punishment in America," *Economist*, Sept. 1, 2007, pp. 20–22. Reflections on the death penalty appear in R.J. Acker, R.M. Bohm, & C.S. Lanier (Eds.), *America's Experiment with Capital Punishment* (Durham: Carolina Academic Press, 2nd ed., 2003).
2. The court ruled in three cases, all involving black defendants, one of them for a robbery–murder, and two for rape; Furman v. Georgia, 408 U. S. 238 (1972). The death penalty is on the statute books of all states except 14—Alaska, Hawaii, Iowa, Maine, Massachusetts, Michigan, Minnesota, New Mexico, North Dakota, Oregon, Rhode Island, Vermont, West Virginia, and Wisconsin. The history of the abolitionist movement is related in M. Meltsner, *Cruel and Unusual: The Supreme Court and Capital Punishment* (New York: Random House, 1973).
3. 428 U.S. 280 (1976).
4. Following the invalidation of North Carolina's mandatory death penalty, James Woodson was resentenced to life in prison. In 1991, he was paroled from prison, and in 1993, he completed his sentence and was discharged from parole. In December 2000, he was a minister of a church in North Carolina.
5. 438 U. S. 586 (1978).
6. 438 U. S. at 604. As a result of the Supreme Court's decision, Sandra Lockett's death sentence was reduced to life imprisonment and, in 2000, she was paroled from prison.
7. 463 U. S. 880 (1983).

8. See P. Appelbaum, "Hypotheticals, Psychiatric Testimony, and the Death Sentence," *Bull. Am. Acad. Psychiat. & Law* 12 (1984): 169; R. Slovenko, "Psychiatric Opinion Without Examination," *J. Psychiat. & Law* 28 (2000): 103. Thomas Barefoot was executed by lethal injection in Texas in 1984.

9. By and large, psychiatrists who testify in capital cases are criticized by psychiatrists who are opposed to the death penalty (the vast majority of psychiatrists), whether or not the psychiatrist testifies on the basis of an examination and not simply on the basis of a hypothetical. See F. D. Master, "Alvaro Calambro: Competency to Be Executed," *Am. J. Foren. Psychiat.* 20 (1999): 17.

10. 463 U. S. at 896. Trial judges continued to appoint Dr. Grigson to evaluate the defendant for the imposition of the death penalty or for competency to be executed. See, e.g., Caldwell v. Johnson, 226 F.3d 367 (5th Cir. 2000); Bennett v. State, 766 S.W.2d 227 (Tex. Cr. App. 1989). In a lengthy dissent in *Bennett*, Judge Teague criticized the appointment of Dr. Grigson, or Dr. Death as he was known. He suggested that whenever Dr. Grigson is appointed, the defendant should stop what he is then doing and commence writing out his last will and testament because he will in all probability soon be ordered by the trial judge to suffer a premature death; 766 S.W.2d at 232.

11. 120 S. Ct. 2214 (2000).

12. On remand to the Texas Court of Criminal Appeals, the court questioned the authority of the attorney general to confess error in the United States Supreme Court and to seek a new sentencing trial.

13. 476 U.S. 1(1986).

14. Ronald Skipper waived his right to jury resentencing and was resentenced by a newly assigned judge to life in prison with the possibility of parole. He was denied parole in 2000.

15. Simmons v. South Carolina, 512 U. S. 154 (1992).

16. 438 U. S. at 604.

17. 438 U. S. at 605.

18. *Ibid.*

19. R.J. Bonnie, A.M. Coughlin, J.C. Jeffries, & P.W. Low, *Criminal Law* (Westbury, NY: Foundation Press, 1997), p. 725; B. S. Ledewitz, "The Requirement of Death: Mandatory Language in Pennsylvania Death Penalty Statute," *Duq. L. Rev.* 21 (1982): 103.

20. Romine v. State, 251 Ga. 208, 305 S.E.2d 93 (1983). In Payne v. Tennessee, 501 U.S. 808 (1991), the Supreme Court, overruling two of its earlier decisions, held that the Eighth Amendment erects no per se bar prohibiting a capital sentencing jury from considering "victim impact" evidence. A state may legitimately conclude that evidence about the victim and about the impact of the murder on the victim's family is relevant to the jury's decision as to whether the death penalty should be imposed; 501 U.S. at 827. See J.R. Acker & D.R. Karp (Eds.), *Wounds That Do Not Bind: Victim-Based Perspectives on the Death Penalty* (Durham, NC: Carolina Academic Press, 2006).

21. 455 U.S. 104 (1982).

22. On remand, after hearing additional evidence, the trial judge again sentenced Monty Eddings to death. In 1984, the Oklahoma Court of Criminal Appeals modified the sentence to life imprisonment because state law did not authorize the remand of a death judgment imposed by a jury for resentencing before a different jury and equal protection required that the same rule apply when the sentence was imposed by a judge; Eddings. v. State, 688 P.2d 342 (Okla. Crim. App. 1984).

23. In general, mitigation evidence can include anything that might persuade the jury against death. The Federal Death Penalty Statute is illustrative of the types of evidence to be considered by the jury to possibly mitigate against a sentence of death. The list of mitigation factors provided for in 18 U.S.C. § 3592 (a) includes the following:

    1. The defendant's capacity to appreciate the wrongfulness of the conduct or to conform conduct to the requirements of the law was significantly impaired.
    2. The defendant was under unusual and substantial duress.
    3. The defendant's participation in the offense was relatively minor.
    4. Another defendant, equally culpable in the crime, will not be punished with death.
    5. The defendant did not have a significant prior history of other criminal conduct.
    6. The defendant committed the offense under severe mental or emotional disturbance.
    7. The victim consented to the criminal conduct that resulted in the victim's death.
    8. Other factors in the defendant's background, record, or character or any other circumstance of the offense that mitigate against imposition of the death sentence.

    The aggravating factors set out in the Federal Death Penalty Act, 18 U.S.C. § 3592 (c)(1)–(16) include the following:

1. Death during the commission of specific crimes including hostage taking, kidnapping, and treason.
2. A previous conviction of a violent felony involving a firearm.
3. A previous conviction of an offense for which a sentence of death or life imprisonment was authorized.
4. A previous conviction of two or more federal or state offenses including the infliction, or attempted infliction, serious bodily injury or death upon another person.
5. Knowingly creating a grave risk of death to one or more persons in addition to the victim of the offense.
6. The murder was committed in an especially heinous, cruel, or depraved manner in that it involved torture or serious physical abuse to the victim.
7. The offense was procured by payment.
8. The offense was committed with the expectation of pecuniary gain.
9. The defendant committed the offense after substantial planning and premeditation.
10. A previous conviction of two or more state or federal felony drug offenses punishable by more than 1 year committed on different occasions.
11. The victim was particularly vulnerable due to old age, youth, or infirmity.
12. A previous conviction of serious federal drug offense under Title II or III.
13. The defendant committed the murder in the course of engaging in a continuing criminal enterprise involving the sale of drugs to a minor.
14. The defendant murdered a high public official, such as the president or a federal judge or law enforcement officer among other public officials.
15. The defendant had a prior conviction of sexual assault or child molestation.
16. More than one person was killed in a single criminal episode.

A study of 153 jurors in 41 South Carolina capital murder trials—22 resulting in sentences of death and 19 resulting in sentences of life imprisonment—explored their understanding of aggravation and mitigation. See S. Garvey, "Aggravation and Mitigation in Capital Cases: What Do Jurors Think?" *Colum. L. Rev.* 98 (1998): 1538. Confirming common assumptions about the most aggravated kinds of murders, the study found several factors to be highly aggravating, especially brutal murders involving torture or physical abuse (75.7%); especially bloody or gory murders (59.1%); murders in which the victim suffered before death (72.5%); murders in which the defendant maimed or mutilated the victim after death (72.2 %); the murder of a child (62.3%); a defendant with a history of violent crime (52.8%); a defendant who might be a danger to society in the future (57.9%); and a defendant who expressed no remorse (39.8%). The study further showed that the overall impact of especially bloody or gory murders, murders involving torture or physical abuse, murders in which the victim suffered before death, future dangerousness, and lack of remorse may be even greater than the findings suggest because a majority of the jurors surveyed believed these factors were present in the cases they had deliberated.

The study presented some findings that may contradict general assumptions about mitigation. While future dangerousness and a history of violent crime are highly aggravating, the fact that the defendant had no previous criminal record (20%) or would be a well-behaved inmate (26.2%) has only some mitigating potential. According to the study, the fact that the defendant has a loving family (18.8%) or that an accomplice received a lesser sentence in exchange for testimony (17.2%) is roughly as mitigating as the fact that the capital murder was an aberration in the defendant's otherwise crime-free life.

According to another study, a critical factor in the jury's decision-making process is the degree to which the jurors can identify with the victim and empathize with the victim's fate. See S. Sundby, "The Capital Jury and Empathy: The Problem of Worthy and Unworthy Victims," *Cornell L. Rev.* 88 (2003): 343. The more the victim is perceived as an innocent or helpless party in the fatal encounter, e.g., a child or an adult chosen at random, the more likely that the jury will bring in a death verdict. By contrast, if the jury believes that the victim had a drug or alcohol problem and was engaging in high-risk or antisocial behavior, or even that the victim was too careless in getting in harm's way, the jury is more likely to vote for a life sentence. The study by T. Eisenberg, S. Garvet, & M. Wells, "Victim Characteristics and Victim Impact Evidence in South Carolina Capital Cases," *Cornell L. Rev.* 88 (2003): 306, found that the introduction of victim impact evidence tended to increase the jury's "admiration" of the victim and that the more the jury admired the victim, the more vicious they thought the murder was. However, the study found no significant relationship among victim impact evidence, jurors' views of "victim admirability," and penalty outcomes.

At least two other studies, however, call into question how much attention jurors actually pay to the penalty phase evidence. See U. Bentele & W. Bowers, "How Jurors Decide on Death: Guilt Is Overwhelming; Aggravation Requires Death; and Mitigation Is No Excuse," *Brooklyn L. Rev.* 66 (2001): 1011; W. Bowers, M. Sandys, & B. Steiner, "Foreclosed Impartiality in Capital Sentencing: Jurors' Predispositions, Guilt-Trial Experience, and Premature Decision Making," *Cornell L. Rev.* 83 (1998): 1476. The former study of capital jurors in six states found that, in deliberating on their penalty decision, the jurors were preoccupied with discussing the evidence of the defendant's guilt, rather than the evidence introduced at the penalty phase. The latter study of capital jurors in 11 states, found that almost half of the jurors thought they knew what the punishment should be during the guilt phase of the trial. The study further established that 3 to 4 of every 10 jurors indicated that the legally irrelevant issue of the defendant's punishment was discussed during guilt deliberations. See N. Rivkind & S.F. Shatz (Eds.), *Cases and Materials on the Death Penalty* (St. Paul, MN: West, 2nd ed., 2005), pp. 549–551.

24. See S.E. Sundby, "The Capital Jury and Absolution: The Intersection of Trial Strategy, Remorse, and the Death Penalty," *Cornell L. Rev.* 83 (1998): 1557.

25. Model Penal Code § 210.6(2) (1980).

26. M. Brick, "Lawyers Make Case for Sparing Killer of 2 Detectives," *New York Times*, Jan. 17, 2007, p. 21. Without exception, the articles in the *Journal of Psychohistory* edited by Lloyd deMause attribute every type of violence (including wars) to child abuse.

27. 456 So. 2d 99 (Ala. Crim. App. 1983).

28. 388 S.E. 2d 816 (S.C. 1990).

29. 388 S.E.2d at 823.

30. See C.M. Sevilla, "Anti-Social Personality Disorder: Justification for the Death Penalty?" *J. Contemp. Legal Issues* 10 (1999): 247.

31. All 15 members of European Union have done away with the death penalty, and the EU now has an official policy of promoting its abolition throughout the world. The United Nations Commission on Human Rights in Geneva for several years in a row has passed resolutions calling for its restriction and eventual abolition. March 1 is observed as International Death Penalty Abolition Day. See R. Hood, *The Death Penalty: A Worldwide Perspective* (New York: Oxford University Press, 1996). When spiraling crime occurred in South Africa, surveys showed that the vast majority of the population wanted the death penalty (and vigilante groups put offenders to death). M. Mathabane, "South Africa's Lost Generation," *New York Times*, June 4, 1999, p. 29. Hundreds of people have protested outside the courts demanding the death sentence for men who rape young children. Rape support groups have called for the death penalty. Some 21,000 cases of child rape were reported to the police in 2000 in South Africa, most committed by relatives of the victims. According to myth, sex with a virgin will protect a man against AIDS or even cure him of it. News release, "Protesters Demand Execution of Rapists," *Detroit Free Press*, Nov. 24, 2001, p. 9.

32. D. O. Lewis et al., "Characteristics of Juveniles Condemned to Death," *Am. J. Psychiat.* 145 (1988): 588.

33. Should the court allow a victim's close relatives to testify at sentencing that they forgive the defendant? The court in Greene v. State, 343 Ark. 526, 37 S.W.3d 579 (2001), answered in the negative. The testimony was deemed not relevant as mitigating evidence because it did not speak to the character or deeds of the defendant. Neither was it relevant as "victim impact" evidence: "We conclude that penalty recommendations from family members of the victim are not relevant as victim impact evidence. Certainly, the penalty recommendation from Edna Burnett that Greene proposes would not counteract mitigating evidence or show the human cost of the murder on the victim's family. But, in addition, if this court permitted forgiveness and penalty recommendations as victim impact evidence, then it stands to reason that it must also allow any evidence of nonforgiveness by the victim's family and any recommendation of a harsher sentence, such as death. We cannot condone either brand of testimony as both would interfere with and be irrelevant to a jury's decision on punishment. Indeed, such testimony would have the potential of reducing a trial to 'a contest of irrelevant opinions.'"

Utah's death penalty statute allows evidence of any relevant aggravating or mitigating circumstances. Section 76-3-207 (2) of the Utah Code states, in pertinent part, "In [capital felony] sentencing proceedings, evidence may be presented as to any matter the court deems relevant to sentence, including ... the defendant's character, background, [and] history." See State v. Lafferty, 749 P.2d 1239 (Utah 1988). See, in general, J.L. Kirchmeier, "Aggravating and Mitigating Factors: The Paradox of Today's Arbitrary and Mandatory Capital Punishment Scheme," *Wm. & Mary Bill of Rights J.* 6 (1998): 345; see also R. Burt, "Disorder in the Court," *Mich. L. Rev.* 85 (1987): 1741; P. Crocker, "Concepts of Culpability and

Deathworthiness: Differentiating Between Guilt and Punishment in Death Penalty Cases," *Fordham L. Rev.* 66 (1997): 21; K.B. Dekleva, "Psychiatric Expertise in the Sentencing Phase of Capital Murder Cases," *J. Am. Acad. Psychiat. & Law* 29 (2001): 58; C. Steiker & J. Steiker, "Let God Sort Them Out?: Refining the Individualization Requirement in Capital Sentencing," *Yale L. J.* 102 (1992): 835. See also the symposia on the death penalty in *Behav. Sci. & Law* 5 (1987): 381–494; *Thomas M. Cooley L. Rev.* 13 (1996): 753–1012; *St. Louis U. Public Law,* vol. 25, no. 2, 2006. Casebooks have been developed for use in courses in law school on the death penalty. R. Coyne & L. Entzeroth, *Capital Punishment and the Judicial Process* (Durham, NC: Carolina Academic Press, 1994); N. Rivkind & S. F. Shatz, *Cases and Materials on the Death Penalty* (St. Paul, MN: West, 2001). See also V. L. Streib (Ed.), *A Capital Punishment Anthology* (Cincinnati, OH: Anderson, 1993).

34. The Arizona Supreme Court explained the state's "especially heinous, cruel or depraved" aggravating factor: (1) whether the killer relished the murder, (2) whether the killer inflicted gratuitous violence on the victim beyond that necessary to kill, (3) whether the killer needlessly mutilated the victim, (4) whether the crime was senseless, and (5) whether the victim was helpless"; State v. Detrich, 932 P. 2d 1328, 1339 (Ariz. 1997). In State v. Martinez-Villareal, 702 P.2d 670, 680 (Ariz. 1985), the Arizona Supreme Court found depravity based upon the defendant's bragging that the killing showed his machismo, but in State v. Graham, 660 P.2d 460, 463 (Ariz. 1983), it found no depravity in the defendant bragging that the victim "squealed like a rabbit." A depravity scale developed by Michael Welner is discussed in Chapter 15 on measuring evil.

35. United States v. Ngyyen, 928 F. Supp. 1525, 1541–1542 (D. Kan. 1996). See R. Slovenko, "Remorse," *J. Psychiat. & Law* 34 (2006): 397.

36. Payne v. Tennessee, 490 U.S. 805 (1989).

37. American Law Institute, Model Penal Code 210.6(4). In Zant v. Stephens, 462 U. S. 862 (1983), the Supreme Court said that it would be constitutionally impermissible to give aggravating effect to factors such as "race, religion, or political affiliation or … conduct that actually should militate in favor of a lesser penalty, such as perhaps the defendant's mental illness"; 462 U. S. at 885.

38. 543 U.S. 551 (2005). The case is discussed, among many other places, in J. Toobin, *The Nine* (New York: Doubleday, 2007), pp. 193–197.

39. 492 U.S. 361 (1989).

40. In national advertisements, Allstate says that teenagers are not to be blamed for the many automobile crashes they are involved in because their brain has not finished developing. See, e.g., Advertisement, *U.S. News & World Report*, Sept. 10, 2007 (back cover). It may be noted that, in the past, when if ever the penalty was actually carried out, the offender was much advanced in years (e.g., Gerald Mitchell was aged 33 when executed on October 23, 2001, for a murder he committed at the age of 17 on June 4, 1984).

41. 543 U.S. at 573.

42. 536 U.S. 304 (2002).

43. For a critique, see J.Q. Wilson, "Executing the Retarded," *National Review*, July 23, 2001, p. 37. One would assume that a mentally retarded individual who meets the test of competency to stand trial would also be competent to be executed. See Chapter 10 on competency to stand trial.

44. In fact, the prosecutor may use the defendant's mental condition as an aggravating factor. See People v. Smith, 107 P.3d 229 (Cal. 2005).

45. S.P. Garvey, "The Emotional Economy of Capital Sentencing," *NYU L. Rev.* 75 (2000): 26; see also W.J. Bowers, M. Sandys, & B. Steiner, "Foreclosing Impartiality in Capital Sentencing: Jurors' Predispositions, Attitudes and Premature Decision Making," *Cornell L. Rev.* 83 (1998): 1476; S.P. Garvey, "Aggravation and Mitigation in Capital Cases: What Do Jurors Think?" *Colum. L. Rev.* 98 (1998): 1538; G. Goodpaster, "The Trial for Life: Effective Assistance of Counsel in Death Penalty Cases," *NYU L. Rev.* 58 (1983): 299; J.S. Liebman & M.J. Shepard, "Guiding Capital Sentencing Discretion Beyond the 'Boiler Plate': Mental Disorder as a Mitigating Factor," *Geo. L. J.* 66 (1978): 757; C. Slobogin, "Mental Illness and the Death Penalty," *Calif. Crim. L. Rev.* 1 (2000): 3, reprinted in *Mental & Physical Disability Law Reporter (MPDLR)* 24 (July/Aug. 2000): 667; L.T. White, "The Mental Illness Defense in the Capital Penalty Hearing," *Behav. Sci. & Law* 5 (1987): 419.

46. Turpin v. Lipham, 1998 WL 804430 (Ga. 1998); Cargle v. State, 909 P. 2d 806 (Okla. Cr. App. 1995). In a PBS documentary, *Expose: America's Investigative Reports* (Sept. 2007), 80 capital cases in four prominent death penalty states were reviewed to see how vigorously defense attorneys investigated their clients' backgrounds as part of the case. In 73 of those cases, the attorneys missed a great deal

of evidence about child abuse, profound mental problems, and defendants with very low intelligence. But should a defendant's life story matter to a jury? Should an awful life history be mitigating? Should justice demand a full life story?

47. Cargle v. State, 909 P. 2d 806 (Okla. Cr. App. 1995). In Payne v. Tennessee, 501 U. S. 808 (1991), the U. S. Supreme Court reasoned that "[v]ictim impact evidence is simply another form or method of informing the sentencing authority about the specific harm caused by the crime in question, evidence of a general type long considered by sentencing authorities." The Court emphasized that the state has a legitimate interest in countering the defendant's mitigating evidence by showing that the victim also is an individual and "a unique loss to society"; 501 U. S. at 825. The Court concluded that it was "now of the view that a state may properly conclude that for the jury to assess meaningfully the defendant's moral culpability and blameworthiness, it should have before it (at the sentencing phase) evidence of the specific harm caused by the defendant"; 501 U. S. at 825. Videotapes about the victims' lives have been allowed. On the other hand, testimony by the victim's relatives forgiving the defendant is barred. See Greene v. State, 343 Ark. 526, 37 S.W.3d 579 (2001), cited *supra* note 33.

48. W.J. Bowers, "The Capital Jury Project: Rationale, Design, and Preview of Early Findings," *Ind. L. J.* 70 (1995): 1043; see also W.J. Bowers, "The Capital Jury: Is It Tilted Toward Death?" *Judicature* 79 (1996): 220. In Weeks v. Angelone, 120 S. Ct. 727 (2000), the U. S. Supreme Court ruled that the trial judge is not obliged to clear up the jury's confusion over the sentencing instruction. The jurors sent the judge a question: If they found [the defendant's] crime to be "outrageously or wantonly vile," or that he was likely to commit other violent acts, was it their "duty" to sentence him to death? Under Virginia law, one such "aggravating circumstance" must be present for a jury to impose the death sentence. The judge referred the jurors to a passage in his written instructions that told them they could impose a death sentence or opt for life imprisonment if they found that death was "not justified." Defense counsel argued that the judge's answer unfairly handicapped their client because it did not clearly point out that they could consider mitigating evidence, such as the defendant's remorse. Justice John Paul Stevens, author of the dissenting opinion, agreed, saying that there was a "virtual certainty" that the jury was confused, as well as "no reason to believe" the judge's answer had resolved the confusion.

49. W.J. Bowers et al., "Foreclosed Impartiality in Capital Sentencing: Jurors' Predispositions, Guilt-Trial Experience, and Premature Decision Making," *Cornell L. Rev.* 83 (1998): 1476.

50. M. Sandys, "Cross-Overs—Capital Jurors Who Change Their Minds About the Punishment: A Litmus Test for Sentencing Guidelines," *Ind. L. J.* 70 (1995): 1183.

51. Out of context, the term *death qualify* might be taken to mean "to qualify (someone) for the punishment of death." A.H. Soukhanov, *Word Watch* (New York: Henry Holt, 1995), p. 183.

52. Kevin Doyle, New York State's capital defender, says: "America divides on the death penalty, but we all agree that the convicted intentional murderer loses virtually all rights to autonomy; society is entitled to set the terms of his (imprisoned) existence for the rest of his life. He may neither judge the fittingness of society's death sentence nor dictate our actions—even to express his remorse, however heartfelt. Morally, therefore, the convicted murderer cannot compel his own execution. He has blood on his hands. He doesn't get to bloody ours." K.V. Doyle (ltr.), "It's Not Up to the Killer," *New York Times*, March 14, 2007, p. 18. See also A. Liptak, "Another Kind of Appeal From Death Row: Kill Me," *New York Times*, March 12, 2007, p. 14.

53. See F. Block, "A Slow Death," *New York Times*, March 15, 2007, p. 25. Georgia State Senator Preston W. Smith, chairman of the Senate Judiciary Committee, opines that the high price of a defense in a capital case is by design rather than necessity. He says, "You're building in an incentive to destroy the death penalty by building in a financial nuclear weapon." Quoted in B. Goodman, "Georgia Murder Case's Cost Saps Public Defense System," *New York Times,* March 22, 2007, p. 16.

54. 477 U. S. 399 (1986).

55. 477 U.S. at 418.

56. The age-old problem of personal identity was raised starkly in Woody Allen's *Zelig*, a "chameleon man" who takes on the characteristics of the people around him. In less dramatic fashion, a person is different from the person he was years earlier. See D. Detmer, "Inauthenticity and Personal Identity in *Zelig*," in M.T. Conard & A.J. Skoble (Eds.), *Woody Allen and Philosophy* (Chicago: Open Court, 2004), pp. 186–202.

57. 339 U. S. 9 (1950).

58. 168 U. S. 398 (1897).

59. 357 U. S. 549 (1958).

60. New evidence regarding a prisoner's mental competence or whether a warden acted in bad faith in not disclosing the new evidence does not constitute grounds for a federal court to alter or amend its judgment upholding a state court's finding that the prisoner is competent when the state court is not first given an opportunity to consider the evidence; Franklin v. Francis, 306 F. Supp. 1009 (S. D. Ohio 1999).

61. 357 U.S. at 552–553.

62. G.B. Melton, J. Petrila, N.G. Poythress, & C. Slobogin, *Psychological Evaluation for the Courts* (New York: Guilford, 3rd ed., 2007).

63. The standards of the American Bar Association, taking an intermediate position, recommend that the indigent condemned be entitled to an independent evaluation of competency, that the condemned be represented by counsel at the competency hearing, and that the burden be on the condemned to show incompetence by a preponderance of the evidence. Commentary to *Criminal Justice Mental Health Standards*, standard 7-5.2 (1984). See also Singleton v. State, 313 S.C. 75, 437 S.E.2d 53 (1993).

64. 616 So. 2d 428 (Fla. 1993).

65. 751 So. 2d 37 (Fla. 1999).

66. 751 So. 2d 597 (Fla. 1999).

67. Provenzano v. Florida, 2000 WL 674703 (Fla. 2000). A dissent stated that Provenzano's delusion that he was going to die because he was Jesus Christ indicated that his mental illness has put him out of touch with reality and made him unfit for execution as he did not know the real reason he was being put to death.

68. 127 S. Ct. 2842 (2007).

69. In this case, the issue was whether the Eighth Amendment permits the execution of an inmate who is factually aware of his impending execution, but has a delusional belief as to why the state is executing him, and thus does not appreciate that his execution is intended to seek retribution for his crime. The Fifth Circuit had held that he nevertheless is competent to be executed. Likewise, in an earlier case, Barnard v. Collins, 13 F.3d 871 (5th Cir. 1994), the Fifth Circuit held that an inmate is competent to be executed if he knows that the state is going to execute him and that the state's ostensible reason for executing him is his conviction for one or more capital crimes. Under this approach, it is irrelevant if the offender is under the delusion that regardless of the state's announced rationale, he, in fact, is being executed for reasons having nothing to do with the crime. Thus, a paranoid schizophrenic who suffers from the delusion that he will be executed not as punishment for his crime, but rather to stop him from preaching the Gospel or to further a conspiracy by space creatures to conquer the Earth would be considered competent for execution. Justice Powell had stated in *Ford* that "one of the death penalty's critical justifications, its retributive force, depends on the defendant's awareness of the penalty's existence and purpose." See the report of the ABA, published in 31:2 *MPDLR* 138 (March/April 2007).

   In the Panetti case, the defendant, Scott Panetti, had a well-documented history of severe mental illness, and though he was floridly psychotic, he was found, in a Texas court, competent to stand trial and was found guilty. He had shaved his head, sawed off the barrel of a shotgun, and driven to his in-laws' home where he killed them in front of his estranged wife and 3-year-old daughter. Then he showered, changed into a suit, and presented himself to the authorities. At his trial he dressed as a cowboy from the Old West and served as his own defense counsel. He subpoenaed John F. Kennedy, Pope John Paul II, Anne Bancroft, and Jesus. He blamed the murder on Sarge, one of four personalities in his delusional mind. "Sarge is gone," he told the jury. "No more Sarge." The jury returned a guilty verdict and the state of Texas sentenced him to death.

   The case went to the Fifth Circuit. Based on Fifth Circuit precedent, Panettti was competent to be executed if he knew the fact of his impending execution and the factual predicate for it. After more than 14 years of legal wrangling, the case came before the U.S. Supreme Court. By 5–4, the Supreme Court ruled that the Fifth Circuit's test was overly restrictive and, thus, unconstitutional under the Eighth Amendment. Expert testimony on behalf of Panetti was to the fact that, although he understood that Texas wanted to execute him for murder, he believed, due to the delusions caused by his mental illness, that the state's assertions were a sham and that it really wanted to execute him to prevent him from preaching. The Fifth Circuit had concluded that such delusions are irrelevant to whether inmates can be executed, so long as they understand that the state has identified a link between their crimes and the proposed punishment. In rejecting the Fifth Circuit's standard, the Supreme Court, in an opinion by Justice Kennedy, responded that such a test ignores the possibility that, even where such awareness exists, delusions based on a severe mental disorder can make inmates so far removed from reality that the reasons for punishing them no longer serve any proper purpose. See R. J. Bonnie, *"Panetti V. Quarterman*: Mental Illness, the Death Penalty, and Human Dignity," *Ohio St. J. Crim. L.* 5 (2007): 257.

70. Missouri now houses its death row inmates among the general population, but this is not the norm. See E. H. Mallett, "Death Row Defense," *Champion*, Aug./Sept. 2000, p. 3. In Texas, the condemned now live in a new high-security unit in Livingston, about 50 miles away from the Huntsville unit of the Texas Department of Criminal Justice.

71. In the novel *The Green Mile* (New York: Simon & Schuster, 1996) p. 250, Stephen King notes similarity between death row and the nursing home.

72. Upon imposing the death sentence on Thomas J. Koskovich, a 21-year-old, Judge Reginal Stanton of New Jersey Superior Court set a deadline of 5 years for the state to carry out the execution, and if the state has not carried it out by then, the judge ordered that the sentence automatically be changed to life in prison. In a statement read in the courtroom, he criticized the nation's courts for delays in executions. "The process has become unacceptably cruel to defendants," he said, "who spend long years under sentence of death while the judicial system conducts seemingly interminable proceedings, which remind many observers of a cruelly whimsical cat toying with a mouse." R. Hanley, "Judge Orders Death Penalty With a Five-Year Deadline," *New York Times*, May 8, 1999, p. 17. Centuries ago, the judge in his sentence directed execution to be performed on the next day. W. Blackstone, *Commentaries* 397. See J.L. Gallemore & J.H. Panton, "Inmate Responses to Lengthy Death Row Confinement," *Am. J. Psychiat.* 129 (1972): 167.

How did the Jewish population of Europe react once it began to dawn upon them that the Germans had decided to murder them? Yehuda Bauer, a prominent scholar of Holocaust studies, writes: "Psychologically, Jewish responses to knowledge of impending destruction were no different from similar responses of other groups. Russian or Polish peasants on the point of execution by German troops, French resistance fighters caught and sentenced to death, Serb villagers confronting Croat or German murderers—people facing inescapable destruction behave in much the same way. The range of reactions extends from numbed fear and hysterical crying to heroic defiance." Y. Bauer, *Rethinking the Holocaust* (New Haven, CT: Yale University Press, 2001), p. 26. The depiction in Truman Capote's *In Cold Blood* of inmates awaiting death is noted in Chapter 19 on posttraumatic stress disorder.

For prisoners executed between 1977 and 1997, the average elapsed time on death row was 111 months from the last sentencing date. U.S. Department of Justice, Bureau of Justice Statistics Bulletin, "Capital Punishment," 1997, p. 12. Supreme Court Justice Clarence Thomas has argued that "[i]t is incongruous to arm capital defendants with an arsenal of 'constitutional' claims with which they may delay their executions, and simultaneously to complain when executions are inevitably delayed"; Knight v. Florida, 120 S. Ct. 459 (1999).

73. See M. L. Radelet, *Executing the Mentally Ill* (Thousand Oaks, CA: Sage, 1993); K. Heilbrun et al., "The Debate in Treating Individuals Incompetent for Execution," *Am. J. Psychiat.* 149 (1992): 596; K. Heilbrun, "Assessment of Competency for Execution? The Guide of Mental Health Professionals," *Bull. Am. Acad. Psychiat. & Law* 16 (1988): 205; D. Mossman, "Assessing and Restoring Competency to Be Executed: Legal Contours and Implications for Assessment," *Crim. Just. & Behav.* 18 (1991): 164; G.B. Leong, J.A. Silva, R. Weinstock, & L. Ganzini, "Survey of Forensic Psychiatrists on Evaluation and Treatment of Prisoners on Death Row," *J. Am. Acad. Psychiat. & Law* 28 (2000): 427; D.H. Wallace, "The Need to Commute the Death Sentence: Competency for Execution and Ethical Dilemmas for Mental Health Professionals," *J. Law & Psychiat.* 15 (1992): 317; B. Ward, "Competency for Execution: Problems in Law and Psychiatry," *Fla. St. U. L. Rev.* 14 (1986): 35.

74. A. Ehrenzweig, "A Psychoanalysis of the Insanity Plea: Clues to the Problems of Criminal Responsibility and Insanity in the Death Cell," *Yale L. J.* 73 (1964): 425.

75. Personal communication.

76. See A.M Freedman & A.L. Halpern, "The Psychiatrist's Dilemma: A Conflict of Roles in Legal Executions," *Austral. & N. Zealand J. Psychiat.* 33 (1999): 629; A.M. Freedman & A.L.Halpern, "The Erosion of Ethics and Morality in Medicine: Physician Participation in Legal Executions in the United States," *N.Y. Law School L. Rev.* 41 (1996): 169; J.C. Schoenholtz, A.M. Freedman, & A.L. Halpern, "The 'Legal' Abuse of Physicians in Deaths in the United States: The Erosion of Ethics and Morality in Medicine," *Wayne L. Rev.* 42 (1996): 1505; see also M.A. Norko, "Reflections on Halpern's Call," *Am. Acad. Psychiat. & Law Newsl.*, April 2000, p. 3. See also Symposium, "Physician Involvement in Capital Punishment," *Mayo Clin. Proc.* 82 (Sept. 2007): 1043–1080; N.J. Farber et al., "Physicians' Willingness

to Participate in the Process of Lethal Injections for Capital Punishment," *Annals Intern. Med.* 135 (2001): 884; A. Gawande, "When Law and Ethics Collide: Why Physicians Participate in Executions," *N. Eng. J. Med.* 354 (March 23, 2006): 1221.

77. The latest challenge before the Supreme Court to the death penalty was whether lethal injection amounts to "cruel and unusual punishment," in violation of the Eighth Amendment. The issue before the Court was the standard by which courts are to evaluate the evidence that lethal injection predictably and with some regularity goes wrong. Litigation over the issue brought executions to a halt in a number of states. Finally, in Baze v. Rees, 128 S. Ct. 1520 (2008), the Supreme Court held that lethal injection is not prohibited as cruel and unusual punishment under the Eighth Amendment, but the issue generated separate opinions from seven Justices. A specific three-drug protocol used in Kentucky was approved in *Baze*, but this approval to other states using somewhat different protocols is unclear. Over the years lethal injections have gone awry in a number of instances. Indeed, it seems that there is a higher rate of botched executions with lethal injection that with earlier methods. See D. Denno, "Getting to Death: Are Executions Constitutional?" *Iowa L. Rev.* 82 (1997): 319. On December 13, 2006, in the carrying out of the death penalty of Angel Diaz, a convicted murderer in Florida, the physician bungled the first set of injections, sliding the needle straight through the vein and pumping the toxic chemicals directly into the underlying flesh. Diaz grimaced and attempted to speak until a second dose killed him. That was 34 minutes later; the execution should take only a fraction of that. Two days later, Governor Jeb Bush suspended all executions in the state. In the summer of 2006, Missouri halted all executions after the physician who supervised them admitted that he was dyslexic and had, on a previous occasion, given an inmate only half the recommended dose of anesthesia.

An electrocution went awry, among other times, in Louisiana *ex rel.* Francis v. Resweber, 329 U.S. 459 (1947), where the attempted electrocution failed due to mechanical difficulties. Francis argued that a second attempt to execute him would be unconstitutionally cruel. The Supreme Court ruled against him, with the dissenting justices asking, "How many deliberate and intentional reapplications of electric current does it take to produce a cruel, unusual, and unconstitutional punishment?"

The Court upheld shooting by firing squad in Wilkerson v. Utah, 99 U.S. 130 (1878). In Fierro v. Terhune, 77 F.3d 1158 (9th Cir. 1998), the Ninth Circuit declared California's use of lethal gas to be cruel and unusual punishment. In Duckworth v. Franzen (1985), Judge Richard Posner, writing the opinion for the Seventh Circuit, concluded that shackled prisoners who were injured during transport when their bus caught fire had not been subjected to cruel and unusual punishment. The intent requirement had not been met because the officers had not intended "maliciously" to cause harm: "Negligence, perhaps ... but not cruel and unusual punishment." What happened was nothing more than "if the guard accidentally stepped on the prisoner's toe and broke it."

See C. Dayan, *The Story of Cruel and Unusual* (Cambridge, MA: MIT Press, 2007); I. Solotaroff, *The Last Face You'll Ever See: The Private Life of the American Death Penalty* (New York: HarperCollins, 2001); S. Trombley, *The Execution Protocol: Inside America's Capital Punishment Industry* (New York: Crown, 1992); D.W. Denno, "When Legislatures Delegate Death: The Troubling Paradox Behind State Uses of Electrocution and Lethal Injection and What It Says About Us," *Ohio State L. J.* 63 (2002): 63. Law professor Victor Streib suggests that if the execution of Jesus of Nazareth had occurred today, the symbol of Christianity might well be lethal injection's hypodermic needle instead of the cross. V. Streib, *Death Penalty in a Nutshell* (St. Paul, MN: West, 2008).

78. The provision adopted by the American Medical Association prohibits physicians from even "attending or observing an execution" or pronouncing death of the prisoner, let alone administering a lethal substance. Pronouncing death is considered unacceptable because the physician is not permitted to revive the prisoner in the event the prisoner is found to be alive. The APA's ethics code calls on APA members to follow the AMA's ethics code. See S.L. Halleck, "Psychiatry and the Death Penalty: A View From the Front Lines," in L.E. Frost & R.J. Bonnie (Eds.), *The Evolution of Mental Health Law* (Washington, DC: American Psychological Association, 2001), p. 181. The following are excerpts from the AMA's Ethics Code:

An individual's opinion on capital punishment is the personal moral decision of the individual. A physician, as a member of a profession dedicated to preserving life when there is hope of doing so, should not be a participant in a legally authorized execution. Physician participation in execution is defined as actions that would fall into one or more of the following categories:

1. An action that would directly cause the death of the condemned.
2. An action that would assist, supervise, or contribute to the ability of another individual to directly cause the death of the condemned.

3. An action that could automatically cause an execution to be carried out on a condemned prisoner.

The following actions do not constitute physician participation in an execution:

1. Testifying as to medical history and diagnosis or mental state as they relate to competence to stand trial, testifying as to relevant medical evidence during trial, testifying as to medical aspects of aggravating or mitigating circumstances during the penalty phase of a capital case, or testifying as to medical diagnoses as they relate to the legal assessment of competence for execution.
2. Certifying death, provided that the condemned has been declared dead by another person.
3. Witnessing an execution in a totally nonprofessional capacity.
4. Witnessing an execution at the specific voluntary request of the condemned person, provided that the physician observes the execution in a nonprofessional capacity.
5. Relieving the acute suffering of a condemned person while awaiting execution, including providing tranquilizers at the specific voluntary request of the condemned person to help relieve pain or anticipation of the execution.

In 2007 the North Carolina Medical Board formalized the national professional standard adopted in 1992, but thereupon, the North Carolina Department of Corrections sued the board to compel retraction of the medical practice guideline. Prison officials have been unable to find a physician willing to risk the board's potential action and take part in an execution. Lawmakers filed bills that would remove the board's authority to punish physicians involved in capital punishments. E. Thompson, "Legislators Say New Law Could Allow State to Resume Executions," *Herald Sun* (Durham), March 14, 2007, p. 7.

Against opposition from the AMA and state medical societies, 35 of the 38 states explicitly allow physician participation in executions. Seventeen require it. To protect participating physicians from license challenges for violating ethics codes, states promise anonymity and provide legal immunity from such challenges. Despite the immunity, several physicians have faced license challenges, though none have lost as yet. See A. Gawande, *Better* (New York: Henry Holt, 2007), pp. 130–153. In North Carolina, Judge Donald Stephens of Superior Court ruled that the State Medical Board overstepped its authority by threatening to punish physicians for participating in executions. News report, "North Carolina: Execution Policy Rejected," *New York Times*, Sept. 22, 2007, p. 12.

Current law restricts prosecutors, in most cases, to asking either for the death penalty or a life sentence, which carries with it a chance for parole after 30 years. Prosecutors may ask for life without the chance for parole only if the defendant has a prior conviction for a violent felony. Giving prosecutors that option would likely reduce the number of death penalty trials. M. King, "Dig Deep Into Death Penalty," *Atlanta Journal-Constitution*, March 4, 2007, p. B-6. Life sentences without the chance of parole make it easier for jurors to oppose death, but it strips those sentenced to that fate of all hope. Corrections officers detest the sentence because it takes away the carrot of possible freedom for good behavior and reduces the stick of additional punishment. And there are practical difficulties in keeping offenders in prison until they die.

79. 498 U. S. 38 (1990) (*per curiam*).
80. In Washington v. Harper, 494 U.S. 210 (1990), the U.S. Supreme Court upheld the constitutionality of involuntary medication for mentally ill prisoners who pose a danger to themselves or others provided such treatment is in their medical interest.
81. State v. Perry, 610 So. 2d 746 (La. 1992). See D. Mossman, "Denouement of an Execution Competency Case: Is *Perry* Pyrric?" *Bull. Am. Acad. Psychiat. & Law* 23 (1995): 269.
82. See Md. Ann. Code art. 27, § 75A(d)(3); Perry v. Louisiana, 610 So. 2d 746 (La. 1992); Singleton v. State, 313 S. C. 75, 437 S. E. 2d 53 (1993). See also M.L. Radelet & G.W. Barnard, "Treating Those Found Incompetent for Execution: Ethical Chaos With Only One Solution," *Bull. Am. Acad. Psychiat. & Law* 16 (1988): 297.
83. The late Dr. Robert D. Miller presented the results of a national survey of attorneys general inquiring about procedures for the determination of competency to be executed and treatment of incompetent condemned prisoners, and discusses the ethical issues involved. R.D. Miller, "Evaluation of and Treatment to Competency to Be Executed: A National Survey and an Analysis," *J. Psychiat. & Law* 16 (1988): 67.
84. Callins v. Collins, 114 S. Ct. 1127 (1994).

85. Colorado district court judge Morris Hoffman argues that despite hype to the contrary, wrongful convictions are exceedingly rare. M.B. Hoffman, "The 'Innocence' Myth," *Wall Street Journal*, April 24, 2007, p. 19. Especially with the advent of DNA.
86. Quoted in M. Sherman (AP news release), "Roberts Hits Stevens in Death Penalty Cases," *Detroit Legal News*, April 30, 2007, p. 43.
87. J. Yardley, "Of All Places: Texas Wavering on Death Penalty," *New York Times,* Aug. 19, 2001, p. WK4.

15
Measurement of Evil

Is it possible to measure evil? In his popular book, *People of the Lie*,[1] the late psychiatrist M. Scott Peck suggested that the word *evil* be given a definite place in the lexicon of psychiatry. He maintained that omission of the word has emasculated the mental health community. He argues that the phenomenon of evil, though a religious construct, can and should be subjected to scientific scrutiny. (In some countries, the forensic expert is actually asked by the court whether the accused is inherently evil.) Although holding a wide readership (he was on the *New York Times* bestseller list for over a decade), Peck is rarely, if ever, mentioned in psychiatric circles. Although he was a psychiatrist, his writings are regarded as spiritual or religious, not psychiatric.[2]

In a chapter titled "Toward a Psychology of Evil," Peck asked why we do not yet have a body of scientific knowledge about human evil. He wrote:

> The concept of evil has been central to religious thought for millennia. Yet it is virtually absent from our science of psychology—which one might think would be vitally concerned with the matter. The major reason for this strange state of affairs is that the scientific and the religious models have hitherto been considered totally immiscible—like oil and water, mutually incompatible and rejecting.[3]

The late Dr. Walter Bromberg, a prominent forensic psychiatrist, wrote that the basic tenet underlying the attempt to therapeutize criminals is the attitude that crime represents misbehavior rather than evil per se: "Although the semantic change from *evil* propensities to *neurotically directed* misbehavior may have sounded trifling to some, it does involve tremendous attitudinal changes of the kind the mental hygiene movement fostered."[4] At one time, the term *moral insanity* was popular in psychiatric circles, but it is not heard today.[5]

If evil is to be named a psychiatric disorder, is it sufficiently unique to stand in a category all by itself or does it fit into one of the already existing categories? Peck said:

> Surprisingly, in view of the degree to which it has been neglected, the present system of classification of psychiatric illness seems quite adequate for the simple addition of evil as a subcategory. The existing broad category of personality disorders currently covers those psychiatric conditions in which the denial of personal responsibility is the predominant feature. By virtue of their unwillingness to tolerate the sense of personal sin and the denial of their imperfection, the evil easily fit into this broad diagnostic category. There is even within this class a subcategory entitled, "narcissistic personality disorder." It would, I believe, be quite appropriate to classify evil people as constituting a specific variant of the narcissistic personality disorder.[6]

In the heyday of psychoanalysis in early 20th century, it was thought, and even today, that psychoanalysis or psychiatry could fix any type of behavior. People who are evil or behave obnoxiously have been assumed to have a treatable psychiatric problem—even Hitler.[7] In 1950, four scholars published an influential study titled *The Authoritarian Personality*.[8] Three of the authors were Jewish. Two of them, including the philosopher Theodor Adorno, were refugees from Nazi Germany. Their goal was to explain Hitler's genocidal anti-Semitism. Based on their evaluation of more than 2,000 American adults, the authors concluded that extreme racist tendencies were associated with an abnormal personality syndrome they labeled *authoritarian*.

Today, Alvin Poussaint, an African-American clinical professor of psychiatry at Harvard Medical School, argues that racism is a mental disorder. A heading of "pathological bias" that may include racism, sexism, and heterosexism is being considered for entry in the *Diagnostic and Statistical Manual of Mental Disorder* (*DSM*), either as a symptom or as a distinct disorder.[9] "The culture influences what you consider pathology," says Poussaint. At one time, when slavery was normative, slaves who deviated from the norm were called mentally ill. In 1851, Dr. Samuel Cartwright, a Louisiana surgeon and psychologist, filed a report in the *New Orleans Medical and Surgical Journal* on diseases prevalent among the black population. Among the various maladies Cartwright described was *drapetomania* or "the disease causing slaves to run away." Though a serious mental illness, drapetomania, wrote Cartwright, was quite treatable. "With the advantages of proper medical advice, strictly followed, this troublesome practice that many Negroes have of running away can be almost entirely prevented." During the days of the Soviet Union, Nikita Khruschev said that anyone who would want to leave communism is mentally ill. President Ronald Reagan called the Soviet Union an "evil empire."

Nazism was mass murder that went hand-in-hand with mass looting. Its crimes were the most abominable in the history of the so-called civilized nations. Hitler turned the country of Bach and Beethoven into the country of Bergen-Belsen and Dachau. What were the mentality and motives of those who implemented or colluded with Hitler? Was it the character of the German people, their circumstances, or booty that led them to swear, "Heil Hitler"? Was it monocausal or multicausal? For Hannah Arendt, as oft-quoted, the years of total war and the murder of millions of Jews revealed not just what Nazis were capable of, but what human beings were capable of. Following the Holocaust, many said such a thing could never happen again, but then came Cambodia, Rwanda, Kosovo, the Sudan, and since 9/11, the threat of international terrorism.[10]

Dehumanization of a people is a common means of breaking down restraints against killing. The process is done in stages. First, a people is demonized, but still retains some human qualities. Later, they are regarded as vermin and completely dehumanized. In the mosques in Gaza and elsewhere in the Muslin world, Jews are referred to as "the brothers of apes and pigs." Hitler in destroying the Jews claimed that it was done in the service of cleansing the nation of vermin. In Rwanda, Hutu first referred to Tutsi as evil, and later began calling them *cafards*, meaning cockroaches—killing cockroaches does not induce guilt feelings, and indeed is laudatory. In the American civil war, Confederate soldiers regarded black troops serving in the Union army as "so many devils" and they were slaughtered or mutilated.

Psychiatric Classification

At the 1993 annual meeting of the American Psychiatric Association, Dr. Allen Frances, chair of the Task Force on *DSM-IV*, stated that 150 suggestions were received recommending new diagnostic categories, but evil was not among them. In any event, it would not be included, he said, because "it would not have clinical utility." He added, "The *DSM* cannot include all human functioning. Evil is beyond the purview of the *DSM*."[11]

Was Jeffrey Dahmer, the Milwaukee anthropophagite, evil or was he mentally ill? He invoked the insanity defense, but unsuccessfully. The defense attorney argued that Dahmer's cannibalistic killings were proof of his insanity because only an insane man would do such things. Can it be that the more terrible the crime, the crazier (and, therefore, the less culpable) the offender? Testifying for the defense, Dr. Fred Berlin, founder of the Johns Hopkins Sexual Disorders Clinic, contended that Dahmer was afflicted with a diagnosable psychiatric disorder (necrophilia) and that he was overpowered by his necrophilic urges. I asked him about evil and mental illness. He responded:

> Historically, all illnesses at one time were attributed, at least by some, to evil forces. People shaking in the midst of a seizure were felt to be possessed. Defining epilepsy as a condition, or illness, possibly amenable to scientific explanation, was in my judgment an important step forward. Jeffrey Dahmer was afflicted with recurrent, intense erotic fantasies and urges about having sex with corpses. His behavior appeared to be a response to these eroticized cravings. Although that observation still leaves much to be understood, appreciating that his behavior was occurring in response to such cravings, rather than as a response to evil within him, in my judgment represents an advance forward. I believe that science and medicine may eventually be able to learn more about how normal and abnormal sexual cravings develop, thereby advancing knowledge in a way that goes well beyond labeling. I have no difficulty concluding that a person is not right mentally (i.e., in labeling him mentally ill) if he recurrently experiences intrusive eroticized cravings about having sex with a corpse.
>
> I am uncertain how to move beyond labeling, at least from the scientific perspective, when the explanation for behavior is some hypothesized phenomenologically unobservable evil force. An abnormal subjective state (whether one is talking about auditory hallucinations or abnormal sexual cravings) can often be reliably described. I am not certain that one can be introspectively observed and described. In my opinion, arguing that behavior is a manifestation of such observable mental phenomena is more explanatory than attributing such actions to ill-defined and unobservable mystical evil forces.
>
> The concept of evil as an explanation is entirely circular. He did it because he is evil. We know he must be evil because he did it. On the other hand, the concept of mental illness as an explanatory aid allows behavior to be tied to subjectively observable mental phenomena (e.g., abnormal erotic cravings). Though only a step, and by no means a full explanation, it is a step forward. It is a step that points the way to further research; research that may help elucidate the etiology of such cravings, thereby perhaps leading to an even more enlightened explanation.[12]

Can psychiatry (or psychology) provide credible information of use to the courts in criminal, civil, employment, or family law cases? The need to standardize mental disorder resulted in the *DSM*, and psychiatrists as expert witnesses offer diagnoses from the *DSM*, though it carries a caveat about applying the *DSM* in the courtroom. In criminal trials, psychiatrists give opinions about diminished blameworthiness; in personal injury cases, they assess degree of suffering; in family court, they discuss the strengths or weaknesses of the parents; and in death penalty cases, they evaluate the likelihood of dangerousness. The caveat notwithstanding, reference is made to the *DSM* in all of these instances.

For several years, psychiatrist Michael Welner of New York, who is often on *Larry King Live*, has been proposing a depravity scale for the clinical assessment of evil behavior and intent in a variety of legal arenas. At the 2001 annual meeting of the American Psychiatric Association, he discussed the proposed depravity scale to an overflow audience (though it was the last session of a 4-day meeting). The depravity scale by its application, Welner suggests, could better rate crimes. Currently, judges use terms such as heinous, atrocious, cruel, outrageous, wanton, vile, or inhuman. Such terms, Welner says, are subjective and depend on the judge or juror's emotions for content. Instead, he wants to develop a consensus morality. He suggests 26 indications, which might be used including: whether the person intended to cause trauma, permanent disfigurement, or to terrorize or target the helpless. Evil actions might include unrelenting attacks or prolonging the victim's suffering. Evil attitudes could include blaming or having disrespect for the victim or taking satisfaction in the pain created. Welner has asked judges, prosecutors and defense attorneys, psychiatrists and theologians to review his criteria and to indicate whether they believe that these are indicators of depravity.[13]

Over 25,000 people from over 50 countries have weighed in to compare the relative significance of different examples of criminal intent, acts, victims targeted, and attitudes about crimes. In an article in *The Washington Post*, Welner reported that crimes that prolong suffering, those that cause grotesque suffering, and crimes of intent to cause emotional trauma drew overwhelming consensus as depraved.[14] Andrea Yates, who drowned her five children, is not rated as depraved because she "did not intend to emotionally traumatize, to terrorize, to show off, or to maximize damage; there was no criminal indulgence or grotesque quality to the suffering, no prolonged agony. She did not desecrate the bodies." On the other hand, John Allen Muhammed, the lead D.C. sniper, charts as depraved because he "intended to maximize destruction, intended to traumatize, targeted because of prejudice, exploited the trust of Lee Boyd Malvo to enlist him in crime, enlisted Malvo in order to have a juvenile to take responsibility, and enlisted and trained Malvo in order to maximize his destructive potential."

What about, say, the O.J. Simpson case? Was the killing of Nicole Brown Simpson and Ronald Goldman depraved? "No," says Welner. "The available evidence from the crime, and the available information about the person believed to have committed it, does not distinguish it from other domestic homicides," he says. "What distinguishes it are dramatic pictures shown to the public and a tragic case of a beautiful woman losing her life, along with a person trying to do her a favor, and a celebrity defendant."[15]

Would the depravity scale assist legislatures in distinguishing blameworthy acts in criminal codes? The criminal law declares what conduct is criminal and prescribes the punishment to be imposed for such conduct. The definition of a particular crime spells out what act (or omission) and what mental state is required for its commission. Furthermore, the definition of a particular crime may require, in addition to an act or omission and state of mind, something in the way of specified attendant circumstances, and with some crimes the definition also requires a specified result of the act or omission. The criminal law sets out what conduct, including what state of mind, is necessary for guilt of murder, rape, burglary, etc.

The depravity scale might be used in sentencing or in the penalty phase of a death penalty case, or in selecting juries, but its introduction as evidence at trial is curtailed by the rule of evidence that provides that any evidence of the defendant's character must first be offered by the defendant. Only then may the prosecutor respond with counterproof. By offering evidence of character, the defendant is sometimes said to "open the door" to character evidence. The accused offers evidence of a pertinent trait of his character to support an inference that he was unlikely to have committed the charged offense. It is called "inconsistent personality evidence" or "propensity evidence."[16]

The definition of a crime at times includes an element of depravity, thereby making the evidence admissible at the outset. Depravity aggravates an assault charge; in New York, "depraved indifference" means circumstances that create a grave risk to human life.[17] Even if no physical injury occurs, depravity warrants a charge of reckless endangerment.[18] Defense attorneys complain that some prosecutors charge depraved indifference, taking advantage of the vagueness of its definition to aggravate the charges against defendants alleged to have committed a variety of crimes.

Nowhere is the standardless standard of depravity more evident than in capital offenses. In these cases, the court is obliged to consider various aggravating and mitigating circumstances. Used time and again are such terms as "especially heinous," "outrageously vile," "wanton," "cruel," "atrocious," and "horrible." In *Arave v. Creech*,[19] a maximum security prisoner pulverized another inmate who had assaulted him with a weapon that consisted of a sock containing batteries. He received the death penalty after being described as a "cold-blooded pitiless slayer." What is cold-blooded? The sentence was challenged on the basis of the decision in *Walton v. Arizona*,[20] which required that aggravating circumstances be defined through objective circumstances. In *Furman v. Georgia*,[21] the Supreme Court ruled that consideration of aggravating circumstances in death penalty cases is unconstitutional if too much discretion is given to the sentencer, or a risk is created that the sentence will be given in too arbitrary a manner.

In *Creech*, Justice Sandra Day O'Connor for the majority wrote, "The facts underlying this case could not be more chilling. ... *Webster's Dictionary* defines 'pitiless' to mean devoid of, or unmoved by, mercy or compassion. ... The lead entry for 'cold-blooded' gives coordinate definitions. One, 'marked by absence of warm feelings.' ... The other ... to mean 'matter of fact, emotionless.'" Justice Blackmun dissented, "In ordinary usage, the nebulous description 'cold-blooded' simply is not limited to defendants who kill without emotion." To illustrate, Justice Blackmun collected news articles from around the country that applied the expression "cold-blooded" to a variety of homicides.

In *State v. Detrich*,[22] the Arizona Supreme Court explained the state's "especially heinous, cruel, or depraved" aggravating factor: (1) whether the killer relished the murder, (2) whether the killer inflicted gratuitous violence on the victim beyond that necessary to kill, (3) whether the killer needlessly mutilated the victim, (4) whether the crime was senseless, or (5) whether the victim was helpless." A few years earlier, in *State v. Martinez-Villareal*,[23] the Arizona Supreme Court found depravity based upon the defendant's bragging that the killing showed his machismo, but a bit earlier, cited in *State v. Graham*,[24] it found no depravity in the defendant bragging that the victim "squealed like a rabbit."

The imprecision in delineating aggravating factors challenges more than just the criminal courts. Personal injury plaintiffs seek punitive damages on the basis of outrageous behavior. There are actions, by virtue of their especial depravity or outrageousness that warrant a more serious monetary penalty. In family court, vile conduct is often alleged in child custody cases.

Yet is the Depravity Scale a misbegotten venture? Dr. Emanuel Tanay, a Holocaust survivor, argues that it is. He says, "In 40 years of practicing forensic psychiatry, I have never been called upon to define evil, and I hope I never will. Evil is a moral concept. The effort to give scientific validity to such concepts as 'atrocious,' 'outrageous,' and 'vile' with an instrument called the Depravity Scale is junk science at its worst. These are concepts that have no place in psychiatric nomenclature."[25]

In ordinary discourse, "evil" translates as that which causes harm, misfortune, or destruction. Evil is not a scientific concept with an agreed upon meaning, to be sure, but the idea of evil is part of a broadly shared human cultural heritage. The essence of evil is the destruction of human beings, not only by killing, but also by the creation of conditions that materially or psychologically destroy people's dignity or happiness. The word developed from Old English *yfel*, meaning bad, wicked, vicious. It means dangerousness or lack of empathy. While those terms are not in the *DSM*, psychiatrists use them time and again in testifying or in their reports.

Endnotes

1. M.S Peck, *People and the Lie/The Hope for Healing Human Evil* (New York: Simon & Schuster, 1983), p. 128.
2. The late Dr. Karl A. Menninger, renowned dean of American psychiatry who also had a bent for religion, lamented the loss of the word "sin" in professional or lay language. See K.A. Menninger, *Whatever Became of Sin?* (New York: John Wiley & Sons, 1995), pp. 275–287. Russian President Boris Yeltsin said the use of the word "sin" by Patriarch Aleksy, the Russian Orthodox Church leader, was unexpected and "cut me to the quick." Aleksy called it a sin not to pay wages and pensions. B. Yeltsin, *Midnight Diaries* (New York: Public Affairs, 2000), p. 75.
3. M.S. Peck, p. 128.

4. W. Bromberg, *From Shaman to Psychotherapist: A History of the Treatment of Mental Illness* (Chicago: Henry Regnery, 1975), p. 225.

5. J. Workman, "Moral Insanity: What Is It?" *Am. J. Insanity* 39 (1882): 334.

6. M.S. Peck, at p. 128.

7. The idea is disabused in R.A. Friedman, "About That Mean Streak of Yours: Psychiatry Can Do Only So Much," *New York Times*, Feb. 6, 2007, p. D-5. See also C.H. Sommers & S. Satel, *One Nation Under Therapy* (New York: St. Martin's Press, 2005); B. Zilbergeld, *The Shrinking of America: Myths of Psychological Change* (Boston: Little, Brown, 1983). Dr. Michael Reznicek of Washington writes: "[H]uman cruelty has too often been pathologized. Our profession has created a mental illness label for just about any behavior. And while this has been a disaster for good manners and social order, we will better serve our public trust, and the truly mentally ill, when we start placing reasonable restrictions on what we call mental illness." M.J. Reznicek (ltr.), "Mental Illness or Human Trait?" *New York Times*, Feb. 13, 2007, p. D-4.

8. T. Adorno, E. Frenkel-Brunswick, D.J. Levinson, & R.N. Sanford, *The Authoritarian Personality* (New York: W.W. Norton, 1950).

9. Critics object to the medicalization of behavior in that it provides excuses. Proclaim "I need help" and go into rehab. Mel Gibson took this route after exploding into an anti-Semitic rant when stopped for drunk driving. So did Michael Richards after being booed off the stage of a comedy club for a racist tirade.

10. See J. Waldron, "What Would Hannah Say?" *New York Review of Books*, March 15, 2007, p. 8; see also T. Judt, "The 'Problem of Evil' in Postwar Europe," *New York Review of Books*, Feb. 14, 2008, p. 33.

11. A. Frances in a comment at the annual meeting of American Psychiatric Association, San Francisco, May 26, 1993.

12. Personal communication (June 13, 1994).

13. M. Welner, "Defining Evil: A Depravity Scale for Today's Courts," *Forensic Echo* 2 (May 1998): 6; A. Liptak, "Adding Method of Judging Mayhem," *New York Times*, April 2, 2007, p. 12; J. McConnaughey, "Psychiatrists Trying to Measure Evil," AP news release, May 11, 2001. Objectifying values is discussed in R. Lepley, *Values: A Comparative Inquiry* (New York: Columbia University Press, 1949). See also cover story, "The Roots of Evil," *Newsweek*, May 21, 2001, pp. 28–37. Through the years there have been efforts at providing assessments of violence or delinquency. See, e.g., S. Glueck & E. Glueck, *Identification of Predelinquents* (New York: Intercontinental Medical Book Corp., 1972); R. Hare, *Manual for the Hare Psychopathy Checklist—Revised* (Toronto: Multi-Health Systems, 1985); J. Monahan & H.J. Steadman, "Violence Risk Assessment: A Quarter Century of Research," in L.E. Frost & R.J. Bonnie (Eds.), *The Evolution of Mental Health Law* (Washington, DC: American Psychological Association, 2001), pp. 195–211.

14. N. Tucker, "Giving Evil the Eye," *Washington Post*, July 23, 2007, C1.

15. Ibid.

16. Federal Rules of Evidence, Rule 404, see Chapter 7.

17. NYS CPL § 120.10.

18. NYS CPL § 120.25.

19. 507 U.S. 463 (1993).

20. 497 U.S. 639 (1990).

21. 408 U.S. 238 (1972).

22. 932 P.2d 1328, 1339 (Ariz. 1985).

23. 660 P.2d 460, 463 (Ariz. 1983).

24. 702 P.2d 670, 680 (Ariz. 1985).

25. E. Tanay (ltr), "Evil Behavior," *Psychiatric News*, Sept. 21, 2001, p. 26. Dr. Phillip Resnick described the depravity scale as "pseudo-science" at the 2007 annual spring meeting of the American Academy of Psychiatry and the Law, Midwest Chapter, in Chicago on April 20, 2007. See R.I. Simon, "Should Forensic Psychiatrists Testify About Evil?" *J. Am. Acad. Psychiat. & Law* 31 (2003): 413; M. Welner, "Response to Simon: Legal Relevance Demands That Evil Be Defined and Standardized," *J. Am. Acad. Psychiat. & Law* 31 (2003): 417. For another critique, see J.L. Knoll, "The Recurrence of an Illusion: The Concept of 'Evil' in Forensic Psychiatry," *J. Am. Acad. Psychiat. & Law* 36 (2008): 105.

PART IV
Sexual Deviation

16

Sex Offender Legislation

Prior to the enactment of the current sexual predator laws more than one half of the states during the period 1930 to 1970 enacted umbrella-type legislation to deal with sex offenders. The legislation—known as the *sexual psychopath* statute—operated in a legal system that already provided criminal sanctions for the same conduct independent of this statute. In addition, civil commitment procedures in all states are applicable to mentally ill persons who might constitute a danger to themselves or others or who are in need of care or treatment.

The Early Sexual Psychopath Legislation

The early sexual psychopath legislation usually provided for the indeterminate commitment of the so-called sexual psychopath. There was, however, no uniformity in the definition of sexual psychopath or circumstances, which called for initiation of the special proceedings. Generally, however, the term *sexual psychopath* was defined as "one lacking the power to control his sexual impulses or having criminal propensities toward the commission of sex offenses."[1] Such a definition involved a prediction or prognosis as well as a diagnosis or description of the current situation.

The statutes reflected the therapeutic optimism of the time. The feeling was that psychiatry could identify and treat potentially dangerous sex offenders. The American Bar Association Criminal Justice Mental Health Standards noted the assumptions underlying this special dispositional legislation:

(1) There is a specific mental disability called sexual psychopathy; (2) persons suffering from such a disability are more likely to commit serious crimes, especially dangerous sex offences, than other criminals; (3) such persons are easily identified by mental health professionals; (4) the dangerousness of these offenders can be predicted by mental health professionals; (5) treatment is available for the condition; and (6) large numbers of persons afflicted with the designated disabilities can be cured.

The statutes were divided into preconviction and postconviction types. The postconviction type applied only to those convicted of sexual crimes; the preconviction type included persons charged with the commission of a specific sexual offense and applied also to those accused of being sexual psychopaths. Here, the law took the position of dealing with status or being, rather than actual doing. It is allegedly an attempt to bridge a legal lag by legislative enactment. But was it a legal advance? How helpful was it? The late Dr. Philip Roche in his Isaac Ray Award Lecture said, "The pursuit of demons disguised as sexual psychopaths affords a glimpse of a 16th-century approach to mental illness."[2]

A law based on being rather than doing tends to defer to psychiatry or psychology, but what are the standards to be used as a measuring device? One might assume that sexual psychopaths or deviates have much in common and form a distinct class. Such homogeneity, however, assuredly does not exist. The terms *sexual psychopath* or *deviate* do not adequately define any legal entity, no more than does the term *offender*, which covers the waterfront. Sexual psychopathy is not a distinct psychiatric category of neurosis or psychosis. Among the deviates, representing the gamut of mental disorders, are neurotics, schizophrenics, schizoid personalities, alcoholics, persons with chronic brain damage, or mentally retarded individuals. It is like the grouping of the jaundices, which brings together strange bedfellows. All that those in the grouping share is a single trait, one that psychiatrists must consider as a symptom.

The American Psychiatric Association's *Diagnostic and Statistical Manual of Mental Disorders* (*DSM*) has a category called *paraphilias*, under the section entitled "Sexual Dysfunction" which includes the following: "exhibitionism, fetishism, frotteurism, pedophilia, sexual masochism, sexual sadism, transvestic fetishism, voyeurism, and not otherwise specified."[3] The essential features of a paraphilia are sexual interests directed primarily toward objects other than people of the opposite sex, sexual acts not usually associated with coitus, or coitus performed under bizarre circumstances, as in necrophilia, pedophilia, sexual sadism, and fetishism. Even though many find their practices distasteful, they remain unable to substitute normal sexual behavior for them.

The label *sexual psychopath* is frequently called into question. There is disagreement as to whether it is a form of mental illness, a form of evil, or a form of fiction.[4] The Group for the Advancement of Psychiatry stated that the term *sexual psychopath* is not a psychiatric diagnosis and has no precise clinical meaning.[5] From a psychiatric point of view, the term is meaningful only descriptively, not psychodynamically. Consequently, the enforcement of the law resulted in a roundup of the vagrant and nuisance type of offender and failed to reach the dangerous, aggressive offender. The late Judge Morris Ploscowe commented, "The sex-psychopath laws fail miserably in this vital task."[6]

The sexual psychopath legislation was not implemented with staff and facilities for treatment, one of the major purposes of the legislation. The justification for deprivation of liberty under the legislation was treatment, but because treatment was lacking, the process failed to measure up to the standard set out in 1966 by the Court of Appeals for the District of Columbia in *Rouse v. Cameron*, which stated: "Had appellant been found criminally responsible, he could have been confined 4 years and the end is not in sight. Because this difference rests solely on the need for treatment, a failure to supply treatment may raise a question of due process of law."[7]

On the day *Rouse* was decided, the same court ruled in *Millard v. Cameron*: "In *Rouse v. Cameron* ... [we] held that the petitioner was entitled to relief upon showing that he was not receiving reasonably suitable and adequate treatment. Lack of such treatment, we said, could not be justified by lack of staff facilities. We think the same principles apply to a person involuntarily committed to a public hospital as a sexual psychopath."[8] A New York court refused to commit a sex offender to a "one day to life" sentence unless it could be "reasonably certain that treatment will be given."[9] The court noted that confinement was based on the expectation of improvement resulting from treatment, which would be impossible because the psychiatric clinic at the institution had been closed down.

Actually the term *treatment* is a holdover from medical training and social usage, and is here misleading because of its medical connotations. The sex offender and some other mentally ill persons are not sick or diseased (unless by "disease" we mean dis-ease, lack of ease or discomfort).[10] Abjuring the language of clinical medicine as prejudicial and confusing, Freud, too, saw health and disease not as clinical entities, but as forms of self-expression. The ego, Freud said, will deform itself to avoid disruptive anxiety.[11]

Special institutions, such as Atascadero State Hospital in California, were established to implement the state's sexual psychopath statute. California, Michigan, and Wisconsin made the most use of their statutes. What was the news about them? To say the least, they did not work out. Indeed, a consensus described these institutions as a hoax.

A special institution is theoretically justified only when there is a homogeneity within the group and when a particular institution can offer a special service for that group. Neither criterion was met. Supposedly, the special proceeding was adopted to detain the dangerous, aggressive offender, but the person usually confined was the mental defective or impoverished farm boy bewildered by city life. The proceeding was designed to offer treatment, but whatever that was supposed to constitute, it assuredly was not available. One court said, "If [hospitals] are to be no more than pens into which we are to sweep that which is offensive to 'normal society,' let us be honest and denominate them as such."[12]

The special proceeding served only to stigmatize. The inmate labeled a *sexual psychopath* lived up to the role and in the institution he himself often placed a sign around his neck, such as, "I am a masturbator," "I am a peeping tom." His self-esteem, low before, became even more abysmal. His troubles with the opposite sex multiplied. Imagine, if you will, his problem when later seeking female companionship. Surely parents would not want their daughter to associate with a sexual psychopath, and surely no employer would likely hire one. No less stigmatizing and dehumanizing are terms such as *sex offender, sexual predator,* or *pedophile.*

Thus sexual psychopath legislation did little more than detain some persons who were regarded as freaks, stigmatize them, and render them forever social outcasts. Nevertheless, it was suggested that the concept of sex crime in sexual psychopath legislation be broadened to include any criminal act in which some type of sexual satisfaction is the motivating force. Some persons with sexual conflicts may obtain sexual stimulation by committing arson, by stealing women's undergarments, or by plunging a knife into a woman's back. A boy with a fetish for motorcycles may steal them to get "sexual" satisfaction out of driving away at high speed. Offenses such as arson, shoplifting (kleptomania), burglary, and murder often have sexually motivating aspects. Breaking and entering by the adolescent is often equated with breaking and entering of the forbidden area of the female (rape). Dr. Karl Menninger observed: "Sexual impulses are frequently involved in compulsive behavior. ... Sexual elements are often transparent in fire setting, kleptomania, addictive gambling, reckless car driving, and various kinds of physical violence. Sometimes, rather than being merely transparently present, the sexual factor is barely conspicuous."[13]

In such cases, however, because the victim has not been sexually assaulted and there has been no use of the sex organs, it could only be inferred that the act might have some sexual significance. The courts that operated on the basis of such inference were soon mired in problems because practically any activity, at some level, could be labeled sexual in nature. As a rule, under the criminal law, motivation (as distinguished from intent) is not an element of a crime. Hate crime legislation that has been proposed would also be mired in ascertaining motivation.

On the other hand, behavior that involves the sexual organs, and which may involve some sexual gratification or overt expression of sexual activity, is not necessarily motivated initially by a desire for sexual satisfaction. The late Dr. Bernard Glueck cited an example of the older man who feels grossly inadequate in his adjustment with other adults, but who does feel relatively comfortable and happy when he is with children. Glueck stated:

> Very often this individual may find himself in a situation that initially has no sexual motivation, but is entirely motivated by a desire for some sort of interpersonal satisfaction. However, in the course of his contact with children, or when the control and judgment faculties are weakened by alcohol, sexual excitement and arousal may develop as an additional pattern, frequently viewed by the individual as an unwanted complication, with the result that some type of prohibited sexual act occurs.[14]

There may be nonsexual motivations in sexual offenses as well as sexual motivations in nonsexual offenses. Hatred and inadequacy more than sexual motivation predominates in most acts of rape. Generally speaking, a rapist might be said to be acting out hostile or destructive rather than sexual impulses. To twist Lord Acton's phrase: powerlessness corrupts, and absolute powerlessness corrupts absolutely. One who is impotent to cope with a situation tends to choose the most primitive way—violence. Even the term *rape* has the nonsexual meaning of pillaging and destroying. Indeed, it is not uncommon for librarians to place "The Rape of Nanking" in the section of the library on sex offenses.

Sexual psychopath legislation was open to the oft-heard criticism that the law looks only at a symptom. Sexual difficulties are, after all, symptoms of personality and relating problems. Sex, being a human-relating experience (potentially the closest one of all), nearly always reflects personality problems. These problems are also reflected in other behavior. The symptom of deviant sexual behavior prompted sexual psychopath legislation; however, interpreting all behavior as sexual in origin in order to overcome the shortcomings and limitations of other statutes was not the way to deal with those who have severe problems relating to other people. The sorry experience in those states that enacted sexual psychopath legislation and established special institutions furnishes ample evidence of the shortcomings of this approach. Michigan's Goodrich Act of 1935, the first sexual psychopath legislation in the country, was enacted to allay public hysteria resulting from the brutal crimes committed by Goodrich.[15] A futile endeavor, it was repealed in 1968.[16] In 1960, 26 states and the District of Columbia had some form of sexual psychopath legislation;[17] in 1992, it was half that number.[18] They were called a "failed experiment." Brakel, Parry, and Weiner explained in their book *The Mentally Disabled and the Law*:

> Growing awareness that there is no specific group of individuals who can be labeled sexual psychopaths by acceptable medical standards and that there are no proven treatments for such offenders has led such professional groups as the Group for the Advancement of Psychiatry, the President's Commission on Mental Health, and most recently, the American Bar Association Committee on Criminal Justice Mental Health Standards to urge that these laws be repealed.[19]

When repealing its sex offender statute in 1981 the California legislature declared: "In repealing the mentally disordered sex offender commitment statute, the Legislature recognizes and declares that the commission of sex offenses is not itself the product of mental disease."

New Sexually Violent Predator Legislation

With the demise of indeterminate sentencing generally, the 1990s witnessed a renewed interest in sex offender commitment. Starting in Washington in 1990, no less than 18 other states have enacted laws for the commitment of sexually violent predators (SVP), to wit: persons (1) convicted of a sexually violent offense, (2) about to be released from confinement, and (3) found to be suffering from "a mental abnormality or personality disorder that makes the person likely to engage in predatory acts of sexual violence."[20] The laws were sparked by cases such as Earl Shriner's rape and sexual mutilation of a 6-year-old boy in Washington, and the killings of Megan Kanka in New Jersey and Polly Klaas in California.[21] In addition, legislation has been enacted in recent years involving (1) the registration of sexual offenders, (2) community notification regarding their whereabouts, (3) zoning restrictions where persons with pedophilia can reside, and (4) chemical or surgical castration.

The SVP laws are different from the early sexual psychopath statutes and from ordinary civil commitment laws in several important respects. First, they do not require a medically recognized serious mental disorder. Second, they do not require any allegation or proof of recent criminal wrongdoing.[22] Third, they require sex offenders to serve their full prison term prior to commitment. Fourth, no *bona fide* treatment program need be in place. The new legislation has no great hopes for treatment, as earlier legislation did, and much more emphasizes incapacitation. Moreover, assessment procedures are controversial.[23] Then, too, it is argued, pedophilia does not necessarily result in harm.[24]

The SVP laws establish civil commitment procedures for individuals with mental abnormality or personality disorder who are likely to engage in predatory acts of sexual violence.[25] In using the concept of mental abnormality, the legislation invokes terminology that can cover a variety of disorders. In challenging Washington's SVP statute, the state's psychiatric association said in an *amicus* brief, "Sexual predation in and of itself does not define a mental illness. It defines criminal conduct." Be that as it may, the Washington Supreme Court, in 1993, upheld its SVP statute against constitutional challenge saying:

> The fact that pathologically driven rape, for example, is not yet listed in the [*DSM*] does not invalidate such a diagnosis. The *DSM* is, after all, an evolving and imperfect document, nor is it sacrosanct. Furthermore, it is in some areas a political document whose diagnoses are based, in some cases, on what American Psychiatric Association leaders consider to be practical realities. What is critical for our purposes is that psychiatric and psychological clinicians who testify in good faith as to mental abnormality are able to identify sexual pathologies that are as real and meaningful as other pathologies already listed in the *DSM*.[26]

The court turned the disclaimer in the *DSM*—that it is intended for clinical purposes, not for purposes of the law—on its head. The court said, "Over the years, the law has developed many specialized terms to describe mental health concepts. ... The *DSM* explicitly recognizes ... that the scientific categorization of a mental disorder may not be 'wholly relevant to legal judgments.'"[27] Indeed, the term *mental abnormality* is no less vague than the definition of mental illness in civil commitment statutes.

In 1994 the Minnesota Supreme Court upheld its statute, but limited its scope to those who exhibit (1) a habitual course of misconduct in sexual matters and (2) "an utter lack of power to control sexual impulses," in addition to (3) proof that the person will attack or otherwise injure others.[28]

Two years later, in 1996 the Kansas Supreme Court ruled its statute, almost identical to the Washington statute, as unconstitutional.[29] The Kansas Supreme Court held that the statute violated substantive due process because the definition of mental abnormality did not satisfy what is perceived to be the definition of mental illness required in the context of involuntary civil commitment. The court did not address double jeopardy or *ex post facto* issues. The court noted that the laws targeted individuals who could not be committed under the general civil commitment law.

In 1997, in a 5–4 decision in *Kansas v. Hendricks*,[30] the U.S. Supreme Court, reversing the Kansas Supreme Court, upheld the statute. The majority opinion, written by Justice Clarence Thomas, held that the Act does not violate the double jeopardy or *ex post facto* prohibitions. Justice Thomas acknowledged that, in addition to dangerousness, "some additional factor" that was causally linked to the dangerous behavior is constitutionally required. However, he wrote, substantive due process does not require that this condition be a mental disorder recognized by treatment professionals: "Not only do psychiatrists disagree widely and frequently on what constitutes mental illness ... but the Court itself has used a variety of expressions to describe the mental condition of those properly subject to civil commitment." He also said, "[W]e have traditionally left to legislators the task of defining terms of a medical nature that have legal significance." Because the statute requires proof that individuals suffer from a volitional impairment rendering them dangerous beyond their control, he concluded, the statute does not allow commitment of individuals based solely on dangerousness.[31]

The majority also concluded that the law was civil in nature rather than punitive in purpose or effect, and thus it did not violate either double jeopardy or *ex post facto* prohibitions. Moreover, being categorized as civil in nature, other constitutional protections associated with criminal proceedings do not apply, such as the Sixth Amendment's provision that "[i]n all criminal prosecutions, the accused shall enjoy the right ... to be confronted with the witnesses against him." [Wisconsin's SVP law provides that "all constitutional rights available to a defendant in a criminal proceeding are available to the person.] An offender does not have a right to an evaluation of competency to stand trial prior to SVP determination—competency is not a prerequisite to either civil mental commitment or civil protective-placement proceedings. Except for Justice Ginsburg, the dissenters agreed with the majority that states have broad authority to define legal mental illness and that the statute's use of mental abnormality satisfies substantive due process. However, the dissenters concluded that the statute was essentially punitive in nature rather than civil, thus violating both double jeopardy and *ex post facto* prohibitions. Under the laws, offenders are committed after they have served virtually their entire criminal sentence, whereas under the earlier sexual psychopath legislation, the prosecutor had to choose between conviction in the criminal system or commitment in the civil system.

The Court suggested *in dicta* that treatability is not a constitutionally required element for commitment, although treatment may be required if the state considers the individual amenable to treatment. The Court observed that the state may be obliged to provide treatment that is available for disorders that are treatable. Moreover, the state can defer such treatment until after the offender had served his full prison term. Justice Thomas wrote, "[U]nder the appropriate circumstances and when accompanied by proper procedure, incapacitation may be a legitimate end of the civil law. ... We have never held that the Constitution prevents a State from civilly detaining those for whom no treatment is available, but who nevertheless pose a danger to others."[32] In a concurring opinion, Justice Anthony Kennedy, who was the swing vote, said, "If the object or purpose of the ... law had been to provide treatment, but the treatment provisions were adopted as a sham or mere pretext, [this would amount to] an indication of the forbidden purpose to punish."

In 1999, acting on a petition for a writ of habeas corpus from Andre Brigham Young, a convicted rapist who had been held under a SVP law for 9 years following his release from prison, the U.S. Court of Appeals for the Ninth Circuit held that he was entitled to a chance to prove his contentions that he was not receiving treatment and that conditions at the state's Special Commitment Center were equivalent to prison or worse. The Ninth Circuit found that if the actual conditions of the offender's confinement appeared to be punitive rather than therapeutic, the extra time could raise double jeopardy and new penalty problems despite the civil designation.[33] In an 8–1 decision, the Supreme Court overturned the Ninth Circuit's ruling, all but ruling out the prospect that additional confinement could ever be challenged in federal court as double jeopardy.[34] In *Hendricks*, it had said that the additional confinement was neither double jeopardy nor an imposition of a new penalty for an old offense.

In *Young*, the majority opinion left important questions unanswered, as Justice O'Connor acknowledged in observing, "We have not squarely addressed the relevance of conditions of confinement to a first instance determination" of whether a statute could properly be called civil in nature. Justices Scalia and Souter, while joining Justice O'Connor's opinion, wrote separately to say that in their view, whether a statute was civil or criminal depended completely on the intent of the legislature. If a civil statute was administered in an unduly punitive way, these two justices said, the remedy was not to invoke the double jeopardy clause, but to sue the administrators in state court. Justice Stevens, the sole dissenter, urged, "If conditions of confinement are such that a detainee has been punished twice in violation of the double jeopardy clause, it is irrelevant that the scheme has been previously labeled as civil without full knowledge of the effects of the statute."

Some years ago, in 1988, the American Psychiatric Association's Council of Psychiatry and Law said that the continued hospitalization of nonmentally ill, personality-disordered persons, who have recovered from their mental illness in a maximum security hospital following acquittal of crime by reason of insanity, is justified on the grounds that "[t]hose who suffer from personality disorders may also benefit from the special management available only in a psychiatric institution where sensitive, comprehensive, unique and imaginative treatment programs can often be developed to assist them in overcoming their destructive behavior."[35]

Of the sexual predator laws that have been enacted, the treatment setting in seven states is a hospital, while in the other states, it is a segregated unit within a correctional facility, or a correctional facility devoted exclusively to sexual predators. In all states, the agencies responsible for providing treatment are the state health services, mental health, or social services department. The ambiguous issue, however, is whether the states must invest sufficient resources in treatment to reach a minimum standard of intervention that could be expected to effect change, and whether the costs will come out of the diminishing mental health budget.

In *amici* briefs, the American Psychiatric Association, as well as its district branches, taking a different position than it did in 1988, and the American Civil Liberties Union, argued against these laws because sex offenders do not necessarily have a mental illness, no curative treatment is yet available for their behavior, and consequently, lifetime preventive detention is likely. They also argued that mental health professionals could not predict future behavior accurately so that some individuals will be committed who would not commit other crimes and others will be set free who will.[36] Past behavior is the best predictor of future behavior. It is also argued that sex offenders would be better dealt with by the criminal justice system, with stiffer criminal sentences for repeat sex offenders.[37] In the absence of mandatory minimums or indeterminate sentences for sexually violent crimes, the SVP laws are seen as the only alternative to protect society.[38]

It may be said that criminal activity ought to be examined with a view to appropriate disposition, but sexual offender legislation is a woefully awkward and misleading way to achieve it. It is moreover an expensive way of achieving social control over a relatively small number of offenders. Sooner or later, it will be realized that the costs in implementing the SVP laws are so exorbitant that they will be abandoned or repealed.

The sorry experience under the earlier sexual psychopath legislation should be a lesson that this approach ought not to be followed. A better approach is indeterminate sentencing of all offenders or heavier sentences for repeat violent sex offenders. A number of states have recently enacted lifetime sentences for repeat offenders who commit violent crimes, including sex offenses. A state commission in Michigan in 1999 recommended longer terms for violent offenders. Under this approach, the need for special sexual psychopath legislation is diminished, but the hypothesis that increased sentences will improve public safety is untested. Suggestions to the contrary have included the possibility that repeat sex offenders may be more likely to kill their victims to avoid discovery as the severity of the sentence increases.

From all reports, psychotherapy serves little, if at all, in changing the behavior of sex offenders. What they learn in psychotherapy is the jargon of psychotherapy. They learn the phrases that will get them past the assessment of being an incorrigible—that they have "recognized the causes" of their behavior, and "seen the offense from the victim's point of view." Evidence is thin, however, that they learn to control their behavior or that they are telling the truth when they say these fine phrases. Behavior therapy is more promising.[39]

What about castration, be it surgical or chemical? Texas not long ago enacted legislation allowing surgical castration of repeat sex offenders. The law makes it voluntary, and those who agree must also agree to take part in a study of sexual behavior after the operation that eliminates testosterone, which is blamed for male sexual aggression. To date, the legislation has not been applied out of concern that it may lead to litigation on the basis that consent under the circumstances is not voluntarily given.[40]

The Michigan Court of Appeals overturned a trial judge's sentence of Depo-Provera® treatment as a condition of probation, finding the condition punitive, unlawful, and coercive, as well as virtually impossible to perform with informed consent.[41] Further the court said that "Depo-

Provera treatment fails as a lawful condition of probation because it has not gained acceptance in the medical community as a safe and reliable medical procedure."[42]

In Germany, where surgical castration is practiced, the recidivist rate is said to have dropped from the 80% range to 3%. Chemical castration (medication), as opposed to surgical castration, has side effects including diabetes and heart problems.[43]

Castration, of whatever type—if it works—may be considered more humane than confinement. The offender is not only free after his sentence is served, but is also freed from the uncontrollable impulses that drive him to violate the freedom of others.[44] Yet a word of caution: Castration may reduce recidivism among offenders who commit a sex crime out of sexual urges, but many sex crimes are carried out as a way to assert power or to express rage or hostility. For these offenders, castration is no remedy.[45]

Sex-Offender Registration and Notification

Sex offenders residing in the community, having served a prison term or having been placed on probation, face registration and notification requirements. Society seems to countenance whatever is proposed for dealing with sex offenders, including sex offender free zones, special license plates, confinement on Halloween, parole ineligibility, etc. All 50 states and the federal government have enacted some type of sex offender registration law since 1994, when young Megan Kanka was beaten, raped, and murdered by a convicted sexual offender who lived near her family's New Jersey home. Compliance with the federal law is one of 17 requirements for states to receive a federal grant that pays for crime prevention and victim's assistance programs. For a grant, states must require sex offenders to register their names and addresses with local authorities for life. The states must require sex offenders who work or attend school in a different state to register with both states.

Whatever the federal law, registration schemes vary from state to state. The following categories have been conceptualized: (1) self-identification model, (2) police discretion model, and (3) police book model. The self-identification model requires the offender to identify himself to the community and the police. The police discretion model provides law enforcement agencies with the discretion over whether to release information to the community about convicted sex offenders. In this model, the community is not notified about all offenders, but rather those who are considered dangerous. The police book model allows members of the community to obtain information from law enforcement upon their request. The statutes focus on sexual assaults, including forcible rape and sexual abuse of children, but several statutes also target promoters of child pornography and child prostitution. Lesser crimes, such as indecent exposure or public indecency are enumerated in some of the statues. A number of states focus their registration statutes exclusively on offenders against children while others focus on habitual sex offenders.[46]

In some states, sexual offenders are currently required to register only for a limited length of time and can ask a court to terminate the registration order. These or other states are at risk of losing grant money if the federal government determines their sex offender registration laws are too weak. Michigan has had a sex registry since 1995 and made it public in 1999. There are now 27,583 offenders on the list, with 1,799 of them tried in juvenile courts. The listing in Michigan stays on the registry for a period of 25 years, Wyoming for 10 years. Failure to register is a felony. Juveniles convicted of a sex crime (those tried in juvenile courts as well as juveniles tried as adults) are listed on the registry.[47]

Some states, to track the whereabouts of discharged offenders, have gone beyond maintaining sex offender registries. They post the information, along with photographs and details of crimes, on Web pages accessible to anyone with access to the Internet. Proponents of the trend, including many state officials, say expanding community notification to the Internet is a valuable and relatively simple way to disseminate information. Critics say online registries, while popular with the public, are a "quick fix" to a complex issue and could stigmatize and victimize marginal offenders and ultimately produce more sex crimes than they prevent. As notification laws become ubiquitous, so have incidents in which ex-offenders have been harassed by neighbors, evicted by landlords, fired from new jobs, or beaten by revenge-minded mobs.[48]

To Sum Up

As each new legal experiment is introduced, perhaps it would be to everyone's advantage if it were tested in the manner of a true experiment, and information gathered about its effectiveness in enhancing community safety and fairness. From such an information base, the next legal steps might have more chance of achieving both. Although the efficacy of sex offender treatment remains inconclusive, its current empirical status may have less to do with its therapeutic soundness than it does with the manner in which treatment is employed or structured within the criminal justice system.[49] There is apparently no evidence that zoning restrictions or community notification has either enhanced the success of treatment or decreased recidivism rates.[50]

Endnotes

1. For example, Minn. Stat. Ann. §526.09 (1947). See D. E. J. MacNamara & E. Sagarin, *Sex, Crime, and the Law* (New York: Free Press, 1977); R. Slovenko (Ed.), *Sexual Behavior and the Law* (Springfield, IL: Thomas, 1965).
2. P.Q. Roche, *The Criminal Mind* (New York: Farrar, Straus & Cudahy, 1958), p. 25.
3. *DSM-IV* (Washington, DC: APA, 2000), p. 522.
4. S.L. Halleck, *Psychiatry and the Dilemmas of Crime* (New York: Harper & Row, 1967), p. 99.
5. Group for the Advancement of Psychiatry, *Psychiatric and Sex Psychopath Legislation: The 30s to the 80s* (Washington, DC: American Psychiatric Association, 1977), p. 840.
6. M. Ploscowe, *Sex and the Law* (New York: Ace Books, 1962).
7. 373 F.2d 451, 453 (D.C. Cir. 1966).
8. 373 F.2d 468, 472 (D.C. Cir. 1966).
9. People v. Jackson, 20 App. Div. 2d 170, 245 N.Y.S.2d 534 (1963).
10. T.S. Szasz, *The Myth of Mental Illness* (New York: Harper & Row, 1961).
11. See *Standard Edition of the Complete Works of Sigmund Freud* 2: 1, 6; 7: 51, 75, 170, 235; 16 :274; 18: 29.
12. Whitree v. State, 56 Misc. 2d 693, 711, 290 N.Y.S.2d 486, 504 (1968). There is, however, a justification for a special institution for sex offenders. In a prison with other offenders they are at the bottom of the totem pole, and they are abused. In prison hierarchy, murderers and professional thieves are "good" criminals. Child abusers, rapists and other sex offenders are not. In the Talinn (Estonia) prison, inmates even refuse to take food from fellow inmates serving in the caféteria whom they believe are sex offenders. "Picky criminals," *Baltic Times*, July 31–Aug. 6, 2008: 1.
13. K. Menninger, *The Vital Balance* (New York: Viking, 1963), p. 191. In a study of Adolf Hitler, *The Psychopathic God: Adolf Hitler* (New York: Basic Books, 1977), the historian Robert Waite suggests that Hitler's use of the extended stiff-arm salute was a substitute for his sexual shortcomings. Indeed, Hitler often boasted that his ability to hold his arm stiff was proof of his masculine power. Likewise, Hitler's lifelong preoccupation with constructing buildings reflected, in Professor Waite's view, behavior designed to quell anxiety about physical defects by making other kinds of structures whole. For all these pent-up fixations, Waite believed, Hitler's rabid anti-Semitism was, for him, a safety valve. In the Jew (and to a lesser extent, minorities such as homosexuals), Hitler found a convenient receptacle for the "displacement and projection" of all that he most feared and loathed about himself.
14. B. Glueck, "An Evaluation of the Homosexual Offender," *Minn. L. Rev.* 41 (1957): 187.
15. The Michigan statute provided: "Any person … suffering from a mental disorder and [who] is not feeble-minded, which mental disorder is coupled with criminal propensities to the commission of sex offenses, is hereby declared to be a criminal sexual psychopathic person."
16. Mich. Stat. Ann. §§ 780.501–509; repealed by Public Act No. 143 (1968).
17. J.F. Grabowski, "The Illinois Sexually Dangerous Persons Act: An Examination of a Statute in Need of Change," *So. Ill. U. L. J.* 12 (1988): 437, 454, n. 106.
18. Colorado, Connecticut, District of Columbia, Illinois, Massachusetts, Minnesota, Nebraska, New Jersey, Oregon, Tennessee, Utah, Virginia, and Washington.

19. S.J. Brakel, J. Parry, & B. Weiner, *The Mentally Disabled and the Law* (Chicago: American Bar Association, 3rd ed., 1985).

20. The states with a SVP law include Arizona, California, Florida, Illinois, Iowa, Kansas, Massachusetts, Minnesota, Missouri, New Hampshire, New Jersey, North Dakota, Pennsylvania, South Carolina, Virginia, Washington, Wisconsin, and a modified version in Texas. California law, for example, defines a sexually violent predator as "a person who has been convicted of a sexually violent offense against two or more victims and who has a diagnosed mental disorder that makes him or her a danger to the health and safety of others … [in that] it is likely that he or she will engage in sexuality violent criminal behavior"; Cal. Welfare & Institutions Code, § 6600.a.1. Not having an SVP law, New York sought to utilize its civil commitment law to commit a sexual offender who was about to be released from prison. The N.Y. State Court of Appeals (the state's highest level of appeal) ruled against it because the individual did not fall within its provisions. State of New York v. Eileen Consilvio, noted in B. Bryant, "Sex-Offender Commitments Hit Legal Roadblock in N.Y.," *Psychiatric News*, Feb. 2, 2007, p. 17. Since then, New York has adopted an SVP law. The adoption of the law is criticized in Editorial, "Wrong Turn on Sex Offenders," *New York Times*, March 13, 2007, p. 18.

21. The new laws are widely known as Megan's Law, named after Megan Kanka, a 7-year-old girl who was raped and murdered by a pedophile who had become a neighbor without the knowledge of her parents. In Russia today many people express a longing for Stalin, saying that he would end the corruption in the country and also the widespread pedophilia. He would confine them in the gulag. *Argument & Fact* (Russian weekly) 31 (July 2008): 5.

22. In *In re* Commitment of Feldmann, 730 N.W.2d 440 (Wis. App. 2007), the Wisconsin Court of Appeals held that the SVP Commitment Act did not violate equal protection as applied to a sex offender who had been released on parole by failing to require proof of a recent overt act or omission to show dangerousness, which is required to support the commitment of mentally or drug dependent persons. The court held that the act was narrowly tailored to the state's compelling interest in protecting the public from sexually violent persons whose mental disorders made them dangerous because of the substantial probability that they would commit future acts of sexual violence. The court noted that treatments of sex offenders and mentally ill persons varied widely, and the state still had the burden of proving that the sex offender who had been released on parole was dangerous. A contrary decision is *In re* Albrecht, 147 Wash.2d 1, 51 P.3d 73 (2002), where the Washington Supreme Court interpreted its SVP commitment statute to require proof of a recent overt act when the person has been released from confinement and into the community after a conviction.

23. Virginia's SVP law includes a tripwire that automatically sets the commitment process in motion if an algorithm predicts that the inmate has a high risk of sexual offense recidivism. Under the statute, commissioners of the Virginia Department of Corrections are directed to review for possible commitment all prisoners about to be released who "received a score of four or more on the Rapid Risk Assessment for Sexual Offender Recidivism" (RRASOR), a points system based on a regression analysis of male offenders in Canada. A score of four or more on the RRASOR translates into a prediction that the inmate, if released, would in the next 10 years have a 55% chance of committing another sex offense. The law is the first law ever to specify the use of a named actuarial prediction instrument and an exact cut-off score on that instrument. The RRASOR system is based on just four factors: the prisoner's number of prior sexual offenses, his age on release, the gender of his victims, and whether or not he was related to them. Since the statute was passed, however, the attorney general's office has sought commitments against only about 70% of the inmates who scored a four or more on the risk assessment. The Virginia law thus channels discretion, but it does not obliterate it. Reported in I. Ayres, "How Computers Killed the Expert," *Financial Times*, Sept. 1–2, 2007, p. 1. A review of assessment procedures appears in T.W. Campbell, *Assessing Sex Offenders* (Springfield, IL: Thomas, 2nd ed., 2007), which argues that these instruments amount to experimental procedures and, therefore, they cannot support expert testimony in a legal proceeding.

    The literature on SVP is extensive and critical. See, e.g., E.S. Janus, *Failure to Protect: America's Sexual Predator Laws and the Rise of the Preventive State* (Ithaca, NY: Cornell University Press, 2007); B.J. Winick & J.Q. LaFond (Eds.), *Protecting Society From Sexually Dangerous Offenders* (Washington, DC: American Psychological Assocation, 2003). A three-part series by Monica Davey and Abby Goodnough in *New York Times*, March 4–6, 2007, raises serious doubts about the SVP laws. See also B.J. Winick & J.Q. LaFond (Eds.), Symposium, "Sex Offenders: Scientific, Legal, and Policy Perspectives," *Psych. Pub. Policy and Law* 4 (March/June 1988); A. Brooks, "The Constitutionality and Morality of Civilly Committing Violent Sexual Predators," *U. Puget Sound L. Rev.* 15 (1992): 709; J. Douard, "Loathing the Sinner, Medicalizing the Sin: Why Sexually Violent Predator Statutes Are Unjust," *Intl.*

J. Law & Psychiatry 30 (2007): 36; A. Horwitz, "Sexual Psychopath Legislation: Is There Anywhere to Go but Backwards?" *U. Pitt. L. Rev.* 57 (1995): 35; S.J. Schulhofer, "Two Systems of Social Protection: Comments on the Civil-Criminal Distinction, With Particular Reference to Sexually Violent Predator Laws," *J. Contemp. Legal Issues* 8 (1996): 69; R.M. Wettstein, "A Psychiatric Perspective on Washington's Sexually Violent Predator Statute," *U. Puget Sound L. Rev.* 15 (1992): 597; H.V. Zonana & M.A. Norko, "Sexual Predators," *Psychiatric Clin. N. Am.* 22 (1999): 109; H.V. Zonana, "The Civil Commitment of Sex Offenders," *Science* 278 (Nov. 14, 1998): 1248.

24. In a controversial article appearing in *Psychological Bulletin*, published by the American Psychological Association, with the rather forbidding title, "A Meta-Analytic Examination of Assumed Properties of Child Sexual Abuse Using College Samples," Bruce Rind (Temple University), Robert Bauserman (University of Michigan), and Philip Tromovitcch (University of Pennsylvania) reviewed and analyzed data from 59 previous studies of college students who reported experiences of childhood sexual abuse. They found that childhood sexual abuse does not generally cause lasting psychological harm. Students who had experienced childhood sexual abuse were, on average, only slightly less well adjusted than other comparable students, and these differences generally disappeared when family environment was taken into account. Noting that the term *abuse* implies that harm is inflicted, the authors argued that classifying behavior as abuse merely because it is considered illegal or immoral, even in the absence of harm, is not scientifically valid. They claim that in many, and perhaps most, cases of sexual activity between an adult and a minor, there is no physical or emotional harm to the child. They suggest that the term *childhood sexual abuse* be restricted to situations in which the sexual activity is unwanted by the minor and is experienced negatively. The North American Man–Boy Love Association, the major pedophilia advocacy group, hailed the report as good news, bolstering their claims that consensual sex between men and boys is not harmful, may be beneficial, and should be legalized. See G.E. Zuriff, "Pedophilia and the Culture Wars," *Public Interest* 138 (2000): 29. The psychologist John Money has been a longtime advocate of this view. See J. Money, *Principles of Developmental Sexology* (New York: Continuum, 1994); J. Money, *Vandalized Lovemaps: Paraphilic Outcome of 7 Cases in Pediatric Sexology* (Buffalo, NY: Promethus Books, 1989). This view, however, is not widely accepted. Michigan Attorney General Mike Cox maintains, "Internet predators pose a clear and present danger to children." He has launched the Michigan Cyber Safety Initiative (Michigan CSI), which educates not only students, but also teachers and parents on how to avoid dangers on the Internet. His office has arrested nearly 150 Internet predators. M. Cox, "State Can't Arrest Its Way Out of Web Predators," *Detroit News*, Oct. 12, 2007, p. 8. One may wonder how many of the Internet predators are without social skills and are unable to form a social bond, so they turn to the Internet. See T. Attwood, *Asperger's Syndrome* (Philadelphia: Jessica Kingsley, 1998); B.G. Haskins & J.A. Silva, "Asperger's Disorder and Criminal Behavior: Forensic-Psychiatric Considerations," *J. Am. Acad. Psychiat. & Law* 34 (2006): 374; J.A. Silva, G.B. Leong, & M.M. Ferrari, "Paraphilic Psychopathology in a Case of Autism Spectrum Disorder," *Am. J. Foren. Psychiat.* 24 (2003): 5.

25. See the symposia on sex offender laws in *Behav. Sci. & Law* 18 (2000): nos. 1–3. See also G.B. Palermo & M.A. Farkas, *The Dilemma of the Sexual Offender* (Springfield, IL: Thomas, 2001).

26. *In re* Young, 122 Wash. 2d 1, 857 P.2d 989 (1993).

27. 857 P.2d at 1001.

28. *In re* Linehan, 518 N.W.2d 609 (Minn. 1994). See also Hince v. O'Keefe, 632 N.W.2d 577 (Minn. 2001). In the Italian comedy film *The Monster*, the psychiatrist is lampooned in his effort to evaluate Loris (Robert Benigni) who is suspected of being a "sex fiend."

29. *In re* Hendricks, 259 Kan. 246, 912 P.2d 129 (1996), ruling on Kan. Stat. Ann. §59-29a01 *et seq.*

30. 117 S. Ct. 2072 (1997).

31. 117 S. Ct. at 2080. In Kansas v. Crane, 534 U.S. 407 (2002), the Supreme Court again reviewed the Kansas law, this time on whether states must prove that offenders cannot control their behavior in order to confine them indefinitely as sexual predators. The case involved Michael Crane who went to prison in 1994 for sexually assaulting a video store clerk and exposing himself to a tanning salon attendant in Kansas City. When he was about to be paroled in 1998, prosecutors went to court to have him committed to a state hospital. The jury agreed to have him committed, following narrow guidelines issued by the judge. He was placed on conditional release after having completed the state's treatment program. The Kansas Supreme Court ordered a new trial, saying that the jury that found him likely to commit another similar crime should also have found him unable to control his behavior. Earlier, in the 1997 case, child molester Leroy Hendricks had admitted he "can't control the urge." In *Crane*, in argument before the U.S. Supreme Court, the state contended that the control requirement is too broad because almost all sexual offenders possess at least some control over their actions. The Supreme

Court ruled that there be a separate finding of inability to control behavior or serious difficulty in controlling behavior. That is, there must be some lack of control determination before one can be civilly committed. The Court considered the constitutional importance of distinguishing a dangerous sexual offender subject to civil commitment from other dangerous persons who are perhaps more properly dealt with exclusively through criminal proceedings; 534 U.S. at 417. During argument, the Justices pressed the attorneys to say specifically how far the Court should go in setting a standard for the proof that states must offer.

32. 117 S. Ct. at 2084.

33. Young v. Weston, 898 F. Supp. 744 (W.D. Wash. 1995). In Sharp v. Weston, 233 F.3d 1166 (9th Cir. 2000), the Ninth Circuit held that persons committed as sexually violent predators have a Fourteenth Amendment right to mental health treatment that gives them a realistic opportunity to be cured and released. The court acknowledged that although the state enjoys wide latitude in developing treatment programs, the courts may take action when there is substantial departure from accepted professional judgment or no exercise of professional judgment at all. The court noted that under Youngberg v. Romeo, 457 U.S. 307 (1982), the decisions made by professionals are presumptively valid, but not conclusive. In Pool v. McKune, 987 P.2d 1073 (Kan. 1999), the question was raised whether convicted sex offenders serving a criminal sentence have a right to privacy under the Fourth Amendment that would preclude required plethysmograph testing in a sexual abuse treatment program, a prison-based 18-month rehabilitation program for sex offenders. The Kansas Supreme Court held that neither the scope of the intrusion, the manner in which the test is conducted, nor the place in which it is conducted outweighs the penological interest in rehabilitating sex offenders.

    Innovations in dealing with sex offenders have often tested constitutional boundaries. In another Kansas case, the U.S. Supreme Court was called upon to decide whether a state violates a convicted sex offender's right against compelled self-incrimination by taking away prison privileges if the inmate refuses to accept responsibility for any previously undisclosed crimes as part of a therapy program. Presumably, by accepting responsibility for past crimes, it would indicate remorse and, hence, a therapeutic gain. The Kansas program uses a polygraph examination to test the completeness and accuracy of an inmate's disclosures. There is no immunity from prosecution for previously undisclosed crimes, although in the years of the program's existence, no inmate has been prosecuted for a confession given in the course of treatment. The case, *McKune v. Lile*, began in 1993 when the inmate, Robert Lile, serving a life sentence for rape and who was approaching his parole date, refused to participate in the sexual abuse treatment program, and as a result he was reduced to the lowest level of the prison's classification system and ordered transferred to a maximum-security prison. L. Greenhouse, "Inmates' Self-Incrimination Debated at Supreme Court," *New York Times*, Nov. 29, 2001, p. 24.

34. Seling v. Young, 531 U.S. 250 (2001). See E. S. Janus, "Sex Predator Commitment Laws: Constitutional but Unwise," *Psychiat. Ann.*, June 2000, p. 411.

35. Council of Psychiatry and Law, American Psychiatric Association, Final Report of the Subcommittee to Review the Insanity Defense (1988), p. 3.

36. There is a continuing debate about whether predictions of dangerousness are accurate enough to support deprivation of liberty. Should risk assessment, which is based on group behavior, be sufficient to establish that a particular individual will be dangerous in the future? For the most part, courts have rejected this argument based largely on public safety concerns. E.S. Janus & P.E. Meehl, "Assessing the Legal Standard for Predictions of Dangerousness in Sex Offender Commitment Proceedings," *Psych., Pub. Policy & Law* 3 (1997): 33. The New Jersey Court of Appeals has ruled that the state met its burden of establishing that under the *Frye* standard, actuarial tools for predicting sex offenders' risk of committing future acts of sexual violence are generally accepted by the scientific community and, thus, are admissible as scientific evidence in SVP commitment proceedings. *In re* Commitment of R.S., 773 A.2d 72 (N.J. Super. Ct. App. Div. 2001). For a critique, see T.W. Campbell, "Sexual Predator Evaluations and Phrenology: Considering Issues of Evidentiary Reliability," *Behav. Sci. & Law* 18 (2000): 111. See D. Boerner, "Confronting Violence: In the Act and in the World," *U. Puget Sound L. Rev.* 15 (1992): 525; A.D. Brooks, "The Constitutionality and Morality of Civilly Committing Violent Sexual Predators," *U. Puget Sound L. Rev.* 15 (1992): 709, G. Gelb, "Washington's Sexually Violent Predator Law: The Need to Bar Unreliable Psychiatric Predictions of Dangerousness From Civil Commitment Proceedings," *UCLA L. Rev.* 39 (1991): 213.

37. B. Bodine, "Washington's New Violent Sexual Predator Commitment System: An Unconstitutional Law and an Unwise Policy Choice," *U. Puget Sound Law Rev.* 14 (1990): 105; see also S.J. Brakel & J.L. Cavanaugh, "Of Psychopaths and Pendulums: Legal and Psychiatric Treatment of Sex Offenders in the United States," *New Mex. L. Rev.* 30 (2000): 69; J.Q. La Fond, "Sexually Violent Predator Laws and the Liberal State: An Ominous Threat to Individual Liberty," *Int. J. Law & Psychiat.* 31 (2008): 158.

38. See, e.g., L. Gigliotti (Ltr.), "A System for Dealing With Sex Offenders," *New York Times*, March 11, 2007, p. WK13.

39. See G.C. Abel, "Behavioral Treatment of Child Molesters," in A.J. Stunkard & A. Baum (Eds.), *Perspectives on Behavioral Medicine* (New York: Erlbaum, 1989), pp. 223–242; R.J. Kelly, "Behavioral Reorientation of Pedophiliacs: Can It Be Done?" *Clin. Psychol. Rev.* 2 (1982): 387.

40. California initiated legislation requiring certain convicted sex offenders as a condition of probation to submit to treatment with the progesterone agent medroxyprogesterone acetate. A number of other states have done the same. The bills do not clearly define what is meant by *chemical castration* other than to list the medication(s) that may be used. See R.D. Miller, "Forced Administration of Sex-Drive Reducing Medications to Sex Offenders: Treatment or Punishment?" *Psych., Pub. Policy & Law* 4 (1998): 175.

41. People v. Gauntlett, 134 Mich. App. 737, at 751 (1984).

42. 134 Mich. App. at 750.

43. During the 17th and 18th centuries, for some 200 years, young males were transformed by surgical castration into mellifluous sopranos. The cause is attributed to the prohibition against women singing in church or appearing onstage. With the invention of Italian opera, a popular style of entertainment, singers with women's voices were required. Until the late 18th century, Italian opera and castrati were indistinguishable concepts. And 70% of male opera singers were castrati. Moreover, throughout history, eunuchs were created for various purposes. They often served in harems, where genitally intact men could not supervise the frustrated women. In the Byzantine and Ottoman empires, they also filled top administrative and military posts, controlling finances and the destinies of entire peoples. Unlike uncastrated men, who had families of their own, eunuchs could be trusted not to intrigue on behalf of the sons they would never have. E. Abbott, *A History of Celibacy* (New York: Scribner, 2000).

44. In 1997, the Texas legislature enacted legislation permitting certain incarcerated sex offenders to request a voluntary orchiectomy as part of a treatment program. The incarcerated sex offenders may obtain an orchiectomy only if the offender has been convicted at least twice as a sex offender and evaluated to be competent, adequately informed, and acting voluntarily. Preliminary evidence is that the lowering of the testosterone level as a result of an orchiectomy (or the administration of drugs, such as Lupron*) enables pedophiles to gain better control of their impulses to seek sexual gratification. See F. Saleh, J. Bradford, A. Grudzinsakas, & D. Brodsky (Eds.), *Sex Offenders: Identification, Risk Assessment, Treatment, and Legal Issues* (New York: Oxford University Press, 2007); W.J. Winslade, T.H. Stone, M. Smith-Bell, & M.D. Webb, "Castrating Pedophiles Convicted of Sex Offenses Against Children: New Treatment or Old Punishment?" *SMU L. Rev.* 51 (1998): 349. See also G.G. Abel & C. Osborn, "Stopping Sexual Violence," *Psychiat. Ann.* 22 (1992): 301; J.V. Becker, M.S. Kaplan, & R. Kavoussi, "Measuring the Effectiveness of Treatment for the Aggressive Adolescent Sexual Offender," *Ann. N.Y. Acad. Sci.* 528 (1988): 215; F S. Berlin & C.F. Meinecke, "Treatment of Sex Offenders With Antiandrogenic Medication: Conceptulization, Review of Treatment Modalities, and Preliminary Findings," *Am. J. Psychiat.* 138 (1981): 601; J.M.W. Bradford & D. McLean, "Sexual Offenders, Violence and Testosterone: A Clinical Study," *Can. J. Psychiat.* 1984: 335; T.A. Kiersch, "Treatment of Sex Offenders With Depo-Provera*," *Bull. Am. Acad. Psychiat. & Law* 18 (1990): 179. See also F.S. Berlin, "Chemical Castration for Sex Offenders," *N. Eng. J. Med.* 336 (1997): 1030; C.L. Scott & T. Holmberg, "Castration of Sex Offenders: Prisoner's Right Versus Public Safety," *J. Am. Acad. Psychiat. & Law* 31 (2003): 502. See B. Engle, "A Study of Castration," *Psychoanal. Rev.* 23 (1936): 363.

45. Randy Thornhill, an evolutionary biologist, and Craig T. Palmer, an evolutionary anthropologist, contend that rape is primarily a crime of sex, not violence and power, as a generation of social scientists and feminist scholars have argued. R. Thornhill & C.T. Palmer, *A Natural History of Rape: Biological Bases of Sexual Coercion* (Boston: MIT Press, 2000), excerpted in "When Men Rape," *Science*, Jan./Feb. 2000, p. 30; critically reviewed in E. Goode, "What Provokes a Rapist to Rape? *New York Times*, Jan. 15, 2000, p. 21.

46. A.R. Bedarf, "Examining Sex Offender Community Notification Laws," *Calif. L. Rev.* 83 (1995): 885. In Connecticut Department of Public Safety v. Doe, 538 U.S. 1 (2003), the petitioner argued that the state's sex offender registry violated the due process clause because registrants were not given a hearing to determine whether they are likely to be currently dangerous. The Supreme Court noted that the

Connecticut registration requirement was based on the fact of a previous conviction, not the fact of current dangerousness; hence, the Court ruled that the law did not violate procedural due process. The Court expressed no opinion as to whether the state law violated substantive due process, and it is not likely to do so. In McKune v. Lile, 536 U.S. 24, 32 (2002), the Court said, "Sex offenders are a serious threat in this nation." In Paul v. Davis, 424 U.S. 693 (1976), the Court held that injury to reputation, even if defamatory, does not constitute the deprivation of a liberty interest.

47. The reason many juvenile records are expunged at adulthood is to give nonviolent offenders the chance to learn from mistakes and start afresh, but that is not reflected when discretion cannot be exercised concerning the sex offender registry. The lengthy registration period in some states (25 years in Michigan) prompts recommendations for separate rules for teen offenders.

48. P. Zielbauer, "Sex Offender Registries on Web Draw Both Praise and Criticism," *New York Times*, May 22, 2000, p. 18. In England, following the murder of 8-year-old Sarah Payne, a campaign began to enact a version of Megan's Law, called Sarah's Law. Rupert Murdoch's *News of the World* carried on a "name and shame" campaign, which resulted in vigilante attacks against suspected pedophiles and the deaths of innocent people, and it was discontinued. E. Vulliamy & N.P. Walsh, "The Paedophile Panic," *Observer*, Aug. 6, 2000, p. 14; A. Gillan, "Paper Relents Over Drive to Shame," *Guardian*, Aug. 5, 2000, p. 1. As a registered sex offender, David Randazzo of Mount Clemens, Michigan, packed up and moved 17 times in a year and a half. He was forced to move so often out of fear because, when his neighbors found him on the Sex Offender Registry, they threatened him and started fights. No employer would hire him. He spends his days at home watching television. He pleaded no contest to fourth-degree criminal sexual conduct for fondling a 13-year-old relative (a no-contest plea is not an admission of guilt, but is regarded as such for sentencing purposes). Under the Michigan Sex Offender Registry, established in 1994, a sex offender may not live, work, or loiter within 1,000 feet from a park, school, or any place where children congregate. First-time violators of the restriction are guilty of a misdemeanor that is punishable by up to a year in jail and a $1,000 fine. Repeat violators are guilty of a felony and face up to 2 years in jail and up to a $2,000 fine. See C. Stolarz, "Sex Offender Wants to Stay Put," *Detroit News*, Oct. 4, 2007, p. B-1. Canada allows anyone who fears on reasonable grounds that some person will commit a sex offense of a minor under the age of 14 may lay information before a provincial court judge. Canada Criminal Code sec. 810.1; discussed in *National Post*, Oct. 21, 2000, p. 9.

49. See J.A. Marvasti (Ed.), *Psychiatric Treatment of Sexual Offenders* (Springfield, IL: Thomas, 2004); W. Edwards & C. Hensley, "Restructuring Sex Offender Sentencing: A Therapeutic Jurisprudence Approach to the Criminal Justice Process," *Int. J. Offender Therapy & Comp. Crim.* 45 (2001): 646.

50. See P.S. Appelbaum, "Sex Offenders in the Community: Are Current Approaches Counterproductive?" *Psychiat. Serv.* 59 (April 2008): 352; F.S. Berlin, "Sex Offender Treatment and Legislation, *J. Am. Acad. Psychiat. & Law* 31 (2003): 510; C.L. Scott & J.B. Gerbasi, "Sex Offender Registration and Community Notification Challenges: The Supreme Court Continues Its Trend," *J. Am. Acad. Psychiat. & Law* 31 (2003): 494.

17
Homosexuality
From Condemnation to Celebration

The history of homosexuality has been one of condemnation punctuated by intervals of celebration. For nearly 2,000 years, homosexuality has been viewed as evidence of moral weakness, criminality, or pathology. These have been the perspectives, in turn, of religion, law, and medicine. Until recently, homosexuality was seen not as the mark of a distinctive, oppressed minority group, but rather as an individual and very personal problem. The development of a homosexual lobby, if you will, had its genesis in 1968 after a riot erupted outside a bar on Christopher Street in New York's Greenwich Village. Homophiles began to mobilize for the first time and soon became a major political and economic force. Taking a cue from the civil rights and feminist movements, the struggle for homosexual rights emerged from obscurity.

In 1985, the Gay and Lesbian Alliance Against Defamation was founded, and in 1987 (the year coincidentally that Rock Hudson died of AIDS), its representatives persuaded the *New York Times* to change its editorial policy and use the word *gay* instead of *homosexual*. The term *gay*, signifying celebration, became common currency. At rallies there were the chants: "Gay is good. Gay is proud. Gay is natural. Gay is normal." "Say it loud, we're gay and proud." "2–4–6–8, gay is just as good as straight." The Gay and Lesbian Alliance Against Defamation is known by its acronym, GLAAD.[1] "Gay pride will rank as one of the great inventions of the 20th century," proclaimed Deb Price, an avowed gay who writes a weekly syndicated column about homosexuality.[2] At the same time, the AIDS epidemic has ravaged the gay (and drug-user) community—it is called another holocaust.[3]

Homosexuality, and society's mainly adverse reaction to it, has a history as long as civilization itself. The people of ancient Sodom proudly proclaimed their homosexuality, but were condemned by the prophet Isaiah, who deemed homosexuality as akin to bestiality.[4] Leviticus 18:22 defined homosexuality as a crime, in biblical language, an "abomination." Leviticus 20:13 went much farther: "If a man lies with a man sexually as with a woman, they have performed an abomination; they shall surely be put to death." The first commandment in the Bible is "be fruitful and multiply."

Homosexuality, however, seems to have flourished in ancient Greece. Greek homosexual love in the 4th century was both passionate and physical. Plato and his friends were overt homosexuals. As far as Plato was concerned, romantic passion was only possible between men and boys. Plato's love for Dion was a model for many ideas about romantic love until the medieval period. The homosexual relationship was cast in the same mold as the modern-day romantic love between men and women.

It would, however, be a mistake to consider homosexual love as the rule in ancient Greece. Although Solon (statesman and lawgiver and believed to be one of the Seven Sages) granted homosexuals civil rights, homosexuality was not condoned by the common populace, and its practitioners were mocked in Aristophanes' plays. The usual justification for homosexuality in Greece was that women were not fit companions for Athenian intellectuals. By and large, women were relegated to a life of obscurity and illiteracy, and were considered boring. There were some sophisticated women, however, such as the poet Sappho, who ran a school for women on the island of Lesbos (from which the term *lesbian* was derived). However, such women were the exception rather than the rule. Demosthenes voiced the typical attitude: "Courtesans we keep for pleasure, concubines for daily [sexual] attendance on our persons, and wives to bear us legitimate children and to be our housekeepers."[5]

Toward the end of the 17th century, religious disapprobation of homosexuality became reinforced by state condemnation, as the sin became a crime. Some penal codes retained the religious abhorrence of homosexuality, describing it as a crime not merely against society, but "against nature."[6] Legal codes in the American colonies set death as the penalty for sodomy, and in several instances courts directed the execution of men found guilty of this act.[7] Although most states abolished the death penalty for sodomy by 1825, all but two (Kansas and Utah) in the mid-20th century still classified it as a felony. Only murder, kidnapping, and rape carried heavier sentences. Although few men and almost no women were punished under such laws, the statutes imposed the stigma of criminality.

The most famous prosecution resulted in the conviction in 1895 of Oscar Wilde, England's celebrated playwright and now a gay icon. Although homosexuality was a criminal offense, Wilde had made little effort to conceal his relations with younger men, particularly Lord Alfred Douglas. Douglas's father, the Marquess of Queensberry, hounded Wilde relentlessly, finally sending him a note calling him a "Sodomite." Wilde sued for libel, a fatal mistake. In the course of the trial, his private affairs were mercilessly exposed, and he lost the case. He was then prosecuted for committing indecent acts, convicted, and sentenced to 2 years at hard labor.[8] He emerged from the degradation of prison a broken and penniless man, and he went to Paris, where he died soon thereafter, at age 46, his health ruined by imprisonment. He died a sad and lonely death, desperately poor and largely abandoned by those he thought his friends. His family changed their surname to Holland to escape the opprobrium surrounding their name.

By the 20th century, prosecution for homosexual activity had grown increasingly rare. Generally speaking, prosecutions for sodomy in the 20th century, even where outlawed, were limited to those involving either gross indiscretion[9] or forceful action.[10] Prosecuting officials and courts would read "notoriety" or "brutality" into the sodomy statutes as essential elements of the offense. The issue in these cases, then, was not really one of homosexuality versus heterosexuality, but rather of the gross violation of social amenities. Writings on the law of homosexuality, as a rule, omit any reference to notoriety or violence and, as a result, they misrepresent the state of enforcement of the law.[11]

The decline in the criminalization of homosexuality was a reflection of the increasing medicalization of it. As early as the 19th century, homosexuality began to be discussed as an illness or disease. It was argued that homosexuals were not so much sinners or criminals as they were mentally ill. In the 1880s and 1890s, doctors debated whether homosexuality was a vice indulged in by weak-willed, depraved individuals; an acquired form of insanity; or a congenital defect that indicated evolutionary degeneracy. By the early 20th century many were saying that homosexuality was hereditary in origin. The advent of Freudian theory in the 1920s, however, changed both the medical explanations and societal perceptions of homosexuality. The Freudian legacy was to focus on early childhood and unresolved Oedipal conflicts. The emphasis shifted from a concern with genetics to psychic conflict. Freud's biographical reconstruction of the life of Leonardo da Vinci suggested that the combination of an absent father and a dominant mother was central in the development of male homosexuality. In contrast, Dr. Irving Bieber and his colleagues in 1962 published data on approximately 100 homosexual males in psychoanalytically oriented therapy that found an abusive father to be the common denominator.[12]

Events surrounding World War II abetted the perception of homosexual behavior as illness. The federal government ordered psychiatric screening of inductees during World War II, leading to an increase in visibility and enhanced prestige for psychiatry. Homosexuals were deemed medically unfit for service. Americans, by and large, came to view sexual behavior not as moral or immoral, but as sick or healthy, with homosexuality falling into the sick category.[13]

In 1948, biologist Alfred Charles Kinsey and his associates entered the scene. In their much-publicized work, they demonstrated that homosexual and heterosexual responsiveness in human beings is not always found in clearly differentiated patterns. They showed that these levels of responsiveness are spread across a continuum that ranges from exclusive heterosexual reactivity to exclusive homosexual reactivity, with various gradations in between. Kinsey suggested a 7-point scale for this continuum based on both overt experience and inner psychological reactions. His study painted a picture of the sexuality of ordinary Americans that was startling. Nothing had challenged the conventional wisdom about homosexuality as much as his finding that 50 percent of males admitted erotic responses to their own sex.[14] Current thinking about gender in the field of sexology challenges the binary conceptualization of gender in categorizing individuals and the resultant pathologizing of gender variance, and promotes the premise of gender as a continuum.[15]

Shortly after World War II, when communism replaced Nazism as a threat to the country, or so it was perceived, President Truman established a loyalty program for federal employees, and in 1950, the Senate produced a report, *The Employment of Homosexuals and Other Sex Perverts in Government*.[16] Some Congressmen argued that *sex perverts* imperiled national security on the grounds that they were vulnerable to blackmail.[17] Kinsey's research caused such commotion that he was denounced as a communist and his research funds were withdrawn.[18]

During the 1960s, the portrayals of homosexual life multiplied in literature and in the mass media. With the growing volume of such material came a new way of seeing the homosexual lifestyle. A significant number of persons began to view homosexuals not as isolated, aberrant individuals, but as members of a group. The militancy of homosexual activists allowed the movement to exploit the sexual permissiveness that characterized American culture in the 1960s. The national debate about sexual matters that was sparked by the Kinsey reports cleared away the residue of proscriptions on sexual discourse that was the legacy of Victorianism. Popular attitudes remained hostile, however, and for the overwhelming majority of homosexual men and women, a retreat to a secret life was preferable to the stigma that openness would bring.

Homosexuals found that they still had to deal with the "sickness" label, which has wider application than the criminal label. While relatively few homosexuals have been convicted of a crime against nature—the vast majority of homosexuals have as spotless a record as heterosexuals—they all fell under the "mental disorder" label of the American Psychiatric Association's *Diagnostic and Statistical Manual of Mental Disorders* (DSM). The first edition of the manual, published in 1952, classified homosexuality as a sexual deviation.[19] The general category within which the sexual deviations appeared was Sociopathic Personality Disturbance, a designation referring to individuals who are ill primarily in terms of society's reaction to them because they fail to conform to the prevailing cultural milieu.[20] In *DSM-II*, the second edition of the manual published in 1968, homosexuality was also classified as a sexual deviation, but sexual deviations were now categorized under Personality Disorders, a group distinguished by deeply ingrained maladaptive patterns of behavior perceptibly different in quality from psychotic and neurotic symptoms.[21]

The "sickness" label backfired on homosexuals. As sickness, it applied broadly, whereas the original label applied only to those who were charged with crime against nature. Government and many private employers justified employment discrimination and other policies by referring to the *DSM*. "Homosexuals are sick," they said, and they were able to point to a respected authority. So, in the early 1970s, homosexuals argued that much of the prejudice confronting them was a product of psychiatric stigmatization. As a consequence, various homosexual activist groups, supported by some psychiatrists, urged that homosexuality should not be considered a form of mental illness. They demonstrated at the annual meetings of the American Psychiatric

Association (APA), disrupted meetings, and stormed the speaker platforms. They cursed Dr. Irving Bieber, who had argued for conversion therapy.

Intimidated, the APA Board of Trustees in 1978 voted unanimously (with two abstentions) to eliminate the general category of homosexuality from the *DSM* and to replace it with a category called Sexual Orientation Disturbance. This designation would apply only to ego-dystonic homosexuality, that is, homosexuals who are either subjectively distressed by or in conflict with their sexual orientation. The APA's Task Force on Nomenclature had recommended that homosexuality be regarded as "a normal variant of human sexuality," but in order to obtain passage, the Board of Trustees changed the wording of the Task Force that homosexuality "by itself does not constitute a psychiatric disorder" to "does not necessarily constitute a disorder."[22] In 1974, APA members voted by ballot to ratify the trustees' decision. The vote was 5,854 (58%) for the trustees' position, 3,810 (37.8%) against, and 367 abstentions. One bemused observer labeled it "the single greatest cure in the history of psychiatry." The APA is mocked, critics saying that its *DSM* cannot be deemed scientific if its diagnoses can be changed by vote.

Under the circumstances, the conclusion is inescapable that the vote was made under compulsion. Dr. Ronald Bayer summarized the events as follows:

> The entire process, from the first confrontations organized by gay demonstrators at psychiatric conventions to the referendum demanded by orthodox psychiatrists, seemed to violate the most basic expectations about how questions of science should be resolved. Instead of being engaged in a sober consideration of data, psychiatrists were swept up in political controversy. The American Psychiatric Association had fallen victim to the disorder of a tumultuous era, when disruptive conflicts threatened to politicize every aspect of American social life. A furious egalitarianism that challenged every instance of authority had compelled psychiatric experts to negotiate the pathological status of homosexuality with homosexuals themselves. The result was not a conclusion based on an approximation of the scientific truth as dictated by reason, but was instead an action demanded by the ideological temper of the times.[23]

Dr. Jon K. Meyer commented,

> At the moment, homosexuality is perhaps the most difficult subject in psychiatry to address. Few conditions affecting the psyche and behavior have been so intensely scrutinized, debated, and politicized. Conceptualization of homosexuality—as a lifestyle, a preference, an illness, a sociopolitical movement, a biological predisposition—is marked by a fundamental lack of consensus.[24]

Homosexuals hailed the change in the APA nomenclature in *DSM-III* as an instant cure.[25] Shortly after the APA vote, the federal government in 1975 eliminated the ban on employment of homosexuals.[26] Then too, the Americans with Disabilities Act of 1990 specifically provided that homosexuality and bisexuality are not impairments and as such cannot constitute disabilities.[27]

In *DSM-III-R* (1987), no mention is made of homosexuality. This edition also shifted gender identity disorder to the pediatric section of the manual ("disorders usually first evident in infancy, childhood, or adolescence"). In *DSM-IV* (1994), Sex and Gender Identity Disorder became an independent category. The drafters of *DSM-IV* removed sexual identity disorders entirely from any kind of perversion section and instead made sexual sadism and masochism subordinate to identity disorders. The World Health Organization, however, still includes homosexuality as a medical diagnosis in the International Classification of Diseases.

The end of the 20th century was marked by unprecedented state-level changes in the law on homosexuality. Today, ironically, homosexuality is constitutionally protected in the United States, but prayer is not. In the year 1999, in state after state, gay rights legislation advanced farther and faster than ever before—thanks to the growing number of openly gay lawmakers, the diligence of statewide gay groups, and the emerging national consensus that gay people should be treated with respect. Various states repealed this ban on gay adoptive and foster parents. Others expanded their hate crimes law to protect gays. California passed a domestic partnership bill that gives unmarried partners—gay or heterosexual—vital benefits, including hospitalization and inheritance rights. The Vermont Supreme Court, on the basis of a 200-year-old clause of the state constitution that government should be "instituted for the common benefit, protection, and security of the people, nation, or community," ordered the state to guarantee the same protections and benefits to homosexual couples that it does to married heterosexuals.[28] Over the past decade, a number of countries have created one form or another of domestic partnership arrangements for the benefit of homosexuals.

The publicity about homosexuality is now pervasive and well nigh inescapable. Homosexuality has gone from condemnation to celebration. It is openly displayed and discussed. It is portrayed on stage and screen and in many publications. Not only offbeat publishers, but mainline publishers and university presses (notably Duke University Press and University of Wisconsin Press) have long lists of books on homosexuality. The *New York Times* in its Sunday edition on its wedding pages carries news, with photos, of gay couples. Guide books on city life include the homosexual scene. Gay study courses are now offered at a number of leading universities in the United States. Tens of thousands of homosexual men and women march in annual Christopher Street Liberation Day parades in major cities. The Victorians would be dismayed.

Recognition of Various Homosexual Rights

Before the 1960s, homosexuals generally feared to speak out about their sexual orientation or to organize groups to secure their legal rights. The few organized groups that did exist used names designed to conceal their homosexual nature so that prospective members would feel less uncomfortable about joining them. Beginning in the 1960s, when the issue came before the courts, it was held rather consistently that advocacy of homosexual rights, even in a state that penalizes private, adult, consensual sodomy, is not advocacy of or incitement to imminent lawless action and is, therefore, protected speech.[29]

Homosexual student service organizations thereupon received university recognition and the benefit of school-run facilities enjoyed by other recognized groups. It was held that a state-run university may not constitutionally reject a student organization whose fundamental purpose is to provide a forum for the discussion of homosexuality. That the presence of such a group may make homosexual behavior more prevalent on campus is not enough, the courts said, to justify a prior restraint on the students' constitutional rights to freedom of association.[30]

A more controversial area concerned the First Amendment rights of homosexual teachers in public schools. It is generally recognized that an adverse employment action is permissible if the controversial speech either falls outside First Amendment protection, or implicates the employee's fitness to perform his or her assigned duties. In *National Gay Task Force v. Board of Education*,[31] the Tenth Circuit Court of Appeals held unconstitutional an Oklahoma statute that permitted public schools to fire teachers for "advocating, soliciting, imposing, encouraging, or promoting public or private homosexual activity in a manner that creates a substantial risk that such conduct will come to the attention of school children or school employees." The United States Supreme Court, in a 4–4 decision with no written opinion, upheld the Tenth Circuit's ruling.[32]

Homosexuals also battled for acceptance in the media. In general, in the absence of any state action, the choice of material that goes into a newspaper is left solely to the editor's discretion. In the broadcasting medium, the Federal Communications Commission compels every broadcast licensee to ascertain the "problems, needs, and interests" of its community and to design informational programming to meet these needs. Such needs are determined through polling the public and interviewing representative leaders of significant groups within the community.[33] Homosexual rights leaders contended that, given the number of homosexuals in the general population (estimates range from 5 to 10% of males and from 2 to 5% of females), they are not properly represented on television. These concerns for a right of access to the media are still in conflict with the discretionary powers of corporate broadcasters.

Today homosexual tabloids are given away free in just about every city and the pages are filled with advertisements directed at the homosexual community. A Gay Financial Network sells financial services products, which recognize the distinct needs of the gay and lesbian community. It publishes a top 50 list of powerful and gay-friendly corporations. The gay and lesbian community is estimated to have over $800 billion in assets, 65% have completed college and they are not necessarily raising families, so their disposable income is greater. The organizing of gays has made it good business to appeal to the homosexual market.

Homosexual organizations have had difficulty in attaining the ultimate symbol of acceptance: tax-exempt status. In general, the Internal Revenue Service (IRS) has denied the applications of homosexual organizations seeking tax-exempt status. Under the Internal Revenue Code, in order to enjoy tax-exempt and tax-deductible status, an organization must generally be operated for one or more of the following purposes: religious, charitable, scientific, public safety, literary, educational, or for the prevention of cruelty to children or animals. Such organizations are prohibited from carrying on propaganda or attempting to influence legislation. Any such group engaged in advocacy of a position must present a full and fair exposition of the issues in order to maintain the exemption.[34]

The military became the last major area of gay intolerance remaining in society. When President Clinton tried to lift the ban on gay service members in 1993, he faced a near-rebellion from the Joint Chiefs of Staff and resounding defeat in Congress. "Don't ask, don't tell" was the compromise that was designed to permit gays to serve without fear of harassment or expulsion as long as they kept their orientation to themselves. John M. Shalikashvili, then chairman of the Joint Chiefs of Staff, supported the "don't ask, don't tell" policy, but now has recommended, as a result of the stretching thin of the military by deployments to the Middle East, a military policy of nondiscrimination based on sexual orientation. At the same time, he urged Congress to debate the issue with sensitivity.[35] Anthropologist Lionel Tiger postulated that the military recruiting crisis is due to the presence of homosexuals and women in the military: "It is no longer macho to be in the military."[36]

On November 4, 2008 the gay rights movement suffered a major setback. Famously, by a margin of 52% to 48%, California's Proposition 8 was passed, which defines marriage as a union between a man and a woman. The measure passed despite advertisements featuring Hollywood tough-guy Samuel Jackson, the backing of Governor Arnold Schwarzenegger and a late surge of donations. The initiative attracted more money than any other campaign in the nation except the presidential one. Similar measures were passed in Arizona and Florida. Some 45 states had already passed what are often called Defense of Marriage Acts, or DOMAs, prohibiting same-sex marriage. There is also a federal DOMA, passed by Congress in 1996 and signed into law by President Clinton, which allows all states to hold against same-sex legal relationships. Scholars agree that DOMA covers same-sex civil unions and domestic partnerships as well as marriage. Many homosexuals in the United States go to Canada where they can marry, even without establishing residence there, but for divorce, residency is required.

Is Homosexuality Contagious?

Restrictions on teachers, media access, and other publicity about homosexuality are rooted in the idea that homosexuality is contagious and should be contained. Are such fears warranted? Is homosexuality contagious? In a sense, yes. All people are capable of homosexuality, though not all have the motivation for it. An individual's personality or behavior is formed, or deformed, by surrounding societal norms and pressures. For example, in the days of the Soviet Union, threats persuaded youngsters to switch to the right hand for important tasks, such as writing. In many societies, left-handers, like homosexuals, have been considered somewhat odd, deceitful, or even evil. As a result, there are few left-handers in such societies. When it is "all right" to be left-handed, there are more left-handers. In the same sense, when it is not considered queer to be a homosexual, their population increases. When the barriers are down, more people go over to "the other side," as homosexuality is called in some countries. People are trisexual; they will try anything. Indeed, the mere description of a condition can make it contagious, be it homosexuality or acrotomophilia (a sexual attraction to amputees).[37]

Jean O'Leary, co-executive director of the National Gay Task Force, conceded that the antihomosexual forces are probably quite right in one respect: "If children understand that one can be a happy and functioning homosexual, perhaps with a beloved teacher as an example, there will be more homosexuals."[38] In a case where homosexuals sought recognition as a student organization on campus, it was argued that formal recognition by the university would tend to "perpetuate" or "expand" homosexual behavior and cause latent homosexuals to become overt homosexuals.[39]

In marked contrast to the United States and other Western countries, there were few overt homosexuals in the Soviet Union (there are now many out in the open). President Mahmoud Ahmadinejad of Iran claimed that there are no homosexuals in his country (and in a speech in 2007 at Columbia University, he was mocked). In every society, some things are assumed to be good and other things are assumed to be bad. In this system of images, the homosexual in the Soviet Union was perceived as evil incarnate. That country uniformly enforced the law against homosexuality with a heavy hand (5 years in a Gulag prison camp). Actually though, it was the stigma associated with homosexuality, far more than the criminal penalty itself, that deterred homosexuality (homosexuals there and elsewhere were called *blue*). It was an utter disgrace to be homosexual in the Soviet Union. It was such a dirty word that no one wanted even to hear it mentioned.[40]

What causes a person to be gay, straight, or bisexual? Homosexual activity is sometimes explained as "compulsive activity," that is, acts that are beyond free choice. Others claim that it is the outcome of a deliberate choice motivated by curiosity, opportunity, or caring for another person of the same sex. Quite often, homosexuality is based more on dependency than on sexuality.[41] Some say that physiological factors, such as sex hormone levels, are at the root of homosexuality. Still others claim that homosexuality begins in the home. In either event, it is asserted that sexual orientation is established at a young age, by 3 or 4, before children enter school. In any case, the propensity is aided or averted by the social matrix. The more negative the stigma associated with certain behavior, the less likely people are to engage in such behavior.[42]

Though the research literature on child-rearing by gays or lesbians is minimal, position statements that they should be allowed to adopt or have custody have been made by the American Psychiatric Association, American Psychological Association, American Academy of Pediatrics, American Academy of Family Physicians, and the American Medical Association. Adolescents with same-sex parents are found not to be disturbed in their psychosocial adjustment, school performance, and romantic relationships. According to the 2000 census data, 25% of same-gender couples are raising children. Florida is the only state by statute that categorically prohibits gay and lesbian individuals from becoming adoptive parents. Heterosexual parents may have gay or lesbian children and, conversely, gay or lesbian parents may have heterosexual children.

Homophobia

Having been identifiably homosexual for 20 years or more, Michael Lassell spent a good deal of time and energy attempting to root out exactly what it is about homosexuals that heterosexuals hate so much. Unable to figure it out, he instead authored a book that sets out 25 reasons to hate heterosexuals.[43] He and other homosexuals are "celebrating," but homosexuality remains, in the judgment of many, the worst fate that could befall a person. Some years ago, in a study of children of the super-rich, Dr. Roy R. Grinker, Jr., found his patients to be bland, bored, and relatively uninvolved; in essence, he found them emotional zombies. Yet, one father, whose daughter at the age of 30 had not one single friend or activity, responded to Dr. Grinker's findings, "Thank God, she's not a lesbian."[44] That, for him, would have been the real tragedy, and that would be the case even today.

Even the use of the word *gay* by homosexuals to identify themselves is an irritant to others. "It saddens me as a word lover that, within a period of 30 years, the fine old Anglo-Saxon word 'gay' has changed its meaning completely," writes "Philologos" in the *Forward*.[45] "'Gay' used to be one of the most agreeable words in the language," the historian Arthur Schlesinger, Jr., observed. "Its appropriation by a notably morose group is an act of piracy."[46] Such is the anxiety provoked by homosexuality that when homosexuals took the word to brighten their image, it dropped from general usage in its other senses. *Gay* as a description of an emotional state has become practically archaic. The chances of being misunderstood, or at the least of provoking amused smiles, are too great to risk using it that way. The new *Encarta World English Dictionary* now gives the primary definition of the word as "homosexual" and reserves "full of light-heartedness and merriment" for its secondary sense, but who would use it in that sense? The result is an impoverishment of the language.

Very few people, if any, would now describe a light-hearted evening as "a very gay time." In New England, the Adam Smith Fish Company, owners of the vessel *Gay Wind*, filed notice with the U.S. Coast Guard that they wanted to rename it. A group of citizens in Knoxville petitioned the city to change the name of its main thoroughfare, Gay Street. If that was unsuccessful, said the group, it would try to persuade homosexuals to give up describing themselves as gay. More than half of the residents of Gay Drive in West Seneca, New York, petitioned for a street name change, and their street became Fawn Trail.[47]

In the 1939 film *Bringing Up Baby*, Cary Grant, naked except for a fur-trimmed gauze negligee and waddling about in bare feet, announced that he was thus attired because he had gone "gay." With this pronouncement, the word *gay* reflected a stereotype: that being "gay" somehow involves dressing up in women's clothing, wishing to be the other sex, and consequently becoming a parody of a woman. To be sure, some gay men dress up in drag, but all transvestites are not homosexual, and all homosexuals are certainly not transvestites. Etymologists have traced the origin of *gay* to Old English, where one of the meanings of the word *gal* was "lustful." Whatever the source, by the early 20th century *gay* was commonly used in English to mean homosexual, male or female gender, but more recently the term *gay* is used for males and *lesbian* for females. Because male homosexuals are called *gay*, it is suggested that female homosexuals be described as "ecstatic." In today's politically correct language, the term for both is "sexually challenged."

Public policy concerning homosexuals has changed in recent years, to be sure, but the feelings of contempt and hostility continue to run deep and are still reflected in many of the laws and attitudes of contemporary society. Dr. Laura Schlessinger, talk radio's top-rated host, called gays "deviants" who "undermine civilization." Harvey Mansfield, a popular professor of government at Harvard, is quoted as declaring that homosexuality would undermine civilization if it was made respectable.[48] Critics call such statements irrational, given that in this day of overpopulation, unlike at the time of Moses, birth control is laudable, and homosexuals through history have made major contributions to the arts and sciences by sublimating their urge for creativity in those directions.

Still others object to the homosexual not out of fear for the threat to their sense of identity, but out of impatience with the hostile and paranoid trends of these often "angry young men." Every group, every society, is concerned about its cohesiveness and does what it can to protect itself; sometimes the dangers are illusory, sometimes not. Behavior, which overtly violates established modes and customs, is a vehicle for unconscious aggressive impulses; the public display of homosexuality involves destructive or self-destructive behavior. The psychic pain of homosexuality is dramatically portrayed in the film *Gods and Monsters* depicting the life of James Whale, director of the famous Frankenstein movies. To deal with the existential pathos, many homosexuals commit suicide, or they drink quite heavily. One in every three LGBT youth (lesbians, gays, bisexuals, and transgenders) will attempt or commit suicide. The late Dr. Karl Menninger, renowned as dean of American psychiatry, described an aggressive nature:

> The fact remains that as we see homosexuality clinically and officially it nearly always betrays its essentially aggressive nature. What passes for love under such circumstances is largely counterfeit. … No amount of euphemism and romanticism can disguise this. … This aggression is often thinly contained. Not only does it overflow in jealous rages or sadistic exploitations, but in backlashes at the despised and despising "normal" environment. Embittered individuals betray these feelings in various subtle or not so subtle ways.[49]

One may wonder whether a reaction is setting in to the celebration of homosexuality, just as 2,000 years ago when the biblical injunction followed an earlier celebration. The noisy "coming out of the closet" may enhance self-esteem, but it seems to be again provoking a backlash in both the United States and abroad. Homosexuality is mocked in television comedies. Homosexuality is cited in crime books on pedophilia and serial murders. The Gay Pride parade is ridiculed as Gay Shame, as for example in Latvia.[50] Truman Capote, who never had any qualms about his homosexuality, suggested a back-to-the-closet movement. But, gays maintain that the "celebration of homosexuality" brought about the political, legal, and social gains the homosexual community has made, though meeting resistance, and they are unlikely to be reversed. While marriage is declining among heterosexuals, homosexuals are enthusiastic for marriage.

Homosexuality—at one time a sin, a crime, and a sickness—may one day be more tolerated and accepted by the heterosexual majority, though likely never wholeheartedly approved of nor afforded the status of heterosexuality. The centuries-old condemnation of homosexuality is not simply a by-product of the taboo in the Judeo-Christian religion. In non-Judeo-Christian countries, too, it is a shameful aberration, even in India where people are quite at ease regarding androgynous qualities. In China, homosexuality has long been regarded as a transgression, as illustrated in Chen Kaige's film *Farewell My Concubine*, widely shown and reviewed in the United States.

In India, homosexuality is generally regarded as a shameful aberration, and is also known to be fairly common in fact but condoned only if practiced in secret.[51] Psychoanalyst Bertram Schaffner on visits to India says that he was cautious whenever he raised the question of homosexuality because he knew it to be a distasteful, controversial subject for Indians, but the men he was interviewing frequently raised the issue on their own. One even said to Schaffner, "There is no homosexuality in India because two men cannot produce a child." Schaffner observed,

> As an analyst, I presume that conscious and unconscious conflicts around sexual orientation must inevitably arise for some Indian men. Perhaps the religious injunction to family formation and parenthood is a powerful factor in suppressing potential homosexual behavior. Indian men are able to carry simultaneous masculine and feminine

identifications without worrying that this is pathological or that this will automatically lead to homosexuality. Because Indians regard it as normal to have both masculine and feminine attributes, in contrast to the Western insistence on two totally distinct gender identities, and "having to be real boys or real girls," androgyny must lead to gender disturbance.[52]

Homosexual Panic

The alleged ringleader in the beating death of college student Matthew Shepard in Wyoming sought to invoke a *homosexual panic* (now called *gay panic*) defense, claiming that he snapped after a sexual advance from Shepard. Then, in Michigan, Jonathan Schmitz claimed that he was humiliated by Scott Amedure, who said on a television taping that he had a crush on him. He went out and got a gun and shot and killed Amedure. These highly publicized cases were just two of the many over the years where in criminal cases the defendant asserts he was provoked by some act or words of the homosexual victim.

Is there any merit at all to claims of homosexual panic? Is evidence of it warranted in a criminal trial? It does not constitute mental illness under an insanity defense and it does not allow a defense of self-defense or provocation as those defenses are based on the behavior expected of a reasonable person. Those defenses are exculpatory.[53] But, what about "diminished capacity" or "diminished responsibility" in jurisdictions that recognize that doctrine? The doctrine is recognized in some states, but not in Wyoming. In diminished capacity or diminished responsibility jurisdictions, evidence of impulsive behavior is admissible to reduce a crime from one requiring specific intent (first-degree murder) to one of general intent (second-degree murder or manslaughter). Schmitz was convicted of second-degree murder. And, in all jurisdictions, various factors about the defendant may be considered in sentencing.

Indeed, in certain individuals, the perceived threat of a homosexual assault may cause anxiety, rage, and fear and may lead to violent acts to ward off the humiliation to masculine pride.[54] Dr. Charles Socarides, clinical professor of psychiatry at New York's Albert Einstein School of Medicine, observed, "The person perceives [the threat of a homosexual assault] as not only physical injury, but a total destruction of one's identity and personality. The panic is an emergency reaction to the threat of shame, embarrassment, and humiliation of the worst kind: destruction of self."[55]

Homosexual panic was first described in 1920 by Dr. Edward Kempf on the basis of a study of 17 individuals who exhibited the panic. Just seeing a homosexual, much less being approached sexually, was found to cause anxiety, sometimes panic, in individuals precariously balanced. A defense of a fragile ego is called *psychological defensiveness*. Some can simply walk away from a sexual advance, but others are stirred beyond control. Shepard's attackers were trying to kill something more than Shepard, something that threatened their equilibrium.

The homosexual reminds us of our struggle for identity, and how tenuous that hold is. The mixed up identity of the homosexual used to be noted by the sobriquet "tutti-frutti," later shortened to "fruit." The homosexual's mixed up identity stirs anxiety, to a more or less degree, and the anxiety is compounded by the culture. Challenging a person's sexuality is usually more disruptive to one's equilibrium than religious or racial insults. That is the reason for homophobia, though there are other reasons as well for bias against gays.[56]

An intriguing incident underscoring the centrality of belief in one's identity is contained in M. Rokeach's book, *The Three Christs of Ypsilanti*.[57] Rokeach was a psychologist at Ypsilanti State Hospital at the time of the writing of the book. One evening Rokeach, to put a stop to a quarrel between his two young daughters, addressed each by the other's name. The quarrel was immediately forgotten in the delight of what the girls interpreted as a new game. Shortly thereafter, however, the younger daughter became somewhat uncertain about whether they still were play-ing and asked for reassurance, "Daddy, this is a game, isn't if?" "No," he replied, "it's for real." They played on a bit longer, but soon both girls became disturbed and apprehensive. Then they pleaded with their father to stop, which he did.

In this incident, which took less than 10 minutes, the father violated his children's belief in their own identities. For the first time in their lives, something had led them to experience seri-ous doubts about a fact they had previously taken for granted, and this sent both of them into a panic reaction. The stimulus that evoked it seemed on the surface trivial enough—it involved nothing more than changing a single word, their name—but this word represented the most succinct summary of many beliefs, all of which together make up one's sense of identity. To have challenged "who I am" is upsetting.

Gay activists charge that the "homosexual panic" defense is designed to use antigay prejudice to win sympathy for defendants. The strategy is simple—the crime victim is the criminal, the defendant is his victim. "All that matters is that you create a foothold, doctrinally, for lawyers to tell the stories about virtuous outlaws and vicious victims," it is said.[58] The introduction of evidence of homosexual panic, or the attempt to introduce it, has become increasingly popular in murder trials, a fact alarming to gay activists. "What's going on here," says Evan Wolfson, staff attorney for Lambda Legal Defense and Educational Fund, "is people relying on or playing to a jury's recoil and horror at the thought of homosexual sex, so much so that they stop seeing the victim as a human and, rather, see the victim as a predator."[59] The gay community seeks to exclude all evidence of the victim's homosexuality or the offender's alleged homosexual panic, yet ironically, they seek the passage of "hate laws" that would draw attention to the homosexual-ity of the victim.[60]

In his book *Rough News, Daring Views*,[61] the late Jim Kepner reports on cases notably during the 1950s when the theory of "homosexual panic" was resorted to as a defense. In the 1980s, it was urged by a defendant in a Louisiana murder trial, who claimed that when the victim touched his leg, it unleashed his "excessive hostility toward and fear of homosexuals." It was urged as a defense in Minneapolis in 1988 by a defendant who claimed his "revulsion from the deceased's homosexual advances elicited a heat-of-passion response." In 1989, in Pennsylvania, a defendant who shot two women, strangers to him, in a campground, reloading his .22-caliber rifle eight times, claimed his "personal abhorrence of lesbians and his surreptitious observation of two women making love" provoked homosexual panic. The defenses in all of these cases proved unsuccessful, but in Toronto, in 1992, a 19-year-old was acquitted of fatally stabbing his boss, claiming he was both in fear for his life and operating out of homosexual panic.[62]

In a 1989 California case, *People v. Huie*,[63] the defendant, charged with murder, claimed that the victim had made a sexual advance toward him and sought to introduce evidence that the alleged advance triggered a violent "pseudohomosexual panic." The trial court excluded the defense. On appeal, defense counsel argued that his experts were not going to testify "that the defendant at the time of this alleged incident was suffering from any mental disease or disorder, defect or illness," but that they were going to address events in his childhood that constituted a "compelling trauma" ostensibly relevant to the formation of the necessary criminal intent. He contended that the expert testimony would show that the defendant "actually lacked the mental state necessary to support the charged offense of murder" as a result of childhood events that bore "directly upon his state of mind at the time of the incident." But because the California Penal Code excluded evidence of mental condition except where it reveals a mental disease, defect, or disorder, the trial court's exclusion of the evidence was upheld.

Reparative Therapy

Psychiatrist Richard Isay, an avowed homosexual, claims that it would be malpractice to convert a homosexual patient into a heterosexual person as "it would create psychopathology."[64] Others are of the same view. "Reparative therapy raises serious ethical concerns for those who practice it and for the psychiatric profession as a whole," writes Jack Drescher, a New York psychiatrist and then chairman of the Committee on Gay, Lesbian, and Bisexual Issues of the American Psychiatric Association.[65] Freud believed (and many of his early disciples agreed with him) that the object of psychoanalysis should not be the "cure" of homosexuality (which he thought was impossible, anyway), but rather, as he said in a letter to an American mother distressed by the homosexuality of her son, to help the homosexual find harmony, peace of mind, and full efficiency.[66] In *Three Essays*, Freud declared that heterosexual intercourse with a loved partner was the ultimate sexual goal.[67] More recently, the prominent psychiatrist Norman Brill wrote: "Psychiatrists who have had the opportunity to treat many homosexuals are convinced that it is not just a variation of normal sexual activity. ... The homosexuality is brought about by unconscious fears that inhibit heterosexual functioning.[68]

In 2000, the Board of Trustees of the American Psychiatric Association agreed to strengthen and expand the APA's 1998 position statement on reparative or conversion therapies. The amended statement is designed to clarify many of the related issues for both the general public and professionals. The statement reiterates the APA's position that homosexuality is not a mental illness and emphasizes that to classify it as such stems from no scientific evidence, but rather "from efforts to discredit growing social acceptance of homosexuality as a normal variant of human sexuality." Moral and political issues have obscured science, the statement cautioned. The amended statement strengthened the APA's stance that "there are no scientifically rigorous outcome studies to determine either the actual efficacy or harm of 'reparative' treatments." What literature does exist on the topic "consists of anecdotal reports of individuals who have claimed to change and then later recanted those claims," the statement noted, and "actively stigmatizes homosexuality."

The statement emphasized that the risks of undergoing therapies aimed at changing sexual orientation are not inconsequential and can include "depression, anxiety, and self-destructive behavior because therapist alignment with societal prejudices against homosexuality may reinforce self-hatred already experienced by the patient." These conversion therapies inevitably fail to inform the patient that he or she "might achieve happiness and satisfying interpersonal relationships as a gay man or lesbian," the statement pointed out.

The statement added a warning to therapists against influencing the course of therapy "either coercively or through subtle influence." Because of an absence of evidence of efficacy after 40 years of studies on the topic, the statement recommended that "ethical practitioners refrain from attempts to change individuals' sexual orientation, keeping in mind the medical dictum to 'first, do no harm.'"[69] Moreover, it is argued, the claim that homosexuality can be "cured" or "repaired" repathologizes homosexuality.[70] In a study of more than 200 people who attended "ex-gay" programs, a majority failed to change sexual orientation, and many reported that they associated harm with conversion interventions. A minority reported feeling helped, although not necessarily with their original goal of changing sexual orientation.[71] Apparently, however, there have been no lawsuits alleging malpractice. Jason Cianciotto, research director of the National Gay and Lesbian Task Force, reports, "'Conversion therapy' providers are able to hide from legal accountability in a number of ways, including the fact that most work within faith-based ministries and are also not licensed medical or mental health practitioners. Additionally, most require prospective clients or their legal guardians to sign a liability waiver. Despite these barriers, Lambda Legal is actively collecting stories from 'conversion therapy' survivors in hopes of finding a case suited for legal action."[72]

In support of reparative therapy," a number of homosexuals who claimed to have converted to heterosexuality as a result of psychotherapy protested at the 1999 annual meeting of the American Psychiatric Association urging the association to reintroduce homosexuality in its manual of mental disorders, saying that it would promote treatment and would caution against the gay lifestyle. The organization NARTH (National Association for Research and Therapy of Homosexuality) maintains that homosexuality is a treatable developmental disorder. The organization, the first of its kind, was founded in 1992 by Drs. Charles Socarides, Benjamin Kaufman, and Joseph Nicolosi. It grew to over 900 mental health professionals and concerned lay people. Gay groups disrupted conventions or pressured hotels into canceling meetings of NARTH and also of the Rev. Louis Sheldon's Traditional Values Coalition. It also campaigned to cancel Dr. Laura Schlessinger's TV show.[73]

At the May 2000 annual meeting of the APA, a panel that planned to discuss whether sexual preference could be changed through therapy was cancelled after two psychiatrists withdrew, saying that the subject was too politically charged for a scientific meeting. The cancellation sparked a protest by a group of self-described former homosexuals who say reorientation therapy can work. They carried placards, "Gays and Lesbians can change ... It's Possible!"[74]

Then, at the May 2001 annual meeting of the APA, Dr. Robert Spitzer, who had spearheaded the move in 1973 to remove homosexuality from the *DSM*, stated that "some people can change from gay to straight, and we ought to acknowledge that." He was prompted to undertake a study on witnessing the demonstrators at the 1999 meeting who claimed to have shifted from gay to straight. The study was met with a barrage of media publicity as well as critiques. Based on telephone interviews with 200 men and women who had undergone help to change their sexual orientation, Spitzer said 66% of the men and 44% of the women had maintained "good heterosexual functioning." Spitzer conceded that the subjects were "unusually religious" and were not necessarily representative of most gays in the United States.[75] It was not noted, but it has long been assumed that the insertor (one taking the male position) in the sexual encounter is more likely to be a better candidate for reparative therapy than the insertee.[76] In undertaking reparative or conversion therapy, pressure from family or society does not vitiate the "voluntary" requirement for an informed consent, but information about the risks of treatment is problematic.

Prior to 1974, clinicians who were behaviorally oriented conducted research to change sexual orientation utilizing deconditioning methods with motivated homosexual patients. Preliminary results indicated some success, but were not conclusive. Following the 1974 APA administrative decision, research in this area virtually ceased. Nonscientific professional and personal attitudes, political concerns, and fear of ethical censure quashed scientific inquiry and research. Instead emotionalism and polemical discussions center on whether it is right to offer strongly motivated homosexual patients an opportunity to change their sexual orientation rather than whether it is possible or beneficial. In any event, the ex-gay movement has become increasingly visible across the country, as evidenced by such organizations as Exodus International, People Can Change, Center for Gender Affirming Processes, LIFE (Living in Freedom Eternally) Ministry, and JONAH (Jews Offering New Alternatives to Homosexuality).

Of increasing frequency are the "late-breaking gays" who abandon their spouse and children for a gay partner. It is depicted in films, in Broadway plays, and on the *Oprah Winfrey* show. Homosexuality is given as a possible answer to the question of why men stop (or never start) having sex with their wives.[77] The popular film *Brokeback Mountain* (2005) put a spotlight on what are now called "brokeback marriages." James McGreevey, the New Jersey governor, announced his resignation after revealing he was gay and had had an adulterous affair with a man; he and his wife divorced. Late-breakers' own needs aside, they transform the world of their spouses and children. According to studies, about 3 million women were or are married to men who partner with other men, and there are about 3.5 million children whose parents came out later in life. Straight Spouses Left Behind members have recourse in the International Straight Spouses Network, which coordinates nearly 80 support groups.[78]

Conclusion

Creatures of every species have a drive to reproduce—that is the usual course of nature, and the diversion of the sex drive from its natural object onto something else, precluding the possibility of procreation, suggests a "biological error," or so says Laura Schlessinger, who holds a doctorate in physiology. Whether it should be considered a sin, mental illness, or amenable to change remains controversial.

Endnotes

1. The struggle to build a gay rights movement in the United States is depicted in D. Clendinen & A. Nagourney, *Out for Good* (New York: Simon & Schuster, 1999).
2. Deb Price writes: "The 20th century brought the gradual dawning of the realization that there's nothing wrong with being gay, that you can't fix what ain't broken. And with that realization came the understanding that what needed fixing was and is society's prejudice. Gay people began coming out the closet—first in a courageous trickle, now in a courageous torrent—to challenge the myths and lies that have triggered beatings, lobotomies, castration, excommunication, firings, murders, ostracism, hatred, and self-hatred." D. Price, "Gay Pride Transforms 20th Century," *Detroit News*, Dec. 20, 1999, p. 13. Deb Price's column was (and is) unique in a family newspaper and began in the *Detroit News*, a once conservative paper until taken over by Gannett.
3. Dr. Ehrenstein, *Open Secret* (New York: Harper Collins, 2000), p. 50. See also K. Mason "Walk This Way," *Out*, Sept. 1993, p. 1. Gay men as well as anyone who has used intravenous drugs or been paid for sex are barred from donating blood. The prohibition is designed to prevent the spread of HIV through transfusions. Before giving blood, men are asked if they have had sex, even once, with another man since 1977, when the AIDS epidemic began in the United States. The Red Cross, the international blood association AABB, and America's Blood Centers have proposed replacing the lifetime ban with a 1-year deferral after male-to-male sexual contact. AP news release, "Drug Agency Reaffirms Ban on Gay Men's Giving Blood," *New York Times*, May 24, 2007, p. 19.
4. Isaiah 3:9.
5. See R. Brain, *Friends and Lovers* (New York: Basic Books, 1976), pp. 65–67.
6. See J. Marmor (Ed.), *Homosexual Behavior: A Modern Reappraisal* (New York: Basic Books, 1980); R. Slovenko, "A Panoramic View: Sexual Behavior and the Law," in R. Slovenko (Ed.), *Sexual Behavior and the Law* (Springfield, IL: Thomas, 1965), p. 81. For example, Oklahoma's statute provided: "Every person who is guilty of the detestable and abominable crime against nature, committed with mankind or with a beast, is punishable by imprisonment in the penitentiary for a period not more than twenty (20) years." Okla. Stat. Ann. tit. 21, § 886 (West 2000). The United States Supreme Court upheld a similar Florida statute against a constitutional challenge of being void for vagueness, saying, in effect, that the meaning of the term "crime against nature" is commonly known; Wainwright v. Stone, 414 U.S. 21 (1973).
7. An English statute of 1533 made "buggery" punishable by death 25 Henry VIII, ch. 6. The "crime against nature" statutes had their origin in this statute and in early Christian writings.
8. See State v. Mortimer, 105 Ariz. 472, 467 P.2d 60 (1970).
9. See R. Slovenko, supra note 6, at p. 81.
10. See State v. Trejo, 83 N.M. 511, 494 P.2d 173 (Ct. App. 1972).
11. See, generally, E. Boggan, M. Haft, C. Lister, J. Rupp, & T. Stoddard, *An ACLU Handbook: The Rights of Gay People* (New York: Avon Books, rev. ed., 1983); W. Barnett, *Sexual Freedom and the Constitution* (Albuquerque: University of New Mexico Press, 1973). For example, a discussion of cases involving gay people dancing together in public places may fail to note evidence that the parties were engaged in intimate fondling while on the dance floor, behavior that would have been illegal for heterosexuals as well. For an omission of this type, see *ACLU Handbook*, at p. 78 (discussing Becker v. New York State Liquor Auth., 21 N.Y.2d 289, 234 N.E.2d 443, 287 N.Y.S.2d 400 (1967)).
12. I. Bieber et al., *Homosexuality* (New York: Basic Books, 1962).

13. It is reported that the sexual psychopath law was applied to "the passing of bad checks by a suspected homosexual," that California's Atascadero State Hospital was known as "Dachau for Queers," and that in the 1960s the *New York Times* referred to homosexuals in Times Square as "promenading perverts." W.N. Eskridge, *Gaylaw: Challenging the Apartheid of the Closet* (Cambridge, MA: Harvard University Press, 1999); reviewed in R.A. Posner, "Ask, Tell," *New Republic*, Oct. 11, 1999, p. 52.

14. A. Kinsey, W. Pomeroy, & C. Martin, *Sexual Behavior in the Human Male* (Philadelphia: W.B. Saunders, 1948).

15. See P.L. Brown, "Supporting Boys or Girls When the Line Isn't Clear," *New York Times*, Dec. 2, 2006, p. 1.

16. S. Rep. No. 241, 81st Cong., 2d Sess. 3-5 (1950).

17. See S. Doc. No. 64, 85th Cong., 1st Sess. 239 (1957); Department of Defense Directive No. 5220 (1966); Note, "Government-Created Employment Disabilities of the Homosexual," *Harv. L. Rev.* 82 (1969): 1738, 1749; Note, "Security Clearance for Homosexuals," *Stan. L. Rev.* 25 (1973): 403.

18. *Star-Ledger* (Newark, NJ), Jan. 20, 1985, p. 45, col. 1.

19. American Psychiatric Association, *Diagnostic and Statistical Manual of Mental Disorders* (Washington, DC: Author, 1952), pp. 38–39.

20. APA, at p. 38.

21. APA, *DSM-II* (Washington, DC: Author, 1968).

22. The APA vote on homosexuality is widely mocked, but the APA sought to appease by coming up with a compromise. It decided not to include homosexuality among the paraphilias (sexual deviations), but wanted to legitimize the treatment of homosexuality, so it created a category called "egodystonic homosexuality," which covers those homosexuals for whom their sexual orientation is a persistent concern. American Psychiatric Association, *Diagnostic and Statistical Manual of Mental Disorders* (*DSM-III*) (Washington, DC: Author, 1980). Individuals who are chronically distressed by their homosexuality can receive a diagnosis of "ego-dystonic homosexuality" under the rubric of Sexual Disorder Not Otherwise Specified. *DSM-IV*, sec. 302.9. To be consistent, however, none of the paraphilias should be considered a mental disorder when ego-syntonic. According to this logic, there would be no mental disorder in the case of a necrophiliac who is not distressed by it. "Distress" is not a factor in the *DSM's* paraphilias. Why is it a factor in homosexuality?

23. R. Bayer, *Homosexuality and American Psychiatry: The Politics of Diagnosis* (New York: Basic Books, 1981), p. 3. See also R. Bayer & R. Spitzer, "Edited Correspondence on the Status of Homosexuality in *DSM III*," *J. Hist. Behav. Sci.* 18 (1982): 32.

24. J.K. Meyer, "Ego-Dystonic Homosexuality," in H.I. Kaplan & B.J. Sadock (Eds.), *Comprehensive Textbook of Psychiatry* (Baltimore, MD: Williams E. Wilkins, 4th ed., 1985), p. 1056. Dr. Harold Voth of the Menninger Foundation noted, "[N]owhere in *DSM-III* is a condition disqualified as a mental disorder if it is ego-syntonic. This provision makes us look like fools." H. Voth, Ltr., *Psychiatric News*, Mar. 18, 1983, p. 2. See S. Lesse, "To Be or Not to Be an Illness: That Is the Question-or-the Status of Homosexuality," *Am. J. Psychother.* 18 (1974): 1. The next edition of the *DSM* (*DSM III-R*) contained a diagnosis of "sexual orientation disturbance" for persons disturbed by, in conflict with, or wishing to change their sexual orientation. The *DSM-IV*, published a year later, in 1994, does not contain any reference to homosexuality as a mental disorder.

25. See R. Restak, "Psychiatry in America," *Wilson Q.* 7 (1983): 95, 119.

26. 42 U.S.C. § 12211(a).

27. See Society for Individual Rights, Inc. v. Hampton, 528 F.2d 905 (9th Cir. 1975); 5 C.F.R. § 731.202; Federal Personnel Manual Supplement 731-33 App. 2.

28. Baker v. State, 744 A.2d 864 (Vt. 1999).

29. See Pickering v. Board of Educ., 391 U.S. 563 (1968). In the 1950s, a closeted homosexual was considered a grave security risk, especially in a high official posting. Homosexuality was thought so alien to the culture that exposure would be ruinous, which meant a homosexual in public life was seen as a candidate for blackmail. It was on such grounds, for instance, that the Marshall–Acheson State Department dismissed some 90 people from the ranks in 1947. M.S. Evans, *Blacklisted by History* (New York: Crown Forum, 2007).

30. See Gay Student Servs. v. Texas A & M Univ., 737 F.2d 1317 (5th Cir. 1984).

31. 729 F.2d 1270 (10th Cir. 1984), *aff'd mem. by an equally divided court*, 470 U.S. 903 (1985).

32. Board of Education v. National Gay Task Force, 470 U.S. 903 (1985).

33. See T. I. Emerson, "Legal Foundations of the Right to Know," *Wash. U. L. Q.* 1976: 1, 10–11.

34. See Big Mama Rag v. United States, 631 F.2d 1030, 1036 (D.C. Cir. 1980). A ruling by the Internal Revenue Service sets out a standard for when a nonprofit homosexual rights organization meets the educational organization standards, to wit, a group which is formed to educate the public about homosexuality in order to foster an understanding and tolerance of homosexuals and their problems qualifies for an exemption under section 501(c)(3) of the Internal Revenue Code. This ruling suggests that a somewhat elaborate factual basis must be demonstrated concerning the organization's educational activities before the tax-exempt status will be granted. Moreover, the ruling emphasized that groups that advocate or seek to convince people that they should or should not become homosexuals will not be granted tax-exempt status.

35. J.M. Shalikashvili, "Second Thoughts on Gays in the Military," *New York Times*, Jan. 2, 2007, p. 19.

36. Personal communication. Of the four services, only the Marines did not experience recruiting problems. It is the only branch of the military that stood fast against the social culture on its military culture. S. Gutmann, *The Kinder, Gentler Military: Can American's Gender-Neutral Fighting Force Still Win Wars* (New York: Scribner, 2000), reviewed in F. Fukuyama, GI Jane, *Commentary*, Feb. 2000, p. 56; C. Stewart & D. Forsmark, Alienating solders may be source of military crisis, *Detroit News*, Dec. 9, 1999, p. 16.

37. See C. Elliot, "A New Way to Be Mad," *Atlantic Monthly*, Dec. 2000, p. 72.

38. *New York Post*, June 10, 1977, p. 29.

39. Gay Lib. v. University of Missouri, 558 F.2d 848, 851 n.7 (8th Cir. 1977).

40. See L. Essig, *Queer in Russia* (Durham, NC: Duke University Press, 1999).

41. L. Ovesey, *Homosexuality and Pseudohomosexuality* (New York: Science House, 1969).

42. See S. LeVay, *Queer Science* (Cambridge, MA: MIT Press, 1996).

43. *The Hard Way* (New York: Masquerade Books, 1995).

44. Address by Dr. Roy Grinker, 130th annual meeting of the American Psychiatric Association (May 3, 1977). The term *homophobia* was introduced almost half a century ago to indicate irrational aversion to nonheterosexual persons and has now become part of everyday parlance. Arguably, its most distressing manifestation is violence, almost always perpetuated by males, and directed against males more frequently than females. See D.M. Huebner, G.M. Rebchook, & S.M. Kegeles, "Experiences of Harassment, Discrimination, and Physical Violence Among Young Gay and Bisexual Men," *Am. J. Public Health* 94 (2004): 1200; R.C. Friedman & J.L. Downey, "Sexual Orientation: Neuroendocrine and Psychodynamic Influences," *Psychiatric Times*, August 2007, pp. 47–52.

45. Philologos, "On Language: Purist or Permissive?" *Forward*, Oct. 15, 1999, p. 12.

46. Actually, in the 19th century, the word *gay* was applied to female licentiousness, from whence it may have gravitated toward its homosexual use. In the 19th century, the "gay life" was prostitution, to "gay" it was to go with whores, a "gay house" was a brothel where whores known as "gay" ladies or girls could be found. R.W. Holder, *The Faber Dictionary of Euphemisms* (London: Faber & Faber, 1987). In the 18th century, the term was often used to refer to a man who was a habitual womanizer, as "he's a real gay Lothario," an expression in Nicholas Rowe's *The Fair Penitent* (1703). Nowadays, of course, *gay* almost always means homosexual.

47. After reading an editorial on the Knoxville street question in the *Montgomery Advertiser*, Benjamin Smith Gay wrote a letter to the editor, "Having lived more than 73 years, bearing my name 'GAY,' I am deeply wounded by the fact that a group of divergents now call themselves Gays," he wrote. "I have not instituted litigation, but when such groups defile one's name, it is justified." When the British ambassador to Ireland was assassinated, his friend Sir Christopher Soames, in a spontaneous radio tribute, said, "He was a gay person. ..." Officials of the BBC were stunned and dropped the word when the tribute was rebroadcast. Other expressions used in the culture of the homosexual have also dropped out of general currency. When is the last time someone said, "I feel like a queen?" And now that *outing* is used to refer to the public exposure by gays of other gays who hitherto had kept their homosexuality private, the word *outing* is rarely used in its "trip to the countryside" sense.

48. L. Richardson, "The Mentor Conservatives Turn to for Inspiration," *New York Times*, Oct. 16, 1999, p. 17. See also H.C. Mansfield, *Manliness* (New Haven, CT: Yale University Press, 2006).

49. K.A. Menninger, *The Vital Balance* (New York: Viking Press, 1963).

50. In Latvia, in the Tallinn Pride gay parades, marchers were pelted with stones and eggs. The parade organizers had hired security guards. J. Alas, "Gay Marchers Hope for Peaceful Parade," *Baltic Times*, Aug. 9–15, 2007. In May 2007, a large truck approached Vilnius, the capital of Lithuania, loaded with promotional material to spread information about antidiscrimination laws, and to commemorate the European Year of Equal Opportunities. However, while the message of tolerance, respect, and the need to combat discrimination is generally supported in Lithuanian society, officials were concerned by the

part of the scheduled events that would have seen a large rainbow-colored "gay pride" flag raised in the central square of Vilnius. The mayor opposed it, and the truck made a detour around Lithuania. In response, the European Commission issued a statement regretting "how much there is still to be done to change behavior and attitudes towards discriminated groups." V. Davoliute, "Unity in Diversity," *Lithuania in the World*, 2007, no. 3, pp. 28–29. Amsterdam, New York, and San Francisco are cities where homosexuals live in large numbers and openly. The Russian weekly, *Komsomolskaya Pravda* (July 13–19, 2007, pp. 12–13), described a "gay pride" parade in Amsterdam as Sodom and Gomorrah. Moscow Mayor Yuri Luzhkov has called gay pride parades "satanic" and said he never will allow one to take place.

51. See W.D. O'Flaherty, *Women, Androgynes, and Other Mythical Beasts* (Chicago: University of Chicago Press, 1980), p. 88.

52. B. Schaffner, "Androgyny in Indian Culture: Psychoanalytic Implications," address at annual meeting of the American Academy of Psychoanalysis in New York on January 8, 2000.

53. See J. Dressler, "When 'Heterosexual' Men Kill 'Homosexual' Men: Reflections on Provocation Law, Sexual Advances, and the 'Reasonable Man' Standard," *J. Crim. L. & Criminol.* 85 (1995): 726; P. Margulies, "Identity on Trial: Subordination, Social Science Evidence, and Criminal Defense," *Rutgers L. Rev.* 51 (1998): 45; R.B. Mison, "Homophobia in Manslaughter: The Homosexual Advance as Insufficient Provocation," *Cal. L. Rev.* 80 (1992): 133.

54. The illustrations of the anxiety provoked by homosexuality are without limit. Lee Iacocca, formerly chairman of Chrysler and earlier with Ford, writes in his autobiography that Henry Ford ordered him to get rid of a certain executive because he is a "fag," "his pants are too tight," "he's a queer," "he's got an effeminate bearing." L. Iacocca, *Iacocca: An Autobiography* (New York: Bantam Books, 1984), pp. 98–99. In football, men dress up as gladiators, and their touching behinds is permissible, but men embracing or walking hand in hand raises eyebrows. M. Slade, "Displaying Affection in Public," *New York Times*, Dec. 17, 1984, p. 14; G. Trebay, "A Kiss Too Far?" *New York Times*, Feb. 18, 2007, sec. 9, p. 2.

Indeed, just calling someone a homosexual may draw gunfire. See AP news report, "Remark About 'Gays' May Have Led to 4 Slayings," *New York Times*, Dec. 19, 1984, p. 17. Killers of gays are unusually conflicted about their own sexual impulses, and the research documented in the PBS *Frontline: Assault on Gay America* (Feb. 15, 2000) is persuasive. Interviewed in prison, where they are serving life sentences for the 1999 murder of Billy Jack Gaither, a resident of a small town in Alabama, Steven Mullins and Charles Butler, Jr., made it clear Gaither never touched them, but his sin, they said, was to "disrespect" them by assuming they would welcome gay sex.

A few years ago a man killed two co-workers and wounded four others because he thought that they were accusing him of being homosexual. He killed himself shortly after the rampage. There was no evidence that the victims even broached homosexual themes, suggesting the possibility that the assailant was delusional regarding his homosexual preoccupation. J.A. Silva, G.B. Leong, & R. Weinstock, "Homicidal Violence in an Ambulatory Public Job Setting: The Role of Delusional Thinking, *Am. J. Foren. Psychiat.* 21 (2000): 57; M. Gold & J. Cox, "Gunman Felt Mocked, Police Say Shooting Worker Yelled, 'I Am Not Gay!' During Rampage, According to Officials," *Los Angeles Times*, June 7, 1997, p. 1.

At one time lawsuits for defamation arising out of an imputation of homosexuality were legion. See, e.g., Nowark v. Maguire, 22 A.D.2d 901, 255 N.Y.S.2d 318 (1964); Buck v. Savage, 323 S.W.2d 363 (Tex. Civ. App. 1959); Hayes v. Smith, 832 P.2d 1022 (Colo. App. 1991). In trials in Texas, when asked on cross-examination about his expulsion from the American Psychiatric Association on account of his testimony in death penalty cases, Dr. James Grigson retorted, "And that's the very same organization that does not consider homosexuality to be a mental disorder." By that retort, his credibility seems to have been enhanced among the jurors.

55. C.W. Socarides, *The Overt Homosexual* (New York: Grune & Stratton, 1968). Dr. Cecil Mynatt, Jr., a state psychiatrist, recanted his testimony against Gerardo Valdez, sentenced to die for a 1989 killing. The psychiatrist said in an affidavit filed with an appeal that new information convinced him that Valdez was temporarily insane when he shot his victim. He said "homosexual panic" brought on paranoia in Valdez at the time of the shooting. J. Thomas, "Help for Mexican on Death Row," *New York Times*, Aug. 24, 2001, p. 12.

56. See R.M. Baird & S.E. Rosenbaum (Eds.), *Hatred, Bigotry, and Prejudice* (Amherst, NY: Prometheus Books, 1999); E. Young-Bruehl, *The Anatomy of Prejudice* (Cambridge, MA: Harvard University Press, 1996), pp. 137–159; R. Slovenko, "Sexual Deviation: Response to an Adaptational Crisis," *U. Colo. L. Rev.* 40 (1968): 222.

57. New York: Knopf, 1964.

58. D. Osborne, "Homosexual Panic," *Lesbian & Gay New York News*, Nov. 4, 1999, p. 4. See also C. Patton (Ltr.), "'Gay Panic': A Specious Defense," *New York Times*, Nov. 4, 1999, p. 26.

59. Quoted in M.R. Keenan, "'Homosexual Panic' Claims Put Gay Activists on the Defensive," *Detroit News*, April 27, 1993, p. C7. See C.P. Chen, "Provocation's Privileged Desire: The Provocation Doctrine, 'Homosexual Panic' and the Non-Violent Unwanted Sexual Advance Defense," *Cornell J. L. & Pub. Policy* 10 (2001): 195; M.A. Smyth," Queers and Provocateurs: Hegemony, Ideology, and the 'Homosexual Advance' Defense," *Law & Soc. Rev.* 40 (2006): 903.

60. Jeffrey Montgomery, a public relations executive, became an activist in Metro Detroit's gay community when his boyfriend was murdered outside a gay bar in 1984 and police refused to investigate it as a hate crime. He and two friends were spurred to establish the advocacy group the Triangle Foundation in 1991. M. Feighan, "Gay Rights Group Leader Bows Out After 16 Years," *Detroit News*, Oct. 11, 2007, p. B3. Hate crime legislation sets out punishment based on motive rather than intention. Normally, the prosecutor has to prove the defendant acted with *mens rea*—that, for example, he acted intentionally, maliciously, or recklessly. In contrast, to prosecute a hate crime, the prosecutor must also prove why the defendant intended to harm. The problem of figuring out "why" is a "can of worms." What if a mugger chooses to victimize disabled people not because of hate, but because they are less likely to fight back? See R. Dooling, "Good Politics, Bad Law," *New York Times*, July 26, 1998, sec. 7, p. 22. Dooling is a lawyer whose most recent novel, *Brain Storm*, dramatizes a hate crime trial. See also F.M. Lawrence, *Punishing Hate: Bias Crimes Under American Law* (Cambridge, MA: Harvard University Press, 1999); S.D. McCoy, "The Homosexual-Advance Defense and Hate Crimes Statutes: Their Interaction and Conflict," *Cardozo L. Rev.* 22 (2001): 629.

61. New York: Harrington Park Press, 1998.

62. See R. Slovenko, *Psychiatry and Criminal Culpability* (New York: John Wiley & Sons, 1995), pp. 111–114.

63. San Francisco Super. Ct., No. 125603, Court of Appeals, 1st App., div. 5, No. A042962, 1989.

64. See R.A. Isay, *Becoming Gay: The Journey to Self-Acceptance* (New York: Pantheon, 1996); see also R.A. Isay, "Remove Gender Identity Disorder in *DSM*," *Psychiatric News*, Nov. 21, 1997, p. 9. For a reply, see H.M. Voth (Ltr.), "Dr. Isay's Proposal," *Psychiatric News*, Feb. 6, 1998, p. 14.

65. J. Drescher, "Reparative or Destructive?" *Clinical Psychiatric News*, March 1998, p. 12. See also M. Luo, "Reining in Desire Proves Complex, at Best," *New York Times*, Feb. 12, 2007, p. 19; "APA Maintains Reparative Therapy Not Effective," *Psychiatric News*, Jan. 15, 1999, p. 1. Protests over "reparative therapy" appear in L. Faderman, *Odd Girls and Twilight Lovers* (New York: Columbia University Press, 1991), pp. 134–138. The 978-page book published in 1996 by the American Psychiatric Press, *Textbook of Homosexuality and Mental Health*, edited by Robert P. Cabaj and Terry S. Stein, starts from the "belief that homosexuality is a normal variation of human sexuality and not mental illness." See also B.J. Cohler & R.M. Galatzer-Levy, *The Course of Gay and Lesbian Lives* (Chicago: University of Chicago Press, 2000); J. Drescher, *Psychoanalytic Therapy and the Gay Man* (Mahwah, NJ: Analytic Press, 1998); T. Domenici & R.C. Lesser (Eds.), *Disorienting Sexuality* (New York: Routledge, 1995).

66. Freud's therapeutic pessimism as well as his acknowledgment that many homosexuals, though arrested in their development, could derive pleasure from both love and work provides the context in which he wrote his compassionate and now famous "Letter to an American Mother" of 1935. He wrote:

> I gather from your letter that your son is a homosexual. I am most impressed by the fact that you do not mention this term yourself in your information about him. May I question you, why you avoid it? Homosexuality is assuredly no advantage, but it is nothing to be ashamed of, no vice, no degradation, it cannot be classified as an illness; we consider it to be a variation of the sexual function produced by a certain arrest of sexual development. Many highly respectable individuals of ancient and modern times have been homosexuals, several of the greatest men among them (Plato, Michelangelo, Leonardo da Vinci, etc.). It is a great injustice to persecute homosexuality as a crime, and cruelty too. If you do not believe me, read the books of Havelock Ellis.
>
> By asking me if I can help, you mean, I suppose, if I can abolish homosexuality and make normal heterosexuality take its place. The answer is, in a general way, we cannot promise to achieve it. In a certain number of cases we succeed in developing the blighted germs of heterosexual tendencies, which are present in every homosexual, in the majority of cases it is no more possible. It is a question of the quality and the age of the individual. The result of treatment cannot be predicted.

What analysis can do for your son runs in a different line. If he is unhappy, neurotic, torn by conflicts, inhibited in his social life, analysis may bring him harmony, peace of mind, full efficiency whether he remains a homosexual or gets changed.

In his first major work with regard to sexuality, "Three Essays on the Theory of Sexuality" (1905), Freud dismantled the connection between the sexual instinct and the object or aim. Hence, if there is no natural object and no natural aim to the instinct, then deviations from genital intercourse cannot be called perverse. But Freud defused this argument by using a Darwinian evolutionary model of psychosexual development that organized all human activity in relation to the survival of the species. By defining "normal" sexuality as procreative, sexuality was essentialized and homosexuality was pathologized.

67. See W. Gaylin, *Talk Is Not Enough: How Psychotherapy Really Works* (New York: Little, Brown, 2000); adapted in "Nondirective Counseling or Advice? Psychotherapy as Value Laden," *Hastings Center Report*, May–June 2000, p. 31.
68. See N.Q. Brill, "Is Homosexuality Normal?" *J. Psychiat. & Law* 26 (1998): 224.
69. "APA Stakes Out Positions On Controversial Therapies," *Psychiatric News*, April 21, 2000, p. 45.
70. M. Kirby, "Psychiatry, Psychology, Law and Homosexuality: Uncomfortable Bedfellows," *Psychiat., Psychol. & Law* 7 (2000): 139.
71. A. Shidlo & M. Schroeder, "Changing Sexual Orientation: A Consumer's Report," *Prof. Psychol., Res. & Prac.* 33 (2002): 249.
72. Personal communication to author (March 1, 2007). Jason Cianciotto and Sean Cahill in March 2006 published *Youth in the Crosshairs: The Third Wave of Ex-Gay Activism* (National Gay and Lesbian Task Force Policy Institute). See also A. Shidlo, M. Schroeder, & J. Drescher (Eds.), *Sexual Conversion Therapy: Ethical, Clinical and Research Perspectives* (New York: Haworth Medical Press, 2001).
73. J. Leo, "Watch What You Say," *U.S. News & World Report*, March 20, 2000, p. 18.
74. E. Goode, "Scientist Says Study Shows Gay Change Is Possible," *New York Times*, May 9, 2001, p. 15; *ibid.*, p. 17.
75. See K.L. Zucker, "The Politics and Science of 'Reparative Therapy'," *Arch. Sexual Behav.* 32 (2003): 399.
76. In the Middle East, homosexual behavior is not automatically labeled deviant. The taxonomy revolves around the roles of top and bottom, with little stigma attaching to the top. A man is not stripped of his masculinity as long as he is in the "top," or active, role. See N. Labi, "The Kingdom in the Closet," *Atlantic Monthly*, May 2007, p. 70.
77. B. Berkowitz & S. Yager-Berkowitz, *He's Just Not Up for It Anymore* (New York: William Morrow, 2008), p. 177.
78. M.J. Penn & E.K. Zalesne, *Microtrends* (New York: Twelve, 2007), pp. 120–122. In a picture book used in a grammar school in Lexington, Massachusetts, *King & King*, a prince, told by his mother Queen to marry, passes over several princesses before falling in love with another prince. The princes kiss on the final page, and a red heart is superimposed on their lips. The parents of Jacob Parker and Joey Wirthlin, second graders, sued in federal court, alleging that because they believe homosexuality is immoral, the school violated their constitutionally protected freedom of religion by introducing their children to the gay-friendly material. A three-judge panel of the U.S. Court of Appeals for the 1st Circuit unanimously ruled in favor of the school's efforts to promote tolerance; Parker v. Hurley, No. 07-1528 (1st Cir. 2008).

PART V
Civil Cases

18
Tort Liability of the Mentally Incompetent and Their Caretakers

The liability of the mentally ill has become a more frequent legal issue due to the increasing numbers of mentally ill in the community and limited community support systems as well as the general increase in litigation. The possibility of a lethal situation is now increased by the widespread use of guns or motor vehicles. The vast majority of tort claims for death or injury involve motor vehicle accidents.

Elements of a Tort

A tort is a civil or private wrong, based on the general principle that every act of man that causes damage to legally protected interest of another obliges him, if at fault, to repair it. The key concepts in this principle are *act, damage, causation,* and *fault.* Etymologically speaking, the word *tort* is derived from the Latin *tortus,* meaning twisted or wrested aside. The metaphor is apparent: a tort is conduct that is twisted or crooked. The word *tort* is used in English as a general synonym for "wrong." Law professor Leon Green described tort law as the "general law for the adjustment of the hurts that result from everyday activities of people."[1]

Tort law is said to have three major goals: (1) to deter harm-causing behavior, (2) to provide compensation to victims, and (3) to provide fairness or justice between the parties. Some scholars and courts have emphasized one goal to the near exclusion of the others. Some focus on the compensation goal, emphasizing the "social insurance" role of tort judgments. Others, by contrast, have emphasized deterrence as the primary goal of tort law, with compensation of the victim merely "a detail," at least from an economic standpoint. But, by and large, courts, practitioners, and scholars routinely have recognized deterrence, compensation, and fairness all as proper goals of the tort system. All would agree that the right of citizens to bring suit for private wrongs, reinforced by widespread knowledge of that right, provides an important outlet for conflict that otherwise might break out into violence. An interesting recognition of this point appears in a federal district judge's comment that recent libel law has restricted the ability of public figures to collect damages to the point that they might have to "resort to fisticuffs or dueling" to get satisfaction.[2]

Act

The beginning point of tort liability is an act, or behavior. A person is not liable for his mere thoughts or for a failure to act (when there is no duty to act). An act is an essential element for liability. In tort, as well as in criminal law, act is defined as a volitional movement or an "external manifestation of the actor's will." Thus, as the American Law Institute's (ALI) *Restatement of Torts* illustrates, "a contraction of a person's muscles, which is purely a reaction to some outside force, such as a knee jerk or the blinking of the eyelids in defense against an approaching missile, or the convulsive movements of an epileptic are not acts of that person. So, too, movements of the body during sleep when the will is in abeyance are not acts." And so, too, if A pushes B against C, knocking C down and breaking his arm, B is not liable because his act was not volitional.[3]

The definition of an act as "a voluntary bodily movement," favored in legal theory since John Austin, generates the problem of defining *voluntary*.[4] W. C. Fields, it may be recalled, quipped that his wife drove him to drink and he did not have the decency to thank her for it. There is general agreement that mental incapacity can compromise voluntariness. The factors that generally influence a clinician's assessment of voluntariness are the nature of the individual's experiential symptoms, the hypothesized causes of those symptoms, and the manner in which they are treated.[5] Acts performed under hypnosis are open to question as to whether they are involuntary. Hypnosis experts claim that it is impossible to make a subject perform an act "which he felt morally unable to do."[6]

As a general principle, one who is stricken by paralysis, has an epileptic seizure, is overcome by poisonous gas, or has lost consciousness under like circumstances is not held liable for what he does or fails to do. Violent behavior following a seizure may stem from an epileptic's misinterpretation of well-meant attempts by bystanders to protect him against the consequences of his confused conduct—and is usually characterized by a clouded consciousness, paranoid ideas, and hallucinations.[7]

Of automatism under the law, it is said: "[I]f a person in a condition of complete automatism inflicted grievous injury, that would not be actionable."[8] The case for no liability rests largely on the proposition that the defendant has done no act at all and, thus, cannot have committed any tort, intentional or otherwise. The result is consistent with the moral basis of tort liability, but not with protecting innocent people from the aggression of others.

George Orwell in an essay, "Such, Such Were the Joys," wrote that in his boarding school days, bed-wetting was looked on as a disgusting crime that the child committed on purpose and for which the proper cure was a beating. Night after night he prayed fervently, "Please God, do not let me wet my bed! Oh, please God, do not let me wet my bed!"[9] In law, the bed-wetting would not be considered an act, there being no volition or consciousness about it.

Damage

The concept of *damage* does not include injury to every known human interest, but only to a legally protected interest. For example, alienation of affections or mental sufferings in various jurisdictions is not such an interest. In law, the terms *hurt*, *harm*, *injury*, and *damage* are used synonymously to refer to an invasion of a legally protected interest. The term *damages* (pl.) is also used to refer to the liability or compensation that the defendant tortfeasor must pay to repair the wrong.

Damages are generally divided into two categories under the law: special damages and general damages. Special damages are past and future medical expenses—hospital and custodial care, therapeutic costs—as well as the loss of earning capacity for life. General damages are for past and future pain and suffering that the individual is going to experience, for life, and for past and future loss of ability to carry on and enjoy life's activities. Many states have placed caps on damages for pain and suffering. "How can you set damages?" The typical response is: "It's awfully difficult to determine. Law is not an exact science."

Causation

In order for there to be liability under the law of torts, there must be a causal relation or nexus between conduct and hurt. The famous ditty in *Poor Richard's Almanac* may be recalled:

> For want of a nail the shoe is lost,
> for want of a shoe the horse is lost,
> for want of a horse the rider is lost.
> For want of a rider the message is lost,

for want of a message the battle is lost—
the war is lost—the fatherland is lost.

As the theory called "sensitive dependence on initial conditions" (chaos, for short) would have it, tiny actions can have enormous unforeseeable consequences. In the culture of popular science, the idea is known as "the butterfly effect." Sometimes big changes follow from small events, and sometimes these changes can happen very quickly. A single sick person can start an epidemic of the flu, a few fare-beaters and graffiti can fuel a subway crime wave, or a satisfied customer can fill the empty tables of a new restaurant.[10] When the effect seems far out of proportion to the cause, it is not deemed a proximate cause in law (though there may be fault). The horseman who had failed to inspect the hooves on his mare was a link in the causal chain, which led to the loss of the fatherland, but it would not be deemed the "proximate cause" required in law. And, of course, correlation is not causation (a joke making the rounds is that the four states that carry out the death penalty by electrocution also happen to have stellar college football teams).

The defendant's act or omission (when there is a duty to act) must be a substantial factor in bringing about the harm. The law is concerned with proximate cause, also called legal cause, that takes a pragmatic view, and not with the "first cause" of philosophy or "field theory" of science. As Judge Andrews put it:

> We cannot trace the effect of an act to the end, if end there is. Again, however, we may trace it part of the way. A murder at Sarajevo may be the necessary antecedent to an assassination in London 20 years hence. An overturned lantern may burn all Chicago. We may follow the fire from the shed to the last building. We rightly say the fire started by the lantern caused its destruction. This would be cause, but not the proximate cause. What we do mean by the word *proximate* is that because of convenience, public policy, or a rough sense of justice, the law arbitrarily declines to trace a series of events beyond a certain point. This is not logic. It is practical politics.[11]

Fault

Another key element of a tort is fault, based on either intent or negligence. The term *intent* denotes the actor's desire to cause the consequences of his act, or his belief that such consequences are substantially certain to result. Intent in the law of torts is limited, wherever it is used, to the consequences of the act rather than to the act itself. Thus, as illustrated in ALI's *Restatement of Torts*, one who fires a gun in the middle of the desert and hits someone who is there without his knowledge does not intend that result.[12] A delusional interpretation of reality does not excuse tort liability.

Intent, for the purposes of determining civil liability, unlike criminal liability, does not presuppose a value judgment or moral culpability. The actor need not know that what he was doing was wrong. Thus, an individual who intends to affect a chattel in a manner inconsistent with another's right of control, though acting in good faith and under a mistake, is liable for a "conversion."[13] Irrespective of good motives, the abducting and deprogramming of a member of a religious cult is a battery and false imprisonment.[14]

In tort law, it is usually irrelevant that an actor intended no harm, or perhaps even intended benefit, to his victim. It requires only that the actor have "substantial certainty" that a battery or other invasion of a legally protected interest will result. The intent required for the tort of battery, for example, is the intent to cause contact, and if it turns out to be harmful or offensive, there is damage and that fulfills the requirements of the tort. A requirement of harm or offense would make this tort inapplicable to many situations in which it might otherwise be applied, such as practical jokes, mistaken identity, or medical treatment.[15] Some courts state that a desire to harm is necessary,[16] but that is not the usual requirement. A surgeon who performs an operation does not desire to do harm—indeed, he desires to help—but without the defense of consent, liability would be for a battery.[17]

Negligence is not defined in terms of state of mind, but as "conduct that falls below the standard of care established by law for the protection of others against unreasonable risk of harm."[18] A person either must act with the care and skill expected of a reasonable, careful, and prudent person under the circumstances or bear responsibility for the resulting damage. The test is not whether the individual acted according to the best of his own judgment.[19]

The *Restatement of Torts* sets out the general rule: "Unless the actor is a child, his insanity or other mental deficiency does not relieve the actor from liability for conduct, which does not conform to the standard of a reasonable man under like circumstances."[20] The *Restatement* gives an example:

> A, who is insane, believes that he is Napoleon Bonaparte, and that B, his nurse, who confines him in his room, is an agent of the Duke of Wellington, who is endeavoring to prevent his arrival on the field of Waterloo in time to win the battle. Seeking to escape, he breaks off the leg of a chair, attacks B with it and fractures her skull. A is subject to liability to B for battery.[21]

Liability Without Fault

Liability without fault (intent or negligence), otherwise known as *strict liability*, was the foundation of tort law until the last half of the 19th century. The principal action was strict liability for trespass, not surprising in a society in which the chief source of wealth was land. A concomitant of the industrial revolution was the concept, urged by entrepreneurs, that there should be no liability without fault. The entrepreneur was held liable to workers only if he was deemed at fault, which happened rarely indeed because risks or hazards involved in carrying on an activity in itself do not constitute fault. There is also reason to believe that the courts found the defense of contributory negligence, along with the concepts of fault and proximate cause, to be a convenient instrument of control over the jury, whereby the liabilities of developing industry were kept within bounds.

Today, in the employer–employee relationship, workers' compensation laws provide that an employee is entitled to compensation for injuries arising in the course and scope of employment, irrespective of any fault, but payment is limited to a fixed schedule. Under no-fault automobile insurance plans, adopted widely, a motorist's insurance company covers his medical and auto damage expenses no matter what caused the accident. In other situations, the foundation of tort liability is fault, except in the situations of ultrahazardous activity or products liability where the principle of strict liability applies.

The Plaintiff's Contributory Negligence

The important public policy that innocent victims be compensated is one reason that mental illness has not been allowed to vitiate tort liability. The central conflict in tort law is whether liability should be based on the moral fault of the defendant and his responsibility for that fault, or whether the focus should be on compensation for the victim.[22] These considerations, however, are not applicable to the issue of a plaintiff's contributory negligence, i.e., conduct contributing as a legal cause to the harm the plaintiff has suffered because it falls below the standard to which he is required to conform for his own protection. The issue of psychiatric status of the plaintiff in a tort suit tends to be of greater importance than in the case of a defendant.

The traditional common law rule denies recovery to a plaintiff who is contributorily negligent, whatever the negligence of the defendant.[23] In most states the doctrine of contributory negligence has been replaced by comparative negligence under which the negligent plaintiff is not completely barred from compensation, but it is reduced by the percentage of his fault.

The courts, while employing an objective standard-of-conduct test for defendant's negligence, tend to employ a subjective standard for the plaintiff's contributory or comparative negligence. The *Restatement* says that the policy factors that disallow insanity of an actor from excusing conduct, which would otherwise be negligence on the part of a defendant, do not have the same force as applied to the plaintiff's contributory or comparative negligence. The subjective standard allows an insane plaintiff's behavior to be measured in relation to his actual competency, which would tend not to defeat his claim.[24] Psychiatric testimony would be material to establish lack of competency.[25]

In response to intentional wrongdoing, it is inconsequential to say that the plaintiff was negligent in failing to avoid harm. Thus, if A intends to strike B, it is no defense to say that B was negligent in failing to avoid the blow.

What about a hypersensitive or idiosyncratic plaintiff? The defendant's knowledge of the plaintiff's special susceptibilities to emotional distress is relevant to the determination of whether a cause of action for intentional infliction of emotional distress is available. In one notorious case, the plaintiff, an eccentric elderly woman, believed that a pot of gold was buried in her backyard and was constantly digging for it. Fully aware of her frailties, the defendant buried a pot with other contents where she would dig it up. When she did so, he had her escorted by a procession in triumph to the city hall, where she opened the pot under circumstances of extreme public humiliation. She suffered mental distress, which further unsettled her and contributed to her early death. In the form of a judgment, her heirs got a "pot of gold."[26]

Defenses of a Defendant

The defenses (or privileges as sometimes called) of a defendant (consent, self-defense, defense of others, defense of property, necessity) depend on the reasonable belief that a fact exists, not a subjective belief. A defendant, believing that the plaintiff is reaching into his pocket for a gun, attacks the plaintiff to defend himself; the plaintiff was actually reaching for his handkerchief. The issue is whether the defendant had reasonable grounds to fear an immediate attack by the plaintiff.[27]

Mental Disability as a Defense

Mental incompetence may be shown under the law to modify contractual obligations, testamentary capacity, and criminal responsibility, but "lunatics usually have been held liable for their torts." The courts almost invariably impose liability on mentally disordered defendants as if they had no such disorder.[28] At least five states have statutorily codified the principle.[29]

This general rule is applied in cases of both negligence and intentional torts. In cases of negligence, an individual is expected to comply with the objective "reasonable person" standard. The rule is also applied with respect to intentional torts, but there is some authority holding an insane person may not have the mental capacity to form the specific intent for certain intentional torts, such as malicious prosecution, misrepresentation, and defamation.[30] In *C.T.W. v. B.C.G.*,[31] the defendant sexually abused his stepgrandchildren. He sought to defend against tort liability on the ground that the sexual abuse was the result of a pedophilic disorder. The court rejected the argument that the defendant should be held only to the standard of "an ordinary prudent person with the mental illness of pedophilia."

Justifications of the general rule that the insane are liable for their torts include the following:

1. The fairness of holding that "where one of two innocent persons must suffer a loss, it should be borne by the one who occasioned it."
2. The encouragement of custodians or caretakers to be vigilant over the care of insane persons.
3. The difficulty of identifying actual mental illness by those feigning insanity to avoid liability for harmful acts.
4. The complications and difficulties of introducing insanity defenses as used in the criminal law into tort doctrine.[32]

As the verdict in criminal cases of not guilty by reason of insanity (NGRI) does not have a counterpart of "not liable by reason of insanity" in tort cases, a person may be found NGRI in a criminal case, but nonetheless may be liable in a tort case.[33] The courts do not inquire in tort cases as they do in criminal cases whether, in the matter at hand, the defendant was able to distinguish right from wrong.[34]

By and large, the decisions adhere to the line set out in 1937 by the Massachusetts Supreme Judicial Court in *McGuire v. Almy*.[35] In this case, the plaintiff, a registered nurse, was employed to take care of the defendant, who was insane. The defendant was "ugly, violent, and dangerous" and injured the plaintiff. The Massachusetts Supreme Judicial Court, reversing the trial court, held for the plaintiff. Of the liability of insane persons, it said:

[T]he law will not inquire … into [a defendant's] peculiar mental condition with a view to excusing him if it should appear that delusion or other consequence of his affliction has caused him to entertain that intent or that a normal person would not have entertained it.

The insane person is deemed capable of having an intent to bring about a specific result, even though the intent is induced by a delusion, and his act is deemed voluntary, even though he may be diagnosed as a pyromaniac or kleptomaniac.[36] For battery resulting in death or wrongful death, the courts on many occasions have held a defendant civilly liable, notwithstanding an earlier acquittal of the criminal charge on account of insanity. The insane have been held liable for trespass to land and conversion of goods. They have been held liable for setting fire to buildings. Imbecility or mental defectiveness is taken into account as a defense only if it has reached an extreme stage.

The traditional rule was again reaffirmed in 1988 by the Connecticut Supreme Court in *Polmatier v. Russ*.[37] In this case, the defendant shot and killed his father-in-law. The defendant told a police officer that his father-in-law was a heavy drinker and he wanted to make his father-in-law suffer for his bad habits. He also told the police officer that he was a supreme being and had the power to rule the destiny of the world and could make his bed fly out of the window. To a psychiatrist, he stated that he believed that his father-in-law was a spy for the Red Chinese, and that he believed his father-in-law was not only going to kill him, but also going to harm his infant child. The psychiatrist testified at both the criminal and civil proceedings, saying that, at the time of the homicide, the defendant was suffering from "a severe case of paranoid schizophrenia" that involved delusions of persecution, grandeur, influence, and reference, and also auditory hallucinations. He did not suggest any malingering. He concluded that the defendant could not form a rational choice, but that he could make "a schizophrenic or crazy choice." He was absolved of criminal liability by reason of insanity, but in the civil action he was found liable.[38]

Commentators trace the majority rule back to the dictum of a 17th-century English case when strict liability was generally the rule. In *Weaver v. Ward*,[39] the English court said, "[I]f a lunatic kills a man, this shall not be a felony because felony must be done *animo felonico* [with felonious intent]. Yet in trespass, which tends only to give damages according to a hurt or loss, it is not so." The majority rule is not, however, without criticism.[40] Professor Bohlen in an article published in 1924 stated:

> [W]here a liability, like that for the impairment of the physical condition of another's body or property, is imposed upon persons capable of fault only if they have been guilty of fault, immaturity of age or mental deficiency, which destroys the capacity for fault, should preclude the possibility of liability. … But so long as it is accepted as a general principle that liability for injuries to certain interests are to be imposed only upon those guilty of fault in causing them, it should be applied consistently and no liability should be imposed upon those for any reason incapable of fault.[41]

Similar views have more recently been expressed by other commentators.[42] One of them characterizes the tort standard as "almost facially unfathomable."[43] Given the conventional wisdom that the mentally ill or mentally retarded constitute a grave threat to society, it should not be surprising, says Professor James Ellis, that "such an atmosphere would foster a rule that refused to absolve such persons from compensating victims for the damage they caused."[44] The criticisms, however, have had little impact on the jurisprudence.

The traditional civil law, in contrast to the common law, holds that a mentally unsound person "cannot commit a fault."[45] The German Civil Code excludes civil responsibility for one who is unable to exercise free will, except where he brought on temporary disability by use of alcohol or similar means.[46] On the other hand, some civil law codes impose liability in at least some cases. The Civil Code of Mexico provides that the incompetent person is liable unless some other person, such as a guardian, is liable.[47]

The most oft-cited U.S. case on standard of care, *Williams v. Hays*,[48] involved a sea captain who had been on duty continuously for 3 days during a storm. During the calm weather following the storm, he permitted his vessel to drift on a shoal and be destroyed. The evidence tended to show that he refused to consider the seriousness of the situation, staggered about the vessel, made irresponsive answers to questions, and appeared to be dazed, drunk, or insane. The day of the wreck, he twice refused the assistance of tugboats offering to tow the disabled vessel. He sought to invoke temporary insanity as a defense. The New York Court of Appeals declared the insanity of the defendant furnished no defense—his acts must be measured by the same standard as that applied to the action of a sane person; however, at the same time the court, contrary to the majority rule, sent the case back for a new trial because evidence had been refused tending to show that the defendant became mentally incompetent by reason of his extreme efforts to save the brig, which, if proved, the court thought would furnish an excuse. The suit was discontinued—a practical victory for the defendant. In light of the decision,, it was uncertain how far an insane person would be held responsible for his acts or omissions.[49]

Under American law, the acts of an epileptic or a person seized with temporary unconsciousness—conditions regarded as involuntary or accidental—are distinguished from the acts of an insane person. Thus, a motorist who suddenly loses control of his car because of a heart attack, a stroke, a fainting spell, or an epileptic seizure, is not liable unless he knew, or should have known, that he was likely to become ill, in which case he is negligent in driving the car at all.[50]

There is some analogy between a motorist going berserk at the wheel and a ship captain going insane during a voyage; the ship captain case has been cited in a number of automobile cases.[51] In a society where nearly everyone drives an automobile, it will not be surprising to find mental illness among drivers. Michael Douglas in the film *Falling Down* (1993) cracks up on a freeway and goes on a rampage.[52] Barbara Bush, the wife of President George H.W. Bush, wrote in her memoirs that she was so deeply depressed in the mid-1970s that she sometimes stopped her car on the highway shoulders for fear that she might deliberately crash the vehicle into a tree or an oncoming auto.[53] State statutes require physicians to report patients with conditions that may affect their ability to drive, and under these statutes, physicians may be held responsible for vehicle accidents caused by their patients.[54] In nonserious cases, no-fault automobile insurance resolves the matter.

Obtaining mental health care does not reduce tort law's expectations of the defendant. Indeed, it may actually increase its expectations of the defendant. Insight gained through diagnosis or treatment may increase the defendant's awareness of the risks that he poses and require him to act with reference to that increased knowledge.[55] An individual may be deemed negligent for failing to seek professional help.[56]

In rare cases where the court has judged that the individual could not foresee an "attack" of mental illness, which played a role in causing injury, the illness is treated somewhat like a physical illness. In this situation, the attack of mental illness is viewed like a heart attack or an attack of epilepsy, e.g., when it occurs while driving. An individual who knew he was subject to epileptic attacks and drove anyway would be liable. Psychiatric testimony may delineate the manner in which mental illness played a role in the accident and provide information as to the possibility that the attack was sudden and unanticipated.[57]

In an oft-cited Wisconsin case, *Breunig v. American Family Ins. Co.*,[58] a psychiatrist testified that the defendant, an insured motorist, believed God took hold of the steering wheel and directed her car. She saw a truck coming and stepped on the gas in order to become airborne. She believed she could fly like Wonder Woman. To her surprise she was not airborne before striking the truck, but she was airborne after the impact. There was evidence that she had been delusional. The appellate court, finding that the defendant had knowledge of her condition, upheld a verdict for the plaintiff. It is only a sudden, first-time breakdown that excuses. The court said that if a situation arises in which the defendant is suddenly overcome without forewarning by a disabling mental disorder, liability will not be imposed.[59] Of course, psychiatrists may say that mental illness compromises cognition and, hence, an insane person may not actually know about his condition or have the ability to make a rational decision.

In a Colorado case, *Johnson v. Lombotte*,[60] the defendant was under observation by court order and was being treated for "chronic schizophrenic state of paranoid type." On the day in question, she escaped from the hospital and found an automobile with its motor running a few blocks from the hospital. She drove off, having little or no control of the car, and soon collided with the plaintiff. Later, she was adjudged mentally incompetent and committed to a state hospital. As in *Breunig*, the Colorado Supreme Court said that this was not a case of sudden mental seizure with no forewarning. The court said, "The defendant knew she was being treated for a mental disorder and, hence, would not have come under the nonliability rule [in cases of sudden attack]."[61]

Liability of Caretakers

Apart from the liability of insane persons, there may be a question of liability of those responsible for their custody and supervision. Even if a mentally ill person is said to lack the ability to form the intent to commit a tort, an action may lie against persons responsible for caring for the mentally ill person, based on negligent supervision.[62] According to circumstances, the plaintiff may sue the hospital, psychiatrist, or the parents or guardian who look after the individual.[63] In the past decade or two, there has been increasing litigation related to psychiatrists' failure to predict that patients will harm themselves or others and subsequent failure to do anything to prevent these harms. The majority of suits imposing liability on the psychiatrist or hospital involves the suicide of a patient in the inpatient setting. The burden of proving fault is on the plaintiff.[64]

Attacks on Caretakers

A number of recent cases have drawn another exception to the general rule that insane persons are liable for their torts. These are cases in which the insane person has been institutionalized and injures a caretaker. More that 100 healthcare workers are killed annually during the course of their work, not to mention the number who are seriously injured. Earlier decisions, as we have noted, imposed liability, holding in favor of the caretaker,[65] but today, the courts tend to say in cases where the defendant is institutionally confined and the injured party is employed to care for or control him, that such imposition of responsibility would serve no purpose in cases involving defendants "with no control over [their] actions and [who are] thus innocent of any wrongdoing in the most basic sense of that term."[66] Even in the case of the killing of a caretaker, there is usually neither a civil nor a criminal proceeding.[67]

Insurers of the Mentally Ill

It is important to determine not only whether the mentally ill will be held liable in tort, but also whether there is a source of compensation. Quite often, the mentally ill are indigent or have no insurance, so a lawsuit would be pointless (though civil commitment or a criminal proceeding may be appropriate). Generally speaking, in the majority of tort cases, damages are not paid by the tortfeasor, but by an insurer, especially in this day of broad coverage for general liability in family insurance policies. Unless the person being sued is cash rich, chances of collecting a judgment are small unless there is liability insurance.

Most litigated cases of torts of the mentally ill involve coverage under their liability or other insurance policy. The standard liability policy language has undergone substantial changes over the past 30 years. Prior to 1966, liability policies generally stated that damage or injury would be covered by the policy only if it was "caused by an accident which occurs during the policy period." Any duty of the insurer to defend or indemnify the insured was restricted by this "accident" requirement, but due to the difficulties in construing the word *accident*—including conflicting opinions on whether the term was to be understood from the viewpoint of the insured or the victim—the National Bureau of Casualty Underwriters and the Mutual Insurance Rating Bureau rewrote the standard policy language in 1966. The revision provided coverage "for damage ... caused by an occurrence," and defined *occurrence* as "an accident ... which results, during the policy period, in bodily injury or property damage neither expected nor intended from the standpoint of the insured."

The revision, defining *accident* from the standpoint of the insured, not the victim, is a position favorable to insurers because it denies coverage to the insured who commit intentional torts. Two lines of cases, however, have developed in the interpretation of this provision.

One line has adopted the view that the insured's subjective intent must be explored in determining coverage. If the insured did not have the specific subjective intent of causing harm to the plaintiff, his acts are deemed accidental, thus falling within the meaning of *occurrence*. The result is a decision in favor of coverage, thereby providing compensation for the victim. Psychiatric testimony is usually involved when a subjective approach is taken.[68] Another line of cases, taking a contrary approach, focuses on an objective analysis of the insured's actions. In so doing, the majority of these courts have found that the intent to inflict injury may be inferred as a matter of law when the insured's actions are of a reprehensible character (such as sexual molestation).[69] Under this objective analysis approach, a finding of no coverage is inevitably the result.[70]

The New Jersey Supreme Court in 1963 handed down a decision, which quickly became the leading case concerning the effect of insanity on the operation of intentional exclusionary clauses in insurance policies. In *Ruvolo v. American Casualty Co.*,[71] a physician, Anthony Ruvolo, shot and killed another physician with whom he had practiced medicine. At the time, Ruvolo had a personal liability insurance policy, which provided that the insurer would pay all sums that Ruvolo "shall become legally obligated to pay as damages because of the death of any person resulting from [his] activities." The coverage was limited by an exclusionary clause providing that the policy did not apply to death "caused intentionally by or at the direction of the insured."

The victim's widow filed a wrongful death suit, which Ruvolo's insurer refused to defend on the ground that the death had been caused by Ruvolo's intentional act. The guardian of the insured then filed a declaratory judgment action against his insurer, seeking to establish that the policy afforded coverage. Relying upon the affidavits of psychiatrists that Ruvolo was insane at the time of the killing and lacked the capacity to form a rational intent, the trial court granted summary judgment for the plaintiff. The trial court held that an act performed under such circumstances could not be considered intentional.

On appeal, the New Jersey Supreme Court concluded that if an insured would have been excused from responsibility under the state's criminal standard (at the time the *M'Naghten* test), then the act was not intentional for the purposes of the insurance policy. The court also provided for a finding of volitional incapacity, like the "capacity to conform conduct" test used in the ALI criminal standards. The Ruvolo case has been followed in a number of other cases.[72]

Disputes over suicide arise in connection with two different types of insurance policies: life insurance policies that exclude benefits for suicide within a certain period of time, and accidental-death policies or double-indemnity riders to life insurance policies.[73] In *Kennedy v. Washington National Ins. Co.*,[74] the insured died through autoerotic asphyxiation when he placed a rope around his neck to reduce the supply of oxygen to his brain to heighten the sexual pleasure during masturbation. In a dispute over a life insurance policy, which included an additional accidental death benefit, the court held that the death was accidental within the meaning of the policy. The court held that the insured's death was not precluded from being accidental because he voluntarily exposed himself to a known high risk of death. Although the insured's act could be considered bizarre or unusual, the court held, there was no evidence that his death was highly probable, expected, or a natural result, because his conduct was solely for the purpose of seeking sexual gratification.

The issue of suicidal intent has been raised as an issue in insurance litigation to recover death benefits under a life insurance policy. Some life insurance policies have a provision precluding recovery of the full value of the policy if death results from "suicide, whether sane or insane." However, it may be argued that the insured did not understand the physical nature and consequences of the act, and, in such a case, the insurer may be held liable for the full amount of the policy.[75] The suicide exclusion has been held not to be applicable in cases of a compulsion or an irresistible impulse to kill oneself.[76] The courts find an irresistible impulse when the decedent acted in a sudden frenzy; on the other hand, the courts find that the decedent had control when a suicide note is written or poison is purchased.[77]

Conclusion

The general rule is that the mentally ill are responsible under tort law, a rule almost invariably applied to both torts of intention or negligence (except when the victim is a caretaker). There is no counterpart of not liable by reason of insanity to the criminal law's not guilty by reason of insanity. However, as a general principle, the courts equate a sudden, unforeseeable mental incapacity with physical causes, such as a sudden heart attack or stroke.

At the same time, while holding the mentally ill responsible under tort law, the courts tend to find coverage under an insurance policy. Holding the mentally ill liable in tort goes hand in glove with holdings of insurance coverage. Moreover, the courts frequently impose liability on psychiatrists and hospitals for negligent supervision or failure to warn or protect third parties.[78]

Endnotes

1. L. Green, "The Study and Teaching of Tort Law," *Tex. L. Rev.* 34 (1955): 3.
2. Quoted in M.S. Shapo, *Tort and Injury Law* (New York: Lexis, 2000), p. 8.
3. *Restatement (Second) Torts,* §2 (Washington, DC: American Law Institute 1964).
4. See H. Morris (Ed.), *Freedom and Responsibility*, (Stanford, CA: Stanford University Press, 1961), chap. 3.
5. S.L. Halleck, "Clinical Assessment of the Voluntariness of Behavior," *Bull. Am. Acad. Psychiat. & Law* 20 (1992): 221; S.L. Halleck, "Which Patients Are Responsible for Their Illnesses?" *Am. J. Psychother.* 42 (1988): 338.
6. Quoted in F.L. Bailey, *The Defense Never Rests* (New York: Signet, 1971), p. 265. In United States v. Fishman, 743 F. Supp. 713 (N.D. Cal. 1990), where the defendant was charged with mail fraud, the court held that the theories of mental health professionals regarding coercive persuasion practices of religious cults were not sufficiently established within the scientific community to be admissible as evidence of the defendant's theory that he was brainwashed by a religious cult. See J.T. Richardson, "Cult: Brainwashing Cases and Freedom of Religion," *J. Church & State* 31 (1989): 451.
7. Interictal aspects that are relevant to the form of epileptic automatism may be the person's natural tendencies, the same psychodynamic factors that determine the content of dreams, the person's social background of violence, and the contents of a person's thoughts immediately before a seizure. P.H. van Rensburg, C.A. Gagiano, & T. Verschoor, "Possible Reasons Why Certain Epileptics Commit Unlawful Acts During or Directly After Seizures," *Med. & Law* 13 (1994): 373. See Lobert v. Pack, 337 Pa. 103, 9 A.2d 365 (1939).
8. Morriss v. Marsden, [1952] 1 All E.R. 925 (Q.B.).
9. G. Orwell, *A Collection of Essays* (New York: Harcourt, Brace, 1950).
10. M. Gladwell, *The Tipping Point: How Little Things Can Make a Big Difference* (Boston: Little, Brown, 2000).
11. Dissenting in Palsgraf v. Long Island R.R. Co., 248 N.Y. 339, 162 N.E. 99 (1928). Consider the case: A man shoots a policeman and injures him so severely that the policeman is paralyzed. The man is convicted of aggravated assault and serves a prison sentence. He gets out on parole, decides he wants to move his life in a positive direction, and even speaks to college students about his efforts to turn his life around. Over four decades after the shooting, the policeman gets an infection and dies. Physicians conclude that the infection would not have happened if not for the shooting many years before. The district attorney charges the man who shot the policeman with murder? Can or should the district attorney do that? The question is asked in M.C. Gordon, "Justice Delayed or Justice Denied?" *Detroit Legal News*, Oct. 10, 2007, p. 3. That fact pattern reflects recent events in Philadelphia in relation to William Barnes who shot Officer Walter Barclay, Jr., back in 1966. See I. Urbina, "New Murder Charge in '66 Shooting," *New York Times*, Sept. 19, 2007.
12. *Restatement of Torts*, §8A. By and large, both in law and custom, one who causes injury without fault is not blamed. Notre Dame coach Charles Weis suffered two torn ligaments in his knee from being hit on the sideline by one of his players. "[The player] must have come to me and apologized four or five times," Weis said. "He felt bad, and he has no reason to feel bad. It wasn't his fault." See J. Carey & A. Gardiner, "Weis Says Knee Surgery Can Wait," *USA Today*, Sept. 15, 2008, p. 14C. Of course, a psychiatrist may say that the action of the player was unconsciously intentional.
13. United States v. Freed, 401 U.S. 601, 607 (1971); Vosburg v. Putney, 80 Wis. 523, 50 N.W.403 (1891).
14. Eilers v. Coy, 582 F. Supp. 1093 (D. Minn. 1984).
15. R.A. Epstein, "Intentional Harms," *J. of Legal Studies* 4 (1975): 391; O.M. Reynolds, "Tortious Battery: Is 'I Didn't Mean Any Harm' Relevant?" *Okla. L. Rev.* 37 (1984): 717.
16. See, e.g., Newman v. Christensen, 149 Neb. 471, 31 N.W.2d 417 (1948); Matheson v. Pearson, 619 P.2d 321 (Utah 1980); Gouger v. Hardtke, 482 N.W.2d 84 (Wis. 1992).
17. See Mohr v. Williams, 95 Minn. 261, 104 N.W. 12 (1905). In Clayton v. New Dreamland Roller Skating Rink, 14 N.J. Super. 390, 82 A.2d 458 (1951), *cert. denied*, 13 N.J. 527, 100 A.2d 567 (1953), the plaintiff fell at a skating rink and broke her arm. Over the protests of the plaintiff and her husband, the defendant's employees proceeded to manipulate the arm in an attempt to set it. They committed a battery.
18. *Restatement of Torts*, §282.
19. "[S]aying that the liability for negligence should be co-extensive with the judgment of each individual … would be as variable as the length of the foot of each individual." Vaughan v. Menlove, 3 Bing. (N.C.) 467, 132 Eng. Rep. 490 (1837). See D.E. Seidelson, "Reasonable Expectations and Subjective Standards in Negligence Law: The Minor, the Mentally Impaired, and the Mentally Incompetent," *Geo. Wash. L. Rev.* 50 (1981): 17.

20. *Restatement of Torts*, § 283B.

21. *Ibid.*, at § 895J, comment c.

22. Professor James, arguing for the latter position, wrote: "[I]f the standard of conduct is relaxed for defendants who cannot meet a normal standard, then the burden of accident loss resulting from the extra hazards created by society's most dangerous groups (e.g., the young, the novice, the accident-prone) will be thrown on the innocent victims of substandard behavior. Such a conclusion shocks people who believe that the compensation of accident victims is a more important objective of modern tort law than a further refinement of the tort principle, and that compensation should prevail when the two objectives conflict." F. James, "The Qualities of the Reasonable Man in Negligence Cases," *Mo. L. Rev.* 16 (1951): 2.

23. *Restatement of Torts*, §467.

24. *Restatement of Torts*, §464. Allowance was made for the plaintiff's inability to exercise the judgment of a reasonable person in Seattle Elect. Co. v. Hovden, 190 Fed. 7 (9th Cir. 1911); Dassinger v. Kuhn, 87 N.W.2d 720 (N.D. 1958). The case of Wright v. Tate, 208 Va. 291, 156 S.E.2d 562 (1967), seems to stand alone in declining to make any allowance for the plaintiff's mental disability and holding him to the standard of the ordinary reasonable person. The court said, "If the rule were otherwise, there would be a different standard for each level of intelligence, resulting in confusion and uncertainty in the law." See W. Seavey, "Negligence: Subjective or Objective?" *Harv. L. Rev.* 41 (1927): 1; Note, "Standard of Care Required of Persons Under Physical Disability," *N. Car. L. Rev.* 34 (1955): 142.

25. In Lynch v. Rosenthal, 396 S.W.2d 272 (Mo. 1965), a child psychologist testified on behalf of the plaintiff, a low moron, who got his hand caught in the defendant's corn picker. The psychologist's testimony dealt with the understanding of the plaintiff. In this case the court used a subjective, rather than the average reasonable person test, in determining whether the plaintiff was contributorily negligent.

26. Nickerson v. Hodges, 146 La. 735, 84 So. 37 (1920). In a criminal case a jury convicted a man of assaulting a woman he rendered helpless by saying the word "sex." The woman, age 39, suffered from conversion hysteria that allegedly caused her to faint at the sound of sex-related words. He took advantage of her condition. S. McLaughlin, "Man, 42, Convicted in 'Sex' Word Assault," *Denver Times* (Reuters), March 12, 1994, p. B7.

27. See, e.g., Keep v. Quallman, 68 Wis. 451, 32 N.W. 233 (1887).

28. See G. Alexander & T. Szasz, "Mental Illness as an Excuse for Civil Wrongs," *Notre Dame Law* 43 (1967): 24; W. Curran, "Tort Liability of the Mentally Ill and Mentally Deficient," *Ohio St. L. J.* 21 (1960): 52; H.J.F. Korrell, "The Liability of Mentally Disabled Tort Defendants," *Law & Psych. Rev.* 19 (1995): 1; S. Morse, "Psychiatric Responsibility and Tort Liability," *J. Foren. Sci.* 12 (1967): 305; R. Sadoff, "Tortious Liability of the Insane: A Psychiatric Evaluation," *Pa. Bar Assn. Q.* 39 (1967): 73; H.L. Silverman & B. Seidler, "Psychological Evaluation of the Law of Torts," *A.B.A.J.* 47 (1961): 180; K.G. Anderson, "Insanity as a Defense to the Civil Fraud Penalty," *Duke L. J.* 12 (1963): 428; R.M. Augue, "The Liability of Insane Persons in Tort Actions," *Dick. L. Rev.* 60 (1956): 211.

    See also W.G.H. Cook, "Mental Deficiency in Relation to Tort," *Colum. L. Rev.* 21 (1921): 333; A.A. Ehrenzweig, "A Psychoanalysis of Negligence," *NW. U. L. Rev.* 47 12 (1953): 855; L.H. Eldredge, "Tort Liability of an Insane Person," *Pa. Bar Assn.* Q. 26 (1955): 176; W.B. Hornblower, "Insanity and the Law of Negligence," *Colo. L. Rev.* 5 (1905): 278; S.I. Splane, "Tort Liability of the Mentally Ill in Negligence Actions," *Yale L. J.* 93 (1983): 153; E.C.E. Todd, "Insanity as a Defence in a Civil Action of Assault and Battery," *Modern L. Rev.* 15 (1952): 486; E.C.E. Todd., "The Liability of Lunatics in the Law of Tort," *Austl. L. J.* 26 (1952): 299; G.B. Weisiger, "Tort Liability of Minors and Incompetents," *U. Ill. L. F.* (1951): 277; W.J. Wilkinson, "Mental Incompetency as a Defense to Tort Liability," *Rocky Mt. L. Rev.* 17 (1944): 38.

29. See Cal. Civ. Code § 41 (West 1990); Mont. Code Ann. § 27-1-711 (1989); N.D. Cent. Code § 14-10-03 (1981); Okla. Stat. Ann. tit. 15 §§ 25,26 (West 1972); S.D. Laws Ann. § 27A-2-4 (1976).

30. In Barylski v. Paul, 38 Mich. App. 614, 196 N.W.2d 868 (1972), the court suggested that insanity might be a defense in cases in which the tort required a specific intent, such as the malice requirement in malicious prosecution, but not in the ordinary battery case.

31. 809 S.W.2d 788 (Tex. App. 1991).

32. These grounds are critically examined in J. Ellis, "Tort Responsibility of Mentally Disabled Persons," *Am. B. Found. Res. J.* (1981): 1079.

33. M. Yancey, "Hinckley May Have to Pay Reagan Guards He Wounded," *Detroit Free Press* (AP news release), Aug. 15, 1992, p. 6.

34. The ALI's *Restatement of Torts*, §283, originally took no position as to the standard to be applied to an insane person in negligence cases, but this was changed in *Restatement (Second) of Torts*, §283B, to state that the mentally ill are to be held in all respects to the standard of the reasonable person who is sane. This is not consistent with the rule on children, but children form a readily discernible category.

    Some oft-cited cases may be noted. In Ward v. Conatser, 63 Tenn. 64 (1874), the defendant, who claimed insanity as a defense to a civil suit, shot and permanently injured the plaintiff. The court charged the jury that "insanity cannot be looked to as a justification of the shooting." In Central Ga. Ry. v. Hall, 124 Ga. 322, 52 S.E. 679 (1905), the court held that mental illness is not a defense to a tort action even when the defendant has been formally adjudged incompetent or committed to a mental hospital.

    In an old but well-known Kansas case, Seals v. Snow, 123 Kan. 88, 254 P. 348 (1927), the widow of Arthur Seals brought a civil action against Martin Snow to recover damages for the death of her husband. The evidence indicated that Snow was insane when he shot Seals and was unable to distinguish right from wrong. The verdict nonetheless was for the plaintiff. Another homicide case applying the majority rule is McIntyre v. Sholty, 121 Ill. 660, 13 N.E. 239 (1887), where liability was imposed on an insane person's estate for the wrongful killing of the plaintiff's wife. As in *McGuire*, the court reasoned: "There is, to be sure, an appearance of hardship in compelling one to respond for that when he is unable to avoid for want of the control of reason. But the question of liability in these cases is one of public policy."

    In Mullen v. Bruce, 168 Cal. App.2d 494, 335 P.2d 945 (1959), the defendant, a patient under treatment for delirium tremens resulting from alcoholism, injured the plaintiff, her special-duty nurse, who was trying to prevent the defendant from leaving; the court imposed liability. In Williams v. Kearbey, 132 Kan. App.2d 564, 775 P.2d 670 (1989), the defendant, a junior high school student, shot and injured two people at his school. The jury found that the defendant was insane at the time of the shootings and because of this fact, the defendant argued that he should not be held civilly liable. The court, following the majority rule, said that a defendant's insanity does not establish a defense to liability. That rule, the court said, reflected a policy decision "to impose liability on an insane person rather than leaving the loss on the innocent victim."

35. 297 Mass. 323, 8 N.E.2d 760 (1937). The court echoed the oft-quoted statement of Justice Oliver W. Holmes: "If, for instance, a man is born hasty and awkward, is always hurting himself or his neighbors, no doubt his congenital defects will be allowed for in the courts of Heaven, but his slips are no less troublesome to his neighbors than if they sprang from guilty neglect. His neighbors accordingly require him, at his peril, to come up to their standard, and the courts which they establish decline to take his personal equation into account." O.W. Holmes, *The Common Law* (Boston: Little, Brown, 1881), p. 108.

36. Note, "Liability of the Insane Defendant," *Cornell L.Q.* 34 (1948): 274. See also S.L. Halleck, "Which Patients Are Responsible for Their Illnesses?" *Am. J. Psychiat.* 42 (1988): 338.

37. 206 Conn. 229, 537 A.2d 468 (1988).

38. An earlier Connecticut case declined to follow the majority point of view. Fitzgerald v. Lawhorn, 29 Conn. Supp. 511, 294 A.2d 338 (Com. Pl. 1972).

39. 80 Eng. Rep. 284 (1616).

40. Bolen v. Howard, 452 S.W.2d 401 (Ky. 1970) (questioning doctrine).

41. F. Bohlen, "Liability in Tort of Infants and Insane Persons," *Mich. L. Rev.* 23 (1924): 9, at 31–32.

42. R.M. Ague, "The Liability of Insane Persons in Tort Actions," *Dick. L. Rev.* 60 (1956): 211; W.G.H. Cook, "Mental Deficiency in Relation to Tort," *Colum. L. Rev.* 21 (1921): 333; W.J. Curran, "Tort Liability for the Mentally Ill and Mentally Deficient," *Ohio St. L. J.* 21 (1960): 52; J.W. Ellis, "Tort Responsibility of Mentally Disabled Persons," *Am. Bar. Found. Res. J.* (1981): 1079; W.J. Wilkinson, "Mental Incompetency as a Defense to Tort Liability," *Rocky Mt. L. Rev.* 17 (1944): 38.

    Defending the imposition of tort liability on mentally disordered defendants: G.J. Alexander & T.S. Szasz, "Mental Illness as an Excuse for Civil Wrongs," *Notre Dame Law* 43 (1967): 24; S.I. Splane, "Tort Liability of the Mentally Ill in Negligence Actions," *Yale L. J.* 93 (1983): 153.

43. D.E. Seidelson, "Reasonable Expectations and Subjective Standards in Negligence Law: The Minor, the Mentally Impaired, and the Mentally Incompetent," *Geo. Wash. L. Rev.* 50 (1981): 17.

44. J. Ellis, "Tort Responsibility and the Mentally Disabled," *Am. Bar. Found. Res. J.* (1981): 1079.

45. In a 1934 Louisiana case, Yancey v. Maestri, 150 So. 509 (La. App. 1934), no longer followed in the state, an insane person seriously wounded the plaintiff who was held to have no cause of action because by Roman and Spanish law alike "an insane person or lunatic or madman" is not responsible for his tort, it being considered an "inevitable accident." Judge Higgins wrote, "The common law considers the effect of the insane person's act, while the civil law regards the cause of it."

46. German Civil Code § 827.

47. Codigo Civil para el Distrito Federal § 1911.

48. 143 N.Y. 442, 38 N.E. 449 (1894), qualified in 157 N.Y. 541, 52 N.E. 589 (1899); discussed in W.J. Wilkinson, "Mental Incompetency as a Defense to Tort Liability," *Rocky Mt. L. Rev.* 17 (1944): 38.

49. Note, "Insane Persons: Tort Liability," *Minn. L. Rev.* 22 (1938): 853.

50. In Cohen v. Petty, 62 App. D.C. 187, 65 F.2d 820 (1933), the plaintiff, a passenger in the defendant's car, alleged that the defendant was at fault in driving his automobile, operating it at an excessive rate of speed, and losing control of it. The car ran off the road and plaintiff was injured in the accident. Defendant claimed he fainted, had never fainted before, was in good health, and had no indication that he might faint. All of a sudden, as the plaintiff acknowledged, he exclaimed, "Oh, I feel sick." His head fell back and his hand left the wheel. On the day in question, he was not feeling bad until the moment before the illness and the fainting occurred. The trial court directed a verdict in favor of the defendant and the appellate court affirmed that verdict, finding the plaintiff had failed to show any fault on the part of the defendant. See J.B. Craig, "Heart Attacks as a Defense in Negligence Action," *Clev.-Mar. L. Rev.* 12 (1963): 59. But see Sauers v. Sack, 34 Ga. App. 748, 131 S.E. 98 (1921), where an epileptic seizure was viewed as similar to insanity and the defendant was held liable. In this case, the defendant was shown to be accustomed to having epileptic or other similar attacks.

51. See, e.g., Sfroza v. Green Bus Lines, 150 Misc. 180, 268 N.Y. Supp. 446 (1934).

52. See M. Arnold, "Driven Mad," *Jerusalem Post*, Oct. 8, 1999, p. 16; A. Martin, "Driving Ourselves Crazy," *Detroit Free Press Magazine*, Aug. 9, 1992, p. 7.

53. B. Bush, *A Memoir* (New York: Scribners, 1994).

54. S.L. Godard & J.D. Bloom, "Driving, Mental Illness, and the Duty to Protect," in J.C. Beck (Ed.), *Confidentiality Versus the Duty to Protect: Foreseeable Harm in the Practice of Psychiatry* (Washington, DC: American Psychiatric Press, 1990), pp. 191–204.

55. See G.H. Morris, "Requiring Sound Judgments of Unsound Minds: Tort Liability and the Limits of Therapeutic Jurisprudence," *SMU L. Rev.* 47 (1994): 1837; D.W. Shuman, "Therapeutic Jurisprudence and Tort Law: A Limited Subjective Standard of Care," *SMU L. Rev.* 46 (1992): 409.

56. In C.T.W. v. B.C.G., 809 S.W.2d 788 (Tex. App. 1991), a pedophile was held negligent for failing to seek professional help and not avoiding situations where he would be alone with children.

57. In Kuhn v. Zabotsky, 9 Ohio St. 2d 129, 224 N.E.2d 137 (1967), a psychiatrist, called by the defense, testified that the defendant was mentally ill and that he was suffering from a psychotic depression reaction, but he did not testify that the defendant had (for the first time) "blacked out" at the time of the accident. Verdict was for the plaintiff. See S.L. Halleck, *Law in the Practice of Psychiatry* (New York: Plenum, 1980), p. 275.

58. 45 Wis.2d 536, 173 N.W.2d 619 (1970).

59. Twenty-four years later, in 1994, in Gould v. American Family Mut. Ins. Co., 523 N.W.2d 295 (Wis. App. 1994) a Wisconsin appellate court said that *Breunig* compelled a conclusion that an individual with a *permanent* mental disability that prevents the individual from controlling or appreciating his conduct cannot be held liable in negligence. In this case, the patient suffered Alzheimer's disease. The court said that to the extent that it prevented him from appreciating or controlling his actions, he could not be held liable in negligence. The patient attacked a member of a health center's staff. Some law professors suggest that Alzheimer's disease be regarded as a physical condition and the standard of care then being "the reasonable person with Alzheimer's." See Memorial Hosp. v. Scott, 261 Ind. 27, 300 N.E.2d 50 (1973) (multiple sclerosis); W.P. Keeton, D.B. Dobbs, R.E. Keeton, & D.C. Owens, *Prosser & Keeton on the Law of Torts* (St. Paul, MN.: West, 5th ed., 1984), p. 175.

60. 147 Colo. 203, 363 P.2d 165 (1961).

61. In a Canadian case, the court found no negligence when a truck driver was overcome by a sudden insane delusion that his truck was being operated by the remote control of his employer and as a result he, in fact, was helpless to avert a collision. The truck driver suffered from syphilis of the brain. He sat transfixed at the wheel, powerless to do anything about the collision, which ensued. Buckley & Toronto Transp. Comm'n v. Smith Transport, 1946 Ont. Rep. 798, 4 Dom. L. Rep. 721 (1946).

62. See Rausch v. McVeigh, 105 Misc.2d 163, 431 N.Y.S.2d 887 (1980); cause of action for negligent supervision against parents of 22-year-old autistic son who attacked his therapist). To encourage individuals to take on the role of guardian, laws in various states provide that a guardian is not liable to third person for acts of the ward. For example, Michigan law provides: "[A] guardian of a legally incapacitated person is responsible for the care, custody, and control of the ward, but is not liable to third persons by reason of that responsibility for acts of the ward." M.L.D. § 700.455 (1). The circumstance of a person being under guardianship as insane does not take away his legal capacity to be sued. Ingersoll v.

Harrison, 48 Mich. 234, 12 N.W. 179 (1882). Not only are guardians not held responsible for the acts of their wards, abuses by guardians of their wards are widespread, and they are rarely held responsible. Nowadays, with families split apart, lawyers and corporation are often named guardian, for a number of people, and they are paid a fee for their service. W. Wendland-Bowyer, "Who's Watching the Guardians?" *Detroit Free Press*, 3-part series, May 24–26, 2000, p. 1.

63. See Tarasoff v. Regents of University of California, 17 Cal.3d 425, 551 P.2d 334, 131 Cal. Rptr. 14 (1976); T.E. Gammon & J.K. Hulston, "The Duty of Mental Health Care Providers to Restrain Their Patients or Warn Third Parties," *Mo. L. Rev.* 60 (1995): 1995; R.I. Simon, "Psychiatrists' Duties in Discharging Sicker and Potentially Violent Inpatients in the Managed Care Era," *Psychiat. Serv.* 49 (Jan. 1998): 62.

64. R.I. Simon, *Clinical Psychiatry and the Law* (Washington, DC: American Psychiatric Press, 2nd ed., 1992), p. 274.

65. See McGuire v. Almy, 297 Mass. 323, 8 N.E. 2d 760 (1937); Van Vooren v. Cook, 273 A.D. 88, 75 N.Y.S. 2d 362 (1947); Mullen v. Bruce, 68 Cal. App.2d 494, 335 P.2d 945 (1959).

66. Anicet v. Gant, 580 So.2d 273 (Fla. Dist. App. 1991); see also Gould v. American Family Mut. Ins. Co., 523 N.W. 295 (Wis. App. 1994); Mujica v. Turner, 582 So.2d 24 (Fla. Dist. App. 1991); Van Vooren v. Cook, 273 App. Div. 88, 75 N.Y.S.2d 362 (1947). In Herrle v. Estate of Marshall, 45 Cal. App. 4th 1761, 53 Cal. Rptr.2d 713 (1996), it was held that a nurse's aide assumed the risk of attack by a patient suffering from Alzheimer's disease. As a consequence of the decision, a dissenter argued that caretakers would be well-advised to use greater force on the patient to avoid injury to themselves. Workers' compensation would provide compensation for employees injured in the course of their employment. See also Creasy v. Rusk, 730 N.E.2d 659 (Ind., 2000).

67. R. Slovenko, *Psychiatry and Criminal Culpability* (New York: John Wiley & Sons, 1995); R. Slovenko, "Violent Attacks in Psychiatric and Other Hospitals," *J. Psychiat. & Law* 34 (2006): 249; S.K. Hoge & T.G. Gutheil, "The Prosecution of Psychiatric Patients for Assaults on Staff: A Preliminary Empirical Study," *Hosp. & Comm. Psychiat.* 38 (1987): 44; R.D. Miller & G.J. Maier, "Factors Affecting the Decision to Prosecute Mental Patients for Criminal Behavior," *Hosp. & Comm. Psychiat.* 38 (1987): 50; M. Privitera et al., "Violence Toward Mental Health Staff and Safety in the Work Environment," *Occupat. Med.* 55 (2005): 480; S. Rachlin, "The Prosecution of Violent Psychiatric Inpatients: One Respectable Intervention," *Bull. Am. Acad. Psychiat. & Law* 22 (1994): 239. See also R. Simon & K. Tardiff (Eds.), *Textbook of Violence Assessment and Management* (Washington, DC: American Psychiatric Press, 2008).

68. See State Farm Fire & Cas. Co. v. Wicka, 474 N.W.2d 324 (Minn. 1991); D.E. Seidelson, "Reasonable Expectations and Subjective Standards in Negligence Law: The Minor, The Mentally Impaired, and the Mentally Incompetent," *Geo. Wash. L. Rev.* 50 (1981): 17.

69. I.N. Perr, "Liability of the Mentally Ill and Their Insurers in Negligence and Other Civil Actions," *Am. J. Psychiat.* 142 (1985): 1414; C.A. Salton, "Mental Incapacity and Liability Insurance Exclusionary Clauses: The Effect of Insanity Upon Intent," *Cal. L. Rev.* 78 (1990): 1027; R.I. Simon, "You Only Die Once—But Did You Intend It? Psychiatric Assessment of Suicide Intent in Insurance Litigation," *Tort & Ins. L. J.* 25 (1990): 650; Note, "Insanity, Intent, and Homeowner's Liability," *La. L. Rev.* 40 (1979): 258.

70. The Washington Court of Appeals in Public Employees Mut. Ins. Co. v. Rash, 48 Wash App. 701, 740 P.2d 370 (1987), held that an insurer is not liable to pay a claim under a homeowner's policy for the insured's sexual assault on a minor in light of the exclusion from policy coverage of injuries caused by insured, which are expected or intended. The court said that the insured's subjective intent or incapability of forming intent is irrelevant in determining whether damage caused by the insured is covered by the policy. See also Germantown Ins. Co. v. Martin, 407 Pa. Super. 326, 595 A.2d 1172 (1992).

71. 39 N.J. 490, 189 A.2d 204 (1963).

72. See George v. Stone, 260 So.2d 259 (Fla. App. 1972); Rosa v. Liberty Mutual Ins. Co., 243 F. Supp. 407 (D. Conn. 1965); Congregation of Rodef Sholom v. American Motorists Ins. Co., 91 Cal. App. 3d 690, 154 Cal. Rptr. 348 (1979); Nationwide Mutual Fire Ins. Co. v. Turner, 29 Ohio App.3d 73, 503 N.E.2d 212 (1986).

73. It was questioned whether Freddie Prinze, the TV star, actually meant to kill himself. Despite the uncontested fact that he shot himself in the presence of a witness, his family and managers tried to prove in court that it was not legally suicide. They had hoped to obtain the $550,000 in insurance— the only big item in Prinze's estate—that two insurance companies refused to pay because of a suicide clause. The family's lawyers pressed two lines of attack, both based on the fact that intent is a key element in suicide. One was that for months before his death, he had been scaring friends by pretending to shoot himself, keeping the safety catch on his gun; he may have tried it the last time unaware the

catch was off. An alternate argument was that use of a depressant drug had rendered him incapable of willing his own death. See G. Schuman, "Suicide and the Life Insurance Contract: Was the Insured Sane or Insane? That Is the Question—Or Is It?" *Tort & Ins. L. J.* 28 (1993): 745.

The courts are divided on their willingness to admit psychological autopsy evidence. At one extreme, a federal court held that a psychological autopsy offered as evidence in a suit over life insurance proceeds was "pure speculation," which did "nothing to assist the trier of fact in the least" in determining whether the deceased had been murdered or committed suicide. Foster v. Globe Life & Acc. Ins. Co., 808 F. Supp. 1281 (N.D. Miss. 1992). At the other end of the spectrum is the decision of a Florida appellate court affirming a child abuse conviction of a woman whose 17-year-old daughter had committed suicide. Its ruling was based in part on a psychological autopsy that found the mother's mistreatment of her daughter, whom she had forced to work as a stripteaser, to be a "substantial contributing factor" in the daughter's decision to kill herself. Jackson v. State, 553 So.2d 719 (Fla. App. 1989). See M. Hansen, "Suicidal Missions," *ABAJ*, March 2000, p. 28.

74. 136 Wis.2d 425, 401 N.W.2d 842, 62 ALR4th 815 (1987).

75. Reviewing a suicide exclusion clause, the U.S. Supreme Court in Mutual Life Ins. Co. v. Terry, 15 Wall. 580, 21 L. Ed. 236 (1873), said: "If the death is caused by the voluntary act of the assured, he knowing and intending that his death shall be result of his act, but when his reasoning faculties are so far impaired that he is not able to understand the moral character, the general nature, consequences and effect of the act he is about to commit, or when he is impelled thereto by an insane impulse, which he has not the power to resist, such death is not within the contemplation of the parties to the contract and the insurer is liable." See also Searle v. Allstate Life Ins. Co., 38 Cal.3d 425, 212 Cal. Rptr. 466, 696 P.2d 1308 (1985).

76. Fuller v. Preis, 35 N.Y.2d 425, 322 N.E.2d 263, 363 N.Y.S.2d 568 (1974).

77. See Brown v. American Steel & Wire Co., 43 Ind. App. 560, 88 N.E. 80 (1909). For a review of the cases, see Grant v. F.P. Lathrop Constr. Co., 81 Cal. App. 3d 796, 146 Cal. Rptr. 45 (1978).

78. The concept of "accident" is disappearing, with blame placed on the alleged wrongdoing, the victim, or a third party. In early 2001 the *British Medical Journal* decided to ban the use of the word *accident*. The *Journal of Accident and Emergency Medicine* also dropped the word and changed its name to *Emergency Medicine Journal*. Ronald Davis, North American editor of the *British Medical Journal*, and Barry Pless, editor of the journal *Injury Prevention*, wrote in a joint editorial, "An accident is often understood to be unpredictable—a chance occurrence or an 'act of God' and therefore unavoidable. However, most injuries and their precipitating events are predictable and preventable. That is why the BMJ has decided to ban the word." Medical sociologists have argued for years about whether the use of the "A" word prejudices public thinking away from prevention and towards fatalistic explanations. Most explanations in contemporary society involve networks of causality without appeal to change. T. Barlow, "You Better Believe It—It's Just an Accident," *Financial Times*, Nov. 3–4, 2001, p. II.

19
Posttraumatic Stress Disorder and Workers' Compensation

The term *posttraumatic stress disorder* (PTSD) refers to a psychogenic disorder following a psychic injury with or without physical injury. It is also known by many other names: traumatic neurosis, neurosis following trauma, neurosis following accident, terror neurosis (schreckneurose), acute neurotic reaction, triggered neurosis, postaccident anxiety syndrome, posttraumatic hysteria, hysterical paralysis, social neurosis, personal injury neurosis, industrial neurosis, accident neurosis, occupational neurosis, litigation neurosis, justice neurosis, compensation neurosis, compensationitis, desire neurosis, unconscious malingering, retirement neurosis, pension neurosis, fate neurosis, and secondary gain neurosis.

Commonly, these terms refer to a disorder developing from an injury caused by another person, which is complicated by factors in compensation and litigation; however, compensation is not an essential element in the etiology of the neurosis. The term *traumatic neurosis* came into use during World War II, a successor to the old term *shell shock*, and more recently, *posttraumatic stress disorder*. In the military situation, other labels include *war neurosis, combat fatigue, combat neurosis, battle stress*, and *stress reaction*. In some measure, the use of a particular descriptive label reflects a particular attitude toward the phenomenon. The terms *malingering* and *goof-off* are commonly used to refer to conscious deception.

No life is without trauma. Otto Rank, a prominent member of Freud's early coterie, in a book *The Trauma of Birth* makes the event of birth itself the crucial fact of life and interprets later psychosexual crises of childhood as variations on the theme of the terror of the issue from the womb and the wish to return to embryonic bliss. From this premise, he reinterprets many of the common Freudian concepts. The painful experience of birth leaves all of us with a measure of "primal anxiety." The universal desire to forget this pain Rank calls "primal repression." Therapy would take 9 months, the time period from conception to birth.[1]

Actually, there is nothing new about PTSD except its name. Willa Cather once observed that if you give people a new word, they think they have a new fact. It has long been known that traumatic events can produce serious emotional reactions. In the 1666 diary of Samuel Pepys, 6 months after he survived the Great Fire of London, he wrote, "It is strange to think how to this very day I cannot sleep a night without great terrors of the fire; and this very night could not sleep to almost two in the morning through great terrors of the fire."[2] In 1871, when Chicago went up in flames, many people came down with PTSD. Veterans of combat in World War I suffered from shell shock; many veterans of World War II had "battle fatigue." Soon the term *traumatic neurosis* came into wide professional, but not official, usage, which lasted until 1980 when the term was officially replaced by *posttraumatic stress disorder*. The attack on September 11, 2001, of the World Trade Center made it an everyday term.

In 1980, with the publication of the *Diagnostic and Statistical Manual of Mental Disorders* (*DSM-II*), PTSD entered the psychiatric nomenclature as a listing under the heading of anxiety disorders. (*DSM-II* had eliminated gross stress reactions, including combat stress, and replaced them with "(transient) adjustment reactions to adult life.") In *DSM-IV*, of 1994, the minimum duration of symptoms of PTSD must be 1 month. The symptoms include free-floating anxiety, muscular tension, irritability, impaired concentration, repetitive nightmares reproducing the accident, and social withdrawal. *DSM-IV* introduced a new diagnosis, "acute stress disorder," when the symptoms occur within 4 weeks of the traumatic event and the symptoms last only for 2 days to a month. It might be considered a brief PTSD or a normal response to trauma. It is listed among anxiety disorders to manifest its association with PTSD.

Although one or another term referring to a psychogenic disorder following a psychic injury has been used and respected in scientific literature throughout the world, none appeared as a nosological entity in the *DSM* until 1980. Some psychiatrists did not and still do not agree that PTSD is an entity. Some see it as a complex of symptoms or scars, not as a disorder. They view most cases as indistinguishable from anxiety, hysterical conversion type, hysterical dissociative type, phobic, obsessive-compulsive, depressive, depersonalization, or hypochondriasis. Other psychiatrists, however, see it as a distinct category of mental disorder that develops in individuals as a result of a specific psychic insult.

A psychiatric diagnostic category is not essential to a cause of action in law, but the listing of stress reactions in the *DSM* has tended to give the claim more legitimacy. Forensic psychiatrists promoted the listing of PTSD in the *DSM*. With the inclusion of PTSD, attorneys on behalf of victims of trauma have increasingly used that formulation in civil as well as in criminal cases. As expert witnesses, psychiatrists embrace PTSD to explain the psychological sequelae of trauma in personal injury cases as well as to formulate opinions regarding criminal responsibility.

Physicians on behalf of war veterans also promoted the listing of PTSD in the *DSM*. Before PTSD appeared in the 1980 *DSM*, veterans at some Veterans Administration hospitals were diagnosed as schizophrenic, so that they could receive benefits, but it was stigmatizing (and dishonest).

The 1994 *DSM-IV* also describes a condition called "posttraumatic stress disorder, delayed type," where the symptoms do not appear until at least 6 months after the trauma. The Veterans Administration authorized compensation and other benefits for PTSD, delayed type. It was the first time since World War I that the Department of Veterans Benefits could consider disorders to be service-connected when the symptoms appeared long after military discharge. The result was a surge of admission to VA hospitals (providing care otherwise not available).[3]

For a diagnosis of PTSD, the *DSM-III* specified a stressor that is "outside the range of usual human experience" that would be markedly distressing to almost anyone. The manual gave examples of "common experiences" that do not qualify for PTSD—simple bereavement, chronic illness, business losses, or marital conflict. Researchers, however, found patients who met symptom criteria for PTSD without meeting the stressor criterion. Dr. Bonnie Green, who served on the advisory committee for the PTSD diagnosis for *DSM-III-R* and on the *DSM-IV* PTSD advisory committee, reports that the most debate regarding this diagnosis centered on the definition of the stressor criterion and also on whether there should be additional diagnoses that reflect responses to traumatic events.[4] *DSM-IV* omits the phrase "outside the range of usual human experience," but like *DSM-III-R*, it requires that the individual "experienced, witnessed, or was confronted with an event or events that involved actual or threatened death or serious injury, or a threat to the physical integrity of self or others." It is an experience that radically alters a person's sense of safety, so that they become dysfunctional.

PTSD is taken as the prototypical environmentally caused disorder, as it allegedly only arises in the aftermath of an environmental insult—the *DSM* suggests that the symptoms of PTSD emerge from an event or events. In a review of the world literature on response to trauma, however, it was concluded that "toxic events are not reliably powerful in yielding a chronic, event-focused clinical disorder such as PTSD."[5] Indeed, with the exception of events such as the Holocaust, most people, it was reported, do not respond to toxic events with persistent symptoms that would rise to the level of a diagnosable disorder such as PTSD. Individuals who do are characterized by preexisting factors, such as long-standing personality traits of emotionality and personal vulnerability, suggesting that their preevent factors contribute more to serious distress disorders than the toxic event.[6]

With the recognition of PTSD in the *DSM*, primary causation was shifted from the individual to the environment, but a growing body of studies raises the important question of whether the symptoms of PTSD are necessarily caused by trauma. Instead, it is noted, the symptom cluster currently attributed to PTSD may be a nonspecific group of symptoms widely observed in individuals with mood and anxiety disorders, regardless of trauma history. Many of the symptoms included in the diagnostic criteria of PTSD, such as intrusive thoughts, emotional numbing, and increased arousal, are similar to those observed in many other mood and anxiety disorders.[7] As Michael First, who is leading the team updating the *DSM*, puts it, "… many different brain states can produce the same mental symptoms, and many different symptoms can arise from the same brain state."[8]

The definition of PTSD in the *DSM* assumes that the event or events that the individual experienced were real, with one of the cardinal symptoms of the diagnosis being that the individual persistently reexperienced this real event. In a study, cases of transplant patients are presented who, while in delirium, experienced delusions and hallucinations of life-threatening events that were later reexperienced as clinically diagnosed PTSD. These cases demonstrate that not only real life-threatening events, but delirium experiences that occur during life-threatening medical crisis or illness, can provoke PTSD. Therefore, it is suggested that PTSD criteria be extended to include both real and psychically induced experiences.[9]

In any event, in tort litigation, PTSD remains a favored diagnosis in cases of emotional distress because it is alleged to be incident specific. The diagnosis tends to rule out other factors important to the determination of causation (vulnerability and resilience). Thus, plaintiffs can argue that all of their psychological problems issue from the alleged traumatic event and not from myriad other sources encountered in life. A diagnosis of depression, on the other hand, opens the issue of causation to many factors other than the stated cause of action. Dr. Alan A. Stone, a past president of the American Psychiatric Association, puts it this way:

> By giving diagnostic credence and specificity to the concept of psychic harm, PTSD has become the lightning rod for a wide variety of claims of stress-related psychopathology in the civil arena. Unlike the diagnostic concept of neurosis, which emphasizes a complex etiology, PTSD posits a straightforward causal relationship that plaintiffs' lawyers welcome. Beyond its significance as an apparent solution to the legal problem of causation, PTSD's greatest importance is that it seems to make matters scientific and objective that the court once considered too subjective for legal resolution.[10]

The diagnostic category is now entrenched in the jurisprudence and also in ordinary language. It has given rise to new schools of psychotherapy, has become the subject (as of May 2006) of more than 10,000 scientific papers, and has spawned a specialty in tort law, which seeks to obtain compensation for individuals reporting symptoms of PTSD. It is asserted that PTSD comes in acute, chronic, delayed, complex, subdural, and even "masked" forms. In *Trial* magazine, it was written: "No diagnosis in the history of American psychiatry has had a more dramatic and pervasive impact on law and social justice than posttraumatic stress disorder."[11] Seeing the mayhem in the film *Saving Private Ryan*, a moviegoer says, "[It] was not a movie; it was an ordeal. I told my husband that I thought I was going to have posttraumatic stress syndrome and wondered if I could sue somebody."[12] Allegedly, jurors listening to gruesome evidence in a murder trial may allegedly suffer PTSD.[13]

The concept of trauma has expanded from a life-threatening event to such stressors as learning about the death of a loved one or to being exposed to obnoxious sexual jokes in the workplace. The more the concept of traumatic stressor is broadened, the less credibly can causal significance be assigned to the stressor, and the more the causal role of preexisting vulnerability must be emphasized.[14]

At trial, psychiatric testimony is offered on the issues of causation and damage. The legal claim of a person who seeks compensation for PTSD may fall into one of the following categories: (1) a tort action for personal injury allegedly inflicted by the fault (intentional or negligent) of the defendant, (2) a workers' compensation claim for disability allegedly due to an accidental injury received in the course and scope of employment, or (3) a claim under a life, health, or accident insurance policy.

There is only limited legal redress for the infliction of mental pain and anguish. It has always seemed quixotic for the law to attempt to secure an emotional or mental state; hence, the courts have afforded legal redress only in the more outrageous types of cases. Wholly aside from the question of how far the law should go in protecting emotional or mental nondisturbance, there are presented difficult evidentiary questions of causation and assessment of harm.

Recovery for emotional distress has long been recognized as an additional or parasitic element of damages in a tort action. Thus, where the actor's tortious conduct results in the invasion of another's legally protected interest, as where it inflicts bodily harm, the ensuing emotional distress may be taken into account in determining the damages recoverable. As a general principle, however, freedom from mental and emotional disturbance has received only limited independent recognition as a legally protected interest.[15]

In a variety of situations where the disturbance is grievous (for instance, in actions for assault, defamation, false imprisonment, invasion of privacy, and malicious prosecution), the law has afforded protection. Gradually, the general proposition developed that one who, without just cause or excuse and beyond all bounds of decency, purposely inflicts mental distress of a serious nature is subject to liability. Thus, a joker who tells a woman that her son has been mutilated in an accident would be liable for her ensuing mental anguish. The tort is called "intentional infliction of mental distress."

In cases of negligence resulting in fright, shock, or other mental suffering, the various jurisdictions have required proof of physical impact or injury. Over the years, the law has been concerned about a flood of litigation or fraudulent claims if compensation were awarded in cases of negligence causing mental distress without accompanying physical impact or injury. As a New York court in 1896 said:

> If the right of recovery [for mental distress in negligence cases without physical impact or injury] should be one established, it would naturally result in a flood of litigation in cases where the injury complained of may be easily feigned without detection, and where the damages must rest upon mere conjecture or speculation. The difficulty which often exists in cases of alleged physical injury, in determining whether they exist, and if so, whether they were caused by the negligent act of the defendant, would not only be greatly increased, but a wide field would be opened for fictitious or speculative claims. To establish such a doctrine would be contrary to principles of public policy.[16]

Likewise, at about the same time, an English court said:

> According to the evidence of the female plaintiff, her fright was caused by seeing the train approaching, and thinking they were going to be killed. Damages arising from mere sudden terror unaccompanied by an actual physical injury, but occasioning a nervous or mental shock, cannot under such circumstances, their Lordships think, be considered a consequence which, in the ordinary course of things, would flow from the negligence of the gate-keeper. If it were held that they can, it appears to their Lordships that it would be extending the liability for negligence much beyond what that liability has hitherto been

held to be. Not only in such a case as the present, but in every case where an accident caused by negligence had given a person a serious nervous shock, there might be a claim for damages on account of mental injury. The difficulty, which now often exists in cases of alleged physical injuries of determining whether they were caused by the negligent act, would be greatly increased, and a wide field opened for imaginary claims.[17]

The theory is that impact or injury affords a guarantee of causal connection and genuineness of harm. But the theory was mocked in a famous Georgia circus case, "impact" being found where one of the performing horses defecated on a spectator's lap, to her great humiliation.[18]

The most frequently cited public policy factors a court will consider when deciding whether liability should not attach to damages caused by a defendant's negligence are

1. The injury is too remote from the negligence.
2. The injury is wholly out of proportion to the defendant's culpability.
3. In retrospect it appears extraordinary that the negligence would have brought about the harm.
4. Allowing recovery places an unreasonable burden on the defendant.
5. Allowing recovery is too likely to open the way for fraudulent claims.
6. Allowing recovery will enter a field having no sensible or just stopping point.

Wholly aside from the questions of how far the law should go in protecting against emotional disturbance, there are difficult evidentiary questions of fault, causation, and assessment of damages. The vulnerability of the victim is considered differently in each of these various elements that together constitute a tort.

Fault

For fault, the risk reasonably to be perceived determines the duty of care. Foreseeability is the traditional test. Thus, a greater duty of care is imposed on a motorist when he sees a handicapped person or child crossing the street. When the vulnerability of a person is not reasonably apparent, the fair assumption is that he is an ordinary individual. Negligence is failing to observe the care expected of a reasonable person in like circumstances.

What about a duty of care to bystanders (e.g., parents who learn of injury to their child)? The *DSM* recognizes that a person who witnesses an event that threatens the physical integrity of others may suffer PTSD. In law, in 1968, a trend began to allow an action for mental distress for bystanders witnessing negligent as well as intentional injury. That year, in the famous case of *Dillon v. Legg*,[19] the California Supreme Court ruled in favor of a mother who saw her infant daughter killed when hit by a car. It set out standards for a bystander action: a close relationship to the person injured, close proximity to the scene, and "sensory and contemporaneous observation" of the accident. The bystander cases in California culminated in the decision in 1989 in *Thing v. La Chusa*,[20] where the California Supreme Court circumscribed the class of bystanders to whom a defendant owes a duty to avoid negligently inflicting emotional distress. In *Thing*, the guidelines in *Dillon* became precise rules. The court set out the limits as follows:

> In the absence of physical injury or impact to the plaintiff himself, damages for emotional distress should be recoverable only if the plaintiff: (1) is closely related to the injury victim, (2) is present at the scene of the injury-producing event at the time it occurs and is then aware that it is causing injury to the victim, and (3) as a result suffers emotional distress beyond that which would be anticipated in a disinterested witness.

Under *Thing*, regardless of foreseeable and actual emotional harm to the plaintiff, the plaintiff would be denied recovery unless actually present and witnessed the injury or threat to a close relation. In *Thing*, a mother who heard her son had been struck by a car, and who rushed to the scene to find her son bloody and apparently dead, had no cause of action for her own distress because she had not been within the zone of danger and had not actually witnessed the injury.[21]

A number of jurisdictions have loosened the requirement that the plaintiff has to be at the scene of the alleged act that caused the mental suffering. In the *Dillon* case, the distressed mother was outside the "zone of danger"; there was no possibility that the mother would be hit by the car that killed her daughter, but she was at the scene. In 1980, the Supreme Judicial Court of Massachusetts allowed a wife and children to sue for mental distress arising out of seeing their injured husband/father at a hospital hours after an accident allegedly caused by the defendant.[22] The Ohio Supreme Court in 1983 suggested a standard of "serious and reasonably foreseeable" that a bystander would sustain emotional injury.[23]

In the famous Buffalo Creek disaster where a dam broke due to the alleged negligence of the defendant, there was a settlement of claims brought by a number of plaintiffs who suffered emotional distress though they witnessed no one in the flood. They were miles away when the water broke through the dam; they heard the news. The 20- to 30-foot tidal wave of rampaging water and sludge, sometimes traveling at speeds up to 30 miles per hour, devastated Buffalo Creek's 16 small communities.[24]

In line with a number of courts that not only require that the bystander witness the event, but also must be closely related to the victim is the decision in *Biercevicz v. Liberty Mutual Ins. Co.*[25] Here, the Connecticut Superior Court held that an automobile accident victim's fiancée was not closely related to the victim so as to allow the fiancée to bring an action for bystander emotional distress. In order for the woman to prevail on her claim, she was required to show, among other things, that she was closely related to the victim (her fiancé), which the defendant argued required a relationship by blood or marriage. The court agreed. It is necessary, the court said, to draw a line to avoid countless other litigants and extend liability on the part of negligent defendants. The fiancée could not prevail on her claim, though other courts have allowed similar claims.

Causation

For causation, the law looks for proximate cause. There is no litmus test for determining proximity, and there may be more than one proximate cause. Some courts use the foreseeability test in determining causation, but usually the courts say it is a question of the objective evidence. For causation, there is the well-known expression, "the tortfeasor must take his victim as he finds him," so that peculiar vulnerability to harm does not excuse. However, it may be argued, sometimes successfully, that the straw that broke the camel's back is not a proximate cause.

The so-called delayed PTSD may be the result of a cumulation of events resulting in a crisis. (In law, the statute of limitations begins when the injury is *made known*.) The approximate cause may arguably be either the earlier or a later event. The term *proximate* has connotations of nearness in time, but that is not its meaning in law. *Legal cause* or *responsible cause* are more appropriate terms, but these terms also leave much room for vagaries in decision making. In a number of cases, the courts have said that the determination of proximate cause is the province of judges not juries, but more often than not, it is a decision left to the jury.

In days gone by, when the term *traumatic neurosis* was used, psychiatrists distinguished between a true traumatic neurosis, where a healthy individual suffers emotional distress as a result of an overwhelming stress, and a triggered neurosis, where a vulnerable individual decompensates as a result of stress that would be quite inconsequential to a healthy individual. For the law, however, the distinction is one without a difference. The argument may prevail, however, that in the case of a triggered neurosis, a triggering event is not a proximate cause.

Trauma, as we have noted, is a relative concept—stimulus in relation to the coping ability of an individual. An individual's response to an injury event may be influenced by preexisting vulnerabilities that facilitate the development and maintenance of symptoms. A prior history of major depression is identified as a significant risk factor for developing PTSD.[26] When a stressor is within the range of common experience, the evidence tends to support a finding that it is not a proximate cause. Also, when a stressor is not outside the range of common experience, suspicion of malingering arises.

The difference in the legal and medical concept of causation results from the differences in the basic problems and exigencies of the two disciplines. In the law of torts, it is said that the tortfeasor is not entitled to complain that his victim was not a perfect specimen. Likewise, in the field of workers' compensation, the employer takes his employee as he finds him. In legal contemplation, if an injury operates on an existing bodily condition or predisposition and produces a further injurious result, that result is deemed caused by the injury.

A number of survivors of Nazi concentration camps, who subsequently suffered serious psychiatric disorders, were denied compensation because certain psychiatric experts appointed by the German Consulate declined to acknowledge a causal connection between the victims' experiences and later mental disorders. In a parallel to Otto Rank's birth trauma theory, these psychiatrists adhered to a theory of constitutional etiology or childhood neurosis, which, coupled with their general approach, made it unlikely that they would recommend compensation for the victims.[27]

Theories pointing to distal causes call to mind the argument that if the injured person had never been born, the injury would not have happened. Therefore, the courts ask whether the wrongful act was the proximate cause. Lord Chancellor Francis Bacon's maxim was, "In law, the near cause is looked to, not the remote one." Testimony of the medical expert witness usually ends up thus:

Q. From everything that you know about this case, Doctor, do you feel there is a causal relationship between the explosion of July 4, and the symptoms that she has shown that you have reported [sudden loss of weight, inability to perform ordinary household duties, extreme nervousness and irritability]?

A. Yes, the trauma was the triggering point for breaking the balance in her. So to speak, the trauma threw her off her rocker.

Q. Trauma?

A. Any trauma. It may be emotional trauma or physical trauma. In this case, it was the explosive sound that she heard and the fears that were aroused by it.

Legal, or proximate, cause may be illustrated by the once-upon-a-time story of the camel that carried loads across the desert for its master. This camel had a weaker back than other camels, but because his master had never loaded him too heavily he had been able to do his job well and was his master's favorite. At the beginning of one trip, the camel was loaded as usual, but while the master's back was turned a prankster put a straw atop the load. The weight of this straw was just enough "to break the camel's back." The prankster's act being the legal cause of the camel's broken back, he is liable to the camel's master for all damages that the master suffers. Thus, the law is interested more in the straw that broke the camel's back than in all the straws already piled on his back.

Consider also the example of a 50-year-old man who, all of his life, has been walking on the brink of a precipice. He has walked close to the brink, but he has kept his footing. Along comes someone who gives this man a push—not much of a push, but just enough to make him lose his balance and plunge him over the edge. It may not have been enough of a push to make a different person lose his balance. But for the purpose of legal causation, it is enough to show that, but for the push, the man could have kept on walking, even if for only one more step. The person who gave the push must pay for all injuries resulting from the plunge.[28] Thus, the court says, "If a man is negligently run over or otherwise negligently injured in his body, it is no answer to the sufferer's claim for damages that he would have suffered less injury, or no injury at all, if he had not had an unusually thin skull or an unusually weak heart."[29]

Law professors like to discuss the case of *Steinhauser v. Hertz Corp.*[30] In this case, the plaintiff, a 14-year-old girl, was riding as a passenger in a car with her parents when it was struck by another vehicle. The occupants did not suffer any bodily injuries. Within minutes after the accident, the plaintiff began to behave in a bizarre manner. After a series of hospitalizations, she was diagnosed as suffering from a "schizophrenic reaction—acute—undifferentiated." Prior to the accident she had a "'prepsychotic' personality" and displayed a predisposition to abnormal behavior. Nevertheless, there was testimony that, had it not been for the accident, she might have been able to lead a normal life and that the accident was the precipitating cause of her psychosis. The trial court did not allow plaintiff's counsel to elicit testimony as to whether the accident could have been an aggravating cause of her condition. In reversing a verdict of no cause of action, the U.S. Court of Appeals for the Second Circuit stated that the evidence made clear that plaintiff had some degree of pathology, which was activated into schizophrenia by the emotional trauma connected with the accident and that she was entitled to have that issue fairly weighed by a jury.

Assessment of Damages

Let us assume the accident was a proximate cause in bringing about the disability. When assessing the amount of damages, the functionings of the plaintiff before and after the defendant's act are compared. The question is: What could the person do before the accident that he could not do afterward? At trial the testimony on "before" and "after" would detail specific instances of change: outgoing versus withdrawn, loving versus indifferent, mild-mannered versus abusive, reliable versus erratic, and clean versus slovenly. The before-and-after testimony would dwell on difference in personality, character traits, and behavior, with the behavior change constituting the better proof because it is more objective and more understandable by the jury. By and large, attorneys prefer before-and-after testimony by lay witnesses to psychological testing. Malingering is always a concern in cases alleging emotional distress, but psychological testing indicating malingering may indicate malingering on the tests rather than in the world outside the testing room.

Damages are not measured in the abstract, for example, by the "value of an eye" as the value of an eye is different for a one-eyed person than it is for a person with normal eyesight. A one-eyed person may be functioning quite well prior to injury, but upon losing the remaining eye, he would be totally incapacitated. However, there may be factors that tend to diminish the value of the interest impaired by the defendant's tort. Thus, in a claim for wrongful death, the value of the deceased's life is assessed in light of relevant factors bearing on its prospective duration, including any disease likely to reduce it.[31]

There is a distinction to be drawn between the issue of negligence and the extent of liability. In seeking to avoid negligent conduct, as we have noted, the reasonable person must consider the effect of his conduct upon ordinary people and, generally speaking, may disregard the possibility of encountering exceptionally sensitive people—to require that one guard against exceptional sensitivity would impose an undue restraint upon conduct. Once it is held, however, that the defendant has been negligent toward the plaintiff, that is, he should have foreseen injury to an ordinary person or because he knew of the peculiar sensitivities of the plaintiff, he is liable for the consequences or injuries resulting from the plaintiff's special sensitivity. An extreme illustration is the case where a milk vendor knowingly left a milk bottle with a chipped top on a customer's doorstep. The customer, without contributory negligence on her part, cut her hand when taking it in, for which the vendor was clearly liable. Unfortunately, the customer suffered from an unusual blood condition that caused blood poisoning and subsequent death. Because a breach of a duty of care to an ordinary person was established, the court imposed liability for the consequential death.[32]

This principle is also applicable where the plaintiff is peculiarly susceptible to nervous shock or neurosis, provided the initial breach of duty owed to him is established. If any injury to a legally protected interest of the plaintiff could be reasonably foreseen, the defendant is liable for all the consequences resulting from his wrongful act.[33] Some courts, however, impose liability only for such damage as could have been foreseen, rather than for all damages that actually resulted. In such cases, the average reasonable person's foresight, rather than the plaintiff's injury, is the measure of recovery.

In many situations more than one person may be legally responsible for a given injury. Frequently concurrent liability results not from any planned action, but from quite independent conduct by two or more tortfeasors resulting in one individual injury to the plaintiff. The acts are said to have concurred or coalesced in causing the injury, as where two negligent motorists collide and hurt a pedestrian or passenger. The acts may be successive in a time sense, though concurrent in their causative effect, as where one person spills gasoline, which later catches fire when a burning match is tossed on it. Neither cause is by itself sufficient without the other to result in the injury; however, it makes no difference if each alone is sufficient, as in the case of two merging fires, either of which could have caused the entire damage. In all these cases, the plaintiff, of course, is allowed but one satisfaction of his loss (he is entitled to reparation, not a bonus), but this does not preclude his seeking a judgment against one or all.

There are cases where it may be feasible to allocate the damages, attributing different injuries to separate causes. For example, if A and B strike C, one injuring his arm, the other his leg, A and B may be held liable for the particular injury that each caused. A similar result may be reached when pollution of a stream can be attributed to several factories in proportion to the volume of discharge. More typical cases, however, are those where the defendant's tortious conduct contributed, together with other responsible causes, to an injury that is not divisible. Often enough, the defendant's share of responsibility may be no greater, perhaps much smaller, than that of other cooperating causes. But if the defendant's conduct is altogether trivial in causal potency, neither necessary nor sufficient to produce the injury because the other coexisting causal factors would by themselves have sufficed, it may fairly be dismissed entirely from consideration. Thus, a person would not be held responsible for having thrown a match that caused a raging fire that subsequently destroyed the plaintiff's home. Proximate cause, which the law requires, must be a substantial factor. If the defendant's act, however, is not trivial in causal potency and if the damages are not divisible, he is liable to the plaintiff for the entire injury and is left to seek contribution from the other tortfeasors.[34]

Discussion of Testimony

In general, testimony concerning emotional disturbance tends to provoke either hostility or ridicule. On the one hand, psychiatric testimony may seem arbitrary, as in the case where psychiatrists failed to make recommendations in favor of concentration camp victims. The testimony in any case must overcome the preconceptions that everyone has about psychological disorders. On the other hand, psychiatric testimony may seem fanciful, bringing into disrepute both law and psychiatry. However accurate these charges may be, there is the important consideration that psychiatric testimony tends to arouse feelings of severe anxiety about one's own mental condition. It may provoke reaction or anxiety in judge or jury—indeed, in anyone—a situation that is handled by denial, laughter, or ridicule.[35]

Overload may break a leg, or it may overwhelm the central nervous system. In view of attorneys and experts, credibility of psychiatric testimony on PTSD is enhanced by discussion of the syndrome. The constellation of key symptoms, essential or near-essential, include free-floating anxiety, varying from mild apprehensiveness to panic ("something is about to happen"), irritability and belligerency, muscular tension ("I just can't seem to relax"), easy fatigability, impaired concentration and memory, insomnia, repetitive frightening dreams (directly or symbolically reproducing the traumatic incident), sexual inhibition or disinterest, and social withdrawal ("peace and quiet at any price").

Often the information must come from the spouse or other family member because the person with disabilities (labeled traumatic neurosis) is often verbally unproductive, unimaginative, and a poor observer of his own feelings and behavior. He is usually the type of person who uses his body to express his feelings and thinks in concrete terms. He tends to think of injury only in physicalistic terms.

For most people, peacetime conditions are less traumatic than those of wartime. But for others, wartime provides a solace. Billy the Kid and his friends always slept better after a "good fight with Indians." The routine of peacetime activities was traumatic for Lawrence of Arabia, the maverick British army officer who became a hero when he led the Arabs against the Turks in the World War I. In the words of Winston Churchill, when he unveiled a memorial to Lawrence at Oxford:

> Lawrence was one of those beings whose pace of life was faster and more intense than what is normal. Just as an aeroplane only flies by its speed and pressure against the air; so he flew best and easiest in the hurricane. He was not in complete harmony with the normal. The fury of the Great War raised the pitch of life to the Lawrence standard. The multitudes were swept forward till their pace was the same as his. In this heroic period, he found himself in perfect relation both to men and events.[36]

Adjustment in any given situation depends on the interaction of an individual's particular makeup with his environment. Every individual has certain emotional strengths and weaknesses. Symptoms of breakdown develop when stresses, internal or external, bear upon the individual's specific emotional vulnerabilities. Hence, no event itself can be described as traumatic. The response to the event may be creative. One-third of the Air Force's Vietnam prisoners of war reported benefits from their POW experience—reprioritized life goals, new view of family importance, etc. Only when the event has a noxious influence, a disorganizing effect on the organism, is the event called traumatic. Preconditions to the nature of the response are constitutional factors, past experience, and the psychic state at the time of the particular stimulus.[37]

The meaning ascribed to an event or what is done is crucial to the outcome of trauma. Religion teaches faith. The potential responses to trauma include (1) thriving—the person may not merely return to the previous level of functioning, but may surpass it in some manner; tragedy is turned into triumph; (2) resilience—recovery or a homeostatic return to the preadversity level of functioning, a return that can be either rapid or more gradual; (3) survival with impairment—the person survives, but is diminished or impaired in some respect; and (4) succumbing—a continued downward slide in which the initial detrimental effect is compounded and the individual eventually succumbs or dies.

What about the trauma of slavery or persecution? It is not a sudden assault against ego integrity or dignity. It is a social condition that gradually molds and forms the person. There is no clear-cut point of beginning and ending. It passes from generation to generation. Some say the effect of trauma is wired in the genes. In a series of books, Richard Dawkins, the evolutionary biologist, charted the natural history of what he called "the river out of Eden"—the flow of information passing down the ages in the genome. Thus, the American Civil War is remembered in successive generations by commemorations, writings, etc. Likewise, in Russia today, there are countless portrayals of the Nazi invasion. The memory of the Holocaust is entwined in the fabric of Jewish life. Saidija Hartman, a descendent of slaves, writes:

I wanted to engage the past, knowing that its perils and dangers still threatened and that even now lives hung in the balance. Slavery had established a measure of man and a ranking of life and worth that has yet to be undone. If slavery persists as an issue in the political life of black America, it is not because of an antiquarian obsession with bygone days or the burden of a too-long memory, but because black lives are still imperiled and devalued by a racial calculus and a political arithmetic that were entrenched centuries ago. This is the afterlife of slavery—skewed life chances, limited access to health and education, premature death, incarceration, and impoverishment. I, too, am the afterlife of slavery.[38]

A Black Manifesto demands that whites pay "reparations due us as people who have been exploited and degraded, brutalized, killed, and persecuted"; Professor Boris Bittker of Yale years ago offered justification in law for the proposition in his book, *The Case for Black Reparation*.[39] A Broadway production performed in 2001 about African Americans suffering PTSD carried the playful but very serious title, *Post-Traumatic Slave Syndrome*.

Then too, there is Posttherapy Stress Disorder that follows psychotherapy (as in the case of the "revival of memory" of child abuse).

Trauma is a relative concept: stimulus in relation to capacity of organism. It involves not just what occurs externally, but the dovetailing of external events and inner psychic organization. What may be traumatic to one person need not be to all others, nor need it adversely affect the same person at a different time. Two passengers in a car accident, for example, while sharing the same experience, may develop different symptoms. Although they are exposed to presumably the same stress experience, the type and extent of psychopathology that develops will be specific for that individual. The sight of female genitalia may result in impairment of one's eyesight; to others, it is a pleasure.

In the aftermath of hurricane Katrina, the federal government funneled more than $50 million to mental health programs in Louisiana, but the money came with strings attached. The money may not be spent on physicians, but instead the money is earmarked for traditional social service workers, what the field calls *crisis counselors*. Meetings are limited to five in number and cannot include anything physicians would label treatment. Outreach workers and counselors recruit people from impoverished areas, they gather for group meetings, and they have muffins.[40]

Not every intruding stimulus is a traumatic one. The common assumption is that the only real ones are the big ones; it is not the particular content of an experience, however, but as Freud in 1933 stated, "The essence of a traumatic situation is an experience of helplessness on the part of the ego in the face of accumulation of excitation whether of external or internal origin."

The movie director Richard Brooks in filming Truman Capote's *In Cold Blood* was intrigued that death-row prisoners are not overwhelmed with anxiety as they go to their execution. Discussing this phenomenon at a staff conference at the Menninger Foundation, the group (including the author) concluded that people are less likely to be overwhelmed by anxiety when they have had an opportunity to prepare psychologically for the event. Thus, a motorist unexpectedly bumped from the rear, though with relatively slight impact, may suffer greater emotional distress than he would in a case of a major frontal collision that was foreseen, though only seconds in advance. Likewise, a shipwreck that is expected results in far less traumatic consequences than one that comes as a surprise. An earthquake is usually traumatic because it is sudden and unpredictable, whereas people prewarned about a fire or a tornado may experience less emotional distress. When there is notice, people can prepare psychologically and, hence, are less helpless. One suffering from traumatic neurosis has repetitive dreams about the event so that he can relive and master it, very much like a child at play or in the re-creation of a traumatic event.

What emerges, then, is a picture of trauma as stimuli over which the person has no control. Overwhelmed by stimuli, the individual seeks seclusion, which accounts for his withdrawal, and through the mechanism of denial, the experience is minimized. Because he feels helpless, it is important that families, physicians, lawyers, compensation board members—all who have any contact with him—do everything they can to foster those factors that emphasize his independence, strength, and capacity for self-sufficiency. His image of himself as an active and effective person should be maintained to the highest possible degree.

Rare is the individual who can function well without the emotional support of sweetheart, wife, or mother. "What should I find to hold onto without you?" Winston Churchill wrote to his wife from the trenches in World War I. Much of lovemaking-fondling and petting—represents a regression. When a deteriorating homelife becomes unbearable, the individual somehow manages to be injured in order to obtain emotional comfort. In need of comfort, a person may become as helpless as a baby; by an accident, he may find himself helped and supported just like one. Injury provides a nonembarrassing way to be cared for and loved in a childlike protected fashion, a need present in everyone. The individual seeks such comfort at his job as well as at home. Workers' compensation, received while debilitated from injury, is often viewed as a dole made up by fellow workers. A *dole* is, according to the dictionary, "a distribution of sustaining or subsidizing contributions." The injured individual may feel, "I never knew before that I had such good friends." Companies with a liberal and supportive policy find that employees quickly return to work following an injury.

Workers' Compensation

Workers' compensation laws are designed to provide employees with compensation against the consequences of employment-related injuries. Injured workers do not have to establish negligence attributable to the employer. They merely have to demonstrate that the condition arose "out of and during the course of their employment." In return for not having to establish negligence on the part of the employer, compensation is limited according to a scale.

The issues in workers' compensation cases are the meanings of the terms "accidental injury" or "personal injury" and "arising out of and in the course of employment." In 1921, in a notable workers' compensation case in Michigan, *Klein v. Darling Co.*,[41] an employee dropped a piece of machinery from a scaffolding and imagined that he had fatally injured a co-worker. It worried him and he died within 3 weeks of the incident. The Michigan Supreme Court held that a worker or his family is entitled to payment even though there was no physical injury or catastrophic event that precipitated the mental anguish.

In 1961, in another landmark case in Michigan, *Carter v. General Motors Co.*,[42] psychiatric testimony was allowed to establish that constant emotional pressures of the job were the cause of the employee's disability. Like Charlie Chaplin in the film *Modern Times*, James Carter was overwhelmed by the assembly line process. The Michigan Supreme Court ruled that psychiatric disability is as much compensable under the workers' compensation law as physical injury.

Employers complained that holding them responsible for psychiatric disabilities would make them hesitant to hire people such as Carter and they threatened to move their operations to another state. The law on workers' compensation, they pointed out, is only one mechanism of carrying out social philosophy of taking care of people who cannot take care of themselves. Alternatives are the guaranteed minimum annual wage and pension plans. Generally, in workers' compensation cases, it is held that nervous or mental breakdown produced solely by the stress or boredom of employment does not constitute an accidental injury within the meaning of the statute.[43]

Michigan revised its workers' compensation law in 1969. In three cases consolidated in *Deziel v. Difco Labs. Inc.*,[44] the question was raised: Under the law enacted in 1969, when and under what conditions are alleged mental disorders compensable? The three plaintiffs believed they were physically unable to work although none of them was *actually* physically unable to work. The facts of these consolidated cases were

1. Mary Deziel handled test tubes, mixtures, and chemicals in the course of her employment. She claimed to suffer headaches, tension, anxiety, and dizziness after dropping a tube of iodine. She had suffered no physical injury.
2. Yusuf Bahu experienced "cultural dissonance" after immigrating to this country. He had assumed "the position of a child" to his wife's position of the de facto parent. He claimed that he was too physically incapacitated for a stressful job at a Chrysler stamping machine.
3. Harold McKenzie became nervous when other workers took defective parts that he was responsible for counting and put them on new vehicles. His compulsive perfectionism allegedly rendered him physically unable to work.

No medical evidence established that the three plaintiffs were physically unable to work. Rather, they subjectively perceived themselves as unable to work because of a mental condition. The statute enacted in 1969 and at issue in *Deziel* provided: "An employee, who receives a personal injury arising out of and in the course of his employment by an employer who is subject to this act at the time of injury, shall be paid compensation as provided in this act. The majority opinion of the Michigan Supreme Court focused on the plaintiff's *own* perception of reality. The majority was not concerned that the statute did not contain the words "an employee who receives *or perceives* a personal injury." The majority held

as a matter of law, that in cases involving mental (including psychoneurotic or psychotic) injuries, once a plaintiff is found disabled and a personal injury is established, it is sufficient that a strictly *subjective* causal nexus be utilized by referees and the WCAB to determine compensability. Under a "strictly *subjective* causal nexus" standard, a claimant is entitled to compensation if it is factually established that claimant *honestly perceives* some personal injury incurred during the ordinary work of his employment caused his disability.[45]

The majority supported its conclusion by reasoning that "a subjective standard is mandated by the requirement that remedial legislation be construed liberally." Moreover, the court stated, the "very general notion of causation was and should always be read progressively or liberally." Further, the court said, "[t]he spirit in which compensation laws were enacted should not be lost in legalistic tort niceties. It is with these equitable concepts in mind that this court adopts the subjective standard in cases involving mental disabilities and injuries."[46] The majority did not identify any ambiguity in the statute itself to justify its resort to liberal construction. As the dissent pointed out, the majority *injected* ambiguity by inventing a vague honest perception standard, which could "only invite confusion, difficulty for the finder of fact and increased arbitrariness."[47]

Following *Deziel*, the Michigan Legislature again amended the state's workers' compensation law, this time to provide that "mental disabilities shall be compensable when arising out of actual events of employment, not unfounded perceptions thereof."[48]

Malingering

Litigation problems tend to discourage recovery and promote malingering. An attempt at social reinvolvement may be detrimental to a legal cause of action in tort or workers' compensation. The courts regard with suspicion a claim that is made in the face of a speedy return to work or low medical bills. As one court expressed it, "In view of his ability to return to work, this seems quite a quick recovery for a person who sued for $193,000 for disability."

The significant increase of personal injury litigation and workers' compensation suits in recent years is indicative of a burgeoning claims consciousness of the public. This phenomenon is due to various factors, including the notoriety accorded successful litigants and their advocates, the paternalistic role of modern-day government, and to some extent, the factor of malingering. With the increased number of claims, it is not surprising that allegations and insinuations of malingering are made ever more frequently.

The widely accepted definition of *malingering* is the "conscious simulation or exaggeration of injury, illness, or disability." The difference between hysteria (or conversion hysteria) and malingering is said to be only one of degree: Malingering is the conscious imitation of illness, whereas hysteria is its unconscious simulation. In malingering, there is deliberate and persistent planning; the conscious mind is a participant in the simulated disorder. Thomas Szasz says, "The significant issue here is knowing the rules of the game. A person who knows nothing about the rules of the sickness game cannot malinger."

Malingering is defined in *DSM-IV* as "the intentional production of false or grossly exaggerated physical or psychological symptoms, motivated by external incentives, such as evading military duty, avoiding work, obtaining financial compensation, avoiding criminal prosecution, or obtaining drugs." *Pure malingering* is the conscious exaggeration of existing symptoms or the fraudulent allegation that prior, genuine symptoms are still present. *False imputation* is the ascribing of actual symptoms to a cause consciously recognized as having no relationship to the symptoms. Surveys of forensic specialists generated estimates of malingering between 7.4% for nonforensic settings and 17.4% for forensic settings.[49]

The courts distinguish "compensation neurosis" from "conscious malingering." Although it is a general principle of law that a claimant has a duty to minimize his damages, an unconscious desire for compensation is not a bar to legal recovery. "'Compensationitis,' curable only by application of a 'greenback poultice,' may constitute a disability compensable under the law." This is the sardonic view as expressed by many courts, and physicians also say, "A good application of 'green poultice' is the best cure known for many injuries."[50]

A plaintiff's lawyer, anticipating the issue of malingering, may decide as a tactical matter to raise the issue himself and deflate it. To do this he examines the psychiatrist testifying on behalf of the plaintiff as follows:

Q. Now, Doctor, when you examined the patient, did you believe that his complaints were imaginary?

A. When you say imaginary, if you mean they didn't exist, no, they were real. That is, to him they were real. It appeared to me that he was suffering from certain symptoms and as far as he was concerned they existed.

Q. Do you mean, Doctor, that these symptoms, even though unsupported by any physical evidence, were present for no reason at all?

A. No, there is a reason for the symptoms, but it is my opinion that the patient is not conscious of these reasons. Therefore, the symptoms became real to him.

Q. Why does the patient exhibit these symptoms?

A. Because he stands to gain a resolution of some unconscious emotional conflict.

Q. Then, Doctor, do you believe that the patient is conscious or aware of the fact that he is demonstrating physical symptoms without physical evidence to support these symptoms? In other words, Doctor, is the patient consciously motivated, say, for instance, by an expectant monetary award, to demonstrate these symptoms you have described?

A. I am of the opinion based on this patient's history, the symptoms I personally observed and from my experience, that this man was not consciously motivated to display these symptoms. The only gain, as some might call it, that he derived from these symptoms was on an unconscious level, and this was somehow an attempt to resolve his inner problems. Also, a person who is malingering usually displays a different set of symptoms than this patient. Most often we see physical symptoms, such as paralysis of a limb or a marked limp. The symptoms this patient displayed were of a psychological nature, extreme anxiety, loss of motivation, dependency, and despondency. I doubt whether this patient had the sophistication to consciously demonstrate these symptoms and expect to gain anything of value.

The possibility of litigation appears to be a significant factor in determining whether pain and perpetuating disability will be exaggerated, be it workers' compensation cases, tort claims, evasion of duty cases, or criminal cases. Years ago, on the extent and detection of malingering, Philadelphia attorney Frederick Lipman said:

> We do not know how frequent malingering is. We do not know what causes malingering. We are not sure of the differential diagnosis of malingering and neurosis. We do not know to what extent a physician's bias affects his diagnosis. The literature in this area is sparse and generally lacks an objective basis. Both the legal and medical professions need more scientific studies to help provide the answer to these and many other unsolved questions.[51]

It appears that medical specialists in fields of the most objective empirical orientation, e.g., neurosurgery, tend to see malingering as being much more prevalent than do those in the most subjective specialty, psychiatry. Perhaps the reason for this disparity lies in the psychiatrist's greater appreciation of the unconscious factors surrounding complaints of injury, an appreciation that seems to militate against a diagnosis of malingering.[52]

The diagnostic tools most useful in detecting malingering are careful physical examination of the claimant, study of the claimant's social and clinical history, and of the physician's clinical experience and knowledge of illness patterns. The diagnostic tools favored by a physician will depend to a large extent on his field of specialization and will vary with the illness or injury to be diagnosed. Some physicians feel that psychological testing is an invaluable aid in the detection of malingering, even if the allegedly injured person has been tested previously and realizes the purpose of the tests. Others feel that such tests are rarely conclusive when the subject is knowledgeable or sophisticated. By and large, the initial suspicion of malingering is often intuitive, like Justice Potter Stewart's oft-quoted description of pornography that, though he may not be able to define it, he knows it when he sees it.

Warning signs to detect PTSD malingering include (1) an excessively idealistic premorbid view of life and functioning; (2) antisocial personality, with criminal history, and job and financial irresponsibility; (3) poor work record; (4) prior claims of "incapacitating" injuries; (5) claims of impairment in work, but not in recreation; (6) evasiveness; (7) inconsistency in symptom presentation; and (8) repetitive, unvarying dreams. Malingering in which the individual is completely fabricating symptoms with no evidence whatsoever of a causal event is much more rare than partial malingering, which involves the exaggerating of legitimate, existing symptoms or the claim that symptoms are still present when, in fact, they are not. There is also a phenomenon of false imputation, in which an individual consciously ascribes symptoms to a cause that he knows is unrelated.[53]

In evaluating the genuineness of alleged PTSD, the clinician considers the reasonableness of the relationship between the reported symptoms and the stressor, the time elapsed between the stressor and development of symptoms, and the relationship between current symptoms and psychiatric problems before the stressor. Phillip Resnick, noted authority on the detection of malingering, points out that malingering individuals may know which symptoms to report, but may be unable to give convincing descriptions or examples from their personal life, or they exaggerate the severity of the stressor. Malingerers are likely to concentrate on telling about reliving the trauma whereas individuals genuinely suffering PTSD focus more on the phenomenon of psychic numbing. In true posttraumatic dreams, the typical pattern is a few dreams that reenact the traumatic event, followed by nightmares that are variations on the traumatic theme in which other elements of the individual's daily life are incorporated into their dreams. Malingerers may claim repetitive dreams that exactly recreate the trauma night after night without variation.[54]

What about the hypochondriac who fervently believes in the reality of his complaints though they cannot be objectively substantiated? That phenomenon, too, is sometimes called unconscious malingering.[55] Apart from the constellation of common symptoms of PTSD, some yardsticks have been suggested that differentiate between the malingerer and the hypochondriac or neurotic. The malingerer is generally unwilling to submit to medical examinations unless he can see material rewards for doing so because he has no pains or disability to be cured by treatment, whereas the neurotic not only searches for treatment due to his discomfort, but is faithful in taking medication and in following any regimen prescribed. A malingerer will often carry on his normal social life, finding pleasure in activities that do not relate to the alleged injury, whereas the neurotic usually is unable to maintain the capacity for either work or pleasure and shows general evidence of increased tension and introversion. The malingerer's history will usually reveal that he has been a social misfit for years. Another yardstick is the manner in which the claim is made. One who tenaciously pursues a claim is unlikely to be very much in depression, an indication of traumatic neurosis. A depressed person would not be much interested in a claim or much of anything else. The content of dreams and the way that the dreams are reported furnish an important clue in detecting malingering. Freud spoke of the dream as "the royal road to the unconscious."

Diagnosis is the Sherlock Holmes dimension of medicine. Indeed, it was a physician—Sir Arthur Conan Doyle—who created the character of that master sleuth, modeled after his former teacher, Dr. Joseph Bell. Sherlock Holmes said he deduced his conclusions, but actually he made inferences, and the inferential process is always open to doubt. Only an accountant is entitled to say, "It's as simple as adding two and two." However, the detective may be more helpful than the physician or psychiatrist (although dressed in a London Fog coat or smoking a pipe) in obtaining evidence to identify malingering. Surveillance by private detective agencies is producing evidence (such as movies) that is frequently used in court to establish malingering. One film of the complainant's activities may disprove or rebut a wealth of medical testimony and expert opinion.

At one time, an expert medical witness was not allowed to express an opinion as to whether a litigant was or was not malingering. The jury was considered as qualified as the witness to form an opinion on that subject. Otherwise put, a diagnosis of malingering very much reflects a moral judgment; it may tell us more about the observer than about the observed.[56]

Endnotes

1. O. Rank, *The Trauma of Birth* (New York: Basic Books, 1952).
2. R.J. Daly, "Samuel Pepys and Posttraumatic Stress Disorder," *Brit. J. Psychiat.* 143 (1983): 64.
3. In *Stolen Valor* (Dallas: Verity Press, 1998), Vietnam veterans B.G. Burkett and G. Whitley provide embarrassing examples of veterans deceiving mental health professionals (or the latter acquiesce in the deception). They attacked the very foundation of the VA's understanding of PTSD, the National Readjustment Study, costing $9 million to complete, that concluded that when lifetime prevalence was added to current PTSD, more than half of male veterans and nearly half of the female veterans had experienced clinically stress reaction symptoms. In an article in 1983, psychiatrist Landy Sparr and psychologist Loren Pankratz were apparently the first to describe the imitators of PTSD. They described five men who said they had been traumatized in the Vietnam War; three said they were former prisoners of war. In fact, none had been a prisoner of war, four had never been in Vietnam,

and two had never even been in the military. L. Sparr & L.D. Pankratz, "Factitious Posttraumatic Stress Disorder," *Am. J. Psychiat.* 140 (1983): 1016. PTSD seems particularly prevalent among war veterans. A service-connected disorder makes veterans eligible for free medical care at VA hospitals, and it also can entitle them to disability compensation. Studies have shown that the result of the VA's cost-free hospital treatment and its disability compensation is that veterans are provided with financial incentives to use impatient psychiatric services frequently and for lengthy periods. Veterans are, in effect, encouraged to be (or appear) ill and unable to work or function socially. See D. Mossman, "At the VA, It Pays to Be Sick," *Public Interest* 114 (Winter 1994): 35; see also S. Satel, "Stressed Out Vets," *Weekly Standard*, Aug. 21–28, 2006, p. 16. The number of Iraq and Afghanistan war veterans seeking treatment for PTSD has jumped by nearly 20,000 in the 12 months ending June 30, 2007. G. Zoroya, "Veteran Stress Cases Up Sharply, *USA Today*, Sept. 20, 2007, p. 1.

4. B.L. Green, "Recent Research Findings on the Diagnosis of Posttraumatic Stress Disorder: Prevalence, Course, Comorbidity, and Risk," in R.I. Simon (Ed.), *Posttraumatic Stress Disorder in Litigation* (Washington, DC: American Psychiatric Press, 1995), pp. 13–29.

5. M. Bowman, *Individual Differences in Posttraumatic Response* (Mahwah, NJ: Erlbaum, 1997).

6. L.D. Pankratz, "Posttraumatic Stress Disorder," *False Memory Syndrome Foundation Newsletter*, Nov./Dec. 2001, pp. 8–9.

7. See the special issue in the *Journal of Anxiety Disorders*, 21 (2007): 161–241, on the controversies over the diagnosis of PTSD.

8. Quoted in S. Begley, "Putting Brains on the Couch," *Newsweek*, Sept. 3, 2007, p. 47. It is now said that the clinical syndrome of PTSD does not require prior exposure to trauma. See J.A. Bodkin, H.G. Pope, M.J. Detke, & J.L. Hudson, "Is PTSD Caused by Traumatic Stress?" *J. Anxiety* 21 (2007): 176.

9. A. DiMartini et al., "Posttraumatic Stress Disorder Caused by Hallucinations and Delusions Experienced in Delirium," *Psychosomatics* 48 (Sept.–Oct. 2007): 436.

10. A.A. Stone, "Post-Traumatic Stress Disorder and the Law: Critical Review of the New Frontier," *Bull. Am. Acad. Psychiat. & Law* 21 (1993): 23, at 29–30.

11. M.J. Pangia, "Post-Traumatic Stress Disorder: Litigation Strategies," *Trial*, Sept. 2000, p. 18.

12. Quoted in T. King, "Just Walk Out," *Wall Street Journal*, Nov. 24, 2000, p. W-1. From Christmas shopping, people suffer "post-traumatic mall syndrome." M. Alvear, "The Christmas That Comes to the Door," *New York Times*, Dec. 25, 2000, p. 21. In the parlance of American couples recovering from adultery, "D-Day" is the day you discover your spouse has been cheating on you. The American Association for Marriage and Family Therapy has warned, "The reactions of the betrayed spouse resemble the post-traumatic stress symptoms of the victims of traumatic events." There are thousands of couples therapists, as well as support groups for wounded spouses. P. Druckerman, "After the End of the Affair," *New York Times*, March 21, 2008, p. 23.

Research studies on PTSD go on and on and on. It appears that just about every university health center has a research study on PTSD. Thus, the Anxiety and Traumatic Stress Program of the Duke University Medical Center advertises in the student newspaper: "Nightmares. Sleep disturbance. Avoidance of reminders. Flashbacks. Trouble concentrating. Feeling edgy. If you have developed some of these symptoms following a traumatic event such as rape, incest, domestic violence, or serious accident or injury, you may be eligible to participate in a research study." Advertisement of March 7, 2007. See S. Satel, "The Trouble with Traumatology," *Weekly Standard*, Feb. 19, 2007, p. 14. Studies explore the effectiveness of a variety of therapeutic approaches and the rate of relapse for PTSD.

13. "Nobody thinks about PTSD coming after a trial," said Howard Varinsky, the prosecution's jury consultant in the murder trial of Scott Peterson. "Marriages are affected, but nobody expects this. People will come away from a trial like this as if they had been in a battle zone. They will be very changed people. These people will become victims when they have to decide on the death of someone." Quoted in G. Beratlis et al., *We, The Jury: Deciding the Scott Peterson Case* (Beverly Hills: Phoenix Books, 2006), p. 17.

14. On the expanding concept of traumatic stress: "Any unit of classification that simultaneously encompasses the experience of surviving Auschwitz and that of being told rude jokes at work, must, by any reasonable lay standard, be a nonsense, a patent absurdity." B. Shepard, "Risk Factors and PTSD: A Historian's Perspective," in G.M. Rosen (Ed.), *Posttraumatic Stress Disorder: Issues and Controversies* (Chichester, UK: John Wiley & Sons, 2004), pp. 39–61. See also N. Breslau & R.C. Kessler, "The Stressor Criterion in *DSM-IV* Posttraumatic Stress Disorder: An Empirical Investigation," *Biolog. Psychiat.* 50 (2001): 699; R.J. McNally, "The Expanding Empire of Posttraumatic Stress Disorder," *Medscape Gen. Med.* 8(2) (2006): 9.

15. See D. Mendelson, *The Interfaces of Medicine and Law: The History of the Liability for Negligently Caused Psychiatric Injury (Nervous Shock)* (Brookfield, VT: Ashgate, 1998).

16. Mitchell v. Rochester Railway Co., 151 N.Y. 107, 45 N.E. 354 (1896).

17. Victoria Railways Commissioners v. Coultas, 13 App. Cas. 222 (P.C. 1888).

18. "[T]he plaintiff was an unmarried white lady, and ... while in attendance as a guest of the defendant at a circus performance given by the defendant for the defendant's guests ... a horse, which was going through a dancing performance immediately in front of where the plaintiff was sitting, [ridden] by the defendant's servant ... [was] caused to back toward the plaintiff, and while in this situation the horse evacuated his bowels into her lap. ... [T]his occurred in full view of many people, some of whom were the defendant's employees, and all of whom laughed at the occurrence, [so] that as a result thereof the plaintiff was caused much embarrassment, mortification, and mental pain and suffering, to her damage in a certain amount. ... [T]he damage alleged was due entirely to the defendant's negligence and without any fault on the part of the plaintiff"; Christy Bros. Circus v. Turnage, 38 Ga. App. 581, 144 S.E. 680 (1928).

19. 68 Cal.2d 728, 441 P.2d 912, 69 Cal. Rptr. 72 (1968).

20. 48 Cal.3d 644, 257 Cal. Rptr. 865, 771 P.2d 814 (1989).

21. In an Alaska case, Kelley v. Kohua Sales & Supply, 56 Hawaii 204, 532 P.2d 673 (1975), the plaintiff, located in California, suffered a heart attack after being informed about the death of her daughter and granddaughter in an automobile accident that occurred in Hawaii. The court denied the plaintiff's claim because she was not located "a reasonable distance from the scene."

22. Ferriter v. Daniel O'Connell's Sons, 381 Mass. 507, 413 N.E.2d 690 (1980).

23. Paugh v. Hanks, 6 Ohio St. 3d 72, 451 N.E.2d 759 (1983).

24. G.M. Stern, *The Buffalo Creek Disaster* (New York: Random House, 1976).

25. 2004 WL 3186225 (Conn. Super.)

26. S.H. Putnam, J.H. Ricker, S.R. Ross, & J.E. Kurtz, "Considering Premorbid Functioning" in J.J. Sweet (Ed.), *Forensic Neuropsychology* (Lisse, the Netherlands Swets & Zeitlinger, 1999), pp. 39–81.

27. The emotional aftereffects of the Holocaust on those of its victims who survived took time to reveal themselves. Immediately after the war everyone had wanted to forget and get on with building new lives. In the late 1950s, when studies found that Holocaust survivors were having problems, the issue of compensation began to arise. The West German government offered reparations to camp victims, but only if a causal link could be established between their current ill health and the traumatic experiences they had undergone. A number of German experts then testified in the German courts that it was "common knowledge that all psychic traumata, of whatever degree or duration, lose their effects when the psychologically traumatizing event ceases to operate." In response, William Niederland, a psychoanalyst in New York, coined the phrase "survivor syndrome." He contended that massive psychic trauma caused "irreversible changes" in the personality. The survivors, he found, suffered from depression, anxiety, and nightmares. An Israeli psychiatrist, Shamai Davidson, believed that "the somewhat stereotyped diagnostic construct" of the survivor syndrome was both too sweeping and too pessimistic. He said, "Each survivor is unique in the individual nature and meaning of his experiences and responses to the shared events in the same situation often had entirely different meanings for different survivors." Chaim Shatan was struck by the resemblance between the emotional aftereffects of extensive Vietnam combat experience, the "homecoming syndromes" of prisoners of war and the "survivor syndromes" of living concentration camp inmates. See H. Krystal (Ed.), *Massive Psychic Trauma* (New York: International Universities Press, 1968); B. Shepard, *A War of Nerves* (Cambridge, MA: Harvard University Press, 2001); K.R. Eissler, "Perverted Psychiatry?" *Am. J. Psychiat.* 123 (1967): 1352.

28. The example is taken with modification from the opinion of Chief Justice Berstein of the Arizona Supreme Court in Tatman v. Provincial Homes, 94 Ariz. 165,382 P.2d 573 (1963).

29. This was the observation in a case where the defendant negligently drove a two-horse van into a tavern and frightened a pregnant woman so badly that she suffered a nervous shock and, as a consequence, a miscarriage. The court held the defendant responsible for this damage. Dulieu. v. White & Sons, [1901] 2 K.B. 669. In Marzolf v. Gilgore, 933 F. Supp. 1021 (D. Kansas 1996), the patient who had been given phenothizine-class drugs for over 14 years was held to have a cause of action against the physician who prescribed the drug for the final 6 months of the long drug-taking period. The early prescription "primed" the patient for the later complications. The final doses, rather than the prior 13½ years, may be deemed the cause-in-law of the patient's tardive dyskinesia (TD). Summary judgment for the physician was denied as the facts created a question for the jury. Thus, under this view, a physician coming on the scene late in the treatment of the patient may be held to have caused a disability (TD) although his prescribed dosage was on the low side.

30. 421 F.2d 1169 (2d Cir. 1970).
31. Value is an estimate of worth at the time and place of the wrong. Hence, an existing disease or a prior accident that reduces the plaintiff's life expectancy limits accordingly the value of his life in an action for wrongful death. Consider the case of a person who is suffering from a fatal illness, such as cancer, which will inevitably shorten his life, and he is negligently killed. The value of his life is measured by his anticipated future earnings, along with other factors. The fact that his disease was certain to get worse is taken into account.
32. Koehler v. Waukesha Milk Co., 190 Wis. 52, 208 N.W. 901 (1926), discussed in G. Williams, "The Risk Principle," *L.Q. Rev.* 77 (1961): 179.
33. Battalia v. New York, 10 N.Y.2d 237, 176 N.E.2d 729 (1961)—Plaintiff was badly frightened when the belt on a ski lift was not locked properly. Slay v. Hempstead, 206 So.2d 718 (La. App. 1968)—Woman during menopause suffered traumatic neurosis after her car was struck in the rear. A number of suits have been brought seeking recovery of damages for emotional distress resulting from racial, ethnic, or religious abuse or discrimination in violation of civil rights legislation. Annot., 40 A.L.R.3d 1290.
34. One court expressed it thus:

    > [I]f there is competent testimony, adduced either by plaintiff or defendant, that the injuries are factually and medically separable, and that the liability for all such injuries and damages, or parts thereof, may be allocated with reasonable certainty to the impacts in turn, the jury will be instructed accordingly, and mere difficulty in so doing will not relieve the triers of the fact of this responsibility. This merely follows the general rule that "where the independent concurring acts have caused distinct and separate injuries to the plaintiff, or where some reasonable means of apportioning the damages is evident, the courts generally will not hold the tortfeasors jointly and severally liable."
    > But if, on the other hand, the triers of the facts ... decide that they cannot make a division of injuries, we have, by their own finding, nothing more or less than an indivisible injury, and the precedents as to indivisible injuries will control. They were well summarized in Cooley on Torts in these words: "Where the negligence of two or more persons concurs in producing a single indivisible injury, then such persons are jointly and severally liable, although there was no common duty, common design, or concerted action."

    Maddux v. Donaldson, 362 Mich. 425, 108 N.W.2d 33 (1961). See also Duma v. Janni, 26 Mich. App. 445, 182 N.W.2d 596 (1971).
35. Extensive nationwide publicity was given a case involving the crash of a runaway San Francisco cable car that allegedly led to "promiscuity and unnatural sex drives." Newspaper headlines: "Crash Stimulated Sex Drive," "Oversexed Woman Blames Cable Car Crash." The woman contended that the crash brought on a sexual need that led to affairs with more than 100 men. Psychiatric testimony supporting the complaint maintained that the accident unlocked memories of her strict disciplinarian father. News reports, *Detroit Free Press*, April 3, 1970, p. 8; *Detroit News*, April 3, 1970, p. 12.
36. Churchill's address appears as the introduction to *The Home Letters of T. E. Lawrence and His Brothers* (New York: Macmillan, 1954), p. xiii. A letter written by T. E. Lawrence months before his death reveals that he was so unhappy with the prospect of leaving the RAF that he considered suicide. The correspondence gives support to those who were not convinced that his death in a motorcycle crash 3 months later was an accident. He ended the letter with the line: "Alas and alas, why must good things end and one grow old? I don't want to grow old ... ever." C. Edwards, "Lawrence of Arabia Wrote Letter Contemplating Suicide," *Sunday Telegraph*, Nov. 18, 2001, p. 13. Another notable example is Vladimir Mayakovsky, whose powerful poetry could not have been sustained under any circumstances except that of the Russian Revolution. With the deceleration of the Revolution, he cropped his hair, Samson-like, and his strength slowly drained; finally he committed suicide. W. Woroszylski, *The Life of Mayakovsky* (London: Gollancz, 1971).
37. See G. Mendelson, *Psychiatric Aspects of Personal Injury Claims* (Springfield, IL: Thomas, 1988); C.B. Scrignar, *Post-Traumatic Stress Disorder* (New Orleans, LA: Bruno Press, 3rd ed., 1996); R.I. Simon (Ed.), *Posttraumatic Stress Disorder in Litigation: Guidelines for Forensic Assessment* (Washington, DC: American Psychiatric Press, 1995).
38. S. Harman, *Lose Your Mother: A Journey Along the Atlantic Slave Route* (New York: Farrar, Straus, & Giroux, 2007), p. 6.
39. For more recent discussion, see R. Robinson, *The Debt: What America Owes to Blacks* (New York: Dutton, 2000). Needless to say, the claim for reparations is highly controversial. Suppose an individual about to board the *Titanic* is unlawfully arrested and as a consequence he is not on the ship when

it sank. Would he not be grateful for the detention? The African-American professor of economics Walter Williams has frequently said that today's black Americans have benefited immensely from the suffering of their ancestors; they have been saved from the horrors of Africa. See K.B. Richburg, *Out of America: A Black Man Confronts Africa* (New York: Basic Books, 1997). Black and Arab involvement in slavery is deeper and of far more duration than that of the United States. Slavery (of which human sacrifice was an important component) has the most solid history within Africa itself and, therefore, the most logical reparations measure ought to come from Africa. Twenty times more Americans have ancestors who went to war to end slavery than ancestors who owned slaves. See J. McWhorter, "Against Reparations," *New Republic*, July 23, 2001, p. 32; see also G. Beauchamp, "Apologies All Around," *American Scholar*, Autumn 2007, pp. 83–93.

40. J. Varney, "Post-Storm Mental Health Plan Comes With a Catch," *New Orleans Times-Picayune*, Oct. 2, 2006, p.1.

41. 217 Mich. 485, 187 N.W. 400 (1921).

42. 361 Mich. 577, 106 N.W.2d 105 (1961).

43. See Special Issue, "Work, Stress, and Disability in the New Millennium," *Int. L. Law & Psychiat.* 22 (1999): 417–616.

44. 268 N.W.2d 1 (Mich. 1978).

45. 268 N.W.2d at 11.

46. 268 N.W.2d at 14–15.

47. 268 N.W.2d at 26.

48. Mich. Comp. Laws Ann. § 418.301(2). In Robertson v. DaimlerChrysler Corp., 641 N.W.2d 567 (Mich. 2002), the Michigan Supreme Court clarified the meaning of this provision and overruled *Deziel*.

49. B.E. McGuire, "The Assessment of Malingering in Traumatic Stress Claimants," *Psychiat., Psychol. & Law* 6 (1999): 163. A number of studies have been published on the use of neuroimaging of PTSD. See, e.g., J.D. Bremmer, "Neuroimaging of Posttraumatic Stress Disorder," *Psychiat. Ann.* 28 (1998): 445. Its use as evidence at trial, however, is questionable (by analogy to the inadmissibility of the lie detector). See D.T. Lykken, *A Tremor in the Blood: Uses and Abuses of the Lie Detector* (New York: Plenum, 1998). It is estimated that 15% of Israel's combat wounded—more than 3,000 vets—suffer from some form of posttraumatic stress. The Defense Ministry has hired private investigators to tail and secretly record PTSD victims to see whether they are faking symptoms. Benefits have been reduced after surveillance. K. Peraino, "How to Increase Paranoia," *Newsweek*, June 4, 2007, p. 8.

50. See, e.g., Miller v. U.S. Fidelity & Guaranty Co., 99 So.2d 511 (La. App. 1957).

51. F.D. Lipman, "Malingering in Personal Injury Cases," *Temp. L. Q.* 35 (1962): 162.

52. Dr. Karl Menninger pointed out the personality deformity of the malingerer thus: "[He] does not himself believe that he is ill but tries to persuade others that he is, and they discover, they think, that he is not ill. But the sum of all this, in the opinion of myself and my perverse-minded colleagues, is precisely that he is ill, in spite of what others think. No healthy person, no healthy minded person, would go to such extremes and take such devious and painful routes for minor gains that the invalid status brings to the malingerer." K. Menninger, *The Vital Balance* (New York: Viking Press, 1963), p. 208.

53. See T.M. Keane, "Guidelines for the Forensic Psychological Assessment of Posttraumatic Stress Disorder Claimants," in R.I. Simon (Ed.), *Posttraumatic Stress Disorder in Litigation* (Washington, DC: American Psychiatric Press, 1995); P.J. Resnick, "Malingering of Posttraumatic Disorders," in R. Rogers (Ed.), *Clinical Assessment of Malingering and Deception* (New York: Guilford Press, 2nd ed., 1997); J.D. Bremmer, "Neuroimaging of Posttraumatic Stress Disorder," *Psychiat. Ann.* 28 (1998): 445; R.D. Miller, "The Use of Placebo Trial as Part of a Forensic Assessment," *J. Psychiat. & Law* 16 (1988): 217; J.W. Schutte & G.A. Barrientos, "Uses and Abuses of PTSD," *Trial Lawyer* 21 (1998): 394; S.D. Wiley, "Deception and Detection in Psychiatric Diagnosis," *Psychiat. Clin. N. Am.* 21 (1998): 869.

54. P.J. Resnick, "The Detection of Malingered Mental Illness," *Behav. Sci. & Law* 2 (1984): 21.

55. See T.S. Szasz, *The Myth of Mental Illness* (New York: Hoeber-Harper, 1961). On the screen Woody Allen, of course, is the undisputed master of hypochondria. He transforms every headache into a sign of terminal illness. In the film *Bandits*, Billy Bob Thornton takes Woody Allen one step farther in playing a compulsively anxious criminal. He becomes so preoccupied with his fictional tumor that he actually collapses. He is well versed in the intimate details of every ailment from tinnitus to partial paralysis.

56. Guidelines for a psychiatric medico-legal report are set out in B. Hoffman, "How to Write a Psychiatric Report for Litigation Following a Personal Injury," *Am. J. Psychiat.* 143 (1986): 164; G. Mendelson, "Writing a Psychiatric Medico-Legal Report," *Austral. Foren. Psychiat. Bull.* 16 (Nov. 1999): 5. The role of PTSD as the basis of a finding of not guilty by reason of insanity or diminished capacity is discussed in Chapters 11 and 12. See also Chapter 8 on syndrome evidence.

20
Duty to Minimize Damages

There's a saying in the law of torts: "A plaintiff may not let the meter run." In other words, there is a duty to mitigate damages, sometimes called the doctrine of avoidable consequences. The rule does not allow damages that the plaintiff could have avoided by reasonable conduct following the wrong committed by the defendant. The rule has an application in the law of contracts as well as in tort law.[1] In criminal law, as we shall note, the doctrine of avoidable consequences may play a role in measuring the degree of the offense.

In the law of torts the rule on avoidable consequences is distinguished from the defense of contributory negligence, which is unreasonable conduct on the part of the plaintiff that contributes to the happening of the injury in the first place. Under a well-established principle of tort law, the plaintiff's contributory negligence that bars recovery must *concur* with the defendant's, whereas the relevant conduct of the plaintiff under the doctrine of avoidable consequences *follows* the defendant's. Both the doctrines of contributory negligence and the doctrine of avoidable consequences, however, rest upon the same fundamental policy of making recovery of damages depend upon the plaintiff's proper care for the protection of his own interests, and both require of the plaintiff only the standard of the reasonable person under the circumstances.

Another problem is presented when the plaintiff's conduct *prior* to the accident is found to have played no part in bringing about the accident, but to have aggravated the ensuing damages. The courts have apportioned the damages, holding that the plaintiff's recovery should be reduced to the extent that they have been aggravated by his own antecedent negligence. In a failure to wear a seatbelt, some jurisdictions by statute provide for a certain reduction of damages.[2] In the case of insurance against vandalism or theft, insurance policies may require that the insured protect and secure the premises, otherwise the insurer provides no coverage for the loss.

The rule on contributory negligence—or as supplanted by comparative negligence—are *fault* apportionment rules, while the rule of avoidable consequences is a *causal* apportionment rule. The distinction is important because if the plaintiff's fault in failing to avoid injury is counted as comparative fault in a modified comparative fault jurisdiction, it might add up to more than 50% and, thus, might bar the plaintiff's claim.[3] If not counted as comparative fault, but as a failure to mitigate damages, the plaintiff's fault then would only bar damages that could be traced to that failure.

In recent years, some courts have ruled that with the advent of comparative fault, as a replacement of contributory negligence that bars recovery entirely, no separate avoidable consequences rules are required. Under these rulings, comparative fault analysis is used, both as to preinjury fault of the plaintiff and postinjury failure to minimize damages.[4] In such jurisdictions, the instruction to the jury is as follows: "If you find that plaintiff failed to mitigate damages, you will include this as part of plaintiff's fault in your comparison of fault."[5] That may be logical when the plaintiff suffers a single indivisible injury, but not when the plaintiff's postinjury negligence causes some separate item of harm.

The avoidable consequence rule reduces damages for discrete identifiable items of loss caused by the plaintiff's fault. Thus, if the plaintiff, after injury, unreasonably refuses to accept medical attention for a foot injury, and as a result ultimately suffers amputation of the foot, which otherwise would have healed, then the avoidable consequences rule would deny recovery for loss of the foot, but would not affect other damages.

Although mitigation of damages is not among the common affirmative defenses listed in court rules, it is recognized as such.[6] The defense is waived if not raised in the defendant's first responsive pleading or by an amended pleading. The defendant also has the burden of proving the plaintiff's failure to mitigate damages. A typical jury instruction states:

> A person has a duty to use ordinary care to minimize his or her damages after (*he or she/ his or her property*) has been (*injured/damaged*). It is for you to decide whether plaintiff failed to use such ordinary care and, if so, whether any damage resulted from such failure. You must not compensate the plaintiff for any portion of (*his/her*) damages, which resulted from (*his/her*) failure to use such care.[7]

The remainder of this chapter is an overview of what has been or has not been required to mitigate damages.

Mitigating Damages

First and foremost, the duty to minimize damages may include a duty to seek and follow medical treatment, including surgery, which does not involve danger to life or extraordinary suffering. There must be a showing that treatment, in fact, would have mitigated the damages.[8] The refusal to undergo surgery is not considered arbitrary and unreasonable when the claimant has a sincere, deep-seated fear of it.[9] The refusal is also not considered unreasonable when the claimant is backed up by a physician's opinion that rebuts the medical recommendation submitted by the defendant.[10]

The duty to mitigate damages applies with equal force in medical malpractice cases. Under this principle, as generally followed, a patient's failure to follow a physician's directions subsequent to the physician's negligent treatment does not relieve against the primary liability, but serves to mitigate the damages.[11] Thus, a patient's neglect of his health following his physician's negligent treatment does not bar all recovery, but may be a reason for reducing damages.[12] In a case where a dentist was negligent, the patient terminated treatment and delayed securing the services of another dentist. A contributory negligence instruction was disallowed, but the jury was permitted to consider the plaintiff's delay as a factor in determining damages.[13]

Following an injury there are times when the individual becomes so despondent that he commits suicide. The question arises: Is the original tortfeasor (or employer in a workers' compensation case) responsible for the death? Could it have been avoided by psychiatric care? Was it an intervening cause? In older cases, courts as a matter of law found that suicide breaks the chain of causation.[14] However, in more recent cases, the question is often left to the jury.[15] In *Fuller v. Preis*,[16] the decedent, a doctor, committed suicide some 7 months after an automobile accident from which he suffered head injury and had experienced many seizures. The theory for recovery of damages was that the automobile crash caused the suicide. The jury found that the doctor was unable to control an "irresistible impulse" to destroy himself as a result of the accident. Most courts find an irresistible impulse only when the decedent acted in a sudden frenzy.[17]

A plaintiff who suffers disfigurement is not obliged to undergo plastic surgery if for no other reason than the plaintiff may be wary of anesthesia. Plastic surgery is considered to be a high benefit procedure, but also high risk in areas of the body where there is limited blood flow. It is not low risk/high benefit that is usually the justification of a requirement to minimize damages. There are perceived as well as known risks even in cosmetic surgery. It is common knowledge that Michael Jackson, the pop star, was hideously disfigured and visibly scared as a result of it.

In workers' compensation cases alleging permanent serious disfigurement, the defense often alleges that the reason the disfigurement is permanent or serious is because the claimant has not bothered to see a physician about having it reduced. The Louisiana Court of Appeals said, "The plaintiff must eventually determine for himself whether he will retain the permanent disfigurement or submit to an operation for its correction."[18]

A constitutional issue arises when a patient has a religious belief about treatment. Christian Scientists and many Pentecostal groups teach that all physical maladies may be cured spiritually. Jehovah Witnesses generally accept medical care, but believe it is a sin to accept blood transfusion even in a life-and-death situation. The Book of Acts (Chapter 5) directs the faithful to "abstain from blood," an admonition the church interprets to proscribe transfusions.[19] A reduction in a tort judgment for failure to mitigate may constitute an undue interference with religious freedom.[20] In an oft-cited case, *Lange v. Hoyt*,[21] the Connecticut Supreme Court applied a reasonable person standard, but instructed the jury to regard the plaintiff's Christian Science beliefs as a relevant factor in its assessment of mitigation efforts. In *Williams v. Bright*,[22] a New York court said that a jury's determination that a Jehovah Witness's rejection of a blood transfusion in surgery as "unreasonable" is an improper judgment as to the soundness of their religion. If a religious-based refusal of medical treatment is permitted, an accompanying issue may be whether all religions, faiths, and equivalent belief systems should be treated similarly.

In criminal cases, whether a battery turns into negligent homicide or murder depends often on medical care, as in the case of Jehovah's Witnesses who refuse a blood transfusion.[23] In an English case, *R. v. Blaue*,[24] the refusal of the deceased, for religious reasons, to accept a blood transfusion, which would have saved her life, did not relieve her assailant of causal responsibility. In this case, it was reasonable to conclude that the act of stabbing was an operative cause of her death and the real issue was whether her subsequent conduct was sufficient to break the chain of causation. The court made reference to the "thin skull" rule: "It has long been the policy of the law that those who use violence on other people must take their victims as they find them. This, in our judgment means the whole man, not just the physical man."[25]

The reference to the thin skull rule was probably unnecessary to the decision, and its extension to psychological conditions questionable. The more problematic cases are those where the conduct of the victim after the assault is under scrutiny. In *R. v. Roberts*,[26] it was stated that such conduct does not break the chain of causation unless it is "daft," that is, it is not an objectively foreseeable consequence of the accused's act nor is it within the range of responses, which might be expected. There might well be convincing policy reasons for considering conduct inspired by religious convictions not to be daft.[27]

In all cases, the availability of emergency medical services is an important factor in homicide or aggravated battery rates. A victim who is near a hospital gets care; another who is far away dies. The intent and behavior of the actor may be the same, but the consequences are often fortuitous.[28] Studies indicate that the differential distribution of medical resources is partially responsible for variation in criminally induced lethality rates.[29] Time and again, in various cases, expert testimony is offered that prompt medical treatment could have saved the victim's life.[30]

In *People v. Webb*,[31] a Michigan case, the deceased had consumed a large quantity of alcohol and gotten into an argument with the defendant at a bar. The defendant struck the deceased repeatedly in the face, and kicked him in the ribs after he had fallen to the floor. Injured and bleeding from the mouth, he went home at which time his wife called paramedics, but he refused treatment. After the paramedics left, he finally agreed he should go to the hospital, but he died moments after the paramedics returned. The medical examiner testified that had he accepted medical treatment promptly, a relatively easy procedure might have avoided the death. The Michigan Court of Appeals, in reversing a dismissal, held that the victim's knowing and voluntary refusal to seek immediate medical treatment was not as a matter of law a supervening cause of death; the issue of causation, the court said, should have gone to the jury.[32]

An accused may be exculpated of a homicide charge if the medical treatment provided the victim was "grossly negligent." In the case of a victim with a nonfatal wound who received medical treatment deemed "grossly negligent," it is said that the treatment breaks the causal link to the resulting death and may exculpate the accused from guilt of a homicide. Mere negligent medical treatment, on the other hand, is deemed a foreseeable event and does not suffice.[33] In the trial of Bernhard Goetz, who gunned down four young men he believed were about to mug him on a New York subway train, the prosecutor sought to blame Goetz for one of the victim's subsequent brain damage, while the defense attorney argued strenuously that it was the result of medical malpractice no one could have foreseen.[34]

In the law of torts there is an old axiom that a defendant must take a plaintiff as he finds him and, hence, may be held liable in damages for aggravation of a preexisting illness.[35] To put it differently, the defendant cannot complain that the plaintiff was not a healthy victim, but he may complain that the plaintiff did not take such preaccident precautions such as wearing a seatbelt, and after the accident, the plaintiff may be obliged to change his style of life in order to mitigate damages. Questions arise: Must the plaintiff stop smoking, drinking, or lose weight in order to mitigate the extent of his injury? His style of life may give him comfort. In a case of an overweight plaintiff who suffered a serious back injury in a collision, the Louisiana Supreme Court said that the plaintiff had an affirmative responsibility to make every reasonable effort to follow medical advice to lose weight in order to mitigate damages—losing weight would have alleviated the stress on her back.[36] In another case, the Minnesota Supreme Court ruled that the plaintiff, a disabled employee, had "an obligation to cooperate with his doctor's directions to achieve weight reduction and thereby improve his condition to the point where employment in another field, possibly after retraining, would be feasible."[37]

What about medical treatment that takes the form of exercise? Is there an element of risk? Whether there has been an unreasonable refusal to exercise depends on the possibility of pain in connection with the exertion, the age of the plaintiff, and the probability of benefit from it.[38]

A plaintiff's failure to obtain treatment may be excused when the failure is a result of the injury itself. In *Botek v. Mine Safety Appliance Corp.*,[39] the plaintiff suffered a posttraumatic stress disorder that was exacerbated by his failure to initiate treatment at an early date. In cases of PTSD, treatment soon after the event usually results in recovery. Experts testified that with counseling and drug therapy, the plaintiff could have achieved a satisfactory result in 3 to 6 months. Instead, by the time the trial began, the plaintiff had endured the effects of the emotional disorder for more than 7 years. He explained that he had made no effort to obtain treatment because he suffered from depression as a result of the incident and was not motivated to seek treatment. The court ruled that where a claimant's rejection of treatment is part of his emotional injuries, he may obtain damages in spite of the failure to receive treatment.[40]

The reasonableness of avoiding treatment can be an issue in cases where a psychotherapist has engaged in "undue familiarity" with a patient. As a result of the undue familiarity, there may be reluctance of the patient to see another therapist. "I have lost all faith in therapists," say patients. One psychiatrist cites the case of a sexually exploited female psychiatric patient who suffered immeasurably as a result of the abuse by her therapist. He writes, "The effects of the affair were disastrous at the time of its occurrence and proved to be a serious complication for subsequent treatment. As a consequence, her illness was aggravated ... and a deep mistrust formed toward subsequent psychiatrists and psychoanalysts."[41] Similarly, a study of 16 female patients of a gynecologist, who conducted internal examinations in a sexually abusive manner, reported their developing an aversion to gynecological healthcare after their experience.[42]

An injured party may have a duty to obtain vocational retraining as part of the duty to mitigate damages. The use of vocational rehabilitation is appropriate in cases where the plaintiff claims to have suffered a loss of work capacity because of injury. Because many public agencies provide rehabilitation services to the disabled, the defense can argue that the individual has not fulfilled his obligation to mitigate his damages by obtaining these services. Vocational rehabilitation expert testimony is helpful in proving that the plaintiff has not mitigated his damages.

It is a matter of fact for the jury to determine whether a reasonable person under the circumstances should have sought vocational retraining as a part of the duty to mitigate damages, just as it is a matter of fact for the jury to determine whether a reasonable person under the circumstances should have undergone medical treatment in order to mitigate damages. Because the determination is a question of fact for the jury, not a matter of law, it is reversible error on the part of a trial judge to instruct a jury that an injured party has a specific duty to obtain vocational training as part of the duty to mitigate damages.[43]

By the way, disability income insurance policies, depending on the policy, may not require training for another occupation in the event of inability to continue in one's field.[44] Thus, one young lawyer who felt harried working in a law office (she called it "a meat grinder") as attested by her psychiatrist is now spending her days gardening at home and collecting disability income insurance. Under her policy, she need not undertake training in a different field.[45] In response to the new stresses of medical practice, many physicians have retired early or have filed for disability insurance and given up their practices.[46]

In a workers' compensation case, a psychiatrist who treated the claimant recommended that he submit to a sodium amytal interview, which would make him drowsy and less resistant and more amenable to suggestion. The purpose would be to overcome by suggestion, the "psychoneurosis conversion hysteria that was superimposed on a minor foot injury." The psychiatrist stated that, if the treatment were successful, a cure could be affected in two or three sessions. The claimant refused to take the treatment, on the advice of his personal physician who stated that he did not believe the psychiatric treatment alone would effect a cure. No doctor testified that the treatment might be harmful or that the claimant's resistance would make the treatment completely ineffectual. The court found, on appeal, that the claimant's refusal to submit to the proposed treatment was unreasonable.[47]

What about electroconvulsive therapy (ECT), or electroshock therapy, as it is also known? Nowadays it is safe and effective (it is low risk/high benefit), but in the public image, it is high risk/low benefit and stigmatizing. Its very name is alarming. A claimant's refusal to submit to ECT is not deemed unreasonable.[48]

In the case of psychiatric treatment, a plaintiff who declines treatment often says: "I don't want to be seen by a psychiatrist." "I hate psychiatrists." "I don't want their medication." Is it a reasonable refusal in view of the side effects?[49] Does the plaintiff have a phobia about psychiatrists? What about the stigma surrounding psychiatric care? Even ex-convicts rank above former mental patients in societal acceptance.[50]

And what about the mitigation of damages in cases where a pharmacist negligently supplies a tranquilizer rather than birth control pills called for by the prescription, as happened in *Troppi v. Scarf*?[51] The defense suggested that parents who seek to recover for the birth of an unwanted child are under a duty to mitigate damages by placing the child for adoption (or obtaining an abortion). If the child is "unwanted," the defendant asked, why should they object to placing the child up for adoption (or aborting), thereby reducing the financial burden on defendant for his maintenance?[52] The court replied:

> [T]o impose such a duty upon the injured plaintiff is to ignore the very real difference which our law recognizes between the avoidance of conception and the disposition of the human organism after conception. This most obvious distinction is illustrated by the constitutional protection afforded the right to use contraceptives, while abortion is still a felony in most jurisdictions [no longer]. At the moment of conception, an entirely different

set of legal obligations is imposed upon the parents. A living child almost universally gives rise to emotional and spiritual bonds, which few parents can bring themselves to break.[53]

A defendant is not likely to raise a failure to mitigate damages when the plaintiff could not afford treatment. The plaintiff would respond, "I didn't have the money for treatment. I couldn't afford it. That's why I went to a lawyer." The jury would likely be moved by sympathy. And, as a matter of law, a claimant may be excused from mitigating damages when lacking sufficient financial resources to do so.[54] In cases where liability is not at issue, and the only question is that of damages, a defendant might cover the expenses of treatment at the outset when injury occurs in order to minimize the damages. It is a common practice in employer–employee and carrier–passenger relationships.[55]

Dispatching teams of counselors (known as *grief workers*) has become commonplace on the occurrence of a traumatic event.[56] Now, shortly after the police, paramedics, and television crews arrive on the scene, grief counselors arrive. The theory of grief work is to work it through and find closure as soon as possible. Early intervention is reputedly the key to recovery following trauma. Psychiatrist Sally Satel cautions, however, that this is not always successful. She writes: "An emphasis on experiencing psychic pain can make some people feel even more vulnerable and out of control. Forced ventilation makes little sense for those whose ordinary coping style is to remain calm, maybe too calm for some people's taste, and spring into purposeful activity."[57] Many of those who undergo stress debriefing develop worse PTSD symptoms than those who deal with the trauma on their own, controlled studies show, probably because the intense reliving of the trauma impedes natural recovery.[58] Then too, communities have long had rituals for coming to terms with calamity.[59] Quite often, when grief workers arrive at the scene of a disaster, they find that survivors do not seek counseling, and the grief workers, feeling unwanted, become depressed and provide therapy for each other.

Endnotes

1. See M.B. Kelly, "Living With the Avoidable Consequences Doctrine in Contract Remedies," *San Diego L. Rev.* 33 (1996): 175; for an application in the employment context, see R. Fraser, "The Unavoidable Doctrine of Avoidable Consequences," *Fla. Bar J.* 54 (1980): 369.
2. Michigan's statute provides: "Failure to wear a safety belt in violation of this section may be considered evidence of negligence and may reduce the recovery for damages arising out of the ownership, maintenance, or operation of a motor vehicle. However, such negligence shall not reduce the recovery for damages by more than 5%." MCL 257.710e(h)(5). See Lowe v. Estate Motors, 428 Mich. 439 (1987); Comment, "Apportionment of Damages in the 'Second Collision' Case,'" *Va. L. Rev.* 63: 475, 1977.
3. About a dozen jurisdictions (e.g., Florida, California, New York, Michigan, and Arizona) and several federal statutes (e.g., FELA, Jones Act) have adopted the pure comparative negligence approach. In those jurisdictions, the plaintiff's recovery is reduced by the percentage fault attributable to the plaintiff. About a dozen jurisdictions (e.g., Georgia, Arkansas, Colorado, Tennessee, and Nebraska) have adopted a modified form of comparative negligence in which the plaintiff's recovery is reduced by the percentage of fault attributable to the plaintiff as long as the plaintiff's fault is "not as great as" the defendant's. If the plaintiff's fault is equal to or greater than the defendant's, the plaintiff is completely barred from recovery. See McIntyre v. Balentine, 833 S.W.2d 52, 56 & n.5 (Tenn. 1992). About 20 jurisdictions (e.g., Wisconsin, Connecticut, Pennsylvania, Ohio, and Illinois) have adopted a modified form of comparative negligence in which the plaintiff's recovery is reduced by the percentage of fault attributable to the plaintiff as long as the plaintiff's fault is "not greater than" the fault of the defendant's. If the plaintiff's fault is greater than the defendant's, the plaintiff is completely barred from recovery. See McIntyre v. Balentine, 833 S.W.2d 52, 56 & n.6 (Tenn. 1992); A.S. Brown & W.L. Gold, "Litigating Comparative Fault and Avoidable Consequences Issues," *New Jersey L. J.* 144: 10 (1986).
4. See Coker v. Abell-Howe Co., 491 N.W.2d 143, 148-149 (Iowa 1992).
5. In Ort v. Klinger, 496 N.W.2d 265 (Iowa App. 1992), that jury instruction was proffered by the defendant, but the trial court did not give it. The Iowa Court of Appeals said that the version that the trial court gave was sufficient. The trial court gave the following instruction in the place of the defendant's

proposal: "If by slight expense and inconvenience a person exercising ordinary care could have thus reduced the consequences of her injury, and failed to do so, she cannot recover for any damage that might have been avoided"; 496 N.W.2d at 268.

6. In Stump v. Norfolk Shipbuilding & Dry Dock Corp., 187 Va. 932, 48 S. e. 2d 209 (1948), a workers' compensation case, an employee refused medication for infected abrasion of skin; the ultimate loss of leg was held not compensable. In Skidmore v. Drumon Fine Foods, 119 So. 2d 523 (La. App. 1960), a claimant with persistent pain following amputation of a finger was required to submit to simple, minor surgery or lose his compensation. See Michigan Court Rules 2.111(f) (3) (a) (not listing failure to mitigate as affirmative defense).

7. Michigan Standard Jury Instruction 53.05.

8. See Miller v. Eichhorn, 426 N. W. 2d 641, 643 (Iowa App. 1988).

9. In Small v. Combustion Engineering, 209 Mont. 387, 681 P. 2d 1081 (1984), a manic depressive claimant refused knee surgery out of fear of detrimental consequences; refusal was held not unreasonable because of mental disorder. See American Asbestos Textile Corp. v. Ryder, 281 A. 2d 53. 56 (N. H. 1971); Zimmerman v. Ausland, 266 Ore. 427, 433–435, 513 P.2d. 1167, 1170-71 (1973); see E. Kelly, "Refusal of Surgery in Mitigation of Damages," Clev.-Mar. L. Rev. 10 (1961): 421; Annot., "Duty of Injured Person to Submit to Surgery to Minimize Tort Damages," 62 A.L.R.3d (1975). The states differ in their approach as to whether the reasonableness of a refusal of treatment be examined objectively or subjectively. See Genuardi Supermarkets v. WCAB, 674 A. 2d 1194 (Pa. 1996); Schwab Construction v. McCarter, 25 Va. App. 104, 486 S. E. 2d 562 (1997); Johnson v. Jones, 123 N. C. App. 219, 472 S. E. 2d 587 (1996); Dorris v. Mississippi Regional Housing Authority, 695 So. 2d 567 (Miss. 1997).

10. In McAuley v. London Transport Executive, [1957] 2 Lloyds Reports 500, the claimant sustained injuries to his hand, severing the ulnar nerve at the wrist. He refused an operation. The defendant's physician advised that it would give him a 90% chance of recovering the gross motor movements to the outer fingers of his damaged hand, and even some chance (35%) of the return of some fine movements to the same fingers. The trial judge held that his refusal was unjustified in the circumstances, and attributed most of his disability to the refusal, rather than to the accident itself. The judge's decision was upheld on appeal. The appellate court ruled that a plaintiff should not disregard the advice of a physician though acting on behalf of the defendants; that the plaintiff was not advised by any doctor not to have the operation; and that, therefore, his refusal was unreasonable. The court said, "[T]he plaintiff, as a reasonable person, ought either to accept that advice, or else go to his own doctor and say: 'Doctor, this is what I have been advised by Mr. So-and-So, the surgeon at Such-and-Such a hospital; what do you think about it?' Of course, the plaintiff here never did any such thing."

11. See Lawrence v. Wirth, 309 S.E.2d 315, 317-18 (Va. 1983); Jenkins v. Charleston Gen. Hosp. & Training School, 90 W. Va.230, 243-44, 110 S.E. 560, 565–66 (1922); H.L. Hirsh, "When a Patient Contributes to His Medical Malpractice Relatively," Med. & Law 4 (1985): 229.

12. Beadle v. Paine, 46 Or. 424, 421, 80 Pac. 903, 906 (1905)

13. Sanderson v. Moline, 7 Wash. App. 439, 499 P.2d 1281 (1972).

14. See Scheffer v. Railroad Co., 105 U.S. 249, 252 (1881).

15. See Stafford v. Neurological Med. Inc., 811 F.2d 470, 473–74 (8th Cir. 1987; allowing jury to decide whether suicide was an "irresistible impulse").

16. 35 N.Y.2d 425, 322 N.E.2d 263, 363 N.Y.S.2d 568 (1974).

17. For a good review of the cases on this issue, see Grant v. F.P. Lathrop Constr. Co., 81 Cal. App. 3d 790, 146 Cal. Rptr. 45 (1978). In Food Distributors v. Estate of Ball, 24 Va. App. 692, 485 S. E. 2d 155 (1997), the court provides a review of the varying approaches taken by the states in the work-related suicide cases.

18. Wilson v. Yellow Cab Co. of Shreveport, 64 So.2d 463 (La App. 1953).

19. Jehovah Witnesses do, however, allow a treatment called auto transfusion in which a "cell saver" is used to remove and filter blood before returning it to the patient.

20. See generally, J. Pomeroy, "Reason, Religion, and Avoidable Consequences: When Faith and the Duty to Mitigate Collide," N.Y.U. Rev. 67 (1992): 1111; Comment, "Medical Care, Freedom of Religion, and Mitigation of Damages," Yale L. J. 87 (1978): 1466. In Mann v. Algee, 924 F.2d 568 (5th Cir. 1991), a wrongful death action, the defense contended that the decedent would have lived had she accepted a blood transfusion and it attacked the sincerity and reasonableness of the decedent's religious beliefs. Over a strong dissent by Judge Rubin, the Fifth Circuit upheld a verdict in favor of the defense.

21. 159 Atl. 575 (Conn. 1932).

22. 1995 WL 619381 (N.Y. Sup.).

23. Time and again a negligent motorist who hits a Jehovah's Witness is convicted of vehicular manslaughter even though a blood transfusion could have prevented the death. In these cases, the defense argues to no avail that "the defendant is responsible for the injury, not for the death," but the courts rule that the car accident was "a proximate cause of the death." See State of Louisiana v. Baker, 1998 La. App. LEXIS 2966; L. Gorov, "Fatality Case in Calif. Melds Religion, Law," *Boston Globe*, Dec. 12, 1998, p.1.

24. [1975] 1 W. L. R. 1411.

25. [1975] 1 W. L. R. 1415.

26. [1971] 56 Cr. App. R. 95.

27. See F. McAuley & J. P. McCutheon, *Criminal Liability* (Dublin: Round Hall Sweet & Maxwell, 2000), pp. 255–256.

28. For a wide-ranging commentary, see N. Rescher, *Luck* (New York: Farrar Straus Giroux, 1995). The U.S. homicide rate is lower than it might otherwise be because of advanced medical therapies available in the United States, which render many attempted homicides unsuccessful. J. Moore (Ltr.), "Trouble in Paradise," *Sciences*, Sept./Oct. 1988, p. 10. The condition of the victim prior to the injury is also a factor in the outcome. The seatbelt defense has been disallowed in criminal negligent homicide cases. See B.D. Fisher & J.H. Fisher, "Use of the Safety Belt Defense in Michigan Negligent Homicide Cases," *Mich. Bar J.*, Feb. 1989: 144. Insurance policies exclude coverage for bodily injuries expected or intended by the insured. In Aetna Cas. & Surety Co. v. Sprague, 163 Mich. App. 650 (1987), the insured unsuccessfully argued that it was his negligence in failing to take his medication and to pursue psychiatric treatment that was the proximate cause of the victim's death. In a criminal trial, the insured had been found guilty, but mentally ill. The Michigan Court of Appeals said that "the complaint is a transparent attempt to trigger insurance coverage by characterizing allegations of tortious conduct under the guise of 'negligent' activity." 163 Mich. App. at 654.

29. See W.G. Doerner & J.C. Speir, "Stitch and Sew: The Impact of Medical Resources upon Criminally Induced Lethality," *Criminology* 24 (1986): 319.

30. "Shaun Gates, 4, could have survived the beating that killed him if he had been taken to the hospital," a pediatrician testified in the trial of Southgate housewife Robin Ryan. Quoted in P. Ross, "Doctor Says Shaun Could Have Lived," *Detroit News*, March 13, 1986, p. B6. "Three-year-old Dominic Mileto bled internally for possibly 3 hours and might have survived a severe beating if he had gotten medical attention," an assistant Wayne County medical examiner testified. News report, "Pathologist Says Beaten Boy Could Have Been Saved," *Detroit News*, April 27, 1988, p. B5.

31. 163 Mich. App. 462 (1987).

32. See 163 Mich. App. at 465 where the court noted that the defendant takes his victim as he finds him, and a severely drunken victim may reasonably be expected to refuse treatment.

33. People v. Robinson, 107 Mich. App. 417, 420, 309 N. W. 2d 624, 626 (1981).

34. See G.P. Fletcher, *A Crime of Self-Defense: Bernhard Goetz and the Law on Trial* (New York: Free Press, 1988).

35. The "eggshell skull" doctrine, also known as the "thin skull" doctrine, holds that a tortfeasor is liable for injuries even when those injuries are heightened by an unforeseeable, preexisting physical condition of the victim. An English court first articulated the rule in Dulieu v. White & Sons, 2 K. B. 669 (1901), stating: "If a man is negligently run over or otherwise negligently injured in his body, it is no answer to the sufferer's claim for damages that he would have suffered less injury, or no injury at all, if he had not had an unusually thin skull or an unusually weak heart"; 2 K. B. at 679. The rule has been applied to cases of preexisting psychological incapacity—the "thin psyche—as well as to explicitly physical conditions. As an English Court put it, "There is no difference in principle between an eggshell skull and an egg-shell personality"; Malcolm v. Broadhurst, 3 All E. R. 508, 511 (Q.B. 1970). In Steinhauser v. Hertz Corp., 421 F.2d 1169 (2d Cir. 1970), the U.S. Court of Appeals for the Second Circuit held that a 14-year-old girl predisposed toward schizophrenia could potentially recover damages for the full-blown psychosis that a car accident allegedly precipitated. See Chapter 18.

36. Aisole v. Dean, 574 So. 2d 1248, 1254 (La. 1991).

37. Fenton v. Murphy Motor Freight Lines, 297 N. W. 2d 294, 296 (Minn. 1980).

38. See Brown v. Premier Mfg. Co., 77 Mich. App. 573, 579 (1977); Blair v. Eblen, 461 S. W. 2d 370, 372 (Ky. 1970). See also Sanderson v. Secrest Pipe Coating Co., 465 S. W. 2d 65 (Ky. 1971; failure to follow a course of exercise); Byrd v. WCAB, 81 Pa. 325, 473 A. 2d 723 (1984; claimant cancelled 8 of 12 physical therapy sessions and suffered second injury because of failure to complete therapy; held unreasonable).

39. 611 A. 2d 1174 (Pa. 1992).

40. 611 A. 2d at 1176-77.

41. H. Voth, "Love Affair Between Doctor and Patient," *Am. J. Psychother.* 26 (1974): 394.
42. A. Burgess, "Physician Sexual Misconduct and Patients' Responses," *Am. J. Psychiat.* 138 (1981): 1335.
43. See Garceau v. Bunnell, 434 N.W.2d 794, 797 (Wis. App. 1988).
44. The State Farm disability income policy provides: "During the first 24 months of Total Disability (Total Disability means complete incapacity) as the result of injury or sickness of the insured to engage in his/her occupation and which requires the regular care of a licensed physician other than the insured. After the insured has been disabled for 24 months, Total Disability means the complete inability to engage in any occupation for which the insured is or becomes reasonably fitted by education, training, or experience."
45. Communication from Dr. Victor Bloom of Grosse Pointe, Michigan (Dec. 4, 1998).
46. J.P. Lassierer (Editorial), "Doctor Discontent," *N. Eng. J. Med.* 339 (Nov. 19, 1998): 1543.
47. Commonwealth, Dept. of Highways v. Lindon, 380 S. W. 2d 247 (Ky. 1964).
48. See, e.g. Dohmann v. Richard, 282 So.2d 789 (La. App. 1973).
49. The courts often point to the negative side-effects of psychotropic medication. See B.J. Winick, *The Right to Refuse Mental Health Treatment* (Washington, DC: American Psychological Association, 1997).
50. In Vitek v. Jones, 445 U.S. 480 (1980), the U.S. Supreme Court noted the "stigmatizing consequences" of a transfer from prison to a mental hospital. See P. J. Fink & A. Tasman (Eds.), *Stigma and Mental Illness* (Washington, DC: American Psychiatric Press, 1992); R. Slovenko, *Psychotherapy and Confidentiality* (Springfield, IL: Thomas, 1998), pp. 503–520. See R.E.T. Corp. v. Frank Paxton Co., 329 N.W.2d 416, 422 (Iowa 1983); Zimmerman v. Ausland, 266 Or. 427, 433, 513 P.2d 1167, 1170 (1973).
51. 187 N. W. 2d 511 (Mich. App. 1971).
52. See S.D. Sayre, "Abortion or Adoption: A Rational Application of the Avoidable Consequences Rule to the Computation of Wrongful Conception Damages," *West. State U. L. Rev.* 12 (1985): 781.
53. 187 N. W. 2d at 519.
54. See R. E. T. Corp. v. Frank Paxton Co., 329 N. W. 2d 416, 422 (Iowa 1983).
55. See Klein Indust. Salvage v. Dept of Industry, Labor & Human Relations, 259 N. W. 2d 124 (Wis. 1977). "We have said that a claimant cannot be said to have unreasonably refused treatment if none was offered by the employer"; 259 N. W. 2d at 126.
56. When a kennel full of pets caught on fire, killing many of them, the veterinarian, before rushing to the scene, telephoned a psychologist, who in turn rounded up three other psychologists, to provide counseling for the pet owners. Counseling sessions were arranged at a nearby church and were led by the psychologist whose specialty was pet loss support. He noted that owners whose pets die in accidents experience the same emotions others feel at the loss of a relative. "It's important to remember," he said, "it's not the object that you attach affection to, it's the intensity of the emotion." C. Christoff, "Trauma Greets Pet Owners at Burned Kennel," *Detroit News*, Nov. 27, 1999, p. 1
57. Pointing out what in other cultures might seem obvious, Dr. Satel writes, "Most people, in fact, are quite resilient and don't need registered experts to deal with anguish. Are our priests and rabbis not up to the task? Are our families' instincts to comfort not keen enough?" S.L. Satel, "An Overabundance of Counseling?" *New York Times*, April 23, 1999, p. 25; see also C.H. Sommers & S. Satel, *One Nation Under Therapy* (New York: St. Martin's Press, 2005); "A Surfeit of Disaster: When Horror Strikes, Does Counseling Help?" *Economist*, May 8, 1999, p. 21. In another critique, Dr. Thomas Szasz writes, "PTSD is now routinely *imputed* to people, especially to children helpless to reject the label. ... Adults, too, are treated as if they could not manage their own grief unassisted by helpers they do not seek. A plane crashes. Relatives and friends of the victims are met by 'grief counselors.' What in the past Americans would have considered ugly meddling, they now accept as medically sound mental health care." T. Szasz, *Pharmacracy: Medicine and Politics in America* (Westport, CT: Praeger, 2001), pp. 150–151.
58. See S. Begley, "Get Shrunk at Your Own Risk," *Newsweek*, June 18, 2007, p.49.
59. See R.A. Haig, *The Anatomy of Grief* (Springfield, IL: Thomas, 1990). Thomas Lynch, a funeral director, observes that TV reporters have become our virtual therapists, trumping "grief facilitators," by dressing public interest and passing curiosity in the needful garb of bereavement. T. Lynch, "Grief, Real and Imagined," *New York Times*, Oct. 30, 1999, p. 27.

21
Child Custody

With the advent of divorce and the demise of the father as master of the children, there arise disputes over child custody. The courts are now asked to determine which of the competing parties is entitled to be named custodian of the child. These disputes divide into three types: parent versus parent, parent versus nonparent, and nonparent versus nonparent. Increasingly, the psychiatrist is asked to provide data and opinion to assist the court in reaching or justifying its decision. The task of the psychiatrist is to uncover and offer testimony relevant to which party should be given custody or visitation.

Approximately one in two marriages in the United States ends in divorce, affecting about one million children per year. Approximately 10% of divorces involve custody litigation. Divorce cases are generally uncontested and raise no custody problem, a fact that is remarkable given that a petition must be filed to obtain a divorce thereby putting the parties in the judicial system and the process is often prolonged and exacerbates the ire of the parties. By and large, businesses negotiate or mediate a dispute without filing a lawsuit, but for marital conflicts, it is necessary to enter the judicial process. Few states promote mediation, and lawyers quite often find it to their interest not to mediate. In any event, litigation (filing a petition for divorce) is necessary and occurs before any mediation of a marital conflict.

Fathers usually contest custody only when they consider the mother grossly unfit or they feel very hostile toward her. Fathers as a rule recognize that the mother can render better care, the children usually wish to be with the mother, and consequently they do not request child custody or possession of the family home in the divorce action. The mother is literally the housekeeper. It is observable among the human and animal species that it is generally the mother who cares for and protects the young. And, of course, as fathers may recognize, a custody dispute is apt to be a futile endeavor. Surveys of sample cases indicate that maternal custody is awarded in 85 to 95% of the cases.[1]

Worldwide, rituals and songs express love and affection for mother, and rarely if ever is father mentioned. Russia is Mother Russia; however, the Germans salute the Fatherland. A popular song in Russia (and translated into other languages) says:

> May there always be sun,
> May there always be sky,
> May there always be momma,
> May there always be me.

In recent years, with the changing role of the mother in modern society, a number of decisions, albeit few in number, have emerged awarding custody to the father. Members of FARCE (Fathers Awareness of Rights and Custody Equality) have picketed at the nation's capitol. Yet, following divorce, the contact of fathers with their children drops off at a staggering rate. Only one-sixth of all children see their fathers as often as once a week after a divorce, and close to one-half do not see them at all. Ten years after a divorce, fathers are entirely absent from the lives of almost two-thirds of these children. About 30% of children are now born to unwed parents. While children of divorce typically have a tie with their fathers that is severed, most children born to unwed mothers never develop this tie at all.[2]

Best Interests of the Child

King Solomon anticipated the modern "best interests of the child" standard by awarding a child to the woman who would give up the child rather than to the woman who would have the child cut in two if she could not get her selfish way. Solomon did not have to determine who the biological mother was. The guiding rule now followed by the courts in child custody disputes is the "best interests of the child." With the emancipation of women, and with divorces becoming more frequent, a parental rights doctrine could hardly resolve custody disputes between parents. The courts came to say, beginning with Justice Cardozo's classic decision in 1925 in *Finlay v. Finlay*,[3] that the prime consideration in child custody disputes is the best interests of the child. Upon examination of the decisions purporting to employ this rule, however, it is seen that the best interests of the child will coincide with a parental rights decision. In effect, courts employ the semantics of the best interest test to achieve a parental rights decision, with the mother usually obtaining custody. Similarly, in disputes between parents and third parties, the child's best interest is usually interpreted to mean custody by a natural parent. The parental right and best interests doctrines are, in effect, opposite sides of the same coin. The fusion of the doctrines results from the generally justifiable view that custody by a natural parent, particularly the mother, is in the best interests of the child.

The phrase "best interests of the child" is magnanimous, but what criteria or evidence do the courts use in reaching such a decision? Cases in which courts spell out their reasoning are very few in number, resulting in criticism reminiscent of Plato's castigation of the poets who would say so many fine-sounding things, yet could not, under questioning, tell precisely what they meant. The best interests doctrine is invoked as though it were a magic formula by which the court, in Solomon-like fashion, would achieve the proper solution in each case. At any rate, the doctrine usually serves to avoid awarding custody to an abusive or drug-addicted parent.

The task of the courts was simple under the parental rights doctrine. The best interests doctrine does open channels of inquiry, but the results usually turn out to be the same. Custody decisions contain amorphous platitudes, but there is a simple rule of thumb that generally governs the cases: Custody goes to the mother.

Assumptions in Deciding Custody

There are certain other assumptions in deciding custody arrangements, however, than just the basic supposition that the mother makes the better custodian, at least for young children: (1) certain types of behavior are so detrimental to a child's welfare that they disqualify a parent as a custodian; (2) the parents' wishes and the child's wishes should be taken into consideration; and (3) the noncustodial parent has no duties in terms of the child's welfare except the payment of support.

Fitness of the party has been the criterion most frequently cited by the court in determining the best interests of a child. This attribute generally refers to the moral climate provided by the party. As one court put it, "As employed by our courts in custody cases, the word 'fit' connotes moral rectitude."[4] Sexual indiscretion known to the children is the most common basis for finding a parent unfit. A separated wife is not required to live in monastic seclusion, but a "calculated and continued public course of misconduct" is regarded as detrimental to the interest and welfare of the children.[5]

In the view of many psychiatrists and other professionals, however, a parent's sexual conventionality or unconventionality has little to do with his or her capacity to function effectively as a parent. They agree that involving the child in such unconventionality is harmful; but there are many women who function effectively as mothers notwithstanding one or more shifts of sexual partners. They do not believe, as do a majority of judges, that the legality of such sexual relationships should be a test of fitness.

Emotional Instability of a Parent

It is within the moral rectitude category that the issue of emotional instability of a parent is raised when evidenced by alcoholism, drug addiction, promiscuity, incest, exhibitionism, or other criminal behavior. Marital fault may be a factor bearing upon the best interests issue. Apart from the aforementioned specific type of evidence, the possibility of emotional harm to a child caused by a mentally disturbed parent is rarely considered in the courtroom. Parental psychosis unattended by such evidence is not sufficient to warrant change of custody, although it is estimated that 15% of children who have a severely mentally disordered parent will themselves become psychotic, and 40 to 50% will develop socially deviant behavior. It is held, though, that a parent who is adjudged incompetent or is a patient in a mental hospital is not a fit custodian.[6]

Allegations of Child Abuse

By legislation, California specifically states that a court-ordered child custody evaluation shall include history of child abuse, domestic violence, substance abuse, and psychiatric illness as well as psychological and social functioning.[7] To affect the outcome in a dispute over custody or visitation, allegations of child abuse are made that are often false. In a large sample of 9,000 families involved in custodial visitation disputes, Thoennes and Tjaden found that the rate of reporting was six times greater than that observed in a national incidence study.[8] Ceci and Bruck concluded that studies generally indicate that approximately one third of all such allegations made in this context are likely false and that as many as 50% or more of such reports in this context are erroneous claims. They further concluded that false reports from preschool children, due to their limited language and nascent symbolizing capacity, and, moreover, due to their similar cognitive limitations in terms of distinguishing reality from fantasy, are significantly more "suggestible" and, hence, less competent at accurately reporting actual occurrences of sexual behavior on the part of their caretakers.[9]

Preference of Child

Most jurisdictions, either by statute or decision, allow the judge to consider the child's preference, giving due weight to his age and maturity. Some state statutes set out the age at which to allow choice. Adolescents often want an advocate to express their desire and viewpoint. The judge often interviews the child or adolescent privately (contrary to the general principle of open proceedings), in an attempt to ensure that neither party is exerting influence upon his choice.

The preference of children is often influenced by what is colloquially called *brainwashing* or what the late Dr. Richard Gardner referred to as *parental alienation syndrome*.[10] Judges are now being asked to decide if children who do not wish to be with or visit their father or mother suffer from clinical alienation or if they are simply expressing a reasonable desire to avoid contact. In Michigan two psychiatrists, Dr. Savitri Bhama and Dr. Rajendra Bhama, were engaged in a prolonged and bitter custody fight over their two young children, almost depleting their assets in legal fees. The mother claimed that her husband alienated the young children from her, hence their desire to be with him, and she sued for intentional infliction of mental distress as well as a change of custody to her. The court found that the father's conduct was "outrageous." The children were returned to the mother, and the suit for intentional infliction of mental distress was allowed.[11]

Psychiatrists question the wisdom of asking a child to make a choice or, for that matter, involving him to any extent in custody proceedings. Discussing cases involving 8, 11, and 14 year olds, they point out that forcing the child to choose the parent with whom he wishes to live is the equivalent to his saying that one parent is good and the other bad, or that one loves him while the other does not.[12] The child often avoids such a predicament by stating that it makes no difference with whom he lives. Conversely, some children may have definite opinions that may be against their own best interests.[13] As a practical matter, custody is awarded in accordance with the preference of adolescents, otherwise they would likely make the custodian's life miserable.

The child, unable to be with both parents together, may perhaps wish to have his time divided equally between his parents; however, awards that alternate custody are not usually made. Alternating custody, while legally possible, was not done even in the day of the parental rights doctrine. The best interests of the child thus prevailed in this respect even when the expressed doctrine was parental rights. Stability in environment and central authority are desiderata in child rearing, but there is something of a trend toward shared custody, so as to maintain a link with the father.

However, an agreement between the parties may provide that the child will be 6 months, for example, with the father and 6 months with the mother, with a change of schools twice a year. Parents and attorneys will sometimes agree to such schedules in order to hurdle the first step— the divorce and settlement—expecting to return to court at a later time. Often, such schedules are then altered in a suit brought by the mother. For the welfare of the child, judges would do well to refuse to accept an agreement that divides the child in such a way between the parents. Moreover, it is usually recommended that siblings not be split up, the custody of some going to the father and others to the mother.[14]

Visitation

The award of custody to one parent is partially counterbalanced by the grant of visitation rights to the other. The noncustodial parent has a right of visitation (also known as *parenting time*) as a matter of course, which is forbidden only in the case of gross unfitness or failure to pay child support. (The noncustodial parent is usually obliged to make support payments, which is considered as a special kind of debt that the courts can enforce through the criminal law or as a civil contempt order.) Psychiatric testimony may be used in the determination of visitation rights as well as custody.[15]

Nowadays, varied and complicated family structures have arisen because of divorce, decisions not to marry, single-parent families, remarriages and step-families, parents who abandon their children to temporary caretakers, and children being raised by third parties because parents are deemed unfit. Given that situation, Washington State enacted a law specifying that "any person may petition the court for visitation rights at any time." Under that law, the court could grant such rights if they served the best interest of the child. The Washington Supreme Court and the U.S. Supreme Court both ruled, however, that the statute was too broad and gave too little deference to the wishes of the parent. The U.S. Supreme Court ruled that these cases should be decided on a case-by-case basis.[16]

Then, too, nowadays people move about often, and when a custodian parent moves to another area, the noncustodial parent's visitation is curtailed as a practical matter as a result of the distance; and the child is uprooted from the old environment. In dealing with a removal petition, the courts frequently rely on the test articulated by the New Jersey Supreme Court in *D'Onofrio v. D'Onofrio*:[17]

1. It should consider the prospective advantages of the move in terms of its likely capacity for improving the general quality of life for both the custodial parent and the children.
2. It must evaluate the integrity of the motives of the custodial parent in seeking the move in order to determine whether the removal is inspired primarily by the desire to defeat or frustrate visitation by the noncustodial parent, and whether the custodial parent is

likely to comply with substitute visitation orders when she is no longer subject to the jurisdiction of the courts of this State.

3. It must likewise take into account the integrity of the noncustodial parent's motives in resisting the removal and consider the extent to which, if at all, the opposition is intended to secure a financial advantage in respect of continuing support obligations.

4. Finally, the court must be satisfied that there will be a realistic opportunity for visitation in lieu of the weekly pattern, which can provide an adequate basis for preserving and fostering the parental relationship with the noncustodial parent if removal is allowed.

The *D'Onofrio* test focuses on what is the best interest of the new family unit, that is, custodial parent and child, and not what is in the best interest of the child; the latter having been decided in the earlier custody hearings (though implicitly the best interests of the child come into consideration under the test). The *D'Onofrio* test recognizes the increasingly legitimate mobility of today's society.[18]

Change of Custody

A custody order is not settled for all time, but may be relitigated. The doctrine of *res judicata* (a matter settled by judgment) does not apply in custody cases. A custody struggle may mean "it's just trial, trial again." In order to obtain a modification of a decree, however, there must be a clear showing of a significant change of circumstances since the time of the prior custody award. The remarriage of the parents, changing employment circumstances, the capacities of the parents, and the actual needs of the child constitute a change of circumstances that may warrant changing the child's custody.[19] It must then be shown that the new circumstances require a change of custody in order to promote the best interests of the child. In cases involving welfare assistance, there may be the testimony of a caseworker, who has the right to make home visits. (A home visitation without a search warrant has been held not to constitute an "unreasonable search" within the meaning of the Fourth Amendment, on the ground that the home visit is not a criminal investigation.)

All too frequently, a claim of changed circumstances represents simply another round in an ongoing battle with the child as the pawn. Some interspousal warfare may be described as "cruel and unusual punishment." Medea acted out her murderous rage on her children to retaliate against Jason. "Holy deadlock" does not end with the divorce. One vindictive tactic may be moving to another locale.

Considerable wardship work of the courts contains an international flavor, and as the number of binational marriages increases, the number of kidnappings outside the country is bound to increase. The 1961 Hague Convention says that disputes over the custody of a child should be handled by the country of the child's "habitual residence," although that may not be in the child's best interests.

Severance of Parental Rights and Adoption

Many cases are presented in which the child has been, for a considerable time, in actual custody of a relative or foster parents who could adopt him. An adoption proceeding places the child in the permanent custody of the adoptive party, who must first satisfy the court as to eligibility, and has the effect of a final decree. It often occurs that after the remarriage of one of the parents, the stepparent seeks to adopt the child. Although adoption is beneficial to the child and would give him a sense of security, it is generally only in cases of abandonment or desertion by the natural parent that the court allows the stepparent to adopt the child. Otherwise, the desire of the natural parent guides the court in permitting adoption.

An order terminating the rights of parents must be justified by conditions that have produced serious, substantial, and continuous damage to the health and welfare of the child. Additionally, there must be evidence that termination will be truly in the best interests of the child. Severance of parental rights is a serious act, affecting not only the rights of parents, but also the rights of children.[20] Yet, unless parental ties are fully severed in appropriate cases, many children would reach adulthood in a succession of foster homes or institutions, temporary placements that become a permanent way of life. Thousands of children live in that interim status of temporary placement, without roots, without family. Often forgotten by their parents and frequently separated from siblings, they are children without identification with a family unit and without the opportunity to form lasting family loyalties. Freeing children from grossly neglectful or abusive parents so that new, constructive, parental relationships may be established with adoptive parents seems a logical measure.[21]

The problem of parental abuse or neglect, whether or not the parents are divorced, raises a basic question as to the rights, duties, and obligations of the community. There is widespread protest over the lack of good, publicly funded child care centers. While not protecting the well-being of children in that way, every state, beginning first in 1963, has enacted legislation requiring a physician to report cases of child (physical) abuse, with failure to report constituting a criminal offense. (The legislation grants immunity from civil and criminal liability to those who report the abuse.) How much right should public officials have in intervening in the parent–child relationship? Out of some deep sense as to the scope of state power, the legislation is limited to physical abuse, as that involves concrete or tangible evidence. In the case of parental psychosis, although ignored by courts of ordinary jurisdiction in deciding custody, the juvenile court may find emotional neglect of the child and remove him from the home.

The concept of child neglect in law, like the concept of mental illness in psychiatry, is built upon limited data and focuses narrowly on the parent or child, apart from the social context in which they live. Like a flashlight in a dark room, investigation of only the individual is narrow in its illumination. Sometimes the light on even that limited area is weak. In an article dealing with family law and the challenge it presents to psychiatry, the late Dr. Andrew S. Watson criticized psychiatry for offering opinions not supported by statistical evidence. Many questions put to psychiatrists by lawyers involve predictions, and, he said, psychiatrists present ambiguous conclusions drawn from shadowy observational data. He writes: "Because of the lack of such basic information in this and most other family law areas, when efforts are made by psychiatrists or social workers to alter custody of a child by means of court procedure, they are quite incapable of responding to the judge's request for some kind of evidence to justify the change."[22] Besides lacking scientific validity, the opinions of mental health professionals concerning dispositions have often been based on data irrelevant to the legal questions in dispute.[23]

Even if the best interests test were in reality to replace the parental right approach, there is the hard problem of determining what the best interests of the child require. Upon the death of the custodial parent, the surviving parent is frequently pitted against a third person. There is fear, albeit infrequently articulated, that application of the best interest doctrine as the real test for custody determination might result in a further undermining of the family. While there is psychological basis for the traditional recognition of the right to custody in the natural parent, there may be times when the importance of the physical relationship is outweighed by other considerations, as in the case where there has been a long, affectionate relationship in a stable environment with another party.

No one can forget Charlie Chaplin's film, *The Kid* (1921), when the mother of the illegitimate child, now suddenly rich, wanted to reclaim her baby from the tramp who had loved and cared for it. In a much publicized case, which came to be known as the Baby Lenore case, Olga Scarpetta gave up her out-of-wedlock child, Lenore, for adoption, though she was of a wealthy family. After the child was placed through a public agency with New York lawyer Nick DeMartino and his wife, the mother changed her mind and, in a successful fight through the New York courts, obtained an order returning the child. (An adoption through an agency is usually anonymous.) The adoptive parents immediately moved to Florida, where the court fight began anew. The New York courts had ruled that the mother's prompt change of mind encouraged it to follow the general rule that a child is better off with its natural mother, especially if she is capable of rearing the child. But the Florida court, noting that the child was now more than two years old, said more damage would be done if Lenore were returned to the mother. The mother then asked the Supreme Court to review the case because of the contradictory rulings of the courts in two states, but she was turned down in a routine order that made no comment on the issues. The adoptive parents then, in 1972, proceeded to complete the legal adoption procedure in Florida.

Another much publicized case rejecting the natural parent occurred in Iowa. Hal Painter placed his 7-year-old son, Mark, with the Bannisters, the maternal grandparents, after the death of the boy's mother and sister in an automobile accident. He had placed Mark first with his own foster parents, who were living in a trailer, and he rented a room in a house where no children were allowed. A request by the foster mother that he pay board for the child precipitated his call to the Bannisters. Four years later, having remarried, he sought custody. Custody, however, was ordered continued with the grandparents, despite the usual presumption that a parent is entitled to custody.[24]

The psychological report submitted to the court indicated that the child's previous relationship with his father was unclear and that he had established a sound relationship with the grandfather, which, if disrupted, could result in emotional damage to the child. Obscuring the report, however, the court commented unfavorably on the father's occupation, freelance photography, and the relative merits of a rural, church-oriented upbringing versus a "more interesting Bohemian life." The decision, allowing another to take the place of a natural parent, provoked a storm of protest.[25]

Guidelines for Determining Custody

Troubled by the criticism, a generation ago Dr. Richard Jenkins came to the defense of the best interests doctrine. As director of the Department of Child Psychiatry at the University of Iowa, Dr. Jenkins daily witnessed the emotional and physical battering of children by parents. Sensitive to their plight, he formulated a position statement on child custody for the American Orthopsychiatric Association, of which he was an active member, that determinations of custody should be based on the best interests of the child. It was adopted unanimously by the Association's Committee on Law and Mental Health (including Slovenko) and approved unanimously by the board, the majority of the Resolutions Committee, and the membership.[26]

The Committee on Law and Mental Health initially reserved adoption of the statement, not because of the best interests principle, which it fully affirmed, but because the committee felt that the real issue was the difficulty in determining what the child's best interests were, and in setting out the issues to be considered in reaching that determination. In the last two decades, several organizations have published standards and guidelines for evaluating child custody disputes: The American Psychiatric Association Task Force on Clinical Assessment in Child Custody (1981), the American Psychological Association (1994), and the American Association of Family and Conciliation Courts (1994). The standards of the American Psychiatric Association and the American Psychological Association provide reference sections that list guidelines from other organizations.

The Uniform Marriage and Divorce Act, which has been adopted in many states, sets out a rather indeterminate approach as to the factors to be considered in a custody dispute. It provides:

The court shall determine custody in accordance with the best interest of the child. The court shall consider all relevant factors including:

1. The wishes of the child's parent or parents as to his custody.
2. The wishes of the child as to his custodian.
3. The interaction and interrelationship of the child with his parent or parents, his siblings, and any other person who may significantly affect the child's best interest.
4. The child's adjustment to his home, school, and community.
5. The mental and physical health of all individuals involved.

The court shall not consider conduct of a proposed custodian that does not affect his relationship to the child.[27]

Trial courts thus are given broad discretion in making child custody awards. The trial court's decision regarding custody will not be upset on appeal "absent a showing of an abuse of discretion or manifest injustice." However, to ensure the court acted within its broad discretion, "the facts and reasons for the court's decision must be set forth fully in appropriate findings and conclusions." The findings must be sufficiently detailed "to ensure that the trial court's discretionary determination was rationally based." "Specificity of findings is particularly important in custody determinations. This is so because the issues involved are highly fact sensitive."[28] In making a custody determination, the trial court is required to "at least consider all statutorily mandated factors," although it "need not make specific findings on each of the factors, as long as determination is based on substantial evidence relating to factors and set forth explicitly in findings."[29] Religion may at times be a factor in determining the child's custody or education.[30]

Michigan's Child Custody Act of 1970 was the first statute to set out criteria of best interests of the child. It defines best interests of the child as the sum total of designated factors to be considered, evaluated, and determined by the court, which include the following:

(a) The love, affection, and other emotional ties existing between the competing parties and the child.
(b) The capacity and disposition of competing parties to give the child love, affection, and guidance, and continuation of the educating and raising of the child in its religion or creed, if any.
(c) The capacity and disposition of competing parties to provide the child with food, clothing, medical care, or other remedial care recognized and permitted under the laws of this state in lieu of medical care, and other material needs.
(d) The length of time the child has lived in a stable, satisfactory environment and desirability of maintaining continuity.
(e) The permanence, as a family unit, of the existing or proposed custodial home.
(f) The moral fitness of the competing parties.
(g) The home, school, and community record of the child.
(h) The mental and physical health of the competing parties.
(i) The reasonable preference of the child, if the court deems the child to be of sufficient age to express preference.
(j) Any other factor considered by the court to be relevant to a particular child custody dispute.[31]

These are sweeping, elastic terms that may say much and at the same time say nothing. Another section of the Act provides that there is a rebuttable presumption that the best interests of the child require that he should remain in the custody of a natural parent as against the claim of a third party. It provides:

> When the dispute is between the parents, between agencies, or between third persons, the best interests of the child shall control. When the dispute is between the parent or parents and an agency or a third person, it is presumed that the best interests of the child are served by awarding custody to the parent or parents unless the contrary is established by clear and convincing evidence.[32]

Significant questions are: To whom does the child turn when hurt or in trouble? In whom does the child confide? For whom does the child behave better and why? The prominent English child psychiatrist D.W. Winnicott suggested an ordinary good-parent concept—to wit, it is possible to be a good-enough parent, and that should give one full legal right to custody without the necessity of determining the psychological better parent by some complicated formula drawn out by behavioral scientists.

Types of Custodial Arrangements

Some unusual custodial arrangements are split custody, joint custody, and custody with one other than a parent. Split custody, separating the siblings, is not favored by the courts; however, joint custody, which places custody equally with both parents, was popular a few years ago. Some custody experts criticized joint custody, others endorsed it. Under joint custody, either spouse as during the marriage may give consent for the medical or other care of the child.[33] Unless the animosity of the parties precludes a joint custody arrangement, it is the one alternative that attempts to use a living pattern and visitation schedule that most approximates the natural family situation. Those who get along ignore whatever the court may have ordered and make their own arrangements. Those who cannot get along have little choice but to turn to the more traditional and unnatural system, which grants sole custody to one parent and sets out in detail each parent's rights and privileges regarding the children's living arrangements and visitation. When "reasonable visitation" is unworkable, the court may render and order such as the following:

> The [mother] shall have custody of the minor children of the parties, and the [father] shall have the right of visitation with the children every Wednesday night from 7:00 p.m. to 9:30 p.m. of the first and third weeks and the first and third weekends from 6:00 p.m. of Friday afternoon to 6:00 p.m. on Sunday afternoon. The [mother] shall have the children on the second, fourth, and fifth weekends. During those weekends, the [father] shall have the children from 7:00 p.m. to 9:30 p.m. on Tuesday and Thursday nights. In the event either cannot exercise visitation, he/she is to notify the other party as soon as practical, but at least an hour before the visitation is to occur.

Under prevailing practice, the noncustodial parent is given access or visitation rights, although, as in joint custody, they may be attacked as perpetuating a relationship that is not in the best interest of the child. Visitation, like custody, is theoretically made in the interest of the child. If there is strong evidence that visitation is creating discord or tension, the court may be persuaded to curtail or bar it entirely. The right of visitation is not linked to the payment of child support. In their book, *Beyond the Best Interests of the Child*,[34] Joseph Goldstein, Anna Freud, and Albert Solnit suggested that when a decision has been made on placement with one parent, there should be no court-required visitation with the other parent. In those situations in which a court order is necessary for the visitation, they say, the visitation is more likely to be unfavorable to the child's development. They believe the court to be too blunt an instrument to rule on the vagaries of child rearing. Most lawyers would argue, however, that a rule leaving the control of visitation to the custodial parent would all too often result in the termination of visitation; even more, they say, the children would be the victims of a continuing feud between the parents. The courts say that the proposal, which would deny the noncustodial parent a legally enforceable right of visitation, represents such a shift in policy that the question of whether it should be adopted should be left to the legislatures. No state has adopted the proposal.

Battle of Experts

No less than in cases of criminal responsibility, a battle of the experts takes place in custody disputes as to what is in the best interests of the child. The controversy on the merits of joint custody is one illustration. Contradictory views are also expressed in cases inquiring whether a homosexual parent should be denied custody or visitation rights. Thus, in one case in which a lesbian mother and her estranged husband battled for custody of their minor daughters, one child psychologist advised the court that the children should remain with the mother, provided her lover move out of the house. A psychiatrist, calling homosexuality a character disorder, recommended that the children be placed in the custody of their father. Another psychologist said the mother's lover should remain in the house if the children were to stay there. In the past, homosexuality was an automatic impediment to gaining custody, and in some parts of the country, it still is.[35]

Decision making in custody disputes is dependent on expert testimony, particularly a court-appointed expert. The court cannot rely on the testimony of neighbors or friends as each side would round up those biased in its favor and the inquiry would not be advanced. There are varying opinions, however, on the scope of the expert testimony.

Some say that mental health professionals should not specifically name the best parent for the child; others say that they should limit themselves to pointing out the person's adequacies or inadequacies as a parent. The court, however, usually expects the expert in such a case to express an opinion on the ultimate issue. In rendering an opinion that one party is more fit than the other to be named custodian, the expert should interview both parties. The expert usually says that both are adequate, but that one is more fit than the other to be named custodian. As the report is seen by the parties, the expert would be well advised not to say, for example, that the mother looks older than her stated age.

Although the adversary system may serve well in criminal proceedings, it is arguably not the best system in family conflicts. Although the introduction of no-fault laws has removed the divorce decision from an adversary proceeding, the conflict over property, alimony, custody, and visitation is still dealt with in the traditional adversarial manner. The issue of fault and the focus of the dispute have been shifted from divorce to that of property and custody and there the parties fight, and they fight over everything—the horse, the saddle, and the manure. When the client has a deep pocket, some lawyers let the meter run; they make motions that have marginal or no relevance or usefulness, but that add to billable hours.

It has been suggested that a system requiring attempts at mediation or arbitration initially and then allowing for adversary resolution when the more conciliatory methods break down would avoid much psychological trauma and result in significant savings as well. Moreover, with court dockets increasing with respect to family breakups, there is a need to look to other ways to handle the issues. Local courts and private organizations in a number of states have marital mediation services in operation.[36]

The child custody dispute is by its nature unsuited to the procedural and evidentiary restrictions of the adversary system. The proceeding is unique because its purpose is not to determine the rights of the parties, but the best interests of the child. Therefore, while the hearsay rule and the right to confrontation provide needed protection in an adversary proceeding, it is argued that they are inappropriate in child custody hearings. The decision that a judge is called upon to make in a custody dispute is more closely analogous to the sentencing stage of a criminal trial than to a determination on the merits and, therefore, it is said, the judge should be given comparable discretion to rely on confidential reports of experts.

Custody Investigation and Reports

Recognizing that "custodial questions have sociological implication," the courts are mindful that "common-law adversary proceedings and social jurisprudence are not entirely harmonious" and that "some reconciliation between them is necessary."[37] This has consequences concerning consent to an investigation and consent to the admissibility and confidentiality of the report.

Statutes in a number of states deal specifically with custody investigation and custody reports. Michigan law provides that the court may utilize the community resources in behavioral sciences and other professions in the investigation and study of custody disputes and consider their recommendations for the resolution of the disputes. Florida authorizes a court investigation in any child-custody case and provides that the court may consider the report that it obtains unrestricted by "the technical rules of evidence." Virginia makes a report admissible even though not authorized by or disclosed to the parties. In the absence of a governing statute, consent of the parties is essential if ordinary rules of evidence and right to cross-examination are to be dispensed with. The general rule is that on factual questions, a court may not consider material which is unknown to the parties. Therefore, the parties are entitled to a copy of the custody report in ample time before the trial and may subject investigators to cross-examination regardless of consent to the investigation.

It is generally agreed that the court may order an independent investigation. Many states have enacted counterparts to Rule 35 of the Federal Rules of Civil Procedure, which provides that, where the "mental or physical condition of a party is in controversy," the court may, upon motion and for good cause shown, order that party to submit to a mental examination by a qualified physician. In any event, obtaining the consent of the parties to allow an investigation is not a major obstacle. There is really no free choice in the matter as consent is given to avoid prejudice. To illustrate, in one case the trial judge stated that, in light of the evidence presented, neither spouse should be awarded custody and requested the parties to consent to an independent investigation. When the plaintiff refused, the judge awarded custody to the defendant.[38]

In a number of jurisdictions, the court often suggests that the parties consult a psychiatrist. The "two hats" syndrome arises when the court order asks the expert to provide therapy as well as an evaluation, or the court sometimes says, "Do an extended evaluation." Wearing two hats—therapist and forensic evaluation—poses ethical questions, including the issue of confidentiality expected in therapy. It allegedly complicates both the therapy and the evaluation.[39]

In cases where the parties consult a psychiatrist to resolve their dispute, they usually accept the recommendation made by the psychiatrist. A result of the psychiatric consultation is that the fight over custody is often displaced to fighting over something like the automobile. However, it is not easy for the parties to locate a psychiatrist who will counsel with them, for many psychiatrists are reluctant to get involved in custody matters. In the event that the matter is not resolved and the dispute goes to trial, the expert often serves as an expert for both sides, the fee divided between the parties. The court hearing is usually very brief, and argument usually has little to do with the best interest of the child or who will be the best parent. As a practical matter, lawyers take few objections or appeals, due in part to the fact that too many lawyers regard divorce and child custody cases as "garbage cases" and do not prepare the case properly. A brief hearing, though, may be preferable to an inappropriate hearing. A court fight may deepen the animosity between the parties and may alienate children called upon to testify.

When both parties recognize that neither is fit and fear that the court will remove the child, they may try to circumvent such a ruling by not contesting custody. The tactic is usually successful. In some cases, commitment to a training school would have been in the best interest of the child. The appointment of an attorney to represent the child as guardian in hearings where custody is disputed or where there is a cause for concern for the child's well-being has been used in a number of family courts. He has the resources of the family court's staff of social workers to make a custody investigation and evaluation. The no-fault divorce law usually provides for the appointment of an attorney to represent the children in the divorce action, but thus far the provision has not been used to any great extent.[40]

In lieu of the formulation of new rules appropriate to the nature of child-custody proceedings, Dr. Lawrence S. Kubie offered a proposal that would oust the court of jurisdiction altogether. Under his proposal, parents upon divorce would agree to joint legal custody of their children and joint resolution of all custodial issues. In case of an impasse, a committee consisting of specialists (psychiatrists or educators) selected by the parties in advance would have the power to make a binding determination.[41] Such an agreement could be useful, despite the fact that courts have complete authority to determine what is in the best interests of the children and that agreements between the parents are not binding upon the court insofar as they relate to children. Such an agreement may well have the effect of causing both parents to submit these questions to a committee, however, rather than resorting to court action. Arbitration agreements respecting custody have been upheld.[42] Apart from the Kubie proposal, the development of the family court offers a way to avoid the uncomfortable atmosphere and procedures of traditional courts.

In child-custody litigation, the options available to the judge, to be sure, are limited. *Fit custodian* is a relative term. Both contestants may be fit, although not ideal, but all too often the question is: Which of the contestants is less unfit?

Changing Social Conditions

One consequence of changing social conditions is that more men, even in cases of illegitimacy, are asking for custody and more judges are granting it. The old order changeth, *o tempora, o mores*. There is a reevaluation of the assumption that the mother is always the better parent.[43] Moreover, while for years husbands have run away from home life, now there is a new runaway: the wife. No accurate statistics exist, but around the country, interviews with marriage counselors, psychiatrists, detective agencies, and women's liberation groups confirm the growth of the phenomenon called the dropout wife, the woman who abandons her family and all responsibility to them.

The no-fault divorce law is also a factor contributing to the rise in child-custody litigation. Under the old fault grounds law, a husband wanting out of marriage would be inclined to take a settlement in terms of support and child custody. This bargaining usually occurred where proof of misconduct was lacking, but one or both parties was through with the marriage. Under the no-fault law, the husband, knowing he will get out of the marriage no matter what, is less inclined to agree in advance to the wife's demands on child custody and property matters.[44]

Comment

Recent years have seen changes that may well make it necessary to think through the problem of child custody again. Few families are families any longer in the old sense. At one time, when divorce was a rarity, the family was an extended one (grandparents, uncles, aunts, cousins) all living together or nearby in a stable community. Today, the family has been reduced to a nuclear one with only two adults, and when there is a divorce, which is commonplace, it is reduced to one, placing an enormous burden on the person bringing up the children.

In an industrialized society, the family is no longer the production labor unit it was in the peasant or artisan family, for example. Its economic function is limited to the organization of everyday activities. With a decreased economic function, the family has been dispersed and, thus, reduced in size, it has not been able to manage adequately other traditional functions. At the same time there has not been a corresponding development of community services to fill the void.

The economy and social structures place a premium on mobility, and the split parents often find themselves in strange and different environments, usually unaided by nursery schools or other facilities for children. While there has been much talk of family assistance, proposed legislation on child development, day care, and education has to date usually been vetoed. Despite a generalized cultural piety about family life, as Daniel P. Moynihan said years ago, the U.S. government has been marked by a lack of social policies in support of the family as an institution.[45] Some young people see communes as the way out of their isolation and as a way of obtaining assistance in rearing their children.

With the nationwide incidence of divorce approaching one divorce for every two marriages, one out of six children has experienced the divorce of his parents. Alvin Toffler, author of *Future Shock*, predicted a subtle but very significant shift to much more temporary marital arrangements and intensification of the present pattern of divorce and remarriage to the point where it will be accepted that marriages are not for life. "I'm not endorsing it," said Toffler, "but I think it's likely to be the case."

The noted British historian Professor Arnold Toynbee, in numerous publications, expressed the view that nations rise or fall in relation to the moral unity of the family and the moral purpose of the state, and he saw a decline in both. On the whole, he was pessimistic, but he hoped that an ethical reformation would come out of the spiritual needs of the contemporary world.

Endnotes

1. Surprisingly, in Nefzger v. Nefzger, 595 N.W.2d 583 (N.D. 1999), the North Dakota Supreme Court held that the wife's continued alcohol use, her three extramarital affairs, and 20-year history of marijuana use did not render her unfit for custody, as she was said to be the primary caretaker of the parties' three children.
2. R. Weissbourd, "Distancing Dad," *American Prospect*, Dec. 6, 1999, p. 32.
3. 240 N.Y. 429, 148 N.E. 624 (1925).
4. State *ex rel.* Tuttle v. Hanson, 274 Wis. 423, 80 N.W.2d 387 (1957).
5. Shrout v. Shrout, 224 Ore. 521, 356 P.2d 935 (1960); mother who had her children bring beer to her while she was in the bedroom with her paramour was held unfit.
6. Annot., "Mental Health of Contesting Parents as Factor in Award of Child Custody," 74 A.L.R.2d 1068 (1960). By and large, the law on custody reaches a result remarkably similar to that advocated by the late Dr. D.W. Winnicott, prominent English child psychiatrist. In a paper dealing with the effects of psychotic parents on the emotional development of the child, Winnicott said:

   > Parental psychosis does not produce childhood psychosis. Aetiology is not as simple as all that. Psychosis is not directly transmitted like dark hair or haemophilia, nor is it passed on to a baby by the nursing mother in her milk. It is not a disease. … [P]sychiatric patients … are people who are casualties in the human struggle for development, for adaptation, and for living. … Parents with [schizoid characteristics] fail in many subtle ways in their handling of their infants (except insofar as they hand over their children to others, being aware of their own deficiency). … [I]n my practice I have always recognized the existence of a type of case in which it is essential to get a child away from a parent, especially a parent who is psychotic or severely neurotic. … [O]ne [must keep] in mind always the stage of development of the infant at the time of the operation of a traumatic factor. The infant may be almost entirely dependent, merged in with the mother, or may be ordinarily dependent and gradually gaining independence, or the child may have already become to some extent independent. … I for one do not want legal power to take children from parents except where cruelty or gross neglect awakens society's conscience. Nevertheless, I do know that decisions to take children from psychotic parents have to be made. Each case needs very careful examination, or in other words, highly skilled casework.

7. California Rules of Court, Rule 1257.3 (1999).

8. N. Thoennes & P. Tjaden, "The Extent, Nature and Validity of Sexual Abuse Allegations in Custody: Visitation Disputes," *Child Abuse & Neglect* 14 (1990): 151.

9. S.J. Ceci & M. Bruck, *Jeopardy in the Courtroom: A Scientific Analysis of Children's Synthesis* (Washington, DC: American Psychological Association, 1995).

10. See M.G. Brock & S. Saks, *Contemporary Issues in Family Law and Mental Health* (Springfield, IL: Thomas, 2008); R.A. Gardner, S.R. Sauber, & D. Lorandos (Eds.), *International Handbook of Parental Alienation Syndrome* (Springfield, IL: Thomas, 2006); see also S. Childress, "Fighting Over the Kids," *Newsweek*, Sept. 25, 2006, p. 25.

11. Bhama v. Bhama, 169 Mich. App. 73, 425 N.W.2d 733 (1988).

12. K.E. Alexander & S. Sichel, "The Child's Preference in Disputed Custody Cases," *Conn. Fam. Lawyer* 6 (1991): 45; J.E. Schowalter, "Views on the Role of the Child's Preference in Custody Litigation," *Conn. Bar J.* 53 (1979): 298; J.M. Suarez, "The Role of the Child's Choice in Custody Proceedings," *Case & Comment,* July–Aug. 1968, p. 46.

13. In a study, youngsters were asked whether they would rather their parents either spent more time at home or earn more money. A mere 20% said they would like to see a bit more of their mother and father; 60% said they would settle for the cash option instead. L. Kellaway, "Working Hard on a Guilt Trip," *Financial Times*, Dec. 20, 1999, p. 12.

14. Annot., "Split," "Divided" or "Alternate" Custody of Children, 92 A.L.R.2d 695.

15. Bowler v. Bowler, 355 Mich. 686, 96 N.W.2d 129 (1959); mother diagnosed as "schizophrenic, paranoid type, chronic, active" and who, according to testifying psychiatrists, should have been in a mental institution, denied visitation as well as custody; In re Two Minor Children, 53 Del. 565, 173 A.2d 876 (1961); mother who had deserted family and lived openly with paramour denied visitation rights notwithstanding expert testimony that she had now become emotionally stable and had a sincere desire to see the children. See also Annot., "Right of Putative Father to Visit Illegitimate Child," 15 A.L.R.3d 887.

16. *In re* Custody of Sara Smith, 137 Wash.2d 1, 969 P.2d 21 (1998); Troxel v. Granville, 120 S. Ct. 2054 (2000). In this case grandparents (parents of the children's father who had committed suicide) petitioned to obtain greater visitation rights. The children's mother did not seek to deny visitation, but did not wish to grant as much as the grandparents wanted. Justice Sandra Day O'Connor, writing the Court's plurality opinion, took care not to disparage the important role of grandparents. She observed that the rise of single-parent households, in which 28% of children are being raised, is making grandparents more important. Judge O'Connor noted that the trial court went so far as to put the burden on the mother to show why expanded visitation was *not* appropriate. The U.S. Supreme Court said the due process clauses of the Fifth and Fourteenth Amendments to the U.S. Constitution have long been held to create "heightened protection against government interference with certain fundamental rights and liberty interests." Ordinarily, however, family law issues, such as visitation and custody, are left to the states, not the federal courts. In a dissent, Justice Antonin Scalia noted that there is no discussion of parental rights in the Constitution.

17. 144 N.J. Super. 200, 365 A.2d 27 (1976), *aff'd*, 144 N.J. Super. 352, 365 A.2d 716 (1976); cited in Henry v. Henry, 119 Mich. App. 319, 326 N.W.2d 497 (1982).

18. The American Academy of Matrimonial Lawyers sets out the following factors in its proposed Model Relocation Act:

    (1) The nature, quality, extent of involvement, and duration of the child's relationship with the person proposing to relocate and with the nonrelocating person, siblings, and other significant persons in the child's life; (2) the age, developmental stage, needs of the child, and the likely impact the relocation will have on the child's physical, educational, and emotional development, taking into consideration any special needs of the child; (3) the feasibility of preserving the relationship between the nonrelocating person and the child through suitable [visitation] arrangements, considering the logistics and financial circumstances of the parties; (4) the child's preference, taking into consideration the age and maturity of the child; (5) whether there is an established pattern of conduct of the person seeking the relocation, either to promote or thwart the relationship of the child and the nonrelocating person; (6) whether the relocation of the child will enhance the general quality of life for both the custodial party seeking the relocation and the child, including but not limited to, financial or emotional benefit or educational opportunity; (7) the reasons of each person for seeking or opposing the relocation; and (8) any other factor affecting the best interest of the child.

    In a comment it is stated:

Unfortunately, while the list of factors is comprehensive, it does little to resolve the dilemma so often presented in litigation. If the contestants are two competent, caring parents who have had a healthy postdivorce relationship with the child, the competing interests are properly labeled "compelling and irreconcilable." The child's custodian may have a compelling interest to move with the child, the noncustodial person may have a compelling competing interest in maintaining the relationship with the child, which may be significantly undermined by the move. The child has a compelling interest in stability—both in the stability of remaining with the custodian and with maintaining frequent contact with the noncustodial parent. In sum, even a perfect list of factors, when applied to decide such a contest, will not resolve the dilemma, i.e., relocation often is a problem seemingly incapable of a satisfactory solution.

See C.S. Bruch & J.M. Bowemaster, "The Relocation of Children and Custodial Parents: Public Policy, Past and Present," *Fam. L. Q.* 30 (1996): 245; J.S. Wallerstein & T.J. Tanke, "To Move or Not to Move: Psychological and Legal Considerations in the Relocation of Children Following Divorce," *Fam. L. Q.* 30 (1996): 305.

19. Prevatt v. Penney, 138 So.2d 537 (Fla. App. 1962).
20. See F.J. Dyer, *Psychological Consultation in Parental Rights Cases* (Washington, DC: American Psychiatric Press, 1999).
21. The best interests doctrine notwithstanding, the guiding maxim adhered to by the courts is that blood is thicker than water. In a contest between a natural parent and a foster parent, the former is generally awarded custody. Parental rights may not be terminated solely on the ground that the child would be better off in another home. S.K.L. v. Smith, 480 S.W.2d 119 (Mo. 1972). See H.H. Foster, "Adoption and Child Custody: Best Interests of the Child?" *Buffalo L. Rev.* 22 (1972): 11.
22. A.S. Watson, "Family Law and Its Challenge for Psychiatry," *J. Family L.* 2 (1962): 71. See P.C. Ellsworth & R.J. Levy, "Legislative Reform of Child Custody Adjudication: An Effort to Rely on Social Science Data in Formulating Legal Policies," *Law & Soc. Rev.* 4 (1969): 167.
23. Psychologist Thomas Grisso has observed:

    Custody cases involving divorced or divorcing parents rarely involve questions of parental fitness, but rather the choice between two parents, neither of whom [is] summarily inadequate [as a parent]. ... Mental health professionals do not have reason to be proud of their performance in this area of forensic assessment. Too often we still evaluate the parent but not the child, a practice that makes no sense when the child's own, individual needs are the basis for the legal decision. Too often we continue to rely on the assessment instruments and methods that were designed to address *clinical* questions, questions of psychiatric diagnosis, when clinical questions bear only secondarily upon the real issues in many child custody cases. Psychiatric interviews, Rorschachs, and MMPIs [Minnesota Multiphase Personality Inventory] might have a role to play in child custody assessments. But these tools were *not* designed to assess parents' relationships to children... [or their] child rearing attitudes and capacities, and *these* are often the central questions in child custody cases. T. Grisso, "Forensic Assessment in Juvenile and Family Cases: The State of the Art" (address at the Summer Institute of Mental Health Law, University of Nebraska–Lincoln, June 1, 1984). The American Psychological Association has published guidelines for child custody evaluations. See *Am. Psychol.* 49 (1994): 677.

24. Painter v. Bannister, 258 Iowa 1390, 140 N.W.2d 152, *cert. denied*, 385 U.S. 949 (1966).
25. See, e.g., *New Yorker*, April 2, 1966, p. 35. The case was also extensively commented upon in the law reviews, e.g., W.H. Poteat, "Iowa Supreme Court v. Wild Oats," *Maine L. Rev.* 18 (1966). The father himself wrote a book, *Mark, I Love You.* Subsequently, during the boy's annual summer visit to California, the father decided to hold onto him and to appeal to a California court. The grandparents agreed to leave the decision to the boy, who chose to stay with his father and stepmother. At this time, the grandfather was in poor health, a matter that presumably influenced Mark's decision. The grandparents made no appearance in the California court action awarding custody to the father; Superior Court, County of Santa Cruz, August 28, 1968.
26. It reads:

    The American Orthopsychiatric Association supports the view that the determining consideration in child-custody cases should be the welfare of the child. Children are not property and should not be regarded as possessions. The rights of a parent to the custody of his child are dependent upon his assuming parental responsibility and functioning as a parent. While there is a strong initial presumption that the custody of a child should rest with his natural parent, the law has long recognized that this presumption may be set aside if the parent is unfit for or fails to assume parental responsibilities.

The Association believes that the presumption in favor of the parent should rest upon the actual existence of a deep bond of mutual attachment between child and parent, such as normally grows out of a parent–child and child–parent relationship. Where such a bond exists, it outweighs all consideration of what advantages a foster home may have to offer because of wealth, education, or social position. Within the range of lawful behavior, it is more important than any value judgment about the family atmosphere. On the other hand, when the natural parent has not functioned as a parent or has been so ineffectual in that functioning that no such mutual bond exists, and when a mutual bond has developed between the child and a foster parent, such a developed relationship is, in the judgment of this Association, also worthy of great respect in the determination of child custody.

In terms of future mental health of our population, the welfare of the child, not the welfare nor interests of the parent nor of the foster parent, should be the determining consideration. The Association will study such issues as the kinds of criteria and evidence that should be useful in deciding what may be in the best interest of the child.

Newsletter, American Orthopsychiatry Association, May 21, 1968, p. 8. It was approved by a mail vote of the membership of 517 yes to 17 no, or 97% approval.

27. Uniform Marriage and Divorce Act § 402, 9A U.L.A. 561 (1987).

28. The quotes are from cases cited in Sukin v. Sukin, 842 P.2d 922 (Utah App. 1992).

29. Brown v. Brown, 600 N.W.2d 869 (N.D. 1999); *In re* Marriage of Converse, 826 P.2d 937 (Mont. 1992); Sukin v. Sukin, 842 P.2d 922 (Utah App. 1992).

30. Religious pressures may adversely affect interspousal disputes, including those over child custody. The judgments of the battling parents may be affected by religious beliefs and possibly affect the future of their fought-over children. See Aldous v. Aldous, 99 S.D.2d 197, 473 N.Y.S.2d 60 (1984); Grayman v. Hession, 84 A.D.2d 111, 446 N.Y.S.2d 505 (1982); Matter of SEI v. JWW, 143 Misc.2d 455, 541 N.Y.S.2d 675 (1989).

31. Mich. Comp. Laws Ann. § 722.23 (Supp. 1972).

32. § 722.25.

33. Noncustodial parents can take a child for emergency medical care, just as anyone can take a child for the treatment of an emergency. The authorization or routine medical care is an area of confusion, however, but the common medical practice is to treat children at the request of noncustodial parents. See W. Bernet, "The Noncustodial Parent and Medical Treatment," *Bull. Am. Acad. Psychiat. & Law* 21 (1993): 1993.

34. J. Goldstein, A. Freud, & A.J. Solnit, *Beyond the Best Interests of the Child* (New York: Free Press, 1973).

35. See D.J. Hutchens & M.J. Kirkpatrick, "Lesbian Mothers/Gay Fathers," in D.H. Schetky & E.P. Benedek (Eds.), *Emerging Issues in Child Psychiatry and the Law* (New York: Brunner/Mazel, 1985). A number of studies find no detriment to children having lesbian mothers. D.J. Kleber, R.J. Howell, & A.L. Tibbits-Kleber, "The Impact of Parental Homosexuality in Child Custody Cases: A Review of the Literature," *Bull. Am. Acad. Psychiat. & Law* 14 (1986): 81. Others find that children of homosexual fathers may be distressed by their father's gay identity. F.W. Bozett, "Gay Fathers," in F.W. Bosert (Ed.), *Gay and Lesbian Parents* (New York: Praeger, 1987).

36. Studies have shown that mediation—whether conducted by lawyers, mental health professionals, or a combination of both—has short-term and long-term benefits. The short-term benefits, which mediation was found to produce, are that (1) it generates user satisfaction and is credited with improving the relationship between former spouses, (2) it creates greater compliance and satisfaction with the agreements that are produced as compared with those coming out of the adversarial system, (3) the parties enjoy more contact with their children through both joint custody arrangements and generous visitation terms, and (4) the cases move through court more rapidly producing modest savings of both time and finances. The long-term benefits credited to the use of mediation, when compared with the adversary system, are that parties who use mediation are (1) more optimistic about being able to resolve future problems with their ex-spouses without returning to court, (2) more satisfied with their court orders, (3) less likely to report serious problems with their orders, (4) more likely to report that their ex-spouse is complying with terms of the order, (5) more likely to report good relationships with the former spouse, and (6) more likely to enjoy joint custody arrangements or greater visitation terms. Parents who used mediation also report a lower amount of filings for subsequent modification. See

J. Pearson & N. Thoennes, "Mediating and Litigating Custody Disputes: A Longitudinal Evaluation," *Family L. Q.* 17 (1984): 497; see also R.M. Coombs, "Noncourt-Connected Mediation and Counseling in Child Custody Disputes," *Family L. Q.* 17 (1984): 469.

37. Kesseler v. Kesseler, 10 N.Y.2d 445, 180 N.E.2d 402 (1962).

38. Withrow v. Withrow, 212 La. 427, 31 So.2d 849 (1947); Comment, "Use of Extra-Record Information in Custody Cases," *U. Chi. L. Rev.* 24 (1957): 349.

39. W. Bernet, "The Therapist's Role in Child Custody Disputes," *J. Am. Acad. Child Psychiat.* 22 (1983): 180. See Chapter 3.

40. R.W. Hansen, "Guardians *Ad Litem* in Divorce and Custody Cases: Protection of the Child's Interests," *J. Family L.* 4 (1964): 181. Professor Levy argued, however, that if the guardian *ad litem* is to serve his function properly, he may feel compelled to make the proceeding more contentious (and so more traumatic) than it would have been without him; and, he said, if there is any area of universal agreement about custody adjudication, it is that adversary procedures do more harm than good. See R.J. Levy, "Treatment of Child Custody Problems in the Family Code," in Proceedings of the Institute on the Family Code Project, Southern Methodist University, mimeo., 1967.

41. L.S. Kubie, "Provisions for the Care of Children of Divorced Parents: A New Legal Instrument," *Yale L. J.* 73 (1964): 1197.

42. Sheets v. Sheets, 22 App. Div. 2d 176, 254 N.Y.S.2d 320 (1964); Note, "Committee Decision of Child Custody Disputes and the Judicial Test of 'Best Interest,'" *Yale L. J.* 73 (1964): 1201.

43. In a case in New York, Family Court Judge Richard C. Delin commented, "The cliché that 'a young child is better off with its mother' has no automatic status in law—nor in human nature—and will be increasingly challenged in a world of working women." *New York Times*, Feb. 23, 1972, p. 44.

44. Under the old law, both parties often arrived at an accommodation as to property settlement, alimony, support, and custody, which was presented to the court for approval. One party then withdrew from the lawsuit, permitting the judge to grant the divorce without an actual contested trial. Under no-fault, however, parties anticipating that they will receive their divorce are often unwilling to make concessions—particularly on property settlements—and the case goes to trial.

45. D.P. Moynihan, "Income by Right," *New Yorker*, Jan. 13, 20, 27, 1973; reprinted in his book, *The Politics of a Guaranteed Income* (New York: Random House, 1973). See also E. Scott, "Rational Decision Making About Marriage and Divorce," *Va. L. Rev.* 76 (1990): 9.

22
Contractual Capacity

Countless legal decisions and commentaries point out that consent, the essence of a contract, must be freely and fully given in order to bind a party. According to theory, a "lunatic," though capable of holding property, is, strictly speaking, incapable of any legal act because "he has no capacity for willing."

In both Roman and early English common law, no agreement could be made if a party was incapable of understanding. Roman law provided that "an insane person cannot contract any business whatever because he does not understand what he is doing." Early English common law said that contracts are based on a "meeting of minds." If a party lacks sufficient "mind," there could be no such meeting. A century ago, voiding a power of attorney given by one confined in a lunatic asylum, the U.S. Supreme Court said:

> The fundamental idea of a contract is that it requires the assent of two minds, but a luna-
> tic, or a person *non compos mentis* has nothing which the law recognizes as a mind, and
> it would seem, therefore, upon principle, that he cannot make a contract, which may have
> any efficacy as such.[1]

The Court noted that just as the lunatic is not amenable to the criminal law because "he is incapable of discriminating between that which is right and that which is wrong," he also may not be held to the provisions of that which purports to be a contract.

Historically, married women, infants, and lunatics had no capacity or limited capacity to contract. Statutes sometimes authorize, as in cases of lunacy, the appointment of guardians for habitual drunkards, narcotic addicts, spendthrifts, aged persons, or convicts. Even without the appointment of a guardian, civil powers of convicts may be suspended in whole or in part during imprisonment.

Lunacy and infancy have usually been equated as to contractual capacity. As one court put it, "Infancy and lunacy are disabilities similar in their effect on the contracts of parties, and we see no good reason why a different role should be applied to the contracts of persons *non compos mentis* from that applied in the case of infants."

However, one's contractual capacity where there has been no ruling of incompetency and, thus, no appointment of a guardian, is a question of fact, depending upon the transaction. The contractual incapacity of a minor is a matter of law. Thus, a minor by operation of law is not bound by a purchase of a car. Parents and schools make decisions on behalf of minors, but as an additional protection, courts are permitted to override decisions that do not appear to be in the minor's interests. At the turn of the 20th century, married women came to have contractual capacity. In the Middle Ages, when commerce was in its formative stage, the doctrine of incapacity did not substantially affect trade because guilds rather than individuals were the trading units. However, with the development of commerce, it was soon recognized that a strict application of the doctrine would prove unfavorable. Consequently, the "meeting-of-the-minds" theory was replaced in large measure by the objective theory of contractual obligation, which merely requires a manifestation of assent. Several statutes, including the Uniform Sales Act, the Uniform Negotiable Instruments Law, and the Uniform Commercial Code have been adopted with a view toward securing transactions. For example, every holder of a negotiable instrument is deemed a *prima facie* holder in due course. Moreover, defenses, such as fraud, duress, and mistake, are not available against a holder in due course.

The outcome of a controversy thus turns very much upon the question whether the transaction involved is a commercial mercantile act. Unlike Anglo-American legal tradition, many civil law countries long ago had two separate codes of law: a commercial code or code of commerce to govern what are called *commercial transactions* (e.g., wholesale purchase of wine), and a civil code to govern what are called *consumer transactions* (e.g., purchase of a bottle of wine). In addition to different applicable laws, separate courts have often been established to handle the two different classes of cases. One example is the commercial court in France where two of the three judges are merchants and a special class of lawyers, called *agréés*, handles the cases.

The morality of business differs markedly from that of sports, which, traditionally a heroic concept, is associated with such moral ideals as fair play, magnanimity in victory, loyalty, and unselfish teamwork. God and sportsmaster are even merged in one image: "And when the last Great Scorer comes/To write against your name,/He'll ask not if you lost or won,/But how you played the game." The condemnation, "It isn't cricket," is not used in the business world, where laissez faire prevails, a doctrine staunchly supported by the law during the 19th century. The precept of W. C. Fields is famous: "Never give a sucker an even break." And he commented, "You can fool some of the people all of the time, and all of the people some of the time, and that's enough to make a good living."

In business, a number of studies have concluded that personality makes or breaks a man as an economic success. Sherlock Holmes describes the Gold King, the famous millionaire in *The Problem of Thor Bridge*: "If I were a sculptor and desired to idealize the successful man of affairs, iron of nerve and leathery of conscience, I should choose [him] as my model. ... Business is a hard game, and the weak go to the wall. I played the game for all it was worth. I never squealed myself, and I never cared if the other fellow squealed."

Increasing legal attention, however, is now being given to the quality of a product—the object of the transaction. This focus often overshadows problems of contractual capacity or of a vice of consent, such as error, fraud, or duress. In ordinary transactions, distributors and retailers and everyone else along the "trail of sale" exercise less discretion than in the past. Apart from the price usually being fixed, the real selling job is done by the manufacturer in mass media advertising. While not called duress or brainwashing, advertising increases demand and seduces the onlooker into a customer. Indeed, the contracting seller and buyer now may be in contact, but not in conversational touch. In large stores, the seller need not even look at the buyer, but only at the article chosen for purchase, the buyer's money, and perhaps his hand. Liberal return or exchange policy (the customer is always right) renders moot contractual remedies based on contractual incapacity or vice of consent. Unless prohibited by law or sanitary regulations, any merchandise will usually be accepted for credit, refund, or exchange. In large transactions where the parties are usually artificial persons, i.e., corporations and governmental agencies rather than natural persons, the tendency of modern legislation is to restrict the defense of *ultra vires*. Flea market concepts are outdated in this age of technology and vast corporate enterprise.

Today, the quality of goods in a bargain is determined more in light of social policy than by natural persons who do not set the terms. Strict liability in tort and implied warranty in contract have ushered in a new era of consumer protection. The doctrine *caveat emptor* (let the buyer beware) is no longer a hallowed precept. A product now carries a warranty implied by law that it will perform its function in a way that one would reasonably expect; in addition, the manufacturer owes a duty to the public to use due care in the design and manufacture of its product or be subject to tort liability. Less than a decade ago, an estimated 50,000 product liability suits were filed. Today, approximately 500,000 suits are filed annually. While it is debatable whether this rash of lawsuits is actually resulting in improved products, they are increasingly successful in compensating injured persons.

Consumer Legislation

During the 1970s, the various states enacted comprehensive consumer legislation. Although the legislation protects all consumers, special emphasis is placed on a consumer's mental condition. The legislation makes it an unfair trade practice to "[take] advantage of the consumer's inability to reasonably protect his interests by reason of disability, illiteracy, or inability to understand the language of an agreement presented by the other party to the transaction who knows or reasonably should know of the consumer's inability."[2] Merchants may argue that the mercantile world is too complex to screen out consumers meeting these criteria. However, a consumer's appearance, actions, and verbal cues should trigger awareness to the possibility that the consumer is mentally deficient. The duty placed on the merchant is not as strict as it may appear, especially considering that the merchant has to meet only a reasonable standard.[3]

The civil law offers other protections. A bargain is not enforceable if either its formation or its performance is criminal, tortuous, or otherwise opposed to public policy. An agreement to commit a crime or tort against a third person is clearly an illegal bargain. An agreement that provides for a greater interest rate than is permitted by law is usurious and illegal (although in practice the prohibition seems to apply to very few transactions). The law on informed consent requires a degree of competence to consent to medical treatment or experimentation.[4] A lawyer who intentionally takes advantage of an elderly or other person with diminished mental capacity to obtain his signature on a document may face disbarment.[5]

Gambling

There is a conflict of authority as to the enforceability of an obligation arising out of a gambling transaction. (Playing the stock market is not considered gambling; the public relations people at the New York Stock Exchange dispel the notion that buying stocks is gambling.) If gambling is deemed against public policy and made unlawful, gambling wins or losses are not recoverable at law. In such jurisdictions, the gambling trade depends to a large extent on trust. English humorist Henry Cecil, who has done for the law what the medical writer Richard Gordon has done for the medical profession, observed:

> Whereas in ordinary transactions everything is normally written down, and often long and (to the laymen) unintelligible contracts are signed in transactions involving only quite small amounts, in the racing world many thousands of pounds are staked by word of mouth only, and the parties are entirely dependent upon one another's honesty.

"Gaming" is the current euphemism for gambling. If it is deemed by the jurisdiction to be within public policy, an obligation of even a chronic gambler is legally enforceable, even though excessive gambling (or gaming) is a form of addiction and free will may be impaired. In *The Gambler*, Dostoevsky describes the compulsive gambling that gripped him. The gambler may have an easy come, easy go attitude, and he and his family may eat beans while he plays in a crap game. Gambling may be the simplest expression of the desire to win money, however illogical, or it may be merely the desire to escape boredom. A character in the film *American Movie* says gambling is preferable to drugs or alcohol because you always lose with drugs or alcohol.

In Dostoevsky's time, a gambling obligation typically arose not at a casino, but at an informal get-together and cash was usually not put up front. The typical scenario now is a gambler with a credit card who gets money from an ATM machine, loses it, and then tries to declare bankruptcy. Not too long ago, state-sanctioned casino gambling in the United States was limited to Nevada and Atlantic City. Today, however, much of the country plays host to some type of gambling. First-generation Las Vegas belonged to Mafia-linked entrepreneurs (such as Bugsy Siegel), but the second was shaped by Wall Street financiers with access to capital markets. Many state legislators, city mayors, and state governors have pushed gambling as a means to stimulate local economies. The social consequence is an increase in the number of people who fall prey to compulsive gambling.

The courts have split on the dischargeability of credit card debt incurred from gambling in bankruptcy. Nonetheless, certain debts are excepted from discharge for policy reasons. The Bankruptcy Code excepts any debt for money, property, services, or credit that was obtained by "false pretenses, a false representation, or actual fraud." Credit card companies have maintained that gambling debts should fall under the fraud exception to discharge, arguing that the debtor did not intend to repay the debt at the time it was incurred.[6]

Compulsive Spending

The law on bankruptcy offers limited protection to another type of addict known as the compulsive spender. Economists view compulsive spending as good for the country (shop til you drop!), but psychiatry often views it as a mental disorder. Inordinate buying (oniomania) is seen as a *forme fruste* of kleptomania. Abraham Lincoln's wife was a depressive who tried to forget her troubles by shopping on a monumental scale, once buying 300 pairs of gloves in 3 months. The inclusion of compulsive shopping was discussed for *Diagnostic and Statistical Manual of Mental Disorders (DSM-IV)*, but not adopted.[7]

Marriage counselors and spouses at or near financial bankruptcy view compulsive spending as tragic, comparable to alcoholism. The psychiatric explanations for compulsive spending vary. One explanation is a need to buy love or objects denied in early life. Other explanations list feelings of worthlessness, deprivation, and lack of self-esteem, the latter especially applicable to those who overspend on others in an attempt to be recognized. Easy credit and charge accounts allow the compulsive spender to spend his salary much in advance. While the bankruptcy law may limit his liability, the outlook is grim. Credit counseling centers, financed by business and lending institutions hoping to avoid the debtor's going into voluntary bankruptcy and extinguishing their claims entirely, have been established in various communities. Some courts have recently allowed recovery for emotional distress or its physical consequences caused by unfair attempts or harassment in collecting a debt. Midnight collection calls or breaking down a door to recoup merchandise sold is prohibited.

Effect of Mental Incapacity

Although limited in application, lunacy, mental illness, or mental incompetence may continue to present problems of contractual capacity. The view that a lunatic has no capacity to contract (making the transaction absolutely void) has given way to the doctrine that a contract is voidable, at the option of the incompetent person or his guardian, if at the time of the contract he did not understand, on account of mental illness or defect, the nature and consequences of the transaction.[8]

The test is twofold, as are other legal tests on mental capacity: (1) the person must be suffering from a mental illness or defect, and (2) the illness or defect affects his understanding of the transaction to the degree stated. In addition to the understanding test, courts sometimes apply an insane delusion test. As there defined, an insane delusion is a belief in the reality of facts that do not exist and in which no rational person could believe, and the delusion is related to and motivates the contract. The test has been applied in such cases as the maker of a promissory note believing that unless he made the note he would be killed or imprisoned,[9] and a husband believing his wife was having an illicit affair deeding his property to his son.[10]

It has been asserted, though, that mental incompetency has no effect on a contract unless other grounds of avoidance are present, such as fraud, undue influence, or gross inadequacy of consideration. Years ago Henry Weihofen, a prominent professor of law and psychiatry, summarized the law of competency to contract: "Was this transaction so foolish or irrational that it shows the person did not adequately understand what he was doing?"[11] Thus, the sale of a truckload of soap to an individual ostensibly needing only a bar may raise the issue of contractual capacity in the form of a vice of consent. The less sophisticated or competent, the more an individual is susceptible to fraud, duress, or error. It is commonly said that an informed consumer is the best protection against fraud or other vice of consent.

To some extent, agreement is an element in civil and criminal procedure as well as in the substantive law of contracts. In the Roman law of civil procedure, the *litis contestatio* entailed a formal contract between the parties agreeing as to the issue in litigation. The criminal law provides a preliminary proceeding known as the arraignment (colloquially known as the *arrangement*) in which the accused is called upon to answer to the indictment. His choice of answer is simple and limited: he may plead guilty, not guilty, or not guilty by reason of insanity. If he says, "Maybe I'm guilty and maybe I'm not," a not guilty plea is entered. At one time a refusal to plead (standing mute) deprived the court of capacity to hear the case, a logical result of the view that the court is an arbitrator entirely disinterested in the litigation. Today standing mute is considered the equivalent of pleading not guilty.[12]

In criminal cases, the question of a defendant's ability to comprehend arises in the areas of plea bargaining, waiver of constitutional rights, and assisting counsel in preparation of defense. Ordinarily, a plea of guilty is the result of plea bargaining between prosecutor and defense counsel. The question of the defendant's ability to comprehend and voluntarily waive his constitutional rights usually centers, not on the plea bargaining stage, but on the issue of whether the police at the time prior to interrogation had advised the defendant of his right to remain silent, that any statements made could be used as evidence against him, and that he has the right to the presence of an attorney, either retained or appointed. The defendant may elect to waive these rights, but such waiver has full force and effect only if made "voluntarily, knowingly, and intelligently."[13] Organic brain disorder, for example, may preclude comprehension of these rights. Thus, a psychiatrist may establish that the defendant is intellectually defective and does not have the "capability of understanding the intricacies of so-called rights."[14]

Is a woman suffering a battered woman's syndrome capable of voluntarily entering into a property settlement agreement with her husband? Is her will constrained by her condition? Is she, in effect, incompetent? Experts say that a temporary interruption in the pattern of battering does not mean that she has recovered sufficiently to freely and voluntarily enter into a settlement agreement without an extended period of therapy. If she has an attorney at the time of making the agreement, the attorney may help to equalize the bargaining positions of the parties. At a court hearing, expert testimony that she was a battered woman may be used to repudiate the agreement.

Basically, the law of contracts, when affected by incapacity or mental illness, involves two conflicting policies. On the one hand is the objective view that seeks to uphold the security of transactions and the reasonable expectations of the contracting parties. On the other hand is the policy of protecting mentally incompetent individuals from the consequences of their own acts and the acts of others. When one party knows of the incompetency of the other, the policy of securing reasonable expectations carries less weight.[15] Likewise, where a mentally incompetent person by contract obtains basic necessities, i.e., shelter, clothes, food, and medical services, the policy of protecting him is less critical, for in such cases there is usually a fair trade.[16] Where necessities have been supplied to an incompetent, as well as a minor, the court raises an "implied contract" against the incompetent or his estate; the law in effect makes the contract for the parties.

There is a crucial proviso to the rule that a contract made by an incompetent or mentally ill person is voidable at his election. The court will declare rescission of the contract provided the other party can be restored to status quo. If the parties cannot be returned to their previous positions, rescission will be denied provided the other party was ignorant of the incompetence and the transaction was fair and reasonable. Otherwise, the rule might easily transform the incompetent's shield to a sword. The incompetent party has the personal option to avoid or ratify, but the power of avoidance is conditioned on restoration of the benefits he has received. The burden of proving incompetence is upon the party alleging it, but once incompetence has been shown, the burden of proving lack of knowledge and fairness is upon the party asking that the transaction be enforced. The determination of the individual's mental status at the time of the making of the contract is made by inferences from historical data and from assessing the individual's current mental condition.

The courts have said that in order to convey land, the grantor must have sufficient mentality to understand and appreciate the nature and consequences of the conveyance upon his rights and interests. A plea of incapacity has usually been successful in upsetting a conveyance only where there is unconscionability or gross inadequacy of the consideration for the conveyance. (Louisiana by statute requires that there be a consideration in land contracts of at least one-half market value.) In one case where the consideration was adequate, the grantor was held capable of executing the deed notwithstanding testimony that at the time of conveyance he ate moldy food, did not bathe, could not carry on a coherent conversation, was jittery, and urinated on the streets of the town and in friends' homes in front of women.[17] The more improvident the transaction, the more likely a court is to find incapacity. The question asked by courts is: Was the transaction so foolish or irrational that it shows the person did not adequately understand what he was doing?[18]

Taking advantage or duping one obviously incompetent, even though an adult, may be a type of fraud that warrants invoking the protective policy of the law. Thus, an incompetent adult would, like the boy in *Jack and the Beanstalk* who sold his mother's cow for some beans, be allowed to recover the cow or its value if the beans turn out to be worthless and not magical. Strictly speaking, the word *fraud* means only "conscious misrepresentation"; but in a broad sense, as Williston said, "It is doubtless a fraud to enter into a contract with an insane person knowing his condition."[19] Thus, the question of a party's mental capacity provides the court with a means to control unfair bargains.

In a transgression of role boundary, therapists at times involve their patients in business deals. The traditional model of psychotherapy assumes a clear separation between the personal and professional roles of the therapist and patient, as essential to proper and effective treatment. Sex between a therapist and patient has been exposed to the public eye, but there are other less publicized boundary violations. Some therapists ask patients to include them in business deals that patients have discussed during the course of therapy. Some therapists are made beneficiaries of large bequests in the patient's will.[20] In a much publicized case, a psychiatrist used a stock tip obtained from a patient during the course of therapy to turn a large profit. The Securities and Exchange Commission learned from the patient of this transmission of "insider" information about a merger, and it charged the therapist with profiting illegally. The therapist neither admitted nor denied the charges, but surrendered the profits and paid a fine of the same amount.[21]

Defects in judgment caused by brain damage or mental deficiency may preclude the understanding deemed necessary for contractual capacity. An insane delusion that motivates contractual action may call for legal protection when there is a substantial degree of divorcement from reality. Many aged persons lose or change their judgment in matters of money, arousing the concern of family members who may seek the appointment of a guardian.[22]

A more difficult case is presented by the hypomanic person who, during the manic or expansive phase of the manic depressive syndrome, engages in all sorts of ambitious schemes. In the hypomanic state, he may accomplish great things because of his tremendous energy output and enthusiasm. (Some of the most effective fundraisers are hypomanics.) A hypomanic may become wealthy in a short time on his ventures, but just as quickly his world may crumble.

During a manic period, relating to others is expanded. There may be a surge of entertainment, incurring great expense. Invitation lists are extended as if there were a need to pack the environment with people. Contacting is accelerated. Long-distance calls are made into all time zones. The telephone bill is many times normal. The telephone company, however, is scrupulously detached in these matters. As one observer put it, theirs is not to wonder why, but only to collect.

Apart from psychogenic factors, there may be a pharmacological explanation for manic behavior. For example, alcohol tends to have an expansive effect on many people. The amphetamines, affecting the frontal lobe, tend to have this result. In the drug culture, amphetamine is called *speed*. Berton Roueche in a case study, *Ten Feet Tall*, describes the overreaching social behavior of a man experiencing a brief manic episode due to the side effects of cortisone treatment. In this case, a New York schoolteacher was treated for periarteritis nodosa, a destructive inflammation of the arteries, which was often fatal before the advent of adrenocorticotropic hormone (ACTH) and cortisone. After a prescription of cortisone, which induced a manic-depressive reaction, the patient began to order costly clothing by telephone to avoid the petty inconvenience of walking from store to store. This was contrary to his usual behavior of shopping cautiously in endless searches to select his clothes.

An investigation by the *New York Times* revealed that Dr. Max Jacobson (called Dr. Feelgood), a general practitioner in New York, over a period of years injected a concoction containing amphetamine into the veins of the country's most celebrated people.[23] Many of the VIPs seen by the doctor insisted—without always knowing what was in the injections—that he helped them achieve success. Most of them said that the shots gave them boundless energy and more productive and pleasurable lives.[24] Following the disclosure of Dr. Jacobson's practice, details of similar practices by other physicians emerged as several former patients and other persons came forward with information.

The individual in a manic or expansive frame of mind has an understanding of his transactions, but his judgment may be grossly impaired, and he may not be able to control his behavior. As one commentator says: "If the understanding test of the law is inadequate, it is so mainly for cases where the person intellectually comprehends the nature and quality of his act, but nevertheless lacks effective control of his actions."[25] With rare exception, though, the courts hold the manic depressive to his contractual obligation because he has the necessary cognitive ability required in law.

An illustrative case is *Beale v. Gibaud*,[26] in which an action was brought to enforce two promissory notes. The defendant had been moderate in his business transactions until, one year, he bought an automobile dealership. His wife said of him then, "He had an exaggerated idea of his business ability and his financial worth." His confidence led him to purchase a second business. After a few months in a sanatorium, followed by a seemingly normal period, he moved to Florida and began trading feverishly in real estate. It was during this period that the promissory notes in dispute were executed. Two psychiatrists testified on behalf of the defendant declaring that he was suffering from a manic depressive illness that had prompted his actions. It was claimed that he was suffering from "an exalted phase of manic-depressive insanity" that caused him to disregard "the impulse of inhibition that a man ordinarily uses in normal health in checking up his transactions," and he was "led by his rosy promise of great success in his transactions." The court found the evidence unconvincing, and, applying the understanding test, was persuaded by testimony on his comprehension of the terms of the contract, the rationality of his conduct, and the regularity of the business transacted.

In *Lovell v. Keller*,[27] in which a similar conclusion was reached, an action was brought to recover the purchase price of stock. The plaintiff, a guardian, claimed that her ward was insane at the time the contract was made. The contract was made and the stock delivered prior to the appointment of plaintiff as guardian of the person and property of the ward. At the trial, the plaintiff testified, in substance, that her ward was extravagant. An eminent psychiatrist was thereupon called to substantiate the contention of the plaintiff that her ward "was at the time of said purported contract and has since remained incompetent to contract, by reason of lunacy." During the course of his testimony, he testified, referring to the ward, that: "She was very much elated, she had a lack of sequels in her ideas, she had ideas that were incompatible with her financial state, she was doing a number of business transactions that seemed unwise. ... She went into tantrums and was a very difficult person in her behavior." It was his belief that "she was suffering from a mild hypomania, that is, a mild mania. Many people have a rhythm of emotion in which they run into depressions that are apt to alternate with periods of elation. All the best work of the world is done by people in a state of elation, but at times it runs into a completely abnormal and pathological situation." The characteristics of hypomania were described as "over elation, lack of proportion, extravagance, violence of behavior." His testimony on direct examination continued further:

Q. Was she, in your opinion, at the time, capable of making a contract and knowing what she was doing?

A. She could make a contract, she would know perfectly well she was making a contract, if that is the whole of your question.

Q. My question is, whether she was capable in your opinion of making a contract and realizing the consequences of what she was doing in that connection?

A. Not realizing the consequences, she would know its nature perfectly, but would not be capable of balancing the facts of the contract.

On cross-examination the attorney for the defendant brought out that the ward was capable of understanding the nature of the contract:

Q. Did I understand you to say, Doctor, that she would understand perfectly the nature of any contract and the full consequences?

A. I believe so.

Q. But she might, mightn't she?

A. I wouldn't trust her.

Q. What?

A. I wouldn't have trusted her.

Q. That is, you wouldn't like to have her transact your business for you?

A. No.

Q. That is about the size of it, isn't it?

A. Right.

Q. But she would know the nature of any contract she entered into?

A. She was quite able to read and understand what she was reading.

Q. And quite able to understand what it was about?

A. Perfectly.

Q. Perfectly?

A. But I believe incapable of judging and balancing wisely.

Q. Balancing wisely; whom do you know that balances them wisely, name me somebody?

A. As wisely—

Q. (Continuing) ... that can know when they make a contract that they are going to profit by it?

A. As wisely as a normal person and as wisely as I think she would have judged had she been all—

Q. (Interrupting) … had she not been afflicted with this elation and depression. But, by affliction with those periods of elation or depression, do you mean to say that she could not enter into a contract under which she might profit?

A. Well, she—

Q. (Interrupting) … well, answer that, won't you?

A. Certainly, she might profit by it.

Q. She might?

A. Yes.

Q. But you do know as a natural matter of fact person suffering in the manner that she suffered at that time could execute a contract and, while it might even be unwise, know what she was doing?

A. Yes. This lady's mind as against her intellectual faculties was clear enough, but she was really suffering in my opinion from an emotional insanity … the instrument in her mind was intact enough, she was being driven like a whirlwind by an abnormal emotional drive, and when the emotional drive is abnormal, the intellect does not work as it ordinarily does.

Upon redirect examination, the following questions were put to the witness, and he was allowed to answer without objection:

Q. Your opinions already expressed, Doctor, were founded upon your observation of the patient?

A. Certainly.

Q. Now, will you tell the jury based upon your entire observations, and having in mind the point [the defense attorney] has brought out, what your present opinion is as to her condition then, whether she was normal or abnormal?

A. I have no doubt whatever that she was abnormal.

Q. You have no doubt?

A. That she was suffering from acute mania.

Q. Was she competent or incompetent?

A. Financially?

Q. To manage her affairs?

A. Incompetent.

The evidence was held insufficient to warrant a holding of contractual incapacity. The court said that the evidence failed to show that the mind of the ward was so impaired at the time the contract was made that she was incapable of carrying on her affairs, as would a reasonable and sensible woman.

These cases occurred in the 1930s, before the wide popularity of psychiatry. Then, in 1963, in apparently the first decision of its kind, a New York court in *Faber v. Sweet Style Mfg. Corp.*,[28] appraising a manic depressive's capacity to enter into a binding contract, allowed him to rescind a transaction for the purchase of land. Testimony revealed that he had been seeing a psychiatrist because he was in a state of depression; that he ceased doing so and within 3 months had entered into numerous business ventures and embarked upon a buying spree. Previously frugal and cautious, he became expansive, began to drive at high speeds, to take his wife out to dinner, to be more active sexually, and to discuss his prowess with others. In this 3-month period, he purchased three expensive cars for himself, his son, and his daughter, began to discuss converting his bathhouse and garage property into a 12-story cooperative, put up a sign to that effect, and discussed the purchase of land for the erection of houses. Against the advice of his lawyer, he purchased the land in question for $41,000 and talked about erecting a 400-room hotel with marina and golf course. Finding him incompetent to enter into the contract because he "acted under the compulsion of a mental disease or disorder, but for which the contract would not have been made," the court granted rescission. This motivational standard of incompetency had never before been applied in a contract case. When, as is generally the case, cognitive capacity is the sole criterion used, the manic is held competent because manic depressive psychosis affects motivation rather than ability to understand. The court gave as its reason for departing from traditional law that "the standards by which competence to contract is measured were, apparently, developed without relation to the effects of particular mental diseases or disorders and prior to recognition of manic depressive psychosis as a distinct form of mental illness."

Faber never reached the appellate level and its effect on the continued validity of the cognitive test even in New York remained uncertain until the 1969 decision in *Ortelere v. Teachers Retirement Board*.[29] In this case, Mrs. Grace W. Ortelere, a teacher for over 40 years in the New York City school system, suffered from a nervous breakdown and went on medical leave of absence. Prior to this, she selected one of the retirement options that made her husband the sole beneficiary of the unexhausted reserve in the pension fund. While still on medical leave and under psychiatric care, however, she wrote to the Retirement System indicating that she planned to retire and asked about the various options available to her. She then executed a retirement application opting for the highest monthly yield without any cash reserve payable to her beneficiary. Shortly thereafter she collapsed from an aneurysm and 10 days later she died. Her husband instituted action to set aside the election of the high-yield option.

The evidence conclusively established that the deceased fully understood her acts, but according to the psychiatric testimony, she was unable to control her conduct. She was under psychiatric treatment for involutional psychosis, melancholia type, and also for cerebral arteriosclerosis. On appeal, the court held, 4–3, citing *Faber*, that a contract may be voided if the party who executed it is laboring under a mental defect that prohibits him from acting in a reasonable manner and the other party has knowledge of the defect. The court restricted its holding by stating that relief would be granted only if two conditions existed: (1) the other party knew or was put on notice about the incompetent's impairment, and (2) the illness that motivated the incompetent's behavior was nothing less serious than medically classified psychosis.[30] In addition, the court implied that it would not allow avoidance if the other party had significantly changed its position in reliance on the contract. The dissent summarized its objections by concluding that the majority's standard would undermine the security of contracts, put excessive emphasis on psychiatric testimony, and encourage frivolous claims.

In *Shoals Ford v. Clardy*,[31] an Alabama case, the court set aside the purchase of a truck by an individual diagnosed as a manic depressive. The wife informed the auto dealer that her husband was in a manic phase and was not capable of making informed decisions about purchasing a vehicle. Nevertheless, the dealer continued to exert pressure on him to complete the purchase. The trial court charged the jury as follows:

> I … charge you that manic depression is a mental illness, but that is not to say that all manic depressives may be classified as legally insane. Some are and some are not. In order to determine if a person is legally insane, you will have to determine whether or not [the individual] in this case, had sufficient capacity to understand in a reasonable manner the nature and effect of the act he was doing. Or put another way, that he had a reasonable perception or understanding of the nature and terms of the contract.

In addition to setting aside the purchase, the jury awarded punitive damages, finding that the defendant auto dealer had acted "wantonly" in coercing the completion of the transaction. The state Supreme Court affirmed.

Depression, at the low end of the manic-depressive syndrome, may also cloud judgment. One lawyer, who for 40 years swung between the highs and lows of manic depression, put it thus: "I enjoyed the manic phases. I was a big shot, on top of the world. I spent not only my own money, but everybody else's I could get my hands on. I bought six suits at a time, a lot of stupid unnecessary things." But in between the highs, on plunges into depression, he dreaded getting out of bed and spent little time at the office. When in a state of depression, innumerable persons have altered their lives to their regret: sold their homes or businesses, quit their jobs, turned away from friends and family, undertaken divorces, even given their children up for adoption. Later, when they felt their old selves, they found their lives wrecked.

Dr. Manfred Guttmacher in his book, *America's Last King*, describes George III as a manic depressive and attributes the loss of the colonies to his condition. According to the National Institute of Mental Health, 125,000 Americans are hospitalized each year with depression, another 200,000 are treated on an outpatient basis, while another 4 to 8 million go without help. Everyone has highs and lows in mood, and grief reaction to a serious loss is a normal part of living, but when the mood swing is exaggerated to the point of impairing function, or grief is prolonged for months at a time, psychiatry labels the condition as depression.

While the legal test applied in *Ortelere* is unique, its adoption has been encouraged by the *Restatement (Second) of Contracts*.[32] The test corresponds roughly to the two-pronged test of cognition or control of the American Law Institute (ALI) test of criminal responsibility.[33] The court in *Ortelere* noted that the change it made regarding the law of contractual capacity paralleled those that have occurred in the law of criminal insanity. The traditional test of criminal insanity, like that of contractual incapacity, has been expressed in the pure cognitive terminology of the *M'Naghten* rule, which holds a person responsible for all actions, even if uncontrollable, as long as he was aware of what he was doing.

Does the person who does not understand what he is doing deserve more sympathy than the person who is unable to control his conduct? The latter type of incompetent person presents a greater danger to the security of contracts because he is more difficult to discover. In *Ortelere*, the Board of Education was aware of the decedent's impairment because of her nervous breakdown that necessitated a leave of absence. In most contracts, the parties are not likely to have known each other intimately enough to evaluate one another's mental health. Hence, situations where the new standard will benefit an incompetent will be few and far between.[34]

Competency of a Multiple Personality

One of the most famous multiple personality cases took an interesting turn when Christine Costner Sizemore, whose life was the basis for the book (by psychiatrists C.H. Thigpen and H.M. Cleckley) and subsequent movie classic (starring Joanne Woodward), *The Three Faces of Eve*, challenged Twentieth Century Fox Film Corporation's claim that it held the motion picture rights to her life story. Actress Sissy Spacek had wanted to co-produce and star in a movie based on a new book by Sizemore, *In Sickness and Health*, but negotiations bogged down when Fox claimed it held the rights to any movies about her. Fox claimed that it owned those rights since 1956, when one of Sizemore's personalities signed over to Fox, "forever," the film rights to "all versions of my life story heretofore published or hereafter published" for $7,000. Sizemore's attorney contended that the original contract proves that Fox knew Sizemore was still deranged—beneath her signature were typed three more names: Eve White, Eve Black, and Jane. (The three faces of Eve were timid Eve White, flamboyant Eve Black, and practical Jane.) In the new book, Sizemore details her life in the years following her development into an integrated personality

—after her real self was distilled from the competing personalities through therapy. She alleged that she was unduly influenced in 1956 into signing away the rights to her life story by her then psychiatrist and author C.H. Thigpen.[35] The case was settled.[36] Following the case, publishers were advised to obtain the consent of all the multiples for the publication of a book by a person with multiple personality disorder (MPD).[37] But, is the fact of several personalities, on the face of it, a sign of incompetency, as Sizemore's attorney claimed?

Effect of Mental Hospitalization

Hospitalization is indicative of contractual incapacity. The determination of competency of patients in mental hospitals, however, is complicated by the unsettled and confused relationship between commitment and legal competency. The Draft Act Governing Hospitalization of the Mentally Ill, adopted in a number of states, specifically provides that every patient in a mental hospital shall retain his civil rights, including the right to contract, unless he has been adjudicated incompetent. The court in *Wyatt v. Stickney*,[38] which, it will be recalled, set out minimum constitutional standards for the treatment of the mentally ill, stated that "no person shall be deemed incompetent to manage his affairs, to contract, to hold professional or occupational or vehicle operator's licenses, to marry and obtain a divorce, to register and vote, or to make a will solely by reason of his admission or commitment to the hospital." Be that as it may, the fact of past or present mental hospitalization will at least raise some doubt concerning competency and will red flag every transaction of a mental patient with the exception of petty cash purchases.

Whether persons who are in need of mental hospitalization as well as those who are committed are necessarily incapable of managing their own affairs is a subject on which there is considerable controversy. Observations such as the following, which was presented at an American Psychiatric Association Mental Hospital Institute, are illustrative: "If they aren't competent to look after themselves outside the hospital, they are not competent to transact business. ... The idea that a person is allowed to sell real estate while he is deprived of the right to walk the streets, I find difficult to comprehend."[39] Mental disabilities, however, are of such variety and degree that concluding one is incompetent from the fact of his hospitalization is without justification. Evidence is needed of incompetency, mental illness, or disability as well as the causal connection between the incompetency and the disability.

In a proceeding for the appointment of a guardian for an alleged incompetent, the superintendent of the hospital testified that the alleged incompetent was of "unsound mind and might dissipate his estate or become the victim of designing persons." He stated that the alleged incompetent suffered from dementia praecox, that he had delusions of persecution, and was convinced that his neighbors had joined in a conspiracy to fill his home with poison gas. The superintendent did not, however, testify to any facts in support of his opinion and admitted that he had not questioned the alleged incompetent concerning the extent of his property, claims against the estate, and the like. The alleged incompetent testified in his own behalf and according to the court "demonstrated an intelligent grasp of his financial situation, recited detailed facts, such as the mortgage arrangements related to his home, and convinced the court he was well familiar with the nature and extent of any property now or heretofore owned by him." In denying the petition, the court stated: "... the criterion is not the mental illness, but rather the inability to manage property by reason of mental illness. Unless the mental illness produces or results in such inability to manage property, the court is not warranted in appointing the guardian for the estate of a mentally ill person."[40]

Responding to an "equal protection of the law" attack on a state statute, which denied trial by jury to persons facing civil commitment but granted it in proceedings to appoint a guardian, a U.S. district court said:

It is true that both the class of persons subjected to involuntary commitment proceedings and the class of persons subjected to the appointment of a guardian may have mental problems. However, it is at that point that the similarity ends. The standards and purposes of the proceedings to commit someone who is mentally ill … are entirely different from the standards and purposes of the appointment of a guardian to one who is found incapable of handling his own affairs … . Assuming arguendo [for the sake of argument] that the classification involved did affect persons similarly situated, we are of the opinion that the difference in treatment is totally justified under the rational basis test. A finding that a person is not capable of handling his own affairs so as to require appointment of a guardian seems to us more susceptible to the practical wisdom of a jury than determining whether a person is mentally ill or an inebriate and dangerous to himself or others. The latter finding may not unreasonably have been thought by the legislature to be beyond the competency of a jury.[41]

Appointment of a Guardian or Conservator

Given the close identity between guardianship and civil commitment criteria, guardianship may be regarded as a less restrictive alternative to commitment. Until the 1970s, most states joined a competency proceeding to a commitment proceeding inasmuch as commitment usually meant commitment for life. In effect, the hospital was made guardian of the individual. Institutionalized persons were presumed incompetent at least until release and perhaps until a court restored them to competency. Today, as a result of short-term commitment, the various states specifically eliminate the presumption of incompetency for institutionalized persons. A number of states still grant hospital administrators some authority over a patient's financial affairs (e.g., disposition of social security benefits) and a few allow other restrictions "necessary for the patient's medical welfare." In *Katz v. Superior Court*,[42] parents of members of the Unification Church obtained at the trial level an order of temporary conservatorship (guardianship) to allow their adult children to be deprogrammed, but the decision was overturned by the California appellate court in a ruling that quelled the growing use of conservatorship laws for such purposes around the country.

In guardianship, a person is appointed by the court to exercise powers over the person of a minor or of a legally incapacitated person. A guardianship is established to provide continuing care and supervision of a proposed ward.[43] A *conservator*, on the other hand, is a person who exercises power over the estate of a minor or legally incapacitated person. The purpose of establishing a conservatorship is to manage the property and affairs of a person who, because of incompetency, mental illness, age or physical infirmity, or other reasons, cannot adequately manage them on his own. (Quite often, the term *guardian* is used to include conservatorship.) They are both fiduciaries to their wards. They act directly on behalf of their wards, they are not agents of their wards.[44] Conservators may also be considered trustees because they exercise the same powers of property management for their wards that trustees exercise on behalf of their settlors and beneficiaries.

When a guardian is sought for a person with assets that may be at risk or need to be managed, a conservator should also be sought as a protection to the ward. The conservator manages and uses the assets for the ward's benefit, must account to the court, and must file a report (whereas a guardian does not). The guardian and the conservator may be the same person; the guardian or the ward might prefer to have another person exercise authority over the assets. The conservator may be an institution, such as a bank or trust company. The factors to consider include the size and complexity of the estate, the inclinations and abilities of those available and willing to serve, and the needs of the ward.

Clear and convincing evidence must show that the adult "is impaired to the extent that the person lacks sufficient understanding or capacity to make or communicate informed decisions concerning his or her person."[45] The impairment might arise from mental illness, mental deficiency, physical illness or disability, chronic use of drugs, chronic intoxication, or other cause. To determine incapacity, the process of decision making is examined, not the outcome of the decision. Whether a decision is responsible or one with which others disagree or feel not to be in the individual's best interest, is not the issue.

Any person interested in the proposed ward's welfare, including the proposed ward in his own behalf, may petition for a finding of incapacity and appointment of a guardian.[46] The petition for guardianship must contain specific facts about the person's condition and specific examples of his recent conduct that demonstrate the need for guardianship.[47] This serves two purposes: (1) it informs the person who is the subject of the petition of specific allegations so that he may prepare a defense, and (2) it can help identify and weed out spurious petitions.

The appointment of a conservator is often not considered necessary unless property of considerable value is involved and is in danger of dissipation. An individual's competence to manage his person or property is not in issue until challenged, usually by a family member who wishes to protect the family or the individual from the consequences of his disability, or who wishes to protect the subject's property, which may soon pass to the petitioner by the statute of descent and distribution.[48] Persons whose property interests require at least some management are increasing in number due to the development of pension plans, veterans' benefits, insurance policies, annuities, and social security.[49]

Important aspects of a diagnostic evaluation include the notion of reversibility versus irreversibility—whether the medical disorder is a potentially curable or reversible one or whether it is a progressive, irreversible process—as well as determining the extent of impairment. In older adults, the most common cause of progressive, irreversible cognitive impairment that may lead to mental incompetence is Alzheimer's disease. The second most common cause is multi-infarct dementia.[50]

After an individual has been formally adjudicated incompetent and a conservator appointed, the theory of the law is that the conservator is vested with control of the ward's property and any contract entered into by the ward is entirely null and void. The ward is legally unable to write or endorse checks, sell property, or enter into business (but he may write a will). Historically, declaration of legal incompetency was an all-or-nothing situation, but now specific or limited guardianship may be ordered.[51]

The laws of the various states provide that a guardian or conservator should be sought and may be appointed for a legally incapacitated adult. This is defined as an adult whose judgment, by virtue of mental illness, deficiency, physical illness, or disability, is impaired to the extent that the person lacks sufficient understanding and capacity to make or communicate responsible decisions concerning his person.[52] A guardian or conservator of a legally incapacitated person has the same powers, rights, and duties respecting the incapacitated adult (ward) that a parent has respecting that parent's unemancipated minor child.[53]

A determination by a psychiatrist that a patient is or is not mentally competent does not necessarily answer the question of whether a patient is legally competent. Legal competency, as a practical matter, is arguably a less stringent standard. Formal medical opinion or evidence may not be necessary, but it may be desired by the court and helps ensure the success of a petition. To avoid any actual or apparent conflict of interest, a hospital employee or staff physician should not act as a temporary or permanent guardian though the hospital or other healthcare provider may initiate guardianship proceedings. As a practical matter, locating an outside individual willing to serve as a guardian is one of the most difficult tasks facing hospitals generally and discharge planners specifically. Some states have a "public guardian," a publicly funded position to represent individuals without family or friends willing to act as a guardian. Even where a patient has a guardian, problems arise where the guardian is, for one reason or another, not properly carrying out his responsibilities and court intervention may be desirable or necessary.

In most states, there are few rules governing who can serve as a guardian or conservator. Frequently, a family member fills the role, but as families become more dispersed, the courts are increasingly appointing professional guardians. Many of them are lawyers, but most states require only that a guardian be an adult and not a felon or ward themselves. During the last decade or so, there has been a rise of guardianship companies, some caring for hundreds of wards at a time. There is no regulation, no licensing, no testing.[54] In Florida, which has a large elderly population and a history of frauds by guardians, the legislature in 1987 enacted a law requiring guardians to be bonded and under training and requiring credit and criminal background checks.[55]

Quite often operators of nursing homes are named as guardian and quite frequently they authorize the "chemical straitjacketing" of residents. Federal legislation has been enacted to guard against the practice.[56] An estimated 1.6 million people in the United States reside in nursing homes. The quality of care varies widely, as does the number of complaints filed. A coalition of advocates for the elderly has called for federal legislation to give patients the right to install a camera in their room and also in other locations, particularly the shower and dining room. Undoubtedly, the cameras would encourage more lawsuits against nursing homes, but that would empower victims and give the nursing home industry an incentive to halt abuses.[57]

What about termination of guardianship or conservatorship? In cases where the guardianship or conservatorship is dormant or where a considerable time has elapsed since the adjudication, the courts tend to hold that the fact of adjudication merely raises a rebuttable presumption of incompetency. A ward actually may have improved and the guardianship may have been allowed to lapse, but the parties neglected to return to court to have the guardianship formally terminated. The courts are usually willing to hear evidence that the ward at the time of the act had recovered sufficiently to be considered competent. Some severe mental illnesses rendering a person incompetent are treatable and over a period of time the individual's competency may be restored. A psychiatrist may be used to help the patient be adjudicated competent and to regain decision-making power.

There being no central statewide registration of incompetents, it is difficult for persons to ascertain whether those with whom they intend to transact business have been declared incompetent.

Impairment of Ability to Fulfill a Contract

And what about an individual's ability to fulfill a contract when becoming mentally ill after entering into the contract? On occasion psychiatrists have been asked to testify about an individual's ability to fulfill rather than to enter into a contract. Mental illness occurring after the time of the making of an agreement—at the time of performance—may excuse a failure to perform the obligations of the contract. The case may arise, for example, of an actor who, during the contract period of his services, suffers a severe depression. An actress may become pregnant and unable to perform. In such events, the mental or physical disability may excuse the obligations of both contracting parties: in the actor's case because of his inability to perform and the employer's because of his failure of consideration.

The longer the term of employment, the greater the possibility of encountering difficulties in fulfilling it. There are limitations, though, on the term period. The free enterprise system would be circumvented were long-term contracts of employment enforced as a matter of course. The Code Napoleon, adopted in the aftermath of the French Revolution, limits the contractual period for personal services to 1 year, the original purpose of the provision being to preclude contracts that would have resulted in a return to serfdom or slavery. The Louisiana Civil Code, steeped in the French code, specifically provides, "A man can only hire out his services for a certain limited time, or for the performance of a certain enterprise." Free enterprise notwithstanding, one proviso everywhere in the United States is that skilled employees who have trade secrets may be barred from working for a competitor; they may leave their jobs only to engage in noncompetitive work or go unemployed.

Many of the early immigrants to America, where "no white man acknowledged a master," bound themselves to service for a period of years after arriving in the land that "flowed with milk and honey." The greater numbers of immigrants were bound to the captain of the ship for their passage to America. On arrival in the port of entry, merchants were on hand to purchase the services of the immigrants who contracted their labors for periods of several years. During that time, they received no salary, only lodging, food, and clothing; their lot was a hard one.

In all jurisdictions, personal performance is discharged by any illness, which makes it "impossible or seriously injurious to health." The excuse makes allowances for the accidents and fragility of human life. A note from the doctor, which is obtained to excuse school attendance, serves other excuses as well. (Football coaches, however, need no excuse; they apparently may quit on a whim.) A number of companies have developed for their employees a "compassionate leave policy." An official of the American Society for Personnel Administration says, however, that the thought of paying for maternity time off repels some employers. "To pay a woman a salary during that period, when maternity is a matter of her choice, grates a little bit." The Equal Employment Opportunity Commission states that pregnancy, miscarriage, abortion, childbirth, and recovery are "temporary disabilities and should be treated as such." On the other hand, while mental or physical disability of an employee may excuse inadequate performance or nonperformance, it is increasingly serving less as a justification for the employer to send him away. Tenure and union practices and the developing concept of a right to a job are restrictions on the employer's rights to dismiss an employee. (The president, though, begins his administration with the "resignations" in hand of his appointments.) Difficulties resulting from old age are generally avoided by mandatory retirement; the inflexibility of the rule, though, is subject to much criticism.

In socialist countries, the right to a job turned into a duty to work. One who did not work was regarded as a parasite. In Soviet ideology, work was seen not only as a material but also as a moral necessity. Checks and counterchecks and various types of stimuli urged the worker to produce more and more, faster and faster. At countless meetings speakers told about superb achievements. In the case of alleged inability to work, a certificate of one physician was obtained to excuse a brief absence and of a three-member panel for a long-term absence. During the days of the Soviet Union, it was quipped, "everyone has a job but no one works."

It may be concluded that while in theory the law of contracts has a role for psychiatry, practice shows that psychiatry has essentially influenced the law of contracts very little. The test of capacity to contract, with a few exceptional cases, has remained essentially the same for centuries. Supervening problems relating to performance are examined in terms of the traditional impossibility concept. Qualitative differences between mental disorders, as related to the type of transaction, and foreseeability of illness or disability are issues that remain relatively unexplored.

Endnotes

1. Dexter v. Hall, 82 U.S. 9 (1872).
2. Mich. Comp. Laws Ann. 445.903(1)(x).
3. D.L. Perkins, "Unfair Trade Practices Under the Michigan Consumer Protection Act: A Movement Toward Uniformity," *Detroit Coll. L. Rev.* (1977): 855.
4. In Zinermon v. Burch, 494 U.S. 113 (1990), the U.S. Supreme Court held that a voluntary admission must be based on "express and informed consent." The individual thought he was entering heaven. Given his condition, the Court concluded that the hospital knew or should have known that he was

incapable of giving informed consent. He should have been given the procedural safeguards required for an involuntary commitment. See B. Winick, "Competency to Consent to Voluntary Hospitalization: A Therapeutic Jurisprudence Analysis of *Zinermon v. Burch*," *Int. J. of Law & Psychiat.* 14 (1991): 169.

5. Committee on Professional Ethics v. Shepler, 519 N.W.2d 92 (Iowa 1994).

6. See E. Drought, "Navigating Scylla and Charybdis: *In re* Briese, Gambling and Credit Card Debt Dischargeability," *Wis. L. Rev.* 1997: 1323. The psychodynamics of compulsive gambling is discussed in E. Bergler, *The Psychology of Gambling* (London: Hanison, 1958).

7. There are a number of national organizations with local affiliates or chapters that provide help for compulsive spenders: Debtors Anonymous, Overcomers Outreach, Shopaholics Limited. Carolyn Wesson's book *Women Who Shop Too Much* (New York: St. Martin's Press), a self-help guide, focuses on the problem of shopping and spending as well as in-depth steps to recovery for compulsive shoppers. It is estimated that one in seven people are hooked on buying items they will not use. See J.B. Twitchell, *Lead Us Into Temptation: The Triumph of American Materialism* (New York: Columbia University Press, 1999); P. Underhill, *Why We Buy* (New York: Simon & Schuster, 1999); T. Serju, "Shopping Addiction Takes Effort to Cure," *Detroit News*, Aug. 14, 1995, p. F-6. "Whoever said money can't buy happiness did not know where to shop," said Gertrude Stein.

8. W.F.H. Cook, "Mental Deficiency and the English Law of Contracts," *Colum. L. Rev.* 21 (1921): 424. Protection is provided against deception in the criminal law as well as in the civil law. The criminal law makes it a crime to misappropriate or take anything of value either without the owner's consent or by means of fraudulent conduct, practices, or representations. In traditional criminal law, however, larceny did not follow from fraud because a type of consent was secured. The current criminal codes usually set out a crime of theft that provides that a defrauder is guilty of theft if the transaction between the parties could be avoided because of fraud. See, e.g., La. Rev. Stat. 14:67(A). Full-time consumer complaint desks have been instituted in many district attorney offices. In the median city, the desk averages between 20 and 30 calls a day. Complaints investigated have been mainly in reference to automobile dealers, home repairs, insurance salesmen, job placement agencies, and real estate agencies.

9. Ellars v. Mossbarger, 9 Ill. App. 122 (1881).

10. Eubanks v. Eubanks, 360 Ill. 101, 195 N.E. 521 (1935).

11. Professor Weihofen wrote:

    [A]lthough the courts formulate the issue in terms of subjective "understanding," they actually rely on more objective standards of behavior because whether a person had a subjective state of mind can never been directly known, it can only be inferred from objective conduct. It is perhaps correct to say that the objective evidence upon which courts place most reliance is the "normality" or "abnormality" of the particular transaction in question. The essential question, as the courts seem to view it, is: Was this transaction so foolish or irrational that it shows the person did not adequately understand what he was doing? This factor is given so much weight that Professor Green called it "the key to an inarticulate standard." The dominant evidentiary factor "is whether the court sees the particular transaction in its results as that which a reasonable man might have made."

    H. Weihofen, "Mental Incompetency to Contract or Convey," *So. Cal. L. Rev.* 39 (1966): 225.

12. E.W. Puttkammer, *Administration of Criminal* (Chicago: University of Chicago Press, 1953), p. 164.

13. "Internal compulsion" does not invalidate a confession. In Colorado v. Connelly, 479 U.S. 157 (1986), the defendant approached a police officer, stating, without any prompting, that he had murdered someone and wanted to talk about it. He was immediately advised of his *Miranda* rights. He said he wished to confess because "his conscience had been bothering him." The next day he said "voices" had come to him. He "followed the directions of voices in confessing." The trial court and the state Supreme Court, affirming, said that an individual's capacity for "rational judgment and free choice may be overborne as much by certain forms of severe mental illness as by external pressure." People v. Connelly, 702 P.2d 722, 728 (Colo. 1985). Reversing the decision, the U.S. Supreme Court ruled that a confession is involuntary only when there is coercive police activity; 479 U.S. at 164.

14. People v. Stanis, 41 Mich. App. 565, 200 N.W.2d 473 (1972).

15. In Kendall v. Ewert, 259 U.S. 139 (1922), the transactor was a common and habitual drunkard, of which the transactee had knowledge and caused the transactor to part with valuable mineral lands for the insignificant sum of $700.

16. Usually, necessities are considered to consist of those things reasonably necessary for the support, maintenance, and comfort of the incompetent person according to his status and condition in life. The term necessities thus includes food and clothing as well as needed medical services and the costs of hospitalization in a mental institution. Chandler v. Prichard, 321 S.W.2d 891 (Tex. Civ. App. 1959)

(medical services including nursing and other usual services rendered a person of unsound mind constitute necessities). But see Woolbert v. Lee Lumber Co., 151 Miss. 56, 117 So. 354 (1928; house is not a necessity).

17. Fortenberry v. Herrington, 188 Miss. 735, 196 So. 232 (1940). An example of unconscionability upsetting a contract is illustrated by Weaver v. American Oil Co., 276 N.E.2d 144 (Ind. 1971), which held unconscionable a lease containing a clause that not only exculpated the lessor oil company from its liability from negligence, but also compelled the lessee to indemnify the lessor for any damages or loss incurred as a result of its negligence. The litigation arose as a result of the oil company's employee spraying gasoline over the lessee, his assistant, and the leased premises, resulting in burns and injuries to each man. The Indiana Supreme Court ruled that the contract was unconscionable, as defined by the Uniform Commercial Code, pointing out that the lessee had left high school after only one and a half years and had spent his time, prior to leasing the service station, working at various skilled and unskilled labor-oriented jobs. "He was not one who should be expected to know the law or understand the meaning of technical terms . ... There is nothing in the record to indicate that [the lessee] read the lease; that the agent asked [the lessee] to read it; or that the agent, in any manner, attempted to call [the lessee's] attention to the 'hold harmless' clause in the lease." The court observed that whenever one party drafts a contract and the other will not read it, the drafter makes an implied warranty to the other party that there is nothing hidden in the fine print that is either unconscionable or unusual; 276 N.E.2d at 145.

18. Stratton v. Grant, 139 Cal. App.2d 814, 294 P.2d 500 (1956). From the original settlers, the Indians got beads and liquor for their land, but, except to the Indians, that is past history.

19. S. Williston, *A Treatise on the Law of Contracts* (New York: Baker, Voorhis, 1936), vol. 1, p. 741 .

20. See J.H. Gold & J.C. Nemiah (Eds.), *Beyond Transference: When the Therapist's Real Life Intrudes* (Washington, DC: American Psychiatric Press, 1993); R.I. Simon, "The Practice of Psychotherapy: Legal Liabilities of an 'Impossible' Profession," in R.I. Simon (Ed.), *Review of Clinical Psychiatry and the Law* (Washington, DC: American Psychiatric Press, 1991), vol. 2, p. 25 .

21. B. Northrup, "Psychotherapy Faces a Stubborn Problem: Abuses by Therapists," *Wall Street Journal*, Oct. 29, 1986, p. 1.

22. "Incompetency Resulting From Senile Dementia," *Am. Jur. & Proof of Facts* 10 (1961): 385.

23. They included author Truman Capote, movie director Cecil B. DeMille, singer Eddie Fisher, President and Mrs. Jack Kennedy, playwright Alan Jay Lerner, Rep. Claude Pepper, movie director Otto Preminger, fashion designer Emilio Pucci, actor Anthony Quinn, and playwright Tennessee Williams.

24. The doctor reported that he gave President Jack Kennedy injections for the summit meeting with Premier Nikita Khrushchev. Movie director Cecil B. DeMille in his autobiography says that he took the doctor along to Egypt as his guest and personal physician during the filming of *The Ten Commandments*. Actor Eddie Fisher often wined and dined the doctor in Hollywood and Las Vegas and, it is said, did not like to open an act without the doctor in the wings. But some of the patients complained of bad reactions and enslaving addictions to amphetamines. According to the Federal Bureau of Narcotics and Dangerous Drugs, which investigated the doctor at different times over almost 5 years, a review of the doctor's records showed that he could not account for a substantial quantity of amphetamines that had been purchased.

25. R.C. Allen, E.Z. Ferster & H. Weihofen, *Mental Impairment and Legal Incompetency* (Englewood Cliffs, NJ: Prentice-Hall, 1968), p. 266.

26. 15. F. Supp. 1020 (W.D. N.Y. 1936).

27. 146 Misc. 100, 261 N.Y.S. 557 (1933).

28. 40 Misc. 2d 212, 242 N.Y.S.2d 763 (1963); noted in *N.Y.L.U. Rev.* 39 (1964): 356.

29. 25 N.Y.2d 196, 250 N.E. 2d 460, 303 N.Y.S. 2d 362 (1969); noted in *Brooklyn L. Rev.* 36 (1969): 145; *N.Y.U. L. Rev.* 45 (1970): 585; *Wayne L. Rev.* 16 (1970): 1188.

30. The court emphasized that "the system was, or should have been fully aware of Mrs. Ortelere's condition." The court emphasized the "special relationship" between a retirement system and its members. See also Keith v. New York State Teachers' Retirement System, 46 A.D.2d 938, 362 N.Y.S. 2d 231 (1974). Many employers found their pension plans through professional insurers, who are not likely to know of an employee's psychosis. In Pentinen v. Retirement System, 60 A.D.2d 366, 401 N.Y.S.2d 587 (3d Dept. 1978), the court held that the widow of a state employee shown to have been suffering a psychosis could not withdraw her election to receive retirement benefits from the State Employees' Retirement System in the form of a life annuity because the incompetency was not known to the system; her grief alone was not enough to give the system notice of the incompetency.

31. 588 So.2d 879, 883 (Ala. 1991).

32. Restatement (Second) of Contracts §15 states a test of contractual capacity in terms of both cognition and volition. The Pennsylvania Supreme Court in McGovern v. Com., State Employees Retirement Board, 512 Pa. 377, 517 A.2d 523 (1986), specifically rejected §15 and appeared to adhere to a cognitive test: "If the benefit contract is freely entered into with an understanding of its terms, the contract cannot be set aside."
33. See Chapter 11 on criminal responsibility.
34. Rescission of contract because of alleged manic depressive state was denied in Fingerhut v. Kralyn Enterprises, 71 Misc.2d 846, 337 N.Y.S.2d 394 (1971); the plaintiff failed to sustain his burden of proof that when he executed the contract he "did so solely as a result of serious mental illness, namely, psychosis." Another case, which was settled without trial, involved a man, about 50 years of age, married, with four children, who suffered from manic depressive periods. He was treated at Lafayette Clinic, Detroit, Michigan, in 1969 for depression. He was a partner in a fur business in a Detroit suburb, and the business was relatively successful. He was conscientious in his business endeavors, but had difficulty during occasional states of depression. In 1972, he became hypomanic for 5 to 6 months. His symptoms included a decrease in sleep, rapid speech, extravagance, distractability, and a general feeling of well-being.

During this period he made three trips to Las Vegas. On the first trip, he spent the money he had brought gambling and then wrote a check payable to the casino for about $2,000. This pattern he repeated on the second trip, when he wrote a check for about $4,000. These two checks were paid upon presentation. On the third trip, the casino extended him credit, after he had lost his cash reserve. After signing a document, he was given chips, totaling many times what he had spent on the previous trips.

Query: Should he be relieved of the responsibilities of fulfilling his contractual obligations, i.e. paying the debt? He understood the transaction in which he had engaged. He was not induced to enter into the transaction by any illegal undue influence, fraud, or overreaching. And the parties can be returned to the status quo, a usual prerequisite to void the contract of an incompetent, only by payment of the money. But this requirement may be excused when one party is aware of the other's incapacity. Las Vegas thrives on people who are in a flamboyant and optimistic state of mind; it does its best to stimulate manic behavior. The illumination of the *Money Game* by Adam Smith is Keynes' observation that the investment game (the stock market) is intolerably boring save to those with a gambling instinct, while those with the instinct must pay to it "the appropriate toll."

A young man proposing marriage tells his girlfriend, "I want to give you all the things you've never had. I think I can get a bank loan." The bank, aware of the purpose of the loan, makes it. Was the transaction the result of mental illness or defect, and was the young man able to act in a reasonable manner in relation to the transaction? See B.D. Lewin, *The Psychoanalysis of Elation* (New York: Norton, 1950). To speak thoughtfully, Thoreau said in *Walden*, we must be far enough apart so that "all animal heat and moisture may have a chance to evaporate." See E.T. Hall, *The Hidden Dimension* (New York: Doubleday, 1966). For the view that the right to make or enforce a contract should not be abridged by the label of mental illness, see G.J. Alexander & T.S. Szasz, "From Contract to Status Via Psychiatry," *Santa Clara L. Rev.* 13: (1973): 537.
35. R.G. Blumenthal, "After All These Years, Here Is the Fourth Face of Eve: Plaintiff," *Wall Street Journal*, Feb. 1, 1989, p. B1; N.J. Easton, "The Real 'Eve' Faces Court Battle Over Biography," *Detroit News*, Feb. 13, 1989, p. B3; D. Van Biema & M. Grant, "Three Faces of Eve Told Her Story, Now Chris Sizemore Is Battling a Major Studio Over Movie Rights and Wrongs," *People*, March 1989, p. 79.
36. "'Faces of Eve' Woman Settles Film Co. Lawsuit," *New York City Tribune*, June 21, 1990, p. 5. Robert K. Ressler, then director of the FBI's Forensic Behavioral Services, mused that the greatest difficulty in inviting Chris Sizemore to speak was that because she had three personalities, they would have to triple their regular honorarium. R.K. Ressler & T. Shachtman, *Whoever Fight Monsters* (New York: St. Martin's Press, 1992), p. 269.
37. *60 Minutes*, CBS, Oct. 22, 1989.
38. 344 F.Supp. 373, 387 (M.D. Ala 1972).
39. D. Blain, *Better Care in Mental Hospitals* (Washington, DC: American Psychiatric Association, 1949), p. 43.
40. Streda Estate, 137 Legal Intel. No. 97, p. 1, col. 3 (Del. Cy. Orphans Ct., 1957); see J. Parry, S.J. Brakel, & B. Weiner, *The Mentally Disabled and the Law* (Chicago: American Bar Foundation, 3rd ed., 1985).
41. French v. Blackburn, 428 F. Supp. 1351, 1361 (M.D. N.C. 1977), *aff'd*, 443 U.S. 901 (1979).
42. 73 Cal. App. 3d 952, 141 Cal. Rptr. 234 (1977).

43. Ordinarily statutes set out the powers and duties of a guardian in a general way and articulated in the court's order of appointment. Frequently, however, statutes specifically withhold certain powers, or require court approval before taking certain actions; Kansas Stat. Ann. 59-3018.

44. Banker's Trust Co. v. Russell, 263 Mich. 677, 249 N.W. 27 (1933).

45. Mich. Comp. Laws Ann. § 700.8(2).

46. Mich. Comp. Laws Ann. § 700.443.

47. Mich. Comp. Laws Ann. § 700.443(1).

48. See E.F. Dejowski, *Protecting Judgment-Impaired Adults* (Binghamton, NY: Haworth Press, 1990); D.J. Sprehe, "Geriatric Psychiatry and the Law," in R. Rosner (Ed.), *Principles and Practice of Forensic Psychiatry*, (New York: Von Nostrand Reinhold, 1994), pp. 501; J.W. Fisher, "Legal Aspects of the Psychosocial Management of the Demented Patient," *Psychiat. Ann.* 24 (1994): 197; W.C. Schmidt & R. Peters, "Legal Incompetents' Need for Guardians in Florida," *Bull. Am. Acad. Psychiat. & Law* 15 (1987): 69.

49. T.S. Szasz & G.J. Alexander, "Law, Property and Psychiatry," *Am. J. Orthopsychiat.* 42 (1972): 610; Response: A.A. Stone, "Law, Property, and Liberty: A Polemic That Fails," *Am. J. Orthopsychiat.* 42 (1972): 627.

50. G.T. Grossberg, "Determining Mental Competence in Older Adults," *Psychiatric News*, Sept. 2, 1994, p. 13.

51. A guardian is sometimes called a conservator, curator, committee, tutor, or fiduciary. The guardian may have limited responsibilities or full control over all decisions. In some states a guardian makes personal decisions, such as whether to place the ward in a nursing home, and a conservator makes financial decisions.

52. See, e.g., Mich. Comp. Laws Ann. § 700.8(2).

53. Mich. Comp. Laws Ann. § 700.455.

54. A durable power of attorney for healthcare and other decisions can also be used if the individual becomes incapacitated. Standards in appointing a guardian are vague. Hearings typically take less than 15 minutes. Supervision of guardians is poor. As a rule, guardians are supposed to notify the court of decisions made on behalf of a ward and in some states they must get permission before making major expenditures or decisions. However, there is usually minimal oversight and a judge may give a guardian's report only a cursory glance.

55. D. Starkman, "Guardians May Need Someone to Watch Over Them," *Wall Street Journal*, May 8, 1998, p. B-1.

56. The legislation, known by its initials OBRA, enacted in 1987, calls for documentation to justify the use of antipsychotic medication.

57. See "Debate, Cameras in Nursing Homes," *USA Today*, Sept. 21, 1999, p. 18.

23
Testamentary Capacity

Unlike contracts, testaments (otherwise called *wills*) require judicial approval; they are admitted to probate. The word *will* originally referred only to bequests of land while *testament* was reserved for bequests from one's personal effects, but today the words are used synonymously or, as in the expression "last will and testament" (the term "dead giveaway" is sometimes used colloquially).

In the event of a challenge of the capacity of the testator to write the will, the capacity must be determined postmortem, the testator being dead at the time of the controversy. Even the most careful lawyer seldom makes a video or tape recording of the execution of the will or calls in a psychiatrist to examine the testator at the time the will is executed, but even that type of evidence is not conclusive.[1]

"Where there is a will, there is a way to break it," it is said, but it occurs only in the exceptional case. Of all wills probated in the course of a year, apparently not more than 3 percent are contested and, of these contests, not more than 15 percent are successful. In view of that slight risk, such precautions as having psychiatrists present at the making of the will are not deemed appropriate. Wills are usually attested before two witnesses, but they are not essential witnesses at the probate of the will; they are present at the making of the will solely to give solemnity to the event.

Our concern is: In what way is psychiatric evaluation of the testator, either at the time of the execution of the will or postmortem, of value to the court in assessing testamentary capacity? Often, the only ground available by which a disappointed heir can contest a decedent's will is an alleged lack of testamentary capacity at the time of the making of the will. To establish either capacity or incapacity, when capacity is challenged, psychiatric testimony is usually summoned.

The tactic usually resorted to when there are no other challenges to the will is to attack the capacity of the testator to make a will. In the inquiry it is asked: Was the testator aware that he was signing his will? Could the testator appraise the quantity and the quality of property? Did he understand who were his legal heirs? Inability to pass that test may be due to, among other things, senile dementia, mental enfeeblement, or delirium. The will, however, may have been made during a lucid interval. It is very difficult for a contestant to establish that the will was not made during a lucid interval.[2]

Eccentricities, unjustified prejudices, or peculiar beliefs or opinions do not of themselves establish lack of mental capacity, although they may be given consideration. The provisions of a will depend on the health, mental condition, and surroundings of the testator. A will rationally made out in a lawyer's office in the testator's prime of life may be thrown aside by the testator during the last days of illness or senility and replaced with a totally different will that is unfair and even ridiculous—unfair in the sense that relatives and lifelong companions and employees are dropped in favor of a new passing acquaintance. In a moment of the testator's senility, vindictiveness, anger, helplessness, or humor, the testament may take a dismaying turn.

According to theory, if an individual has testamentary capacity, freedom of testation allows his will to be as unjust and capricious as his desires may dictate. "One has the right to make an unjust will, an unreasonable will, or even a cruel will."[3] This freedom of testation is quite in contrast with prior history.

Real property (land), the principal source of wealth, was not in early history subject to testamentary disposition. All land was held on behalf of the lord, and it was laid down as a rule of law that land was not subject to a devise. A medieval feudal lord might occasionally permit his tenant to make a post obit gift (as he might also acquiesce in an *inter vivos* alienation), but the devisee was obligated to pay the lord a heavy price to obtain possession. As obligations owed to the lord were ancillary to the possession of land, he was cautious about a change of tenants. Among the lord's rights was the *jus primae noctis* (right of the first night); a diversion of the land from the heirs to a stranger by devise would tend to weaken or undercut feudal obligations. Thus, in the case of realty, the common law evolved a strict rule of primogeniture, which may be called a principle of "first come, first served," whereby a tenant's land, on his death, would descend to his eldest son. Feudal society was a fixed society.

The ecclesiastical courts had sole jurisdiction over deathbed gifts of personal property (personalty), but were allowed no rights over realty. The church instilled the fear of a spiritual ban by refusing absolution to those who died intestate and, thus, encouraged testamentary dispositions of personalty. There was a close connection between the last will and the last confession, fostered by the church, which asserted the right to control and force gifts by will for pious purposes. In primitive times, the possessions of a deceased person went to whoever got there first and grabbed them. The family and others often hovered around like a flock of vultures. Later in the course of history, clergymen called in to perform the last rites were asked to write down the wishes of the dying man. By the 13th century, wills of personal property had developed from mere deathbed distributions into wills in the modern sense. Wills became ambulatory, that is, they included property acquired after, as well as before, the making of the will and were revocable at any time before the testator's death. The will was not required to be in any particular form.

With the passing of time, public interest increasingly demanded that land be freely alienable, and the claims of the lord had to give way. During the 15th and early part of the 16th centuries, it became a common practice of a tenant to convert property to a friend to hold it for use and benefit of the tenant or third party in order to avoid certain feudal incidents. After enactment of the Statute of Uses in 1535, legal title was vested in the party for whom the use of the land was created. A consequence of this statute was a loss of the power, which had developed to transmit a use estate through wills. Shortly thereafter, in 1540, the enactment of the Statute of Wills allowed a limited power to devise land by an instrument in writing. Since then, there has been an almost unbroken policy in favor of freedom of testation. It is interesting to note that such testaments are designated as wills, indicating freedom of determination.[4]

The policy underlying the prohibition against the transfer of land, while strengthening the institution of feudalism, also protected the heir against dissipation of the inheritance by the ancestor. Along with the rule of free testation were developed means to avoid the so-called unnatural disposition. Some jurisdictions provided that a certain portion of the estate must go to children, who were called forced heirs. Most reliance was placed, though, on the concepts of testamentary capacity and undue influence. Life insurance, though, is not governed by testamentary concepts and may even circumvent forced heirs.

Criteria for Testamentary Capacity

The statutes of the various states usually provide that in order to be capable of making a will, the person must have a "sound and disposing mind and memory," leaving to the courts the determination of capacity in each case. Only Georgia by statute defined testamentary capacity and the effect of specific mental aberrations. Its statutory provisions begin by stating that "every person may make a will, unless laboring under some legal disability arising either from a want of capacity or a want of perfect liberty of action."[5] The subsequent sections stated:

The amount of intellect necessary to constitute testamentary capacity is that which is necessary to enable the party to have a decided and rational desire as to the disposition of his property. His desire must be decided, as distinguished from the wavering, vacillating fancies of a distempered intellect. It must be rational, as distinguished from the ravings of a madman, the silly prating of an idiot, the childish whims of imbecility, or the excited vagaries of a drunkard.

Infants under 14 years of age are considered wanting in that discretion necessary to make a will.

An insane person generally will not make a will. A lunatic may, during a lucid interval. A monomaniac may make a will, if the will is in no way the result of or connected with his monomania. In all such cases, it must appear that the will speaks the wishes of the testator, unbiased by the mental disease with which he is affected.

Eccentricity of habit or thought does not deprive a person of the power of making a will; old age and weakness of intellect resulting therefrom do not of [themselves], constitute incapacity. If that weakness amounts to imbecility, the testamentary capacity is gone.

In cases of doubt as to the extent of this weakness, the reasonable or unreasonable disposition of the [person's] estate should have much weight in the decision of the question.

Conviction of crime shall not deprive a person of the power of making a will.

A person deaf, dumb, and blind may make a will, provided both the interpreter and the scrivener are attesting witnesses thereto and are examined upon the petition for probate of the same. In such cases, strict scrutiny into the transaction should precede the admission of the paper to record.

The very nature of a will requires that it should be freely and voluntarily executed; hence, anything which destroys this freedom of volition invalidates a will, such as fraudulent practices upon testator's fears, affections, or sympathies, duress or any other influence, whereby the will of another is substituted for the wishes of the testator.

A will procured by misrepresentation or fraud of any kind, to the injury of the heirs at law, is void.[6]

These provisions of the Georgia law were taken from a very long opinion in an 1848 case in which the main authority cited was *Shelford on Lunacy* written in 1833.[7] Interestingly enough, articles on testamentary capacity that have been written in recent years by psychiatrists or others offer essentially the same observations, with some change in terminology.

In the various jurisdictions, where the criteria are made by a judge, the courts uniformly state that at the time the testator makes his will, he must be capable of knowing, without prompting, (1) the nature of the act he is making, (2) the nature and extent of his property, and (3) the natural objects of his bounty and their claims upon him. In deciding whether these criteria have been met in a particular case, the court is guided by the individual facts of the case, hence, unlike in constitutional law, for example, the cases do not lend themselves to deep legal analysis.

While the specific requirements for mental capacity to make a will are minimal, the necessary capacity requires a greater mental competency than is required for marriage. A person may have insufficient capacity to make a will on the same day as the person has sufficient capacity to marry.[8] Thus, an old man suffering from cerebral arteriosclerosis may be able to marry, but not make a will. Marriage alone will give the surviving spouse a share of the senile spouse's estate, even though he has no capacity to devise it to her.[9]

1. *Nature of act*: The testator must know he is executing a will. This does not mean that the testator comprehends the possible legal effects of the words he employs, but that he realizes the import of the act. In usual practice, the lawyer writes the will and reads it to the testator, who thereupon signs it. Most vengeful wills are written by the testator by hand, without benefit of a lawyer, and are probably written in the heat of anger. A testator who was toxic, confused, or did not recognize anyone at the time of the writing very possibly did not appreciate the nature of the act he was performing. This requirement is of particular importance in the case of the deathbed will where the testator may not have consciousness of what he is signing.

2. *Nature and extent of property*: The omission by a testator from his will of important parts of his property might indicate such a lack of memory as to constitute testamentary incapacity. The capacity to dispose of an estate may depend upon its size and complexity.

3. *Natural objects of bounty*: The natural objects of the testator's bounty usually include his blood relatives, but may include others as well. The old notion of bequeathing a child a penny anticipates a future effort to contest the will on grounds of testamentary capacity. A testator's failure to mention a child could be deemed lack of memory. According to this notion, the protection of the family afforded by the testamentary capacity limitation lies not so much in preventing the testator from pauperizing his family as in preventing his pauperizing them without first considering them. The testator mentions his child: "My child married without my consent. I consider her as though she was never born." The film star Joan Crawford disinherited her children "for reasons known to them"; she left her fortune to charity. By noting their existence, she indicated that she was aware of the natural objects of her bounty, but she chose to disinherit them.

Failure to have knowledge of the elements—nature of act, knowledge of property, and natural objects of bounty—constitutes, in the usual rhetoric, lack of sound and disposing mind and memory. Sometimes, instead of using these three elements as the criteria of a sound mind, a court may say that the lack of knowledge must be the product of an unsound mind (whatever that is) in order for there to be testamentary incapacity. The mere fact of the testator having used drugs of the type that could influence the functioning of the mind would not necessarily deprive the testator of testamentary capacity or would not necessarily render him susceptible to undue influence.

The concept of *lucid interval* is used as a defense of a will that is contested when the testator is known to have been severely demented or mentally ill for some time. For instance, if the testator was schizophrenic, the court will probably find the will valid if written during a lucid period, but not if it was related to a delusion. To determine whether the will was written during a lucid or delusional period, the expert, in order to be persuasive, must interview people who had contact with the testator at the time of the writing of the will—say, neighbors or the clerk at the bank— and also other evidence, such as a diary.

Given the criteria for testamentary capacity, what type of questions may properly be asked of an expert concerning the capacity of a testator to make a will (or a grantor involving a deed)? The principle is that it is improper to ask an expert for an opinion of a party's "mental capacity to make a will" because the answer would constitute a legal conclusion or would not be helpful to the court. The issue of capacity to make a will is one for the jury. Moreover, a question phrased in those terms is improper because it assumes that the expert is aware of the legal standard of competence required to execute a will. Thus, it is improper to ask the expert: "Do you think the testator has sufficient mental capacity to declare his last will and testament and dispose of his property?"[10] In addition to expert testimony, the mental capacity of the testator is often addressed by having lay witnesses describe the testator's behavior at the time of signing of the will.[11]

By and large, the courts disallow answers to questions that involve a direct answer as to an individual's capacity to execute a will or a deed. Incorporating one or more phrases of the legal definition of capacity has resulted in a host of inconsistent decisions. As a rule, answers to questions phrased in terms of the legal definition of testamentary capacity are held to be admissible because such questions do not require the witness to base his conclusions on anything other than the question asked and his knowledge of the testator's mental condition.

Conditions Affecting Capacity

The following conditions are discussed in court opinions in determining whether the testator was of unsound mind.

Organic Brain Damage

Brain injuries, syphilitic infection, chronic encephalitis, congenital brain anomalies, and epilepsy may render a testator incompetent to execute a will. Organic brain damage interferes with one's cognitive capacity. Wills of the elderly are most subject to challenge, usually on the basis of organic brain disease. Old age has traditionally prompted charges of senility from disgruntled heirs and would-be beneficiaries.[12] While senility is not purely a chronological fact, common infirmities of old age are Alzheimer's disease, senile psychosis or senile dementia, and cerebral arteriosclerosis. These syndromes are characterized by impairment of memory, symptoms of confusion and disorientation, and paranoid delusions. There may be fluctuating levels of consciousness or, as the courts put it, "lucid intervals" or "glimmers of reason" that may sustain capacity.

Bodily Infirmity or Disease

Any injury or disease, of sufficient severity, is capable of causing at least temporary derangement. Psychotic conditions frequently follow toxic conditions of the blood stream, such as uremia. Severe infections, such as typhoid fever and pneumonia, may result in delirium. Testimony by the testator's physician about his bodily conditions is thus relevant on the issue of testamentary capacity.

Mental Deficiency

Mental deficiency may impair the testator's ability to know the natural objects of his bounty or to recall the nature and extent of his property. Illiteracy may be probative of mental deficiency.

Alcohol or Drug Condition

Hallucinations or paranoid delusions may result from alcohol or drug intoxication. Excessive use of alcohol or drugs over an extended duration may produce permanent degeneration of the brain. Psychological effects are also produced by drugs administered to alleviate pain in terminal patients. In all these cases, delusions may influence the provisions of a testament.

Psychological State of Mind

Belief in witchcraft, spiritual influences, religious fanaticism, or eccentricity does not in itself render the testator incapable of executing a valid will.[13] W.C. Fields, who hated Christmas, used to say menacingly to his relatives, "Nobody who observes Christmas will be mentioned in my last testament."

Of the many cases involving an eccentric testator is the famous 1944 Michigan case, *In re Johnson's Estate*,[14] where the testatrix, a spinster, willed her estate to the Humane Society for the care of cats and dogs. Her nephew, who was expressly left out of the will, claimed that the testatrix lacked testamentary capacity and that he was omitted from her will because she had an insane delusion and false belief that he was a worthless character and was trying to get her money and property. No medical testimony was given as to the mental condition of the testatrix. The evidence tendered to defeat the will indicated only that the testatrix lived and conducted herself in a rather eccentric and abnormal manner. To sway the court that the testatrix was under an insane delusion, the nephew entered into evidence her eccentricities: she kept numerous animals in her house, spent time in jail for her role in political suffrage, smoked cigars, and in the winter wore male long underwear and boots. In the later years of her life, her principal interest appears to have been in dogs and cats, which were given free use of her home and premises.[15]

In the aforecited case, the Michigan Supreme Court, quoting authority, said: "An eccentric person may make a will, and eccentricity of conduct is not sufficient, of itself, to invalidate a will. Singularity should not be confounded with insanity, and eccentricities, bad manners, and grotesque conduct, generally, are not evidence of insanity, especially where they are normal to the testator." The court went on to rule that the testatrix was not suffering from an insane delusion regarding the nephew. The testatrix's opinion that the nephew was a worthless person may have been erroneous, the court said, but it was not an insane delusion affecting her testamentary capacity.

Many people, especially as they grow older, lose patience with those around them. An incidental occurrence may take on larger and larger proportions, until the testator concludes that the action had great significance. The testator may then retaliate by cutting the alleged offender out of his will. This situation may ultimately lead to a will contest based on the testator's capacity. The challenger claims the belief is an insane delusion and attempts to void the will.

Insane Delusion

As a general rule, courts do not reform or invalidate wills because of mistake, whereas they do invalidate wills resulting from an insane delusion. Suppose, for example, that the testator falsely believes that her son has been killed and therefore executes a will leaving all her property to her daughter. In fact the son is alive. The testator is mistaken, not under an insane delusion, and the will is entitled to probate.[16]

Long ago, in 1896 in *Rivard v. Rivard*,[17] the Michigan Supreme Court set out different examples of an insane delusion that would invalidate a will: Where a testator disinherits a daughter in the belief that she is a bad woman or that she is not his own offspring, or a son in the belief that he is a drunkard, or his grandchildren in the belief that their father (the testator's son-in-law) has threatened to kill him. The court went on to discuss that if there is no foundation in fact for such beliefs, then they are delusions, and the will is void. This is true even if the testator is entirely sane on all other subjects, and fully competent to manage his life and business affairs.

How is a delusion distinguished from a mistake? As commonly put, a delusion, unlike a mistake, is not susceptible to correction when the individual is told the truth; it is not subject to a reality check. One who is not delusional *possesses* an idea, while one who is delusional is possessed *by* an idea. Among those suffering mental disorder, schizophrenics are most likely to be delusional. The *Diagnostic and Statistical Manual of Mental Disorders* (*DSM*), drawing on the work of Karl Jaspers, defines a delusion as:

> A false personal belief based on an incorrect inference about external reality and firmly sustained, in spite of what almost everyone else believes, and in spite of what constitutes incontrovertible and obvious proof of evidence to the contrary. The belief is not one ordinarily accepted by other members of the person's culture or subculture.[18]

The law uses the term *insane delusion* (not simply *delusion*). The Michigan Supreme Court, citing earlier cases, provided the following definition:

An insane delusion exists when a person persistently believes supposed facts that have no real existence, and so believes such supposed facts against all evidence and probabilities and without any foundation or reason for the belief, and conducts himself as if such facts actually existed. … If there are any facts, however little evidential force they may possess, upon which the testator may in reason have based his belief, it will not be an insane delusion, though on a consideration of the facts themselves his belief may seem illogical and foundationless to the court; for a will, it is obvious, is not to be overturned merely because the testator has not reasoned correctly.[19]

This concept has been dubbed the "any facts" test, meaning that if there is any factual basis or reason for the alleged insane belief, there will be no finding of an insane delusion.

The determination of falsity is easy when the delusion is clearly bizarre and arises from internal morbid processes, as in the case of the old childless woman who believed that her baby was being withheld from her in the hospital ward refrigerator. The determination is also easy when the interpretation on which the delusion is based is clearly autistic, as in the case of the man who mentioned that when he entered a public bathroom he saw a piece of soap on the basin and understood that it meant that he himself was a piece of soap.[20]

Once the presence of a delusion has been confirmed, the next evaluative step is the determination of the degree of influence of the delusion on the behavior or, in other words, the measurement of the motivational capacity of the delusional idea. To what extent and in what way does the delusion affect the testator's perception of reality, judgment, and behavior in relation to the will? Proof of the existence of a delusion at the time of making the will does not *ipso facto* establish a causal relationship between the delusion and the content of the will. The question is whether the delusion distorted the testator's cognitive skills in relation to preparation of the will (as, e.g., a testator has the delusion that his wife seeks to poison him and so leaves her out of his will).[21] Only that part of the will caused by the insane delusion fails; if the entire will was caused by the insane delusion, the entire will fails. Insane delusion cases often involve some false belief about a member of the family.

Delusional thinking may destroy testamentary capacity when it causes a disposition different from that which it might reasonably be found that the testator otherwise would have made. Delusions of grandeur ("I own the world") or poverty ("I own nothing") may render the testator incapable of knowing the extent of his property for the purpose of making a valid will. A delusion of marital infidelity, especially prone to occur in the involutional and senile psychosis, may result in a will, which seeks to disinherit the spouse or the child, who is believed by the testator not to be his and, thus, not the "natural object of his bounty."[22]

A review of decisions of insane delusion indicates that there must be a great deal of proof that the suspicions or beliefs of a testator are completely unfounded before they can be held to be an insane delusion. In a Florida case, a testator, believing that his son was out to kill him, disinherited him. The rule that the testator was acting out of a delusion, the Florida Court of Appeals said, "The conception must be persistently adhered to against all evidence and reason."[23]

In a Michigan case, it was alleged that the testatrix disinherited her son because she believed her daughter-in-law was immoral and the latter's mother ran a house of ill fame. The court said, "Contestant had the burden of proving that testatrix believed her statements, she had no reasonable information or evidence supporting them, and, but for such belief, she would not have disinherited him."[24]

In a New Jersey case, the testatrix, a militant feminist, regarded men as a class with an insane hatred and she left her male relatives out of her will. She looked forward to the day when women could bear children without the aid of men and all males would be put to death at birth. She never married. She once wrote: "My father was a corrupt, vicious, and unintelligent savage, a typical specimen of the majority of his sex. Blast his worm-stinking carcass and his whole damn breed." The court held that she lacked testamentary capacity.[25]

In a Missouri case, the testatrix was so angry with her child that instead of seeing the child she saw a grotesque phantom and did not include her in her will. The jury upheld the will. A physician who treated the testatrix testified: "Well, if we are to be practical about this thing, I think she was of sound mind. … She seemingly had her faculties so far as conducting her business. She made no statements that would make me feel that she was of unsound mind."[26]

In a Maryland case, it was held that the fact that a testator falsely believed his son had stolen his money, based on the father's belief that the son had done something wrong by sending the father to a nursing home, did not mean the father had an insane delusion when he disinherited the son. The court ruled that there had to be evidence that the belief was a product of a mental disease. The court found that the father had a delusion that his son had stolen his money, but that the delusion was not an insane delusion. Although it was false that the son had done something wrong and prompted the father to disinherit him, the court said it was not an inexplicable delusion that only could have come into being as the product of an insane mind.[27]

Vindictive disinheritance is not equated with insane delusion, though that is the contention when the will is challenged. Vindictive disinheritance is usually based on longstanding differences between parents and children, parental displeasure with the children's way of life, and accusation that the children have been disrespectful. It is possible to infer that writing a will gives parents one of their only opportunities for getting their animosity off their chest. Invariably, when rage motivates the provisions of a will, the will is used as a weapon to express hostility. One mother wrote in her will, "My only son, Roger, is not to have a penny from my estate. During his whole lifetime since he attained majority, he has been disobedient, ungrateful, and a constant source of anxiety, humiliation, and sorrow."

A wealthy banker cut two family members from his will with a stinging codicil: "To my wife and her lover, I leave the knowledge I wasn't the fool she thought I was. To my son, I leave the pleasure of earning a living; for 25 years he thought the pleasure was mine."

Not infrequently, suicide notes have instructions for the disposition of property. The state of mind necessary to carry out a suicide is probably incompatible with a thoughtful consideration of one's circumstances. What is remembered tends to be only slights, disappointments, and grievances. Thus, it was written in a suicide note: "Don't let that rotten son of a bitch so-and-so get his hands on my car."[28]

Undue Influence

Undue influence, as that concept has come to be known, is the kind of influence which comes from the outside, as contrasted with motivations that originate within the testator's own mind, and which is applied unfairly with the intent of benefiting the person who exercised the influence. Questions arise most often when someone in constant attendance is made the beneficiary of a changed will. The psychiatrist is called upon to testify as to the susceptibility of the testator to undue influence. Undue influence is urged as a challenge to a will in cases where the testator has capacity to make a will. Where testamentary capacity is lacking, the issue of undue influence need not be broached.[29]

One of the extreme examples of undue influence or lack of testamentary capacity occurred in *In re Lande's Estate*.[30] In this case, a doctor who was the sole beneficiary of his bachelor brother's will kept him in a private room under the influence of drugs, such as morphine, for some time prior to his death. He allowed no one else to see the testator during the last 10 days of illness when the will was made that excluded from inheritance another brother who was kept ignorant of the testator's illness. As shown by the record, the Minnesota Supreme Court said, an overdose of morphine is "destructive to the mental condition. It shatters reason and dethrones the will.

The rascally doctor 'substituted his own will for that of the testator.'" The court ruled that the will was obtained by undue influence and it could also have said that the testator lacked testamentary capacity.[31]

In the book *Undue Influence: The Epic Battle for the Johnson & Johnson Fortune,* David Margolick calls that will contest "the largest, costliest, most spectacular, and most conspicuous in American history."[32] On one side was Barbara Plasecka Johnson, a farmer's daughter who had only $200 when she left Poland in 1967. On the other side were Mrs. Johnson's six grown step-children—the progeny of J. Seward Johnson, who lavished more attention on his prize Holsteins than on his unhappy family. The grand prize: the $402,824,971 that Johnson left behind when he died in 1983. His children wanted more than what they got; Mrs. Johnson was the principal beneficiary and had sworn not to give them "the dust off half a penny." The children claimed that Mrs. Johnson and her attorney had, in effect, brainwashed the dying Johnson. A last-minute settlement netted the children a larger sum as well as $10 million for their attorney.

When one is at death's doorstep, one may be particularly susceptible to the overreaching influence of others. The concept of coveted result includes obtaining for oneself or another a benefit such person would normally not receive. Bequests to physicians and ministers attending the patient during the terminal illness are suspect. The law places an evidentiary burden on a fiduciary who has been left a bequest to establish that no undue influence was exercised.[33]

Some eight factors have been identified as tending to establish undue influence:

1. Whether the person accused of undue influence has made any fraudulent representations to the deceased.
2. Whether the will was hastily executed.
3. Whether such execution was concealed.
4. Whether the person benefited was active in securing the drafting and execution of the will.
5. Whether the will was consistent with prior declarations of the decedent.
6. Whether the provisions were reasonable rather than unnatural in view of the decedent's attitudes, views, and family..
7. Whether the decedent was susceptible to undue influence.
8. Whether there existed a confidential relationship between the decedent and the person allegedly exerting the undue influence.[34]

The transference that develops in the psychiatrist–patient relationship may constitute undue influence jeopardizing a bequest made by the patient to the psychiatrist or clinic. The law places the burden of proof on a fiduciary who is left a bequest to establish that no undue influence was exercised. In Louisiana, undue influence is not recognized as grounds for invalidating a will, but the principle of the doctrine is recognized, at least in part, by the limitation upon bequests to physicians and ministers attending the patient during the terminal illness. A presumption of undue influence arises "when there is a confidential relationship between the testator and a beneficiary who actively participates in preparation and execution of the will and unduly profits therefrom."[35]

Guardianship

An incompetency proceeding and the appointment of a guardian may be considered necessary when a member of the family is dissipating the family's assets. The guardianship process may be used when property is in danger of dissipation in the case of, say, the aged, the retarded, alcoholics, and psychotics. The issue is whether the person is capable of managing his own affairs; however, a guardian appointed to take control over property of one deemed incompetent cannot make a will for the ward. An adjudication of insanity or the appointment of a guardian does not necessarily indicate a lack of mental capacity to make a will, but it may give rise to a presumption of incompetence.[36]

Discussion

It is commonly said, "You cannot take it with you," but to whom do you leave it, and under what conditions, and for what reason? To be remembered lovingly, or to get even posthumously? Testaments reveal emotions of love and gratitude, of spite and hate. Time and again, people have used their last bequests to redress wrongs committed by them in life, to gain revenge, and, most manipulative, to control events after they are gone.[37] Charles Atlas bequeathed part of his body-building fortune to his son with the stipulation that he be baptized a Roman Catholic. Groucho Marx supposedly said, when asked if he intended to leave a large amount of money to his heirs, "Why should I, what did the future generation ever do for me?"

W.C. Fields, who left an estate of $800,000 in 1946 (a large sum at the time), bequeathed only $10,000 to his wife (they were married in 1900 and estranged, but never divorced) and $10,000 to his son. A heavy drinker, Fields recuperated in several sanatoriums. The wife and son contested the will and overrode many of the comedian's last wishes. In an attempt to deter any contest of the will, Fields included the following provision: "I wish to disinherit anyone who in any way tries to confuse or break this will or who contributes in any way to break this will." Fields' famous statement, "Never give a sucker an even break," turned out, in this instance, with Fields looking like the sucker, and his wife and son getting the break.[38]

The question is posed: "We are writing a will and want to leave all our money to our two children. One is very rich and the other lives almost hand to mouth. Do we divide equally or give the poorer one a greater proportion?" In the *New York Times*, the ethicist Randy Cohen responded:

> Why give the money to either of them? It's yours to enjoy as you choose; it is not their fortune to be held in trust. You're free to bequeath it to a home for incorrigible cats or squander it on riotous living. Parents are not obliged to enrich their adult children.
>
> Perhaps the most ethical approach is to ask how the money will do the most good, a question that leads some people to donate their savings to a cause they believe in rather than keep it in the family. Indeed, this might be asked at any point in one's life, not just when drawing up a will.[39]

In actual fact, the real basis of the testamentary incapacity or undue influence action is the alleged unfairness of a distribution that excludes close members of the family; however, it is a legally unacceptable means of challenge and the claim, therefore, is based on incapacity or undue influence. There may be real cases of incapacity and undue influence, but more often than not these are artificial bases of the claims of contestants. Because the accumulation of an estate is the result of the efforts of the entire family, directly or indirectly, it is unfair economically to disinherit those members who have participated in what might be called a joint venture. Moreover, if helpless dependents will become public charges, disinheritage is unfair to the interests of society generally. A parent is under a duty to provide for the support and maintenance of his children during the period of their dependence.

The societal interest in testaments is unlike the sanctity of contracts. For example, an individual on the same day that he executed a will may have purchased stock or an automobile. If he later attempts to void the contract on the basis of contractual incapacity, the court will likely decide against him in the interest of commerce. On the other hand, if at the time of his death his will is contested on the ground of testamentary capacity, the court, in the interest of family maintenance, is unlikely to uphold the will if he has pauperized a helpless member of his family. The societal interest in testaments is unlike the sanctity of contracts, which also may be undone for reasons of incapacity of the contracting party. The interest of commerce underlies the sanctity of contract; the interest of family maintenance underlies the societal interest in testaments. Testaments, unlike contracts, require passage in the courts as a matter of course.

The suggestion that decisions are usually based on the unnaturalness or abnormality of the disposition rather than on the testator's understanding is also supported by the fact that the court examines the dispositive elements of the will by admitting the will in evidence in the contest. Strictly speaking, though, the terms of the will are irrelevant to the issue of mental competency. Because the lawyer usually prepares the will, it does not provide a sample of the testator's handwriting, except for the signature, which may be evidence of incompetence.[40]

An examination of the cases seems to reveal that, by and large, the validity of a will depends on the extent it affords family protection. Societal notions of fairness usually seem to prevail, regardless of the evidence tending to prove the existence or lack thereof of testamentary capacity or undue influence. The courts are more likely to overturn a will when close relatives are disinherited and left penniless than when a nondependent relative challenges the will. At one time or another Louisiana in its civil code and some other states limited the disposable portion of an estate in the event of children; also, a spouse as a matter of law is one-half owner of community property. In an article on the role of mental competency, Law Professor Leon Green stated:

> It is submitted that in determining the issue of mental incompetency, more frequently than otherwise, courts are passing upon the abnormality of the transaction rather than on the ability of the alleged incompetent to understand the transaction.[41]

Philadelphia lawyer Edwin Epstein put it this way:

> The attack on the testator's mental competency is often a mere litigative trapping that the contestants assume to give them a pretext for challenging the will, because the law presently provides no procedure by which they can argue the real basis of their claim, i.e., that the will is unfair to them and they are unhappy with the provisions made for them in it. Although this economic dissatisfaction underlies almost every will contest, the contestants must artificially base their case on lack of capacity or on the other presently legally acceptable bases for challenge.[42]

The unfairness rationale may be shown by comparative cases in which the courts have given differing weight to evidence of testamentary incapacity.[43] The term *testamentary capacity* is a rubric to equalize distribution. In the Institutes of Justinian, that famous Roman emperor tells us that if a child is disinherited by a parent, he may impeach the will by "the pretext that the testator was of unsound mind at the time of the execution. This does not mean that he was really insane, but the will, though legally executed, bears no mark of that affection to which the child was entitled."

Sometimes a will is executed during the relatively early years of the testator's life, when he is sound and hearty, and he may not have written another will, although subsequently there may have been significant family changes that would ordinarily dictate it. The testator in his later years may have been psychotic, but to upset the will, the doctrine of testamentary capacity is unavailing because the time of the making of the will is the determining one. The law here comes to the rescue of the family in a different way. Under the common law, and expressly by statute in a number of states, wills are held to be revoked by operation of law by certain changes in the domestic relations of the testator. Many states provide by statute that a subsequent marriage revokes a will, that a subsequent divorce impliedly revokes a testamentary gift to the wife, or that children born subsequent to the writing of the will are included within it.

The source of this doctrine of implied revocation is attributed to the Roman law. Cicero in his *De Oratore* wrote: "For who is it that would seek to inherit under this will which the father of the family made before his son was born? Nobody; because it is agreed that a will is broken through lack of knowledge." The Louisiana Civil Code expressly provides that a testament is revoked by the later birth of a legitimate child or the subsequent adoption of a child by the testator. Usually a testamentary gift is made to a class, such as children or grandchildren, which would include members of the class who are born after the execution of the will or would exclude those who may predecease the testator.[44]

It is highly unlikely that a testament will be upset by a claim of a collateral or distant relative, irrespective of the testamentary capacity of the testator. As one judge caustically observed: "A man without parents, wife, or children, can scarcely be said to have natural objects of his bounty; and when he has been permitted to go through life attending to his own affairs, and taking good care of his estate, it is too late, after he has made his will and died, for collaterals to discover that for 6 or 8 years his mind has been under a cloud, and that it passed into total eclipse just at the moment of their disappointment."[45]

The idea of testatorial absolutism must be taken with a grain of salt. There is a deep-seated aversion to the power of arbitrarily diverting the natural course of the devolution of property. Generally speaking, the interests of society in family maintenance are greater than its interests in the protection of the freedom of testation. In order for that preference to be given priority, it is necessary for a will contestant to allege, in effect, that the testator was crazy. Will contests based upon a testator's supposed lack of testamentary capacity are simply "litigatory trappings that the contestants assume."[46]

Endnotes

1. See *In re* Bottger's Estate, 14 Wash. 2d 676, 129 P.2d 518 (1942); Note, "Psychiatric Assistance in the Determination of Testamentary Capacity," *Harv. L. Rev.* 66 (1953): 1116.
2. See G.W. Beyer & W.R. Buckley, "Videotape and the Probate Process: The Nexus Grows," *Okla. L. Rev.* 42 (1989): 43. In *In re* Dokken, 604 N.W.2d 487 (S.D. 2000), the testator did not have contractual capacity, a guardian had been appointed, and when he failed to take medication, he had psychotic episodes that involved beating on and talking to trees and disposing of his clothing in the garbage. He was held to have testamentary capacity. The court said, "[I]t is not necessary that a person desiring to make a will should have sufficient capacity to make contracts and do business generally nor to engage in complex and intricate business matters. ... The testator may lack mental capacity to such an extent that according to medical science he is not of sound mind and memory, and nevertheless retain the mental capacity to execute a will"; 604 N.W.2d at 491.
3. *In re* Willits' Estate, 175 Cal. 173, 165 Pac. 537 (1970).
4. See W.J. Spaulding, "Testamentary Competency: Reconciling Doctrine With the Role of the Expert Witness," *Law & Hum. Behav.* 9 (1985): 113. In Russia, where feudalism lasted until 1862, Peter the Great in 1714 issued a decree on the law of inheritance that provided the following: (1) Immovables were not to be alienated, but were to remain in the family. (2) Immovables were to pass from a testator to one of his sons, selected by the testator. Movables were to be divided by the testator as he wished among the remaining children. Failing sons, the same system was to be applied to daughters. In cases of intestacy, immovables were to go to the eldest son, failing whom, the eldest daughter, and movables were to be divided equally among the other children. (3) A child testator could leave his immovables to "any member of his family he pleased" and could dispose of his movables as he liked, either to relations or to strangers. In cases of intestacy where there were no children, the immovables went to the nearest relative and the movables were to be divided "in equal parts to whomsoever may be thought proper." Decree of March 3, 1714. In this way noble families would not be extinguished "but would continue to be illustrious and eminent," whereas the division of estate would lead to the ruin of noble families and turn them into simple countrymen "of which there are already numerous examples in the Russian people." V. Klyuchevsky, *Peter the Great* (New York: Vintage Books, 1958), p. 106.
5. Ga. Code Ann., tit. 113, § 201.
6. Ga. Code Ann., tit. 113 §§ 202–209.
7. In this case, the testator was about 90 years old, was rendered almost speechless by age and the loss of his health, was bedridden, and on account of his bodily infirmities at least, if not mental, was rendered pretty much incapable of attending to and managing his ordinary business. The Court said,

"All attempts to draw the line between capacity and incapacity have ended where they began, namely, in nothing. All agree that there must be a sound and disposing mind and memory, but to define the precise quantum, *hoc opus, hic labor est.*" Potts v. House, 6 Ga. 324 (1848).

8. See Estate of Park, [1953] 2 A11 E.R. 408. In contrast, an oft-cited case in Scotland, *Blair v. Blair*, stands for the principle that a marriage (then indissoluble) could not be made by a person defective in reason (though showing some little sense), while a revocable one like a last will and testament could. J. Erskine, *An Institute of the Law of Scotland* (Edinburgh: Bell & Bradfute, 5th ed. 1812), vol. 1, p. 158; R. Houston & U. Frith, *Autism in History: The Case of Hugh Blair of Borgue* (Oxford, UK: Blackwell, 2000), p. 93.

9. Various states in the United States have legislation prohibiting persons without capacity from entering into contracts for marriage. Michigan law, for example, in relevant part states: "No insane person, idiot, … shall be capable of marriage"; MCL 551.6. The statute is a means by which a marriage engineered by a predator could be voided after the death of the deceased person. The Michigan case of Almond v. Hudson, No. 99-918792 (Jan. 26, 2000) involved a paraplegic requiring 24-hour care who was the prey of a day care aide. Almond had been under full guardianship and adjudged incapacitated by a probate court. Against the guardian's explicit instructions, the day care aide took him out of his home to the clerk's office where she obtained a marriage license and marriage. Almond left a substantial estate to be distributed when he died. His mother (guardian) contested the marriage to the short-term day care giver. Because one of the parties to the alleged marriage was already deceased, the issue was whether the marriage, "a civil contract," was *void ab initio*. Because "marriage is a civil contract" like any other civil contract requiring capacity, a void contract for marriage is one that, in effect, was never formed. The statute was the basis for annulment of the marriage. See also Evasic v. Evasic, No. 215875 (Feb. 4, 1999). The Michigan senate recently passed Bill 0067 repealing MCL 551.6, and it also initiated Bill 0273 that would allow a court to grant a guardian power to consent to a ward's decision to marry only if it finds by clear and convincing evidence that the individual lacks capacity to marry and is unlikely to ever regain that legal capacity. If enacted, the only way to protect the vulnerable individual would be a ruling on testamentary or contractual capacity. B. Callahan (Ltr.), "Marriage Laws Discriminate Against the Disabled," *Mich. Bar. J.,* June 2001, p. 10. In Hoffman v. Kohns, 385 So.2d 1064 (Fla. App. 1980), where a housekeeper married a senile man, a will made one day later was set aside, but the marriage was held valid.

10. It is sometimes allowed, however. In a New Mexico will contest, a psychiatrist, claiming that he was familiar with the standard of competency necessary to execute a will, was allowed to testify that the testatrix was probably competent at the time she signed the will. Lucero v. Lucero, 884 P.2d 527 (N.M. Applicant 1994). Allowing the psychiatrist to testify to the legal consequences of the testatrix's state of mind is criticized in L. A. Frolik, "Science, Common Sense, and the Determination of Mental Capacity," *Psychol., Pub. Policy, & Law* 5 (1999): 41. See Carr v. Radkey, 393 S.W.2d 806 (Tex. 1965).

11. The witnesses on behalf of a contestant to a will must offer testimony that the testator did not (1) understand the nature of his acts, or (2) know the extent of his property, or (3) understand the proposed disposition of it, or (4) know the natural objects of his bounty. In Nebraska Methodist Hosp. v. McCloud, 155 Neb. 500, 52 N.W.2d 325 (1952), the court noted that all of the witnesses for the contestant simply testified that in their opinion the testator was "not of sound mind" or "not really of sound mind," but not one question was asked, nor any answer of the witnesses, that revealed any mental quality upon which testamentary incapacity could be predicated. Thus, the issue of testamentary capacity became a question of law for the court. See also *In re* Estate of Ellis, 9 Neb. App. 598, 616 N.W.2d 59 (2000).

One of leading cases in the law of evidence on hearsay, Wright v. Tatham, 112 Eng. Rep. 488 (Exch. Ch. 1837), involved testamentary capacity. The case involved a contest over the will of John Marsden, an English gentleman who left his estate to his steward. Marsden's relative, Admital Tatham, contested the will, claiming that Marsden was mentally incompetent. In support of Marsden's competency, the steward offered into evidence several letters that had been found in Marsden's effects. All had been written to Marsden by third persons. These letters were written in language suggesting that the writers believed Marsden to be mentally competent; otherwise they would not have written to him in the way that they did. The steward wanted the court to infer the writers' belief in Marsden's competence from the letter, and to infer from the belief that the fact believed was true. The Privy Council held them to be hearsay, holding that conduct, even when not intended as assertive, is hearsay when offered to show the actor's belief and, hence, the truth of the belief. In the United States, on the other hand, implied assertions are not classified as hearsay. See Rule 801, Federal Rules of Evidence.

12. *In re* Ver Vaecke's Estate, 327 Mich. 419 (1923; property willed to housekeeper); see J.P. Rosenfeld, *The Legacy of Aging: Inheritance and Disinheritance in Social Perspective* (Norwood, NJ: Ablex, 1979); W.F. Gorman, "Testamentary Capacity in Alzheimer's Disease," *Elder L. J.* 4 (1996): 225; M. Houts, "Alzheimer's Disease and Testamentary Capacity," *Trauma* 26 (1985): 2; D.C. Marson, "Loss of Competency in Alzheimer's Disease: Conceptual and Psychometric Approaches," *Intl. J. Law & Psychiat.* 24 (2001): 267; J.P. Rosenfeld, "Bequests From Resident to Resident: Inheritance in a Retirement Community," *Gerontologist* 19 (1979): 594.

    Not long ago, for a time, the Division of Neuropsychology of Henry Ford Hospital in Detroit had a Testamentary Capacity Assessment Program to protect the rights of older adults to distribute property by documenting and understanding their abilities and suggesting compensatory strategies when indicated. It provided a focused and concise evaluation of cognitive and emotional processes targeted at addressing the client's decision-making ability, awareness, and knowledge of personal assets. The evaluation included an extensive, in-depth clinical interview, a battery of paper-and-pencil neuropsychological tests and functional measures, and assessment of depression and general mental health. It provided a detailed report with recommendations, if needed, and the staff was available if expert testimony would be required.

13. Religious fanaticism marked the will of Joseph Lieberman's uncle, Bernard Manger, who left an estate of $40 million. He disinherited two of his four children because they had married people who were not born Jewish. As he grew older, Manger became more and more concerned that intermarriage was threatening the existence of the Jewish people. P. Kuntz & B. Davis, "A Beloved Uncle's Will Tests Diplomatic Skills of Joseph Lieberman," *Wall Street Journal*, August 25, 2000, p. 1. Some courts hold that religious or other beliefs held too intensely can destroy testamentary capacity. Religious beliefs may become, on some level, insane delusions that render invalid will provisions affected by them. The question, of course, is how to determine whether a belief has become a delusion and, if so, whether the delusion caused the testator to make a challenged disposition. On this question, courts disagree. J.B. Baron, "Empathy, Subjectivity, and Testamentary Capacity," *San. Diego L. Rev.* 24 (1987): 1043.

14. 308 Mich. 366, 13 N.W.2d 852 (1944).

15. While millions of people are mired in poverty, large bequests are often made for the care of a pet. When pets are not provided for, they often go to a shelter with other discarded animals; those that are not adopted end up euthanized. But bequests of millions of dollars for the care of a pet? The late Leona Helmsley, the hotel magnate known as the Queen of Mean, left a $12 million trust fund for her dog, named Trouble. She left nothing to two of her grandchildren. M. Fernandez, "Newly Minted Millionaire Can't Buy Herself a Friend," *New York Times*, Sept. 3, 2007, p. 14. Tobacco heiress Doris Duke left $100,000 to care for her Shar-Pei named Rodeo. And the singer Dusty Springfield left a bequest that covered a lifetime of imported baby food for her cat, Nicholas. "This is becoming an increasingly common practice," says a tax expert in Detroit. "I am working on a will now that leaves $1 million to a pet." Quoted in B. O'Conner, "When Fortunes Go to Dogs," *Detroit News*, Sept. 1, 2007, p. B1. At a gathering at the home of Michigan Probate Judge Frank Szymanski, I asked him whether he ever probated a will naming a pet as beneficiary. "Yes," he said, "a million dollars was left to a dog." I asked, "Where is the dog?" "Upstairs, in the bedroom," the judge smiled.

16. See Bowerman v. Burris, 138 Tenn. 220, 197 S.W. 490 (1917). The Uniform Probate Code §2-302(c) (1990) gives a child an intestate share where the testator mistakenly believes the child is dead. See J. Dukeminier & S.M. Johanson, *Wills, Trusts, and Estates* (Boston: Little, Brown, 5th ed., 1995).

17. 109 Mich. 98, 66 N.W. 681 (1896).

18. See K. Jaspers, *General Psychopathology* (Manchester, U.K.: Manchester University Press, 1963), pp. 95–96.

19. *In re* Solomon's Estate, 334 Mich. 17, 53 N.W.2d 597 (1952).

20. This was an Israeli case. *Soap* is an Israeli slang term for fool. See R. Mester, P. Toren & N. Gonen, "The Delusion Based Will: The Question of Validity," *Med. & Law* 13 (1994): 555.

21. As it is said, a person possessed by a delusion can make a valid will unless the will was the "offspring of the delusion." The court in State v. Jones, 50 N.H. 369 (1871), said that a man "who labors under a delusion that his legs are made of glass, or that he is charged with controlling the motions of the planetary system, but is in other aspects sane," need not be deemed incapable of making a valid will. A man may believe he is the supreme ruler of the universe, but if that delusion does not affect any provisions in his will, it is deemed to be a valid will. Fraser v. Jennison, 42 Mich. 206, 3 N.W. 882 (1880).

22. Tawney v. Long, 76 Pa. 106 (1874); see G. L. Usdin, "The Physician and Testamentary Capacity," *Am. J. Psychiat.* 114 (1957): 249.

23. Estate of Hodtume v. Nora Casesaree Harmony Lodge, 267 So.2d 686 (Fla. App. 1972).

24. Jackson City Bank & Trust Co. v. Townley, 268 Mich. 340 (1934).

25. *In re* Strittmater's Estate, 53 A.2d 205 (N.J. 1947). Assuming this hatred of men was an insane delusion, did it cause the bequest? The court assumed it did. The testatrix devised her property to the National Women's Party. Some cousins, whom she saw very little in the last years of her life, contested the will on the ground of insanity. The court, probably out of male bias, assumed that her hatred of men was irrational. The case would likely today not be decided the same way. The testatrix did not cut off close relatives who supported her during her life.

26. Hardy v. Barbour, 304 S.W.2d 21 (Mo. 1957).

27. Dougherty v. Rubenstein, 914 A.2d 184 (Md. App. 2007).

28. Suicide notes, of course, vary. They are categorized into five types: (1) notes that blame someone, (2) notes that deny that an obvious reason is the cause ("I did not kill myself because my wife left me"), (3) notes that blame and deny ("My wife is to blame, but I did not kill myself because she left me"), (4) notes that contain an insight ("Perhaps I gave her reason to leave me"), and (5) notes that contain no explanation at all and have only instructions for the disposition of property. See A. Wilkinson, "Notes Left Behind," *New Yorker*, Feb. 15, 1999, p. 44.

29. The essential elements of "undue influence" are as follows: a testator is a person who is or can be influenced by reason of advanced age, physical infirmities, mental condition, fear, or for any other reason would yield to the desire or will of another person or persons; the opportunity for a person or persons to exert it; the fact of improper influence exerted or attempted; a will showing the effect of such influence. A typical jury instruction on "undue influence" is as follows: "General influence, however strong or controlling, is not undue influence unless it is brought to bear directly upon the act of preparing the will and imposes another person's plans or desires upon the testator. If the will, as finally executed, expresses the free and voluntary plans and desires of the testator, the will is valid, regardless of the exercise or influence." The jury is also typically instructed: "Undue influence sufficient to invalidate a will is that which substitutes the plans or desires of another for those of testator. The influence must be such as to control the mind of the testator in the making of his will, to overcome his power of resistance, and to result in his making a distribution of his property, which he would not have made if he were left to act freely and according to his own plans and desires." See Ohio Jury Instructions, sec. 363.05.

30. 236 N.W. 705 (Minn. 1931).

31. See generally, D.J. Sharpe, "Medication as a Threat to Testamentary Capacity," *No. Car. L. Rev.* 35 (1957): 380.

32. New York: William Morrow, 1993. See also B. Goldsmith, *Johnson v. Johnson* (New York: Knopf, 1987).

33. See, e.g., Jahn v. Harmes, 249 N.W.2d 638 (Iowa 1977); Flemming v. Hall, 374 Mich. 278, 132 N.W.2d 35 (1965); Totorean v. Samuels, 216 N.W.2d 429 (Mich. App. 1974); *In re* Estate of Garfield, 222 N.W.2d 369 (Neb. 1974).

34. J.D. Lewis, "Will Contests," *Ariz. Atty.*, March 21, 1990; D.J. Sprehe & A.L. Kerr, "Use of Legal Terms in Will Contests: Implications for Psychiatrists," *Bull Am. Acad. Psychiat. & Law* 24 (1996): 255. See also L.A. Frolik, "The Strange Interplay of Testamentary Capacity and the Doctrine of Undue Influence: Are We Protecting Older Testators or Overriding Individual Preferences?" *Intl. J. Law & Psychiat.* 24 (2001): 253. In a study of cults, Dr. Margaret Singer identifies six factors that make up the components for a person to exercise undue influence over another: isolation, creating a siege mentality, dependency, sense of powerlessness, sense of fear and vulnerability, and keeping the person in ignorance by manipulating the environment. M.T. Singer, "Undue Influence and Written Documents: Psychological Aspects," *Cultic Stud. J.* 10 (1993): 19. Evidence that the party benefiting by a will made no attempt to keep others from seeing and conversing with the testator tends to show the absence of a disposition to exert undue influence. *In re* Estate of Ellis, 9 Neb. App. 598, 616 N.W.2d 59 (2000).

35. *In re* Estate of Madsen, 535 N.W.2d 888 (S.D. 1995).

36. Estate of Goddard, 164 Cal. App.2d 152, 330 P.2d 399 (1958); *In re* Higbee Will, 365 Pa. 381, 75 A.2d 599 (1950).

37. See N. Roth, *The Psychiatry of Writing a Will* (Springfield, IL: Thomas, 1989). An old Jewish tradition, fallen into disuse, is the "ethical will" used to convey feelings to close ones. One illustration: "there's nothing more precious than time—use it wisely." Another: "For the sake of a father who took a wrong turn, take the right one." See R. Slovenko, "Deathbed Declarations," *J. Psychiat. & Law* 24 (1966): 469. For compilations of vindictive wills, see F. Thomas, *Last Will and Testament* (New York: St. Martin's, 1972); R.S. Menchin, *The Last Caprice* (New York: Simon & Schuster, 1963). On humorous wills, see

F.L. Golden, *Laughter Is Legal* (New York: Pocket Books, 193); De Morgan, "Wills: Quaint, Curious and Otherwise," *Green Bag* 13 (1901): 567; J.M. Gest, "Some Jolly Testators," *Temp. L. Q.* 8 (1934): 297; E.M. Million, "Humor in or of Wills," *Vand. L. Rev.* 11 (1958): 737.

38. H.E. Nass, *Wills of the Rich and Famous* (New York: Warner Books, 1991). The woman who stood by Fields for the final 15 years of his life, and figured prominently in his will, was Carlotta Monti, who was at his bedside on Christmas Eve, 1946, as he fought a losing battle to retain consciousness. The battle over Fields' money was fought in the courts for 4 years. Under California's community property laws, Fields' estranged wife claimed half of everything. In the end she settled for $65,000. Another of Fields' last wishes was ignored. Though he joked that he loathed children, he requested in his will the establishment of a "W.C. Fields College for orphan white boys and girls" and stipulated that "no religion of any sort is to be preached." Between the court squabbles and lawyers' fees, nothing ever came of the nondenomination, if racist, orphanage. C. Panati, *Browser's Book of Endings* (New York: Penguin, 1999), pp. 68–69.

39. R. Cohen, "Heir Unapparent," *New York Times Magazine*, Dec. 12, 1999, p. 58. The estate of another famous comedian, Groucho Marx, was embroiled in controversy over testamentary capacity. See S. Kanfer, *Groucho: The Life and Times of Julius Henry Marx* (New York: Knopf, 2000).

40. Before drafting a will, a lawyer does not have a duty to investigate the mental capacity of a client, though he may appear rather bizarre. In Gonsalves v. Superior Court, 19 Cal. App. 4th 1366, 24 Cal. Rptr.2d (1993), the lawyer-drafter was sued by the disinherited heir, charging that the lawyer should have known of the testator's alleged incompetence. The court held that a lawyer is not required to investigate the client's condition and may rely on his own judgment regarding capacity or lack thereof.

41. L. Green, "Proof of Mental Incompetency and the Unexpected Major Premise," *Yale L. J.* 53 (1944): 271.

42. E.M. Epstein, "Testamentary Capacity, Reasonableness and Family Maintenance: A Proposal for Meaningful Reform," *Temple L. Q.* 35 (1962): 231.

43. In Matter of Arnold's Estate, 16 Cal.2d 573, 107 P.2d 25 (1940), the evidence of psychosis was fairly extensive (loss of memory as a result of chronic alcoholism); however, the case reflects the general hesitancy of courts to overturn a testamentary disposition where the testator has provided for the natural objects of his bounty. In Matter of Gilbert's Estate, 148 Cal. App. 2d 761, 307 P.2d 395 (1957), the testatrix's will, which left her entire estate to educational institutions and charities, was contested by her cousins. (Charitable and religious organizations strive to develop good will—and good wills!) The court, in holding that the decedent was competent, minimized the extent and weight given to testimony that she was "very frantic looking, very wild looking." In cases where the disinherited contestant is a member of the testator's more immediate family, however, the courts are more impressed with this type of evidence. Thus, in Matter of Kirk's Estate, 161 Cal. App.2d 145, 326 P.2d 151 (1958), where the testator's two disinherited sons contested a will, which left the major part of the estate to the testator's brother, sister-in-law, and grandchildren, the court held that the testator's psychosis with cerebral arteriosclerosis was such as to evidence clearly a lack of testamentary capacity. In Matter of Bourguin's Estate, 161 Cal. App.2d 289, 326 P.2d 604 (1958), the testatrix left the bulk of her estate to a Christian Science rest home in which she died. In so doing, she neglected her son. The court relied heavily on evidence of physical debility in finding a lack of testamentary capacity. The court in Matter of Alexander's Estate, 111 Cal. App. 1, 295 Pac. 53 (1931), is unusually candid in alluding to the fact that the reasonableness or unreasonableness of the provisions of the will is used in determining the question of testamentary capacity. The court in Hutchins v. Barlow, 221 Miss. 811, 74 So.2d 870 (1954), said that where it appears that a will is inconsistent with the duties of the testator in regard to his family, the proponents of the will must give a reasonable explanation thereof. See P. Aries, "Wills and Tombs: The Rise of Modern Family Feeling," *New Society*, Sept. 25, 1969, p. 473.

44. E. Durfee, "Revocation of Wills by Subsequent Change in the Condition or Circumstances of the Testator," *Mich. L. Rev.* 40 (1942): 406; W.A. Graunke & J.H. Beuscher, "The Doctrine of Implied Revocation of Wills by Reason of Change in Domestic Relations of the Testator. *Wis. L. Rev.* 5 (1930): 387; T.H. Leath, "Lapse, Abatement and Redemption," *No. Car. L. Rev.* 39 (1961): 313.

45. Stevenson's Executor v. Stevenson, 33 Pa. 469 (1859). The determination of whether a will is unnatural depends on the circumstances of each case. *In re* Estate of Velk, 192 N.W.2d 844 (Wis. 1972). It has been more acceptable for a wife to bequeath nothing to her husband than vice versa. One wife had a provision in her will, which was probated, that provided: "Whereas I have been a faithful, dutiful, and loving wife to my husband, and whereas he reciprocated my tender affections for him with acts of cruelty and indifference, and whereas he has failed to support and maintain me in that station of life which would have been possible and proper for him, I hereby limit my bequest to him to one dollar"; Loetsch v. N.Y. City Omnibus Corp., 291 N.Y. 308, 32 N.E.2d 448 (1943).

46. See R.M. Bedard & E.G. Mart, "Practical Assessment of Testamentary Capacity and Undue Influence in Wills," *Am. J. Foren. Psychol.* 25 (2007): 7; J. Spar & J.D. Garb, "Assessing Competency to Make a Will," *Am. J. Psychiat.* 149 (1992): 169.

LAW IN PSYCHIATRY

PART I
Hospitalization of the Mentally Ill

24

Civil Commitment

Views held by the medical profession and the surrounding culture about insanity (or *mental illness*, as now called) and what to do about it have changed over the years. For centuries the idea of "demonic possession" reflecting the biblical explanation of insanity held sway. In the late 18th and early 19th centuries insanity came to be regarded as a disease rather than as divine retribution or demonic possession. At that time, a convergence of popular indignation, growing medical interest, and several examples seemed to prove that, with humane treatment, insanity could be cured. In this context laymen and physicians developed a system that they called moral treatment. It was considered revolutionary in the history of psychiatry.[1]

Most prominently, two years after the French Revolution, Philippe Pinel in 1791 in France introduced humanitarian principles in the care and treatment of the mentally ill. As director of two psychiatric hospitals in Paris, he ordered the unchaining of the inmates. He advocated "moral medicine," directed at the mind and emotions, advising physicians to approach patients with "gentleness" and "consoling words, the happy expedient of reviving the hope of the lunatic and gaining his confidence." No longer would the devil be beaten out of a person (as was done to King George III). In the early years of the 19th century, Jean-Etienne-Dominique Esquirol, Pinel's disciple, and others demanded an end to bleedings and purgings, which were standard treatments for mental illness.

In America, Dr. Benjamin Rush, the renowned political leader of the Revolutionary War period and the father of American psychiatry championed this philosophy of moral treatment. Later, during the 1800s, Dorothea Dix, who carried on a campaign to build state institutions after it had become generally apparent that private philanthropy could not cope unaided with so large a burden, took up the cause of moral treatment for the mentally ill.[2]

The philosophy of moral treatment espoused by these pioneers prevailed in the United States in the early part of the 19th century. At that time, in part reflecting the positive results of humane treatment of the mentally disordered and in part reflecting the stresses arising out of the burgeoning industrial era, there was considerable social pressure to take care of the mentally ill on a larger scale. Palatial manors to house the mentally ill were built at considerable expense in rustic, attractive (though remote) parts of the states. Constructed at a cost unparalleled in the world, these facilities were designed with the premise that madness might be soothed in a setting of architectural and environmental beauty. This progressive thinking as well as the building efforts it engendered became a model for the whole world.[3]

In Europe, before the 18th century, only a small proportion of individuals deemed to be mentally ill were put in a special institution. People who were a menace to others or utterly incapable of looking after themselves were taken care of by their family, or by charity, or by their parish, or occasionally locked away in a jail. Systematic confinement of the mentally ill instigated by the state developed in France from the mid-17th century as part of the "great confinement" of troublemakers launched by Louis XIV's absolutism. In England, the biggest growth sector for the confinement of the mentally ill before the 19th century lay within the market economy, where a "trade in lunacy" grew up, centered on the private madhouse. These institutions might be run by physicians or laymen; some were big, others small, all of a private nature. They were accused of shady practices, above all, the iniquitous confinement of sane people. Daniel Defoe among others alleged that they were tailor-made for husbands who wished to put away their wives. As historian Roy Porter observed, "It is not surprising then that so many of the earliest autobiographical writings of English 'mad people' raise a howl of protest against the private asylum and its abuses."[4]

In 1842, Charles Dickens noted approvingly that American mental hospitals were supported by the state, a fact that made the government, in his view, a merciful and benevolent protector of people in distress.[5] With increasing numbers of the seriously mentally ill on the streets and in the jails, the various state governments in the United States came to accept full responsibility for their care and built the large public mental hospitals. The constitutions of the various states mandated state-sponsored care of the mentally ill.[6] In England, on the other hand, where public charity was minimal, the government offered the mentally ill, as Dickens said, "very little shelter or relief beyond that which is to be found in the workhouse and the jail."[7]

This era of moral treatment in America, however, soon came to an end. As the population increased with the influx of immigrants, the public mental hospitals were turned into welfare institutions. Previously, every state hospital had a farm or dairy that provided meaningful work and activity for the residents. Beginning in the late 19th century, business interests seeking to sell supplies to these big institutions, however, effectively pressured to have the farms and dairies closed. As a result, once meaningful work experiences in the hospital were replaced with a state of idleness. The hospital degenerated into the "snake pit," a place of chaotic disorder and distress; its motto became: "Abandon hope, all ye who enter here."

During this period Mrs. E.P.W. Packard (Elizabeth Parsons Ware) began her crusade for the enactment of laws on the hospitalization of the mentally ill as well as laws for the protection of patient rights.[8] Her crusade had its genesis in her hospitalization. Her husband, the Reverend Theophilus Packard, stating that he could not "manage" her at home, had her committed, utilizing a state statute, which provided that married women could be involuntarily committed on the request of the husband without the evidentiary standard applicable in other cases.[9] Upon her discharge, she went on a crusade for the adoption of mental health codes that became the foundation of modern codes.[10] She claimed that sane persons were illegally incarcerated and maltreated. Her attacks, along with exposés by other former patients, resulted in the passage of legislation that would more effectively safeguard the rights of patients and circumscribe the powers of hospital officials.

At the turn of the 20th century, a second revolution in psychiatry was brought about by Sigmund Freud. Like Pinel, Freud engendered hope and enthusiasm in the treatment of the mentally ill. On the basis of the new learning, laws were enacted on sexual psychopathology, alcoholism, and drug addiction that would divert individuals out of the criminal law process and into the hospital system. These behaviors came to be regarded as mental illness rather than as crime.[11] Much of the impetus for these new laws came from the success achieved in treating battle-fatigued soldiers during World War I.

Following World War II, in the 1950s, a third revolution in psychiatry occurred with the development of psychotropic medication. These chemical agents resulted in a decrease in the use of physical restraints, psychosurgery, electroshock, hydrotherapy, insulin coma, and other physical means of treatment. These chemical agents would control the voices and delusional thinking of schizophrenia and the mania of manic-depressive psychosis. For the first time, the number of persons admitted to mental hospitals declined.

With this decline, a new philosophy began to emerge, which had as a goal the abandonment of state mental hospitals altogether. First of all, proponents of this philosophy argued, hospitalization while reducing stress produces "institutional dependency," which offers not mental health, but mental death, and robs the individual of all incentive. Sociologist Erving Goffman, who had worked for a time as an occupational therapist in a large mental hospital, crystallized this thinking. He wrote that "chronic schizophrenia" is merely an adaptation to the social system of the hospital. In his 1961 book *Asylums*, Goffman presented a scathing critique, not only of the conditions prevailing in mental hospitals, but also of the basic philosophical premises on which such institutions were founded.[12] Thereafter, the word *asylum* became a derogatory term.

In fiction, in the novel *One Flew Over the Cuckoo's Nest* , Ken Kesey described the hospital staff as a tyrannical, sadistic group that forced patients into total submission.[13] In still another dramatic view, Thomas Szasz in his book *The Manufacture of Madness* drew a parallel between the persecution of witches in the 13th through the 17th centuries and what he termed our persecution of people labeled mentally ill in the 20th century.[14] In his view, repeated in many books, modern psychiatry has led not to more enlightenment, but only to different victims for persecution.[15]

During the tumultuous 1960s and 1970s, Bruce Ennis, an attorney for the American Civil Liberties Union, led the Mental Health Bar in litigation to close all mental hospitals. These efforts were unlike those of Packard who, a century earlier, sought hospital safeguards and regulations instead of outright closings. In 1972, Ennis and three other young attorneys (Charles Halpern, Paul Friedman, and Margaret Ewing) formed the Mental Health Law Project (MHLP), which rapidly became—and has remained (it changed its name in 1993 to the Bazelon Center for Mental Health Law)—the ideological and logistical center of the mental patient liberation bar, as it was called. They were abolitionists, not reformers, who challenged every assumption of the mental health system.[16] An observation by the U.S. Supreme Court in 1972 in a criminal case gave impetus to litigation on the commitment power of the state: "Considering the number of persons affected, it is perhaps remarkable that the substantive constitutional limitations [on a state's commitment] power have not been more frequently litigated."[17] On another occasion, the Supreme Court commented that there is more stigma to mental hospitalization than to imprisonment.[18]

Ennis wrote a polemic against mental hospitalization, *Prisoners of Psychiatry*, which also appeared in 1972.[19] In a preface, Szasz praised Ennis for recognizing "that individuals incriminated as mentally ill do not need guarantees of treatment but protection against their enemies—the legislators, judges, and psychiatrists who persecute them in the name of mental health." In this book, Ennis portrayed psychiatry as a means to control or dispose of people who annoy others. As Ennis wrote: "How would we tame our rebellious youth, or rid ourselves of doddering parents, or clear the streets of the offensive poor, without it?" For Ennis, hospitals were places "where sick people get sicker and sane people go mad." In 1974, in an interview published in *Madness Network News*, Ennis stated: "My personal goal is either to abolish involuntary commitment or to set up so many procedural roadblocks and hurdles that it will be difficult, if not impossible, for the state to commit people against their will."[20]

Ironically, in the 1960s and 1970s, with some notorious exceptions, mental hospitals were at their best in staffing and conditions since the era of moral treatment of the early 1800s.[21] In the 1960s, when the allegations of abuse at mental health facilities began to mount, Senator Sam Ervin (later of Watergate fame) held hearings and uncovered no cases of "railroading."[22] The American Bar Association also commissioned a field investigation of mental hospitals in six states, and it concluded that railroading was a myth.[23] In general, a patient in a mental hospital who wanted to leave simply had to put one foot in front of the other and walk out. As Professor Gerald Grob, the prizewinning historian of mental hospitals, has written, hospitals provided an asylum nowhere else available.[24]

With liberty said to be at stake, the MHLP urged that the substantive and procedural due process requirements of criminal justice be applied to the civil commitment process, which would make it more difficult to achieve a commitment. For the substantive criterion, the police power of the state (dangerousness) rather than *parens patriae* (need of care) would become the primary focus of civil commitment.[25] By 1985, dangerousness became the prevailing necessary prerequisite that involves prediction, and prediction is always problematical.[26] Massachusetts's legislation requires that the harm necessary to justify commitment must be manifested by behavior that is suicidal, is homicidal, or places others in reasonable fear of serious physical harm.[27] With community-based services, it became difficult to justify, except in the case of dangerous individual, the institutionalization of the "gravely disabled" or of those unable to render a competent judgment for the need of treatment. In any event, quite often, rather than leave it to the court to decide on commitment, psychiatrists prejudge whether an individual is committable under what they understand about the "dangerousness" criterion, and do not certify, though the tendency of courts is to commit when the family appears in court pleading for hospitalization of a distraught family member.

Another restriction on hospital commitment has been the development of the concept of the least restrictive alternative (LRA), also known as the least restrictive environment. Under this doctrine, state intervention resulting from commitment is to take place in the least restrictive manner. The basis for the doctrine is the constitutional requirement that the state may restrict the exercise of fundamental liberties only to the extent necessary to effectuate the state's interest.[28] Under this scheme, the state hospital is posited as the most restrictive environment, with community-based services and outpatient care seen as less restrictive.

Thinking in terms of liberty, proponents of LRA did not use the phrase "most beneficial alternative." Under the LRA concept, any feasible alternative must be implemented in lieu of involuntary hospitalization. The trial court must find "by clear and convincing evidence that alternative treatment is not adequate or hospitalization is the least restrictive alternative."[29] The first enunciation of LRA in the law on civil commitment was in 1966 in a case involving Catherine Lake, a 60-year-old woman who wandered about in the downtown crime-ridden district of the nation's capital, appearing disoriented, and carrying her worldly possessions around with her in a shopping bag.[30] She was placed in a mental hospital. In assessing a *habeas corpus* petition brought on her behalf, the D.C. Circuit Court of Appeals ruled that whatever is done should not exceed the minimum necessary to ensure the patient's protection. Writing for the majority, Judge David Bazelon, with Warren Burger (later to become Chief Justice of the Supreme Court) dissenting, ruled that the trial court is to make the determination, not the department of mental health.[31]

In a case that came before the U.S. Supreme Court, *Addington v. Texas*,[32] the MHLP sought to invoke the "proof beyond a reasonable doubt" procedural standard of criminal justice in the civil commitment process.[33] The case involved a man whose mother filed a petition to have him involuntarily committed to a state mental hospital. Writing the opinion of the Court, Chief Justice Burger wrote that to require proof beyond a reasonable doubt of the "mental illness" or "dangerousness" criteria of civil commitment would be well-nigh impossible, and thereby would do away with involuntary commitment.[34] In the opinion, handed down in 1979, he said that the criminal law "beyond a reasonable doubt" standard was inappropriate because, "[g]iven the lack of certainty and the fallibility of psychiatric diagnosis, there is a serious question as to whether a state could ever prove beyond a reasonable doubt that an individual is both mentally ill and likely to be dangerous."[35] However, he called for a clear and convincing evidence standard in commitment hearings, which is more than the preponderance of the evidence standard of the ordinary civil case and less than proof beyond a reasonable doubt of criminal cases.[36]

Over the years, mental health associations have urged voluntary mental hospitalization in preference to involuntary commitment, while recognizing that there are times (as with suicidal or violent mentally ill individuals) when an involuntary commitment is in order. Admission practices were promoted by these associations that would encourage individuals to sign themselves into the hospital as voluntary patients (some were known as *coerced voluntaries*). That process would lessen the stigma of civil commitment. In recent years, however, the courts have tilted in the direction of hospitalization by way of a judicial proceeding. In 1990, in *Zinermon v.*

Burch,[37] the U.S. Supreme Court ruled that patient competency must be considered in regard to hospital admission as well as to treatment. The Court said that, "even if the state usually might be justified in taking at face value a person's request for admission to a hospital for medical treatment, it might not be justified in doing so without further inquiry as to a mentally ill person's request for admission and treatment at a mental hospital."

The case involved Darrell Burch who was seen bruised and bloodied wandering on a Florida highway, and was brought by a concerned citizen to a community mental health service. He was hallucinating, confused, and disoriented. At the hospital, he thought he was entering heaven. He signed a form for voluntary admission and another authorizing treatment. After 3 days of treatment with psychotropic medication, he was transferred to Florida State Hospital where he again signed voluntary admission and treatment forms. As a voluntary patient, he was free to leave at any time. He remained there for about 5 months.

Upon discharge, he complained that he had been improperly admitted to both facilities and, thus, had been confined and treated against his will. He was brought to the hospital; he did not appear there on his own motion. He claimed that because he had not been competent to sign any legal documents, he had a constitutional right to a judicial commitment before being admitted and treated, and that because there was no such hearing, he had been deprived of his liberty without due process of law. The Supreme Court agreed. In a 5–4 ruling, the Court held that before being admitted and treated he was entitled to a judicial hearing, or at least some other hearing, that would be a safeguard against arbitrary action by the state, to determine either that he was competent to consent to admission or that he met the statutory standard for involuntary commitment. The Court acknowledged that persons who are mentally ill and incapable of giving informed consent to admission would not necessarily meet the statutory standard for involuntary placement, which requires either that they are likely to injure themselves or others, or that their neglect or refusal to care for themselves threatens their well-being. The Court said:

> The involuntary placement process serves to guard against the confinement of a person who, though mentally ill, is harmless and can live safely outside an institution. Confinement of such a person not only violates Florida law, but also is unconstitutional. ... Thus, it is at least possible that if Burch had an involuntary placement hearing, he would not have been confined at FSH. Moreover, even assuming that Burch would have met the statutory requirements for involuntary placement, he still could have been harmed by being deprived of other protections built into the involuntary placement procedure, such as the appointment of a guardian advocate to make treatment decisions, and periodic judicial review of placement.[38]

As a result of the decision, a psychiatric facility faces liability for false imprisonment if it admits an individual of questionable competence on a voluntary basis without providing some procedure, possibly an adversarial judicial hearing. Most patients brought to a psychiatric facility are in such a condition that their competence to admit themselves voluntarily or to consent to treatment is questionable. Actually, while it may be argued that he was deprived of his liberty without due process, there was little in the way of damages to Burch, and he had been helped by his hospitalization. Accordingly, a nominal settlement was negotiated, giving Burch some money and making a contribution to his lawyer.[39] In practice, the decision is honored more in its breach than in its observance.

Why burden hospital admission with a courtroom procedure? Though cumbersome, it is advantageous that a patient enter a hospital via the judicial route because a voluntary patient does not enjoy the same due process protections as an involuntary patient. In *Kennedy v. Schafer*,[40] the Eighth Circuit ruled that a teenage patient who committed suicide while under treatment at a state psychiatric facility did not have a constitutionally protected liberty interest in a safe and humane environment under the due process clause of the 14th Amendment. Because the patient was voluntarily admitted to the state facility by her parents, the court held that she was not entitled to the same due process right to a safe and humane environment as would be a patient under the same circumstances who had been involuntarily committed to the facility. Her parents brought suit for infringement of rights conferred by the Constitution.[41]

The due process clause of the 14th Amendment ensures that "[n]o *State* shall ... deprive any person of life, liberty, or property, without due process of law," (emphasis added). Thus, the Eighth Circuit said: the "deprivation of liberty" that triggers "the protection of the Due Process Clause" is "the State's affirmative act of restraining the individual's freedom to act on his own behalf—through incarceration, institutionalization, or other similar restraint of personal liberty."[42] Thus, from the perspective of both the hospital and the patient, the judicial route becomes preferable, but one may wonder about it. In these cases, the judicial commitment process is usually a rubber-stamping. Assuredly, Darrell Burch (and the others) would have been committed had he been presented to a court, but he got a monetary award because he was not.

Passage of Commitment laws

Elizabeth P.W. Packard, outraged by her experience, persuaded the various states to enact broad commitment laws, not simply to do away with the commitment power of a husband. Were the laws warranted, distinguishing the care of the mentally ill from that of the physically ill? Was she railroaded? (She was literally put on a train.) In the book *The Private War of Mrs. Packard*, Barbara Sapinsley contends that Mrs. Packard's husband, a rigid, fundamentalist clergyman, had her confined in an insane asylum because she questioned his beliefs, but the evidence indicates that she was in need of hospitalization. According to the historian Albert Deutsch, Mrs. Packard claimed to be the mother of Christ and the Third Person of the Blessed Trinity.[43] Her doctor at the hospital, Andrew McFarland, was driven to despair treating her, and he vowed never again to treat a woman (he later committed suicide).

As a general principle, under the common law, there is no duty to come to the aid of another, but family members owe a duty of providing care to each other, and anyone may come to the assistance of the mentally ill. Unwarranted intermeddling, however, could result in a tort action for false arrest or false imprisonment.[44] In 1869 Isaac Ray, the prominent forensic psychiatrist, suggested that families should be left to their own "sense of duty and affection" in determining appropriate care for ill relatives.[45] The early laws in America focused on need for care under *parens patriae*.[46]

Until the 1990s, Poland did not have commitment laws. Individuals went or were brought into a mental hospital no differently than into other hospitals. There were no complaints as the care was fairly decent, particularly if a *lapowka* (payment under the table) were given the doctor. But the history of the misuse of psychiatry in the former USSR, just as it had an impact on commitment laws in the United States, prompted the enactment of commitment laws in Poland though it did not have a history of abuse of psychiatry. The law in Poland was pushed by Dr. Stanislaw Dabrowski who was in tune with U.S. laws. In many countries, for better or worse, the United States has become the model (though it has millions of homeless mentally ill).

In reaction to the misuse of psychiatry, Russia has now enacted commitment laws similar to those in the United States.[47] Actually, the crucial issue was really not *how* something was accomplished, but rather *what* was accomplished. The political dissidents who were put in a mental institution could have readily been prosecuted under its criminal laws. For some dissenters, the worst penalty was the psychiatric hospital; for others, the labor camp; for still others, exile to the West. The issue was the quashing of dissent, not how it was done. There is a saying, "If your intention is to beat a dog, you can always find a stick," but psychiatrists worldwide were concerned about the misuse of psychiatry and their image, not about other ways of quashing dissent. Like a man looking through the wrong end of a telescope, psychiatrists, with some exception, indulged in what might be called a perspective fallacy.

The Soviet Union's use of psychiatric hospitalization as a means of social control gave impetus to the view in the United States that the population of American mental hospitals is composed of social or political critics. Indeed, the antipsychiatry movement in the 1960s and 1970s claimed that schizophrenics are, in fact, social dissenters. That was implicit in the statement in 1973 by Jerome J. Shestack, Chairman of the American Bar Association Commission on the Mentally Disabled, that the United States must prevent "the kind of situation that is developing in Russia in which a diagnosis of antistate conduct is equated with being deviate and subject to commitment to a mental institution."[48]

The result was a change in focus of civil commitment in the United States from *parens patriae* to police power. Criminal justice criteria were invoked in civil commitment, mental hospitals were closed, and jails housed the mentally ill.[49] The concern over the misuse of psychiatry ignored various safeguards in the United States that did not exist in the Soviet Union. In the United States, the state is not the only source of employment for psychiatrists: an outside (privately employed) psychiatrist may evaluate a patient, there is judicial review by writ of *habeas corpus*, an unfounded or malicious petition may result in liability, and volunteers and relatives and friends who may visit in mental hospitals may report any abuses.

With the economic collapse of the country, and now privatization, Russia's health care deteriorated. As in the United States, the mentally ill now sleep on the streets, and shout in public places, or they are jailed. Many do not know who or where they are. And no one seems to care. A family seeking help will likely be told that under the new commitment laws nothing can be done when an individual resists going to a hospital. Moreover, hospital staff is not interested in treating an uncooperative patient. Why bother, when there are many others needing care?

There has been a rash of suicides in Russia committed by jumping in the paths of subway trains. In St. Petersburg, just after there were three deaths on the subway rails within a period of 12 days, the head of the subway police said, "I would not recommend that anyone commit suicide on the subway rails. If it is urgent, jumping from a tall building is better. Death under a train is not necessarily a quick one, and can be very tortuous."[50] What else could have been suggested? To suggest social services or psychiatric care would have been fanciful, given their disappearance.

The Massacre at Virginia Tech University

The massacre at Virginia Tech University on April 16, 2007, carried out by Seung-Hui Cho that took the lives of 32 students and faculty was the worst peacetime shooting in U.S. history. It followed many other deaths in the United States by gunfire, but it was the worst. In the aftermath of the massacre, explanations were sought: Was it the availability of lethal weapons,[51] mental illness of the offender,[52] closure of mental hospitals along with restrictive commitment laws,[53] or violence in the media?[54]

Had lethal weapons not been available, Cho would have killed fewer people, or perhaps none at all. Deranged people exist in every society, but they do not have easy access to weapons of awesome destructive power. Are homemade bombs in the offing?

Given easy access to weapons, focus is put on the mental illness of individuals and the question is asked whether the individual should be committed to an institution or ordered to take medication. Privacy taken as a holy grail, however, is a barrier.[55]

To lessen the stigma of mental illness, mental health organizations promote the idea that psychiatric patients are not more dangerous than the general population, but that is true only if they are taking medication.[56] Of course, not all mentally ill individuals are dangerous, but the dangerous are often mentally ill. Whether the individual is dangerous depends on the type of diagnosis, the nature and severity of the symptoms, whether the individual is receiving treatment, if there is a past history of violence, the co-occurrence of antisocial personality disorder, and substance misuse, and the social, economic, and cultural context in which the individual lives.

A district court found reason to believe Cho mentally ill and "an imminent danger to self or others" and ordered him to undergo a psychiatric evaluation, but it found "his insight and judgment were normal" and he was discharged. Dr. Robert Hare, who created one of the most authoritative models for detecting psychopathy, commented, "Diagnoses are ill advised if they are made too quickly. Most warning signs often stand out only in retrospect, and many of Cho's traits were not all that uncommon."[57] One may wonder about the utility of a psychopathy checklist.

Having greater exposure to Cho, teachers and students saw him as disturbing and menacing.[58] He was a stalker; wrote morbid, violent, hate-filled plays; set fire to his room; and even frightened professors and students to the point of being barred from class. One professor was so shocked by his classroom manner that she asked for help from her department head, but because Cho had not made any direct threats, officials said that there was little that they could do.[59] As Philip K. Howard, the author of *The Death of Common Sense,* said, "The legal system has substantially disabled the judgment of the people with responsibility."[60] Samuel Jan Brakel, one of the authors of the American Bar Foundation's *The Mentally Disabled and the Law,* commented, "To make a police operation out of the state's efforts to provide needed care and treatment is misguided, as is the adversarial inclination to exploit the already excessive criminal law protections that surround the process in an effort to keep as many people from obtaining treatment as possible."[61]

Those who were behind the movement to close mental hospitals and to render it difficult to hospitalize have yet to apologize. They continue to believe that they "emancipated" the mentally ill.

The Value of Commitment Laws

Who really benefits from commitment laws? For one thing, they provide a rationale not to provide care when the individual does not meet the standard of involuntary commitment (now essentially based on dangerousness). For another, they stigmatize, as they regard the mentally ill as though they were criminals. Moreover, in a country such as the United States where malpractice litigation is commonplace, commitment laws more or less provide a safeguard against liability, now that sovereign immunity has generally fallen by the wayside.[62] In that regard, commitment laws are a plus for the hospital staff, not the patient. For patients, the writ of *habeas corpus* and tort remedies provide a better safeguard in the case of malicious confinement.

The bill of rights in U.S. mental health codes, a section of the code following provisions on admission and discharge, actually adds nothing to the law. Commitment to a hospital is neither a determination of incompetency nor a deprivation of civil or political rights. At one time, when hospitalization was lifelong, an incompetency proceeding was joined with a commitment proceeding, in effect rendering the hospital the legal guardian of the patient. Without an adjudication of incompetency, the status of a mental patient is, or should be, the same as that of any individual, and the patient should have all the rights listed in the mental patient's bill of rights without their enumeration. Indeed, a special bill of rights implies that the mental patient has only these rights and no more. Safeguards against inappropriate treatment lie in the writ of *habeas corpus,* a malpractice action, or the appointment of an ombudsman.

The focus on commitment laws may draw attention to the conditions of institutions, but lest the tail wag the dog, it must be emphasized that the quality of institutions determines public attitudes, the commitment laws, and their interpretation. In cases of an involuntary hospitalization, the individual almost always in a few days is grateful for it, so one must question the merit of a judicial proceeding. Posttreatment reports of changed beliefs by patients in their need for hospitalization and their saying "thank you" would indicate that excessive value ought not to be placed on an initial refusal of hospitalization.[63]

A number of courts have pointed out certain benefits that accrue to a proposed patient in delaying a judicial determination on hospitalization. They note that the stigma of a court record is avoided when treatment can begin immediately, and the length of hospitalization is shortened.[64] At least until the 1970s, when control of the commitment process was taken over by the courts, two physicians (including a psychiatrist) who had no financial interest in the treatment of the patient or the medical examiner had authority, for all practical purposes, to admit a mentally disordered person to an institution. Before the 1970s, physicians and families would usually call the medical examiner (the coroner in Louisiana) who when appropriate would take the disturbed individual to a hospital. Nowadays they do not know whom to call, perhaps emergency or the police, who would take the individual in a paddy wagon, likely to jail. By and large, when encountering a person acting out because of mental illness, the police find that trying to get the person into treatment means taking hours away from other vital work to transport the person and fill out paperwork, and it does not guarantee the person will be admitted, so they take the person to jail, and book him for a criminal offense.[65] Nowadays, with the closure of mental hospitals, the police may have no alternative but to take the mentally disordered person to jail. There are 600,000 to 700,000 seriously mentally ill individuals booked into local jails every year.[66]

Mental health and criminal justice systems often deal with the same groups of chronically troubled and troublesome individuals. In practice, however, the two systems of social control rarely exchange cases, information, and resources. The lack of systems coordination is especially apparent in the area of aftercare services. Many seriously mentally ill persons in jail receive psychiatric services during their incarceration, but are usually discharged with no referrals to community treatment.[67]

In any event, the development of pharmacological drugs and community-based programs cause laws on commitment to a hospital to be regarded as archaic vestiges of a bygone era. With deinstitutionalization, the various states either under the doctrine of least restrictive alternative or by enactment of outpatient commitment laws require the taking of medication as a condition for living in the community.[68] However, as in the case of institutional care, these states tend to require that the individuals be an "imminent danger" to themselves or others before they can be involuntarily treated. Psychotic individuals who are merely making threats against others or eating out of garbage cans are not usually considered as meeting the criteria for outpatient commitment. Once again, police power rather than *parens patriae* has become the guiding principle of the commitment.

As history shows, nothing could be more meaningless than commitment laws when there are no hospitals, and when there are decent hospitals there is usually no need to turn to the law. The need for commitment laws is in inverse proportion to the quality of care. By and large, when there are decent hospitals, people seek admission. In any event, the terms in civil commitment statutes—*mental illness, need of treatment, danger to self or to others*—cannot be defined with the realistic precision necessary to allow application in a general fashion. They are as elastic as a rubber band. Sympathetic judges can (and do) interpret *dangerousness* when it is the only criterion for commitment to include the "gravely disabled" or those who lack the capacity to make an informed decision concerning treatment. In the case of physical illness, a physician cannot formulate a general rule stating when a person should be admitted to a hospital. Likewise, in the case of emotional disorder, the decision has to be on a case-by-case basis, after consideration of the degree and kind of disability and the effect the individual will have on the people around him as well as the resources available at the hospital. Many jurisdictions have enacted legislation that protects those responsible for committal if they have acted in good faith and with reasonable care. The role of counsel is an important factor in the disposition of civil commitment cases; some lawyers take a "best interest" approach while others litigate as though it were a criminal case (Minnesota and Wisconsin lead the country in the number of appellate decisions involving civil commitment).

Community Mental Health Centers

The emergence of the community mental health center (CMHC) laid the groundwork for a fourth revolution in the care of the mentally ill.[69] The CMHCs were designed to maintain patients in the community, thereby sparing them the allegedly dreadful consequences of institutionalization.[70] California's commitment law, the Landerman–Petris–Short (LPS) Act,[71] was regarded as the "outstanding accomplishment of the California legislature in its 1967 session."[72] It was designed to keep hospital population down by limiting commitment, thus saving liberty while saving money. The LPS Act was hailed as a model to which all other states could look, and it was even called "the Magna Carta" of the mentally ill. The act was designed to "protect the civil liberties of persons alleged to be mentally ill" and to accelerate the trend toward community treatment of the mentally ill as an alternative to hospitalization in remote state institutions. Presumably, the mentally disturbed would be willing to come to the center with small problems before they became big ones, thus shifting the state's role from custodial to preventive.

President John Kennedy was impressed with the Report of the Joint Commission on Mental Illness and Health, *Action for Mental Health*. He endorsed it, and made funds available for its implementation (his sister Rosemary had been lobotomized with harmful results).[73] The CMHC program had the support of both the political right and left. The right wanted to close the mental hospitals to save money, and the left thought it was freeing prisoners of snake pit psychiatric bureaucracy.

At the time, there was little or no support among policy makers for mental hospitals. Many legislators and judges were persuaded by both the legal and psychiatric professions that mental hospitalization was both outdated and expensive. The state hospitals became expensive because they were no longer run by the patients, but rather by the civil servants who were paid prevailing wages; the courts had held that patients could not work without compensation because that was interpreted as exploitation rather than rehabilitation.[74] The community mental health program was sold to legislators on the basis of saving money—and no argument is more appealing to a legislator's heart. The legislators after whom the California commitment law was named (Lanterman–Petris–Short) were members of the Ways and Means Committee—a finance committee—and were, therefore, probably concerned about the state getting its moneys' worth.

The change in the treatment of mental patients precipitated the change in funding sources for mental healthcare facilities from the states to the federal government. In 1963, when CMHCs were first funded and deinstitutionalization had just begun, the total amount of public funds spent on the mentally ill was approximately $1 billion per year. An estimated 96% of these funds came from the states. Following passage of the CMHC Act, the configuration of fiscal responsibility changed. The first change was a liberalization of rules making mentally ill individuals living in the community eligible for federal benefits under the Aid to the Disabled program. This program was subsequently incorporated into the federal Supplemental Security Income (SSI) program for individuals who did not qualify for Social Security benefits, and into the Social Security Disability Insurance (SSDI) program for those who did qualify. In addition, a federal Food Stamps program, which could also be used by mentally ill individuals in the community, was enacted in 1966.

At the same time, other federal programs were enacted that paid part of the costs for mentally ill patients in nursing homes and in the psychiatric units of general hospitals, but provided relatively little for such patients in state mental hospitals. These programs were Medicaid, enacted in 1965, and Medicare, in 1966. Medicaid and SSI require states to provide some funds to match the federal subsidy, whereas Medicare and SSDI do not have this requirement. Even with the matching funds, however, states saved at least 50% of the costs of inpatient and outpatient psychiatric care by the use of such federal programs. As a result of the shifting fund base, the 552,150 beds occupied nationwide in 1955 in state mental hospitals have been reduced by over 85%.[75]

Given that economics was the primary motivation in the deinstitutionalization of the mentally ill, the tax dollars not spent on hospitalization did not follow the patient into the community.[76] During these changes, no one seemed to ask about the "community" in mid-20th century America. In places that might be considered a community, the reaction to the CMHC program has been expressed in an acronym, NIMBY (not in my backyard).[77] The mental hospital may not be a rose garden, but compared to urban America, it smells and looks a whole lot sweeter. Since the 1950s, the saying, "Abandon hope, all ye who enter here," applies more appropriately to the inner cities than to the mental hospitals. The sprawl of the suburbs has encroached upon and enhanced the value of the land of the historic asylums resulting in their demolition. The new domicile of mental patients is the jail or the abandoned inner city.

Ironically, when mental hospitals were known as asylums, the environmental pattern of the communities from which the individuals came was close-knit, small-scaled, and personalized. At one time, service and amenity facilities were in pedestrian proximity, but today, when the mental hospital is no longer regarded as an asylum, the environmental pattern of the so-called community is loose-knit, large-scaled, and depersonalized. Service and amenity facilities are only in automobile proximity. For survival, the denizen in today's so-called community must exercise his constitutional right to bear arms and to negotiate the hazards of an expressway in order to get around.[78]

The grounds of any state hospital offered more freedom of movement than the streets of the inner cities of America. In 1996 in *Lake v. Cameron*,[79] regarding the community placement of Mrs. Lake, the "bag lady," Judge Burger (later Chief Justice of the Supreme Court) dissented, saying, "This city [the nation's capital] is hardly a safe place for able-bodied men, to say nothing of an infirm, senile, and disoriented woman to wander about with no protection except an identity tag advising police where to take her." The state of the cities remains essentially the same, but the process of deinstitutionalization proceeds apace.

In 1999, in *Olmstead v. L.C.*,[80] a divided U.S. Supreme Court held that under Title II of the Americans with Disabilities Act (ADA), institutionalized persons with mental disabilities have a right to be placed in a community setting if (1) the state's treatment professionals have determined that community placement is appropriate, (2) the transfer from institutional care to a less restrictive setting is not opposed by the affected individual, and (3) the placement can be reasonably accommodating, taking into account the resources available to the state and the needs of others with mental disabilities. Title II of the ADA states that "a public entity shall administer services, programs, and activities in the most integrated setting appropriate to the needs of qualified individuals with disabilities."[81]

The decision in *Olmstead* stemmed from a 1995 lawsuit brought by Lois Curtis and Elaine Wilson, two women with mild retardation and mental illness who had been housed in the Georgia Regional Hospital in Atlanta. The two women, known as L.C. and E.W., complained through a legal attorney that Georgia's failure to place them in community-based treatment was a violation of ADA. Appealing an adverse decision, Tommy Olmstead, then commissioner of Georgia's health department, asked the Supreme Court to decide whether the ADA requires states to provide patients with community mental health services when appropriate treatment can also be delivered in institutions.

With the aforementioned qualifications, the majority of the Court embraced the principle that undue institutionalization is a form of prohibited disability discrimination, but, in any case, a decision is iffy given the qualifications. The first qualification requires the reasonable exercise of professional judgment. The second qualification calls for a decision on placement by the affected individual, but if incompetent to make a decision, who if, anyone, is to make it? The third qualification provides that the states may take into account the "resources available" and the needs of others with mental disabilities when making decisions to deinstitutionalize.

Justice Kennedy, with Justice Breyer, while concurring in the judgment, commented that "[i]t would be unreasonable, it would be a tragic event ... were the [ADA] to be interpreted so that States had some incentive, for fear of litigation, to drive those in need of medical care and treatment out of appropriate care and into settings with too little assistance and supervision." They quoted from Dr. E. Fuller Torrey's book *Out of the Shadows*: "For a substantial minority ... deinstitutionalization has been a psychiatric Titanic. Their lives are virtually devoid of 'dignity' or 'integrity of body, mind, and spirit.' 'Self-determination' often means merely that the person has a choice of soup kitchens. The 'least restrictive setting' frequently turns out to be a cardboard box, a jail cell, or terror-filled existence plagued by both real and imaginary enemies."[82]

Mandatory outpatient treatment laws, which have been adopted in most states and the District of Columbia, would seem superfluous in light of the doctrine of least restrictive alternative. It strains logic to draw a distinction between hospitalization followed by conditional discharge and outpatient commitment straightaway.[83] The outpatient commitment law is usually enacted following a heinous crime committed by a mentally ill person who was not taking medication; the enactment of the law tends to put the public at ease. To implement the law, however, there is rarely any appropriation of new funds to pay the costs of intensive treatment. A subcommittee on mandatory outpatient treatment of the American Psychiatric Association Council on Psychiatry and Law has published a Resource Document that recommends mandatory outpatient treatment for those patients who are unlikely to comply with "needed treatment," even if these individuals would be deemed legally competent. According to the Resource Document, the enactment of mandatory outpatient treatment may prompt the legislature to provide the funding needed to provide enhanced community services for all patients, whether or not they are subject to a commitment.[84] That has not happened, and as a result, the laws are usually considered a dead letter. People resist medication that has adverse side-effects, and who is to verify that the medication is taken?

What will substitute for the structure and support afforded in the hospital? Medication? Actually, in appropriate cases, the ADA may be invoked to call for mental hospitalization as the reasonable accommodation for the individual.[85] Psychiatric medication was condemned when used in the hospital, but now its use is even greater in the outpatient setting. The medication is proclaimed to alleviate symptoms and to make possible resocialization, remotivation, rehabilitation, and reemployment. Actually, it may indeed reduce symptoms, but in fact it may not improve effectiveness in living. It causes sedation, and it causes weight gain with an increased risk of diabetes. It increases the rate of morbidity and mortality. Life span is reduced. Patients on medication typically die 10 to 15 years earlier.[86]

Due to relapse, 300,000 patients are rehospitalized annually (it is a revolving door), and often, with every relapse, there is brain damage.

The CMHC was supposed to bring about an era without snake pits, without exploitation of patients, and without deprivation of liberty. Unfortunately, it has not turned out that way, and has resulted in high costs to families and society as well as to the individual. As Los Angeles Superior Court Judge Eric Younger put it: "Crazy people are now everywhere. Modern notions of civil liberties and fiscal considerations have combined to produce a population of very disturbed people in every city in America. The notion of local treatment alternatives for mentally incapacitated citizens is a cruel hoax. It is clear that the vast majority of dangerously impaired people are out there on the streets."[87]

The shift from large institutions to nursing home care or other facilities is not deinstitutionalization, but reinstitutionalization—a new custodialism replete with its own failures and shortcomings. In 1984, John Talbott, as president-elect of the American Psychiatric Association, pointed out that more than 50% of nursing homes were populated by persons with primary or secondary diagnoses of mental disorder; thousands of disturbed persons were wandering the urban landscape without housing; and legions were inhabiting welfare hotels, board and care homes, and adult residences.[88]

Many of the chronic mentally ill, who previously were housed in state hospitals and working on hospital farms or in laundries, kitchens, and housekeeping services, functioned better, had greater feelings of self-esteem, and contributed more to their own existence than they do now in the so-called community system. Today, time and again, the complaints are countless about the mentally ill running amok in public housing or nursing homes.[89] Now these patients are on their own and they are given low priority in the CMHCs. A hospital bed often is not available when needed and with increasing frequency these chronic, rejected, and displaced patients end up in jail. Years of progress in state hospital care have been reversed by penal custody, which has often become the treatment of choice.

Those who originally advocated deinstitutionalization and community treatment programs supported the claim that not only would their programs be better (more effective), but that CMHCs would cost less. Now, these advocates bemoan the lack of adequate funds and attribute their failures to it. Their vision of a system of clinics, halfway houses, day-care centers, nursing homes, skilled nursing facilities, general hospital beds, and residential facilities would require, by far, a budget that would exceed previous costs.[90] The trend now is to permit "for profit" companies to bid against public mental health agencies to provide care to the mentally ill and developmentally disabled and drug and alcohol abusers.

The asylum concept has been abandoned, and there is little or no mention of therapeutic community. The CMHC system is basically a nonmedical system without commitment to research or interest in developmental and familial factors. Instead of treating the seriously ill, the CMHCs have turned into counseling centers for marital problems, existential crises, adolescent turmoil, and general unhappiness. The physical disorders of many patients go either unrecognized or untreated, which is evidenced by the fact that many CMHCs do not even have an examining room. Separating psyche from soma, they dichotomize the treatment of sick people. Dr. Donald G. Langsley, past president of the American Psychiatric Association, was prompted to ask, "Does the community mental health center treat patients?"[91]

Often to the dismay and fear of families, neighbors, and others in the community, thousands of psychotic individuals have been discharged from hospitals. In the oft-quoted words of Dr. Donald A. Treffert, these patients are left to die with their rights on.[92] There are crippling limitations of mental illness that do not yield to current treatment methods. Apathy, withdrawal, submissiveness, and passivity may not be the result of hospitalization as many have claimed in promoting deinstitutionalization, but symptoms of the illness itself. Patients with these conditions are pushed into communities less able to care for them than the hospitals. The result is a situation where not only the rights of others are ignored, but where patients' rights too have diminished.

In some instances, families, when assisted by the CMHC, have been helpful in the rehabilitation of the patient. Such success is more apt to be with the less severely ill and less disturbed individuals whose behavior is less bizarre and where contact with reality is less impaired. These patients do not impose as much of a burden on families as those who are much sicker, more regressed, more bizarre, more out of contact, and more out of control, but who, despite the severity of their symptoms, were discharged from hospitals because they were not considered homicidal or suicidal and presumably were able to take care of themselves.[93]

In cases where institutionalization is needed, admission to a private hospital under Medicare has often been denied by a hospital utilization review committee, contrary to medical opinion.[94] Other mentally ill patients who seek voluntary treatment in state hospitals may be turned away because there are no beds available. We have come nearly full circle to the days of Patrick Henry.

When in 1775, he uttered the famous words, "Give me liberty or give me death," he had his wife, a mother of six, confined in a basement room; she was disturbed and disturbing, and he had no other recourse. His biographer has written:

> An insane asylum had just been established at Williamsburg, but it was hardly a place where Henry would have confined his wife. It does seem that she was kept in the basement with a Negro woman attendant; probably the kindest fate for the unhappy woman, considering the horrors in store for the mentally ill in the 18th century, whose families were unable to care for them.[95]

The family physician wrote, "Whilst his towering and master-spirit was arousing a nation to arms, his soul was bowed down and bleeding under the heaviest sorrows and personal distresses. His beloved companion had lost her reason, and could only be restrained from self-destruction by a strait-dress."[96]

Once again, for lack of care and treatment, families lock up a disturbed or disturbing member, or he wanders the streets. The Ik, the mountain people of north Uganda described by Colin Turnbull, put their defective members on mountain tops to be destroyed by the elements.[97] The state hospitals have been often maligned, but they filled a vital need. Even with the best community support system, there are individuals who need an asylum. The critics of the hospital system in the 1960s and 1970s were acclaimed, but by the end of the 1970s, the failures of deinstitutionalization had become all too apparent.

The families of chronic patients are protesting. In the 1950s and 1960s, they were loosely organized, but in the 1970s, they formed political action associations with chapters in virtually every state and they remain active in seeking legal reform to make involuntary commitment easier and they want increased public funding and services for the mentally ill.[98] The overall population of state psychiatric hospitals has been reduced from 559,000 in 1955 to less than 80,000 today. In Michigan, 15 of the state's 21 mental hospitals have been closed, with only one for children still operating.[99] Nationwide, the state of affairs is similar.[100] With the virtual demise of public psychiatric hospitals as the caring and treating agency for individuals with debilitating mental illness, many of the seriously mentally ill now walk the streets or sit in jails.[101]

Specialty Courts

Specialty courts have a long history for adjudicating bankruptcies, labor relations, tax cases, or other commercial matters. At the turn of the 20th century, juvenile courts and later family courts were established. With the return of the mental hospital not on the horizon, though it is often suggested,[102] resort is increasingly being made to specialty courts that mandate treatment for the mentally ill who commit minor offenses. Noncompliance with treatment results in imprisonment. Gone is the day of "right to refuse treatment." There are now mental health courts as well as drug courts or therapy courts devoted to drugs and spousal abuse.[103] Residents in psychiatry are often employed by these courts. It has become a cottage industry. More recently, a gambling treatment court has been established.[104]

In these mental health courts and drug courts, the judge conducts a hearing on whether to divert the individual to treatment, weighing factors, such as the nature and seriousness of the alleged crime, prior criminal record, and the likelihood of benefiting from mental health services. The prosecutor has the right to determine who participates in drug courts— the decision is very discretionary.[105]

Fueled by federal grants, drug courts have swept the country (federal funds are available only for start-up programs). The first was introduced in 1989 in Miami-Dade County, Florida. As of the end of 2006, there were 1,665 drug courts operating in the United States with 386 more in the planning phase.[106] Several studies indicate that the recidivism rates for drug court participants are lower than for offenders who do not take part in the drug court system. Research also suggests that drug courts save money, increase retention in treatment, and provide affordable treatment to drug offenders.[107]

There is, however, dissenting opinion. In a 97-page article, Colorado District Judge Morris Hoffman concludes, after surveying the research on drug courts, that there is little evidence that drug courts reduce recidivism and substantial evidence that they create profound operational and institutional problems. Citing Thomas Szasz's writings, he maintains that courts should not be in the business of forcing medical treatment on people convicted of crime as a condition of a favorable sentence. They most certainly should not, he says, be in the business of forcing treatment on defendants who have not yet been convicted as a condition of being released on bail.[108]

Endnotes

1. See J. S. Bockhoven, *Moral Treatment in American Psychiatry* (New York: Springer, 1963); N. Dain, *Concepts of Insanity in the United States, 1789–1865* (New Brunswick, NJ: Rutgers University Press, 1964); A. Deutsch, *The Mentally Ill in America: A History of Their Care and Treatment From Colonial Times* (New York: Doubleday, 1973); L. Gamwell & N. Tomes, *Madness in America* (Ithaca, NY: Cornell University Press, 1995); D.J. Rothman, *Discovery of the Asylum: Social Order and Disorder in the New Republic* (Boston: Little, Brown, 1990); J.S. Bockhoven, "Moral Treatment in American Psychiatry," *J. Nerv. & Ment. Dis.* 124 (1956): 167; E.T. Carlson & N. Dain, "The Psychotherapy That Was Moral Treatment," *Am J. Psychiat.* 117 (1960): 519.

2. R.B. Caplan, *Psychiatry and the Community in Nineteenth-Century America* (New York: Basic Books, 1969).

3. G.N. Grob, *Mental Institutions in America: Social Policy to 1875* (New York: Free Press, 1973); see also G.N. Grob, "Mental Health Policy in America: Myths and Realities," *Health Affairs* 11 (1992): 7; G.N. Grob, "Mental Health Policy in the Liberal State: The Example of the United States," *Int. J. Law & Psychiat.* 31 (2008): 89.

4. R. Porter, *A Social History of Madness* (New York: Weidenfeld & Nicolson, 1987), p. 168.

5. C. Dickens, *American Notes and Pictures from Italy* (1842) (New York: Oxford University Press, 1957), p. 28.

6. For example, Michigan's Constitution, as revised, provides the following: "Institutions, programs and services for the care, treatment, education or rehabilitation of those inhabitants who are physically, mentally, or otherwise seriously handicapped shall always be fostered and supported"; Mich. Const. Art. VII, § 8. The words "programs and services" were added in 1963. (Convention comment).

7. C. Dickens, *op. cit supra* note 5.

8. B. Sapinsley, *The Private War of Mrs. Packard* (New York: Paragon House, 1991); reviewed in R. Morantz-Sanchez, "Not Mad, but Plenty Angry," *New York Times Book Review,* August 25, 1991, p. 9.

9. See S.J. Brakel, J.W. Parry, & B. Weiner, *The Mentally Disabled and the Law* (Chicago: American Bar Association, 3rd ed., 1985); J.C. Mohr, *Doctors and the Law: Medical Jurisprudence in Nineteenth-Century America* (Baltimore, MD: Johns Hopkins University Press, 1993).

10. E. Packard, "Modern Persecution or Insane Asylums Unveiled: My Abduction," in C.E. Goshen (Ed.), *Documentary History of Psychiatry: A Source Book on Historical Principles* (New York: Philosophical Library, 1967), pp. 640–665; M.S. Himmelhoch & A.H. Shaffer, "Elizabeth Packard: Nineteenth Century Crusader for the Rights of Mental Patients," *J. Am. Studies* 13 (1979): 343. The writ of *habeas corpus* (brought by her son on her behalf) obtained her release not from the hospital, where she stayed 3 years, but from the bedroom where her husband confined her after her discharge.

11. See K.M. Bowman & B. Engle, "Sexual Psychopath Laws", in R. Slovenko (Ed.), *Sexual Behavior and the Law* (Springfield, IL: Thomas, 1965), p. 757.

12. E. Goffman, *Asylums* (New York: Doubleday, 1961). The logical corollary to Goffman's conclusion that most of the patients' behavior was a reaction to being hospitalized, not a result of their illnesses, was that one needed only to open the gates of the hospital and let the patients go free, no strings (or medication) attached, and they would live happily ever after. Calling Goffman's book one of the worst books on schizophrenia, Dr. E. Fuller Torrey, clinical and research psychiatrist specializing in schizophrenia, says that one only wishes today that Goffman could be given a mattress under a bridge or freeway in any American city so that he could observe how deinstitutionalization has worked out. E.F. Torrey, *Surviving Schizophrenia* (New York: HarperCollins, 4th ed., 2001), p. 428.

In a highly influential book, *Madness and Civilization* (1961), Michel Foucault indicted the modern West for its treatment of the "insane." According to Foucault, Western societies built an institutional quarantine against madness; the madman must not roam freely through town and country as he did during the Middle Ages. Instead, Foucault claimed, the insane were thrown into cells with other dissidents from the rising bourgeois moral order: the poor, the criminal, and the licentious. M. Foucault, *Madness and Civilization: A History of Insanity in the Age of Reason* (New York: Vintage Books, 1965; French edition, 1961); reviewed in B.C. Anderson, "Madness and Enlightenment," *Pub. Interest* 138 (2000): 104.

13. Ken Kesey, *One Flew Over the Cuckoo's Nest* (New York: Viking Press, 1962). Made into a popular movie, Kesey's *One Flew Over the Cuckoo's Nest* was a fictional version of Goffman's *Asylums*. (Russian President Putin called the film his favorite.) Kesey, working for a time as a night attendant on the psychiatric ward of a veterans' hospital, became convinced that the patients were locked into a system that was the very opposite of therapeutic. The book describes a man called McMurphy who feigns mental illness to evade a prison sentence, but whose presence proves so cheering to the inmates and so disruptive to the regime of the mental hospital that he is lobotomized. Kesey became well known not only because of his book, but also as the hero of Tom Wolfe's famous nonfiction book about psychedelic drugs, *The Electric Kool-Aid Acid Test*. Kesey with a group of like-minded friends, self-styled Merry Pranksters, went around the country in a vintage school bus decorated with polychromatic swirls intended to evoke the effects of LSD. Kesey's life is depicted in an obituary by Nicholas Foulkes, "Ken Kesey," *Financial Times*, Nov. 17–18, 2001, p. xxvi, and also by Christopher Lehmann-Haupt, "Ken Kesey, Author of 'Cuckoo's Nest' Who Defined the Psychedelic Era, Is Dead at 66," *New York Times*, Nov. 11, 2001, p. 34. Torrey calls Kesey's book another of the worst books on schizophrenia, and he observes, "Kesey was a guru of psychedelic drugs at the time, and his story also has an hallucinatory ring to it." E.F. Torrey, *op. cit. supra* note 12.

14. T. S. Szasz, *The Manufacture of Madness* (New York: Harper & Row, 1970). Torrey opines that Szasz has produced more erudite nonsense on the subject of serious mental illness than any writer alive. He wonders whether Szasz has ever seen a patient with schizophrenia. E.F. Torrey, *op. cit. supra* note 12 at p. 431.

15. See, e.g., T.S. Szasz, *Psychiatric Slavery* (New York: Free Press, 1977). On the occasion of Dr. Thomas Szasz's 80th birthday, on April 15, 2000, Dr. Abraham Halpern commented, "Indoctrinated by centuries-long teachings that involuntary hospitalization was warranted to isolate or treat persons who were believed to be mentally ill, psychiatrists failed to appreciate the primacy of freedom as a value to be prized in a democratic society. The influence of Thomas Szasz on psychiatrists over the past 37 years has been enormous and has led to the abandonment of involuntary hospitalization of hundreds of thousands of nondangerous persons seeking psychological help, and to a meaningful respect for fundamental human rights in many countries, especially in the United States." Szasz has repeated his contention that mental hospitalization is psychiatric slavery in many articles and over 20 books, the latest being *Coercion as Cure: A Critical History of Psychiatry* (New Brunswick, NJ: Transaction, 2007). For a rebuttal, see R. Slovenko, "On Thomas Szasz, the Meaning of Mental Illness, and the Therapeutic State: A Critique," in J.A. Schaler (Ed.), *Szasz Under Fire: The Psychiatric Abolitionist Faces His Critics* (Chicago: Open Court, 2004), pp. 139–158.

16. R.J. Isaac & V.C. Armat, *Madness in the Streets* (New York: Free Press, 1990).

17. Jackson v. Indiana, 406 U. S. 715 at 737 (1972).

18. Vitek v. Jones, 445 U. S. 480 (1980).

19. (New York: Harcourt, Brace & Jovanovich, 1974).

20. L.R. Frank, "An Interview with Bruce Ennis," in *Madness Network News Reader* (1974), p. 162.

21. G.N. Grob, *Mental Institutions in American Social Policy to 1875* (New York: Free Press, 1973). To add to the irony, Bruce Ennis later became legal counsel for the American Psychological Association and Joel Klein, who was allied with Ennis in the Mental Health Law Project, became counsel for the American Psychiatric Association. Thus, in a turnaround, these outspoken attorneys found themselves responding to their own allegations. One might say that Ennis and Klein created their own jobs.

22. *Constitutional Rights of the Mentally Ill*, Hearings Before the Subcommittee on Constitutional Rights of Comm. on the Judiciary, 87th Cong., 1st Sess. (1961). Allegedly unjustified hospitalization came to be called "railroading" following the case of Mrs. Packard who was put on a train when sent to the hospital.

23. R.S. Rock, M.A. Jacobson, & R.M. Janopaul, *Hospitalization and Discharge of the Mentally Ill* (Chicago: University of Chicago Press, 1968), p. 77.

24. G. Grob, *op. cit. supra* note 21; see also G.N. Grob "Rediscovering Asylums: The Unhistorical History of the Mental Hospital," *Hastings Center Rep.* 7 (1977): 4, 33. See also L.H. Gold, "Rediscovering Forensic Psychiatry," in R.I. Simon & L.H. Gold (Eds.), *Textbook of Forensic Psychiatry* (Washington, DC: American Psychiatric Publishing, 2004), pp. 3–36.

25. In Lessard v. Schmidt, 349 F. Supp. 1078 (E. D. 1972), the court prohibited commitment unless the person is found to be dangerous "based upon findings of a recent overt act, attempt or threat to do substantial harm," and it called for the full panoply of criminal justice procedure and rules of evidence in civil commitment. See B.A. Weiner & D.M. Wettstein, *Legal Issues in Mental Health Care* (New York: Plenum, 1993); Symposium, "Civil Commitment," *Behav. Sci. & Law* 6 (1988): 3–148.

26. In a publication in 1978, Dr. Seymour Halleck wrote:

    > Psychiatrists in most states are now required to present evidence of the patient's dangerousness to self or others before initiating commitment. Dangerousness to self is difficult enough to predict; dangerousness to others is almost impossible. The new legal approach to civil commitment has forced us to pretend an illegitimate expertise. We cannot predict dangerousness and we cannot even give reasonable probability statements as to the likelihood of dangerousness. As a result, much psychiatric energy is devoted to obsessing about predictions we are incapable of making. The new laws also hurt patients. In most jurisdictions the new laws are not substantial enough to allow for the involuntary confinement and treatment of an individual who is desperately ill and who would respond to treatment; such a patient cannot be treated because there is no proof of dangerousness to self or others.

    S.L. Halleck, "Psychiatry and Social Control: Two Contradictory Scenarios," in S. Smith (Ed.), *The Human Mind Revisited* (New York: International Universities Press, 1978), p. 433. Though the observation was made in 1978, it remains the state of affairs notwithstanding the development of risk-assessment scales in recent years. Hare Psychopathy Checklist as revised has been found to be among the best predictors of risk for offending.

    The term *dangerousness* is taken to include four elements: (1) magnitude of harm, (2) probability that harm will occur, (3) frequency with which harm will occur, and (4) imminence of harm. "Magnitude of harm" is further divided into harm to the person (further subdivided into physical and mental harm) and harm to property. A.D. Brooks, *Law, Psychiatry, and the Mental Health System* (Boston: Little, Brown, 1974), pp. 680–682. In regard nonphysical danger to others, a few states explicitly permit commitment of a person who may cause "emotional" or "psychic" harm to others. See, e.g., Iowa Code Ann. 229.1 (2)(b). Kenneth Donaldson's "delusions" caused psychic pain to his parents and he was committed and was institutionalized for 15 years. O'Connor v. Donaldson, 422 U. S. 563 (1975). Some states also explicitly include harm to property as a commitment criterion. A mentally ill person who threatens to kill pets belonging to others could face retaliation and thus the "danger to self" criterion under the commitment statute would be satisfied. However, the court in Suzuki v. Yuen, 617 F. 2d 173 (9th Cir. 1980), said, "Under the current Hawaii definition of 'danger to property,' a person could be committed if he threatened to shoot a trespassing dog. The state's interest in protecting animals must be outweighed by the individual's interest in personal liberty." In regard frequency of harm, no state statute explicitly requires that the fact finder assess the frequency of the anticipated harm perhaps because frequency is an integral part of magnitude-of-harm analysis. See C.J. Fredrick (Ed.), *Dangerous Behavior: A Problem in Law and Mental Health* (Washington, DC: Government Printing Office, 1978); G.H. Morris, "Defining Dangerousness: Risking a Dangerous Definition," *J. Contemp. Legal Issues* 10 (1999): 61.

27. Mass. Gen. Laws Ann. Ch. 123, § 1 (West Supp. 1999). See also N.Y. Mental Hyg. Law § 9.01 (McKinney 1996).

28. The doctrine developed originally in cases involving the First Amendment. See Shelton v. Tucker, 364 U.S. 479 (1960).

29. *In re* J.K., 599 N.W.2d 337 (N.D. 1999).

30. Lake v. Cameron, 364 F.2d 657 (D.C. Cir. 1966).

31. 364 F.2d at 660. The court remanded the case to the lower court for consideration under the least restrictive means analysis. 364 F.2d at 661. See also Lessard v. Schmidt, 349 F. Supp. 1078 (E.D. 1972).

32. 441 U.S. 418 (1979).

33. 441 U.S. at 427.

34. 441 U.S. at 428-31.

35. 441 U.S. at 429.
36. 441 U.S. at 433.
37. 494 U.S. 113 (1990).
38 494 U.S. at 133–134.
39. In the event of guardianship, a guardian may not under prevailing law with exception of a couple of states admit the ward into a mental hospital. A guardian is not allowed to bypass the commitment law. Ordinarily, a guardian has the same powers, rights and duties respecting the ward that a parent has regarding a child; Mich. Comp. Laws Annot 700.455. A proposal would authorize a limited guardian or other independent decision maker to make decisions about hospitalization for the incompetent person. J.C. Beck & J.W. Parry, "Incompetence, Treatment Refusal, and Hospitalization," *Bull. Am. Acad. Psychiat. & Law* 20 (1992): 261.
40. 71 F.3d 292 (8th Cir. 1995).
41. Suit was brought under the Civil Rights Act, 42 U.S.C. §1983.
42. Quoting DeShaney v. Winnibago County Dept. Soc. Servs., 489 U.S. 189, 200 (1989). In Wilson v. Formigoni, 832 F. Supp. 1152 (N. D. Ill. 1993), the court upheld a mental patient's claim that the failure to have her involuntarily committed harmed her by preventing her inclusion in due process protections. She was deemed incompetent to make a decision to remain voluntarily.
43. *The Mentally Ill in America: A History of Their Care and Treatment from Colonial Times* (New York: Doubleday, 1937), pp. 424–425.
44. Carter v. Landy, 163 Ga. App. 509, 295 S.E. 2d 177 (1982); Note, "Civil Liability of Persons Participating in the Detention of the Mentally Ill," *Wash. U. L. Q.* 1966: 193. Texas law provides: "All persons acting in good faith, reasonably and without negligence in connection with examination, certification, apprehension, custody, transportation, detention, treatment or discharge of any person, or in the performance of any other act required or authorized by [the Mental Health Code], shall be free from all liability, civil or criminal, by reason of such action"; Tex. Rev. Civ. Stat. Ann. art. 5547–18. In James v. Brown, 637 S.W.2d 914 (Tex. 1982), a suit for damages against three psychiatrists arising out of an involuntary hospitalization, the plaintiff alleged libel, negligent misdiagnosis, medical malpractice, false imprisonment, and malicious prosecution. The Texas Supreme Court rejected a blanket immunity from all civil liability for mental health professionals testifying in mental health proceedings. The court declined to allow a defamation claim for the testimony prior to the hearing. The court noted that "[the plaintiff] is not prevented from recovering from the doctors for negligent misdiagnosis—medical malpractice merely because their diagnoses were later communicated to a court in the due course of judicial proceedings."
45. I. Ray, "The Confinement of the Insane," *Am. L. Rev.* 3 (1869): 193.
46. For example, a Connecticut law adopted in 1702 provided:

> [W]hen and so often as it shall happen, any person to be naturally wanting of understanding, so as to be incapable to provide him, or herself; or by the Providence of God, shall fall into Distraction and become *Non Compos Mentis*, and no Relations Appear, that will undertake the care of providing for them; or that stand in so near a degree, as that by law they may be compelled thereto; in every such case the selectmen or overseers of the poor of the Town, or Peculiar, where such person was born, or is by law an Inhabitant, be, and hereby are empowered and required, to take effectual care and make necessary Provision, for the relief, support, and safety, of such impotent or distracted person. Acts and Law of His Majesties Colony of Connecticut in New England (1702).

47. See S.V. Polubinskaya, "Law and Psychiatry in Russia: Looking Backward and Forward," in L.E. Frost & R.J. Bonnie (Eds.), *The Evolution of Mental Health Law* (Washington, DC: American Psychological Association, 2001), pp. 113–125.
48. Quoted in *New York Post*, Dec. 8, 1973, p. 4. See also G.M. Carstairs, "Revolutions and the Rights of Man," *Am. J. Psychiat.* 134 (1977): 979.
49. A.B. Johnson, *Out of Bedlam: The Truth About Deinstitutionalization* (New York: Basic Books, 1991); R. Slovenko, "Criminal Justice Procedures in Civil Commitment," *Wayne L. Rev.* 24 (1977): 1.
50. Cover Story, *Itogi* (Russian weekly), July 21, 1998, pp. 38–48. In recent years 60,000 Russians commit suicide annually. Cover story, "Russians Are Killing Themselves," *Newsweek* (Russian edition), September 3–8, 2007, pp. 40–49.
51. "America's Tragedy," *Economist*, April 21, 2007, pp. 11, 27–29.

52. B. Healy, "A Path to Mental Health," *U.S. News & World Report*, May 7, 2007, p. 68; N.R. Kleinfield, "Before Deadly Rage, A Lifetime Consumed by a Troubling Silence," *New York Times*. April 22, 2007, p. 1.

53. J. Kellerman, "Bedlam Revisited," *Wall Street Journal*, April 23, 2007, p. 17.

54. M. Cieply, "After Virginia Tech, Testing Limits of Movie Violence," *New York Times*, April 30, 2007, p. C-1; M. White, "Making a Killing," *New York Times*, May 2, 2007, p. 17.

55. E. Bernstein, "Colleges' Culture of Privacy Often Overshadows Safety," *Wall Street Journal*, April 27, 2007, p. 1; M. Luo, "Privacy Laws Slow Efforts to Widen Gun-Buyer Data," *New York Times*, May 2, 2007, p. 14. See also Ltrs., "Colleges Should Not Hide Behind Privacy Act," *Wall Street Journal*, Oct. 1, 2007, p. 21. Chancellor Phillip Clay of MIT is quoted as saying, "Privacy is important. Different students will do different things that they absolutely don't want their parents to know about. Students expect this kind of safe place where they can address their difficulties, try out lifestyles and be independent of their parents." Quoted in S. Wolbarst (ltr.), "A Son's Death Spotlights Student Privacy Policies," *Wall Street Journal*, Sept. 14, 2007, p. 11. In the face of the Federal Protection Law, a number of colleges offer waivers that let parents see their children's records, but will they sign? E. Bernstein, "Families Grapple With Student Privacy," *Wall Street Journal*, Sept. 20, 2007, p. D-1. Cornell has begun taking advantage of a rarely used legal exception to student-privacy rights: It is assuming students are dependents of their parents, allowing the school to inform parents of concerns without students' permission. At some universities, e.g., DePaul, any student who is disruptive must see a mental health professional. See E. Bernstein, "Bucking Privacy Concerns, Cornell Acts as Watchdog," *Wall Street Journal*, Dec. 28, 2007, p. 1.

    Finally, the Federal Education Department set out new regulations to clarify when universities may release confidential student information. The new regulations were prompted by concerns that universities were overemphasizing the students' privacy rights under the Family Educational Rights and Privacy Act to not intercede with young people who appear troubled. The new regulations actually provide no major substantive changes, but they are deemed important to the extent that they stop administrators from invoking the privacy act as an excuse for inaction. A federal report in June 2007 found widespread confusion over the laws. "Colleges and universities tend to be very law abiding and sometimes go too far to be sure they are in compliance," said Ada Meloy, general counsel of American Council on Education. T. Lewin, "After Campus Shootings, U.S. to Ease Privacy Rules," *New York Times*, March 25, 2008, p. 16.

    In response to the Virginia Tech shootings, Virginia enacted changes in its mental health law. The old standard for civil commitment emphasizing "imminent danger" to self or others is replaced by "a substantial likelihood that, in the near future, he or she will cause serious harm to himself or herself or another person" or "will suffer serious harm due to substantial deterioration of his or her capacity to protect himself or herself from such harm or to provide for his other basic human needs." But, with the extensive cutback in psychiatric facilities, where will the individuals be hospitalized? See A. Levin, "Virginia's Commitment Law Raises Many Questions," *Psychiatric News*, April 4, 2008, p. 21.

56. E.F. Torrey, "Commitment Phobia," *Wall Street Journal*, April 27, 2007, p. 17. See also G. Ghornicroft, *Shunned* (New York: Oxford University Press, 2006), p. 139. Time and again, Law Professor Michael Perlin has decried "sanism," an irrational prejudice, due to a person's mental or emotional disability, that is based predominantly upon stereotype, myth, superstition, and deindividualization. See M.L. Perlin, *The Hidden Prejudice* (Washington, DC: American Psychological Association, 2000).

57. Quoted in J. Schwartz & B. Carey, "Experts Shy From Instant Diagnosis of Gunman's Mental Illness, but Hints Abound," *New York Times*, April 20, 2007, p. 16.

58. As Holman W. Jenkins Jr. writes, "Psychologists make a professional habit of saying that violence can't be predicted, perhaps true in the clinical setting. In the workplace and the normal encounters of everyday life, however, others do get glimpses of the personality and external circumstances that sometimes combine to produce such mass shootings. One of our enduring frustrations is that—after we've waded through the predictable thickets of adjectives describing the killer as 'quiet' and the killings as 'senseless'—it turns out warning signs were present, that co-workers, neighbors or family members had seen the culprit clearly enough to be afraid." H.W. Jenkins, "The Mass-Shooting Puzzle," *Wall Street Journal*, April 18, 2007, p. 16.

59. B. Carey, "When the Group Is Wise," *New York Times*, April 22, 2007, sec. 4, p. 1; I. Urbina & M. Fernandez, "University Defends the Return of Troubled Students," *New York Times*, April 20, 2007, p. 17. There is a presumption against treatment. "It is not enough that a person would benefit from treatment; the person must require treatment. To establish that a mentally ill person requires treat-

ment, there must be convincing evidence that the person poses a serious risk of harm if left untreated." Interest of I.K., 2003 N.D. 101, 663 N.W.2d 197, 199 (2006). See also A. Levin, "Liability Concerns Shouldn't Guide Decisions About Troubled Students," *Psychiatric News*, June 8, 2008, p. 10.

60. Quoted in Editorial, "Caught in the (Legal) Crossfire," *Wall Street Journal*, April 20, 2007, p. W13.

61. S.J. Brakel, "Searching for the Therapy in Therapeutic Jurisprudence," *N. Eng. J. Crim. & Civil Confine.* 33 (2007): 498–499. See also E. Tanay, "Virginia Tech Mass Murder: A Forensic Psychiatrist's Perspective," *J. Am. Acad. of Psychiat. & Law* 35 (2007): 152. Query: Could it be that the patient-advocate in mental institutions is a vestige of another time? Do they often not serve the best interest of the patient, the family, or society? For example, the patient-advocate did not help the Bruces. Aided by a patient-advocate, William Bruce was discharged from a psychiatric hospital, over the objection of his parents, and he killed his mother. See E. Bernstein & N. Koppel, "A Death in the Family," *Wall Street Journal*, Aug. 16–17, 2008, p. 1; Ltrs., "The Mental Health Advocates Didn't Help the Bruces," Ibid., Aug. 23–24, 2008, p. 16. I asked Brakel for his opinion. He responded with an emphatic "yes" that the patient-advocate is a vestige of another time: "The concept was founded at a time when mental hospitals were often snake pits and treatment for mental disorders was largely unavailing, and more importantly, continues to be practiced on the false perception that nothing has changed in this regard." Personal communication (Sept. 3, 2008).

62. Failure to follow the statutorily prescribed involuntary commitment standards is evidence of negligence for a fact finder to consider, and not negligence per se. See Fair Oaks Hosp. v. Pocrass, 628 A.2d 829 (N.J. Super. 1993); Moore v. Wyoming Medical Center, 825 F. Supp. 1531 (D. Wyo. 1993). In some countries, and also in some states in the United States, legislation protects persons responsible for the committal if they acted in "good faith." See A. Alston, "Wrongful Committal," *Psychiat., Psychol. & Law* 7 (2000): 71.

63. W. Gardner, C.W. Lidz, S.K. Hoge, J. Monahan, M.M. Eisenberg, N.F. Bennett, E.P. Mulvey, & L.H. Roth, "Patients' Revisions of Their Beliefs About the Need for Hospitalization," *Am. J. Psychiat.* 156 (1999): 1385; A. Wertheimer, "A Philosophical Examination of Coercion for Mental Health Issues," *Behav. Sci. & Law* 11 (1993): 239. The civil commitment hearing is defended in B.J. Winick, "Therapeutic Jurisprudence and the Civil Commitment Hearing," *J. Contemp. Legal Issues* 10 (1999): 37. Predictably, civil libertarians challenge outpatient commitment as intrusive of the rights of people. See, e.g., B.J. Winick, "Outpatient Commitment: A Therapeutic Jurisprudence Analysis," *Psychol. Pub. Policy & Law* 9 (2003): 107.

64. French v. Blackburn, 428 F. Supp. 1351 (M.D. N.C. 1977); Logan v. Arafeh, 246 F. Supp. 1265 (D. Conn. 1972), *aff'd*, Briggs v. Arafeh, 411 U.S. 911 (1973).

65. Nationally, almost 10% of police calls and 10% of arrests involve persons with flagrant mental disorders. Despite the frequency of contact with emotionally disturbed persons, police officers often lack adequate training on how to deal safely and effectively with such individuals. Many of these incidents are written off as "a nut with a knife" or "suicide by cop." J. Meyer & S. Berry, "Lack of Training Blamed in Slayings of Mentally Ill," *Los Angeles Times*, Nov. 8, 1999, p. 1. A symposium on police encounters with persons with mental illness appears in *J. Psychiat. & Law* 28 (2000): 325–347. See also S. S. Janus, B.E. Bess, J.J. Cadden, & H. Greenwald, "Training Police Officers to Distinguish Mental Illness," *Am. J. Psychiat.* 137 (1980): 228.

66. J. Abrahms, (AP news release), "Congress Approves New Treatment Program for Mentally Ill Criminals," *Detroit Legal News*, Oct. 27, 2000, p. 18.

67. A.J. Lurigio, J R. Fallon, & J. Dincin, "Helping the Mentally Ill in Jails Adjust to Community Life: A Description of a Postrelease ACT Program and Its Clients," *Int. J. Offender Ther. & Compar. Criminol.* 44 (2000): 532

68. Nearly all the states and the District of Columbia have adopted outpatient commitment laws. Outpatient commitment does not guarantee patients' compliance with taking medication, but it is considered that it improves patients who are discharged from general hospital psychiatric units but who the treatment team knows will probably not be compliant with their medication and other treatment modalities. M. Kohl, "New York State Moves Toward Involuntary Residential Commitment of the Mentally Ill," *Psychiatric Times*, Sept. 1999, p. 30. See R. Miller, *Involuntary Civil Commitment of the Mentally Ill in the Post-Reform Era* (Springfield, IL: Thomas, 1987). Outpatient commitment is related to the old idea of "paroling" mental patients from the hospital or giving them trial discharges. Patients unable to manage in the community would be recalled to the hospital without further legal proceedings. In its new guise, it is not limited to former inpatients but can serve as a disposition of choice at a commitment hearing (under the theory of least restrictive alternative). However, under Florida's outpatient commitment law, effective January 2005, only 71 orders for outpatient commitment have been issued

in 3 years, even though during that period 41,997 adults had two or more 72-hour involuntary emergency examinations under Florida's civil commitment law. Statutory criteria make filing a petition for outpatient commitment difficult, as well as a lack of community treatment resources and enforcement mechanisms. J. Petrila & A. Christy, "Florida's Outpatient Commitment Law: A Lesson on Failed Reform?" *Psychiat. Serv.*, 59 (Jan. 2008): 21.

69. See P.S. Appelbaum, *Almost a Revolution* (New York: Oxford University Press, 1994).
70. L. L. Bachrach, *Deinstitutionalization: An Analytical Review and Sociological Perspective* (Washington, DC: U. S. Government Printing Offfice, 1976).
71. Calif. Welfare & Institutions Code chap. 1, § 5000.
72. R. J. Isaac & V. C. Armat, *op. cit. supra* at chap. 6.
73. H. R. Lamb (Ed.), *The Homeless Mentally Ill* (Washington, DC: American Psychiatric Press, 1984).
74. R. Cancro, "Functional Psychoses and the Conceptualization of Mental Illness," in R.W. Menninger & J.C. Nemiah (Eds.), *American Psychiatry After World War II* (Washington, DC: American Psychiatric Press, 2000), pp. 413–429.
75. G.N. Grob, "Mental Health Policy in Late Twentieth-Century America," in R.W. Menninger & J.C. Nemiah (Eds.), *American Psychiatry After World War II* (Washington, DC: American Psychiatric Press, 2000).
76. M.J. Mills & B.D. Cummings, "Deinstitutionalization Reconsidered," *Int. J. L. & Psychiat.* 5 (1982): 271.
77. S. Sandler, "The Westside Has Lost Patience," *New York Times*, Nov. 7, 1992, p. 15.
78. R. Slovenko, "Mobilopathy," *J. Psychiat. & Law* 12 (1984): 293.
79. 364 F.2d 657 (D.C. Cir. 1966).
80. 119 S. Ct. 2176 (1999).
81. 42 U. S. C. § 12101. See S. Stefan, "The Americans with Disabilities Act and Mental Health Law: Issues for the Twenty-First Century," *J. Contemp. Legal Issues* 10 (1999): 131.
82. 119 S. Ct. at 2191. See S. Fishman, "*Olmstead v. Zimring*: Unnecessary Institutionalization Constitutes Discrimination Under the Americans With Disabilities Act," *J. Health Care Law & Policy* 3 (2000): 430.
83. Professor Michael Perlin contends that the "least restrictive alternative," the roots of which justified outpatient commitment, was originally seen as a way of limiting the numbers of persons under state control in public psychiatric hospitals, but is now frequently suggested as a means of exerting control over more individuals in community settings. (Address at the annual meeting of the Association of American Law Schools on January 6, 2001, in San Francisco.) Studies have shown that the clientele of community treatment centers includes few chronic patients and is comprised mostly of a new class of patients who formerly either did not seek treatment or received it from the private sector. See R.D. Miller, "Clinical and Legal Aspects of Civil Commitment," in C.P. Ewing (Ed.), *Psychology, Psychiatry, and the Law: A Clinical and Forensic Handbook* (Sarasota, FL: Professional Resource Exchange, 1985), pp. 149–180. See also K. Kress, "An Argument for Assisted Outpatient Treatment for Persons With Serious Mental Illness Illustrated With Reference to a Proposed Statute for Iowa," *Iowa L. Rev.* 85 (2000): 1269.
84. J.B. Gerbasi, R.J. Bonnie, & R.L. Binder, "Resource Document on Mandatory Outpatient Treatment," *J. Am. Acad. Psychiat. & Law* 28 (2000): 127. Stirring the most controversy is the stance of the American Psychiatric Association on reserving mandatory outpatient treatment for those who meet the long-standing "dangerousness" measure. The Resource Document broadens the criteria defining which patients are eligible for outpatient commitment to include those who simply are "unlikely to seek or comply with needed treatment unless a court enters an order." "Resource Document on Mandatory Outpatient Treatment Reviewed," *Psychiatric News*, Oct. 6, 2000, p. 16. The American Psychiatric Association has also published a special section on outpatient treatment in the March 2001 issue of its *Psychiatric Services*. An additional resource is a RAND study, completed for the California legislature, "The Effectiveness of Involuntary Outpatient Treatment."

In a challenge to New York's outpatient commitment law (known as Kendra's law), in Urcuyo v. James D. and Trachtenberg, King's County New York Supreme Court Justice Anthony Cutrona upheld the law on constitutional grounds. The law was attacked as amounting to summary arrest. Under the law, the court noted, the individual must have a history of a lack of compliance with mental health treatment, causing the individual to be hospitalized at least twice in the preceding 36 months. Also, the individual must have received services from a forensic or other mental health unit of a correctional facility or have a history of mental illness that has resulted in one or more acts of serious violent behavior, or threats or attempts at serious physical harm, to self or others. The individual must be found, by clear and convincing evidence, to be unlikely to participate voluntarily in a recommended treatment plan. Additionally, in light of the individual's treatment history and current behavior, the individual must be found in need of assisted outpatient treatment to prevent a relapse or deterioration that would likely result in serious harm to the individual or others. Under Kendra's law the court may order the patient to self-administer psychotropic medication or accept the administration of such medication by authorized personnel as part of an assisted outpatient treatment program. Such treatment may be ordered for periods of up to one year; N.Y. Ment. Hyg. L. § 9.60(K). Forced medication has been aptly described as the "core of outpatient commitment." S. Stefan, "Preventive Commitment: The Concept and Its Pitfalls," *Ment. & Phys. Dis. L. Rep.* 11 (1987): 288. On the closing of the Northville Regional Psychiatric Center, one of the last mental hospitals in Michigan, medication that "helps control mental illness" was cited as the chief reason behind the hospital closing. C. Garrett, "Michigan Will Sell Last Mental Hospital," *Detroit News*, Nov. 9, 2001, p. D-1. Under Kendra's law, a patient who fails or refuses to comply with a treatment plan authorized by the court cannot be held in contempt of court, but can be transported to a hospital and held up to 72 hours to determine if the individual is in need of "involuntary care and treatment"; N.Y. Ment. Hyg. L.§ 9.60(N).

85. In Helen L. v. DiDario, 46 F. 3d 325 (3d Cir. 1995), the Third Circuit ruled that a state welfare department regulation that forced certain patients to receive required care services in a nursing home rather than through a community-based attendant care program violated the ADA. In Kathleen S. v. Dept. of Public Welfare, 10 F. Supp. 2d 476 (E. D. Pa. 1998), the Pennsylvania Department of Public Welfare sought a stay enforcement of an order requiring acceleration of the integration into the community of patients at a state mental health facility. The federal district court held that the department failed to satisfy the requirements for a grant of stay, namely, that granting of the stay would inflict substantial injury on the patients in community placement and would not be in the public interest.

86. In a lengthy article, Dr. Douglas Mossman argues that the introduction of atypical medications in 1994 should result in less hesitation in imposing treatment as they do not produce the extrapyramidal side effects of the typical antipsychotics. D. Mossman, "Unbuckling the 'Chemical Straitjacket': The Legal Significance of Recent Advances in the Pharmacological Treatment of Psychosis," *San Diego L. Rev.* 39 (2002): 1033. See also S.J. Brakel & J.M. Davis, "Overriding Mental Health Treatment Refusals: How Much Process Is 'Due'?" *St. Louis Law J.* 52 (2008): 501. But, the atypicals place patients at more risk of developing troublesome metabolic conditions, including obesity, alterations in lipid metabolism, and diabetes mellitus. See P.R. Breggin, *Medication Madness* (New York: St. Martin's Press, 2008); G.H. Morris, *Refusing the Right to Refuse: Coerced Treatment of Mentally Disordered Persons* (Lake Mary, FL: Vandeplas, 2006). See also E. Mattison, "Commentary: The Law of Unintended Consequences," *J. Am. Acad. Psychiat. & Law* 28 (2000): 154; B. Carey, "Study of Newer Antipsychotics Finds Risks for Youths," *New York Times*, Sept. 15, 2008, p. 17.

87. Quoted in N. Q. Brill, *America's Psychic Malignancy* (Springfield, IL: Thomas, 1993), p. 113.

88. J.A. Talbott, "Psychiatry's Agenda for the 80's," *JAMA* 251 (May 4, 1984): 2250.

89. Ltrs., "Patient Cry for Help; System Cries for Reform," *Detroit Free Press*, Oct. 12, 2000, p. 10.

90. A study in Massachusetts reports that 27% of those discharged from state psychiatric hospitals became homeless within 6 months; a similar study in Ohio found the figure to be 36%. And, an increasing number of mentally ill people are in jails and prisons. See also R. Blumenthal, "Emotionally Ill Pose Growing Problem to Police," *New York Times*, Nov. 16, 1989, p. 1.

91. D.G. Langsley, "The Community Mental Health Centre: Does it Treat Patients?" *Hosp. & Commun. Psychiat.* 31 (1980): 815.

92. D.A. Treffert, "Dying With Your Rights On," *Prism* (Socio-Econ. Magazine of AMA) 2 (1974): 49.

93. G.N. Grob, "Mental Health Policy in America: Myths and Realities," *Health Affairs* 11 (1992): 7.

94. W. Chittenden, "Malpractice Liability and Managed Health Care: History and Prognosis," *Torts & Ins. L. J.* 26 (1991): 451.

95. R.D. Meade, *Patrick Henry: Patriot in the Making* (Philadelphia, PA: Lippincott, 1957), p. 281.

96. *Ibid.*

97. C.M. Turnbull, *The Mountain People* (New York: Simon & Schuster, 1972). In China parents put their mentally ill children in a cage in their home. N. Zamiska, "Caged in China: Parents Grapple With Mentally Ill," *Wall Street Journal*, Jan. 16, 2008, p. 1.

98. J.Q. LaFond & M.L. Durham, *Back to the Asylum: The Future of Mental Health Law and Policy* (New York: Oxford University Press, 1992); J.T. Carney, "America's Mentally Ill: Tormented Without Treatment," *Geo. Mason U. C. R. L. J.* 3 (1992): 18; D.H.J. Hermann, "Barriers to Providing Effective Treatment: A Critique of Revision in Procedural, Substantive, and Dispositional Criteria in Involuntary Civil Commitment," *Vand. L. Rev.* 39 (1986): 83.

99. P. Chodoff (ltr.), "Jails and Mental Illness," *Psychiatric News*, Dec. 4., 1992, p. 2; see N. Sinclair, "Mentally Ill Crowd Metro Area Jails," *Detroit News,* Aug. 29, 1999, p. 1; see also A. Mullen, "Death in the Lockup," *Detroit Metro Times*, Sept. 15, 1999, p. 14; N. Sinclair, "Disturbed Kids Abandoned," *Detroit News*, Aug. 30, 1999, p. 1.

100. In Oregon, for example, while the state's population has increased substantially, commitment rates have dropped by 50%. Dr. Joseph Bloom, dean emeritus of the Oregon School of Medicine, writes, "There are many possible factors that have contributed to this decline in commitment rates, including a stricter functional definition of 'danger to self or others,' but perhaps the most significant reason is the shortage of the acute psychiatric beds that are essential in the commitment process. It is hard not to conclude that civil commitment in this state is headed toward functional extinction." J.D. Bloom, "Civil Commitment Is Disappearing in Oregon," *J. Am. Acad. Psychiat. & Law* 34 (2006): 534. See also P. Earley, *Crazy: A Father's Search Through America's Mental Health Madness* (New York: G.P. Putnam's Sons, 2006).

101. According to a report by the Pew Center on the States (2008), the U.S. prison population, the world's largest, has grown nearly eightfold over the past 35 years and now costs taxpayers at least $60 billion a year, up from $11 billion in 1987. More than one in every 100 American adults is in jail or prison, and that does not count the hundreds of thousands of people who are on probation and parole. Michigan, with one of the nation's highest incarceration rates, spends $2 billion a year on corrections, or 20% of its general fund, more than it spends on all of its universities of higher education (as do Connecticut, Delaware, Oregon and Vermont). Of the 600,000 in prison in Michigan, some 50 to 75% are seriously mentally ill. As elsewhere in U.S. prisons, unlike in Stalin's gulag, the inmates do very little productive work. Editorial, "One Nation, Behind Bars," *Detroit Free Press*, March 6, 2008, p. 18. A year-long examination of prison health by the *New York Times* revealed repeated instances of medical care that has been flawed and sometimes lethal. P. Zielbauer, "As Health Care in Jails Goes Private, 10 Days Can Be a Death Sentence," *New York Times*, Feb. 27, 2005, p. 1. See Symposium, "1950–2000: Reflections on the Past Fifty Years of Psychiatric Services," *Psychiat. Serv.* 51 (Jan. 2000): 70–118.

102. See, e.g., J.Q. LaFond & M.L. Durham, *Back to the Asylum: The Future of Mental Health Law and Policy* (New York: Oxford University Press, 1992); Ltrs, "Is It Time to Return the Truly Mentally Ill to Psychiatric Hospitals? *Wall Street Journal*, May 2, 2007, p. 19. See also A.B. Klapper, "Finding a Right in State Constitutions for Community Treatment of the Mentally Ill," *U. Pa. L. Rev.* 142 (1993): 739.

103. See R.D. Schneider, H. Bloom, & M. Heerema, *Mental Health Courts* (Toronto: Irwin Law, 2007); Special Issue, "Specialty Courts," *Int. J. Law & Psychiat.* 16 (Jan./Feb. 2003): 1–110; Special Issue, "Mental Health Tribunals and Decision Making," *Psychiat., Psychol. and Law* 10 (2003): 1–198; G. Fields, "U.S. Mental-Health Courts Offer Some Defendants a Way Out of Jail," *Wall Street Journal*, Aug. 23, 2006, p. 12; Michigan has 37 DWI (Driving While Impaired) or Sobriety Court programs, about 10% of the nation's total. R.M. Gubbins, "Michigan a Leader in Number of Sobriety Courts," Detroit Legal News, Sept. 1, 2008, p. 1. New York has a court, the only one in the country, for military veterans who fall into addiction, mental illness and crime. M. Daneman, "Court in N.Y. Gives Vets Chance to Straighten Out," *USA Today*, June 2, 2008, p. 3.

104. K. Belson, "In Gambling Treatment Court, Help Is Stressed Over Penalties," *New York Times*, May 1, 2007, p. 1.

105. See State v. DiLuzio, 121 Wash. App. 822, 90 P.3d 1141 (2004). Prosecutors are even given discretion whether to seek the death penalty.

106. The number of new drug courts in Michigan, for example, has increased every year since 2002. In 2002, there were 24; in 2003, 36; in 2004, 49; in 2005, 56; in 2006, 59. In the program run by Novi Judge Brian MacKenzie, alcohol and drug tests are given twice a day for 60 straight days, then once a day for another 7 months. A single positive test results in the defendant going to jail. Judge MacKenzie mainly funds his $150,000-a-year program with a $135 fee that every person convicted of drunken driving must pay (that raised $135,000 in 2006). J. Chambers, "Cutbacks Hit Drug Courts Hard," *Detroit News,* Oct. 25, 2007, p. 1.

107. See S.L. Satel, *Drug Treatment: The Case for Coercion* (Washington, DC: American Enterprise Institute, 1999); E.L. Jensen & C. Mosher, "Adult Drug Courts: Emergence, Growth, Outcome Evaluations, and the Need for a Continuum of Care," *Idaho L. Rev.* 42 (2006): 443; T. Oram & K. Gleckler, "An Analysis of the Constitutional Issues Implicated in Drug Courts," *Idaho L. Rev.* 42 (2006): 471. A reduction from 42 to 18% for drug-related offenses and from 63 to 38% for all offenses is reported in D. Eisman, "Drug Courts: Changing People's Lives," *Advocate* 46 (2003): 16. See also D. Banks & D. Gottfredson, "The Effects of Drug Treatment and Supervision on Time to Re-arrest Among Drug Treatment Court Participants," *J. Drug Issues* 33 (2003): 385; A. Kaplan, "Mental Health Courts Reduce Incarceration, Save Money," *Psychiatric Times*, July 2007, p. 1; A. Levin, "Mental Health Courts: A Strategy That Works," *Psychiatric News*, Sept. 21, 2007, p. 6.

108. M. Hoffman, "The Drug Court Scandal," *No. Car. L. Rev.* 78 (2000): 1437. See also L.B. Erlich, *A Textbook of Forensic Addiction Medicine and Psychiatry* (Springfield, IL: Thomas, 2001).

25

Failure to Treat and Related Issues

In general, nonfeasance does not result in liability unless there is a duty to act. With some exception, there is no duty to render assistance to another who is in peril, no matter how easily aid might be furnished, and regardless of whether the failure to act is inadvertent or intentional. The expert swimmer, with a boat and a rope at hand, who sees another drowning, is not required to do anything at all about it, but may sit on the dock and watch the man drown. Thus, under this principle, a physician is under no duty to answer the call of a stranger who is dying and might be saved.[1]

This common law "no-duty" rule was articulated in a New Hampshire case in 1897 where the court said, "With purely moral obligations, the law does not deal. … For example, suppose A, standing close by a railroad, sees a 2-year-old baby on the track and a car approaching. He can easily rescue the child with entire safety to himself, and the instincts of humanity require him to do so. If he does not, he may, perhaps justly be styled a ruthless savage and a moral monster, but he is not liable in damages for the child's injury."[2]

Deeply rooted in the law of torts is the distinction between *nonfeasance* and *misfeasance*, but during the last century liability for nonfeasance has been imposed in a limited group of relations, in which public sentiment and views of social policy have led the courts to find a duty of affirmative action. A special relation between the parties has afforded a justification for the creation of a duty. Notably, upon the formation of a physician–patient relation, there comes about a duty on the physician to care for the patient. A carrier is required to take reasonable affirmative steps to aid a passenger in peril, and an innkeeper to aid its guests. It also is recognized that if the defendant's own negligence has been responsible for the plaintiff's situation, a relation has arisen that imposes a duty to make a reasonable effort to give assistance and avoid any further harm. Moreover, when a duty of care is voluntarily undertaken, as when one comes to the rescue of another, the rescuer assumes a duty to use proper care in the performance of the task. Just when the duty is undertaken, when it ends, and what conduct is required are nowhere clearly defined, and perhaps cannot be.

Once therapy is undertaken, the physician–patient relationship continues until (1) it is terminated by mutual consent, (2) it is ended by the patient, (3) the services are no longer needed, or (4) the physician withdraws after giving the patient reasonable notice. As a matter of good practice, if not law, a physician who wishes to terminate a patient in need of further care should at least offer to refer the patient to another therapist. A physician who abandons a patient who later harms himself or another could be held liable for malpractice.

As hereinafter discussed, an action for failure to treat may arise out of the inpatient or outpatient setting.

Institutionalized Patients

In the case of an individual who has been institutionalized, the right to treatment is generally claimed on the basis of provisions of the commitment statute, which premise involuntary commitment on the patient's need for care and treatment. While not common, it has been held that an involuntarily committed patient may recover damages for inordinate length of confinement resulting from a lack of proper psychiatric care. The claim may be based on a violation of an individual's constitutional right to freedom. In *O'Connor v. Donaldson*,[3] the U.S. Supreme Court ruled that "a State cannot constitutionally confine without more [i.e., without treatment] a non-dangerous individual who is capable of surviving safely in freedom by himself or with the help of willing and responsible family members or friends." Donaldson was awarded both compensatory and punitive damages.

In another much discussed case, *Whitree v. State*,[4] the state of New York was held liable for confining and failing to treat a patient who had been committed because of incompetence to stand trial.[5] The patient was confined for over 14 years; he was a patient only in the sense that he was "patient." Had he received the maximum sentence for the theft alleged, he would have been in jail for 3 years. His expert testified that with proper care his competence to stand trial could have been restored within 3 to 6 months after admission. His diagnosis at commitment was chronic alcoholism with paranoid features, whereas upon discharge he was found to be "a schizoid personality with paranoid features, but not in such a state of idiocy, imbecility, or insanity as to be incapable of understanding or contributing to his defense." The court commented that the hospital record "was about as inadequate a record as we have ever examined."

Earlier, in the right-to-treatment case of *Rouse v. Cameron*,[6] Judge Bazelon had intimated that failure to supply treatment may "raise a question of due process of law," may "violate the equal protection clause," or may "be so inhumane as to be 'cruel and unusual punishment.'" The remedy afforded in *Rouse* was discharge from the hospital on a writ of *habeas corpus*; the remedy afforded in *Whitree* was discharge and money damage.

The standard of care applied by the court in *Whitree* is the general rule applicable in malpractice cases: careful treatment "consonant with medical standards." The court concluded that careful examination was totally lacking and that no competent professional judgment had been made. Clearly, the total absence of diagnostic investigation is inconsistent with any standard of rehabilitative care. The decision was indicative of the public concern over the inadequacies of state mental institutions and the treatment furnished there.

Failure to Seek Hospitalization

An aspect of failure to treat is failure to seek hospitalization of a patient in need of such, particularly in the case of a suicidal patient. On the one hand, negligent certification can lead to liability in torts of malpractice (negligence), defamation, or assault and battery. On the other hand, though it does not often occur, a therapist may be held responsible in not seeking the hospitalization of a patient or providing other treatment.[7]

An illustration is a Wisconsin case, *Shuster v. Altenberg*.[8] A patient, who was diagnosed as a manic depressive and was taking medications that carry warnings not to drive while under their influence, within an hour of seeing her therapist drove into a tree at 60 mph, killing herself and leaving her 17-year-old daughter a paraplegic. The complaint alleged that the therapist, a psychiatrist, was negligent in his management and care of the patient "in failing to recognize or take appropriate actions in the face of her psychotic condition, including failure to seek her commitment, to modify her medication, to alert and warn the patient or her family of her condition or its dangerous implications."

For the purposes of addressing the legal sufficiency of the complaint, the Wisconsin Supreme Court categorized the allegations as follows: (1) negligent diagnosis and treatment, (2) failure to warn the patient's family of her condition and its dangerous implications, and (3) failure to seek the commitment of the patient. Generally, once a court determines that a claim has been stated as to one particular theory, it will not proceed to determine what additional theories are valid, but in this case the court, upon the request of both parties and in the interest of judicial economy, ruled on all three theories, finding them all legally sufficient. For one, the court said, a therapist may be held liable in negligence for failure to warn of the side effects of a medication if the side effects were such that a patient should have been cautioned against driving because it was foreseeable that an accident could result, causing harm to the patient or third parties if the patient drove while using the medication. For another, the court said, if it is ultimately proven that it would have been foreseeable to a psychiatrist, exercising due care, that by failing to warn a third person or by failing to take action to institute detention or commitment proceedings someone would be harmed, negligence will be established. The pleadings established grounds upon which a jury could find negligence and could further find such negligence to have constituted the cause-in-fact of the injury.[9]

In an article oft-quoted by the courts, Victor Schwartz, then a law professor, wrote:

First, it seems clear that liability could be imposed upon a psychiatrist for a gross error in judgment with respect to whether a patient should be confined. Giving full ambit to psychological justifications for not confining patients unless absolutely necessary, suicidal symptoms may be so apparent that a psychiatrist of ordinary skill would order confinement. For example, if an individual has made serious suicidal attempts, has been deeply depressed, has suffered loss of sleep, appetite, and in effect is almost unable to function in society, but his psychiatrist has declined to have him placed in a hospital, the psychiatrist might be held liable for the individual's subsequent suicide.[10]

Yet, suicide prediction is notoriously unreliable, with suicide prediction resulting in numerous "false positives," that is, prediction that individuals will commit suicide when, in fact, they would not. The courts recognize that the widespread use of civil commitment to prevent suicide would result in numerous patients who are not suicide risks being subjected to a loss of freedom.[11] In the commitment and release context, the courts tend to indulge professional judgment in the assessment of risks versus benefits because aberrant behavior, such as suicide and homicide, occurs only infrequently and is not amenable to reliable prediction.[12]

In a Florida case, Linda Kay Paddock went to a wooded area, took a butane cigarette lighter from her purse, and set her blouse on fire. She suffered serious burns over most of her body, but she survived and she brought a malpractice action against her psychiatrist, Dr. Chowallur Chacko, claiming that he should have had her hospitalized before she burned herself. She saw Dr. Chacko just once before setting herself on fire. The psychiatric testimony at trial was extensive, taking 793 pages of transcript. Her experts testified that she was suicidal and that Dr. Chacko should have sought her hospitalization. After deliberating for 13 hours, the jury concluded that Dr. Chacko had been negligent, and that his negligence had caused Paddock's injuries. The jury further concluded that Paddock had not been contributorily negligent. They awarded Paddock $2.15 million, twice the largest malpractice award in Orange County, Florida.

The Florida Court of Appeals reversed the judgment, saying that there is no legal duty to commit a patient to a hospital involuntarily, at least not in Florida. Such an obligation, the court said, would "create an intolerable burden on psychiatrists and the practice of psychiatry."[13] The court commented, "The science of psychiatry represents the penultimate grey area. Numerous cases underscore the inability of psychiatric experts to predict, with any degree of precision, an individual's propensity to do violence to himself or others. ... A substantial body of literature suggests that the psychiatric field cannot even agree on appropriate diagnosis, much less recommend a course of treatment."[14]

One study argues that hospitalization does not prevent suicide, and indeed it may add pressure to commit suicide. There is little conclusive evidence to suggest that being placed on a psychiatric unit reduces a person's chance of committing suicide in either the short or the long term.[15] Yet, according to estimates of malpractice claims against psychiatrists, some 20% are based on suicide or attempted suicide.

Premature Discharge

Premature discharge is another aspect of failure to treat. The psychiatrist and hospital are caught between the Scylla of tardy discharge of a patient and the Charybdis of premature discharge. The former may constitute malpractice or false imprisonment; the latter may result in the patient's assault upon a third person or suicide. The psychiatrist and hospital are clearly in a quandary in determining when to release a patient who has been involuntarily committed because of possible dangerousness. Liability is imposed if a patient who causes harm was negligently released. The intervening criminal act of the patient does not, per se, break the chain of causal connection so as to insulate the psychiatrist or hospital from liability. A negligent party may be held liable for harm caused by the reasonably foreseeable criminal acts of third persons, in this case, the acts of the patient.

Thus, in one case, an injured party obtained a substantial judgment against a private sanatorium and a psychiatrist for premature release of a patient with aggressive tendencies. The patient, having attacked his wife, had been committed to a state mental hospital and shortly thereafter transferred to a private sanatorium, where he stayed for 4 months. Both his confinements were uneventful and the patient, according to the hospital, appeared to have recovered. Shortly after discharge, however, during a conference with the plaintiff, who was his wife's attorney, the patient leaped across the desk, grabbed the attorney's head, and actually bit off a substantial part of his nose, apparently to spite his face.[16]

Insurance or managed care limitations may pose obstacles to treatment resulting in a failure to treat. A physician may have an obligation to assist patients in obtaining payment of healthcare. At a minimum, a physician must be aware of reimbursement constraints, so that he can promptly advise the patient. A physician may be obliged to engage in bureaucratic infighting, when a utilization review process has rejected his recommendation.[17] The courts have held external utilization review bodies liable for negligent review if a patient suffers harm through denial of care, but that depends on an adequate presentation by the physician.[18]

Withdrawing from Providing Treatment

Once there is a professional relationship, which establishes a duty of care, the right to withdraw is contingent upon giving the patient reasonable notice so that he may secure other services. The condition of the patient, the size of the community, and the availability of other services are factors that determine the reasonableness of a withdrawal notice. In undertaking a service, a special agreement may be made that the engagement is limited to a particular treatment or procedure.

In the wake of litigation imposing liability on a psychiatrist on the ground of abandonment, the American Psychiatric Association's Managed Care Help Line received numerous calls about terminating relationships with patients. As a result it provided a sample letter to patients which states:

> This is to inform you that I believe it is necessary to terminate our professional relationship. [Psychiatrist may, but is not required to, specify reason.]
>
> I have been serving as your psychiatrist since [specify date] and am currently treating your for [indicate diagnosis] with a program of [specify treatment mode, including any drugs].
>
> In my view, you [would/would not] benefit from continued treatment.
>
> If you wish to continue to receive treatment, you are, of course, free to contact one of the following [psychiatrists/facilities], [who/which] may be willing to accept you as a patient: [indicate specific referrals here]. If you find that none of these choices is acceptable, please contact me; I will make every effort to suggest additional alternatives. If you do decide to obtain treatment from one of these psychiatrists or facilities, or from any other psychiatrist or facility of your choice, I will be happy to forward your clinical records to your new doctor on your written authorization.

Finally, be assured that I will be available to treat you until [specify date]. (The following factors, among others, may be used to determine what is "reasonable" in a particular situation: condition of the patient, length of the psychiatrist–patient relationship, availability of other psychiatric services in the community, reason for termination, and amount of money owed, if any.)

The APA Office of Healthcare Systems and Financing also advised: "Although 30 days notice is generally considered appropriate, in a rural or other underserved area, it may be necessary to provide longer notice. When terminating a relationship with a patient it is also necessary to give proper instructions concerning any medication the patient is taking (e.g., if stopping medication abruptly could cause injury)." The office also advised that it is never appropriate to sever a treatment relationship when a patient is in an emergency situation unless the patient agrees to see another clinician or is hospitalized.

Faulty Diagnosis

A physician who makes a diagnostic mistake or error in judgment does not incur liability, whatever the harm, provided the error is one that other similarly trained physicians would have made under comparable circumstances, and provided that all necessary diagnostic means were utilized. A mistaken or missed diagnosis does not in itself constitute fault or malpractice. A physician is not a warrantor of cures. The patient must establish that a wrong diagnosis resulting in inappropriate treatment was caused by the physician's failure to exercise ordinary diligence and skill and that it led to untoward consequences. Whenever doubt exists in the physician's mind and the differential diagnosis includes potentially serious conditions, a record that notes that the doubt was considered is persuasive exculpatory evidence. Good faith or honesty alone does not excuse a faulty diagnosis.

The faulty diagnosis upon which suit is premised in psychiatric malpractice usually involves interpreting as psychological a problem, which is essentially physical in origin. James Thurber tells about a male adult who was seeing double, and he went to a psychiatrist, who decided that the man's problem lay in his inability to make up his mind as to which one of two girls he was in love with. The distracted fellow then called on an ophthalmologist who cleared up the condition with eye drops.

Organic (bodily caused) syndromes can mimic functional (mind caused) disorders in their symptomatology. The emotional responses may be identical. Thus, neurological disorders, such as brain tumors, various forms of epilepsy, general paresis (the late stages of syphilis), traumatic brain damage (concussion, subdural hematoma), multiple sclerosis, and the diseases of aging (such as arteriosclerosis) often produce neurotic or psychotic symptoms. Endocrine disorders, such as pituitary disorders, hyperthyroidism, and hypothyroidism, may produce neurotic and psychotic symptoms. Numerous general medical conditions, such as colitis and vitamin deficiency, may masquerade as a psychic disorder. It is often charged that physicians tend to overlook the dynamic factors of disorders while psychiatrists, notwithstanding their medical training, tend to overlook organic factors. The philosophy that history-taking or a physical examination might interfere with transference or might be considered a seduction has at times had tragic results.

Generally, there is no duty to ask for a consultation. However, the fact that psychiatrists are medically trained does not obviate the need to obtain a consultation in certain cases. An example is the negligent diagnosis of a veteran suffering from organic brain damage who was diagnosed at a Veterans Administration Hospital as psychosomatic and was so advised and released without having received proper treatment. The patient, wounded in combat, had experienced blackouts, unaccountable falls, and severe head pains. The court held the hospital liable in negligence because of the presence of manifest neurological symptoms indicative of organic brain damage, which were either overlooked or not understood. The court found the hospital negligent both in the manner of its examination and in failing to make necessary diagnostic tests.[19]

Let us assume negligent failure to properly diagnose with the result of inappropriate treatment. Then there are questions of (1) proximate causation and (2) resultant damages. The defense always is that *even if* proper diagnosis had been made and resultant treatment undertaken, the treatment would have been futile and impossible or both. The failure to diagnose cancer is the most common of misdiagnosis-type cases. In the cancer case, one can expect to hear that the failure to diagnose cancer, even if true and tantamount to malpractice, would not have made any difference. In other words, "So what?"

This brings us to an evidentiary question: What amount of proof is necessary to show the loss of a chance, and does it have any real value if it is proven? *What* caused a loss is a separate question from what the *nature* and *extent* of the loss are. The "lost chance" doctrine could create an injustice. Healthcare providers could find themselves defending cases simply because a patient fails to improve or where serious disease processes are not arrested because another course of action could possibly bring a better result.[20] A patient who has been in psychotherapy for over 12 years claims that it was a waste of time and it resulted in the loss of her child-bearing years. Assuming the therapist was negligent in not obtaining a consultation, or in not using medication, the necessary proof that would sustain a theory of lost chance is a controversial issue.

Assume that an individual was negligently detained and was delayed in boarding the *Titanic*. The wrongful detention would turn out to have saved the individual's life. Some commentators who have considered the "doomed steamer" example have concluded, on a visceral level, that the threat to the ship was simply too remote and contingent to be introduced into a loss valuation. Law professor William Prosser wrote that "if such factors as these are to be considered as reducing value, they must be in operation when the defendant causes harm, and so imminent that reasonable men would take them into account."[21]

In Poland during the time of martial law, as the story goes, a soldier shoots a man on a Warsaw street one evening at 10 minutes before 11. "But curfew doesn't start until 11," a bystander protests. "Yes," says the soldier, "but I know where that man lived. He never would have made it on time."

Protecting Patients from Injury

What of injury inflicted by an assaultive patient on another patient? Patients in institutions are entitled to such reasonable care and attention as will ensure the safety of themselves and others in light of their known mental and physical conditions.[22] This duty of care not only includes prevention of improper direct acts by hospital personnel, but also protection from all conditions that may create danger of injury to the patient. Depending on the circumstances, injury to one patient at the hands of another may be a breach of the duty of reasonable care and may lead to liability on the part of the hospital or the psychiatrist.[23] The administrative personnel have general responsibility for overall operation of the hospital, supplies, facilities, supervision, and hiring of staff.

Thus, a patient in one case brought an action against the hospital for a physical beating received at the hands of a fellow patient, who was suffering from delirium tremens. The hospital was aware of his violent nature and posted a female nurse in his room as a guard. The hospital was found negligent, however, for having breached its duty to provide safe conditions because one female nurse was deemed insufficient protection for the other patients.[24]

Overcrowding or understaffing in an institution is no defense. In an action brought by a patient in a state mental hospital for injuries suffered from an attack by a fellow patient, the court recognized that the hospital was 38% overcrowded and that sufficient funds were not available to employ an adequate staff; however, it was held that the state was negligent in not having an adequate number of personnel to provide their patients with the safety that was due them. Insufficiency of attendants in a mental institution is an act of negligence.[25]

To hold either a hospital or a psychiatrist liable, it must be shown that they were in fact negligent and that this negligence was the proximate cause of the injuries sustained. Neither is an insurer of a patient's well-being, but is held only to a duty of reasonable care to protect against foreseeable occurrences. Thus, the hospital was found not liable in a case where a patient, while in a work party of 17 patients supervised by only one attendant, was struck by a fellow patient and suffered the loss of one of his eyes. The court found that the hospital had no knowledge of the violent character of the assailant and that the act had occurred so suddenly that even additional attendants would have been unable to prevent the injury.[26]

An issue that occasionally arises in these cases is contributory negligence. As a general principle, a plaintiff's contributory negligence bars his recovery in an action based on the negligence of the defendant, even though the plaintiff's negligence may be much less serious than that of the defendant. However, the defense of contributory negligence may be untenable when the plaintiff's mental condition places him beyond the sphere of responsibility for his acts.[27]

Nonprofit Hospitals

In return for providing charitable services, hospitals receive numerous benefits, including exemption from federal and state income taxes and property and sales taxes. Nationwide each year these hospitals receive $12.6 billion in tax exemptions. About 3,900 of the nation's short-term, acute care hospitals, or 62%, are nonprofit. Another 20% are government hospitals and 18% are for-profit. The Northeast and Midwest have the highest concentrations of nonprofit hospitals; the South has the least. Generally, charity care, or free care, is offered to those who meet federal poverty guidelines. That determination varies from hospital to hospital.

The Emergency Room Situation/EMTALA

The emergency room situation provides a wide area of litigation. Even a private hospital may be held liable for refusing to care for an individual in an emergency situation on the theory that the public is led to believe that it is available to the general public in the case of emergency. Frequently, emergency rooms are understaffed, lack facilities, and turn away persons in need of attention. As a general practice, the police tend to take emergency cases to public rather than to private hospitals.

Because the states largely failed to require hospitals to provide emergency care to the poor, Congress in 1946 enacted the Hill–Burton act requiring hospitals, as a condition of receiving federal funds for construction or modernization, to treat and stabilize all emergency patients. However, the requirement proved to be ineffective for several reasons. First, the Department of Health and Human Services failed to enforce the indigent patient requirement. Second, the term *emergency* was not effectively defined, thus allowing hospitals to disregard the requirement. Third, there were no punitive remedies for violation of the statute. Then, too, most patients were unaware of any rights and remedies under the statute.[28]

In 1986, the Emergency Medical Treatment and Active Labor Act (EMTALA) was enacted as part of the Consolidated Omnibus Budget Reconciliation Act of 1985 to require hospitals to screen and stabilize patients who come to an emergency room in need of medical attention.[29] New regulations went into effect in 2003 to clarify the applicability of EMTALA.[30] It is estimated that some 45 million people in the United States are without health insurance and many more millions have poor coverage. President George Bush has said that these people without insurance can get treatment in an emergency room, but many studies have shown that people without insurance postpone treatment until a minor illness becomes worse, harming their own health and imposing greater costs.[31]

EMTALA requires hospitals that receive federal Medicare funding and have emergency facilities to provide a medical screening examination to "any individual regardless of diagnosis, financial status, race, national origin, or handicap." While the statute's applicability is dependent on a hospital's participation in the Medicare program, its protections extend to all persons and not solely to Medicare recipients who present to the emergency department of a Medicare-funded hospital. Patients are personally responsible for any treatment that they receive, but a patient who is indigent or lacks health insurance is unlikely to be able to pay an emergency care bill.

An "emergency medical condition" is defined as:

(A) A medical condition manifesting itself by acute symptoms of sufficient severity (including severe pain) such that the absence of immediate medical attention could reasonably be expected to result in: (1) placing the health of the individual (or, with respect to pregnant women, the health of the woman or her unborn child) in serious jeopardy, (2) serious impairment to bodily functions, or (3) serious dysfunction of any bodily organ or part, or (B) with respect to a pregnant woman who is having contractions: (1) that there is inadequate time to effect a safe transfer to another hospital before delivery, or (2) that transfer may pose a threat to the health or safety of the woman or the unborn child.[32]

In order to trigger the applicability of EMTALA, the individual must (1) "come to" an emergency department of a qualifying hospital and (2) request treatment. The term *come to* means that the individual requesting treatment is on hospital property or in a hospital-owned ambulance. An individual in an ambulance not owned by or affiliated with the hospital does not "come to" the emergency department until the ambulance reaches the hospital property, even if paramedics have called and received prior permission to deliver the patient.[33] An individual in an ambulance who comes somewhere other than at the dedicated emergency department of the hospital must request examination or treatment of what may be an emergency medical condition in order to trigger EMTALA.[34]

EMTALA imposes an obligation to stabilize a patient once the hospital determines through screening that a bona fide emergency condition exists. If the screening does not indicate an emergency, the hospital has no further duty under EMTALA. However, if a bona fide emergency exists, stabilization is both the minimum and maximum duty owed by the hospital.[35] Once the patient is stabilized, the hospital may "dump" him. *To stabilize* means "to provide such medical treatment of the condition necessary to assure, within reasonable medical probability, that no material deterioration of the condition is likely to result from or occur during the transfer of the individual."[36] A patient who is suicidal is considered stabilized under EMTALA "if he is no longer a threat to himself or others."

A patient under EMTALA can be transferred provided he is properly stabilized, but there are exceptions: (1) the patient requests a transfer, or (2) a physician certifies that the medical benefit of the transfer would outweigh the attendant risks.[37]

Both hospitals and physicians are subject to substantial penalties for violating the provisions of EMTALA. Physicians who participate in the wrongful discharge of an unstabilized patient can not only be fined, but can also be excluded from federal and state medical reimbursement programs for "gross and flagrant" or repeated EMTALA violations. The Centers for Medical and Medicare Services along with the U.S. Department of Health and Human Services (HHS) are responsible for investigating complaints of alleged EMTALA violations and reporting actual violations to the HHS Office of Inspector General for imposition of civil monetary fines.[38] Moreover, liability under EMTALA does not foreclose liability under state medical malpractice laws. EMTALA actions are brought in federal court and are not subject to the limitations under state malpractice actions. Expert testimony is generally not required in an EMTALA action as it is not a malpractice case.[39]

EMTALA differs from a traditional state medical malpractice claim principally because it requires *actual* knowledge by the hospital that the patient is suffering from an emergency medical condition and because it mandates only stabilizing treatment, and only such treatment as can be provided within the staff and facilities available at the hospital. EMTALA thus imposes liability for failure to stabilize a patient only if an emergency medical condition is actually discovered, rather than for negligent failure to discover and treat such a condition. In addition, EMTALA imposes only a limited duty of medical treatment: A hospital need provide only sufficient care, within its capability, to stabilize the patient, not necessarily to improve or cure the patient's condition. The purpose of EMTALA is to eliminate patient dumping and not to federalize medical malpractice. EMTALA penalties are available in addition to the liability that may be imposed under state liability law.

The courts tend not to impose EMTALA liability involving claims of psychiatric emergency care. In the definition in EMTALA of "medical emergency," it is difficult to show that a psychiatric condition qualifies as an "impairment to bodily functions" or "serious dysfunction of an organ." For that reason, nearly every EMTALA case claiming a psychiatric emergency involves suicide.[40] The cases denying liability even in those instances far exceed those granting it.[41]

EMTALA remains a controversial statute leading to much debate and concern from healthcare providers and hospitals claiming overcrowded emergency departments and delays due to people coming to the emergency department for nonurgent services as well as uncertainties of obligations. According to the HHS, an "overarching" concern among hospital officials and physicians is uncertainty about the extent of their responsibilities under EMTALA.[42]

Special Relationships

The *special relationship* concept in the law of torts has impacted on the common law doctrine that there is no duty to aid others in the absence of an explicit agreement to do so. The common law "no duty" rule has been widely criticized, causing it to be eroded by exceptions, most notably by that of a special relationship that prevails between the plaintiff and the defendant. Initially, in the common law, the special relationship concept was limited in the types of relationships where a duty to aid was imposed. A carrier was required to take reasonable affirmative steps to aid a passenger in peril, and an innkeeper to aid a guest. The relationship of husband and wife or parent and child called for the same conclusion.

In the 20th century, the concept of special relationship was expanded to impose a duty of aid upon a shopkeeper to a business visitor, upon a host to a social guest, and upon a jailer to a prisoner. Subsequently, it was ruled that landlords owed a duty to protect their tenants from criminal acts by intruders, businesses owed a duty to protect customers on their premises from foreseeable criminal acts, and educational institutions owed a duty to protect their students from foreseeable criminal assaults.[43]

The special relationship concept is now ever expanding with the courts seemingly applying the concept whenever they seek a desired result. When the physician is the defendant, the rules on medical malpractice (such as the requirement of expert testimony) are sometimes applied, sometimes not.

By virtue of the special relationship that a therapist has with a patient, the therapist also has a duty of care to third parties who might be injured by the patient. That was the holding, as is discussed in Chapter 36, in the 1976 decision of *Tarasoff v. Regents of the University of California*,[44] where the California Supreme Court said: "Although under the common law, as a general rule, one person owed no duty to control the conduct of another nor to warn those endangered by such conduct, the courts have carved out an exception to this rule in cases in which the defendant stands in some special relationship *to either the person whose conduct needs to be controlled or in a relationship to the foreseeable victim of that conduct*" (emphasis added).[45]

Then comes the application of the special relationship concept in situations where physicians or psychiatrists undertake evaluations on behalf of employers or insurance companies. When performing evaluations that are not intended or reasonably construed to be therapeutic, a therapist–patient relationship—the hallmark of a malpractice action—is normally not created or legally implied. Usually one of two circumstances will result from an allegedly negligent evaluation: Either the individual is denied initial or continued employment, or the physician fails to discover a significant condition that might have been treated had it been diagnosed or had the examinee been informed of his or her condition. Over the years, the courts have held that in the absence of a physician–patient relationship no duty of treatment is owed to the person who was examined.[46] In *Reed v. Bojarski*,[47] the New Jersey Supreme Court observed, "Courts throughout the nation have been grappling with the question of the obligation owed by a physician to a patient [sic] in the preemployment screening setting. … Most jurisdictions adhere to the traditional malpractice model in which the absence of a classic physician–patient relationship results in the physician owing no duty to the examinee to discover and disclose abnormalities or conditions, let alone report them."[48]

Forensic examiners take it for granted that they do not owe those whom they evaluate the general duty of physicians to advance their examinee's interests and not cause harm, yet when it is apparent that the examinee is in need of medical treatment, it would be common decency to say to the evaluee, "I am not your physician, but you should see a physician." The courts now have begun to apply the special relationship concept (as well as the *Tarasoff* duty to warn a threatened individual) to cases of examinations. The Ninth Circuit, while declining to set out the "exact contours" of an examinee's duty to disclose, found persuasive expert testimony given at trial "that, at a minimum, the radiologist should have notified [the examinee] of [an] abnormality."[49] In recent years, a number of courts have imposed a duty of care to make reasonable and timely efforts to discover and communicate to the examinee any findings that pose an imminent threat to his or her well-being.[50]

In *Stiver v. Parker*,[51] the Sixth Circuit Court of Appeals assessed the duties that surrogacy brokers and other professionals owed to the participants of a surrogate parenting program. In this case, a physician, a psychiatrist, and a lawyer evaluated the proposed surrogate mother. The surrogate mother gave birth to a child with severe birth defects that were caused by prenatal exposure to a virus. She brought suit, alleging that the sperm donor's semen was the source of her exposure to the virus. The district court granted the defense's motion for summary judgment because the plaintiff had failed to present expert witnesses as to the appropriate standard of care, which was required for a medical or legal malpractice case. On appeal, the Sixth Circuit rejected the district court's characterization of the case as a malpractice action and, framing the decision in terms of general tort law, concluded that expert testimony was unnecessary and that it was for a jury to decide whether the broker and other professionals had acted with "the kind of care commensurate with the exercise of a high degree of diligence in protecting the parties from harm."[52] The court found that the relationship between the surrogacy professionals and the contracting parties shared many of the same features that courts have traditionally used in negligence cases to find that a special relationship existed, giving rise to affirmative duties of protection. Thus, by holding that the surrogacy broker and assisting professionals had a special relationship with the participants in the program, the court ruled that they had an affirmative duty to provide protection from foreseeable harm.

The *Stiver* decision has been urged as precedent for the application of a duty resulting from a special relationship in tobacco litigation as well. In *City and County of San Francisco v. Phillip Morris*,[53] the plaintiffs alleged that the defendants falsely represented to the public at large and to them, specifically, that they would assume a special duty to undertake all possible efforts to learn the facts and disclose the truth about smoking and health. The plaintiffs relied on *Stiver* to contend that the court may apply a special duty to impose liability. However, as the plaintiffs had stated claims for fraud and misrepresentation, the court ruled that the claim of breach of a special duty was simply a restatement of their fraud cause of action.

In research, clinical trials pose the issue of the legal obligations of researchers to subjects. What are these obligations? Research is fundamentally different from ordinary clinical treatment in that it is designed to produce generalizable knowledge. As we have noted in an earlier chapter, the researcher's job is not the betterment of any particular subject. Thus, to require researchers to adhere to the same therapeutic obligations as treating physicians would be tantamount to a prohibition of clinical trials. The researcher–subject relationship is not fiduciary in nature, as the purpose of the relationship is not to promote the best interests of the subject.[54]

In research, the investigator cannot in good faith promise fidelity to doing what is best medically for the patient subject.[55] How then may vulnerable individuals be protected? In a lengthy opinion in *Grimes v. Kennedy Krieger Institute*,[56] the Maryland Supreme Court ruled that researchers conducting a study on lead paint poisoning in inner city households had a duty based on the "special relationship" that "normally exists between research and subject" to warn children in the households when blood tests revealed that the children had elevated lead levels.[57] The court said, "This duty requires the protection of the research subjects from unreasonable harm and requires the researcher to completely and promptly inform the subjects of potential hazards existing from time to time because of the profound trust that participants place in investigatory institutions, and the research enterprise as a whole, to protect them from harm."[58] This duty is independent of consent, although obtaining consent is one of the duties a researcher must perform. The court added, "The determination as to whether a 'special relationship' actually exists is to be done on a case-by-case basis."[59]

Regarding the imposition of a duty of care, the Hawaii Supreme Court had the following to say:

> In considering whether to impose a duty of reasonable care on a defendant, we recognize that duty is not sacrosanct in itself, but only an expression of the sum total of those considerations of policy, which lead the law to say that the particular plaintiff is entitled to protection. … The question of whether one owes a duty to another must be decided on a case-by-case basis. However, we are reluctant to impose a new duty upon members of our society without any logical, sound, and compelling reasons taking into consideration the social and human relationships of our society.[60]

The ever-expanding role of "special relationship" in large measure now makes us our brother's keeper. Moreover, a number of recent cases have indicated that, in clinical trials of drugs, there may be a "fiduciary duty" on the part of the manufacturer to continue to provide the medication after the termination of the clinical trial, unless the contrary is made clear at the outset.[61]

Endnotes

1. W.P. Keeton, D.B. Dobbs, R.E. Keeton, & D.C. Owen, *Prosser and Keeton on the Law of Torts* (St. Paul, MN: West, 5th ed., 1984), pp. 375–382.
2. Buch v. Amory Mfg. Co., 69 N.H. 257, 44Atl. 809 (1897).
3. 422 U.S. 563 (1975).
4. 56 Misc. 2d 693, 290 N.Y.S.2d 486 (Ct. Cl. 1968), noted in *Harv. L. Rev.* 82 (1969): 1771.
5. The award, in the amount of $300,000, included compensation for moral and mental degradation, physical injuries, pain and suffering, and loss of earnings during the period.
6. 383 F.2d 451 (D.C. Cir. 1966).
7. In Kockelman v. Segal, 61 Cal. App.4th 491, 71 Cal. Rptr. 552 (1998), a wrongful death action, the surviving wife alleged that the defendant psychiatrist and clinic were negligent in treating her husband for his chronic depression, and that this negligence was a proximate cause of her husband's suicide. The trial court granted summary judgment in favor of the defendants, finding as a matter of law that there was no duty owed to the decedent because he was being treated as an outpatient rather than in

a hospital setting. The Court of Appeals reversed, concluding that this is not the law. The court said, "Whether [the psychiatrist] acted within the duty of care in the circumstances of this case involves factual determinations, which must be resolved by the opinions and specialized knowledge of experts in the field ... [T]he trial court erred in ruling that [the decedent's] status as an outpatient decided the issue of duty as a matter of law"; 71 Cal. Rptr. at 561. See also Bellah v. Greenson, 81 Cal. App.3d 614, 146 Cal. Rptr. 535 (1978).

The lower federal courts are in conflict as to whether the Americans with Disabilities Act (enacted in 1990) mandates that police departments provide their officers with specialized training on how to deal with persons with psychiatric disabilities. While the Supreme Court has yet to rule on the issue, some lower courts have ruled that a claim may be made against a municipality for failing to provide their police officers with that special training. A claim may also be brought under the Civil Rights Act, § 1983. See Gohier v. Enright, 186 F.3d 1216 (10th Cir. 1999); Schorr v. Borough of Lemoyne, 243 F. Supp.2d 232 (M.D. Pa. 2003). But see Thompson v. Williamson County, 219 F.3d 555 (6th Cir. 2000); Buchanan v. Maine, 417 F. Supp. 45 (D. Me. 2006). See T.M. Green, "Police as Frontline Mental Health Workers: The Decision to Arrest or Refer to Mental Health Agencies," *Int. J. L. & Psychiat.* 20 (1997): 469; L.A. Teplin & N.S. Pruett, "Police as Streetcorner Psychiatrist: Managing the Mentally Ill," *Int. J. L. & Psychiat.* 15 (1992): 139.

8. 424 N.W.2d 159 (Wis.1978).
9. See also Freese v. Lemmon, 210 N.W.2d 576 (Iowa 1973); Duvall v. Goldin, 139 Mich. App. 342, 362 N.W.2d 275 (1984); Kaiser v. Suburban Transportation System, 65 Wash.2d 461, 401 P.2d 350 (1965); Annot., 43 A.L.R.4th 153 (1986).
10. V. Schwartz, "Civil Liability for Causing Suicide: A Synthesis of Law and Psychiatry," *Vand. L. Rev.* 24 (1971): 217; cited in Adams v. Carter County Memorial Hosp., 548 S.W.2d 307 (Tenn. 1977).
11. It was so stated in Johnson v. United States, 409 F. Supp. 1283 (M.D. Fla. 1976).
12. Schrempf v. State, 66 N.Y.2d 289, 496 N.Y.S.2d 973, 487 N.E.2d 883 (1985). The standard of care is evaluated in terms of the therapist's specialty. Stepakoff v. Kantar, 393 Mass. 836, 473 N.E.2d 1131 (1985).
13. Paddock v. Chacko, 522 S.E.2d 410 (Fla. App. 1988). The case is discussed at length in J.L. Kelley, *Psychiatric Malpractice* (New Brunswick, NJ: Rutgers University Press, 1996).
14. 522 So.2d at 413.
15. J.A. Chiles & K.D. Strosahl, *Clinical Manual for Assessment and Treatment of Suicidal Patients* (Arlington, VA: American Psychiatric Publishing, 2005).
16. Vassalo v. Halcyon Rest Hosp., cited in *Medical World News*, Oct. 14, 1966. See also Merchants National Bank & Trust Co. v. United States, 272 F. Supp. 409 (D.C. No. Dak. 1967), where Veterans Administration hospital doctors ignored indications of the seriousness of a mental patient's illness and placed the patient at a ranch, from which the patient departed and killed his wife. See also Underwood v. United States, 356 F.2d 92 (5th Cir. 1966). This case involved the negligent release of a mentally ill airman who had been hospitalized and had been known to have attacked his estranged former wife; the Air Force then assigned him to duty where he had access to firearms with which he shot and killed his former wife. In Higgins v. State, 43 Misc. 2d 793, 252 N.Y.S.2d 163 (1964), negligence was found in allowing a state hospital patient to leave the hospital grounds without permission, and such negligence was deemed the proximate cause of injuries sustained by a young boy, who was beaten by the patient.

On the other hand, no liability is imposed for an honest error in judgment in releasing a patient into the community. Thus, in a New York case, the state was not held culpable for the violent actions of a state mental hospital patient on leave, inasmuch as qualified physicians of the institution had judged the patient to be sufficiently controlled to be able to go home for a specified period; Orman v. State, 37 App. Div. 2d 674, 322 N.Y.S.2d 914 (Sup. Ct. 1971).
17. Wickline v. State, 192 Cal. App.3d 1630, 239 Cal. Rptr. 810 (1986).
18. Wilson v. Blue Cross of Southern California, 271 Cal. Rptr. 876, 222 Cal. App.3d 660 (1990). The following communication was sent by Dr. Lillian Robinson of New Orleans to an insurance company, with copies to the state insurance commissioner and the attorney general, and it resulted in a successful resolution to an appeal, with the claim paid in full:

> The following is in response to your letter of reconsideration dated ... regarding Ms. : In this letter you state that your retrospective review of her hospitalization concluded that her admission was "medically unnecessary."

I have reviewed the medical records, and this case has also been submitted to our in-hospital uti-lization review committee. All of the medical personnel who have looked at this case are in agree-ment that this patient clearly meets the criteria for inpatient treatment due to her well-documented suicide risk.

Since the information substantiating her need for hospital treatment is so well established in the chart, we are concerned that your refusal to honor your obligation to pay for her treatment con-stitutes either a serious breach of professional standards, or is simply an act of bad faith. Since you have also refused to provide us with utilization review criteria employed to justify this decision, as well as refused to provide the name of the physician involved with the retrospective review, we have no choice but to refer this matter to the Louisiana State Insurance Commissioner and to the office of the Attorney General. Recent revisions in the Louisiana Medical Practice Statutes require that any physician who makes judgments regarding medical necessity must have a license to practice in this state. Your failure to provide documentation of this licensure implies that you are potentially in knowing violation of this statute.

In addition, we will file official complaints with the appropriate legislative and licensure authorities in Texas and Arkansas.

This matter can be resolved quickly if you wish by simply honoring your obligation to provide decent service to your beneficiary. Or you can continue to attempt to justify your actions before the appropriate regulatory bodies. Please contact this office if you wish to provide additional clarifica-tion of your position.

19. Hungerford v. United States, 307 F.2d 99 (9th Cir. 1962), overruled on other grounds, Ramirez v. United States, 567 F.2d 854 (9th Cir. 1967). In another case, a psychiatric resident's emergency room diagnosis of viral sore throat and "hysterical reactions" (when the patient actually had a rare staphylo-coccal infection that ultimately caused his death) led to a $200,000 settlement against the hospital. As well as maintaining that the psychiatric resident was not competent to examine the patient, the plain-tiffs (patient's wife and three children) alleged that he had been negligent in diagnosing the breathing difficulties as hysterical in origin and in not calling for a consultation because the symptoms were out of his field of expertise or knowledge. It was alleged that he should have kept the patient under observation at the hospital, where a tracheotomy could have been performed. The hospital claimed that the patient had a disease that was very rare in adults, that all patients with sore throats cannot be hospitalized, and that no consultation was required in view of the known symptoms; Weinshenk v. Kaiser Foundation Hosp., Cal. Super. Ct., Alameda Cy., Docket No. 40027, 1971.

20. In Delaney v. Cade, 255 Kan. 199, 873 P.2d 175 (1994), the Kansas Supreme Court, while recognizing a cause of action for the lost chance for a better recovery due to malpractice, expressed a caveat:

In adopting and applying the loss of chance theory to medical malpractice cases, it must always be kept in mind that the practice of medicine and the furnishing of appropriate health care is not an exact science. In many, if not most, instances there is more than one acceptable approach to treat-ment, and the fact that one doctor selects one method as opposed to another does not in and of itself mean that one method is better than or preferable to another. For every treatment there are undoubtedly other doctors who might have performed or used a different one. Courts should use extreme caution in second-guessing the methods used by medical care providers, particularly in an area as nebulous as the loss of a chance for a better or more satisfactory recovery.

873 P.2d at 187. See R.B. Stuart, *Trick or Treatment: How and When Psychotherapy Fails* (Champaign, IL: Research Press, 1970).

21. W. Prosser, *Handbook of the Law of Torts* (St. Paul, MN: West, 4th ed., 1971), p. 321; discussed in J.H. King, "Causation, Valuation, and Chance in Personal Injury Torts Involving Preexisting Conditions and Future Consequences," *Yale L. J.* 90 (1981): 1353.

22. Wood v. Samaritan Institution, 26 Cal.2d 847, 161 P.2d 556 (1945); G. Garcetti & J. M. Suarez, "The Liability of Psychiatric Hospitals for the Act of Their Patients," *Am. J. Psychiat.* 124 (1968): 961. Likewise, in group therapy the therapist has a duty to protect patients in the group from a member who poses a danger. Moreover, under tort law on the responsibility of owners or lessees of property, there is a duty to safeguard those on the premises. However, in a Michigan case, the Court of Appeals in a 2–1 decision (wrongly) applied the *Tarasoff* doctrine to reverse a judgment in favor of members of the group who were injured. Dawe v. Bar-Levav, Oakland Circuit Court, No. 269147 (July 10, 2008); reported in D. Eggert, "Michigan Court Reverses Office Shooting Verdict," *Detroit Legal News*, July 15, 2008, p. 3.

23. A Texas appellate court held that a patient who was assaulted at a hospital operated by the Texas Department of Mental Health & Mental Retardation may sue the department for violating the patient bill of rights promulgated under the Texas Health & Safety Code; Texas Dept. of Mental Health & Mental Retardation, 2000 WL 550822 (Tex. App. 2000).

24. Univ. of Louisville v. Hammock, 127 Ky. 564, 106 S.W. 219 (1907). See Annot., 48 *A.L.R.3d* 1288 (1972).

25. Luke v. State, 253 App. Div. 783, I N.Y.S.2d 19 (1937). See also Rossing v. State, 47 N.Y.S.2d 262 (Ct. Cl. 1944); Gould v. State, 181 Misc. 884, 46 N.Y.S.2d 313 (Ct. Cl. 1944).

26. DiFiore v. State, 275 App. Div. 885, 88 N.Y.S.2d 815 (1949). See R. Slovenko, "Violent Attacks in Psychiatric and Other Hospitals," *J. Psychiat. & Law* 34 (2006): 249.

27. Gould v. State, 181 Misc. 884, 46 N.Y.S. 2d 313 (Ct. Cl. 1944); DeMartini v. Alexander Sanitarium, 192 Cal. App. 2d 442, 13 Cal. Rptr. 564 (Ct. App. 1961).

28. K.I. Treiger, "Preventing Patient Dumping: Sharpening the COBRA's Fangs," *N.Y.U. L. Rev.* 61 (1986): 1186.

29. 42 U.S.C. § 1395dd.

30. Special Responsibilities of Medicare Hospitals in Emergency Cases, 42 C.F.R. § 489.24 (2003).

31. See Editorial, "World's Best Medical Care?" *New York Times*, August 12, 2007, p. 18.

32. 42 U.S.C. § 1395dd(e)(1). See Bryant v. Adventist-Redbud Hosp., 289 F.3d 1162 (9th Cir. 2001).

33. 42 C.F.R. § 489.24(b). See Arrington v. Wong, 237 F.3d 1066 (9th Cir. 2001). Hospitals can designate themselves as being on "discretionary status" when they temporarily have reached their treatment capacity, and do not have the staff to treat additional patients.

34. In Preston v. Meriter Hospital, 700 N.W.2d (Wis. 158), the personal representatives of the estate of an infant born severely premature filed suit alleging violation of EMTALA. Summary judgment was entered for the hospital because the infant arrived through the hospital birthing center, not the emergency room. The plaintiff argued, in vain, that it is a ridiculous distinction, one which places form over substance, to state that the care a patient receives depends on the door through which the patient walks; 700 N.W.2d at 167.

35. For example, in Gerber v. Northwest Hospital Center, 943 F. Supp. 571 (D. Md. 1996), a patient told her physician that she contemplated killing herself because of her pain. Two days after she was released, she tried to commit suicide by shooting herself in the head. The court dismissed her EMTALA claim because her physical complaints were addressed in a medical screening examination and she was discharged in stable condition.

36. 42 C.F.R. § 489.24(b). There is no duty under EMTALA to provide stabilization treatment to a patient with an emergency medical condition who is not transferred; Harry v. Marchant, 291 F.3d 767 (11th Cir. 2002).

37. 42 U.S.C. § 1395dd(c)(1).

38. 42 U.S.C. § 1395dd(d)(1)(A).

39. In Coleman v. Deno, 813 So.2d 303 (La. 2002), the Louisiana Supreme Court held it was error for the lower court to find intentional patient dumping where the patient's cause of action against the physician was based solely on a claim of medical malpractice. The court found that the gravamen of the plaintiff's claim was that the physician failed to properly diagnose and treat the plaintiff's condition. The court held that while claims of medical malpractice and patient dumping can overlap, here the treatment decision was inseparable from the transfer decision. In Smith v. Botsford General Hosp., 309 F. Supp.2d 927 (E.D. Mich. 2004), an action under EMTALA tried to a jury under Michigan's Wrongful Death Act, the court limited the award damages to the Michigan cap on noneconomic damages in a medical malpractice action. The action stemmed out of the patient's transfer to another hospital before being stabilized.

40. See, e.g., Card v. Amisub, 2006 WL 889430 (W.D. Tenn. 2006), where an individual who attempted suicide after discharge from an emergency room was allowed to pursue an EMTALA as well as a medical malpractice claim against the hospital. The court concluded that the individual had set forth in his petition an issue of material fact as to whether the hospital had actual knowledge of his emergency medical condition and had failed to stabilize his condition prior to discharge. Similarly, the court ruled that the individual could pursue his medical malpractice claim, which would focus on the adequacy of the care he had been provided at the hospital.

41. For discussions of EMTALA, see B. Furrow, "An Overview and Analysis of the Impact of the Emergency Medical Treatment and Active Labor Act," *J. Legal Med.* 16 (1995): 325; L.D. Hermer, "The Scapegoat: EMTALA and Emergency Department Overcrowding," *J. Law & Policy* 9 (2006): 695; T.M. Lee, "An EMTALA Primer: The Impact of Changes in the Emergency Medicine Landscape

on EMTALA Compliance and Enforcement," *Loyola Univ. Ann. Health Law* 13 (2004): 145; S.J. Saks "Call 911: Psychiatry and the New Emergency Medical Treatment and Active Labor Act (EMTALA) Regulations," *J. Psychiat. & Law* 32 (2004): 483.

42. Emergency room protection proposals appear to be a new legislative trend surfacing in the states. These proposals shield hospitals and physicians from all claims made by anyone entering the hospital via the ER, unless a plaintiff can show "gross negligence" by "clear and convincing evidence." Proponents know that it will be almost impossible for a patient to meet this most difficult burden of proof. In effect, it would grant immunity from liability. Once a hospital initially "evaluates or treats" the patient in the ER, this shield follows the patient wherever the patient goes in the facility. In 2005, Georgia and South Carolina enacted such a provision. Arizona defeated such a proposal in 2006.

43. In Samson v. Saginaw Professional Bldg., 242 N.W.2d 843 (Mich. 1975), the Michigan Supreme Court held that an office building landlord owed a duty of protection to a person who suffered injuries from an attack by a mental patient in an elevator. Noting that common areas are under the landlord's control, the court held that the landlord is responsible for ensuring that these areas are "reasonably safe for the use of tenants and invitees."

44. 17 Cal.3d 425, 131 Cal. Rptr. 14, 551 P.2d 334 (1976).

45. 551 P.2d at 343.

46. See, e.g., Keene v. Wiggins, 69 Cal. Rptr. 3 (Cal. App. 1977); Tolisans v. Teton, 550 N.Y.2d 450, 551 N.Y.S.2d 197 (1989). Of course, the examiner may be held liable for infliction of emotional distress, e.g., by verbally abusing the examinee. See Harris v. Kreutzer, 271 Va. 188, 624 S.E.2d 24 (2006).

47. 166 N.J. 89, 764 A.2d 433 (2001).

48. 764 A.2d at 437.

49. Daly v. United States, 946 F.2d 1467 at 1470 (9th Cir. 1991).

50. See, e.g., Green v. Walker, 910 F.2d 291 (5th Cir. 1990); Webb v. T.D., 287 Mont. 68, 951 P.2d 1008 (1997).

51. 975 F.2d 261 (6th Cir. 1992), noted in *Harv. L. Rev.* 106 (1993): 951; *Mo. L. Rev.* 67 (2006): 421.

52. 975 F.2d at 272.

53. 1998 WL 230980 (N.D. Cal.).

54. W.A. Gregory, "The Fiduciary Duty of Care: A Perversion of Words," *Akron L. Rev.* 38 (2005): 181.

55. H. Brody & F.G. Miller, "The Clinician-Investigator: Unavoidable But Manageable Tension," *Kennedy Inst. Ethics. J.* 13 (2003): 329.

56. 366 Md. 29, 782 A.2d 807 (Md. 2001).

57. The ruling in Grimes v. Kennedy Krieger Institute is in marked contrast to rulings in Ande v. Rock, 256 Wis.2d 365, 647 N.W.2d 265 (2002) and Goodman v. United States, 298 F.3d 1048 (9th Cir. 2002), where the courts reasoned that since there was no physician–patient relationship and no fiduciary duty, the duties of the researcher did not go beyond ordinary negligence. See C.H. Coleman, "Duties to Subjects in Clinical Trials," *Vand. L. Rev.* 58 (2005): 387; K. Gatter, "Fixing Cracks: A Discourse Norm to Repair the Crumbling Regulatory Structure Supporting Clinical Research and Protecting Human Subjects," *UMKC L. Rev.* 73 (2005): 581; see also F. Miller & H. Brody, "A Critique of Clinical Equipoise: Therapeutic Misconception in the Ethics of Clinical Trials," *Hastings Center Rep.,* May–June 2003, p. 19.

58. 782 A.2d at 851.

59. *Ibid.* at 858.

60. McKenzie v. Hawaii Permanente Medical Group, 98 Haw. 296, 47 P.3d 1209 (2002).

61. See Suthers v. Amgen, 372 F. Supp.2d 416 (S.D. N.Y. 2005); Abney v. Amgen, 372 F. Supp.2d 416 (S.D. N.Y. 2005).

PART II
Psychiatric Malpractice

26

Malpractice, Nonmedical Negligence, or Breach of Contract?

Not every lawsuit against a professional involves malpractice, that is, professional negligence. Intentional wrongdoing as well as ordinary negligence (such as defective premises) or a contractual undertaking fall outside the purview of malpractice.[1] Yet, protective of the medical profession, behavior that ordinarily might be considered intentional wrongdoing or nonmedical negligence quite often has been considered as malpractice and subject to malpractice limitations of which there are several. Malpractice actions are curtailed by a 2-year statute of limitations (prescription) rather than 3 years in the case of nonmedical negligence (7 year in the case of an intentional tort and 6 years for breach of contract). Malpractice actions require expert testimony (except in obvious cases of wrongdoing as where a surgeon amputates the wrong limb).[2] There are other differences. The professional liability insurance policy covers malpractice, not intentional wrongdoing or ordinary negligence or contractual obligations (having a single carrier covering both malpractice and ordinary negligence avoids a conflict as to coverage).[3] Moreover, judgments attributable to negligence, medical or nonmedical, are discharged in bankruptcy, but not those attributable to intentional wrongs; punitive damage are usually awarded in the case of intentional wrongs.

Malpractice

Professional negligence, or malpractice, includes all professionals—they must possess and apply the average skill or knowledge of other professionals in like circumstances.[4] However, when a person speaks of a malpractice action, it is presumed that it is about a lawsuit against a physician rather than about the negligence of a member of any other professional group. Indeed, there are special laws on medical malpractice. *Malpractice* is even defined in some dictionaries as "improper treatment or culpable negligence of a patient by a physician."[5]

The medical profession has been successful in persuading various state legislatures to alleviate an alleged medical malpractice crisis. The legislation varies considerably among the states. (Michigan legislation hereinafter will be set out.) Caps have been imposed on awards for pain and suffering and limitations on expert testimony. Many states now require submitting the case to a screening arbitration, and others impose restrictions on contingent fees. Then, too, the political rhetoric and media publicity about a "medical malpractice crisis" affect the outcome of cases (during the 2004 presidential campaign, the issue of medical malpractice reform was raised almost daily). By and large, jurors are compromised.

In 2004, the U.S. Supreme Court handed down, in what is called a groundbreaking decision, *Aetna v. Davila*,[6] in which it addressed federal preemption of state law claims against health maintenance organizations (HMOs). The Court held that the Employee Retirement Income Security Act (ERISA) completely preempts state law medical malpractice claims challenging health benefits decisions made by HMOs. In doing so, *Davila* marked a turnaround in recent Supreme Court decisions that seemed to have eroded ERISA's preemptive effect. It also resolved a split among the circuit courts as to whether health plan members can sue their HMOs for making negligent medical decisions. Instead of making a claim under state law, plan participants must enforce their rights to benefits under the federal ERISA statute, which provides various remedies designed to protect the participant's claim to benefits. However, the chief criticism of ERISA has been not so much the nature of the remedies provided as much as the type of relief that is unavailable under ERISA, such as much lower punitive damages. ERISA limits recovery to the benefits due under the plan or injunctive relief to secure them. Other than possibly obtaining attorney's fees, the consequential damages caused by ERISA violations—including wrongful benefit denials—are not recoverable.[7]

One argument against allowing a malpractice action against an HMO is that, strictly speaking, it is not practicing medicine. A physician–patient relationship is usually a prerequisite to a professional malpractice suit against a physician. Traditionally, a physician's duty of care has been limited to persons with whom a physician–patient relationship has been established.[8] A court-ordered medical examination of a claimant does not give rise to a physician–patient relationship. (The medical examiner also enjoys a qualified tort immunity as an expert witness.[9]) In performing evaluations on behalf of employers or insurance companies that are not intended or reasonably construed to be for purposes of treatment, no physician–patient relationship is normally created or legally implied.[10] Thus, when a physician employed by an insurance company examines an individual for the purpose of qualifying him for insurance coverage, the usual rule has been that the physician owes no duty to the individual to treat or to disclose problems discovered during the examination (subject to the developing concept of "special relationships" discussed in Chapter 25).[11] Likewise, preemployment physicals do not give rise to the relationship, given the absence of a therapeutic purpose,[12] nor do examinations by an insurer's physician of a claimant against the insurer as the result of injuries from an accident.[13] Experimentation or nontherapeutic research, i.e., where there is no intention of directly benefiting a subject, does not create a physician–patient relationship, but there often occurs a "therapeutic misconception" where the subjects do not comprehend that the research might not be beneficial to them.[14] A line of cases holds that the presence or absence of a physician–patient relationship is simply a factor to consider in determining the type or nature of the duty owed, if any, to the nonpatient.[15] The courts hold that a research subject has no recourse under medical malpractice law (though a number of courts hold that there is a "special relationship" calling upon the researcher to at least inform the subject of a disability.)[16]

In general, there is no duty to come to the aid of a stranger, but once aid is undertaken, be it by a physician or other person, that individual then owes a duty of care. In the case of a physician coming to the aid of another, there is a physician–patient relationship that continues until ended by the parties' mutual consent, revoked by dismissal of the physician, or until the physician determines that the services are no longer beneficial to the patient, and the patient is given a reasonable time to procure other medical attention.

Every state in the United States has enacted a so-called Good Samaritan statute, which provides that a physician (or other medical professional) who in good faith aids another at the scene of an emergency is not liable for any harm caused by the aid unless "gross negligence" or willful and wanton misconduct can be proven.[17] While the Good Samaritan statutes do not create a duty to act (in contravention of the tort principle of no duty to aid in the absence of a preexisting special relationship), the legislatures sought to provide incentives for physicians (or other medical professionals) to aid by removing the threat of civil liability. Those not listed in the Good Samaritan statute who come to the rescue of another are measured by what would be expected of the average reasonable person, not by a measure of what might be considered gross negligence.

When enacting Good Samaritan statutes, the legislatures by and large had a specific scenario in mind: the roadside accident. The statutes were passed in order "to encourage physicians and other healthcare providers who have no preexisting duty to assist, and who in good faith believe that a person is unconscious, ill, injured, or in need of assistance, to come as a volunteer to the aid of that person without fear of litigation should the physician's care fall beneath a reasonable standard, so long as that care is not grossly negligent."[18] The care must be rendered without charge (or in some states without even the intention of charging).[19]

The various states exclude from Good Samaritan immunity physicians and others who provide emergency care as part of the normal course of their work. Michigan, for example, extends protection only to professionals whose "actual hospital duty does not require a response to an emergency situation."[20] Be that as it may, one of the most litigated issues involving Good Samaritan statutes has been whether the immunity covers emergencies in the hospital setting. The statutes range from providing immunity only for emergencies outside the hospital to providing immunity for emergencies inside the hospital. As mentioned, the scenario that legislatures had in mind when passing these statutes (especially those that were passed early on) was the roadside accident scenario, where a physician is without the equipment, assistance, and general support available in a hospital setting. As the New Jersey Supreme Court put it: "Good Samaritan immunity under [New Jersey's Good Samaritan Act] encompasses only those situations in which a physician (or other volunteer) comes, by chance, upon a victim who requires immediate emergency medical care, at a location compromised by lack of adequate facilities, equipment, expertise, sanitation, and staff. A hospital or medical center does not qualify under the terms of the Good Samaritan Act."[21] The decision disturbed physicians practicing in New Jersey.[22]

This is not always the state of affairs nationwide, however. Elsewhere it is said that the legislative purpose behind the Good Samaritan statute is broader than the roadside scenario. In the words of a California court, the intent behind the statute is "to induce physicians to render medical aid to individuals who, though in need of such care, were not receiving it" and further was "directed towards physicians who, by chance and on an irregular basis, come upon or are called to render emergency medical care."[23] Michigan is one of at least six states where the law explicitly covers emergencies within the hospital or medical center setting.[24] In these jurisdictions, the most frequently litigated issue is whether it was truly an emergency and whether there was already a preexisting duty to render aid. The courts have been generous in their definition of emergency.[25]

When do physicians or psychotherapists owe a duty to persons other than their patients? It is an axiom that good medical care involves consideration not only of the patient, but also to others. As a legal matter, should the duty to others, if any, be considered as falling under medical malpractice or as nonmedical negligence? In the famous case of *Tarasoff v. Regents of University of California*,[26] the California Supreme Court held that by virtue of the "special relationship" that a therapist has with a patient, there results a duty of care to third parties who might be injured by the patient. It is immaterial whether the treatment of the patient falls below standard of care or whether there is a causal nexus between the treatment and the injury to the third person.

In determining whether the patient is a danger to others, the judgment of the therapist is to be measured by a "professional standard of care, requiring the therapist to exercise the 'reasonable degree of skill, knowledge, and care ordinarily possessed and exercised by members of his professional specialty.'" That, of course, is a malpractice standard. To establish what the defendant should have known, expert testimony regarding the standards of the profession is required. (But what can be said when professional guidelines are ill-defined or nonexistent?) With danger known or knowable, the therapist is obliged to use reasonable care to protect the potential victim. The adequacy of the therapist's conduct in dealing with the danger is to be measured according to the traditional negligence standard of "reasonable care under the circumstances," that is, without expert testimony, just as negligence is measured in ordinary accident cases. Many states by legislation have provided that the duty imposed on the therapist is dischargeable by a simple warning to the potential victim.

The court in *Tarasoff* reached its result by analogy to common law cases imposing liability on a physician who misdiagnoses a communicable disease to the detriment of those coming into contact with the patient.[27] The lawsuit by the plaintiff, though not a patient, is sounded in malpractice with the result that the limitations on malpractice actions apply. At least one state—Louisiana—calls it ordinary negligence, not malpractice, thereby avoiding the limitations of malpractice actions.

Many statutes that prescribe specific conduct and impose a criminal penalty for violation do not mention tort law consequences, but the courts often apply these statutes in tort cases as a specific rule of conduct. For example, in an action against a physician for failure to diagnose and report battered child syndrome as required by statute, the California Supreme Court held that the child as plaintiff (whether or not a patient) stated a cause of action in malpractice, thus requiring expert testimony.[28] If reporting had been done, the child may have been saved from further abuse.

What about failure to obtain the consent of the patient for treatment? Liability arising out of medical treatment where consent is lacking can rest on one of two theories: battery (an intentional tort) or negligence. Typically, an action based on battery occurs where the physician obtains the consent of the patient for the performance of a particular procedure, but thereafter performs a different procedure for which consent was not obtained. On the other hand, when consent is given for a procedure, but injury results due to an undisclosed risk, the theory in such a case is usually negligence. It could be said that lack of informed consent also results in a battery, but the various states by court decision or statute have deemed lack of informed consent to constitute malpractice, not battery. Unlike in a case of battery, expert testimony is required to establish the elements of an action based on lack of informed consent: competency, disclosure, and voluntariness. As lack of informed consent is a negligence—not intentional—tort action, proof of damages is necessary. A complaint of battery, on the other hand, may be based solely on an insult to bodily integrity.

Likewise, it would be assumed that "undue familiarity" with a patient is an intentional tort, but the courts have held that because it occurs with some frequency in psychotherapy, it is a risk of psychotherapy. It is said to occur when the therapist mishandles the so-called transference phenomenon, resulting in sexual attraction between therapist and patient. An allegation of "intentional" misconduct would result in malpractice carriers disclaiming coverage for the behavior. In recent years, however, with the increasing numbers of claims of sexual misconduct, malpractice carriers now routinely disclaim coverage in their policies. Consequently, sexual misconduct cases now often allege intentional tort, and seek punitive damages as well.

An allegation of improper restraint or seclusion in a mental or other institution could be classified as an intentional tort (false imprisonment), but is nonetheless classified as malpractice. In *Youngberg v. Romeo*,[29] the U.S. Supreme Court said in a lawsuit alleging false imprisonment and constitutional deprivation: "The decision, if made by a professional, is presumptively valid [and] liability may be imposed only when the decision by the professional is such a substantial departure from accepted professional judgment, a practice or standard as to demonstrate that the person responsible actually did not base the decision on such a judgment." Further, the Court defined "professional" broadly and pragmatically, encompassing "a person competent, whether by education, training, or experience to make the particular decision at issue."

Concurrent with the trend of categorizing alleged physician wrongdoing as malpractice came rules making malpractice litigation more difficult and expensive. No one change was a watershed event, but the cumulative effect has been to diminish the chances of proceeding against a physician or holding the physician liable for malpractice. In recent years, legislation in various states has dramatically altered the law governing medical malpractice actions.[30] In particular, Michigan sets out numerous hurdles to bringing a malpractice lawsuit, and then it is rare to obtain a judgment against the hospital or physician, and in the event that a judgment is obtained, it is likely to be reversed on appeal.[31]

As a practical matter, lawyers for plaintiffs are mindful of the liability insurance coverage of the defendant. There is no point in filing suit if the defendant has no assets or is judgment-proof by virtue of a transfer of assets. Then, too, a settlement is more likely if there is insurance. But when filing an action alleging malpractice, which is covered by insurance, the plaintiff's attorney is faced with an increasing number of obstacles (as illustrated by the Michigan legislation). The courts in various states at times are mindful of the obstacles facing a plaintiff alleging malpractice, so a bypass occurs by a holding (based on a pleading) that the scenario is one of nonmedical negligence. To demonstrate, during World War II, the Germans went around the Maginot Line that the French thought would protect them from invasion.[32]

Michigan is a notable exception. Without question, Michigan nowadays is more protective of the medical profession than other states. The Michigan Supreme Court is accused of being aligned with the legislature in providing that protection.[33] Not only is it very difficult to make out a case of medical malpractice in Michigan, but just about anything that occurs in a medical setting, except possibly slips and falls, are categorized as falling under the limitations of a malpractice action.[34] Unlike in many states, the Michigan Supreme Court has upheld against constitutional objection the caps on damages enacted by the legislature. The qualifications of an expert are more difficult to establish than in other states.[35] Michigan is one of the few states that expand Good Samaritan immunity to include hospital care.[36]

Nonmedical Negligence

In a New Hampshire case, *Powell v. Catholic Medical Center*,[37] a phlebotomist was injured when a patient attacked her as she was attempting to draw blood. She brought action against the hospital and doctor, alleging that they breached their duty to warn her of the patient's potentially assaultive behavior. The New Hampshire Supreme Court held that expert testimony was not required because determining whether a patient posed a risk and whether a warning was necessary were in the purview of average jurors. The court said that this case was an ordinary duty of care case. It is only fortuitous that one of the defendants is a physician, the court said, and the court declined to follow *Tarasoff* where it was held that expert testimony was essential in establishing a duty to protect.

In a case in Alaska, *D.P. v. Wrangell General Hosp.*,[38] a schizophrenic patient brought a negligence action against a hospital and nurses, alleging that she was inadequately supervised. As a result, she left the hospital and had sexual relations with a man whom she delusionally believed was either Jesus or a prophet. The Alaska Supreme Court said that the facts of the case did not raise medical malpractice issues, and therefore, the patient was not required to present expert medical testimony. The plaintiff did not allege that the defendants failed to appreciate her mental health status, to recognize a risk of harm to her, or to order reasonable precautions. She instead faulted the defendants' failure to follow the ordered precautionary measures. There was a strong dissent.

The defendants in *D.P.* relied primarily on cases discussing whether the healthcare provider failed to recognize the suicidal or elopement tendencies of the patient or failed to order appropriate precautions.[39] On the other hand, most courts characterize cases in which the plaintiff alleges a failure to adequately supervise and safeguard the patient as involving ordinary negligence issues.[40] In *Meier v. Ross General Hosp.*,[41] the California Supreme Court concluded that the scenario supported instructions on both ordinary negligence and medical malpractice. In this case, the patient jumped through an unbarred second story window of a hospital. Issues relating to improper medical diagnosis and chemotherapy treatment required an instruction on the professional standard of care. But, the court concluded that an instruction on ordinary negligence was appropriate on the question of whether it was negligent to allow the decedent, who was depressed and had previously slashed his wrists, to wander freely around a hospital where there were no bars on the windows.

By characterizing the conduct in question as ministerial rather than medical, the traditional expert testimony approach to the liability of healthcare providers is avoided. For example, in an Iowa case, *Kastler v. Iowa Methodist Hosp.*,[42] a psychiatric patient brought a negligence action after falling while taking a shower. The court characterized this activity as involving "routine" care and held that the plaintiff was not required to produce expert testimony as to the standard of care. On the other hand, in a Pennsylvania case, *Saltzer v. Reckord*,[43] a patient fell from a stool after he had stated that he felt faint following a blood test. The fall caused a sterilizer to spill, burning the patient. The court held that this was a malpractice case and not one that could be maintained on a premises liability theory.

In another Iowa case, *Campbell v. Delbridge*,[44] the patient brought suit against his treating doctor and hospital seeking damages for reinfusing the patient's own blood following surgery. The plaintiff alleged negligence, failure to obtain informed consent, breach of contract, medical battery, and invasion of privacy. The defendant moved for summary judgment on the ground that, without expert testimony, the plaintiff could not make a prima facie showing of any of his theories of recovery. The Iowa Supreme Court held that (1) evidence concerning the lack of communication between the doctor and the hospital nurses, the possible mix-up in patient charts, and the doctor's admission of error were capable of being resolved by a fact-finder without the testimony of experts; and that (2) expert testimony was not necessary to sustain the patient's claim of emotional distress.

Then, too, proof of a medical standard of care is not required in cases where the injury resulted from a doctor's misrepresentation or breach of contract. In *Osborn v. Irwin Memorial Blood Bank*,[45] parents wanted to arrange to donate their own blood and that of friends for the benefit of their child who was to undergo surgery. The defendant's employee erroneously told them they could donate blood, but could not reserve it for their child's use. Accordingly, other blood was used in transfusions. The child contracted the AIDS virus from the blood transfusions. The court said these facts would show negligent misrepresentation that would be actionable if it is a proximate cause of harm.

The result of misrepresentation may be a battery claim. In *Duttry v. Patterson*,[46] the plaintiff underwent surgery performed by the defendant for esophageal cancer. A leak later occurred along the surgical site, requiring emergency surgery, and as a result the plaintiff allegedly developed a respiratory disease rendering her unable to work. Plaintiff said "she questioned Dr. Patterson about his experience and he advised her he had performed this particular procedure on an average of once a month." In fact, the plaintiff alleged, "he had performed it only five times in the preceding 5 years." The court rejected defendant's assertion that the plaintiff had to have expert testimony to prove her claim. The court said, "In this type of claim where the plaintiff alleges the physician did not have her informed consent to perform the surgery because she was misinformed of his qualifications, the theory of recovery is battery and the plaintiff need not establish negligence."

Breach of Contract

Sometimes the patient can allege injury from a breach of contract or some specific promise distinct from any implied promise to conform to the medical standard of care. Proof of breach of a specific promise may suffice without expert testimony. In *Hull v. Ratino*,[47] the allegation was that the plaintiff contracted for a breast reduction operation, but that the doctor actually augmented her breasts. "[T]he standard of care required that [the doctor] perform the procedure he agreed to perform," the court said, so the question was not medical custom, but whether he deviated from that agreement and whether the plaintiff suffered harm.

In an early Michigan case, in 1971, *Guilment v. Campbell*,[48] the Michigan Supreme Court confirmed an award against a surgeon who had been sued for both malpractice and breach of contract. The jury found no showing of malpractice, but concluded that he had breached his contract. There was evidence that the claimant, who suffered from a bleeding ulcer, in conversations with the physician had been assured that a vagotomy would "take care of all your troubles" and that the operation would incapacitate him for only "about 2 or 3 weeks." The evidence also indicated that the physician said he would "be a different man" after the operation. There were, however, substantial complications following the surgery, including a perforated esophagus and hepatitis. Because the patient had not recovered as he had been "promised," the physician was found to have committed a breach of contract.

As a general principle of law, a physician is not a guarantor of a cure, does not warrant a good result, is not an insurer against mishaps or unusual consequences, and is not liable for honest mistakes of judgment. Generally speaking, a contract for medical services is not relegated to the level of a commercial transaction, where assurances are construed as warranties. Medicine or psychiatry is not an exact science. It is a different matter, however, if the physician makes a guarantee. "It is well settled," the Michigan Supreme Court said in the 1971 case, "that a physician or surgeon *may* bind himself by an express contract to perform a cure or obtain specific results by treatment." "What we are saying," the court explained, "is that under some circumstances the trier of fact might conclude that a doctor so speaking did contract to cure a patient." At the trial, the physician had contended that the conversations reported were typical expressions of reassurance and comfort generally employed by all physicians, and that to interpret reassurance as a promise to cure would chill the practice of medicine. The court ruled, however, that "what was said, and the circumstances under which it was said, always determine whether there was a contract and if so what it was." In a concurring opinion, three members of the court went to some lengths to point out that "every assurance by a physician does not constitute a contract to cure, but that the particular statements in this case did."[49]

Types of contract claim include (1) contracts for a specific result, (2) contracts for specific procedures, and (3) contracts to perform services. A contract for a specific result is illustrated by the aforementioned case, *Guilmet v. Campbell*. An action for breach of contract may arise when the physician contracts to use a specific procedure and fails to do so. An action for breach of contract also may result when it is agreed that a particular physician will perform the services, and the physician fails to do so.

A number of prominent law professors have advocated reconceptualizing medical malpractice law in terms of contract rather than tort.[50] Contract theory might be based on advertising or promotional statements. Once a rarity in medicine, now there is a glut of advertising in newspapers, on billboards, and on television touting the quality of various medical institutions. Even if these assertions cannot be taken as warranting specific results from particular procedures, they can be argued to heighten the ordinary standard of care. Many physicians include in the informed consent form a statement that specifically denies any guarantee of results and asserts only that the physician will use his professional skills in the accepted manner.

Traditionally, a profession has been distinguished from a business, but increasingly the practice of medicine is being regarded as a business. The physician is called a *provider* and the patient is called a *consumer* of healthcare. In a number of states (e.g., Oregon), what might be considered as malpractice is made actionable under "bad practices" legislation. The recoverable damages, however, are less than in a malpractice action.

Framing a case may depend on the time that has elapsed since the alleged wrongdoing. Breach of contract is governed by a 6-year prescriptive period, 3 or 4 years more than an action for malpractice or nonmedical negligence and 5 years more than an action for an intentional tort. The damages recoverable for breach of contract, however, are limited to those within the contemplation of the defendant at the time the contract was made, and in contract actions there can ordinarily be no recovery for mental suffering. Generally speaking, the tort remedy is likely to be more advantageous to the injured party in the greater number of cases, if only because it will often permit the recovery of greater damages, but when prescription has run on a malpractice action, breach of contract or nonmedical negligence may be the only viable alternative for the complainant.

Endnotes

1. Thus, in Self v. Executive Committee of Georgia Baptist Convention, 245 Ga. 548, 266 S.E.2d 168 (1980), where a hospital patient slipped and fell because the hospital left a slippery substance on the floor, the court held that this was not a claim of medical malpractice and, hence, did not require expert testimony.
2. In an Iowa case, Oswald v. LeGrand, 453 N.W.2d 634 (Iowa 1990), the Iowa Supreme Court ruled that a fact-finder could evaluate the propriety of a doctor's early departure from the hospital—he knowingly had left the patient unattended in a hospital corridor screaming hysterically that she was about to give birth. In a similar case, a New Jersey court held that a woman claiming medical malpractice based on an "utter lack of attendance" at her delivery in a hospital need not produce expert testimony in order to overcome a motion for summary judgment. The court said in its ruling: "The question of malpractice in that regard would appear to be within the province of the jury of laymen, depending upon the proofs submitted. 'There are basic aspects of childbirth procedure within the common knowledge of laity.' (Citation omitted) Attendance of a patient in labor at or near the moment of giving birth would seem to be an aspect particularly within that knowledge"; Friel v. Vineland Obstetrical & Gynecological Prof. Assn, 166 N.J. Super. 579, 400 A.2d 147 (1979).
   In Runnells v. Rogers, 596 S.W.2d 87 (Tenn. 1980), a physician failed to remove a wire that was embedded in a patient's foot. The patient's foot turned blue, and then black, and oozed "some sort of liquid substance." The Tennessee Supreme Court was livid in its judgment that one need not present expert testimony in such a situation: "Even a barefoot boy knows that when his foot is infested by a sticker, splinter, thorn, pin or other foreign object, it must be removed. Most assuredly this lies within the ken of a layman"; 596 S.W.2d at 90.
   It is said that jurors, as a general matter, are better able to understand the sorts of decisions that physicians make, by contrast with those that lawyers make. Failure to present expert testimony is usually fatal to a plaintiff's legal malpractice action (giving rise to the belief that courts are more likely to be more protective of lawyers than physicians). See Barth v. Reagan, 139 Ill.2d 399, 564 N.E.2d 1196 (1990). In any event, where the plaintiff is relieved of the burden of producing expert testimony, the other restrictions on a malpractice action remain in place.
3. Protection in cases of ordinary negligence is provided by the standard homeowner's policy and by personal liability insurance, sometimes referred to as an umbrella policy because it sits on top of other coverage. An umbrella liability policy also covers libel and slander, which are not covered by standard policies.
4. In Rehabilitative Care Systems of America v. Davis, 73 S.W.3d 233 (Tex. 2002), a physical therapist was allegedly negligent in supervising a rehabilitation exercise, with the result that the plaintiff was further injured. The Texas Supreme Court said that "physical therapist malpractice suits are no different than any other medical malpractice," and that, therefore, expert testimony would be required.
5. C.T. Jones (Ed.), *The Shorter Oxford English Dictionary* (Oxford: Clarendon Press, 3rd ed., 1965). It is also to be noted that in common parlance *malpractice* is often equated with liability. Legally speaking, "malpractice" means fault, and for liability there must be a causal nexus between the fault and the harm.
6. 124 S. Ct. 2488 (2004).
7. See M. Kolosky, "*Aetna v. Davila*: A New Look at ERISA Preemption of Medical Malpractice Claims," *The Brief* (American Bar Association) 34 (Spring 2005): 34.
8. Hospital records or other evidence tending to indicate some direct contact between the physician and patient have been held to preclude summary judgment on the issue. See Easter v. Lexington Mem. Hosp., 303 N.C. 303, 278 S.E.2d 253 (1981); Willoughby v. Wilkins, 65 N.C. App. 626, 310 S.E.2d 90 (1983).
9. See, e.g., Hafner v. Beck 916 P.2d 1105 (Ariz. App. 1995).
10. See B.R. Furrow, T.L. Greaney, S.H. Johnson, T.S. Jost, & R.L. Schwartz, *Health Law* (St. Paul, MN: West, 2nd ed., 2000), p. 260; R.I. Simon, *Clinical Psychiat. and the Law* (Washington, DC: American Psychiatric Press, 2nd ed., 1992), pp. 3–19.

11. Pelrosky v. Brasner, 718 N.Y.S.2d 340, 279 A.D.2d 75 (2001); Saari v. Litman, 486 N.W.2d 813 (Minn. App. 1992).
12. Ney v. Axelrod, 723 A.2d 719 (Pa. Super. Ct. 1999).
13. Martinez v. Lewis, 942 P.2d 1219 (Colo. App. 1997).
14. P.S. Appelbaum, L.H. Roth, & C.W. Lidz, "The Therapeutic Misconception: Informed Consent in Psychiatric Research," *Int. J. Law & Psychiat.* 5 (1982): 319; J. Katz, "Human Experimentation and Human Rights," *St. Louis L. J.* 38 (1993): 7.
15. See, e.g., Daly v. United States, 946 F.2d 1467 (9th Cir. 1991); Reed v. Bojarski, 166 N.J. 89, 764 A.2d 433 (2001); Meena v. Wilburn, 603 So.2d 866 (Miss. 1992).
16. In Ande v. Rock, 256 Wis.2d 365, 647 N.W.2d 265 (2002), the Wisconsin Supreme Court denied the research subject's malpractice claim on the ground that there was no physician–patient relationship. The project was designed to test out the physician's theory that treating the nutritional needs of children with cystic fibrosis prior to the arrival of their symptoms would reduce impairment to their overall health. The plaintiff's child fell within the placebo group, thus they were not told their child tested positive. The plaintiffs sued on grounds of malpractice claiming that had they been informed of their child's positive results, they would not have conceived their second child. Yet another case where the individual participating in a clinical trial is injured and uncompensated is Goodman v. United States, 298 F.3d 1048 (9th Cir. 2002). On the other hand, in Grimes v. Kennedy Krieger Institute, 782 A.2d 807 (Md. 2001), the Maryland Supreme Court held that "the very nature of nontherapeutic scientific research on human subjects, can and normally will, create a special relationship out of which duties arise." See also Kernke v. Menninger Clinic, 172 F. Supp.2d 1347 (D. Kansas, 2001); see C.H. Coleman, "Duties to Subjects in Clinical Research," *Vand. L. Rev.* 58 (2005): 387; K. Gatter, "Fixing Cracks: A Disclosure Norm to Repair the Crumbling Regulatory Structure Supporting Clinical Research and Protecting Human Subjects," *UMKC* 73 (2005): 581.
17. Some statutes protect all Good Samaritans, without regard to their profession. See Perkins v. Howard, 283 Cal. Rptr. 764 (Cal. App. 1991). The District of Columbia provides immunity for midwives and nurses providing obstetrical care; D.C. Code §2-1345.
18. See Colby v. Schwartz, 144 Cal. Rptr. 624 (Cal. App. 1978); cited in S.R. Reuter, "Physicians as Good Samaritans: Should They Receive Immunity for Their Negligence When Responding to Hospital Emergencies?" *J. Legal Med.* 20 (1999): 157.
19. McIntyre v. Ramirez, 109 S.W.3d 741(Tex. 2003).
20. Michigan Compiled Laws §691.1502(1).
21. Velazquez v. Jimenez, 172 N.J. 240, 798 A.2d 51 (2002).
22. R. Porter, "New Jersey Good Samaritan Law Does Not Immunize Emergency Room Doctors," *Trial* 38 (Aug. 2002): 74.
23. Colby v. Schwartz, 144 Cal. Rptr. 624 at 628 (Cal. App. 1978).
24. The Michigan statute provides: "If an individual's actual hospital duty does not require a response to the emergency situation, a physician ... who in good faith responds to a life threatening emergency or responds to a request for emergency assistance in a life threatening emergency within a hospital or other licensed medical care facility is not liable"; Michigan Compiled Laws § 691.1502.
25. In Pemberton v. Dharmani, 188 Mich. App. 317, 469 N.W.2d 74 (1991), *interlocutory appeal*, 207 Mich. App. 522, 525 N.W.2d 497 (1994), the plaintiff Denise Pemberton decided to undergo a voluntary tubal ligation. After beginning the surgery, Dr. Sheila Dharmani noticed several pelvic adhesions causing her difficulty locating the left fallopian tube. Dr. Dharmani rang for assistance, but no Ob/Gyn doctors inside the hospital were available to respond. Dr. B.N. Zarewych, who had an office near the hospital, left a patient in his own office and responded to the emergency. After the surgery, it was discovered that part of Ms. Pemberton's colon had been accidentally removed instead of the fallopian tube. In the ensuing suit against Dr. Zarewych for malpractice, the main issue was whether it must be established that a life threatening emergency actually existed, or whether a good faith subjective belief that a life threatening emergency existed at the time of the initial response was enough to trigger Good Samaritan immunity. Ultimately, the court concluded that a good faith, subjective belief when initially responding to an emergency was enough to warrant Good Samaritan protection. It was not necessary to establish that a life threatening emergency actually existed as long as the physician responded with the belief that a life threatening emergency was present. The court felt that, if it adopted the position that the plaintiff suggested, it might actually delay responses from physicians. A physician responding to an emergency might want assurance that the emergency was indeed life threatening before coming to render aid and this would simply delay the assistance, defeating the purpose of the statute altogether, and could result in the worsening of patient conditions.

26. 17 Cal.3d 425, 131 Cal. Rptr. 14, 551 P.2d 334 (1976).

27. See, e.g., Bradshaw v. Daniel, 854 S.W.2d 865 (Tenn. 1993).

28. Landeros v. Flood, 17 Cal.3d 399, 131 Cal. Rptr. 69, 551 P.2d 389 (1976).

29. 102 S. Ct. 2452 (1982); discussed in D.B. Wexler, "Legal Aspects of Seclusion and Restraint," in K. Tardiff (Ed.), *The Psychiatric Uses of Seclusion and Restraint* (Washington, DC: American Psychiatric Press, 1984), pp. 111–124.

30. See R. Blumenthal, "After Texas Caps Malpractice Awards, Doctors Rush to Practice There," *New York Times*, Oct. 5, 2007, p. 21.

31. The Michigan legislature (MCL § 600.2169) has enacted the following:

    - Criteria and qualifications to be used in order to determine whether an expert witness is entitled to testify on the appropriate standard of care in a medical malpractice case.
    - Requirement that all medical malpractice lawsuits go through a mediation process.
    - A $280,000 cap on plaintiffs' recovery for noneconomic damages in medical malpractice actions.
    - Establishing a burden of proof whereby plaintiffs must prove that it is more probable than not that injuries were caused by the negligence of a health professional.
    - Limitation on a plaintiff's recovery by disallowing recovery for loss of an opportunity to survive or of an opportunity to achieve a better result unless the opportunity was greater than 50%.
    - A requirement that a plaintiff give 182 days written notice of the intent to file a medical malpractice action and setting forth the requirements for the contents of the notice, and that both parties provide access to medical records and requiring a written response by the potential defendant within 154 days after receipt of the initial notice.
    - Authorizing the defendant in a medical malpractice action to file a certificate of noninvolvement with the court, which certifies he or she was not involved in the occurrence alleged in the complaint, and unless the certificate is opposed by the plaintiff or another co-defendant, the defendant is entitled to dismissal of the action against him or her.
    - Mandating that a plaintiff file an affidavit of merit along with the complaint, which is signed by a health professional who meets the qualifications for an expert witness;
    - Requiring the defendant to file an affidavit of meritorious defense within 91 days of the plaintiff filing his or her affidavit of merit, also to be signed by a health professional that satisfies the expert witness qualification standard.
    - Automatic waiver of the physician–patient privilege by plaintiff's filing of a medical malpractice action with regard to any events, persons or other related elements that are part of the basis of the plaintiff's claim.
    - Altering the time the standard 2-year statute of limitations starts to run in some situations, and altering the statute of limitations tolling periods for malpractice actions in others.
    - Amending the rules governing joint liability.

32. In religion as in law, circumventions are often accomplished by a recategorization. A Jewish joke tells about a religious Jew who on the Sabbath sees a large sack of money lying on the street. Jews are not allowed to handle money on the Sabbath. He prayed and prayed and suddenly, it was Tuesday.

33. Trial attorneys representing plaintiffs in Michigan are outraged by the current holdings of the Michigan Supreme Court. For example, J. Martin Brennan, Jr., a trial attorney and former candidate for the court, says, "Since the conservative majority has taken over the court, the decisions have tendentiously favored … insurance companies, doctors [and] hospitals." J.M. Brennan (ltr.), "State's High Court GOP," *Detroit Free Press*, May 18, 2005, p. 10. It is not at all unusual for Michigan physicians—even those in high-risk specialties—to carry only $200,000 or even $100,000 in liability coverage. "It is time to start counting paperclips or reducing how much coffee you order every month for your office," says Thomas Peters, chairman of the negligence law section of the Michigan State Bar. *Quarterly of the Negligence Law Section*, Winter 2008, p. 1. This state of affairs in Michigan was depicted in CBS's *60 Minutes*. The 2008 election produced the unseating of the chief justice.

34. The definitive opinion in Michigan distinguishing medical malpractice from ordinary negligence is Bryant v. Oakpointe Villa Nursing Centre, 471 Mich. 411, 684 N.W.2d 864 (2004). In this case, plaintiff Denise Bryant, personal representative of the estate of her deceased aunt, alleged that the defendant

Oakpointe Villa Nursing Centre, was responsible for the death of her aunt, who died from positional asphyxiation while in the defendant's care. The plaintiff alleged that the defendant was negligent in several distinct ways: (1) by failing to train its certified evaluated nursing assistants to recognize the risk of positional asphyxiation posed by bed rails, (2) by failing to take adequate corrective measures after finding the aunt entangled in her bedding on the day before her asphyxiation, (3) and by failing to inspect the aunt's bed arrangements to ensure that the risk of positional asphyxia did not exist for the aunt. The Michigan Supreme Court, in a 5–2 decision, held that the plaintiff's failure-to-train and failure-to-inspect claims sounded in medical malpractice. However, the court held that the plaintiff's claim that the defendant failed to take action after its employees found the aunt entangled in her bedding on the day before her asphyxiation sounded in ordinary negligence. In a dissent, Justice Marilyn Kelly contended that all of the plaintiff's claims sounded in ordinary negligence. Justice Kelly observed, "The danger here was similar to that experienced by an infant in a crib whose mattress is too small and whose rails allow the baby to slip through. Those caring for such a child would quickly recognize the danger, and an expert would not be required to point it out. Similarly, ordinary jurors can assess whether defendant's caregivers here should have recognized the danger and acted with due care"; 471 Mich. at 441.

In *Bryant*, the Michigan Supreme Court provided a two-pronged test for determining ordinary versus professional negligence. The test is (1) whether the claim pertains to an action that occurred within the course of a professional relationship, and (2) whether the claim raises questions of medical judgment beyond the realm of common knowledge and experience. *Bryant* essentially affirmed the prior holding of the court in Dorris v. Detroit Osteopathic Hospital, 460 Mich. 26, 594 N.W.2d 455 (1999). In *Dorris*, the court stated that the plaintiff's allegations "concerning staffing decisions and patient monitoring involve questions of professional medical management and not issues of ordinary negligence that can be judged by the common knowledge and experience of a jury"; 594 N.W.2d at 465-466. The court went on to say: "The ordinary layman does not know the type of supervision or monitoring that is required for psychiatric patients in a psychiatric ward"; 594 N.W.2d at 466.

Despite the relative clarity of the court's analysis in *Bryant* and the two-pronged test it enunciated, factual patterns continue to challenge the notion that ordinary negligence can be readily discerned. In *Bryant*, Justice Stephen Markham offered advice: "[I]n future cases of this nature, in which the line between ordinary negligence and medical malpractice is not easily distinguishable, plaintiffs are advised as a matter of prudence to file their claims alternatively in medical malpractice and ordinary negligence within the applicable period of limitations"; 684 N.W.2d at 876. Plaintiffs are also well advised to file a motion for summary disposition and obtain a definitive court ruling on this issue as soon as possible.

Bryant has been repeatedly discussed and interpreted in the numerous court of appeals cases that have followed it. In Harrier v. Oakwood Skilled Nursing Center Trenton, an unpublished opinion issued on March 27, 2007 (Docket No. 273729), the Michigan Court of Appeals held that nursing home personnel who were aware that the plaintiff was at great risk of falling, but failed to act were liable in ordinary negligence. The court said: "We find that no expert testimony is necessary to show that defendants acted negligently by failing to respond appropriately to the knowledge that Anne Harrier was prone to falling and that the aide was negligent by abandoning her patient in the face of that known danger."

In Karwoski v. Barnabei & University of Michigan Hospital, Washtenaw County Circuit Court, No. 05 1012 NH (March 18, 2007), a $3 million verdict was rendered in a claim against the University of Michigan Hospital arising out of the mislabeling of slides by a clerk in the pathology lab. As a result of the error, plaintiff underwent a partial mastectomy as well as lymph node mapping, dissection, and removal. The defendant argued that the clerk's conduct was malpractice. The court rejected the argument and held that the conduct was ordinary negligence. The judge said: "Putting the wrong identification sticker on a sample is no different from putting a document in the wrong file, depositing a check in the wrong account, placing a letter in the wrong mailbox. It is simple human error that can be evaluated by jurors on the basis of their common knowledge and experience."

35. S.S. Schwartz, "Where's Dr. Waldo?" *Mich. Negligence Law Sect. Q.*, Spring 2004, p. 3.
36. It is also to be noted that Michigan was the only state in the United States that shielded pharmaceutical companies from liability if the drug was approved by the Food and Drug Administration (patients could obtain damages only if they prove a company withheld or misrepresented information about a drug that would cause the FDA to not give or withdraw its approval). See M. Orey, "How Business Trounced the Trial Lawyers," *Business Week*, Jan. 8, 2007, pp. 44–50. In 2008 repeal of the provision was proposed.

In 2008 the U.S. Supreme Court ruled that makers of medical devices such as implantable defibrillators are immune from liability for personal injuries as long as the Food and Drug Administration approved the device before it was marketed and it meets the agency's specifications. In *Riegel v. Medtronic,* 128 S. Ct. 999 (2008), the Court ruled that federal power under the Constitution's Commerce Clause preempted state product liability laws. Following the Dalkon Shield fiasco and growing number of state laws contradicting FDA statutes, Congress passed the Medical Device Amendments (MDA) in 1976, which established a single national standard. The law's language precludes states from imposing "any requirement that is different from, or in addition to, any requirement under this chapter." An exception is granted to "claims premised on a violation of FDA regulations," such as improper manufacture or concealing real risks. Editorial, "Medical Double Jeopardy," *Wall Street Journal*, March 1–2, 2008, p. 8.

The Civil War ended the confederacy and diminished states rights. Increasingly, over the years, federal law has preempted state law. Most recently, in Cipollone v. Liggett Group, 505 U.S. 504 (1992), the Supreme Court shielded cigarette makers from lawsuits from smokers who claimed they were not truly warned of the dangers. The federal cigarette warning label act required tobacco companies to put warnings on each pack of cigarettes, but it also said "no requirement or prohibition" may be added by the states. In Rowe v. New Hampshire Motor Transport Association, 128 S. Ct. 989 (2008), the Court shielded delivery services, such as FedEx and UPS, from state laws requiring that they check with an adult before dropping off cigarettes at a residence. In Preston v. Ferrer, 128 S. Ct. 978 (2008), the Court ruled that the Federal Arbitration Act preempts conflicting state laws. The U.S. Chamber of Commerce welcomes the rules for recognizing the conflict faced by businesses that operate nationally. They want one set of national regulations, not a patchwork of inconsistent state and local requirements. D.G. Savage, "Trumping the States," *ABAJ*, May 2008, p. 26.

What about drug makers? Drug and device makers are governed under separate standards. Shortly after its decision in *Riegel*, the Supreme Court in Warner-Lambert v. Kent, 128 S. Ct. 1168 (2008), was faced with the question whether a state trial court is the proper jurisdiction to adjudicate fraud that a pharmaceutical company allegedly committed during FDA review. As a result of a tie vote, 4 to 4, the Supreme Court automatically affirmed the lower court's judgment. In this case, the federal appeals court in New York had rejected the company's argument that the reasoning of a 7-year-old Supreme Court precedent barred individual damage suits that are based on the claim that the drug manufacturer obtained FDA approval through fraud. Affirmance by a tie vote resolves only the particular dispute, without setting a precedent for other cases. Chief Justice John Roberts, Jr., recused himself from the case because he owned stock in the defendant pharmaceutical company. L. Greenhouse, "Court Allows Suit Against Drug Maker," *New York Times*, March 4, 2008, p. 21.

More recently, in Wyeth v. Levine, No. 06–1249, the Court was faced the question whether *Riegel* protection applied to drug companies. The case presented the issue of whether FDA drug approval is grounds to preempt common law tort claims based on the manufacture and labeling of the drug. While *Riegel* involved a medical device governed by the MDA, which has a preemption clause, *Wyeth* is governed by the Federal Food, Drug and Cosmetic Act (FDCA), which contains no preemption clause. In *Wyeth*, a Vermont patient contended that the warning label on the antinausea drug Phenergan® was not specific enough about its risks.

In an amicus brief, the editors of the *New England Journal of Medicine* argued that lawsuits can serve as "a vital deterrent" and protect consumers if drug companies do not disclose risks. Donald Kennedy, editor emeritus of *Science* and former commissioner of the FDA, says: "(1) the FDA is badly underfunded, and (2) the nature of the FDA's standard process makes it unable to make a secure guarantee of safety." D. Kennedy, "Misbegotten Preemptions," *Science* 320 (May 2, 2008): 585. Nonetheless, the Bush administration supported Wyeth's position. Solicitor General Paul D. Clement wrote in the administration's brief, "FDA considers and approves specific labeling for a drug, and the drug manufacturer is generally barred from making unilateral changes to the FDA-approved labeling." Yale law professor Peter H. Schuck says, "[A] seldom-discussed advantage of the FDA (and of agencies more generally) when compared with common law tort litigation is the FDA's vastly superior capacity to learn from its environment and correct its policy mistakes in a timely fashion. The common law proceeds slowly and incrementally, driven by opportunistic legal entrepreneurs who tend to act in largely uncoordinated, unsystematic ways." P.H. Schuck, "FDA Preemption of State Tort Law in Drug Regulation: Finding the Sweet Spot," *Roger Williams U. L. Rev.* 13 (2008): 73 at 97.

The Supreme Court's decision in *Wyeth* is pending.

37. 145 N.H. 7, 749 A.2d 301(2000).

38. 5 P.3d 225 (Alaska 2000).

39. See, e.g., Rudy v. Meshorer, 146 Ariz. 467, 706 P.2d 1234, 1236-38 (App. 1985) (requiring expert testimony to show that psychiatrist "was negligent in his determination that [decedent] was not suicidal"); Dimitrijevic v. Chicago Wesley Mem'l Hosp., 92 Ill. App.2d 251, 236 N.E.2d 309 (1968; requiring expert testimony to determine "whether defendant doctors failed to exercise ordinary skill and care in not characterizing decedent as a suicidal risk"); Kanter v. Metropolitan Med. Ctr., 384 N.W.2d 914 (Minn. App. 1986; recognizing that expert testimony would assist trier of fact in determining whether nurse should have recognized patients' "potential [suicidal] tendencies"); Reifschneider v. Nebraska Methodist Hosp., 222 Neb. 782, 387 N.W.2d 486 (1986; where emergency room patient fell from hospital cart, court refused to find that laypersons could determine whether hospital had duty to restrain or supervise patients on carts).

40. See Paulen v. Shinnick 291 Mich. 288, 289 N.W. 162 (1939) (where patient leapt from window, "Whether [attendant] should have locked the screen ... or taken some other precaution to prevent plaintiff's escape, is not a question on which a jury requires the advice of trained psychiatrists"); Staliman v. Robinson, 364 Mo. 275, 260 S.W.2d 743 (1953) (where decedent hanged herself with her nightgown, expert testimony not required to determine "whether the patient was reasonably safeguarded and protected, in the circumstances in view of her known condition" because the case was not "strictly speaking a malpractice case"); Kent v, Whitaker, 58 Wash.2d 569, 364 P.2d 556 (1961) (action was not a malpractice case where patient with known suicidal tendencies strangled herself with plastic tubing while unattended in unlocked room because it did not concern "improper diagnosis or negligent treatment" but rather "failure of the specific duty of exercising reasonable care to safeguard and protect a patient with known suicidal tendencies from injuring herself').

41. 69 Cal.2d 420, 71 Cal Rptr. 903, 445 P.2d 519 (1968).

42. 193 N.W.2d 98 (Iowa 1971).

43. 179 Ad. 449 (Pa. 1935)).

44. 670 N.W.2d 108 (Iowa 2003).

45. 5 Cal. App.4th 234, 7 Cal. Rptr.2d 101 (1992).

46. 741 A.2d 199 (Pa. Super. 1999).

47. 12989 WL 128492 (Tenn. App. 1989).

48. 385 Mich. 57, 188 N.W.2d 801 (1971).

49. Breach of contract is frequently alleged in cosmetic surgery cases. In the leading case of Sullivan v. O'Connor, 363 Mass. 579, 296 N.E.2d 183 (1973), the plaintiff recovered on an express warranty theory after alleging that the defendant plastic surgeon had promised to enhance her beauty and improve her appearance. Nevertheless, the court cautioned: "Statements of opinion by the physician with some optimistic coloring are a different thing, and may indeed have therapeutic value. But patients may transform such statements into firm promises in their own minds, especially when they have been disappointed in the event." See A.R. Holder, "Plastic Surgeon's Liability in Cosmetic Surgery Cases," 22 Am. Jur. Proof of Facts 2d 721; K. Tierney, "Contractual Aspects of Malpractice," Wayne L. Rev. 19 (1973): 1457. See also S. Dennehy, "Mirror, Mirror, on the Wall," Trial, August 2006, p. 54. See generally S.L. Gilman, Making the Body Beautiful (Princeton, NJ: Princeton University Press, 1999); A. Kuczynski, Beauty Junkies (NY: Doubleday, 2006); E. Gorbis & Y. Kholodenko, "Plastic Surgery Addiction in Patients with Body Dysmorphic Disorder," Psychiatric Times, Sept. 2005, p. 79. By plastic surgery at least one woman has changed the size of her breasts depending on the desires of her boyfriends as they change. C. Lesesne, Confessions of a Park Avenue Plastic Surgeon (New York: Gotham Books, 2005). To raise revenue for government initiatives such as health care for poor children, various states have considered taxing certain cosmetic surgery procedures, including face-lifts, tummy-tucks and Botox injections. R. E. Silverman, "The Nose-Job Tax," Wall Street Journal, June 1, 2005, p. D-1. Any physician can practice plastic surgery.

50. See, e.g., J. Epstein, "Contracting Out of the Medical Malpractice Crisis," Perspect.in Biol. & Med. 20 (1977): 228; J. Epstein, "Medical Malpractice: The Case for Contract," Am. Bar Found. Res. J. 1976: 87; C.C. Havighurst, "Altering the Applicable Standard of Care," Law & Contemp. Prob., 49 (1986): 265.

27

Establishing Malpractice Liability

It is textbook knowledge that in any negligence or malpractice action the aggrieved party must establish by a preponderance of the evidence (1) that the defendant has failed to conform to a certain standard of conduct, (2) that there is a reasonable cause-and-effect relationship between that failure and the alleged injury, and (3) that the loss or injury is of a type of concern to the law. The substantive law and the rules of evidence govern the admissibility of evidence at trial, but licensing or administrative boards are not bound by the rules of evidence.[1]

Standard of Care

The public expects that the performance of a professional or a specialist will measure up to the standards of the profession or specialty. A person avowing professional or specialty status is held to the degree of skill claimed by that profession or specialty. The public relies on it. Hence, the test of fault or breach of duty in malpractice cases is determined not by reference to the traditional reasonable or prudent man's standard (as in ordinary personal injury cases), but by whether there was a departure from customary professional conduct. Thus, the legal standard of care for a lawyer is that of the "reasonable and prudent lawyer." The legal standard of care for a doctor is that of "reasonable and prudent doctor." The legal standard of care for a nurse is that of the "reasonable and prudent nurse." And so on.

On national standard of care expert testimony, the District of Columbia Court of Appeals set out the following: (1) it is insufficient for the expert to merely recite the words *national standard of care*, (2) the expert's testimony may not be based on his or her personal opinion, nor on mere speculation or conjecture, and (3) the expert's opinion must reflect some evidence of a national standard, such as attendance at national seminars or meetings or conventions, or reference to published materials, when assessing a medical course of action or treatment.[2]

But what in the mental health field is the standard of care? What is the competence, avowed or otherwise, of the various practitioners? There are now reportedly over 200 varieties of psychotherapy that range from classical psychoanalysis to procedures administered in cult-like surroundings reminiscent of techniques used by preliterate peoples. They are called a *psychotherapy jungle*.[3] Indeed, there are books on psychotherapies resembling travel guides.[4]

As a general rule, a practitioner is liable for failure to refer when the circumstances are such that the duly careful practitioner should have known that a problem existed that he was not equipped to handle. Good sense, the law, and professional ethics would all maintain that one should not undertake services in a matter outside of one's competence. And where it turns out services are undertaken by not one competent for it (and does not expect to become qualified), there is an affirmative duty to seek qualified assistance. With the advent of specialization, a practitioner may not be able to defend against the imposition of higher standards of care by pleading insufficiency of knowledge or lack of expertise in a given area.

Most patients with depressive disorders are seen in primary care settings; only about 10% of depressed patients are referred and seen in the mental health specialty sector. Depressed patients come to primary care physicians with such complaints as headaches, fatigue, or gastrointestinal distress, so detection of the depression is thus delayed or missed, sometimes resulting in suicide. In recent decades, the treatment of depressive disorders has progressed from being a mystery and an art to being an array of effective, practical approaches, yet less than 50 percent of patients with depression are properly recognized and adequately treated by practitioners. The primary care physician is today the major dispenser of psychiatric medication, but whether they are properly used is subject to question. Busy primary care practices are not organized to provide the necessary social and psychotherapeutic interventions that may be appropriate.[5]

Every physician or therapist does what he knows best, we may suppose, but, in the practice of psychiatry, should the therapist's forte be applied to one and all in distress? Surely, one would say no, but in the mental health field, questions abound. For example, what is the link, if any, between psychiatric diagnosis and treatment modality?[6] When is there a need to consult or refer to one more competent or specialized?[7] Who is the specialist? What skill does the therapist hold himself out to the public as having? What can the public expect? When may it be said that a psychological problem is caused by a physical problem, and a medical doctor ought to be consulted? What difference does the etiology or pathogenesis of a disorder make as to whether the therapy should be somatic or psychological? How do the therapist's feelings or personality enhance or interfere with the process of psychotherapy? When may it be said that the diagnosis is improper, the prognosis faulty, or the treatment plan inappropriate? Stated differently, is there a statistically preferred treatment? Is psychotherapy, on the other hand *ad hoc* or true to nothing but uncertainty, like politics or religion? Psychiatry, like medicine, is known as "the healer's art," but it is also said that there is a "science to the art of healing." Just about every public lecture in psychiatry begins with the introduction, "Welcome to this *scientific* meeting" (emphasis theirs).

The following is read at the beginning of the monthly meetings of the Michigan Society for Psychoanalytic Psychology (MSPP), a chapter of the Division of Psychoanalysis of the American Psychological Association:

> MSPP holds the position that psychoanalysis is not a monolith in theory, scholarship, practice or educational format. MSPP further holds the position that in all things psychoanalytic there are legitimate, long-standing and valid differences of opinion and that all such positions are part of the discourse of psychoanalysis. MSPP maintains that there is no single, correct and "scientific" psychoanalysis and no single pathway toward becoming a competent professional. It is also our view that the public and professional communities are best served by knowing this and being thus encouraged to think about different perspectives within psychoanalysis, including the differing perspectives about the location of psychoanalysis among the disciplines. This knowledge will allow for informed choices. MSPP welcomes as members people of all disciplines with an interest in psychoanalysis.

In general, as we discuss, the courts tend not to pass judgment on the appropriate therapy or the efficacy of different forms of treatment. Thus, the courts decline to consider which of two equally reputable methods of psychiatric treatment—psychotherapy as against a physiological approach—would prove efficacious in a particular case.[8] The issue of negligence may be raised, however, where anachronistic therapeutic modes have been applied to psychiatric disorders where newer and more effective therapies are available.

The doctrine that a malpractice action properly lies only where the practitioner has fallen short of the generally accepted standard of the profession itself is a deference to and a reflection of the old Durkheimian insight that each occupational group possesses its own morality.[9] Thus, a practitioner is held to a standard of care that is really defined by his own profession. The standard of the profession is the measuring rod of the standard of care. To put it differently, one's own profession does the fingering.[10] In the usual negligence action, say, in a collision case, the standard of care to which the defendant must conform is that degree of care, which, in the jury's view, a reasonable person of ordinary prudence would have exercised in the defendant's place in the same or similar circumstances, but in professional negligence (malpractice) actions the standard of care is that degree of skill and learning, which is ordinarily possessed and exercised by members of that profession in good standing.[11] It follows the practice of the early common law when merchants were judged by the custom of their trade. Hence, an action for malpractice usually requires the plaintiff to produce an expert to establish the standard and that there was a deviation from it.[12]

Negligence theory presupposes some objective standard (it is not the best of which the defendant is capable). Thus, a physician is expected to act in accordance with an objective standard of care. In determining the appropriate standard by which to measure the action or inaction being considered. The particular facts and circumstances of the situation will be taken into consideration. Generally, a physician must act as similar professionals would act in the same or similar circumstances. Thus, a board-certified surgeon will be held to the same standard as other board-certified surgeons of like training and background under similar facts and circumstances. This standard may vary from state or from community to community.

The rationale of the traditional "locality rule" was that physicians in small or rural communities lacked opportunities to keep abreast of advances in the profession and would usually not possess the most up-to-date facilities and equipment for treating patients. That rule has either been modified or done away with entirely. The Massachusetts Supreme Court in 1968 stated:

> The proper standard is whether the physician, if a general practitioner, has exercised the degree of care and skill of the average, qualified practitioner, taking into account advances in the profession. In applying this standard, it is permissible to consider the medical resources available to the physician as *one* circumstance in determining the skill and care required. Under this standard some allowances is thus made for the type of community in which the physician carries on his practice.[13]

The court also stated that "one holding himself out as a specialist should be held to the standard of care and skill of the average member of the profession practicing the specialty, taking into account the advances in the profession. And, as in the case of the general practitioner, it is permissible to consider the medical resources available to him."[14]

The treatment or technique provided the patient need not be the best; it need be acceptable only by respectable professional authority, provided the standard is not a careless one. As Judge Learned Hand of the Second Circuit wrote in an oft-quoted passage, which summarizes the law in this area: "[I]n most cases reasonable prudence is in fact common prudence, but strictly it is never its measure; a whole calling may have unduly lagged in the adoption of new and available devices. It never may set its own tests, however persuasive be its usages. Courts must in the end say what is required; there are precautions so imperative that even their universal disregard will not excuse their omission."[15]

To be sure, negligence is not established simply by proof that the technique used in the particular case was not effective,[16] or that it is not regarded as the best or optimal one by other professionals.[17] Were it otherwise, it might be said that a medical student who does not graduate with a grade of 100 is something of a murderer.[18]

In determining standard of care, the courts take into account the various schools of therapy as well as the many techniques and modes of therapy within each school. Hence, a psychiatrist is entitled to be judged according to his school and the mode of therapy. He may show that his conduct conformed to a minority school within the profession even if most practitioners would not follow his technique.[19] However, this has been somewhat limited by the requirement that "the school ... be a recognized school of good standing, which has established rules and principles of practice for the guidance of all its members, as respects diagnosis and remedies, which each member is supposed to observe in any given case."[20] A single practitioner adhering to a certain theoretical framework would not constitute a school.[21]

It is not enough for a practitioner to say (in effect), "I belong to the school of mumbo jumbo, and I apply mumbo jumbo therapy." The school may be repudiated at law. Some "schools" repudiated by the courts include the spiritualist or clairvoyant school, magnetic healers, and Chinese herb doctors.[22] On one occasion, the court was called on to decide the question whether one who holds himself out as a clairvoyant physician should be held to the standard that is applicable to ordinary physicians.[23] The court concluded that, there being no recognized school of clairvoyant medicine, the defendant was held liable on the ground that, having held himself out as other physicians, he had not met the requirements of the rule of law applicable to them.[24] So, also, another court held that a magnetic healer was liable to a patient to whom he had administered treatment that, in the opinion of ordinary physicians, could not be justified by the rules of recognized schools, though they knew nothing of the principles of magnetic healing.[25]

Christian Science has fared better. In one of a number of cases,[26] the plaintiff, through her interest in the doctrines of Christian Science and the cures that the defendant professed to be able to perfect through the agency of prayer, was induced to employ him to cure her of an attack of appendicitis. He undertook the cure for a reward, but, the malady growing worse, the plaintiff went to a surgeon, had an operation, and was cured. She then brought action against the defendant for damages for malpractice. The court said that one who holds himself out as a Christian Science healer and is employed to give treatment by the methods adopted by such practitioner is required to possess only the knowledge and exercise the care and skill of the ordinary Christian Scientist. Christian Science being a recognized school, the defendant is to be judged by the standard of care, skill, and knowledge of the ordinary Christian Scientist, insofar as he confined himself to those methods.[27]

With the veritable smorgasbord of accepted theories in the mental health field, the defendant will likely always find support from a colleague. A psychiatrist of one school may testify against a psychiatrist of another school. However, may a psychiatrist of whatever school testify against a psychologist or social worker, or vice versa, as to standard of care or need for referral? Though separately licensed, they all now fall under the rubric of mental health professionals, but there is among these professionals an intense sibling rivalry that tends to prejudice their testimony. Under the school rule, one may testify about another school when the methods of treatment for a particular ailment are generally the same in both schools.[28]

Observers wonder if there is, or ought to be, a uniform standard for mental health care extending beyond the psychiatrist to the traditional clinical disciplines of psychology and social work, perhaps even embracing pastoral counseling, transactional analysis, or Erhard seminar training.[29] At one time the psychiatrist did the treating, the psychologist did the testing, and the social worker collected the data, but now they are all engaged in the practice of what is called psychotherapy.

The issue that arises of the qualification of the expert may be illustrated by a malpractice action in Illinois against a podiatrist. Taking a restrictive view, the Illinois Supreme Court held that the standard of care owed by a podiatrist to a patient may not be established by offering the testimony of a physician or another expert other than a podiatrist.[30] Some other courts have taken a similar position.[31]

In the past, and still in some states, the plaintiff could turn to one outside a school provided that person was familiar with the practice of the school. Apparently prompted by continued assertions of a "conspiracy of silence" in malpractice cases, the courts in many jurisdictions allowed the testimony of experts of other schools. Thus, the court has permitted an orthopedic surgeon to testify as an expert against a psychiatrist who had allegedly negligently administered electroshock. The orthopedist, though he had not ever given electroshock, was familiar with the literature on the subject, had talked with specialists in that field, and had treated fractures sustained in that treatment.[32]

No rule of law is without exceptions. Here, too, in establishing standard of care, there are exceptions to the rule requiring expert testimony. One exception is where the nature of the alleged negligent conduct is such that inferences to be drawn from the facts are within the range of common experience.[33] A similar exception is where "the very nature of the acts complained of bespeaks improper treatment." *Res ipsa loquitur*—the thing speaks for itself.[34] Thus, a sponge is not ordinarily left in an abdomen in the absence of negligence. This theory was employed in *Hammer v. Rosen*,[35] where ironically the patient's name was Hammer and the psychiatrist (Dr. John Rosen) used beatings as part of his therapy with catatonic patients. His technique was well known in professional circles. The court held that expert testimony was not necessary to establish negligence in such a case because the treatment used bespoke negligence. Actually, "beating the devil out of the afflicted" is an old therapy, but it was not recognized by the court. The court left open the possibility that such a therapy could be properly used if there was evidence that showed that the beatings constituted proper treatment.[36]

Still another exception to the rule requiring expert testimony is where a statute formulates a standard of care, one example is the use of narcotics in violation of an antinarcotics statute. Under the law of torts, the violation of a statute constitutes negligence. Also, standard of care may be shown by published standards, drug manufacturers' instructions, and under the Federal Rules of Evidence and in many states, by medical treatises.[37]

The underlying premise of mental health and other health agencies in seeking to extend care to a larger number of people is that "supervision" safeguards or improves the standard of care.[38] It is said that even paraprofessionals can play an important and increasing role in healthcare if they have "appropriate training and supervision."[39] The supervisor would establish the overall tone and direction of the agency, develop new treatment programs, and work closely with staff to make sure patients are properly evaluated and treated.

The nature and structure of the outpatient psychiatric clinic (OPC) that prevailed at one time in Michigan warrants examination regarding standards and potential abuses to be found in that pattern of care. Under it, the services of psychologists and social workers were reimbursable only if they were supervised by psychiatrists. Psychiatrists, reasonably enough, expected payment for their services. In many cases, however, what this meant was that the psychologist or social worker actually did the work of treating the patient while the psychiatrist, though spending little time supervising, obtained a substantial portion of the fee that the insurer paid for the therapy. Some called it duplicity, others called it fraud and abuse, yet others called it protection money. For the fee, the psychiatrist signed payment forms.

But even assuring that the psychiatrist indeed acted as a supervisor, it was asked, was the supervision needed at all? The Michigan Psychiatric Society took the position that there must be a psychiatrist as medical director who has responsibility for all patients as well as for the quality of their care. On the other hand, the psychologists and social workers argued that each profession should be independently responsible for the mental health personnel in its discipline.[40] They said, supervision by one who merely carries the title of psychiatrist served no useful purpose. They would prefer, if needed, the facade of supervision to the actual supervision, as they claimed the latter would be merely a waste of time. In the best operating OPCs, the arrangement in practice was collegial, not hierarchical; supervision in such cases was essentially an exchange of ideas.

The position of a resident in training changes gradually from that of a novice to that of a professional colleague, and in the latter role he is free to use his own style and orientation.[41] Completion of residency training is something like a Bar Mitzvah, where the rabbi tells the young lad: "Beginning today you are old enough to be responsible for your own sins. Your father no longer takes them on his shoulders. Today you are a man." In law, a parent is not responsible for the acts of a child arising out of failure of supervision when the child is capable of appreciating a duty of care. But those supervised in the OPC—professionals and paraprofessionals alike—never achieved this level of freedom; they remained supervisees forever. In a psychiatric residency-training program, a psychologist may be a teacher or supervisor, but upon completion of the training, a psychiatrist ranked over the psychologist in the OPC hierarchy. After a long struggle, psychologists in Michigan, claiming that they performed equally well in the practice of psychotherapy, obtained legislation requiring insurance companies to pay them on the same basis as they pay psychiatrists. Such laws, called "freedom of choice" laws, have been enacted in a number of states. Licensed psychologists have been recognized as independent providers in CHAMPUS, CHAMPVA, FEHBA, Aetna insurance programs, Medicaid, some BCBS plans, etc.

The hierarchy set up in the OPC was the source of controversy. Even more disconcerting was the inadequacy of guidelines and statements concerning the actual providers of services. There was want of delineation of the educational preparation, amount of experience, and kind of quality of training of the providers of services. Within this nonstructure some service providers were prepared, others were not. Inadequately trained persons were allowed to perform services on the theory that supervision would remedy any deficiencies. This expectation placed the supervisor in the role of educator, a role for which the supervisor may or may not have been prepared.[42] There have been many expressions of surprise, given the large number of people who have been treated in these clinics and given the litigiousness of the times, that no lawsuits alleging malpractice were brought against the OPCs.

The Michigan OPC operation points out the potential impact of third-party payment programs. It makes for exploitation of mental health professionals and paraprofessionals, and for poor quality care. It is not a happy picture of cost effectiveness and is another example of the corruption of the medical profession by insurance. It sharply poses several questions that have been raised for some time:

1. Who shall be considered a mental health professional?
2. Should there be a hierarchy among the mental health professions?
3. What were the practical guidelines that might be offered insurance carriers?
4. Without practical or just guidelines, should there be insurance coverage of outpatient psychotherapy at all?
5. Is hospitalization the alternative to outpatient psychotherapy (hospital practice has the economic attraction—for the physician—of allowing "head in the door" visits)?
6. What is truly the best way of containing costs yet providing best care?[43]

Considering, as data seems to suggest, that the mental health professions themselves are not clearly differentiated in terms of professional functions when it comes to psychotherapy, funding agencies and administrators at all levels would have difficulty deciding which professional should engage in which function.[44]

Psychiatrists say that as physicians, only they are capable of recognizing physical illnesses that mimic mental disorders; a person with a physical illness seen by a psychologist might be in useless therapy while the real illness goes untreated. Moreover, only they, as physicians, can prescribe medication or other somatic therapy that is sometimes needed in the treatment of mental illness. On the other hand, psychologists argue that the overwhelming majority of people with symptoms of mental illness do not have physical diseases and that requiring psychiatric supervision to screen out the few is an unwarranted expense. Furthermore, they contend, the problem can be solved more cheaply and more effectively by having the client get a physical examination from an internist before psychotherapy begins; a client who needs drugs can then be referred to a psychiatrist or family doctor for a prescription and he can return to the psychologist for continued therapy.[45]

The controversy continues. The class system in some measure prevails and with it, the concept of supervision. With that regime prevailing, litigation involving supervisors has been called the "suit of the future." Profiting from an enterprise, the supervisor, like a corporate officer or director, must also bear its perils. That is the underlying principle of vicarious responsibility, "let the superior rely."

For the treatment of many mental disorders, various studies recommend combining psychotherapy and medication (it may be required by the health plan). In carrying out this approach, the treatment is often split between a psychiatrist, who provides the medication, and a non-medical therapist, who provides the psychotherapy. Managed health plans, however, call for that split.[46] It is a variation of the defunct OPC practice in Michigan. As the patient may assume that the therapists are working together in providing treatment, the legal result may be joint and several liability, i.e., each therapist is fully liable for any wrongdoing.[47] To avoid this outcome, patients are advised (often by written contract) of separate responsibility of the therapists. However, when two therapists are involved in the treatment of a mental patient, though acting independently, they may be hard put to argue in the case of the suicide of the patient that they should not be regarded as jointly and severally liable, just as in the case where a patient is seen by, say, an internist and orthopedist. In any event, joint and several liability has given way in many states to several liability, under which each defendant is responsible for only his share of the total damages, usually defined in terms of causal negligence.[48] In medical practice, a consultant simply proves input, a supervisor oversees and directs all aspects of the treatment, and, in a collaborative relationship, all of the clinicians are usually joined as defendants. The plaintiff optimizes the chances of a settlement by citing as many defendants as possible and thereby obtaining a contribution from the various insurers that cover the therapists. The term *nuisance value of a lawsuit* describes the amount insurers pay to settle even though they believe there is no merit to the lawsuit. Practitioners who are involved in shared treatment would do well to have a hold-harmless/indemnification agreement.

All states (except Florida) and the District of Columbia recognize a privilege against disclosure of peer review of performance. There is no peer review privilege in federal law. Thus, peer reviews may be disclosed to plaintiffs in federal discrimination and antitrust cases.[49]

Causation

How is causal relationship established between a psychiatric treatment and patient deterioration? Beyond doubt, it is extremely difficult in a malpractice action to establish causation when a significant segment of the psychiatric community is espousing various treatment modes, albeit solely on an impressionistic basis. This difficulty in establishing causation would particularly characterize the talking therapies where the influence of therapist on patient, whether pernicious or therapeutic, would be virtually impossible to concretize to a court. Many conditions, particularly a psychiatric condition, may have a deteriorating course without treatment, so deterioration in therapy does not of itself establish negligent treatment or causation, but the continuation of a form of treatment over years in the face of deterioration or the absence of improvement may prove to be a case of liability.

As a practical matter, it is often necessary to see a pattern of behavior in order to establish malpractice, or fraud. The testimony of one psychiatric patient is often not credible in the eyes of a jury. The testimony is likely to be considered the product of an unstable or infirm mind. Thus, to establish a case, or to impeach credibility, it is often crucial to show a pattern of behavior, but to do this the complainant would have to obtain the name of other patients.

Consider, for example, the suit by Julie Roy against her psychiatrist, Dr. Renatus Hartogs. She claimed that Dr. Hartogs lured her into sex under the guise of therapy. The doctor, denying it, asserted that she was delusional and further testified that he was impotent during the last 10 years due to a physical condition. The climax of the trial came when other women, reading about the case in the newspapers, came forward and testified that during this period of time they too were patients of the doctor and that he had had sexual intercourse with them.[50] Without the testimony of these other women, the complainant probably would have been laughed out of court. Suppose instead of publicity that produced other witnesses, the plaintiff had requested the names of other women treated by the doctor in order to interview them? Could their names be obtained? Would their evidence be admissible?

At times, only a pattern may reveal incompetence or abuse, or lack of credibility on the part of the defendant. For example, there may be something amiss when a male psychiatrist at a hospital quickly discharges patients of his sex, but holds onto young women for unusually long stays. The tendency to keep a harem would not be revealed by studying the case of a single individual who complains of unnecessary treatment or hospitalization.[51]

Also, only a pattern might establish that a therapist is incompetent to deal with particular classes of people, e.g., women, homosexuals, or suicidal individuals. It may be significant, were it known, that an unusually large number of patients of a particular therapist obtain divorces or commit suicide. It may also be significant that an unusually large number of a therapist's patients are pushed onto other therapists. The custom of a profession is admissible evidence to establish standard of care, but generally speaking, to establish either fault or causation, the law on evidence leaves the admissibility of similar fact evidence involving the defendant to a case by case determination.

The law on evidence of past acts or pattern of conduct of the defendant requires convincing proof that the previous acts occurred; a careful comparison of the prior acts with present circumstances, especially with regard to similarity; a clear showing of relevance to a material issue; a showing of necessity; and a weighing of prejudice against probative value. In particular, the prior acts of the defendant must be of "like character." Assuming that the test is met, the evidence is weighed in the calculus of probative value versus prejudice or confusion of issues,[52] and, more often than not, it is excluded, but, questions of probative value versus other dangers can be resolved only on a case-by-case basis and not by any rigid rule.[53]

A situation of high probative value of similar incidents was presented in *Carter v. Yardley & Co.*,[54] where the plaintiff alleged that her skin was damaged by the defendant manufacturer's cosmetic. One of the defenses was that any skin damage resulted from a source or cause other than the defendant's product. To establish what had caused the skin condition, the court allowed the plaintiff to show that two other users of the defendant's preparation sustained similar skin damage. To obtain similar fact evidence, the complainant usually would need to confer with other patients. In the few cases on discovery of the names of other patients, disclosure appears obtainable to establish fiscal fraud,[55] but not malpractice.[56] However, the testimonial privilege covers the content of a communication, and not the fact of the relationship; indeed, a relationship must be established in order to claim the benefit of a privilege. As it turns out, the testimonial privilege does not provide an adequate guideline as to whether a physician or psychotherapist, without the consent of patients who are not a party to litigation, may be compelled to respond to an inquiry in a legal proceeding that would reveal their identity.[57]

An "off-label" use of drugs or medical products may be the basis for suit against the physician who prescribed it, or it may come up as a defense on the part of the manufacturer. An off-label use is one that is not included in FDA-approved labeling for the products. The recent fen-phen (fenfluramine/phentermine) diet drug litigation is an example of off-label use on an enormous scale. Information that a use is one that is not approved by the FDA or is regarded as experimental may be relevant to a patient's decision regarding treatment options. The FDA has made it clear that while it licenses drugs and devices, it does not purport to regulate the *practice* of medicine. In the agency's view, physicians are free to exercise their medical judgment in prescribing drugs and devices. However, major departure from package insert instructions could be the foundation for a strong malpractice case, especially for failure to obtain informed consent. Patients have a right to be informed not only of the risks associated with off-label prescribing, but also that the drug was not approved for its prescribed use.[58]

In cases alleging improper use of medication resulting in tardive dyskinesia (TD) or other serious side-effects, the patient must offer proof that the side effect occurred more probably than not as the result of the physician's prescription (in law, there must be proximate cause, but there may be more than one proximate cause, any one of which may justify liability). On the difficulty of proof of causation in TD cases, the *Diagnostic and Statistical Manual of Mental Disorders IV* states, "although [movement disorders] are labeled 'medication induced,' it is often difficult to establish the causal relationship between medication exposure and the development of the movement disorder, especially because some of these movement disorders also occur in the absence of medication exposure."[59]

Even before the advent of the neuroleptic medication that causes TD, TD was not unknown. Schizophrenia is a neurologic disease that has a motor component. Without any exposure to neuroleptics, patients may develop spontaneous neurologic disorder associated with schizophrenia, and at a lower rate with other disorders. On the other hand, with exposure to neuroleptics, there is a greater risk of developing TD in the case of mood disorders. In the case of patients with disorders other than schizophrenia, the emergence of a movement disorder is almost always the result of neuroleptics.[60]

In the case of a particular patient with schizophrenia, it is not possible to determine whether the involuntary movement was due to the schizophrenia and not neuroleptic induced. So, in either case, the courts tend to rule that the appearance of an involuntary movement is the result of medication.[61] The courts have grappled with the subject of epidemiology and what it means to establish causation. The burden of proof in civil cases is typically "preponderance of the evidence" (i.e., "more likely than not.") In a case where radiation was alleged to be the cause of cancer, the court provided an analysis of statistical significance in establishing causation:

> In a case where a plaintiff tries to establish a factual connection between a particular cause and a delayed, nonspecific effect, such as cancer or leukemia, the strongest evidence of relationship is likely to be statistical in form. Where the injuries are causally indistinguishable, and where experts cannot determine whether an individual injury arises from culpable human cause or nonculpable natural causes, evidence that there is an increased incidence of the injury in a population following exposure to defendant's risk-creating conduct may justify an inference of "causal linkage" between defendant's conduct and plaintiff's injuries.[62]

Sometimes the proximate cause of the patient's TD can be attributed to the patient (or the family). Thus, summary judgment was granted in favor of a psychiatrist because the patient had failed to inform him of side effects she was experiencing until it was too late for him to effectively treat them. The court noted that, as under traditional law, the plaintiff has a duty to exercise ordinary care for her own protection by keeping her physician informed of problems she might be having with the prescribed treatment.[63]

There are apparently no direct reports of TD occurring as a result of therapy with the tricyclic antidepressant drugs alone. A few instances have been noted of TD that have occurred in patients who were taking tricyclic antidepressants and antipsychotic medication concurrently. In most of these reports, the antipsychotic drugs were the phenothiazines. However, the medications associated with the development of TD are not limited to the neuroleptics. TD can be caused or influenced by other pharmacologic agents, or it may occur spontaneously. Several drugs have been identified that exacerbate TD.

A study by the research department of the Carrier Foundation reported a significant prevalence of TD among elderly residents of nursing homes who have never received neuroleptics. This study strongly suggested that aging either alone or in combination with senile brain disease may produce a syndrome that may be called *spontaneous dyskinesia*, and that neuroleptics cannot be held solely responsible for dyskinesia.[64] What seemed to be TD, by description, was noted already by Kraepelin in the 1890s in elderly (chronic) patients diagnosed with dementia praecox. This was long before the pharmacologic revolution.

Damage

Not every human interest or concern has legal protection. The law differentiates between the various kinds of interests for which individuals may claim protection against injury by others. Until the 1960s and 1970s, the courts ruled that there was no liability in negligence actions causing emotional distress without physical injury or impact. In a famous dissent, Justice Musmanno of the Pennsylvania Supreme Court protested the continued application of the physical injury or impact rule in a case in which the litigant suffered fright and shock on being chased by a straying bull owned by the defendant. As the bull did not strike or touch the complainant, the suit was dismissed, prompting Justice Musmanno to say he would "continue to dissent from [the logic of such cases] until the cows come home."[65]

The courts in various states in recent decades have been holding that psychic impairment is compensable without physical injury or impact as a rule of law, but still today, as a practical matter, judges or juries are skeptical of a claim of emotional distress standing alone. In negligence actions, proof of emotional disturbance or of causal connection is considered highly speculative.

It is a matter of common experience that the *ad damnum* clause or prayer of a pleading usually does not bear any logical relationship to the amount of any recovery. The plaintiff's attorney fixes the demanded damages for a variety of reasons. The demand may be set unreasonably high for the psychological impact upon a defendant. It may be set high to hedge against future inflation, increases of verdicts in like cases, and the desire to avoid amendment of the prayer. It may be calculated when the attorney has little or no understanding of the extent of injuries for which his client lays claim. In any event, the prayer causes the defendant to suffer anxiety out of concern that a verdict will exceed insurance coverage. It prompts a settlement. By way of illustration: a group of people, denied the use of a Vic Tanny Health Club in Michigan because they refused to adhere to the exercise room color code in clothes, sued the place for $7.3 million. Mike Wallace of CBS's *60 Minutes* was sued for defamation for $125 million. The demands make headlines.

In most states punitive damages may be awarded in addition to compensatory damages. The Restatement (Second) of Torts (Section 908) states:

(1) Punitive damages are damages other than compensatory or nominal damages awarded against a person to punish him for his outrageous conduct and to deter him and others like him from similar conduct in the future.

(2) Punitive damages may be awarded for conduct that is outrageous because of the defendant's evil motive or his reckless indifference to the rights of others. In assessing punitive damages, the trier of fact can properly consider the character of the defendant's act, the nature and extent of the harm to the plaintiff that the defendant caused or intended to cause, and the wealth of the defendant.

The key words are "outrageous conduct ... because of defendant's evil motive or his reckless indifference to the rights of others." The purposes are to punish and to deter. The wealth of the defendant may be shown so as to punish. Some five states—Louisiana, Massachusetts, Nebraska, New Hampshire, and Washington—ban or severely limit punitive damages on the rationale that private lawsuits brought by injured people should have only the goal of compensation for a loss, and that punishments should be meted out only by the criminal justice system. In wrongdoing in a nursing home, however, the individuals suffer no economic loss (no loss of wages), and the only remedy or deterrence is a punitive award. In some countries, criminal and civil proceedings are combined—the prosecutor makes out a case and an award is made to the victim.

In a number of states, a liability insurance policy may not cover punitive damages as well as damages arising out of an intentional tort. That would be considered against public policy. Moreover, those judgments are not dischargeable in bankruptcy. As far as the award to the victim, the tax code's exclusion as income applies only to compensatory damage awards, which are those that serve to reimburse the plaintiff for injuries actually incurred. Then, too, a tort judgment against a physician may result in suspension or loss of a license to practice.

Statute of Limitations

The statute of limitations, or prescription, may be suspended as a result of the mental incompetency of the claimant. The "insanity provision" in the statute of limitations allows an insane person to bring a claim usually within one year after the disability is removed. The insanity savings provision applies to medical malpractice cases as well as to other types of cases.

Discussion

It would appear that a psychiatric patient should be told what treatment modalities are available for his particular disorder, how they work, and then be given some approximation of what they may require in time and money. In departing from published standards of care including drug manufacturers' instructions, the doctor should indicate to the patient that he is doing so. In some instances the patient's cognitive capacity may be so impaired that the information will have to be imparted to a legally responsible member of the family. For example, if a therapist opts to treat a major psychosis like acute schizophrenia with psychotherapy alone because of some strong antidrug conviction, he is entitled to do so. At the same time he should inform the family what the current consensus of psychiatric literature has to say about results, undesirable consequences, etc., when various treatment modes are compared. Similarly, if a patient consults a therapist because of acute anxiety related to some stressful life event, he should have the information that will enable him to choose between the intensive long-term psychotherapies and the brief methods, in terms of what he may expect from them and what each will demand of him.

But, properly speaking, let us hasten to ask, can or should accountability of psychiatrists and related professionals be approached in a vacuum? Consider, for example, the state mental health organization. The psychiatrist and other mental health workers are at the bottom of a long chain of authority. What is the responsibility of the legislature, the executive, the judiciary, and the public generally? What type of programs will they support? Economic accountability very much controls the nature or type of treatment. More and more, the fiscal third-party controls "who gets what." The third-party payer looks for ways to pay less and less (and, if possible, not to pay a claim at all). The psychoanalytic or long-term approach is under attack by the AMA with its pill or surgery medicine, and by government and insurance companies because it is cheaper to control symptoms with drugs.

Economic accountability is increasingly determining the length of treatment, the length of hospitalization, and the kinds of treatment. One California insurer concocted a list of various diagnostic categories that are matched with treatment. This "standard of treatments" was formulated by Blue Shield in consultation with psychiatrists selected by them (not by any psychiatric organization). There are rigid details of what constitutes indications for psychotherapy and hospitalization. This latter includes specifications when a patient must be discharged. For depression, it is stated that "chemotherapy and electric shock therapy are the treatments of choice." Psychotherapy might be indicated in some cases, but has to be justified.

Psychiatric treatment veering to the cheapest means symptom control with electroshock or drugs (without psychotherapy), patients dumped on the community, treatment programs that are gestures of doing something rather than meaningful treatment.[66] Rapid bed turnover has resulted in patients being released before they are stabilized.

And many sick patients are not being accepted in a general hospital psychiatric unit for two reasons: they are viewed as malpractice fodder and they create problems for the staff that is inadequate for the needs of such patients. Patients are being refused admission because their insurance standing is clouded, and retrograde denial of claims leaves hospitals without payment if they admit them. There are families torn apart because the patient member refuses treatment and there is nothing the family can do to protect itself.

Conclusion

In a psychiatric malpractice action, with the exclusion of similar fact evidence, establishing fault or causation is problematical. The outcome is often like a lottery. And at the same time, tort law fares poorly as a certification service as it essentially deals with a performance in a particular situation and not with competency to perform a particular function. It is quite chancy whether the competent or the incompetent practitioner is tagged. The board-certified psychiatrist is as often sued and found liable as is the nonboard-certified. The biggest game of chance is not in Las Vegas, but in a courtroom.[67] And so—given the litigious nature of the times, the number of lawyers, and the availability of insurance—lawsuits now are to be considered as an ordinary unavoidable part of the cost of doing business or carrying on a profession. One must guard against it with insurance as best as one can, as one would guard against a flood or tornado.

Endnotes

1. See Federal Rules of Evidence, Rule 1101; State *ex rel.* Lucas v. Board of Education, 277 N.W.2d 524 (Minn. 1979).
2. Hawes v. Chua, 769 A.2d 797 (D.C. App, 2001).
3. S. Lesse, "Editorial: Caveat Emptor? The Cornucopia of Current Psychotherapies," *Am. J. Psychotherapy* 33 (1979): 325; Special Section, "The Psychotherapy Jungle: A Guide for the Perplexed," *Saturday Review*, Feb. 21, 1976, p. 12.
4. See, e.g., J. Kovel, *A Complete Guide to Therapy: From Psychoanalysis to Behavior Modification* (New York: Pantheon, 1976); R.B. Stuart, *Trick or Treatment: How and When Psychotherapy Fails* (Champaign, IL: Research Press, 1970); D. Sobel, "Freud's Fragmented Legacy: A Bewildering Choice of Therapies for the Anxious American," *New York Times Magazine*, Oct. 26, 1980, p. 28.
5. D.A. Adler & K.M. Bungay, "Treating Depression in Primary Care: 'Best of Times and Worst of Times,'" *Medicine & Behavior*, Oct. 1999, p. 24. When, if ever, should a general practitioner refer to a specialist, say, in a case of appendicitis? What is the standard of care? Does the public expect a different one in such cases? To incur liability, it must appear that breach of duty to refer to a specialist, in fact, caused patient's injury, and this can be shown only if treatment the plaintiff received was in some way inferior to the treatment he would have received from a specialist; Larsen v. Uelle, 246 N.W.2d 841 (1976).
6. Symposium, "Diagnosis and the Difference It Makes," *Bull. Menninger Clin.* 40 (1976): 411; P. Williams, "Deciding How to Treat—The Relevance of Psychiatric Diagnosis," *Psycholog. Med.* 9 (1976): 179.
7. In Bogust v. Iverson, 10 Wis.2d 129, 102 N.W.2d 228 (1960), a troubled student sought help from the college guidance counselor (a professor of education with a doctor of philosophy degree). After 5 months of sessions, the interviews were terminated on the suggestion of the counselor. Six weeks later, the student committed suicide, and her parents brought a claim against the guidance counselor and the college. The court stated that, although the individual defendant was a guidance counselor, he could not "be charged with the same degree of care ... as a person trained in medicine or psychiatry." Considering the counselor as a nonexpert, the court found that no facts were alleged that would have apprised him of the student's suicidal tendencies. The court further indicated that even a sufficiently alerted guidance counselor, conceded to have a duty to take some affirmative steps to prevent the

suicide of a student, would not be civilly liable for causing suicide unless the suicide was committed in a way that would suggest negligence on the part of the counselor; 10 Wis. 2d at 137, 102 N.W.2d at 232. In a critical comment, Victor Schwartz (then a law professor) wrote that if a college provides a counselor to assist students with personal problems as it did in *Bogust*, it should make sure that the counselor "has sufficient training to recognize suicidal symptoms. If the college's psychiatric facilities are overburdened, there should at least be a duty to refer students to other sources for psychiatric assistance." V.E. Schwartz, "Civil Liability for Causing Suicide: A Synthesis of Law and Psychiatry," *Vand. L. Rev.* 24 (1971): 254. See Chapter 28.

8. See, e.g., United States v. Klien, 325 F.2d 283 (2d Cir. 1963).

9. C. Bock, *Forgive and Remember: Managing Medical Failure* (Chicago: University of Chicago Press, 1979), p. 5.

10. E.D. Shapiro, "Medical Malpractice: History, Diagnosis and Prognosis," *St. Louis U. L. J.* 22 (1978): 469. See, generally, F. James & D.K. Sigerson, "Particularizing Standards of Conduct in Negligence Trials," *Vand. L. Rev.* 5 (1952): 697; C. Morris, "Custom and Negligence," *Colum. L. Rev.* 42 (1942): 1147. One exceptional case is Helling v. Carey, 83 Wash.2d 514, 519 P.2d 981(1974), where the court rather than the profession in a malpractice action set the standard of care for an ophthalmologist.

11. The standard of conduct is what a reasonably careful person engaged in a particular activity, trade, occupation or profession would do or would refrain from doing under the circumstances then existing. Moreover, medical malpractice must be pled more specifically than other types of negligence. It is not sufficient for a plaintiff to simply describe what a physician did or failed to do and then allege that the action or omission was negligent. The plaintiff must allege the proper or accepted method of diagnosis and treatment; Simonelli v. Cassidy, 336 Mich. 635, 59 N.W.2d 28 (1953). The diversity of practice, however, challenges the concept of standard of care. See S. Brownlee, *Overtreated* (New York: Bloomsbury, 2007); J. Groopman, "A Knife in the Back: Is Surgery the Best Approach to Chronic Back Pain?" *New Yorker*, April 8, 2002; expanded in *How Doctors Think* (New York: Houghton Mifflin, 2007). But, as lawyers are well aware, time-honored buzz words and phrases are used to describe medical due care. "Standard of care" is one of them.

12. Bivins v. Detroit Osteopathic Hosp., 258 N.W.2d 527 (Mich. App. 1977). However, in a case where there is no informed consent, it is often not necessary to have expert testimony for the simple reason that such a case hinges on the fact that had the plaintiff been informed of the risks and hazards he would have not agreed to the treatment. The fact that the treatment was properly or improperly performed is immaterial.

13. Brune v. Belinkoff, 354 Mass. 102, 235 N.E.2d 793 at 798 (1968).

14. 235 N.E.2d at 798.

15. T.J. Hooper, 60 F.2d 737 (2d Cir. 1932). This case involved the question of whether it was negligent for a tugboat not to have a wireless radio on board to get weather reports. The tugboat sank with the plaintiff's cargo during a predicted storm that the tugboat could easily have avoided had the captain listened to weather forecasts. The practice in the tugboat industry was not to carry wireless radios, but the court rejected the "nobody does it" defense. Specifically, with respect to healthcare, the courts have held that "conformity with established medical custom practices by minimally competent physicians ... while evidence of performance of the duty of care, may never be conclusive of such compliance"; Hall v. Hilbun, 466 So.2d 856 (Miss. 1985). See also Darling v. Charleston Community Memorial Hosp., 33 Ill.2d 326, 211 N.E.2d 253 (1965).

16. A choice of therapy is not subject to criticism simply because it was not effective in a particular case. Hindsight is always 20–20. Negligence is based not on whether a particular choice of treatment brings about a cure, or was in fact the "right treatment" with benefit of hindsight, but rather on whether the treatment chosen, based on facts available at the time of treatment, was reasonable. T.F. Campion & J.A. Peck, "Ingredients of a Psychiatric Malpractice Suit," *Psychiat. Q.* 5 (1979): 236. See A.H. Tuma & P. May, "And If That Doesn't Work, What Next ... ? A Study of Treatment Failures in Schizophrenia," *J. Nerv. Ment. Dis.* 167 (1979): 566.

17. H.B. Rothblatt & D.H. Leroy, "Avoiding Psychiatric Malpractice," *Calif. West. L. Rev.* 9 (1973): 260.

18. "In medical school, I was transformed or transformed myself into a straight A student. I had the conscious and continuing thought that, if I failed to learn or comprehend this matter or that, I might kill a patient because of my ignorance. This view was fostered by my teachers. Our professor of pharmacology, for example, began each of his classes with a 10-question written quiz, each requiring knowledge of the current dosage of drugs. There were only two grades, written on our quiz papers in bold red letters—either 100% or MURDER." Quip by Dr. John L. Schimel, "Accountability in Psychiatry," *J. Psychiat. & Law* 8 (1980): 191.

19. P.S. Cassidy, "The Liability of Psychiatrists for Malpractice," *U. Pitt. L. Rev.* 36 (1974): 108.

20. B.R. Furrow, "Defective Mental Treatment: A Proposal for the Application of Strict Liability to Psychiatric Services," *Boston U. L. Rev.* 58 (1978): 408.

21. In Abraham v. Zaslow, 26 Citation 169 (Cal. Super. Ct., Santa Clara Co., 1972), a psychologist was found liable in the use of an experimental "rage reduction therapy," which resulted in physical and mental injuries to the patient. Note, "Psychiatric Negligence," *Drake L. Rev.* 23 (1974): 640. In a practice regarded as highly unusual, the eminent Dr. Harold Searles turned to psychotherapy in the treatment of the severely chronic schizophrenic. H. Searles, *Collected Papers on Schizophrenia and Related Subjects* (New York: International Universities Press, 1965). See also C.R. Rogers, *The Therapeutic Relationship and Its Impact: A Study of Psychotherapy with Schizophrenics* (Madison: University of Wisconsin Press, 1967); J.S. Strauss et al. (Eds.), *The Psychotherapy of Schizophrenia* (New York: Plenum, 1980).

22. Hansen v. Pock, 57 Mont. 51,187 Pac. 282 (1920; herb doctor). In an incident making the news, one spiritualist suggested to a wife that she beat her husband, and she did, in order to save their floundering marriage. *Detroit Free Press*, Jan. 18, 1980, p. 3. One may find a parallel in what is called witchcraft in other countries. B. van Niekerk, "A Witch's Brew From Natal: Some Thoughts on Provocation," *So. Afr. L. J.* 89 (1972):169. Exploitation of the elderly, we know, is commonplace. Members of Washington's House Select Committee on Aging have heard countless reports about quacks peddling fake medical cures to older citizens, along with tales of their physical and mental abuse. Various states have enacted legislation that provides for mandatory reporting of the neglect as well as exploitation or abuse of elderly persons, and grant anonymity and immunity to those investigating or reporting. See N.J. Mehlman, "Quackery," *Am. J. Law & Med.* 31 (2005): 349. Years ago, Dr. Tichenor's antiseptic was popular. In response to my question, "What is it good for?" the salesman answered, "Last year, a million dollars."

23. Nelson v. Harrington, 72 Wis. 599, 40 N.W. 228 (1888).

24. In this case, the court was asked by the defendant to charge that if, at the time the defendant was called to treat the plaintiff, both parties understood that he would treat him according to the approved practice of clairvoyant physicians, and that he did so treat him, with the ordinary skill and knowledge of the clairvoyant system, plaintiff could not recover. The court refused the charge. Instead of the words, "with the ordinary skill and knowledge of the clairvoyant system," the instruction properly was, "with the ordinary skill and knowledge of physicians in good standing."

25. Longan v. Wellmar, 180 Mo. 322,79 S.W. 655 (1904). See also Ellis v. Newbrough, 6 N.M. 181, 27 Pac. 490 (1891; misrepresentation); see A. Hill, "Damages for Innocent Misrepresentation," *Colum. L. Rev.* 73 (1973): 679; L.H. Rubenstein, "Criminal Aspects of Faith Healing," *N. Eng. J. Med.* 224 (1941): 239.

26. Spread v. Tomlinson, 73 N.H. 46, 59 Atl. 376 (1904).

27. The Christian Science practitioner's usual defense is constitutional religious freedom. However, if the practitioner violates the state medical practice act (making a medical diagnosis or manipulating the limbs and body), that defense cannot prevail. L.H. Rubenstein, "Malpractice Against Christian Science Practitioners," *Med. Trial Techni. Q.*, Spring 1979, p. 372. "I often wonder," says a character in a novel by Michael Crichton, "about what medicine would be like if the predominant religious feeling in this country was Christian Scientist. For most of history, of course, it wouldn't have mattered; medicine was pretty primitive and ineffective. But, supposing Christian Science was strong in the age of penicillin and antibiotics. Suppose there were pressure groups militating against the administration of these drugs. Suppose there were sick people in a society who *knew* perfectly well that they didn't have to die from their illness, that a simple drug existed that would cure them. Wouldn't there be a roaring black market in these drugs? Wouldn't people die from home administration of overdoses, from impure, smuggled drugs? Wouldn't everything be an unholy mess." M. Crichton, *A Case of Need* (New York: Penguin Books, 1968), p. 31.

28. See Wemmett v. Mount, 134 Ore. 305, 292 Pac. 93 (1930); H.H. Strupp & S.W. Hadley, "Specific vs. Nonspecific Factors in Psychotherapy," *Arch. Gen. Psychiat.* 36 (1978): 1125.

29. B.R. Furrow, *Malpractice in Psychotherapy* (Lexington, MA: D.G. Heath, 1980).

30. Dolan v. Galluzzo, 396 N.E.2d 12 (Ill. 1979).

31. See, e.g., Daniels v. Finney, 262 S.W.2d 431 (Tex. Civ. App. 1953). Legislation has been enacted in various states that expert witnesses in malpractice actions must teach or practice in the same medical specialty as the physician who is being sued. The avowed goal of the legislation is to cut down on the testimony of "professional hired guns." In a criticism of the legislation, Dr. Emanuel Tanay said, "The legislation is designed to protect physicians from malpractice litigation, and one can only be dismayed by its results. I am reminded of a case in Cleveland where a severely depressed patient was admitted to

a clinic operated by a nutritional chiropractor. The treatment essentially consisted of starvation. After a few days, the patient committed suicide. It was argued that I could not testify in that case because I was not a nutritional chiropractor, whatever that is. The situation in another case is even more bizarre in my opinion. A dermatologist or a psychiatrist would know that under the facts of the case, a sigmoidoscopic examination was indicated. To exclude the opinion of a gastroenterologist because he is not a colorectal surgeon is unreasonable on the face of it." Dr. Tanay adds, "The subspecialization in medicine is growing exponentially. A group practice of ophthalmology where I have been a patient for years has at least half a dozen subspecialties. If my ophthalmic surgeon failed to diagnose my glaucoma, could I use a general ophthalmologist as an expert witness? I believe that any physician should be able to testify that failure to test for glaucoma when doing any type of eye examination is negligent." Personal communication (Sept. 27, 1999).

32. Quinley v. Cocke, 183 Tenn. 428, 192 S.W.2d 992 (1946). See the discussion in Chapter 2 on obligations and responsibilities of lawyers and experts.
33. "Expert testimony is generally necessary except where the matters in issue fall within the area of common knowledge and lay comprehension." Olfe v. Gordon, 286 N.W.2d 573 (Minn. 1980); see also Orozco v. Henry Ford Hospital, 290 N.W.2d 363 (Mich. 1980); Christy v. Salterman, 288 Minn. 141, 149 N.W.2d 288 (1970).
34. Comment, "The Application of *Res Ipsa Loquitur* in Medical Malpractice Cases," *Nw. U. L. Rev.,* 49 (1966): 852.
35. 7 N.Y.2d 376, 165 N.E.2d 756, 198 N.Y.S.2d 65 (1960).
36. 198 N.Y.S.2d at 67. However, another New York court ruled against the patient even though allegations of beatings by the therapist were essentially not contradicted. The court states that the lower court improperly substituted its judgment for that of the physicians and that there was no medical evidence showing improper procedure; Morgan v. State, 337 N.Y.S.2d 536 (App. Div., 1972).
37. See comment, "Substantive Admissibility of Learned Treatises and the Medical Malpractice Plaintiff," *Nw. U. L. Rev.* 71 (1976): 678.
38. W.S. Bell, "Medico-Legal Implications of Recent Legislation Concerning Allied Health Practitioners," *Loyola L. A. L. Rev.* 11 (1978): 379.
39. See E.G. Poser, "The Effect of Therapists' Training on Group Therapeutic Outcome," J. *Consult. Psych.* 30 (1966): 283; H.H. Strupp & S.W. Hadley, "Specific vs. Nonspecific Factors in Psychotherapy," *Arch. Gen. Psychiat.* 36 (1979): 1125; P.G. Bourne (ltr.), *Am. J. Psychiat.* 135 (1978): 1113. "Mothers Good Candidates as Counselors," *Clinical Psychiatry News,* Oct. 1979, p. 32.
40. "Psychology: Clinicians Seek Professional Autonomy," *Science* 181 (1973): 117.
41. S.E. Greben, E.R. Markson, & J. Sadovy, "Resident and Supervisor: An Examination of Their Relationship," *Can. Psychiat. Assn. J.* 18 (1973): 473.
42. R. Slovenko, "Legal Issues in Psychotherapy Supervision," in A.R. Hess (Ed.), *Psychotherapy Supervision: Theory, Research and Practice* (New York: John Wiley & Sons, 1980), p. 453.
43. P. Chodoff, "Psychiatry and the Fiscal Third Party," *Am. J. Psychiat.* 135 (1978): 1185.
44. W.C. House, S.I. Miller, & R.H. Schlachter, "Role Definitions Among Mental Health Professionals," *Comprehen. Psychiat.* 19 (1978): 469.
45. J.P. Brady & H.K.H. Brodie (Eds.), *Controversy in Psychiatry* (Philadelphia: Saunders, 1978); J.R. Neill & A.M. Ludwig, "Psychiatry and Psychotherapy: Past and Future," *Am. J. Psychother.* 34 (1980): 39.
46. In a retrospective study, one HMO found it actually spent less money when it did not split the treatment. W. Goldman et al., "Outpatient Utilization Patterns of Integrated and Split Psychotherapy and Pharmacotherapy for Depression," *Psychiat. Serv.* 49 (1998): 477. See also A.N. Sabo & L. Havens (Eds.), *The Real World Guide to Psychotherapy Practice* (Cambridge, MA: Harvard University Press, 2000).
47. P.S. Appelbaum, "General Guidelines for Psychiatrists Who Prescribe Medication for Patients Treated by Nonmedical Therapists," *Hosp. & Comm. Psych.* 42 (1991): 276; J. Melonas, "Split Treatment: Does Managed Care Change the Risk to Psychiatrists?" *Psych. Prac. & Managed Care* 5 (May–June 1999): 5; D.J. Meyer & R.I. Simon, "Split Treatment: Clarity Between Psychiatrists and Psychotherapists," *Contemp. Psychiat.* 29 (1999): 327; L.K. Sederer, J. Ellison, & S. Keyes, "Guidelines for Prescribing Psychiatrists in Consultative Collaborative and Supervisory Relationships," *Psych. Serv.* 49 (1998): 1197; "Split Treatment: A New Set of Malpractice Risks," *Psychiatric News,* August 24, 2000, p. 9; W.A. Imperio, "Bridging the Professional Divide in Split Therapy," *Clinical Psychiatry News,* August 2000, p. 25.
48. See e.g., Kan. Stat. Ann. 60257a(d), as interpreted and defended in Brown v. Keill, 580 P.2d 867 (Kan. 1978).

49. See Adkins v. Christie, No. 06-13107 (11th Cir. 2007); Viramani v. Novant Health Inc., 259 F.3d 284 (4th Cir. 2001); Memorial Hosp. v. Shadur, 664 F.2d 1058 (7th Cir. 1981).

50. Roy v. Hartogs, 381 N.Y.S.2d 587 (Sup. Ct. N.Y. 1976); see L. Freeman & J. Roy, *Betrayal* (New York: Stein & Day, 1976), W.C. Gentry, "Psychiatric Liability: Abuse of the Therapist–Patient Relationship," *Trial*, May 1980, p. 26; L. Siskin, "Sexual Relations Between Psychotherapists and Their Patients: Toward Research or Restraint," *Calif. L. Rev.* 67 (1979): 1000.

51. H.M. Silverberg, "Protecting the Human Rights of Mental Patients," *Barrister*, Fall 1974, p. 46.

52. Federal Rules of Evidence, Rule 403.

53. G.C. Lilly, *An Introduction to the Law of Evidence* (St. Paul, MN: West, 1978), p. 146; D. Worm, "Similar Facts Evidence: Balancing Probative Value Against the Probable Dangers of Mission," *U. Calif. Davis L. Rev.* 9 (1976): 395.

54. 319 Mass. 92, 64 N.E.2d 693 (1946); see Annot., 42 A.L.R.3d 780 (1972).

55. But see Hawaii Psychiatric Society v. Arilyshi, 481 F. Supp. 1028 (D. Hawaii 1979).

56. Division of Med. Quality v. Gherardini, 156 Cal. Rptr. 55 (Cal. App. 1979).

57. R. Slovenko, *Psychotherapy and Confidentiality* (Springfield, IL: Thomas, 1998).

58. The American Medical Association estimates that 40 to 60% of prescriptions are for unapproved uses. Off-label prescribing is especially common in the field of pediatrics; most drugs are tested and approved based upon research conducted in adults, not children. And off-label prescribing has become commonplace in mainstream medicine. Off-label use has proven effective in treating cancer patients, and off-label, antiretroviral combination therapists have prolonged the lives of AIDS patients. One of the drugs most often prescribed for schizophrenia—valproate—has never been approved by the FDA for that purpose.

    "Off-label" use does not mean that the medication is experimental. It means that no studies have been submitted to the FDA for approval of the medication for that particular use. The FDA requires that each medication target a specific diagnosis in order to receive approval. As seeking approval from the FDA is an expensive and time-consuming procedure, pharmaceutical companies do not submit studies for approval for more that one or two diagnoses. As a result, clinical practice does not correspond to what the *PDR* publishes. Off-label use in psychiatry is more the rule than the exception. Psychiatric diagnoses do not fit into the narrow categories of the *DSM*. Individuals do not suffer in the same way from both a biochemical and psychological standpoint. See C. Sherman, "Off-Label Anticonvulsants Useful in Schizophrenia," *Clin. Psychiatry News*, Aug. 2000, p. 17. On liability, see P.D. Rheingold & D.B. Rheingold, "Offense or Defense? Managing the Off-Label Use Claim," *Trial*, March 2001, p. 52; see also S.R. Salbu, "Off-Lable Use, Prescription, and Marketing of FDA-Approved Drugs: An Assesssment of Legislative and Regulatory Policy," *Fla. L. Rev.* 51(1999): 181.

59. (Washington, DC: American Psychiatric Association, 1994), pp. 678–679.

60. With the appearance of the atypical medications, the neuroleptics have fallen markedly in use. The development of the atypicals was prompted by the occurrence of TD in the use of the neuroleptics. The reduced risk of TD that accompanies the use of the atypicals is seen by many practitioners as the standard of care for schizophrenia, although the issue has apparently not yet been tested in the courts. Would a "respectable minority" of the profession justify the use of neuroleptics in view of the new medication? There may be no reason to turn to new medication when old medication has proved therapeutic without serious side effects and is less expensive. Then, too, the new medication is not without its side effects. The federally funded Clinical Antipsychotic Trials in Intervention Effectiveness trial found that older and less expensive schizophrenia medications were just as good as newer, more expensive (and many believe far more tolerable) atypical antipsychotic drugs. This finding has made little impact on medical practice because few physicians believe the study is credible. See S. Gottlieb, "The War on (Expensive) Drugs," *Wall Street Journal*, Aug. 30, 2007, p. 11; see also ltrs., "Best Drug, or Best Money Maker?" *New York Times*, May 13, 2007, p. WKII.

61. Accardo v. Cenac, 722 So.2d 302 (La. App. 1998).

62. Allen v. United States, 588 F. Supp. 247 (D. Utah 1984), *reversed on unrelated grounds*, 816 F.2d 1417 (10th Cir. 1987), *cert. denied*, U.S. 1004 (1988).

63. Tisdale v. Johnson, 177 Ga. App. 487, 339 S.E.2d 764 (1989).

64. D.E. Casey, "Managing Tardive Dyskinesia," *J. Clin. Psychiat.* 39 (1978): 748; see also R. Slovenko, "Update on Legal Issues Associated with Tardive Dyskinesia," *J. Clin. Psychiat.* 61 (2000): 45 (supp. 4).

65. Bosley v. Andrews, 393 Pa. 161, 142 A.2d 263 (1958). In Christy v. Continental Insurance Co., 274 N.W.2d 679 (Wis. 1979), the Wisconsin Supreme Court ruled that a claim of negligence for mental injuries without accompanying physical injury is barred by public policy. On another occasion, the

Wisconsin Supreme Court (quoting 64 A.L.R.2d 113) said: "The contention that because of the nature of evidentiary problems involved, the judicial process is not well adapted to distinguishing valid from fraudulent claims in this area, has been recognized as probably the most substantial of the reasons advanced for denying recovery for mental distress or its physical consequences." Bogust v. Iverson, 10 Wis.2d 129, 102 N.W.2d 228 (1960). See R. Slovenko, "Causation in Law and Psychiatry" in I. Freckelton & D. Mendelson (Eds.), *Causation in Law and Medicine* (Burlington, VT: Ashgate, 2002), pp. 357–378.

66. Dr. Jonas Robitscher in his Isaac Ray Award Lectures said, "The doctor who has a choice of therapies, but picks electroshock because the patient's Blue Cross coverage allows for only 21 days of in-hospital care, and electroshock can easily be accomplished in that period, will never be criticized for his therapy choice." But in a non sequitur, Robitscher blamed psychiatry for not being good psychiatry, and for abusing its power. J. Robitscher, *The Powers of Psychiatry* (Boston: Houghton Mifflin, 1980), p. 409.

67. E. Osborne, "Courts as Casinos? An Empirical Investigation of Randomness and Efficiency in Civil Litigation," *J. Legal Studies* 28 (1999), p. 187.

28

An Overview of Psychiatric Malpractice

Psychotherapists and nonpsychotherapists alike have expressed concern about the quality of services rendered in the name of treatment. Therapists know about inept or abusive treatment of patients either from other therapists or from their own patients who were treated by a previous therapist. But, in either case, little or no remedial action is taken. One of a number of law review articles (one of which carries the title, "The Song Is Ended But the Malady Lingers On") concludes that the solution, if there is one, lies with the judicial system.[1] With regulatory legislation (licensing or certification) said to protect the interests of a professional group rather than those of the public, the tort suit is increasingly looked to as a type of decertification of competency. Settlements as well as judgments are (supposedly) reported to the National Data Bank.

To be sure, there is another dimension to litigation. In these litigious times nearly every human or social ill, real or imagined, finds its way to the courthouse. Just about every human problem is now turned into a legal one. And then, too, there is the big payoff. The public pays for the courts, the attorneys (should they be willing) subsidize the costs of litigation, and the loser does not pay the other's costs; so, from the viewpoint of the litigant, why not take a chance at a winning? Approximately one of nine malpractice suits is a judgment rendered against the physician, so the chances are somewhat better than the lottery or the stock market. When asked why he robbed only banks, Willie Sutton replied, "Because that's where the money is." Now, instead of robbing banks, one sues, for that's where the money is.

The word *lawsuit* scares physicians almost as much as their bill scares patients. Being sued evokes unnerving images of grim courtrooms, austere judges, rigid formality, esoteric talk, aggressive lawyers, a hostile complainant, biased witnesses, unknowledgeable jurors, and—win or lose—stigma and loss of time and money. In defending against a claim, it is necessary to devote considerable time to interviews with investigators, meetings with attorneys, depositions before trial, and attendance in court, and notwithstanding all this, judgment may be unfavorable and could exceed insurance coverage.

The ideal behind medical and psychiatric service, like that of other services, is often realized. The individual comes on his own (except in civil commitment), follows a prescribed regimen, and obtains results that he feels justify the trust and the fee. But there are points of tension. The individual may not know of his need for service, or knowing of his need, he may not want service, or obtaining it, he may find his situation worsened.

In the usual case, medical or psychiatric tort liability is premised on negligence. There are few instances of intentional wrongdoing. Negligence is conduct that falls below the standard of care established by law for the protection of others against unreasonable risk of harm. Compliance with custom, or what is commonly done, is strong evidence of reasonable conduct, but is not conclusive. The standard of care is a hypothetical, objective standard by which the law may necessitate more care, or the use of new procedures or devices that are not commonly used. The narrow and restrictive test using the community in which the defendant practices, or a similar locality, as the measure of the applicable standard of care has been replaced by a national standard for the specialty. The standard is not found in a Gallup poll or in a fashion page, but from logic and experience. In the last analysis, as Judge Learned Hand said, it is for the court to determine the standard.[2]

Definition of Professional Negligence

Professional negligence in general is the adjudged failure of a professional person, evidenced in the results of his activity, to possess the average skill or knowledge of other professionals in like circumstances, or, if he does possess average skill and knowledge, his failure to use it. It is a departure from "good, accepted, proper practice." If negligence is proved, there is an obligation to compensate for the damage caused.

The physician's legal responsibility could accurately be termed professional tort liability, but the terms "medical malpractice" or simply "malpractice" are embedded in both legal and medical literature and habit of thought. When a person speaks of a malpractice action, it is presumed that it is about a lawsuit against a physician rather than about the negligence of a member of any other professional group. Malpractice is even defined in some dictionaries solely as "improper treatment or culpable negligence of a patient by a physician."[3]

The word *malpractice* is misleading because from *mal* comes the tendency to think of other words like malicious, malevolent, or malfeasance. It makes the physician sound like a villain. Actually, malpractice has to do with negligence, not deliberate or planned wrongdoing. Less significantly, from the practice portion of the word, there may be the tendency to think that one is learning; in common parlance, physicians (and lawyers) have a practice whereas other people work. The term *professional liability* would be preferable to malpractice.

Rate of Malpractice Suits

The rapid increase in the number of medical malpractice suits, to use the prevailing language, following World War II has corresponded with the changing patterns of medical practice and physician status. Criticism is widespread that American medicine is swiftly degenerating into a hurried and depersonalized form of production-line service. A department store is said to take better care of its merchandise than a hospital does of its patients. As Dr. Donald Berwick, chief executive of Institute for Healthcare Improvement, say, "In almost no other field would consumers tolerate the frequency of error that is common in medicine."[4] Medical mistakes kill anywhere from 44,000 to 98,000 hospitalized patients in the United States a year, says a report from the Institute of Medicine, which called the errors stunning and demanded major changes in the nation's healthcare system to protect patients.[5] At the same time, medical costs are sky-high, and the popular symbol of medicine has become the dollar sign, equating medicine with business. A number of patients try to get out of their financial burden by filing bankruptcy or by suing for malpractice.

The scene has markedly changed since the time when Robert Louis Stevenson wrote his eulogy of the doctor, which said: "There are men and classes of men that stand above the common herd; the soldier, the sailor, and the shepherd not infrequently; … the physician almost as a rule. He is the flower (such as it is) of our civilization." The patient no longer believes, as he did at that time, that the physician can do no wrong. As a consequence, while once a relative rarity, malpractice suits are now common throughout the United States. According to the American Medical Association, one fourth of all United States physicians will be sued for malpractice before the end of their careers.

Factors that stimulate claims, with or without regard to the issue of negligence, are severity of injury and indirect influences of an economic, psychological, or sociological nature, which include the following:

Interpersonal problems between provider and patient leading to a breakdown in rapport during the course of therapy.

Frustration with the manner in which specific complaints about ongoing or proposed modes of treatment, including complications, are handled or not handled.

Unrealistic expectations by patients regarding the outcomes of medical treatment, based
in part on misinformation and in part on problems of communication between patient
and physician (including problems related to obtaining consent for surgery).

A growing national trend toward suit consciousness, healthcare consumerism, and other
sociological stimuli to litigation.

Those most likely to be sued are anesthesiologists, orthopedists, surgeons, and obstetricians. The
bond between them and their patients tends to be thin, and their errors tend to be self-evident.

At the other end of the spectrum has been the psychiatrist, the talking doctor, who stands in
contrast to the surgeon, the cutting doctor. For a long time, almost anything seemed acceptable
in talking. In *The Making of a Psychiatrist*, Dr. David Viscott said that it was a standing joke in
medical school that it did not matter whether a psychiatrist was a quack because psychiatrists
did so little it was unlikely that they could do any harm. It was not, he said, until you were out
practicing psychiatry for a while that you really knew how bad psychiatrists could get.[6] In a
review of the book, Thomas Lask of the *New York Times* quipped that he would not go so far as
to say that one has to be out of his mind to go to a psychiatrist for help, but it evidently makes
it easier.[7]

In the past, most litigation involving psychiatrists resulted from physical and not psychic
damage to the patient. Nowadays, and to some extent in the past, litigation involving psychiatrists allege physical or psychic damage resulting from faulty diagnosis, improper certification
in commitment proceedings, failure to exercise adequate suicidal precaution, breach of confidentiality, "revival of memory" of abuse, failure to report a patient who poses a danger, improper
administration of medication or of electroshock treatment, and sexual relations with patients.
Claims reported by the Psychiatrists Purchasing Group (2005) are as follows: Incorrect treatment
(33%), attempted or completed suicide (20%), incorrect diagnosis (11%), improper supervision
(7%), improper commitment (5%), breach of confidentiality (4%), unnecessary hospitalization
(4%), and undue familiarity (3%).

Unless injury to the patient is physical or there has been obvious misconduct, as in the cases
later discussed, the patient is in a difficult position to associate the harm with the therapy and,
even if the patient does establish causality, to establish negligence. And a cause of action based
on breach of contract would also be difficult to sustain because the psychiatrist, when treatment
commences, makes a point of promising nothing. An extralegal consideration of undoubted
importance dissuading a lawsuit is the reluctance to reveal one's personal life in a courtroom.
Moreover, researchers who seek to study psychiatric malpractice may be denied access to the
necessary data. To illustrate, investigators seeking to identify the factors associated with suicides
at a mental institution are likely to find that necessary records are labeled confidential or have
been lost and that relevant personnel are unavailable.

Until the 1980s, the number of lawsuits against psychiatrists was miniscule compared with
suits against other physicians (psychiatrists compose about 6% of all physicians). A nationwide
study by the National Association of Insurance Commissioners found that of 71,778 malpractice
claims filed against all physicians between 1974 and 1978, only 217 (0.3%) were against psychiatrists, but in 1985 an insurance underwriter reported that "the number of lawsuits filed against
mental health practitioners has skyrocketed in recent years."[8] From 1985 through 1998, more
than $13.3 million was paid out in psychotherapy-related claims against psychiatrists, accord-
ing to a report from the Physician Insurers Association of America, which analyzed data from
20 large malpractice insurers nationwide. Overall, psychiatry ranked 20th in number of claims
reported and 23rd in the amount of money paid out for claims among the 28 specialties surveyed. As a consequence, psychiatrists pay much less than other medical specialties for malpractice coverage.

Studies show that psychiatrists who have high-volume practices (more than 25 patients in a day) or who practice at a number of locations are at an increased risk of being sued. Specialization (such as geriatrics) has developed in the field of psychiatry and that increases the risk of a malpractice suit particularly when the psychiatrist practices outside his specialty.

Another explanation for the relative increase in malpractice complaints is that restrictions have made it more difficult to hospitalize patients, and those who are hospitalized tend to be discharged more rapidly, so psychiatrists are dealing with sicker people on an outpatient basis. Another explanation for the increase in malpractice complaints is that many insurance plans or managed care engage psychiatrists only for medication management and then contract with nonphysicians for psychotherapy. Dr. Paul Appelbaum said, "To the extent that you're seeing people for medication, your risk is increased both because you don't know these patients as well and are not as able to make good judgments about them, and also because there is less coordination of care when there are two caregivers."[9]

Recent years have seen growing attention in the legal and psychiatric literature to the nature of psychotherapy, and to "mal-psychotherapy." The number of books and journal articles on the subject is now considerable. The thought at one time that talk therapy could do no harm has been abandoned. The very concept of therapy would suggest that the therapist exerts some kind of influence or impact, benign or malignant, on the patient. In this connection, Dr. Abraham Kardiner wrote in *My Analysis with Freud*, "Freud was always infuriated whenever I would say to him that you could not do harm with psychoanalysis. He said, 'When you say that, you also say that it cannot do any good. Because if you cannot do any harm, how can you do good?'"[10] Others say the chief danger is wasting the patient's time and money, diverting him from effective treatment, and that may be malpractice. Philip Rieff in his 1966 book *The Triumph of the Therapeutic* claimed that the real danger to humanity in our time is not socialism, but therapy.

A fundamental purpose of professional tort liability is to provide a remedy for a wrong, and also to provide something of a certification service for the public. There is a popular saying: "For a wrong, there ought to be a remedy," but is everything permissible in the name of psychotherapy? A therapist when in New York had a spare room, and his father (a retired railroad engineer) said to him, "I can do what you are doing, let me use that room, let me have the patients for whom you don't have the time." The therapist son would have none of that, but on moving to California, and seeing what passed there for therapy, he mused that his father would not have, by any stretch of the imagination, engaged in such shenanigans.

Yet what is the standard of care in psychotherapy? Therapists differ on what is important, and what is of no moment. For example, how often should a patient be seen? For how long? Should the patient lie on a couch? Should the patient be seen individually or in a group? Should medication be used? Should therapy be "split" between a therapist who provides medication and another who provides psychotherapy? Should a patient who is suicidal be asked to promise that he will call for help rather than act out suicidal thoughts or impulses? Should inquiry about trauma be made before transference has developed? Should an interpretation be made without corroboration by external information? Should a patient keep a diary during the course of therapy? What is a boundary violation? Should there be any physical touching of a patient? What if anything should the therapist reveal to the patient about himself? Is it necessary for the therapist to know about the cultural background of the patient? Should the therapist consult with the patient's family? What should be said about confidentiality? Should a therapist testify on behalf of a patient? How should a therapist react to a changing marketplace? Is recordkeeping essential for psychotherapy? To what extent, if any, does the therapist interfere or help in the patient's daily life? Is therapy case-specific and very little can be said about a standard of care?

An extraordinary and unprecedented number of psychotherapeutic techniques have emerged in recent decades. Actually, it is not surprising. The human organism can get out of balance in innumerable ways, and there are innumerable ways to regain one's equilibrium. But questions arise. Is the treatment of choice largely a matter of fashion? Which techniques help? Which present dangers? For depression, one might ask, should it be psychotherapy, electroshock, pills, plastic surgery, comedy films, jogging, chasing girls, or a job? Dr. Stephen Appelbaum, when with the Menninger Foundation, crisscrossed the United States to take a firsthand look at various therapies, including primal scream, est, Silva Mind-Control, Rolfing, transcendental meditation, biofeedback, bioenergetics, macrobiotic dieting, and Alexander technique—about 20 new forms of treatment. He found much that was constructive, but he also saw much that dismayed him. He observed, "An unfortunate fact of our time is that poorly trained and untalented people do all kinds of things purporting to be therapeutic, and do so under the imprimatur of glittering titles and institutional affiliations."[11]

The history of psychiatry may be divided into roughly three periods: the asylum period of the years 1770 to 1870, in which biological concepts were dominant; the psychotherapy period of the years 1870 to about 1970, in which Freud's doctrine of psychoanalysis came increasingly to the fore; and the second biological period, from the 1970s to the present, in which biology has prevailed, with psychotherapy being practiced by psychologists rather than psychiatrists. Edward Shorter, professor of the history of medicine at the University of Toronto, writes, "The past 40 years have seen the virtual death of one of the great intellectual paradigms that guided psychiatry—psychoanalysis—and its replacement by a starkly different kind of paradigm, one emphasizing brain biology in the understanding of illness and psychopharmacology as the leading edge of treatment."[12]

The development of guidelines that has occurred is part of a movement toward "evidence-based" practice, but there are many different models of it. One is to base practice upon evidence of change. Another is the "empirically supported treatments" movement, which focuses on the degree of evidence for specific treatments for specific disorders. These models adopt a medical model perspective on psychological dysfunction and its remediation, and are focused on symptom removal.[13] On the other hand, many approaches to psychotherapy do not hold that effectiveness in psychotherapy is homologous to effectiveness of a drug. For one thing, a therapy could be said to be efficacious if it provides a certain kind of opportunity or experience to make a variety of personal changes, none of which is connected in a linear or mechanistic way with what the therapist does. The effectiveness of the therapy is in terms of how it allows individuals to explore their lives and find more meaningful ways of engaging in their existence.[14] As Dr. Sidney Blatte of Yale University says, "Research clearly indicates that the personality of the patient and the ability of the therapist to establish a therapeutic alliance are what determine treatment outcomes. So, much of the effort to identity evidence-based treatments is misguided because it focuses on the techniques rather than relationship."[15] That is particularly true in the case of psychotherapy.

Focus in Tort Cases

Faulty performance or no, in tort law, in considerable measure, the tail (damages) often wags the dog (the other rules). The extent of injury—or insurance coverage—may compromise the element of fault. Given insurance coverage, some theory more or less is developed to provide an avenue of recovery. As a practical matter, there is a link, more or less, between tort claims and insurance coverage. Thus, the availability of insurance coverage for pastoral counseling encouraged suits against pastoral counselors.

Even a single suit, given publicity, triggers litigation in the area. It is what is known as a vicious circle: a lawsuit occurs, it is given publicity, insurance companies advertise the risk (to promote insurance), the insurable become targets of litigation, more litigation ensues, premiums mount, more litigation, and more of the same. In short, one event builds on the other.[16]

On top of that, there is the increasing public demand for accountability—an aspect of the movement called consumerism. The phenomenon is growing in the field of medicine, including psychiatry.[17] The development of third-party payment, the pressure of insurance reimbursement for psychotherapy, and federal and state supervision of mental health programs have sharpened the issue. Pushed by the scrutiny that must come with public funding, those in the mental health field are being asked to demonstrate (through extensive forms) what it is that is being treated, what kind of treatment is being offered, what the outcome of the treatment is, and who is doing the treatment.[18] Recent legislation mandates specific physician disclosure standards prior to treatment, pretreatment peer review and review, and recordkeeping systems.[19] Legislation or judicial decisions also regulate the administration of "intrusive therapies."[20]

Recent legislation also seeks to make every physician something of a supervisor over other physicians, though they are not in his employ (the development is on the horizon for other professions as well). A number of states have enacted mandatory reporting statutes requiring a physician to report a colleague's professional misconduct, subject to being charged with misconduct for having failed to report witnessed acts.[21] Several states make it unlawful to withhold information from licensing boards about doctors with debilitating problems and make those who knew or should have known liable for the actions of their colleagues. These reporting statutes provide immunity from suit for the complaining doctor—the fear of a defamation suit has been a concern—but it is doubtful whether these statutes, like peer review, have proven to be of much consequence. Surveys indicate that while 38 percent of physicians could identify colleagues who were experiencing debilitation problems, very few say they would discuss this with the individual involved or report the problem to the appropriate authority. And so there is increasing reliance on the malpractice action to weed out incompetency (though the competent physician is apparently sued no less frequently than the incompetent).

Most insurance carriers have placed psychiatrists in the same "risk rating category" as general practitioners, even though the loss ratio of psychiatrists is not as high. The exclusions in a professional liability policy usually provide that the policy does not apply to such risks as injury arising out of the performance of a criminal act, sexual relations with a patient, injury caused by a person while under the influence of intoxicants or narcotics, liability assumed by the insured under an agreement guaranteeing the result of any treatment, electroshock therapy (unless specifically included in the policy at an additional premium), and liability of the insured as the proprietor or executive officer of a hospital or sanitarium.[22]

A plaintiff is more likely to be successful in litigation when a hospital is a party defendant. As a matter of trial tactics, it is generally not advisable to name a nurse or aide as a party defendant, even if she is the one primarily responsible for the harm, as juries still equate her with Florence Nightingale. A physician still cuts a somewhat appealing figure and juries hesitate to find him liable, but an institution is amorphous. Hence, the hospital is invariably sued alone or with the physician whenever there has been hospitalization. In an earlier day, charitable or governmental immunity protected nonprofit hospitals from liability, but now that the immunity defense has fallen by the wayside, a public or private hospital is liable for its wrongful acts or omissions to act.

Any comment on tort liability must necessarily be tinged with the observation that the law of torts has come to perform a significant function of providing social security. This role was thrust upon it as the result of changes in the social and economic environment, especially the rise of liability insurance. Tort liability originally served as an incentive to procure liability insurance, but now that liability insurance is so very common, it influences the pattern of tort liability. The function of tort law in the larger scheme of social security is open to debate, but beyond the scope of this work.

Vulnerable Psychiatrists

The thrust of malpractice litigation into psychiatry appears to be directed at those practitioners who treat the more seriously mentally ill within an institutional setting. The institutional psychiatrist is vulnerable when he uses involuntary commitment procedures to hospitalize a potentially dangerous patient, and he faces a similar hazard when he chooses to discharge that patient. His vulnerability increases when he utilizes electrotherapy or the psychotropic drugs. He is less in danger when he simply sits and listens, only occasionally responding with a supportive or insightful comment. Whenever he acts in a manner that cannot be concretized in relatively simple and understandable cause-and-effect terms, as, for instance, the effect of a drug in producing a noxious, compensable side effect, the psychiatrist need not be overly concerned about malpractice insurance.

The state hospital psychiatrist, often foreign-born and educated, requires the broadest insurance protection because he struggles with an enormous caseload consisting of the most severe psychoses in an understaffed and inadequately financed institution. The psychiatrist in private practice, on the other hand, has chosen to treat, in the comfortable isolation of his office, those patients with less serious mental illnesses, despite the fact that he may be better trained. The economic and therapeutic rewards of private practice far outweigh those offered by a state hospital system. His patients are communicative and manageable, and he rarely has to make the decisions or utilize the therapeutic modalities that later form the basis for a malpractice action.

The private practice psychiatrist encounters litigation for negligent psychotherapy primarily when he assumes a role forbidden to him by society. It is even possible for such a role to have therapeutic consequences, as in the case of Dr. John Rosen, who struck some schizophrenic patients in order to make them more communicative and accessible, a form of therapeutic behavior that will, upon occasion, resolve an acute psychosis.[23] Yet doctors are not supposed to strike patients, and such a corporeal role cannot be accepted by the court or society.

Overall, the fact that relatively few instances in which psychotherapy has been deemed by a court to be negligent is remarkable, considering the number of individuals who have been treated by psychotherapy. As Dr. Abraham Kardiner wrote in *My Analysis of Freud*, if communication can be therapeutic, driving sick people sane, then the negative is also possible. That psychiatrists powerfully influence the lifestyles, values, and attitudes of their patients would seem beyond doubt (e.g., the number of divorces or changes in employment of persons in therapy is disproportionate to the average). That such influence could be contrived to work for the benefit of the psychiatrist and to the detriment of the patient is quite another matter and most difficult to establish in a court of law.

Revival of Memory Cases

Recent years have witnessed the development of the "revival of memory" of childhood sexual abuse, which has been the subject of intense controversy. Patients have come out of therapy convinced that their parents or stepparents had sexually abused them when they were children, and they blame their lifelong difficulties on the abuse. In bringing suit against their parents, they claim delayed discovery that would suspend the statute of limitations because they had "psychologically dissociated and buried their memories of childhood sexual abuse." Approximately half of the states rushed to extend the statute of limitations in the past decade or two.

Many patients later retracted these allegations, but the damage had already been done; families were divided, and parents were defamed and stigmatized. Finding that professional organizations and licensing boards were of little or no assistance, consumers of mental health services organized. Pamela Freyd, an educational psychologist accused, along with her husband, of unspecified abuse of her estranged daughter, led the way in forming the False Memory

Syndrome Foundation (FMSF) in 1992. Hundreds of parents joined. With an advisory board of scientists and scholars, the FMSF gained almost immediate credibility in the media. (Disclosure: The author is a member of the Advisory Board.)

In 1995 in Minnesota, multimillion-dollar jury decisions were returned in false memory cases brought by former patients and their parents against the therapists.[24] For the first time, awards for malpsychotherapy paralleled those for malsurgery. Treatment in the cases involved the diagnosis of multiple personality disorder, otherwise called *dissociative identity disorder*. The therapist used hypnosis, guided imagery, and sodium amytal to help the patients recover memories, some of which involved belief in a satanic ritual abuse cult.[25]

Therapists who uncover dissociative identity disorder have claimed that its genesis is child-hood abuse, so in every case of dissociative identity disorder, they have said, an allegation of child abuse is warranted. In a 1988 article in *Psychiatric Annals*, Daniel Hardy, a psychiatrist who also holds a law degree, wrote, "The psychiatrist or therapist must be alert to the potential danger of a malpractice suit arising from failure to diagnose multiple personality disorder."[26] As it turned out, just the opposite has happened, to wit, diagnosing or uncovering dissociative identity disorder may be regarded as malpractice, which follows the proposition that dissociative identity disorder is treatment-created or sometimes the result of self-hypnosis. Dr. Paul McHugh, director of the Department of Psychiatry and Behavioral Science at Johns Hopkins, wrote, "[Dissociative identity disorder] is an iatrogenic behavior syndrome, promoted by suggestion and maintained by clinical attention." He noted that multiple identities disappear when the therapist does not ask about them, take notes about them, or otherwise take an interest in them.[27] Clinics specializing in the treatment of dissociative identity disorder have closed their doors.

Belatedly, in a position statement issued in March 2000 by the Board of Trustees of the American Psychiatric Association, it was said, in part: "When asked to provide expert opinion involving memories of abuse, psychiatrists should refrain from making public statements about the historical accuracy of individual patients' reports of new memories based on observations made in psychotherapy."[28]

As a result of the backlash against therapies that try to elicit suppressed recollections, insurers excluded "revival of memory" from coverage. For lawyers, the "dinner bell" sounded. With the news of the large judgments, law firms began holding conferences exploring the potential of suing psychotherapists. Apart from "undue familiarity" with patients, nothing has done more to discredit psychotherapy than revival of memory of childhood sexual abuse. In the conclusion of a study of revival of memory cases, psychologist Terence Campbell wrote, "The incompetence of legions of psychotherapists amounts to a public health hazard, and decisive action is warranted as a result."[29] The tide has turned against revival of memory therapy (but many families remain angry about it).[30] The revival of memory phenomenon in the mid-1980s peaked in the early 1990s and declined rather sharply by the late 1990s.[31]

Psychotherapy Versus Chemotherapy

As we point out in the discussion on torts, the determination whether in a specific case a defendant will be held liable is a matter of policy and involves the consideration of a number of factors, including the foreseeability of harm to the plaintiff, the degree of certainty that the plaintiff suffered injury, the closeness of the connection between the defendant's conduct and the injury suffered, the moral blame attached to the defendant's conduct, and the policy of compensating injured persons and preventing future harm. Causation is very much a matter of practical politics and, for that reason, the issue does not lend itself to a ready and easy solution.

Psychotherapy is no longer the dominant form of treatment in psychiatry today. The influence of psychoanalysis has diminished as advances have been made in biological psychiatry. But more than in any other specialty of medicine, psychiatrists devotedly and cultistically follow certain leaders, conceptual systems, and therapeutic rituals. One criterion that a court may apply in determining whether a professional person is negligent is the obligation "to keep abreast of progress in the profession."

If psychiatry purports to deal with human conflict, it is, indeed, a specialty, which is itself torn by internecine conflict. Generally speaking, psychiatrists can be categorized into two groups: directive-organic and analytic-psychological. The directive-organic group is medically oriented, utilizing such physical therapies as electroshock and drugs, and approaching their patients with firm suggestion and environmental manipulation. The analytic-psychological group prefers to do only psychotherapy, seeing patients several times weekly. It expresses an abhorrence for the physical therapies. It views drugs as a chemical straitjacket and electroshock as the ultimate form of barbarism.[32]

The courts tend not to pass judgment on the appropriate therapy or the efficacy of different forms of treatment. This reflects Judge Benjamin Cardozo's observation that the law treats medicine with diffidence and respect. Thus, the courts refuse to consider which "of two equally reputable methods of psychiatric treatment" (psychoanalysis as against a physiological approach) would prove most efficacious in a particular case.[33] In *Youngberg v. Romeo*,[34] which involved the training or "habilitation" of a mentally retarded individual at a state institution, the U.S. Supreme Court noted, "It is not appropriate for the courts to specify which of several professionally acceptable choices should have been made." It went on to say, "[L]iability may be imposed only when the decision by the professional is such a substantial departure from accepted professional judgment, practice, or standards as to demonstrate that the person responsible actually did not base the decision on such a judgment."

In 1982, Dr. Rafael Osheroff ignited a controversy when he initiated a lawsuit against Chestnut Lodge, a private psychiatric hospital in suburban Maryland. Although the case was settled without court adjudication, it generated widespread discussion on the growing controversy between psychotherapy and pharmacotherapy and whether the courts would play a role in that controversy.[35] The central issue in the case was whether Chestnut Lodge committed malpractice in relying exclusively on psychotherapy. After the case was settled and even before, when it was pending, Dr. Osheroff waged a public campaign, talking to reporters and peppering professional journals with letters and phone calls about his case. Soon, the entire profession was talking about *Osheroff v. Chestnut Lodge*. He discussed his treatment before a large audience at an annual meeting of the American Psychiatric Association, where it was the subject of a 3-hour panel discussion featuring Osheroff and six psychiatrists, including an official from Chestnut Lodge, and it was debated at an annual meeting of the American Psychiatric Association and in the pages of the *American Journal of Psychiatry* by Dr. Gerald L. Klerman and Dr. Alan A. Stone.[36]

The treatment of Dr. Osheroff during his 7-month stay at Chestnut Lodge was intensive psychotherapy. In accordance with the practice at Chestnut Lodge, he received no medication. He showed no improvement, instead, he showed distinct deterioration. For months he spent nearly every waking moment—sometimes 16 hours—trudging an estimated 18 miles a day up and down the hall of a locked ward in the hospital. The soles of his feet blistered, ulcerated, and turned black. He lost 40 pounds and stopped bathing and shaving. He could not sit still long enough to eat with a knife and fork; instead, he would snatch food off a plastic tray as he paced. He repeatedly asked for medication, but "forget drugs," his hospital psychiatrist told him, they would only obscure his real problem—a narcissistic personality disorder rooted in his relationship with his mother. Prior to his hospitalization at Chestnut Lodge, a psychiatrist gave him medication for depression to no avail.[37]

His family, appalled by his deterioration, moved him from Chestnut Lodge to Silver Hill, a private hospital in Connecticut, where with chemotherapy, he showed substantial improvement and was discharged after a 3-month stay. At Silver Hill, Osheroff made a point of noting, he was addressed as "Dr. Osheroff," not "Ray," as he was called at Chestnut Lodge. In his lawsuit against Chestnut Lodge, Osheroff claimed that the hospital and the two psychiatrists responsible for his treatment committed malpractice by misdiagnosing his biologically based depression and treating it with intensive psychotherapy alone, when effective and widely prescribed medication was available. He also alleged that the Lodge failed to obtain his informed consent about the probable duration and method of treatment. The Lodge contended that Osheroff was actually suffering from a narcissistic personality disorder for which drugs are not the appropriate therapy. The Lodge's treatment, it contended, was endorsed by a respectable minority of psychiatrists and, therefore, it was not malpractice. "Breakdown is breakthrough," it is oft said. One of the few things on which everyone agreed is that when Osheroff signed himself in at the Lodge, he appeared to be suicidally depressed.

Klerman, who was scheduled to be one of the experts on behalf of Osheroff in the litigation, argued that a patient has a right to "effective treatment," and he said, "there was no scientific evidence for the value of psychodynamically oriented intensive individual psychotherapy." In response, Stone said that effective treatment is used as a way to promulgate ideas about using uniform scientific standards of treatment in the psychiatric field and about a consensus regarding efficacious treatment. Klerman postulated that efficacious treatment should be measured solely by the results of controlled clinical trials and because psychopharmacology has more supportive studies than psychotherapy, it is the more effective mode of treatment. Klerman challenged the "respectable minority" doctrine, which holds that if a minority of respected and qualified physicians approve of and practice a standard of care, this would constitute a sufficient defense to a malpractice claim.[38]

The tradition of using psychoanalysis on patients with major mental illnesses rooted itself firmly in the Washington–Baltimore area thanks to Adolf Meyer, an early member of the American Psychoanalytic Association and a large presence in the local Washington–Baltimore society. It was there that two private clinics—Chestnut Lodge in Rockville, Maryland (founded in 1910 by Ernest Luther Ballard) and the Sheppard and Enoch Pratt Hospital in Towson, Maryland (opened in 1891 as the Sheppard Asylum)—became the flagship hospitals for applying psychoanalysis to gravely ill patients. In 1922, Harry Stack Sullivan, perhaps the most famous figure in the psychoanalytic treatment of psychoses, arrived at the Sheppard.

Following the *Osheroff* litigation, Chestnut Lodge and other institutions turned to the use of drugs for nearly all of its patients. One member of the Chestnut Lodge staff commented, "The days of drug-free treatment at the Lodge are a thing of the past, yet pressures toward conformity rob our field of the opportunity to use individual clinical judgment, particularly with refractory cases, such as the Lodge specializes in treating."[39]

For panic disorder, treatment of choice is said to consist of pharmacotherapy, psychotherapy, or both; for posttraumatic stress disorder (PTSD), cognitive behavior therapy; for bulimia nervosa, cognitive behavior therapy; for general anxiety disorder, pharmacotherapy, psychotherapy, or both; for major depression, cognitive behavior therapy or behavioral therapy; for schizophrenia, pharmacotherapy; and for bipolar disorder, pharmacotherapy. Dr. Daniel Casey of the U.S. Veterans Hospital in Portland, Oregon, a prominent researcher in psychopharmacology, had this to say about psychopharmacology as a standard of care:

> The principle forms of treating mental illnesses should be primarily through psychopharmacology. However, if someone's life is a mess and the needed changes do not occur once the psychopharmacological treatments have provided their full benefits, then psychotherapy aimed at improving the functioning lifestyle seems reasonable. However, this does not necessarily require a medical degree or psychoanalytic training. The central issue is whether psychological approaches could be of meaningful value in helping a person

gain greater function in their life after medicines have also been given their best chance at helping the patient.

I would consider it malpractice to fail to offer lithium to a case of bipolar disorder. Some patients will not take medicine during an episode of bipolar illness and then one's options are considerably more limited. However, to fail to offer at any time or to fail to continue to offer on a timely schedule access to lithium (or other effective antibipolar drugs) would not meet the current standards of practice.[40]

"Evidence-based medicine" (EBM, a concept that developed in the late 1990s) is now at the forefront of professional thinking. Terms such as *validation* are being determined by and used by insurance companies and various regulatory agencies to set standards of care and practice. It is no surprise that EBM draws strong support from governments that seek uniform standards to assess performance and cost effectiveness, and it is being urged as standard of care in malpractice suits. Important questions arise as to what the nature of *evidence* is, who is to determine what appropriate evidence is, and by what measures and standards a practice should be judged? EBM, in the opinion of critics, is like a recipe book. It ignores the clinician's experience. Moreover, how does a provider of care manage the many studies that could qualify as producing data for evidence-based care? Then, too, as many as half of the disorders and possible treatments that could be prescribed have not even been studied adequately.

In view of the various approaches in psychiatry to therapy, is it suitable, as Klerman suggested, that courts pass judgment on the appropriate therapy or the efficacy of different forms of treatment? In some instances, the courts or legislatures step in and impose a standard of care. The duty to report a patient who poses a danger and child abuse-reporting statutes are impositions of a duty to warn and protect. The "informed consent" doctrine imposes a duty to advise patients of the risks of treatment.

Yet another notable example of a duty of care imposed by a court is *Helling v. Carey*.[41] In this case, the undisputed expert testimony was that the standard of care of ophthalmology did not require pressure tests for glaucoma in patients under 40 years of age in cases of similar circumstances to that of the plaintiff. The court rejected the professional norms and determined that an ophthalmologist's failure to perform a simple, noninvasive test that would have prevented the patient's blindness was negligence. The decision changed the practice of ophthalmology. Ophthalmologists now routinely give glaucoma tests to patients in young adult age groups. In any event, *Helling* does not translate well to psychiatry. In psychiatry, there are no tests comparable to an eye pressure test.[42]

Electroshock Therapy

In every type of case, the lawyer becomes something of a specialist on the particular matter in issue. He draws books from the library and reads whatever he can about the subject. To be sure, he is a dilettante; however, on the issue in dispute, he stands ready to do battle with the experts. It is with a slow dismay that he realizes that psychiatrists themselves do not know exactly what happens when a person is given electroshock (also known as electroconvulsive therapy, or ECT). All they have are unverified theories and the knowledge that it gets results.[43]

Electroshock is an approved, though not a preferred, method of treatment by all clinicians. In the 1950s, with the development of less risky means of preventing spinal fractures, ECT had become "the treatment of choice," as Dr. Lothar Kalinowsky put it, for manic depressive illness and major depression.[44] It was found to be more effective than other therapies, and it acted swiftly. In the 1950s and 1960s, many psychiatrists devoted a considerable amount of their practice to "buzzing patients." These psychiatrists were held in low regard and were frequently referred to as *shockiatrists*, despite the fact that ECT was an established treatment.[45]

In 1959, the antipsychiatric movement was about to bring ECT to an end, at least for a period of time. Quite a number of specialists as well as many patients contended that it was "barbarous, unscientific, and dangerous and ought to be outlawed."[46] Before the advent of phenothiazine tranquilizing drugs, ECT was used as a punishment for violating institutional rules in mental hospitals and prisons.[47] While the evidence on this is mostly anecdotal, it suggests that the practice was widespread. In Ken Kesey's popular novel *One Flew Over the Cuckoo's Nest*, Big Nurse's first effort to transform the hero, McMurphy, into a good patient was by means of ECT.[48] Those who make out a Psychiatric Advanced Directive (PAD) and are familiar with *One Flew Over the Cuckoo's Nest* tend to exclude ECT as a treatment. In 1950, in an article in the *Journal of the American Psychiatric Association*, Dr. Mervyn Shoor and Dr. Freeman Adams wrote about ECT as a management technique. "Our goals were not curative. … We had in mind the management of chronic disturbed psychotic patients, free of restraint, seclusion, and sedation."[49] They selected patients for ECT on the basis of need for control.

In the 1960s, I often listened to Dr. Karl Menninger, renowned dean of American psychiatry, rail against electroshock. Each year at graduation exercises at the Menninger School of Psychiatry, he condemned its use. Years later, in 1980, I asked him what he then thought of the widely controversial views about ECT. He responded:

I spent many years of my younger professional life fighting electroshock therapy. It came to be very widely used by some and also very disapproved of by others. Patients usually develop an indescribable fear of it. They sometimes improve after it, especially in cases of depression. Some are made worse. I remember a case in which I was called as a consultant after a very fine university professor [a woman] had failed to respond to all the [other] treatments in the books, including hard work and long and expectant idle waiting. They had, however, scrupulously avoided giving her shock therapy. I said I was not an advocate of it, but occasionally it seemed to do a lot of good. They gave her one or two shocks and she recovered pronto! Everybody (well, *some* people) thought I was a wizard, including her.

It probably has definite and considerable value in treating depression, but I do not know if we feel very certain about the criteria for its elective use. I do feel certain that it has been greatly abused, overused, oversold, and over inflicted on the patients and it not infrequently injures memory. Because it is a machine effect and so easily produced and so impressive whether or not successful, on the whole I think it is a dangerous modality for psychiatry.[50]

Over the years, countless patients have voiced complaints about ECT. Some patients have perceived ECT as a terrifying experience (at least initially), some regarded it as an abusive invasion of personal autonomy, some have experienced a sense of shame because of the social stigma they associated with ECT, and some reported extreme distress from persistent memory deficits.[51] Here is one complaint:

Electroshock convulsions resulted in my brain being "taught" to have convulsions. In other words, I am now epileptic. This side effect is not super common, but has been documented since the 1940s.[52]

In the early days of ECT, fractures and mortality were a significant problem. The commonly quoted overall mortality rate in the first few decades was 0.1%, or 1 per 1,000. Over the years, safer methods of administration were developed, including the use of short-acting anesthetics, muscle relaxants, and adequate oxygenation. Present mortality is very low. In the least favorable recent series reported, there were 2.9 deaths per 10,000 patients. Overall, the risk is not different from that associated with the use of short-acting barbiturate anesthetics. Nonetheless, ECT remains controversial. Its opponents play up its risks, and to this day, they call ECT a "gruesome treatment."[53] Its advocates play down the risks. Medicine is a highly regulated profession, and ECT is the most regulated psychiatric treatment.[54]

The psychiatrist may be liable if he fails to make a reasonable disclosure to the patient of the significant facts and the more probable consequences and difficulties inherent in the treatment, including the risk of fractures. Depending on the circumstances, severity of the need and urgency, the psychiatrist is obliged to communicate with and advise the spouse or other family members who are available and competent to advise or speak for the patient.[55]

ECT has involved at least three considerable dangers (reflected in the premium for insurance policies covering ECT, which usually carry a 25% surcharge). Fractures and dislocations have been a hazard; over the years new methods have been developed to diminish the risk. Apnea or cessation of breathing is a danger that must be guarded against by artificial respiration.[56] Following the treatment, the patient will suffer memory impairment and find himself in a severe state of confusion, which may result in loss of self-control.

The most numerous cases in litigation have involved fractures resulting from the convulsion induced during the treatment, but these cases are of an earlier time. Next most frequent are cases in which the patient is left unattended during the posttreatment period and injures himself in some way. Another series of cases involves the psychiatrist's failure to disclose the possible hazards of the treatment, and in some cases the psychiatrist's assurance that no harm could possibly result.[57]

The doctrine of *res ipsa loquitur*, justifying a presumption of negligence, does not apply to injuries resulting from electroshock treatment. The *res ipsa* doctrine, although invested with an esoteric aura, means nothing more than that certain events bespeak negligence. In a common-sense view, the event implicates the defendant: "The thing speaks for itself." The aura surrounding the phrase, though, prompted Lord Shaw of the House of Lords to say, "If that phrase had not been in Latin, nobody would have called it a principle."

In the seminal case on the *res ipsa* doctrine, a barrel of flour falling from a warehouse onto a passerby in the street was deemed more consistent with negligence on the part of the warehouseman than any other explanation. The phrase, found in Cicero's prose, was used in the case by Chief Baron Pollock, an English gentleman with a classical education.[58] When applicable, *res ipsa* means simply that rather than the plaintiff proving defendant negligent, the defendant is forced to produce evidence that he was not. Much the best observation was made by the Mississippi Supreme Court when it said in a classic case, "We can imagine no reason why, with ordinary care, human toes could not be left out of chewing tobacco, and if toes are found in chewing tobacco, it seems to us that somebody has been very careless."[59]

In the cases involving fractures during ECT, the courts have noted that since their occurrence is not dependent on the lack of care in administering the treatment, the doctrine has no bearing on the injury. Fractures occur during treatment even when it is properly administered; therefore, the injury cannot in and of itself denote negligence. Fractures are part of the "calculated risk of the treatment."[60] The plaintiff must show that the treatment was not administered in consonance with the usual electroshock method employed by the usual skilled practitioner.

In a leading case on negligent ECT, the plaintiff suffered a compression fracture of his ninth thoracic vertebra during the first treatment. He complained of pain in his back after the treatment. Successive shock treatments nevertheless were administered and the injury was aggravated. The psychiatrist failed at any time to take x-rays. The plaintiff was allowed to use as evidence the *Standards of Electroshock Treatment* prepared by the American Psychiatric Association. Among the standards is one that states, "If the patient should complain of pain or impairment of function, he should receive a physical examination, including x-rays, to ascertain whether he suffered accidental damage." The court held that the defendant psychiatrist could be held to the published standards and was negligent in not taking an x-ray.[61]

In cases centering on the problem of posttreatment observation, someone, usually one on the hospital staff, has failed to keep watch over the patient who is in a state of confusion and in some way causes injury to himself. In some cases, he falls out of bed, in others he falls down a flight of stairs. Generally deciding in favor of the plaintiff, the courts take the view that failing to observe the patient in his confused state constitutes negligence. The psychiatrist is held liable when he fails to direct that the patient be attended,[62] and the hospital is held liable when it fails to exercise reasonable safeguards.[63]

The most difficult cases concern the alleged lack of consent on the part of the patient, or an inadequate consent due to a failure on the part of the psychiatrist to disclose fully the nature and hazards of the treatment (see Consent to ECT form).[64] It is usually argued that the very fact that electroshock is recommended, at least the initial treatments, indicates that the patient, on account of his agitation or depression, is not in a condition either to consent or not consent. In one noted case, the court began its opinion with the stringent statement concerning disclosure and consent as generally applied to physicians: "[A patient] must have full and frank disclosure by a physician of all pertinent facts relative to his illness and treatment prescribed or recommended; otherwise, any consent obtained from the patient for administration of such treatment is ineffectual." But having said that, the court then went on to say that complete and full disclosure when dealing with a mental patient may not always be the rule. In cases where, as the court put it, the patient is overwhelmed with anxiety, the physician may not be required to make a complete disclosure. In this particular case the defendant psychiatrist not only failed to inform the patient of the dangers of electroshock, but in fact told him no harm could result, so as to reassure and calm him.[65]

Undertaking ECT does not fall within the obligation of a plaintiff in a personal injury case to minimize his damages, although ECT may alleviate the plaintiff's suffering. As the Louisiana Court of Appeal put it, "[A] plaintiff's refusal to submit to electroshock therapy is [not] unreasonable."[66] In the case of an involuntarily committed patient, ECT (like psychosurgery) is deemed an intrusive therapy that will not be imposed against the patient's will.

It is highly unusual for a medical treatment to become the subject of local legislation, but just such an event occurred in California in regard ECT. The California legislature in 1973 sought to interdict entirely the use of ECT (along with lobotomy and psychotropic drugs). The law was challenged in court and enjoined as an unlawful restriction on medical practice.[67] The legislature revised the law to set consent and reporting requirements and to limit the use of ECT in patients under the age of 12. Other states also restricted the use of ECT.[68] It has become statutorily regulated with strict procedures for its application on incarcerated or committed individuals. However, even in the many states that by law permit the use of ECT, the departments of mental health in many states do not allow it, and as a result, it is not available in state-run hospitals or in many of the smaller community hospitals that serve the uninsured, members of minority groups, and the more severely ill. Thus, ECT is not done in state hospitals in Michigan, but patients may be referred to the private sector for the treatment. Liability insurance premiums for the use of ECT remain relatively high, so that is a disincentive to its use.

Following passage of the legislation in California, the American Psychiatric Association in 1975 established a Task Force on Electroconvulsive Therapy. The task force surveyed members of the association, reviewed the published accounts, and held public hearings in order to get a picture of the then contemporary ECT practice. Their report supported the use of ECT for patients with major depressive disorders, particularly for those whom psychotropic drugs had not helped.[69] ECT is supported as well for patients with mania or who are suicidal, as ECT is quick acting, unlike medication that takes a long time to take effect. Its use is also supported for the treatment of patients who are catatonic, schizophrenic, or in a state of delirium (independent of the cause of the delirium). Its use is also supported in the treatment of women during the early trimester of pregnancy (avoiding the side-effects of medication). There is growing use in the treatment of children, as it calls for a low threshold of electricity and they are physically able to undergo ECT.

The controversies over ECT, however, have taken a toll. The availability of ECT is uneven and sparse, though making a comeback. Henry Ford Hospital, the major hospital in Detroit, reinstituted it in 2000. ECT is now an ambulatory treatment, but insurers tend not to cover ECT unless administered in a hospital, so the patient is unnecessarily hospitalized. As a result of the outcries against ECT, the FDA has put a cap on the amount of electricity, but practitioners often exceed it in order for it to be effective. Risk factors are brain lesions, cardiovascular problems, or unstable heart.

The name *electroshock* is frightening, but it is no longer the fearsome treatment pictured in films. The term is a carryover from the time when the procedure was indeed frightening because it was used without general anesthesia and was often abused. It has been suggested that it now be called a "stimulation" procedure. Anesthesia, controlled oxygenation, and muscle relaxation make the procedure so safe that the risks are less than those that accompany the use of some psychotropic drugs, and, for the elderly, the systemically ill, and pregnant women, ECT is now a safer treatment for mental illness than any alternative.[70] Indeed, it is the most effective treatment in all of medicine, yet it is slighted. Dr. Keith Russell Ablow had this to say:

> Unlike medications, ECT is not profitable to the industry. If it were, there might be a flurry of industry-supported research to document its effectiveness and reduce its stigma. Psychiatrists would get the same hard-sell educational materials on ECT as we do on anti-depressants. Maybe even some pens, pads of paper, and briefcases with little lightning bolts or something, just like the ones we get with drug logos. But it's the power company that is paid for electrical current, not a pharmaceutical manufacturer.[71]

When ECT is properly administered, about 85% of patients with serious depression respond to it. In 2003, assessing the effectiveness of ECT in a series of depressed Israeli patients, Barnard Lerer, director of the Biological Laboratory of Hadassah University Hospital in Ein Karem, Israel, said to a journalist, "Have you ever asked yourself how it is that a treatment with such a terrible stigma, a treatment that the public is afraid of and is said to be primitive and unhelpful, has, despite all this, survived into the 21st century, and not in obscure little places, but in the world's most advanced centers? The answer is simple. Because it works."[72]

Researchers now recommend that ECT should be considered more frequently as the treatment of choice for depressed patients with delusions, patients at high risk for suicide, older patients who cannot tolerate tricyclic antidepressants and whose history shows them to be poorly responsive, severely depressed patients without delusions, and those with limited insurance coverage.[73] FDA has approved ECT for depression, mania, and catatonia, and there are an increasing number of new brain stimulation therapies, including focal electrically administered seizure therapy (FEAST), magnetic seizure therapy (MST), vagus nerve stimulation (VNS), transcranial magnetic stimulation (TMS), and deep brain stimulation (DBS). Neuropsychiatrists take out patents on the place of the brain to be stimulated. Too much electricity kills (as in the death penalty), but a little electricity is shown to be curative. In an address at the American Psychiatric Association Institute on Hospital and Community Psychiatry, Dr. John Nardini observed:

> I am sure that most of you in the field have known many patients who certainly would have been dead long since had they not had the benefit of shock treatment. Furthermore, prolonged hospitalization and the economic distress to the individual and his family would have been so much more extreme without that benefit. It is a mystery to me how shock treatment has come to be so ill-regarded. The antipathy for shock exists in various ways

and at various levels and it has resulted in the deprivation of prompt and effective treatment for many individuals. One of the things that has made me feel earlier intervention of shock treatment is indicated is, of course, the high index of suicide and suicidal potential. I have known many patients who would have been alive for many years thereafter had they had shock treatment instead of other approaches.[74]

"That many people have negative things to say about electroshock is not surprising," says Dr. Max Fink, a longtime advocate of ECT. He says, "Most people have negative things to say about their doctors and how they failed to cure them. All humans die; everyone of us is a medical failure; and blaming the doctor or his treatment is fair game." And he says:

What is surprising about electroshock is its remarkable efficacy and extraordinary safety. It is antidepressant, antipsychotic, antimanic, and anticatatonic; a breadth of action not matched by any other treatment for mental disorders. And, now that we have been through 65 years of experiments, it has become remarkably safe; in patients with systemic disorders, it is the safer option when compared to the risks of medicines. The increased use of ECT, now estimated at 100,000 patients in the U.S. annually, is due to one fact: the repeated failure of medicines to help these patients, and the success of ECT when medicines fail. It is for pharmacotherapy failures that ECT has been resurrected. However, many hospitals owned by insurance schemes do not have facilities for electroshock. From their point of view, the need for pre-ECT medical evaluations, the charges by anesthesiologists, the paucity of trained psychiatrists, and the hospital rules that often require in-patient care, all make the initial cost too high for them to encourage its use. The return of electroshock is not due to any managed care effect.[75]

During the 1990s, though a time of resurgence of the use of ECT, there has been little litigation involving ECT.[76] Indeed, a suit for malpractice for suicide was brought when ECT was *not* given. In an unreported wrongful death action, the psychiatrist was sued because 13 years earlier the patient had been helped by him with ECT. The widow claimed that the patient, her husband, had gone to him again for ECT, but had received medication without success. The court held for the psychiatrist, apparently on the theory that the court would not mandate a course of therapy when the treatment given meets standard of care.

What about the right of a voluntary patient in a state hospital to opt for ECT? In this situation, the California Court of Appeals said, "Where informed consent is adequately insured, there is no justification for infringing upon the patient's right to privacy in selecting and consenting to the treatment. The state has varied interests that are served by the regulation of ECT, but these interests are not served where the patient and his physician are the best judges of the patient's health, safety, and welfare."[77]

Professional Guidelines on Treatments

The American Psychiatric Association, through its American Psychiatric Press, in 1989 published the monumental 3,000-page, 4-volume *Treatment of Psychiatric Disorders* (prepared by the Task Force on Treatment of Psychiatric Disorders). The prepublication infighting spilled a lot of professional blood. Those opposing an "official treatment manual" believed it would spur malpractice suits against psychiatrists. They said it would provide contentious or dissatisfied patients and their attorneys with ammunition in the form of an allegedly authoritative checklist of standards against which treatment would be measured in a courtroom.[78] It was also said that it would promote a cookbook mentality. A clinician providing therapy other than that mentioned in the "official treatment manual" would have difficulty in justifying his or her actions.

When expert witnesses at trial are in disagreement (as is often the case), practice standards play a particularly important, if not determinative, role in the outcome of the case.[79]

The treatment efforts of psychiatrists are indeed graded by the manual not only for malpractice or professional competency questions, but also for reimbursement. Because payment for healthcare today comes mainly by way of a third-party payer and is distributed among a variety of health service providers, evaluation and regulation of practice are increasingly practiced by the payers. The "informed consent" doctrine requires practitioners to inform patients of the various treatment alternatives, but the reimbursement policy influences what will be treated, how it will be treated, and who will do the treating. In making such an assessment, the third-party payer looks to authoritative guidelines. The treatment manual was generated, in large measure, to satisfy the health care payer.

Several psychiatrists launched a petition drive aimed at compelling the APA to cancel publication of the work. Clinical experience encourages therapists to use their own intuitive impression when selecting and applying treatment methods. They eschew the appropriateness of standardized treatments, insisting that they should be able to use their creative thinking and professional judgment. In the end, the APA issued a disclaimer, saying that the book is not official policy, but rather an "approved" task force report. In the disclaimer, the APA states that the work contains information on evolving knowledge, does not encompass all approaches, is not intended to impose rigid methods, and leaves final assessment up to the practitioner.[80] The term *guidelines* is used rather than *standards* to suggest flexibility in treatment.[81] It is nonetheless argued by attorneys in the courtroom as state-of-the-art and in clinical circles psychiatrists are warned, "When we depart from the APA guidelines, we become vulnerable to a lawsuit."[82]

The issue of negligence is rarely raised, however, where anachronistic therapeutic modes are applied to psychiatric disorders, notwithstanding the availability of newer and more effective therapies. In this area, the issue of informed consent may well be applicable. It would appear that a psychiatric patient should be told what treatment modalities are available for his particular disorder and how they work, and then be given some approximation of what they may require in time and money. In some instances, his cognitive capacities may be so impaired by psychosis that the information will have to be imparted to a legally responsible member of the family. For example, if a therapist opts to treat a major psychosis like acute schizophrenia with psychotherapy alone because of some strong antidrug convictions, he is entitled to do so. At the same time, he should inform the family what the current consensus of psychiatric literature has to say about results, undesirable consequences, etc., when various treatment modes are compared. Similarly, if a patient consults a therapist because of acute anxiety related to some stressful life event, he should have the information that will enable him to choose between the intensive long-term psychotherapies and the brief methods.

Increasingly, psychiatry has been called upon to define its methods and results to the consuming public. In addition to the courts, the leaders of major labor unions and the health insurers have looked at the results of the psychiatric therapies with understandable concern about the return on the insurance dollar. Beyond a doubt, it would be extremely difficult within the definition of malpractice to prove negligence when the efficacies of utilized psychiatric treatment modes have never been fully established and a significant segment of the psychiatric community is espousing their use, albeit solely on an impressionistic basis. This difficulty in establishing negligence would particularly characterize the talking therapies where the influence of doctor on patient, whether pernicious or therapeutic, would be virtually impossible to concretize to a jury. The continuation of a form of treatment over years, however, in the face of deterioration or the absence of improvement may prove to be a more easily demonstrable matter.

When a patient does not improve or his status deteriorates, as in the case of Osheroff, it should occasion referral for consultation and a reevaluation of diagnosis, psychodynamics, and therapeutic technique. The consultant should probably have a conceptual orientation somewhat at variance with the referring psychiatrist to avoid a validation and simple mirroring of his views. Such consultative help will not only be useful to the patient, but to the psychiatrist as well, should a malpractice defense ever be necessary.

Managed Care

A current phenomenon that affects the standard of care in the psychiatric treatment and choice of treatment is the role of managed care. It is no secret that the overall purpose of managed care is to reduce the cost of medical care. This can be in direct contradiction to providing the most appropriate psychiatric care that is available to the patient. By determining treatment choices based on economic incentives, HMOs have succeeded in establishing new standards of care, often to the detriment of the patient.

This situation has perhaps affected psychiatry more than other specialties. Over the past 15 years, mental health expenditures have skyrocketed to 10% of overall health costs. In reaction, it is now quite common for employers to contract with HMOs to administer mental health benefits with control over the choice of mental healthcare provider, treatment, and length of therapy. Patients enrolled in managed care organizations may not have access to new, effective, but expensive, drugs or information about them from their physicians, who may be implicitly prohibited from discussing expensive therapies. The managed care physician has divided loyalties: to the patient, who deserves good care, and to the organization, which may demand that corners be cut at every opportunity. Under capitation plans, the less the physician does, the more he or she earns. The result of managed care is "a complete separation between economic concerns and therapeutic standards."

A backlash has occurred. Physicians now seek to form unions to safeguard their interests (under the law, only physicians who are employees may form a union). The Clinton administration endorsed a consumer's medical bill of rights, which included the repeal of gag clauses that prevented doctors from disclosing financial incentives of treatment decisions and an appeal process if needed care is denied. The proposal was not adopted on the federal level.

Until recently, the argument that HMOs do not make medical decisions but only insurance decisions provided them with some medical malpractice protection. In scores of lawsuits around the country, HMOs have asserted that they have no legal liability for negligence or medical malpractice because they are administering employee benefit plans. Under the 1974 Employee Retirement Income Security Act (ERISA), a person in an employer-sponsored health plan may recover the benefits in questions and can get an injunction clarifying the right to future benefits, but courts have repeatedly held that the law does not allow compensation for lost wages, death or disability, pain and suffering, or other harm that a patient may suffer as a result of the improper denial of claims. But things are changing.

In 1997, Texas became the first state to allow medical malpractice suits against HMOs. Missouri achieved a similar result by making it clear that HMOs practice medicine. Approximately 20 other states are considering similar laws, including New Jersey, Rhode Island, Connecticut, Washington, New York, and California. Proposals have also been made at the federal level. Some courts have ruled that recipients of healthcare may bring an action against HMOs on the grounds of "bad faith" just as they may against insurers on that ground. The Illinois Supreme Court held that a patient's HMO may be held vicariously liable for negligence of its independent-contractor physicians under agency law. A few states (New York, for example) have enacted a bill of rights for managed care patients that states that a managed care organization must provide the number of consumer grievances it has received each year and the number of grievances decided in favor of the consumer.

New Restrictions on Bringing a Malpractice Claim

Restrictions on bringing a medical malpractice claim have multiplied, notwithstanding the developments of HMOs restricting care. The medical profession has been successful in persuading various state legislatures to alleviate the medical malpractice crisis. Lobbyists placed much of the blame for the crisis on the law of negligence, and various modifications of the law were rushed through the legislature of almost every state.

The legislation varies considerably. Caps have been imposed on awards for pain and suffering and limitations on expert testimony. Many states now require submitting the case to a screening board before filing an action, others require submission to arbitration, and others impose restrictions on the contingent fee. Many commentators say the reform has deformed tort law. The restrictions are under challenge. Trial lawyers have leveled a wide array of constitutional salvos against the "doctors' legislation."

In some measure, the counterattack has been successful. Several state supreme courts have held that the right to recover damages for injury is a fundamental right, thereby requiring strict scrutiny of equal protection review. The restrictions also are called an "unconstitutional limitation on access to the courts." The Missouri Supreme Court declared its state's mediation plan unconstitutional on grounds that it violates the right to seek immediate redress in the courts. Constitutional guarantees of substantive due process ensure that legislation or other governmental actions will not deprive any citizen of "life, liberty, or property without due process of law." Laws that diminish tort rights are subject to challenge as constituting a taking of the injured persons' property, the right to sue, without due process of law. Many state constitutions contain a prohibition against special legislature.

Then, too, there is an end-run that may be made around the restrictions. To avoid the cap on compensatory damages, allegations are made that would allow punitive damages. Several states allow punitive damages awards in medical malpractice upon a showing of gross negligence.

The National Practitioner Data Bank

As part of the Health Care Quality Improvement Act of 1986 (HCQIA), which included provisions granting limited immunity to persons or organizations participating in peer review activities, Congress established the National Practitioner Data Bank (NPDB).[83] It became operational in 1990. Under it, state medical and dental licensing boards are required to report to the NPDB certain disciplinary actions taken on grounds related to the professional competence or professional conduct of the licensed professional. Denial of privileges to a hospital must be reported to the NPDB, and also judgments and settlements (judgments or settlements over $25,000 remain permanently in the record). Hospitals must query the NPDB at least every 2 years for each member of their medical staff, state licensure boards are not required to make a query of the NPDB, but may do so. The general public does not have access to the information in the data bank, although consumer organizations have lobbied for access. Attorneys for plaintiffs in malpractice suits can access the NPDB only if the plaintiff can prove that the defendant healthcare entity failed to make a query on the practitioner defendant. Neither malpractice insurers nor third-party payers are given access to the data bank, but apparently these entities are requiring physicians to request and turn over their own records to the NPDB as a condition of receiving coverage or reimbursement.

Physicians may request their own records from the NPDB and are to receive a copy from the data bank of each report at the time it is made. They may dispute any report made against them (but space is limited to 600 characters). They may circumvent any report to the NPDB by using their P.C. (professional corporation) as the named party in any litigation or in settling a case. Attorneys for plaintiffs want to posture a case so that it will be settled, and realizing that a practitioner will be reluctant to settle if it will be reported to the NPDB, they only name the hospital as party defendant in cases where a mishap occurred in a hospital. Then, too, a disciplinary action that is longer than 30 days is to be reported, but the loophole is to make it less than 30 days. Moreover, insurance companies draft the information that goes to the data bank, and they tend to spin it in favor of the physician. The federal General Accounting Office has issued a report that is critical of the accuracy of the information contained in the NPDB, including the information that is provided by state medical boards.[84]

According to published reports, the well-intentioned regulations intended to enforce the HCQIA have been largely ignored and the NPDB system, which was intended to alert healthcare employees to problems with physicians, has failed. According to reports, 54 to 60% of hospitals and 84% of HMOs have never reported a single adverse action taken against physicians to the NPDB.[85] In part, this low level of reporting to the NPDB can be traced to the retaliatory lawsuits filed by physicians who are reported to the NPDB. These lawsuits include claims for defamation, antitrust violations, tortuous interference with business advantage, and constitutional violations. Rather than report an adverse event taken against a physician to the NPDB, healthcare entities often choose to ignore the mandate of the HCQIA in an effort to avoid the possibility of costly litigation. The fear of liability is rather unfounded as HCQIA expressly provides that a hospital or HMO is immune from liability so long as the report it makes to the NPDB is accurate. The issue for purpose of immunity is whether the healthcare entity accurately reported the action that it took, not whether the action that it took was justified.[86]

Electroconvulsive Therapy (ECT) Consent Form

Name of Patient: _____

My doctor, _____, has recommended that I receive treatment with electroconvulsive therapy (ECT). This treatment, as well as the risks and benefits that I may experience from it, have been fully described to me. I give my consent to be treated with ECT.

Whether ECT or an alternative treatment, like medication or psychotherapy, is most appropriate for me depends on my prior experience with these treatments, the features of my illness, and other considerations. Why ECT has been recommended for me has been explained.

ECT involves a series of treatments, which may be given on an inpatient or outpatient basis. To receive each treatment, I will come to a specially equipped area in this facility. The treatments are usually given in the morning. Because the treatments involve general anesthesia, I will have had nothing to eat or drink for several hours before each treatment. Before the treatment, a small needle will be placed in my vein so that I can be given medications. An anesthetic medication will be injected that will quickly put me to sleep. I will then be given another medication that will relax my muscles. Because I will be asleep, I will not experience pain or discomfort, nor will I remember the procedure. Other medications may also be given, depending on my needs.

To prepare for the treatment, monitoring sensors will be place on my head and body. Blood pressure cuffs will be placed on an arm and a leg. This monitoring involves no pain or discomfort. After I am asleep, a carefully controlled amount of electricity will be passed between two electrodes that have been placed on my head.

I may receive bilateral ECT or unilateral ECT. In bilateral ECT, one electrode is placed on the left side of the head, and the other on the right side. In unilateral ECT, both electrodes are placed on the same side of the head, usually the right side. Unilateral ECT (electrodes on the right side) is likely to produce less memory difficulty than bilateral ECT. However, for some patients bilateral ECT may be a more effective treatment. My doctor will carefully consider the choice of unilateral or bilateral ECT.

The electrical current produces a seizure in the brain. The amount of electricity used to produce the seizure will be adjusted to my individual needs, based on the judgment of the ECT physician. The medication used to relax my muscles will greatly soften the contractions in my body that would ordinarily accompany the seizure. I will be given oxygen to breathe. The seizure will last for approximately 1 minute. During the procedure, my heart, blood pressure, and brain waves will be monitored. Within a few minutes, the anesthetic medications will wear off and I will awaken. I will then be observed until it is time to leave the ECT area.

The number of treatments that I will receive cannot be known ahead of time. A typical acute course of ECT is 6 to 12 treatments, but some patients may need fewer and some need more. Treatments are usually given three times a week, but the frequency of treatment may also vary depending on my needs. I understand that this consent form covers a maximum of 12 treatments to be administered in a series over several weeks. If additional treatments are needed, a new consent form will be obtained.

My illness is expected to improve with ECT. However, I understand that I may recover completely, partially, or not at all. After ECT, my symptoms may return. How long I will remain well cannot be known ahead of time. To make the return of symptoms less likely after ECT, I will need additional treatment with medication, psychotherapy, or ECT. The treatment I will receive to prevent the return of symptoms will be discussed with me.

Like other medical treatments, ECT has risks and side effects. As with any medical treatment, people who receive ECT differ considerable in the extent to which they experience side effects. To reduce the risk of complications, I will receive a medical evaluation before starting ECT. The medications I have been taking may be adjusted. However, in spite of precautions, it is possible that I will experience a medical complication.

- The minor side effects that are frequent include headache, muscle soreness, and nausea. These side effects usually respond to simple treatment.
- ECT may result in irregularities in heart rate and rhythm. These irregularities are usually mild and short lasting, but in some instances can be life threatening.
- With modern ECT technique, dental complications are infrequent and bone fractures or dislocations are very rare.
- ECT very rarely results in serious medical complications, such as heart attack, stroke, respiratory difficulty, or continuous seizure.
- As with any procedure using general anesthesia, there is a remote possibility of death from ECT. The risk of death from ECT is very low, about one in 10,000 patients. This rate may be higher in patients with severe medical conditions.

If serious side effects occur, I understand that medical care and treatment will be instituted immediately and that facilities to handle emergencies are available. I understand, however, that neither the institution nor the treating physicians are required to provide long-term medical treatment. I shall be responsible for the cost of such treatment whether personally or through medical insurance or other medical coverage.

When I awaken after each treatment, I may be confused. This confusion usually goes away within an hour. During the treatment course, I may have new difficulties in attention and concentration and other aspects of thinking. These problems rapidly go away after completion of ECT.

I understand that memory loss is a common side effect of ECT. The memory loss with ECT has a characteristic pattern, including problems remembering past events and new information. The degree of memory problems is often related to the number and type of treatments given. A smaller number of treatments is likely to produce less memory difficulty than a larger number. Shortly following a treatment, the problems with memory are greatest. As time from treatment increases, memory improves.

I may experience difficulties remembering events that happened before and while I received ECT. The spottiness in my memory for past events may extend back to several months before I received ECT, and, less commonly, for longer periods of time, sometimes several years or more. While many of these memories should return during the first few months following my ECT course, I may be left with some permanent gaps in memory.

For a short period following ECT, I may also experience difficulty in remembering new information. This difficulty in forming new memories should be temporary and typically disappears within several weeks following the ECT course.

The majority of patients state that the benefits of ECT outweigh the problems with memory. Furthermore, most patients report that their memory is actually improved after ECT. Nonetheless, a minority of patients report problems in memory that remain for months or even years. The reasons for these reported long-lasting impairments are not fully understood.

Because of the possible problems with confusion and memory, I should not make any important personal or business decisions during or immediately following the ECT course. During and shortly after the ECT course, and until discussed with my doctor, I should refrain from driving, transacting business, or other activities for which memory difficulties may be troublesome.

The conduct of ECT at this facility is under the direction of Dr. _____. I may contact him/her at _____ if I have any further questions.

I am free to ask my doctor or members of the ECT treatment team questions about ECT at this time or at any time without prejudice during or following the ECT course. My decision to agree to ECT is being made voluntarily, and I may withdraw my consent for further treatment at any time.

I have been given a copy of this consent signed form to keep.

_____   _____
Patient (or appropriate guardian) Signature   Date

_____   _____
Signature of Person Obtaining Consent   Date

The patient is unable to consent because_____

_____

and I, as his/her legally authorized representative, therefore consent for the patient.

_____   _____

Legally Authorized Representative   Date

_____   _____

Signature of Person Obtaining Consent   Date

This consent is valid until the date of _____

Endnotes

1. J. Freiberg, "The Song Is Ended But the Malady Lingers On: Legal Regulation of Psychotherapy," *St. Louis U. L. J.* 22 (1978): 519. See also T.E. Shea, "Legal Standard of Care for Psychiatrists and Psychologists," *West. State U. L. Rev.* 6 (1978): 71. Liability without fault (strict liability) has been urged in the case of psychiatric care. B.R. Furrow, *Malpractice in Psychotherapy* (Lexington, MA: Lexington Books, 1980).

2. T.J. Hooper, 60 F.2d 737 (2d. Cir. 1932); noted in Chapter 27.

3. C. T. Onions (Ed.), *The Shorter Oxford English Dictionary* (Oxford: Clarendon Press, 3rd ed., 1965). Approximately one third of the states have statutes of limitations specifically applicable to malpractice actions, usually providing a shorter period of time (generally 2 years) in which the action must be instituted. (The statutes of limitations usually provide a 3-year period for a negligence action and 1 year for intentional torts.)

4. Quoted in R. Abelson, "In Push for Better Care, a Heart-Surgery Warranty," *New York Times*, May 17, 2007, p. 1.

5. For a critique of the report, see S.B. Nuland, "The Hazards of Hospitalization," *Wall Street Journal*, Dec. 2, 1999, p. 22. For patient safety, the traditional approaches include credentialing of healthcare professionals, morbidity and mortality conferences, peer review when incidents occur and are reported, tort liability, and criminal liability. The focus is generally on injuries, meaning little attention is paid to near misses. Mary R. Anderlik of the University of Houston Law Center writes:

   At the center of attention are events of professional negligence, i.e., incidents of substandard or below average performance by a professional resulting in patient injury. A system intended to compensate for negligent injury may be a poor proxy for periodic competency testing for health care professionals or a structure of sanctions and rewards linked to the development and dissemination of best practices by organizations. The threat of liability for negligence may promote mediocrity rather than innovation to improve safety.

   "Introduction to Patient Safety," *Health Law News* (University of Houston Health Law and Policy Institute), March 2000, p. 3.

6. D. S. Viscott, *The Making of a Psychiatrist* (New York: Arbor House, 1972). Sharon Begley writes: "No one bats an eye when a drug for a severe mental illness such as schizophrenia or depression causes serious side effects such as nausea, weight gain, blurred vision or a vanishing libido. But what few patients seeking psychotherapy know is that talking can be dangerous, too—and therapists have not exactly rushed to tell them so." And she adds, "For treatments that come in a bottle, the Food and Drug Administration requires proof of safety and efficacy. For treatments that come from the lips of psychologists and psychiatrists, there's no such requirement. ... Too many clinicians practice 'psychoquackery.'" S. Begley, "Get Shrunk at Your Own Risk," *Newsweek*, June 18, 2007, p. 49; see also Ltrs., *Newsweek*, July 2–9, 2007, p. 20.

7. Attorney Donald Dawidoff, a Harvard graduate, was one of the first to argue for a cause of action against a psychiatrist not only for malpractice in improperly rendering electroshock or drug therapy, but also for faulty or negligent rending of psychoanalysis and psychotherapy. See D.J. Dawidoff, *The Malpractice of Psychiatrists* (Springfield, IL: Thomas, 1973). Dawidoff's own history with psychiatry

is sadly depicted by his son in N. Dawidoff, "My Father's Troubles," *New Yorker*, June 12, 2000, p. 58. See also N. Dawidoff, *The Crowd Sounds Happy* (New York: Pantheon Books, 2008); reviewed in S. Stephenson, "Safe at Home," *New York Times Book Review*, June 1, 2008, p. 39.

8. Quoted in J.L. Kelley, *Psychiatric Malpractice* (New Brunswick, NJ: Rutgers University Press, 1996). See also R. Bonnie, "Professional Liability and the Quality of Mental Health Care," *Law, Med. & Health Care* 16 (1988): 299; P.F. Slawson, "Psychiatric Malpractice: Ten Years' Loss Experience," *Med. & Law* 8 (1989): 415; P.F. Slawson, "Psychiatric Malpractice: A Regional Incidence Case Study", *Am. J. Psychiat.* 126 (1970): 1302; Notes, "Medical Malpractice: The Liability of Psychiatrists," *Notre Dame Law* 48 (1973): 693; "Psychiatric Malpractice—A Survey," *Washburn L. J.* 11 (1972): 461.

9. Quoted in J. Frieden, "Psychotherapy Problems Top Malpractice Complaints," *Clinical Psychiatry News*, Feb. 2000, p.1.

10. A. Kardiner, *My Analysis with Freud* (New York: Norton, 1977), p. 69. On deterioration in therapy, see R.B. Stuart, *Trick or Treatment: How and When Psychotherapy Fails* (Champaign, IL: Research Press, 1970); D. Tennov, *Psychotherapy: The Hazardous Cure* (New York: Doubleday, 1976); H.H. Strupp, "The Performance of Psychiatrists and Psychologists in a Therapeutic Interview," *J. Clin. Psychol.* 14 (1958): 219; D. Hartley, H.B. Roback, & S.I. Abramowitz, "Deterioration Effects in Encounter Groups," *Am. Psychol.* 31 (1976): 241.

11. S.A. Appelbaum, *Out in Inner Space: A Psychoanalyst Explores the New Therapies* (Garden City, NY: Doubleday, 1979), p. 66. In searching for a cure for his mentally ill brother, the writer Jay Neugeboren traveled the country looking at a variety of treatment programs, and it brought him up against a heated controversy: therapy versus drugs, which matters most? J. Neugeboren, *Transforming Madness* (New York: Morrow, 1999), reviewed in T. Parks, "In the Locked Ward," *New York Review of Books*, Feb. 24, 2000, p. 14. In *Selling Serenity: Life Among the Recovery Stars* (Boca Raton, FL: Upton Books, 1999), Andrew Meacham calls into question addiction treatment programs. In a blurb of the book, Thomas Szasz says, "It is a superb account of Americans' irrepressible faith in humbug, now masquerading as a combination of medicine and religion, therapy and virtue."

   A parody of regression therapy is the unorthodox New Age treatment called "rebirthing therapy," which is supposed to overcome "reactive attachment disorder" in which children resist forming loving relationships and become unmanageable and violent. Wrapped in a flannel blanket meant to represent the womb, the child is pushed against with pillows and urged to fight his way out and become reborn. In a nationally publicized incident in Colorado, a child died of asphyxiation. Colorado does not require therapists to be licensed, though they must register with state. C. Caldwell, "Death by Therapy," *Weekly Standard*, May 28, 2001, p. 20; A. Cannon, "From Mumbo Jumbo to a Child's Death," *U.S. News & World Report*, Sept. 18, 2000, p. 36. See M.T. Singer & J. Lalich, *'Crazy' Therapies* (San Francisco: Jossey-Bass, 1996). The history of medicine is full of quacks who believed in the effectiveness of their harmful therapeutic methods. See, e.g., R. Gordon, *Great Medical Disasters* (New York: Stein & Day, 1983); W.H. Helfand, *Quack, Quack, Quack* (New York: Grolier Club, 2002); E.S. Valenstein, *Great and Desperate Cures: The Rise and Decline of Psychosurgery and Other Radical Treatments for Mental Illness* (New York: Basic Books, 1986); M.J. Mehlman, "Quackery," *Am. J. Law & Med.* 31 (2005): 349. See Chapter 37 on regulation of psychotherapy.

12. *A Historical Dictionary of Psychiatry* (New York: Oxford University Press, 2005), p. vii.

13. Maia Szalavitz, a senior fellow of a media watchdog group, writes, "[M]ental health care is often entirely disconnected from evidence. Some therapists argue that the human mind is too complex and variable to allow for standardized treatments. But shouldn't they at least start with approaches known to work for the largest number of patients?" "When the Cure is Not Worth the Cost," *New York Times*, April 11, 2007, p. 23. Ignac Semmelweis is remembered for the importance of empirical proof. See S.B. Nuland, *The Doctors' Plague* (New York: W.W. Norton, 2003).

14. Not surprisingly, "evidence based" practice draws strong support from government and insurance companies that seek uniform standards to assess performance and cost effectiveness. According to law professor Marc Rodwin, "evidence based" practice puts experts trained in social science, public health, epidemiology, and economic analysis on par with physicians and "breaks the lock hold" the profession has over how medicine is practiced and compensated. Quoted in B. Healy, "Who Says What's Best?" *U.S. News & World Report*, Sept. 11, 2005.

15. Ltr., *New York Times*, April 16, 2007, p. 22 (in response to Maia Szalavitz).

16. In a Texas case, a minister advised the wife to seek separation from the husband, due to their marital problems. She followed this advice. The husband later, in a state of rage, shot her, seriously injuring her. The couple later reconciled and then jointly sued the minister for his counsel and advice. They prevailed. The case sent clergymen scurrying to insurance companies. (Correspondence from Robert

M. Plunk, Vice President of Preferred Risk Mutual, to author.) Following the Texas case, a number of alienation of affection suits were filed against ministers, and there have been other types of cases. UPI news report, "Ministers Taking Out 'Peace of Mind' Policy," *Chicago Sun-Times,* Oct. 19, 1980, p. 30; "Suing Clergymen for Malpractice," *Time,* Jan. 12, 1981, p. 75. A new crop of insurance policies was spawned to guarantee that, when doling out advice, men of God have more than God on their side. See AP news release, "Malpractice Insurers Are Finding a New Market Among Ministers," *New York Times,* May 18, 1980, p. 49; Editorial, "Suing the Clergy," *Detroit News,* May 15, 1980, p. 22.

17. A.R. Somers, "Accountability, Public Policy, and Psychiatry," *Am. J. Psychiat.* 134 (1977): 959. See also T.G. Gutheil, *The Psychiatrist in Court: A Survival Guide* (Washington, DC: American Psychiatric Press, 1998).

18. Congress has been asking: Does psychotherapy work? Does it work well enough to be paid for out of public funds? B.S. Herrington, "Congress Asks: Does Therapy Work?" *Psychiatric News,* March 21, 1980, p. 1; "Therapy Efficacy Test Bill Finally Introduced," *Psychiatric News,* Sept. 19, 1980, p. 3. In a study some years ago, University of Minnesota Psychology Professor William Schofield surveyed a randomized sample of 377 psychologists, psychiatrists, and psychiatric social workers, and uncovered what he called the "YAVIS Syndrome," an overwhelming preference for patients who are "young, attractive, verbal, intelligent, and successful." They are, on balance, healthier in the first place—a ready-made success package. In effect, the psychiatric profession has abandoned the psychotic or seriously disturbed individual. See E. Ames, "What Your Shrink Really Thinks of You," *New Yorker,* April 7, 1980, p. 40.

19. R. Slovenko, "On the Need for Recordkeeping in the Practice of Psychiatry," *J. Psychiat. & Law* 7 (1980): 399.

20. E.L. Hodgson, "Restrictions on Unorthodox Health Treatment in California: A Legal and Economic Analysis," *U.C.L.A. L. Rev.* 24 (1977): 647; M.J. Karson, "Regulating Medical Psychotherapists in Illinois: A Question of Balance," *John Marshall J. Pract. & Proced.* 11 (1978): 601; R. Plotkin, "Limiting the Therapeutic Orgy: Mental Patients' Right to Refuse Treatment," *Nw. U. L. Rev.* 72 (1977): 461; J.E. Smith, "Electroconvulsive Therapy: The Patient's Right to Consent in Utah," *J. Contemp. L.* 5 (1979): 233.

21. Michigan law provides that the duty of a physician to report an impaired physician does not apply to a physician who is in a "bona fide health professional–patient relationship" with the impaired physician; MCL § 333.16223.

22. What about the discharge of a tort judgment in bankruptcy? In Kawaauhau v. Geiger, 523 U.S. 57 (1998), the U.S. Supreme Court held that debts arising from recklessly or negligently inflicted injuries do not fall within the willful and malicious injury exception to discharge under bankruptcy law. The decision affirmed the Eighth Circuit's opinion and is contrary to earlier holdings of the Sixth and Tenth Circuits. Relying on the words of the bankruptcy law and other statutory indications, the U.S. Supreme Court held that a typical malpractice judgment is not a debt for "willful and malicious injury." The high court's opinion relied on a doctrine learned by first-year law students in their course on torts: Garratt v. Dailey, 279 P.2d 1091 (Wash. 1955), to wit, intended acts that cause injury are distinguishable from acts done with intent to cause injury or with knowledge to a substantial certainty that injury will occur.

23. Hammer v. Rosen, 7 N.Y.2d 376, 198 N.Y.S.2d 65 (1960).

24. The duty of therapists in "revival of memory" cases to parents or other relatives of the patient is discussed in Chapter 36 on the duty of therapists to third parties.

25. See J. Acocella, *Creating Hysteria* (San Francisco: Jossey-Bass, 1999); M. Johnson, *Spectral Evidence* (Boston: Houghton Mifflin, 1997); R. Ofshe & E. Watters, *Making Monsters: False Memories, Psychotherapy, and Sexual Hysteria* (New York: Scribner, 1994). In 1995, Christopher Barden, an attorney and psychologist, began circulating to federal and state legislatures a proposal for a new law, the Truth and Responsibility in Mental Health Practices Act. A key sentence states: "No tax or tax exempt moneys may be used for any form of healthcare treatment, including any form of psychotherapy, that has not been proven safe and effective by rigorous, valid and reliable scientific investigations and accepted as safe and effective by a majority of the relevant scientific community." The words "tax exempt" would exclude coverage of such therapies not only by public programs but also by private insurers because the insured write off the cost of health insurance. The law would also include requirements for informed consent. In 1997, in response to the lobbying efforts of Tom Rutherford, whose daughter had a "revival of memory" in therapy of childhood sexual abuse, the Indiana state legislature passed a law requiring that mental health providers obtain informed consent from any prospective patient that would inform the patient of the "risks and relative benefits of proposed treatments and alternative treatments." Barden's proposal was signed not just by him, but by a number of respected psychologists and psychiatrists. The argument is made that any psychotherapeutic technique, which

cannot be scientifically proven to be effective, constitutes "an experimental and dangerous procedure" mandating informed consent for experimentation. See J. Cannell, J.I. Hudson, & H.G. Pope, "Standards for Informed Consent in Recovered Memory Therapy," *J. Am. Acad. Psychiat. & Law* 29 (2001): 138.

Professor Alan Scheflin and Dr. David Spiegel write, "Strange as it may sound, psychiatrists today are probably safer from legal liability for authorizing psychosurgery that, despite its highly controversial history in medicine and law, is now making a comeback, than they are from simply talking with a patient about memories of the past." A.W. Scheflin & D. Spiegel, "From Courtroom to Couch: Working With Repressed Memory and Avoiding Lawsuits," in D.A. Tomb (Ed.), *Diagnostic Dilemmas* (Philadelphia: Saunders, 1998), p. 847. Dr. Paul Fink, a former president of the American Psychiatric Association, organized a Leadership Council consisting of a group of therapists, lawyers, etc., who promote the validity of repressed memories, recovered memory therapy, dissociative memories, and multiple personality disorders. It was organized in reaction to recovered memory therapists' being sued by former patients who have recanted these memories. The group included Dr. Richard Kluft, Dr. David Speigel, Professor Alan Scheflin, and Dr. Bessel Van der Kolk. See L. Alison et al., "Considerations for Experts in Assessing the Credibility of Recovered Memories of Child Abuse," *Psych. Pub. Policy & L.* 12 (2006): 419; R.T. Reagan, "Scientific Consensus on Memory Repression and Recovery," *Rutgers L. Rev.* 51 (1999): 275. Multiple personalities allegedly made Herschel Walker successful as a football player. H. Walker, *Breaking Free: My Life with Dissociative Identity Disorder* (New York: Simon & Schuster, 2008). The statute of limitations in "recovered memory" cases is discussed in the above cited article by R.T. Reagan at p. 283.

Assuming the historical reality, what abuse results in trauma? Psychologically speaking, abuse is very much in the eyes of the beholder. Sexual abuse that is revealed by "revival of memory" and that is alleged to be traumatic ranges from petting to penetration. Bettina Aptheker claims that her father, Herbert Aptheker, the Marxist historian of slavery, traumatized her by sexually molesting her when she was a child. She estimates that from the age of 3 or 4 until the age of 13, her father induced her to play "choo-choo train" on the rug of their apartment. In this game, she alleges, he would press against her back, hold her tight, rock back and forth, and shudder, leaving her "wet and sticky." See C. Phelps, "Father of History," *The Nation*, Nov. 5, 2007, p. 24.

26. "Multiple Personality: Failure to Diagnose and the Potential for Malpractice Liability," *Psych. Ann.* 18 (1988): 543. Books by therapists treating (or creating) multiple personality as well as by patients abound. Psychiatrist Richard Baer tells about treating a woman with 17 personalities in *Switching Time* (New York: Random House, 2007); reviewed in A. Underwood, "Inside Karen's Crowded Mind," *Newsweek*, Oct. 29, 2007, p. 42.

27. "Psychiatric Misadventures," *Am. Scholar*, Autumn 1992, p. 497; reprinted in P.R. McHugh, *The Mind Has Mountains* (Baltimore: Johns Hopkins University Press, 2006), pp. 3–17. See also P.R. McHugh, *Try to Remember* (Washington, DC: Dana Press, 2008); reviewed in T. Dalrymple, "Destructive Delusions," *Wall Street Journal*. Nov. 20, 2008, p 19.

28. "APA Stakes Out Positions on Controversial Therapies," *Psychiatric News*, April 21, 2000, p. 45.

29. T.W. Campbell, *Smoke and Mirrors: The Devastating Effect of False Sexual Abuse Claims* (New York: Insight Books, 1998). Psychology professors Kelly Lambert and Scott O. Lilienfeld maintain that dredging up painful and buried memories might itself traumatize patients and require more treatment to deal with the consequences. "Brain Stains," *Scientific American Mind* (Oct. 2007), reported in *Wall Street Journal*, Oct. 12, 2007, p. B-5. In *Therapy's Delusions* (New York: Scribner, 1999), Ethan Watters and Richard Ofshe claim that, over the years, talk therapy has masqueraded as a scientific discipline and has cost patients time, money, and their mental well being. See also S. Taub (ed.), *Recovered Memories of Child Sexual Abuse* (Springfield, IL: Thomas, 1999).

30. That attitudes about "revival of memory" therapy have changed is indicated by the award given in June 2001 by the American Psychological Society to Dr. Elizabeth Loftus, who for over a decade was criticized for her work debunking revival of memory. The award states, "As a result of her pioneering scientific work as well as her activity within the legal system, society is gradually coming to realize that such memories, compelling though they may seem when related by a witness, are often a product of recent reconstructive memory processes rather than of past objective reality."

31. In 1997, the directors of FMSF began discussing its future at their board meetings. Why 1997? By that year so much had changed in the memory wars that some of them believed (naively, as it turned out) there would soon be no need for the FMSF. In those 5 years, excellent books that explained the FMSF had been published, scholarly papers showed how false memories could develop, and numerous excellent documentaries had appeared on television. Articles in the general media had begun to show caution about abuse claims based solely on recovered repressed memories. Indeed, former recovered-

memory patients had even won million-dollar awards. Several well-known leaders of the recovered memory movement had been disgraced; the vast majority of people were becoming skeptical about bizarre claims of satanic ritual abuse; some families reported that their lost children were returning; and far fewer people contacted the FMSF for help. Still today, however, FMSF remains active. Partly, the clergy abuse scandals have kept claims of recovered repressed memories alive. Mostly, however, the directors of FMSF underestimated the depth of popular belief in recovered memories and the intensity with which people would justify their beliefs about recovered memories. Giving up recovered memory beliefs turns out to be hugely more difficult than it was accepting them. Research shows that it takes retractors significantly longer to give up the false memories than it did to acquire them. Although people who made accusations based on recovered-memory beliefs can usually understand that they were especially vulnerable when they were encouraged to redefine themselves as "incest survivors," they still must accept responsibility for the harm they caused their families. The difficulty of resolving the cognitive dissonance that retraction requires probably accounts for the fact that so many families have still not reunited and that the majority of those who do return to their families do not want to talk about what happened.

32. See T.M. Luhrman, *Of Two Minds: The Growing Disorder in American Psychiatry* (New York: Knopf, 2000).

33. United States v. Klein, 325 F.2d 283, 286 (2d Cir. 1963). In this case Judge Kaufman commented about disagreements among psychiatrists on treatment: "Mental disorders being what they are, it is not surprising that eminent psychiatrists differ as to methods of treatment. Here, [one psychiatrist] believed that [the accused] would respond to a psychoanalytic form of therapy; [the government psychiatrist] favored a more physiological approach. Courts of law, unschooled in the intricacies of what may be the most perplexing of medical sciences, are ill equipped to choose among such divergent but responsible views." Although cognitive therapy is the best-studied form of psychotherapy, its effectiveness compared with antidepressant medication remains controversial. See E.S. Friedman, "Cognitive Therapy: What Is Its Role in Depression Treatment?" *Psychiatric Times*, Sept. 2007, p. 1. For an aching back (a common ailment), Lisa Gubernick consulted eight different specialists—an osteopath, chiropractor, acupuncturist, psychiatrist, homeopath, physiatrist, neurologist, and a celebrity doctor—and got eight different diagnoses and recommended treatments. L. Gurernick, "'Have I Got a Cure for You!'" *Wall Street Journal*, Oct. 6, 2000, p. W1.

34. 457 U.S. 307 (1982).

35. A challenge to procedures followed by the Maryland Health Claims Arbitration office appears in Osheroff v. Chestnut Lodge, 62 Md. App. 519, 490 A.2d 720 (Md. App. 1985).

36. G. L. Klerman, "Implications of *Osheroff v. Chestnut Lodge*," *Am J. Psychiat.* 147 (1990): 419; A.A. Stone, "Law, Science, and Psychiatric Malpractice: A Response to Klerman's Indictment of Psychoanalytic Psychiatry," *Am. J. Psychiat.* 147 (1990): 419. See also J.L. Kelley, *Psychiatric Malpractice* (New Brunswick, NJ: Rutgers University Press, 1996); J.G. Malcolm, *Treatment Choices and Informed Consent: Current Controversies in Psychiatric Malpractice* (Springfield, IL: Thomas, 1988). Stone later wrote, "Psychoanalysis is losing favor as part of psychotherapeutic treatment as the Freudian paradigm is replaced by scientific advancements." A.A. Stone, "The Decline and Fall of Psychoanalysis: And What It Means to Physicians," *TEN* 3 (2001): 48. There is an extensive literature on psychopharmocology versus psychotherapy in the treatment of mental illness. See, e.g., T.M. Luhrman, *Of Two Minds: The Growing Disorder in American Psychiatry* (New York: Knopf, 2000); R.R. Slavney & P.R. McHugh, *Psychiatric Polarities* (Baltimore, MD: Johns Hopkins University Press, 1987); E.S. Valenstein, *Blaming the Brain: The Truth About Drugs and Mental Health* (New York: Free Press, 1998); see also J. Acocella, "Three Cheers for Psychotherapy," *New Yorker*, May 8, 2000, p. 112; L. Luborsky, B. Singer, & L. Luborsky, "Comparative Studies of Psychotherapies," *Arch. Gen. Psychiat.* 32 (1975): 995.

37. G. Boodman, "A Horrible Place & a Wonderful Place, *Washington Post Magazine*, Oct. 8, 1989, p. 18.

38. Subsequently, Stone expressed disillusionment with psychoanalysis (but not psychotherapy), and he wrote that "the social and intellectual history of psychoanalysis involves opening our eyes to sordid facts and gaining new understanding." A.A. Stone, Book Review, *Am. J. Psychiat.* 155 (1998): 851. See also A.A. Stone, "Where Will Psychoanalysis Survive?" *Harvard Magazine*, Jan./Feb. 1997, p. 34. Psychologist Carol Tavris says, "No one knows why medication helps some people but has no effect on others. No one knows why psychotherapy helps some people and has no effect on others. And when medication or therapy do work, no one knows why they do." C. Tavris, "The Know-Nothing Healers,"

Times Literary Supplement, Oct. 27, 2000, p. 10. Some find a therapeutic element to the martial arts that helps children with attention deficit disorder cope. S. Saulny, "Using Martial Arts for Attention Disorders," *New York Times*, Dec. 2, 2000, p. 16.

39. Personal communication.

40. Personal communication.

41. 83 Wash.2d 514, 519 P.2d 981 (1974).

42. A. Gawande, "No Mistake: The Future of Medical Care: Machines That Act Like Doctors, and Doctors Who Act Like Machines," *New Yorker*, March 30, 1998, p. 74.

43. There was at one time a psychoanalytic theory that ECT was a punishment that assuaged guilt and, thus, was curative of depression. The best-selling 1946 autobiographical novel by Mary Jane Ward, *The Snake Pit*, and the famous 1948 film based on it, told of the experiences of a woman in a crowded mental hospital where therapy for schizophrenia included being wrapped in wet, cold sheets, boiled in a bathtub, and given electroshock treatment. The snake pit of the title referred to the medieval practice of lowering the mentally ill into snake pits in the belief that a fright that would unhinge a sane person would cure an insane one. See G.J. Alexander & A.W. Scheflin (Eds.), *Law and Mental Disorder* (Durham, NC: Carolina Academic Press, 1998), pp. 981–1001.

44. L.B. Kalinowsky, "Convulsive Shock Treatment," in S. Arieti (Ed.), *American Handbook of Psychiatry* (New York: Basic Books, 1959), vol. 2, pp. 1499–1520, quote at p. 1510.

45. See D.S. Viscott, *The Making of a Psychiatrist* (New York: Harbor House, 1972); see also R. Cancro, "Functional Psychoses and the Conceptualization of Mental Illness," in R.W. Menninger & J.C. Nemiah (Eds.), *American Psychiatry After World War II* (Washington, DC: American Psychiatric Press, 2000).

46. See E. Shorter, *A History of Psychiatry* (New York: John Wiley & Sons, 1997).

47. In a fictional story by Chinese-born writer Ha Jin, a young, gay man in China, is sent to a mental hospital where a doctor confides that homosexuality is not a disease and cannot be cured, but still he says, "Electrotherapy is prescribed by the book—a standard treatment required by the Department of Public Health. I have no choice but to follow the regulations." H. Jin, *The Bridegroom* (New York: Pantheon, 2000).

48. Ken Kesey's *One Flew Over the Cuckoo's Nest*, published in 1962, had a marked impact on regulation of ECT and attitudes about it, and they very much remain though ECT now poses little risk of harm. The novel was republished as a Viking Compass Edition in 1964 and Penguin Books in 1976. In it, Kesey wrote:

> The Shock Shop ... is jargon for the EST machine, the Electro Shock Therapy. A device that might be said to do the work of the sleeping pill, the electric chair, and the torture rack. It's a clever little procedure, simple, quick, nearly painless it happens so fast, but no one ever wants another one. Ever ...
>
> You are strapped to a table, shaped, ironically, like a cross, with a crown of electric sparks in place of thorns. You are touched on each side of the head with wires. Zap! Five cents' worth of electricity through the brain and you are jointly administered therapy and a punishment for your hostile go-to-hell behavior, on top of being put out of everyone's way for six hours to three days, depending on the individual. Even when you do regain consciousness you are in a state of disorientation for days. You are unable to think coherently. You can't recall things. Enough of these treatments and a man could turn out like ... drooling, pants-wetting idiot at thirty-five. Or turn into a mindless organism ..."

(New York: Penguin, 1976), p. 59.

49. M. Shoor & F.H. Adams, "The Intensive Electric Shock Therapy of Chronic Disturbed Psychotic Patients," *Am. J. Psychiat.* 107 (1950): 279.

50. Letter of Jan. 17, 1980, quoted with permission.

51. It is well-known that ECT may be responsible for retrogressive amnesia, but what has not been clearly defined is the effect of ECT on autobiographical versus interpersonal memories. Reporting on research, Dr. Frank J. Ayd, Jr., points out that bilateral ECT causes more marked amnesia for events and details than right unilateral ECT, especially for impersonal memories. The results indicate that the amnestic effects of ECT are greatest and most persistent for knowledge about the world, compared with distinctly remote events and for less salient events. Bilateral ECT produces more profound amnestic effects than right unilateral ECT, particularly for memory of impersonal events. F.J. Ayd, "Reading and Reflections," *Psychiatric Times*, Aug. 2001, p. 5. Leonard Roy Frank of San Francisco edited and published a book, *The History of Shock Treatment* (1978), that is highly critical of ECT. The periodical *Madness Network News*, also published in San Francisco, takes aim at ECT.

In a sexual abuse malpractice claim, McNall v. Summers, 25 Cal. App. 4th 1300, 30 Cal. Rptr.2d 914 (1994), the trial judge commented on the expert testimony of Dr. Maria Lymberis, a psychiatrist: "Dr. Lymberis said that women do not like orgasms because it's the same to them as electroshock therapy. And, still, when I go home and I am listening to the radio and I get Dr. Toni Grant or some of these on, there are women calling in all the time wondering how they can achieve orgasm. And here's a woman who says that women do not want it because it's just the most horrible experience that they could possibly have next to electroshock therapy." Dr. Dmitri Dosrtzev, embryologist at Wayne State University School of Medicine, points out that not infrequently women who suffer having an orgasm compare it to ECT. Personal communication (Nov. 11, 1999).

52. Personal communication (Oct. 29, 1999). Ernest Hemingway underwent two series of ECT treatments for depression. Following the treatments, he apparently experienced significant memory loss. He stated: "What these shock doctors don't know is about writers and such things as remorse and contrition and what they do to them. They should make all psychiatrists take a course in creative writing so they'd know about writers. … What is the sense of ruining my head and erasing my memory, which is my capital, and putting me out of business?" Quoted in A.E. Hotchner, *Papa Hemingway* (New York: Da Capo Press, 2005).

53. See P.R. Breggin, *Electroshock: Its Brain-Disabling Effects* (New York: Springer, 1979); P.R. Breggin, *Toxic Psychiatry* (New York: St. Martin's Press, 1991), pp. 184–215; J. Horgan, *The Undiscovered Mind: How the Human Brain Defies Replication, Medication and Explanation* (New York: Free Press, 1999).

54. The regulations or statutes in the various states are set out in V. Harris, "Electroconvulsive Therapy: Administrative Codes, Legislation, and Professional Recommendations," *J. Am. Acad. Psychiat. & Law* 34 (2006): 406. Under California legislation, ECT treatment may not be performed on minors under the age of 12. Minors between the ages of 12 and 16 may be treated with ECT if it is an emergency situation considered necessary to save the life of the minor. The legislation requires that any facility that performs ECT must designate a committee to review all ECT treatments and "verify the appropriateness and need for such treatment"; Calif. § 5326.8.

55. Mitchell v. Robinson, 334 S.W.2d 11 (Mo. 1960).

56. Whether psychiatrists are qualified to give anesthesia for ECT is controversial. See T. Pearlman, M. Loper, & L. Tillery, "Should Psychiatrists Administer Anesthesia for ECT?" *Am. J. Psychiat.* 147 (1990): 1553.

57. See S. Taub, "Electroconvulsive Therapy, Malpractice, and Informed Consent," *J. Psychiat. & Law* 15 (1987): 7.

58. Byrne v. Boadle, 2 H.& C. 722, 159 Eng. Rep. 299 (1863).

59. See D.B. Dobbs, *The Law of Torts* (St. Paul, MN: West, 2000), pp. 370–381.

60. Farber v. Oklon, 40 Cal.2d 503, 253 P.2d 520 (1953); Quinley v. Cocke, 183 Tenn. 428, 192 S.W.2d 992 (1946); Foxluger v. State, 23 Misc. 2d 933, 203 N.Y.S.2d 985 (Sup. Ct. 1960); Johnson v. Rodis, 151 F. Supp. 345 (D.C. 1957), *rev'd on other grounds*, 251 F.2d 917 (D.C. Cir. 1958).

61. Stone v. Proctor, 259 N.C. 633, 131 S.E.2d 297 (1963); see *Standards for Electroshock Treatment* (Washington, DC: American Psychiatric Assn., 1953).

62. Brown v. Moore, 247 F.2d 711 (3d Cir. 1957).

63. Quick v. Benedictine Sisters Hosp. Assn., 257 Minn. 470, 102 N.W.2d 36 (1960); Adams v. Ricks, 91 Ga. 494, 86 S.E.2d 329 (1955).

64. In Wilson v. Lehman, 379 S.W.2d 478 (Ky. 1964), the court held that where there is no evidence of any false representations, a patient's consent to electroshock treatment will be presumed from his voluntary submission to it. Samuel Jan Brakel says: "The principle of informed consent is widely subverted in practice to make it impossible for patients, much less their guardians, to assent to effective, accepted treatment modalities, such as Electroconvulsive Therapy (ECT) (considered the most or only effective treatment for those suffering from severe mood disorders in particular)." S.J. Brakel, "Searching for the Therapy in Therapeutic Jurisprudence," *N. Eng. J. Crim. & Civil Confine.* 33 (2007): 455, at 463.

65. Woods v. Brumlop, 71 N.M. 221, 377 P.2d 520 (1962).

66. Dohmann v. Richard, 282 So.2d 789 (La. App. 1973); discussed in Chapter 20 on duty to minimize damages.

67. Aden v. Younger, 57 Cal. App.3d 662, 129 Cal. Rptr. 535 (1976); Northern California Psychiatric Society v. City of Berkeley, 223 Cal. Rptr. 609 (1986).

68. In obtaining an informed consent, some states require that the patient be told that the risks of ECT are (1) confusion, (2) impairment of memory, and (3) fracture of bones. It is difficult enough to get a patient or family to consent but mentioning the risk of fracture frightens them away. See the standard form that appears herein.

69. According to the American Psychiatric Association, "ECT is the most effective and most rapidly acting treatment available for severe major depression." ECT is also used to treat mania, schizophrenia, bipolar disorder, schizoaffective disorder, catatonia, and Parkinson's disease. *Task Force Report, Electroconvulsive Therapy* (Washington, DC: American Psychiatric Association, 1978).

70. L. Cammer, *Up from Depression* (New York: Simon & Schuster, 1969). In response, Joe Kennedy Adams, PhD, wrote: "Dr. Leonard Cammer, one of electric shock treatment's most outspoken advocates, has tried to allay public fear concerning its use. He believes the 'shock' scares a lot of people and calls the procedure 'electric-stimulation treatment.' I don't believe the word 'shock' in this case scares people nearly enough, and propose that this technique be called 'electric shock torture.'" "You're In for the Shock of Your Life," in S. Hirsch (Ed.), *Madness Network News Reader* (San Francisco: Glide, 1974), p. 84. See also C.H. Kellner & D. Ramsey (ltr.), "Please No More 'ECT,'" *Am. J. Psychiat.* 147 (1990): 1092.

71. See M. Fink, *Electroshock: Restoring the Mind* (New York: Oxford University Press, 1999); D. Smith, "Shock and Disbelief," *Atlantic*, Feb. 2001, p. 79.

72. Quoted in E. Shorter, *A Historical Dictionary of Psychiatry* (New York: Oxford University Press, 2005), p. 95. Kitty Dukakis, in her book about her experience with ECT, strives to counter ECT's negative image among the public. She is the wife of former Massachusetts governor and 1988 Democratic presidential nominee Michael Dukakis. See K. Dukakis & L. Tye, *Shock: The Healing Power of Electroconvulsive Therapy* (New York: Penguin, 2006); see also G. Borzo, "Electroconvulsive Therapy Undergoes Renaissance," *Clinical Psychiatry News*, Sept. 2000, p. 11. At an invited lecture at the American Psychiatric Association's 2007 annual meeting, Dukakis said she was grateful that ECT was her "anniversary gift" (she received her first treatment with ECT on the morning of her 38th wedding anniversary). L. Lamberg, "Dukakis Grateful That ECT Was Her Anniversary Gift," *Psychiatric News*, July 8, 2007, p. 4.

    More than 100,000 people undergo ECT annually in the United States, with about 80% receiving it for depression. Those in the public eye who have received ECT include Judy Garland, Thomas Eagelton, Connie Francis, Jimmy Piersall, Francis Farmer, Janet Frame, Cole Porter, Tammy Wynette, Gene Tierney, Martha Manning, Leonard Roy Frank, Vladimir Horowitz, Ernest Hemingway, Sylvia Plath, William Styron, and Dick Cavett. Reported in Jeffrey Geller, Book Review, *Psychiat. Serv.* 58 (August 2007): 1133. In *People* (Aug. 3, 1992), Dick Cavett wrote that thanks to ECT, he could say, "Goodbye darkness." Psychosurgery, too, is making a comeback in the treatment of obsessive-compulsive disorder (OCD) when not responsive to medication or other treatment. For its use in the treatment of chronic fatigue, see T.M. Burton, "Surgery on the Skull for Chronic Fatigue? Doctors Are Trying It," *Wall Street Journal*, Nov. 11, 1999, p. 1.

73. The National Institute of Mental Health stated in a report: "Given a diagnosis for which the efficacy of ECT has been established, the immediate risk of suicide (when not manageable by other means) is a clear indication for the consideration of ECT. Acute manic episode—especially when characterized by clouded sensorium, dehydration, extreme psychomotor agitation, high risk for serious medical complications or death through exhaustion, and nonresponse to pharmacological interventions—are also clear indications for ECT. The severe and unremitting nature of the patient's emotional suffering, or extreme incapacitation, are also important considerations." "Electroconvulsive Therapy," *Consensus Development Conference Statement*, 1985, vol 5, no. 11. See also J. Markowitz, R. Brown, J. Sweeney, & J.J. Mann, "Reduced Length and Cost of Hospital Stay for Major Depression in Patients Treated With ECT," *Am. J. Psychiat.* 144 (1987): 1025; S. Squire, "Shock Therapy's Return to Respectability," *New York Times Magazine*, Nov. 22, 1987, p. 78; G. Stone, "When Prozac Fails ... Electroshock Works," *New Yorker*, Nov. 14, 1994, p. 55. A consumer-oriented mental health organization, however, insists that the NIMH report presents an incomplete picture of ECT and overlooks serious problems." "Consumer Group Criticizes Unpublished ECT Report," *Psychiatric News*, Nov. 5, 1999, p. 1.

74. Quoted in *Roche Report/Frontiers of Psychiatry*, March 1, 1980, p. 1.

75. Personal communication (Nov. 9, 1999). See M. Fink, *Electroshock: Restoring the Mind* (New York: Oxford University Press, 1999); see also M. Fink (ltr.), "Treating Depression," *New York Times*, Oct. 8, 1999, p. 30. Dr. Fink has a Web site dedicated "to helping both psychiatrists and patients better understand electroconvulsive therapy and how best to take advantage of its benefits." The Web site is: www.electroshock.org

76. Some litigation may be noted. In Shafran v. St. Vincent's Hospital, 694 N.Y.S.2d 641 (N.Y. App. 1999), the patient suffered status epilepticus that lasted for several hours, she lapsed into a coma for approximately 10 days, and sustained permanent injuries including bilateral deafness, memory loss, and seizure disorder. These injuries persisted until she died six years later. At trial the jury returned a verdict

in favor of the defendants, but the appellate court reversed, remanding the case for a new trial, on the ground that the trial judge had improperly excluded defense experts. In McNall v. Summers, 25 Cal. App. 4th 1300, 30 Cal. Rptr.2d 914 (1994), the trial court ruled that the 3-year statute of limitations for commencing suit had run out on a claim that ECT was negligently administered. The appellate court reversed, remanding for a new trial, on the ground that memory loss suspended the running of the prescriptive period. In Andre v. Mecta Corp., 186 A.D.2d 1, 587 N.Y.S.2d 334 (1992), the patient brought a products liability claim against the manufacturer of the ECT machine, claiming inadequacy of warnings about memory loss. The court held that the manufacturer is not liable to a patient for any failure to warn the hospital or its staff of the side effects of the treatment with the machine. The court noted that the side effect of memory loss was well known to the hospital staff and even appears as one of the "rare or uncommon side effects" in the printed consent form signed by the patient.

77. Aden v. Younger, 57 Cal App.3d 662, 129 Cal. Rptr. 535 (1976); see M. Shapiro, "Legislating the Control of Behavior Control: Autonomy and the Coercive Use of Organic Therapies," S. Cal. L. Rev. 47 (1974): 237.

78. D. Goleman, "Psychiatry: First Guide to Therapy Is Fiercely Opposed," New York Times, Sept. 23, 1986, p. C1.

79. To illustrate, in James v. Woolley, 523 So.2d 110 (Ala. 1988), the Alabama Supreme Court upheld a finding of negligence in the choice of a vaginal delivery rather than a cesarean section by relying, in part, on the physician's failure to comply with the American College of Obstetrics and Gynecologists' guidelines recommending a cesarean delivery for infants estimated to weigh more than 4 kilograms. In Pollard v. Goldsmith, 572 P.2d 1201(Ariz. App.), the Arizona Court of Appeals found evidence of a violation of the standard of care in failing to follow the guidelines set by the American College of Surgeons' Prophylaxis Against Tetanus and Wound Management, which require that patients with wounds indicating an overwhelming possibility of tetanus be given human immune globulin. D.W. Shuman, "The Standard of Care in Medical Malpractice Claims, Clinical Practice Guidelines, and Managed Care: Towards a Therapeutic Harmony?" Cal. West. L. Rev. 34 (1997): 99.

80. The American Psychiatric Press advertises the second edition of Treatments of Psychiatric Disorder as "the treatment companion to DSM-IV. It is a compendium of state-of-the-art treatments of all major psychiatric disorders." In the editor's words, it offers "useful approaches" rather than "rigid guidelines."

81. Guidelines are meant to improve medical care by codifying what panels of experts deem to be best practice in a given field, but the problem is that many physicians are unaware of any number of guidelines, and those who read them often fail or refuse to follow their recommendations. M.D. Cabana et al., "Why Don't Physicians Follow Clinical Practice Guidelines? A Framework for Improvement," JAMA, Oct. 20, 1999, p. 1458; M. Sherman, "Study Finds Lapses on Medical Guidelines," New York Times, Nov. 2, 1999, p. D-10.

The term practice parameters, as used by the American Medical Association, encompasses (1) standards, which are generally accepted principles for patient management; (2) guidelines, which are recommendations for patient management that may identify a particular management strategy or a range of strategies; and (3) other patient management strategies, such as practice options and practice advisories. As a rule, a practice parameter may be introduced as evidence of the standard of care in malpractice litigation, provided that it is relevant to the clinical issues involved and meets certain indicia of reliability. E.B. Hirshfeld, "Should Practice Parameters Be the Standard of Care in Malpractice Litigation?" JAMA 266 (Nov. 27, 1991): 2886.

82. Comments of Dr. R. N. Bhavsar, Director of Education at Northville State Hospital, at conference on March 19, 1998.

83. 42 U.S.C.A., §§11101-11152.

84. "National Practitioner Data Bank: Major Improvements Are Needed to Enhance Data Bank's Reliability" (GAO-01-130, Nov. 30, 2000). See also J. Aske, "Disciplinary Actions: Report to the National Practitioner Data Bank Constitutes Defamation," Am. L.L. & Med. 27 (2001) 147, M. Kadzielski, "The National Practitioner Data Bank: Big Brother or Paper Tiger?" HealthSpan (July/Aug. 1992), p. 8; J. Lovitky, "The National Practitioner Data Bank: Coping with the Uncertainties," J. Health L. 33 (2000): 355; J. Reichert, "Researchers Questions Reliability of National Practitioner Data Bank," Trial 35 (Nov. 1992): 102.

85. R. Pear, "Incompetent Physicians Are Rarely Reported as Law Requires," New York Times, May 29, 2001.

86. Malpractice judgments and settlements must be reported to the medical license board as well as to the NPDB. Hospital and managed care organization disciplinary actions must also be reported to the medical license board as well as to the NPDP. Then too, anyone can file a complaint with the Board of Medicine. Medical license sanctions are required to be reported by the physician to all hospitals where the physician has privileges, to the physician's employer, in many instances to all the physician's

patients, and to the NPDB. It is not unusual for a license sanction, even a minor one such as a fine, or a managed care termination or some other negative event, to result in many inquiries for insurers, managed care programs and hospitals that can often lead to suspension or termination of participation or privileges. Moreover, an action in one state can lead to an action in another state where a physician is licensed.

In Estate of Phuoc Fazaldin v. Englewood Hosp. & Medical Center, (N.J. Super. App. Div., Docket No. A-4948-04T34948-04TC), decided in 2007, the court was faced with the question of the responsibility of a hospital and its department chair for failure to report in accordance with the NPDP and the state licensing authorities. The alleged result was the death of the plaintiff's decedent at the hands of an incompetent physician. The court held that failure to report could give rise to liability. The case was remanded for an evidentiary hearing.

29

Admission or Apology in Liability Prevention

Admissions play a role as proof of fault in all types of cases, but they have special importance in cases of malpractice (professional negligence). Unlike in ordinary negligence cases, expert testimony is required as a matter of law to prove a case of malpractice. An admission obviates that requirement.[1] A party is in no position to complain that when making the statement, he was not under oath or subject to cross-examination. After all, it is that person's own statement. "Anything that you say may be used against you," according to the familiar phrase.[2]

When, if ever then, should a physician make an admission of wrongdoing or of an error or to express sorrow? Should the physician always send a bill because failure to do so might indicate culpability? Should the physician ever say to a patient, "I'm sorry?" Good manners are essential for social life, but given the risk of litigation, one must be wary. A Tokyo office worker, reminiscing about living for a while in New York, said that Japanese friends in that city had advised her not to apologize too readily to Americans when confrontations arose. In the United States, they warned, saying "sorry" could be taken as an admission of wrongdoing, inviting legal action. The Japanese are a people who apologize profusely.[3]

A Miami attorney, Samuel J. Powers, Jr., had this to say in an address to a medical association:

> Some things that happen in your practice have a severe emotional impact on you. It's only natural to sympathize with a patient. Some physicians, emotionally overwrought under such conditions make statements to the effect that they're sorry this or that happened, as though they hoped to lessen its impact on the patient or on his relatives, but all they are really doing is digging their own graves. People nowadays are conscious of the fertility of this field of malpractice suits, and they remember those statements when you go to trial.[4]

To be courteous is to let down one's guard and invite disaster. The word *sorry* in conjunction with other language or circumstances may constitute an admission.[5] From experience, one physician writes, "In today's legal climate, doctors grieve, and apologize, at their own peril."[6] In an Oklahoma case, the doctor diagnosed the patient's condition as a tumor, but when he operated, he found that she was pregnant. The doctor then told the woman and her husband, "I'm sorry, I should have done more tests on you." The only witnesses at the trial were the plaintiff and her husband, who testified as to this statement, and the doctor, the defendant, who was only asked his qualifications. The Oklahoma Supreme Court ruled that the remark was sufficient to make a prima facie case of malpractice, and it remanded the case to be tried before a jury.[7]

Was the doctor's statement an admission of negligence? Apart from this statement, and the harm done, there was no evidence to show that the doctor's conduct was unskillful and not in accord with the work of physicians of good standing. Suppose an attorney loses a case and says to his client, "I'm sorry. I lost your case. I should have done more research." Will this statement alone be sufficient to take the case against the attorney to the jury even though the attorney may have in reality done much more than the average attorney in the community might have done?[8] Bob Eaton, then Chairman and CEO of Chrysler Corporation, observed, "There's a disconnect between what we were taught in civics class and the way the adult world really works. And the word for that disconnect is cynicism. ... [Y]ou can't say 'I'm sorry' anymore."[9]

Concerned by what might be said, lawyers advise doctors not to go to the funeral of a patient. Physicians at funerals are heard to say, "We did the best we could." But how good was that? Does it, in fact, measure up to the standard of care?

The statement "I'm sorry" should not be sufficient to establish fault, says one commentator in a law review article, "for this is what every decent human would say when the desired result was not accomplished even though he performed at his highest capability, which might be far above that of his colleagues in his community. ... On the other hand, one should not have to spell out everything that the law requires in order to hold the defendant doctor negligent."[10]

Two leading authorities on the law of evidence, Stephen Saltzburg and Kenneth Redden, are not very reassuring in a lengthy comment in their manual on the Federal Rules of Evidence about the effect of an apology.[11] Massachusetts in 1986 enacted a so-called sorry law that excludes an expression of sorrow as an admission. It provides: "Statements, writings, or benevolent gestures expressing sympathy or a general sense of benevolence relating to the pain, suffering, or death of a person involved in an accident and made to such a person or to the family of such a person shall be inadmissible as evidence of an admission of liability in a civil action."[12] Beginning in 1999, the legislatures in some 34 states, including California, Florida, Georgia, Ohio, Oklahoma, Oregon, Texas, and Wyoming, have enacted legislation patterned after that in Massachusetts, and Vermont made a similar change via a judicial opinion.

Paul Appelbaum and Thomas Gutheil have urged regional professional societies to promote the enactment of similar legislation in other states.[13] In 2006, Senators Hillary Rodham Clinton and Barack Obama introduced legislation, the Medical Error Disclosure and Compensation Act, laying out a two-apology approach whereby expressions of sympathy would be made immediately to patients and expressions of remorse and discussions of accountability would be offered only after a full investigation, but the bill did not make it out of committee. In any event, the legislation and judicial opinions that have come about only ensure freedom to say one is sorry, but not other types of admissions. Thus, if someone says, "I'm sorry, this is all my fault, I was yelling at my wife on my cell phone and wasn't looking," everything after "I'm sorry" is admissible in evidence as an admission. Florida's legislation expressly preserves the admissibility of statements that acknowledge fault.[14] Colorado's statute allows medical providers to apologize to the patient or family and include not just words of benevolence and sympathy, but a full admission of fault. (One might wonder why the sorry legislation is limited to the health care industry.)

Legal departments of companies are concerned about the legal impact of an apology, so they provide an apology that does not really say anything.

Trial lawyers are wary of legislative efforts that might too broadly define the apology to include other evidence, such as medical records or nurses' testimony. The legislation has to be narrowly crafted, they argue, so as not to include evidence of negligence that would otherwise be admissible and discoverable.

Are physicians between a rock and a whirlpool? On the one hand, admissions or even an apology may be used against the physician as evidence in a malpractice suit, while on the other hand, the physician is told that the physician–patient relationship is improved by leveling with the patient and thereby lessening the risk of a malpractice suit. Countless times we hear doctors or others advising doctors: "People sue when they are angry, so say you are sorry."[15] "A warm relationship with a patient is the best defense against malpractice. You don't have a warm relationship when you regard the patient as an adversary."[16]

In an article in the *Washington Lawyer*, it is noted that the apology has now taken on a near-mythic quality in the healthcare arena, owing in no small part to the national movement to break through the secrecy shrouding hospitals after an adverse medical event occurs or a medical error comes to light.[17] As a part of this movement the "Sorry Works! Coalition," a Glen Carbon, Illinois, group is made up of physicians, lawyers, mediators, and government officials, who promotes a swift apology and early settlement negotiation. But apologies have become so ubiquitous in healthcare and elsewhere that their meaning and value are easily diminished by sheer volume.

Several states, e.g., Florida, Nevada, New Jersey, New York, Pennsylvania, and Vermont, now require that hospitals or physicians disclose to patients that an adverse outcome has occurred, usually within 7 days of the occurrence or discovery of the event.[18] Years earlier, Joan Vogel and Richard Delgado in a law review article urged the enactment in law of an affirmative duty on the physician to disclose medical mistakes or malpractice. In support of that enactment, they said that if the primary physician and other members of the treatment team conceal malpractice, the patient might believe that his pain, debilitation, or loss of function is merely unfortunate results of the operation or procedure. A duty to disclose malpractice is necessary, they contended, because the medical profession does not regulate itself effectively, discourages the reporting of malpractice to patients, and erects formal and informal barriers to a patient's access to information. This proposed duty to disclose malpractice is consistent, they said, with current trends in tort law, such as the development of the doctrines of informed consent, collective responsibility, duty to warn, and duty to supervise. It would remedy a serious imbalance in the physician–patient relationship, as well as enable some victims of malpractice to obtain relief who would otherwise be unable to do so, and would give tangible expression, they said, to the moral imperative that professionals who injure their clients must inform them of the injury.[19]

The Patient Safety and Quality Improvement Act of 2005[20] seeks to encourage healthcare providers to voluntarily report medical errors to patient safety organizations. The concept is that the compilation and analysis of such data will identify trends and assist in the development of methods to prevent future medical errors. The database will not identify specific patient or provider information. Patients will not be permitted to use the data as evidence in medical malpractice lawsuits or other litigation and the accrediting bodies or governmental or nongovernmental regulators will not use the data to take action against providers.[21]

The National Practitioner Data Bank (NPDB), adopted in 1990, is designed to share information about physicians' performance with medical facilities and state licensing and credentialing organizations, but it is not open to the public.[22] The confidentiality of the peer review process, however, is going by the board. Florida in 2006 gave patients "a right to have access to any records made or received in the course of business … relating to any adverse medical incident," including incidents "reported to or reviewed by any … peer review, risk management, quality assurance, credentials, or similar committee."[23] Federal law does not shield the peer review process.

Of course, physicians who misrepresent the nature, outcome, or prognosis of a completed procedure, or who either by silence or reassurance willfully conceal the state of the patient's condition, may be liable for fraud.[24] Physicians have an obligation to tell the truth about a patient's condition, even if that would reveal one's own or a prior physician's negligence.[25] In such cases, unless disclosure is made, the statute of limitations will be tolled as to fraud, and if other physicians are involved, conspiracy as well. Therefore, writes Dr. Robert M. Wettstein, a patient with tardive dyskinesia (TD), who comes to the physician for diagnosis or treatment, should be told he has the condition, regardless of whether he inquires specifically about it or whether it is a consequence of present or past negligence. Dr. Wettstein says, "The physician should not deny, if the patient asks, and arguably should volunteer if the patient does not ask, that the TD is a result of negligence, if the clinician believes this to be the case."[26]

C. G. Schoenfeld, the late book editor of the *Journal of Psychiatry & Law*, said that he filed a negligence suit against a hospital "only because it wouldn't say it was sorry." His mother was dropped by nurses in transferring her from a stretcher to a bed, fractured her hip, and she then died from complications following the injury. The jury awarded him $176,000. He said, "If they had just faced up to what they did and sat down with me and said, 'We're sorry,' I would never have sued. They did the one thing that you never do to a man who has suffered the terrible loss of a loved one—they insulted my intelligence with tortured explanations."[27]

A television documentary, *Diagnosis: Malpractice*, began with a patient saying, "I was forced to sue. No one came to me and said, 'We're sorry, we made a mistake.'"[28] The viewpoint is often heard that patients often sue physicians or hospitals not so much for the original mistake, as for the lack of openness and honesty and the wish to see the physician called to accountability. In a study, when patients were asked whether "once the original accident had occurred, could anything have been done that would have meant you did not feel the need to take legal action?" Forty-one percent (not 100%) of the respondents replied, "yes," and gave as the most important reason, "explanation and apology."[29]

Studies of institutions that have adopted policies of disclosure or apology, and quick settlement of claims that are determined to have merit, have been done notably at the Veterans Affairs Medical Center in Lexington, Virginia, and at the University of Michigan Health System. They report that as a result of the policy, cases settle more quickly, self-reporting of errors by the medical professionals has increased, the hospital has received positive publicity, and litigation costs have declined. The VA hospital in Lexington was in the top 20% of facilities in terms of the amount of total payments. At the University of Michigan Health System, its policy of encouraging full disclosure of errors and apologies to patients when warranted reportedly resulted in a drop from 260 claims in 2001 when the policy was implemented to fewer than 100 pending in 2007.[30] The University of Michigan has not released data on the average payment under its program.

However, a number of factors make it problematical to generalize from the experience in Lexington and the University of Michigan to healthcare settings more generally. The VA is not subject to punitive damages, federal government cases are determined by a judge instead of a jury, the personal liability exposure of the providers in the system differs from that of providers in the private sector, and the patients are not representative of the broader population and may have access to additional sources of compensation.[31] And the decline at the University of Michigan Health System must be considered in the context of medical malpractice actions generally in Michigan, where as a result of the decisions of the state Supreme Court and legislation, it is rare for a patient to succeed in a malpractice action. Many trial lawyers in Michigan specializing in malpractice have abandoned the practice in droves.

By and large, the expression of sympathy may lead to some form of utterance which, in the hands of a skillful lawyer, might be turned into an "admission" of wrongdoing. It is like walking a tightrope to express sympathy and concern without its being turned into an admission of liability.

Should one attempt it, or should one act as a motorist involved in an accident, adopt bludgeoning tactics and blame the other party? Are good manners incompatible with the law, or with insurance coverage? Insurers are often blamed for much of the lack of courtesy because, as a rule, most liability insurance policies will have a provision saying that after an accident, one must not make any admission of liability. The following clause is typical: "The insured shall not, except at his own cost, voluntarily admit his liability, or offer or promise any payment, assume any obligation, or incur any expense other than for first aid to others at the time of the accident." Premiums, if not coverage, will be affected.

Liability insurance companies consider an admission by the insured party that he has done something wrong as failure of cooperation, voiding insurance coverage. Insurers insert cooperation clauses into insurance policies in an attempt to prevent any collusion and to eliminate any connivance between the insured and a third-party claimant. An admission of liability would detrimentally affect the insurer's ability to conduct an effective defense against the claim. Therefore, before a physician should ever state to a patient that he did something wrong, he needs to be aware of what effect such a statement might have on his insurance coverage. Thus, in a pragmatic sense, there are definite reasons why a physician should refrain from stating that something is or is not his fault unless he has cleared it with his insurance company.

Consider what others do. When a street criminal commits a crime, he remains silent or says, "I didn't do it." When large companies are charged with violating the law, its spokesmen turn to gobbledygook, or they have no comment: "The charges are so ridiculous that they are unworthy of comment." Or they pass the buck: "Under normal conditions, our product is accident-proof, but we can't guarantee it when the consumer doesn't follow the instructions."

Lawyers and negotiators do not make admissions, but they do not lie; they dissemble. A law professor says, "In representing a client, lawyers can be dishonest. They can twist and bend because everyone knows that's what they do."[32] "Just remember that lying can get you into a lot of trouble if not done properly," advises a lawyer. That was in a cartoon, but many would say it is true to life.[33]

Lawyers understand the importance of never admitting to anything—it's the lawyer's commandment. It is most important, at least from a legal perspective, to say nothing; particularly, to admit no guilt or responsibility whatsoever. In a discussion on automobile accidents, a commentator on national television advised: "Don't apologize. Don't say anything about it."[34] That is typical lawyer advice. "If you start explaining or apologizing to the victim," says a lawyer specializing in insurance cases, "you will be giving him crucial evidence for a suit against you."[35]

There is a classical parable (about the M'raglim [spies]) that describes the process of becoming lost. One does not suddenly find himself in the depths of a dark, trackless forest, but instead, one deviates from the familiar, broad roadway a step at a time. Gradually and imperceptibly, one strays farther and farther from the road until one ends up lost in the forest.

A woman, whose husband was negligently killed by a third party, confessed her feelings to a friend, "The freedom is wonderful. I'm enjoying life now as never before. I'm glad he's dead." Being completely honest about one's feelings may be healthy, confession may be good for the soul, but in a wrongful death action, the value of the case is jeopardized by introduction of this evidence.[36]

The compulsion to confess—or boast, if you will—has resulted in crucial evidence in criminal as well as in civil cases. "People love to spill their guts, and they hang themselves."[37] Ernesto Miranda, whose name is given to the warning that police must give a suspect before questioning, was in the end convicted on the basis of statements he made to a girlfriend about the crime.[38] James Earl Ray boasted while imprisoned in London of participating in a conspiracy to kill civil rights leader Martin Luther King, Jr. A London policeman, who overheard Ray make the comments after his arrest, was the lead-off witness in the hearings.[39]

Many times a physician ends up with a result that is not satisfactory and there is always a question as to what caused the detrimental outcome. While it is important for the physician to be open and honest with the patient about the patient's problem or condition, it is not necessary, however, for the physician to tell a patient what might constitute legal fault for any adverse development. Apart from other considerations, there is a very real risk that such an opinion will later be proven to be wrong. In many cases, a physician thinks he is responsible for a problem (or, probably more often, he feels some other physician or entity is responsible for the problem) when later, after all the evidence has been gathered, it becomes clear that someone else is responsible. During or immediately following treatment, it is usually premature for physicians to attribute fault when indicating to a patient what has happened. For example, if a sponge has been left in during surgery, the patient should be told about this problem (the patient will likely find out about it anyway), but the doctor need not make a determination as to who is to blame for it. It might have been a nurse's fault, or a doctor's fault, or both.

As a result, physicians ought not to admit fault, regardless of what may have occurred. This may not comport with the ideal of physician–patient rapport, but it is appropriate, given the complexities of the legal ramifications of the relationships. While a physician has a duty to say, for example, the ureter was injured during surgery, he does not have an obligation to tell the patient whether that injury was or was not the result of his negligence. To be sure, a physician provokes a lawsuit when he is dismissive of a patient or lacks empathy, but it is one thing to say, "I'm sorry this turned out badly," and quite another to admit negligence.[40]

As a matter of practice, the physician usually does not say, "Sorry, I gave you the wrong medicine," but rather, "I'm going to change your prescription." Because the physician seldom admits either a mistake or malpractice, it makes it more precious for the lawyer to latch onto any statement, where in front of third persons, in court, or in his own hospital records, the doctor confesses he goofed. The situation is a *tabula in naufragio* (a plank in a shipwreck). Hospital or other medical records as well as depositions are an important source of admissions. That is why the plaintiff's attorney goes over the records or deposition with a fine-tooth comb, and why doctors and other personnel must be careful about what is noted. Nowadays, many law firms have nurses or other medical personnel on their full-time staff just to study and advise on material in medical records.

The altering of records (or other conduct of that ilk) is commonly regarded as an admission. The courts often speak of a "presumption" against the spoliator. By resorting to wrongful devices, the individual is said to give ground for believing that he thinks his case is weak and not to be won by fair means. Accordingly, a party's false statement about the matter in litigation, whether before suit or on the stand; his fabrication of false documents; his destruction or concealment of relevant documents or objects; his undue pressure, by bribery or intimidation or other means, to influence a witness to testify for him or to avoid testifying; his attempt to corrupt the jury; and/or his hiding or transferring property in anticipation of judgment are all instances of admission by conduct.[41]

Statements made by the physician to his attorney are protected by the attorney–client privilege, but what about statements made by the physician to an investigator of his own insurer? Are these communications privileged? In law, there is no insurer–insured privilege similar to that of the attorney–client privilege. Is the insurer's investigator to be considered an agent of the attorney, though the investigator is not in the employ of the attorney, thus entitling communications to be the work product of the attorney? By and large, the courts say that the statements are in preparation for trial within the meaning of the work product rule and, therefore, the plaintiff must show prejudice, hardship, or injustice, and good cause in order to obtain a production order. As this can usually be shown, these statements are subject to discovery.[42]

Some physicians, when sued, call the suing party or attorney, telling them it is all a misunderstanding and asking to drop the lawsuit. Caught up in the emotional side of litigation, they fail to see how the legal system works, and they make statements often to their detriment.

Some lawyers representing a complainant will, as part of the investigation of the case, consult with the treating doctor to get his side of the story. Doctors often decry the abuse of the legal process, including the filing of a suit without interviewing them, but when that is done, it may inure to the disadvantage of the doctors. What he says (except in the course of a settlement negotiation) can be used against him. Many lawyers, it must be noted, consider it unethical to "get the doctor's side of the story" without the doctor having legal assistance, for that would be an underhanded way of getting admissions.[43] As discussed in Chapter 30 on confidentiality, the Health Insurance Portability and Accountability Act (HIPAA), where applicable, precludes *ex parte* communications between defense attorneys and plaintiff's treating physicians.

One lawyer who defends the practice of consulting with the treating doctor, but telling him that he may wish to have his lawyer present, says: "Invariably there are two sides to every story. Should I wait until filing a complaint to find out just what are the basic facts? I say to the doctor, 'We want to have your version. We want to truly find out what happened.'" If the doctor replies,

"I'm not going to talk to you," the lawyer at trial (if put into evidence) may argue to the jury, "We tried to talk with the doctor, we asked for an explanation, but he wouldn't talk to us."[44]

What about utterances not intended for the outside world, as in an internal report or where one makes entries in a secret diary, or in process notes, or where one is overheard talking to oneself? Are they admissible in evidence?

Organizations of every type, be it a hospital or a television company, have to be able to take a look back at their own work when questions arise so that they can correct mistakes, but members of the organization will likely not be candid about their failures if they know those reports might later be used against them or the organization. Legally, however, internal investigative reports are generally not shielded from discovery.[45] Most jurisdictions do not recognize a "self-critical analysis" privilege. Thus, to take an example, the evaluation and recommendation portion of a report prepared by a chemical company's employees concerning a tank car derailment, which gave rise to a lawsuit, was not exempt from discovery.[46] Peer review reports, however, are privileged, except in Florida.

In a complaint against a physician, the patient has a right to discover process notes as well as the records of the physician. Process notes (or information in a computer) may be analogized to a diary. Notes in a diary may be used not withstanding the ordinary expectation of privacy. A seizure of a diary does not violate the Fourth Amendment's prohibition of "unreasonable searches and seizures." John W. Hinckley Jr.'s diary was used as evidence against him.[47] In a child custody case, a diary in which the father recorded his feelings about the child was used against him. As stated in the Advisory Committee's notes to the Federal Rules of Evidence, "[A] party's books or records are usable against him, without regard to any intent to disclose to third persons."[48]

Even statements made in prayer may be used as evidence. A case that went to the British Columbia Court of Appeal involved an accused who, in his cell, slid off his chair, fell to his knees, raised his hands and prayed, "Oh, God, let me get away with it just this once." The room was equipped with a video camera and concealed microphone. The supplication was offered as evidence. Though he was speaking to God, the appellate court allowed the introduction of the evidence as an admission. A dissent would have excluded the statement on the grounds that it was made in complete privacy.[49]

Given the negative consequences in law of an apology or admission, the crucial question becomes: Does the apology or admission so enhance the physician–patient relationship that litigation is put out of mind? Is it really helpful to therapy to be apologetic or to admit mistakes? Or does it just get the doctor into more difficulty? And what does it do to the magic in the art of healing?

And do we say "I'm sorry" because we truly feel remorse for a wrongdoing we have done, or is it merely a way to ease our conscience between now and the next time we hurt someone? Some neurotics, whether they cause harm or not, are always saying they are sorry. Psychiatrists recognize it as masochism.[50] On the other hand, some people are so ill-mannered that they do not apologize or admit wrongdoing whatever the circumstances.

Actually, the failure to admit error or to express sorrow is only one form of irritation that may prompt a lawsuit. Apart from psychoanalysts, physicians tend not to be mindful about the time that patients spend waiting in the office. Airlines overbook, infuriating passengers, and physicians schedule several patients for the same time, and they do not apologize when they are late. Patients consider it unprofessional, if not unethical, and they become angry, ready to sue on any pretext.[51] There is always the hope of hitting the jackpot in the litigation lottery.

One might suggest that if there is a positive transference, the patient will recognize that the physician is only human and makes mistakes, but if there is a negative transference, the admission or apology will just fuel the discord. In Erich Segal's *Love Story*, love means not having to say you're sorry.[52] But what a thin line separates love from hate. People will slap you on the back one day and feel like slapping your face the next. A taxi driver says, "Lovers come in my cab and leave as enemies."[53] But be that as it may, patients know that the real defendant in a malpractice suit, the one who will be paying the judgment, is not the doctor, beloved or not, but the insurance company.

At a recent annual meeting of the Association of American Trial Lawyers, an organization of lawyers representing plaintiffs, word got around that physicians were urging colleagues to confess errors to their patients. They exclaimed, "That's wonderful!"

In a recent article in the *New England Journal of Medicine*, it was observed, "Overall, disclosure probably will not have the chilling effect on litigation that some advocates have claimed. Although disclosure may quell some patients' interest in litigation, it will ignite interest in others, particularly those who would never have known of their injury in the absence of disclosure."[54]

Empirical research that has been done suggests that apologies have the potential to facilitate the settlement of healthcare disputes. The effect of apologies, however, is likely to be complex and dependent on a variety of factors including the nature of the apology, the situation, and the parties involved.[55]

Endnotes

1. Illustration may be noted of the physician's statement justifying the case going to the jury without the necessity of expert testimony. "Oops, I cut in the wrong place," was the evidence used against a surgeon in Orozco v. Henry Ford Hosp., 408 Mich. 248, 290 N. W. 2d 263 (1980). In Hill v. McCartney, 590 N. W. 2d 52 (Iowa App. 1998), a dentist's statement that he "did something freaky" was held to be enough of an admission to stand as patient's expert testimony for trial. In Sheffield v. Runner, 163 Cal. App. 2d 48, 328 P. 2d 828, 830 (1958), where the patient died in her home from pneumonia, the doctor said, "I should have put her in the hospital." In Wickoff v. James, 159 Cal. App. 2d 664, 324 P. 2d 661 (1958), where the patient's intestine was torn during a sigmoidoscopic examination, the doctor said, "Boy, I sure made a mess out of things." In Pappa v. Bonner, 268 Ala. 185, 105 So. 2d 87 (1958), involving damage to a young child's central nervous system, the doctor admitted the child was not given proper postoperative care. In Lashley v. Koerber, 26 Cal. 2d 83, 156 P. 2d 441 (1945), the physician admitted he should have x-rayed and said that it was his own fault. In Stickman v. Synhorst, 243 Iowa 872, 52 N. W. 2d 504, 506 (1952), involving catastrophic hemorrhage, the doctor said, "I don't know whether I can perform that operation [on another person] after the mess I made out of you." In Wooten v. Curry, 50 Tenn. App. 549, 362 S. W. 2d 820 (1961), noted in *NACCA L. J.* 28 (1961–62): 163, a malpractice action for failure to make a postoperative examination to prevent a patient's vagina from closing following a hysterectomy, the doctor said he was sorry it happened and could probably have avoided it if he had made the proper postoperative examinations. See D. W. Louisell & H. Williams, *Medical Malpractice* (Albany, NY: Matthew Bender, 1969), vol. 1,§ 11.28.90; T.F. Lambert, "Law in the Future," *Trial*, Aug. 1983, p. 62. But cf. Locke v. Pachtman, 446 Mich. 216, 521 N. W. 2d 786 (1994).
2. F.W. Cleary (Ed.), *McCormick on Evidence* (St. Paul: West, 3rd ed., 1984), p. 774.
3. C. Haberman, "Japan, Land of a Million Mea Culpa's," *New York Times*, Oct. 4, 1986, p. 4.
4. "'Witless Pedantry' Is Blamed in 90% of Malpractice Suits," *Medical Tribune*, Dec. 7, 1962, p. 12.
5. Giangrasso v. Schimmel, 190 Neb. 228, 207 N. W. 2d 517 (1973). In Peterson v. Richards, 73 Utah 459, 272 P. 229 (1928), the doctor said that he was sorry about the condition of the patient's hand. The patient's fingers were in some manner injured in the hospital. In a malpractice action, the doctor's statements were used against him as an admission. In Wojcik v. Hutzel Hospital, Circuit Court for Wayne County, Michigan, case no. 84-420-030, the doctor said to the patient in the presence of several witnesses that "different doctors perform this surgery in different ways" and that he was "sorry."
6. A.J. Dajer (ltr.), "Physicians and Fate," *New York Times*, April 24, 2001, p. D-3.
7. Greenwood v. Harris, 362 P. 2d 85 (Okla., 1961).
8. Following a collision, a motorist says, "Thank God I've got insurance." It is debatable whether it is an admission of fault. See Wilbur v. Tourangeau, 71 A. 2d 565 (Vt. 1950); A.H. Travers, "An Essay on the Determination of Relevancy Under the Federal Rules of Evidence," *Ariz. St. L. J.* 1977: 327. In some cases the physician admits his error, says he will not send a bill, and indeed, announces that he will pay for the second or subsequent corrective surgery. Barrette v. Hight, 353 Mass. 268, 230 N. E. 2d 808 (1967). Under Rule 409 of the Federal Rules of Evidence, evidence of furnishing or offering or

promising to pay medical, hospital, or similar expenses occasioned by an injury is not admissible to prove liability for the injury. The rule is designed to encourage people to help others when a problem arises for which one party may feel some responsibility, even if not legal responsibility.

9. "No Joking Matter" ("My Turn" column), *Newsweek*, Sept. 23, 1996, p. 20. 10.

10. Note, *Okla. L. Rev.* 15 (1962): 476.

11. S.A. Saltzburg & K. R. Redden, *Federal Rules of Evidence Manual* (Charlottesville, VA: Michie, 3rd ed., 1982), p. 199.

12. Mass. Gen. Laws, c. 233, s. 23 D.

13. P.S. Appelbaum & T.G. Gutheil, *Clinical Handbook of Psychiatry and the Law* (Philadelphia: Lippincott Williams & Wilkins, 4th ed., 2007) pp. 147–148. In Australia, every state and territory has introduced legislation that promotes the making of apologetic statements in civil proceedings. A. Allan, "Apology in Civil Law: A Psycho-Legal Perspective," *Psychiat., Psychol. & Law* 14 (2007): 5.

14. Fla. Stat. Ann. 590, 4026 (2) (1995).

15. Communication by Dr. Bruno Bettelheim to Ralph Slovenko (July 26, 1983).

16. Comment by Dr. Gene L. Usdin in 1986 Distinguished Lectureship, "The Stress and Gratification of a Physician," at Tulane University School of Medicine. Admissions or apologies are recommended in S.S. Kraman & G. Hamm, "Risk Management: Extreme Honesty May Be the Best Policy," *Ann. of Intern. Med.* 131 (1999): 963; S. Keeva, "Does Law Mean Never Having to Say You're Sorry?" *ABAJ*, Dec. 1999, p. 64; D.W. Shuman, "The Role of Apology in Tort Law," *Judicature* 83 (2000): 180; A.W. Wu, T.A. Kavanaugh, S.J. McPhee, B. Lo, & G.P. Micco, "To Tell the Truth," *J. Gen. Intern. Med.* 12 (1997): 770; D. Grady, "Doctors Urged to Admit Mistakes," *New York Times*, Dec. 9, 1997, B-15.

17. S. Kellogg, "The Art and Power of the Apology," *Washington Lawyer*, June 2007, p. 21.

18. See, e.g., S. Kershaw, "In Bid for Transparency, New York City Puts Data on Hospital Errors Online," *New York Times*, Sept. 7, 2007, p. 26.

19. J. Vogel & R. Delgado, "To Tell the Truth: Physicians' Duty to Disclose Medical Mistakes," *U.C.L.A. Law Rev.* 28 (1980): 52.

20. PL 109-41.

21. The American Medical Association and the American Hospital Association have vehemently opposed mandatory reporting of errors. They contend that if doctors and hospital employees fear being sued, they will be reluctant to discuss the lessons that could be learned from their mistakes. R. Pear, "Clinton Order Steps to Reduce Medical Mistakes," *New York Times*, Feb. 22, 2000, p. 1.

22. There have been efforts to open the National Practitioner Data Bank to the public. The NPDB, established in 1990 by the U. S. Department of Health and Human Services, contains information on malpractice payments made by physicians as well as disciplinary actions taken by local and state medical boards and hospitals. Currently, only HMO's, hospitals and healthcare organizations have access to the NPDB. S. Barlas, "Pressure to Make Data Bank Public," *Psychiatric Times*, May 2000, p. 56. See Chapter 31 on informed consent.

23. Fla. Const. Art. X, § 25 (2006). See I.N. Moore, J.W. Pichert, G.B. Hickson, C. Federspiel, & J.U. Blackford, "Rethinking Peer Review: Detecting and Addressing Medical Malpractice Claims Risk," *Vand. L. Rev.* 59 (2006): 1175.

24. See, e.g., Baum v. Turel, 206 F. Supp. 490 (D.C.N.Y. 1962).

25. See T.K. LeBlang, "Disclosure of Injury and Illness; Responsibilities in the Physician–Patient Relationship," *Law, Med. & Health Care* 9 (1981): 4.

26. R.M. Wettstein, "Tardive Dyskinesia and Malpractice," *Behav. Sci. & Law* 1 (1983): 91. In a subsequent communication, Dr. Wettstein said, "I don't think I definitely have formed my opinion at this point about a doctor telling a patient he was negligent in prescribing medication and can see good arguments for either side." Communication from Dr. Robert M. Wettstein to Ralph Slovenko (July 15, 1987).

27. After the verdict was announced, the jurors called Schoenfeld into the deliberation room to talk about how they reached the decision. A juror suggested to Schoenfeld that he finance a hospital fund in his mother's memory for patients who cannot afford private nurses. Schoenfeld seized on the idea and said he would organize the fund with a substantial portion of the $176,000. C. Lachman, "He Wins 176G Suit & Will Give It Away," *New York Post*, Nov. 25, 1981, p. 9.

28. American Broadcasting Co., Dec. 27, 1986.

29. S.S. Kramen & G. Hamm, "Risk Management: Extreme Honesty May Be the Best Policy," *Ann. of Intern. Med.* 131 (1991): 963; K. Sack, "Doctors Start to Say 'I'm Sorry' Long Before 'See You in Court,'" *New York Times*, May 18, 2008, p. 1; Ltrs., What to Say After a Medical Mistake?" *New York Times*, May 26, 2008, p. 18.

30. L. Landro, "Doctors Learn to Say 'I'm Sorry,'" *Wall Street Journal*, Jan. 24, 2007, p. D5.

31. See J.K. Robbennolt, "What We Know and Don't Know about the Role of Apologies in Resolving Health Care Disputes," *Ga. State Univ. L. Rev.* 21 (2005): 1009.

32. Comment by Prof. James J. White, "Effective Negotiation Techniques for Lawyers," Institute of Continuing Legal Education, Southfield, Michigan, June 10, 1987.

33. "Pepper and Salt," *Wall Street Journal*, Sept. 4, 1986, p. 23. In the congressional hearings on the Iran-Contra affair, Secretary of State Schultz testified without a lawyer at his side, prompting a cartoon in the *Oregonian* that said, "I guess that means he's telling the truth."

34. T. Coleman, *Money Matters*, NBC, Oct. 15,1982.

35. Comment by Alan J. Schnurman of New York, quoted in K. Johnson, "You Can Get Sued, Even at Home," *New York Times*, Jan. 10, 1982, p. F15.

36. Quoted in *Detroit Free Press*, April 26, 1978, p. C3. San Francisco attorney Richard Brown says, "Families don't realize when they pour out their souls to an insurance adjuster or company employee that their words might later be used against them." Brown handled a Delta airline crash case in which a distraught family member remarked to a sympathetic adjuster that the victim, a married man, had been having an extramarital affair. "They threw it back at us in settlement talks and really took us by surprise," says Brown. Quoted in B. Bean, "Damage Control," *Wall Street Journal*, Nov. 7, 1986, p. l.

37. Comment by attorney William E. Wisner, "Handling the Personal Injury Case," Institute of Continuing Legal Education, June 18, 1987 in Southfield, Michigan.

38. Miranda v. Arizona, 384 U. S. 436(1966).

39. *Wall Street Journal*, Nov. 10, 1978, p. 1.

40. See T.H. Gallagher et al., "Choosing Your Words Carefully: How Physicians Would Disclose Harmful Medical Errors to Patients," *Arch. Intern. Med.* 166 (2006): 158; A. Lazare, "Apology in Medical Practice an Emerging Clinical Skill," *JAMA* 296 (2006): 1401. There are programs such as "Apology in Medical Practice: An Emerging Clinical Skill," at DePaul University College of Law, April 19, 2007.

41. F.W. Cleary (Ed.), *McCormick on Evidence* (St. Paul: West, 3rd ed., 1984).

42. Federal Rules of Evidence, Rule 408. See also Note, "Agents' Reports and the Attorney-Client Privilege," *U. Chi. L. Rev.* 21 (1954): 752; Annot., "Insured-Insurer Communications as Privileged," 55 ALR 4th 336 (1987).

43. The American Bar Association Code of Professional Responsibility and Code of Judicial Conduct provides in Disciplinary Rule 7-103 on communicating with one of adverse interest: "During the course of his representation of a client, a lawyer shall not: (1) communicate or cause another to communicate on the subject of the representation with a party he knows to be represented by a lawyer in that matter unless he has the prior consent of the lawyer representing such other party or authorized by law to do so; (2) give advice to secure council, if the interests of such person are or have a reasonable possibility of being in conflict with the interests of his client."

Informal Opinion No. 908 of the Standing Committee on Professional Ethics of the American Bar Association (Feb. 24, 1996) provides that it is not unethical behavior for a potential plaintiff's attorney to interview a potential defendant so long as the latter knows that the statement is being taken by the lawyer in his status as attorney for the plaintiff. Once a complaint has been filed, a lawyer is prohibited from giving the other party any advice other than the advice to secure a lawyer; W.T. Grant Co. v. Haines, 531 F. 2d 671 (2nd Cir. 1976). Professor Harry Cohen of the University of Alabama School of Law, founder and editor of the *Journal of the Legal Profession*, observed,

> I believe that if there is any doubt that a person could be a defendant, the lawyer who interviews him without more, could be guilty of breach of the new A.B.A. Model Code Section 4.3 dealing with a lawyer contacting another who is not explicit about a situation where there is no "adverse party." However, I believe that where it is reasonable to assume that a doctor (or other person) could be a defendant, the lawyer must be very careful when implying that the lawyer is disinterested in the matter. The cases generally say that the lawyer must not approach one whom the lawyer believes will be an adverse party without telling that person that he or she should hire a lawyer and cautioning them that they should not say anything against their own interests. This is especially true where the person is ignorant or unaware of their involvement in the situation. See Lyons v. Paul 321 S. W. 2d 944 (Tex. Ct. Civ. App. 1959). It is true that the cases deal with parties to suits but as I read them and the ethics opinions they seem to deal with all adverse parties. In the doctor cases, I believe that a caution to the doctor before his lawyer talks to him or her would cause the doctor to call his lawyer. The lawyer who would talk to the doctor to get his side of the story without a strong cautionary statement could well be in breach of A.B.A. Model Code Section 4.3.

Communication from Professor Harry Cohen to Ralph Slovenko (July 6, 1987).

44. Texas attorney Wayne Fisher in 1986 ABA Program on Medical Malpractice for Attorneys, Physicians, and Risk Managers.

45. J. Friendly, "Decision in CBS Cases Raises New Concerns," *New York Times*, April 30, 1983, p. 48. Here are interrogatories put to defendant(s) that they are obliged to answer: "Please state whether or not any committees or hearings were held by Defendant Hospital with respect to the care and treatment of Plaintiff during confinement to said Hospital, and if so, please state with particularly what action, if any, was taken by Defendant Hospital, or on its behalf, in the regular course of business or in preparation for litigation, concerning any matters relating to the occurrence complained of in this action? Were any statements obtained by Defendant Hospital or on its behalf from any person concerning any matter relating to Plaintiff's decedent's condition?"

46. Peterson v. Chesapeake & Ohio Ry. Co., 112 F. R. D. 360 (W. D. Mich. 1986).

47. S. Taylor, "Hinckley Lawyers Urge Federal Judge to Bar Use of Some Evidence," *New York Times*, Oct. 28, 1981, p. 11. In the correctional institute where he was held for psychiatric examinations, Hinckley wrote daily in a diary labeled "The Diary of a Person We Know." The guards routinely read the diary and other papers, except for correspondence with lawyers, while Hinckley was out of his cell. Hinckley's lawyers sought to suppress the material because it contained "Mr. Hinckley's most private (if not secret) thoughts about his legal situation." They argued that under the Fourth Amendment, Hinckley "has a reasonable expectation that his handwritten papers would not be read by prison guards." S. Taylor, "Hinckley's Notes Discussed in Secret," *New York Times*, Oct. 22, 1981, p. 15.

48. Advisory Committee's Notes to Rule 801(C), Federal Rules of Evidence.

49. UPI news report, *New Orleans Times-Picayune*, Sept. 11, 1980, p. 3.

50. L.H. Farber, "I'm Sorry, Dear," in L.H. Farber, *The Ways of the Will* (New York: Basic Books, 1966); reprinted in L.H. Farber, *Lying, Despair, Jealousy, Envy, Sex, Suicide, Drugs and the Good Life* (New York: Harper & Row, 1976) p. 123. Russell Baker writes amusingly about apologies in "Never Say Sorry," *New York Times Magazine*, Jan. 10, 1982, p. 19. See also A. Lazare, *On Apology* (New York: Oxford University Press, 2004); R. Slovenko, "Remorse," *J. Psychiat. & Law* 34 (2006): 397.

51. G. Kolata, "Remedy for Waiting: A Special Report," *New York Times*, Jan. 4, 2001, p. 1.

52. E. Segal, *Love Story* (New York: Harper & Row, 1970).

53. M. Rose, "Taxi Passengers Are No Bargain," *New York Times*, June 26, 1987, p. 27.

54. T.H. Gallagher, D. Studdert, & W. Levinson, "Disclosing Harmful Medical Errors to Patients," *N. Eng. J. Med.*, June 28, 2007, pp. 2713–2719.

55. See J.K. Robbennolt, "What We Know and Don't Know About the Role of Apologies in Revolving Health Care Disputes," *Ga. State U. L. Rev.* 21 (2005): 1009; S. Jauhar, "Explain a Medical Error? Sure. Apologize, Too?" *New York Times*, Jan. 1, 2008, p. D5.

30
Breach of Confidentiality

Just as claims are made over geographical territory, individuals by natural impulse make claims controlling information about themselves. Ethologists call the geographical claim a *territorial imperative*, and a set of facts, which are of several varieties, a territorial-like *information preserve*. This preserve includes the content of one's mind or biographical facts about the individual. There is also, akin to the information preserve, as ethologists put it, a *conversational preserve*. Control over these preserves is threatened by a summons to talk, by being overheard, or by queries that are seen as intrusive or untactful. They are protected in law, more or less, by various procedural and substantive principles.

The legal duty of professional confidentiality or secrecy refers to the obligation not to release information about a client or patient without his permission, except when divulgence is required by law. The concept of privileged communication, which is discussed in Chapter 5, involves the right to withhold information in a legal proceeding—testimonial privilege statutes establish when a therapist must or must not testify concerning patient information in a judicial or administrative proceeding. Outside a judicial proceeding, the duty of professional confidentiality is in essence a restriction on the volunteering of information.

A professional person is bound, legally as well as ethically, to hold in confidence all information that is revealed to him or discovered as a result of his relationship with his client or patient. To a considerable degree, the law regulates the extent to which information confided by a patient is actually nondisclosable. Reporting laws, such as those for child abuse or the duty to warn the potential victim of a dangerous patient, require therapists to make disclosures of patient information.[1] That notwithstanding, the management of confidentiality on a daily basis is much more a matter of professional ethics than of legal requirements.[2]

The usual case of breach of confidentiality by psychiatrists outside the judicial process occurs in response to a request for information that they believe to be warranted either on moral or legal grounds. Nonetheless, the disclosure may be improper and may result in an adverse judgment based on defamation, invasion of privacy, or breach of confidentiality. Only an action for defamation is subject to the defense of truth. A breach of secrecy, even if the statement is true, may result in a claim in tort for invasion of privacy or in contract for breach of a fiduciary duty. These actions, of course, are not limited to physicians or psychiatrists. They also include the lawyer and other professionals who enjoy a confidential relationship. A number of states provide that the willful betrayal of a professional secret constitutes unprofessional conduct justifying, in addition to sanctions in tort or contract law, suspension or revocation of the right to practice. Few actions have been brought under these statutes, however. In some countries, breach of professional confidence constitutes a criminal offense.

The professional's duty to keep information confidential did not arise full-blown and has never been an absolute principle. When Hippocrates urged medical secrecy, he and his followers were in a minority; medical secrecy apparently was not the rule in his day. In the time of the Roman Empire and in the Middle Ages, physicians disclosed all manner of things about patients. As the role of a physician approached that of a priest, the concept of confessional secrecy spread through Catholic countries during the 16th century to include the physician. The spirit of the French Revolution and its concern with individual liberty stirred interest in this area and inspired a provision in the French Penal Code of 1810. In the 19th century, the idea of absolute medical secrecy, as well as other absolutes, gained ground. In the 20th century, there has been a return to the view that medical secrecy is relative, which was, in effect, the view of Hippocrates.[3]

The ethical and legal prohibitions are designed not to deter each and every breach of confidentiality but those deemed unjustified. According to the Hippocratic oath, still administered at most medical schools at graduation, the physician pledges that "whatsoever I shall see or hear in the course of my profession as well as outside my profession in my intercourse with men, if it be what should not be published abroad, I will never divulge, holding such things to be holy secrets." The oath, however, helps the physician little in deciding when, and to whom, he should reveal what he has seen or heard with regard to a patient because the proscription gives no criteria for determining that which ought to be spoken. An oath, like any ritual text, serves not a literal but a symbolic meaning. Its essential point is that, as a general principle, the physician will preserve the confidence of his patient, but there may be exceptions.

The most significant contribution to ethical history subsequent to Hippocrates was made by Thomas Percival of England, a physician, philosopher, and writer, who in 1803 published his Code of Medical Ethics, which bears his name. It is clear from the records and the preface to the American Medical Association's first-adopted Code of Ethics, in 1847, that it was based on Percival's Code. Through the years, while there have been revisions to reflect the temper of the time and the desire to express basic concepts with clarity, the language and concepts of the original Code adopted in 1847 have generally remained the same. The version adopted in 1957 states in pertinent part: "A physician may not reveal the confidence entrusted to him in the course of his medical attendance or the deficiencies he may observe in the character of his patients, unless he is required to do so by law, or unless it becomes necessary in order to protect the welfare of the individual or of the community." This principle of the AMA carries the comment: "Sometimes a physician must determine whether his duty to society requires him to employ knowledge, obtained through confidences entrusted to him as a physician, to protect a healthy person against a communicable disease to which he is about to be exposed. In such instance, the physician should act as he would desire another to act toward one of his own family in like circumstances."

Principles of medical ethics are not laws but standards. In the discharge of his professional obligations, the physician must look to the nature of his profession and the place it holds in society. For the general welfare of society, lawmakers in approximately a dozen situations demand that the physician under penalty come forward and make known information about a patient. Statutes in most states require the physician to report contagious and infectious diseases, to file certificates of birth, and to certify causes of death on certificates of death or stillbirth, along with such medical data as can be furnished. The physician has the same duty as any other citizen to render aid and assistance in enforcing the criminal laws. It is generally a criminal offense for any individual who knows of treasonous activities to fail to notify the proper authorities, but there is no duty to report other offenses. Several states have statutes that require physicians who treat persons suffering injuries, such as gun and knife wounds, which may have been received in an unlawful manner, to report the facts to the police. The various states have statutes that require reporting of parents who are thought to physically abuse their children. In various states, a therapist has a duty to warn others that a patient may pose a danger.[4]

Legislation requires physicians to report or allow the inspection of their records if they prescribe, administer, or dispense any scheduled drugs, including barbiturates and amphetamines. Various states require physicians to report to the commissioner of the state department of health the full name, address, and date of birth of every person who, in the opinion of the physician, is dependent upon controlled drugs. Another section of the law immunizes physicians from civil or criminal liability for such reporting and provides that their reports will not be admissible as evidence in trials against the drug abuser and that they "shall be held confidential" by the commissioner.[5]

When an investigation of medical practice is at issue, the law provides an exception to the rules controlling privacy. When the patient does not give permission to disclosure, the government must have a "compelling interest" in obtaining the records that "outweighs the patient's privacy interest." The burden of proof lies with the government. In *City of New York v. Bleuler Psychotherapy Center*,[6] a New York state court ordered a psychotherapy center to provide the medical records of a former patient, Andrew Goldstein, who killed Kendra Webdale by pushing her from a subway platform into the path of an oncoming train. The Department of Mental Health (DMH) had subpoenaed the records, but the center declined to produce them. The court in ordering the center to produce the records cited the New York Mental Hygiene Law, which provides that a court can order the release of documents if it finds "that the interest of justice significantly outweigh the need for confidentiality." The director of the DMH stated that its responsibilities include reviewing local services and facilities for persons with mental disabilities in the city and determining whether (1) there are any gaps in the system, (2) more services are needed, (3) the quality of services is adequate, and (4) other types of services are necessary. Consequently, the court ruled that the DMH needed the records in order to determine whether Goldstein's treating mental health providers acted properly in the past and to see what steps could be taken to minimize the occurrence of similar incidents. The court noted that the disclosure would be to an agency that has a statutorily mandated responsibility to investigate, and, furthermore, the court noted, the agency must keep the information confidential.

Obviously, there is no liability for invasion of the right of privacy or defamation when one does what the law requires. It is the promiscuous nontestimonial disclosure of information that leads to liability. Thus, in one case, a complainant was allowed recovery against her physician on a theory of breach of contractual relation because of disclosure made to her husband concerning her diagnosis and statements made by her while in psychotherapy.[7] Likewise, the protection of society does not include warning a prospective bride that her prospective husband (patient) is a psychopathic personality and has a poor character.[8] Further, invasion of privacy by unwarranted disclosure of information resulting in the patient's loss of employment has been recognized and given redress.[9]

Given that work constitutes a major part of one's life, it is not surprising to find psychiatrists discussing their patients during their leisure time. Many of us prefer shop talk to small talk. In some cases, the psychiatrist may be attempting to deal with his own anxieties about a patient or to obtain free supervision and support. When the patient is a VIP, a very important person, the psychiatrist in revealing the patient's identity may be bragging or trying to gain prestige; however, this is the patient who is probably most harmed by nothing more than a disclosure that he is seeing a psychiatrist. As it is, it is difficult to get a VIP to undertake treatment in a community where he is well known. The press has a gentlemen's agreement not to publish a politician's sex life and drinking habits unless it hits a police blotter, but it will disclose his history of medical or psychiatric treatment. One notable exception was that of Richard Nixon, who before becoming president was seen over an extensive period of time by Dr. Arnold Hutschnecker, a specialist in psychosomatic medicine—a fact that was referred to openly in British newspapers, although not so openly in the United States.

The Group for the Advancement of Psychiatry in its report, *The VIP With Psychiatric Impairment*, pointed out that one prominent psychiatrist in Washington, D.C., in his long experience has never been able to maintain a member of Congress in psychotherapy for more than a few months. The VIP fears that disclosure about his treatment would jeopardize his status and position. The disclosure of Senator Thomas Eagleton's history as a mental patient and the type of treatment (electroshock) resulted in his being dropped as the Democratic vice-presidential candidate and set back George McGovern's campaign for the presidency.[10] In all these cases, omission of identifying material in discussing patients would lessen the hazard of invasion of privacy.[11]

Writing About a Patient

The prominent physician–author William Carlos Williams in 1926 wrote about a patient without concealing his identity. He should have known better. The patient brought a lawsuit against Dr. Williams that was settled for $5,000, an amount that equaled his annual salary, and he never made that mistake again.[12] In writing about a patient, the nonpsychiatric physician usually has no difficulty because the configuration of the body can be discussed without anyone recognizing the patient. Psychiatrists, on the other hand, are obliged to disguise their clinical data, even though it is detrimental to the scientific value of the material, in order to avoid the recognition of the patient. Freud in his "Notes Upon a Case of Obsessional Neurosis" pointed out that the case history was not easy to compose, not only because of the inevitable compression, but also because of the need for greater discretion in print. His powers of presentation were taxed as the patient was well known in Vienna. Freud said, "How bungling are our attempts to reproduce an analysis; how pitifully we tear to pieces these great works of art Nature has created in the mental sphere." In his opening remarks, Freud explained how it is that intimate secrets could be more easily mentioned than the trivial details of personality by which a person could be readily identified, and yet it is just these details that play an essential part in tracing the individual steps in an analysis.

Freud published six case histories, now classic in psychoanalytic literature. The first of these, a case of hysteria, was turned down by the editor of the first journal to whom he sent it, apparently on the ground that it was a breach of discretion. In the fourth study, the actual name of the subject was used, but in this case, Freud had never seen him. He based his study almost entirely on an autobiographical book. In this study, Freud apparently was unconcerned about public reprimand or a defamation suit, notwithstanding the fact that the subject, Dr. Daniel Paul Schreber, was a paranoid—the most litigious type of personality—and was the presiding judge in a division of an Appeals Court in Saxony and a member of a distinguished family. Freud's other case histories are referred to as "The Case of Dora," "The Little Hans Case," "The Man with the Rats," "The Wolf-Man," and "A Case of Female Homosexuality."[13] As a precautionary measure, psychiatric journals usually advise contributors of articles that "where case presentations are submitted, it is the author's responsibility to disguise the identity of the patient."

About Freud himself, Drs. Ernest Jones and Max Schur, with permission, each published some information of his private life, but the Freud Archives promises to keep secret material on his boyhood for 50 years. Public figures are held to have lost, to some extent at least, their right of privacy. Thus, there is no liability when they are given additional publicity as to matters within the scope of the public interest they had aroused.

Dr. Martin Orne was criticized in 1991 when it was revealed that he had allowed a biographer of Pulitzer Prize-winning poet Anne Sexton access to audiotapes of his therapy sessions with her in the 1960s. Sexton, who committed suicide in 1974, wrote confessional poetry, much of which was drawn from her troubled life that included more than 20 hospitalizations, 10 suicide attempts, and extramarital affairs. When she entered therapy with Dr. Orne, who was then on the faculty at Harvard, she was a Boston housewife. He encouraged her to write poetry as part of her therapy and taped their sessions to help her remember their content and advance her treatment. Sexton wrote a poem to him in 1962, in which she said, "But you, my doctor, my enthusiast, were better than Christ; you promised me another world to tell me who I was." Dr. Orne released the tapes only after 5 years of prodding by the biographer, Diane Wood Middlebrook, and with the blessing of Sexton's daughter and literary executor, Linda Gray Sexton. He was heavily criticized by mental health professionals, who believed that his action set a dangerous precedent and violated widely adopted guidelines that confidential medical records not be made public without the patient's explicit permission. He was even attacked in a *New York Times* editorial, which accused him of betraying Sexton and dishonoring his profession. He responded in an opinion piece in that newspaper: "Sharing her most intimate thoughts and feelings for the benefit of others was not only her expressed and enacted desire, but the purpose for which she lived."

Frederick Wiseman's film *Titicut Follies*, containing scenes at Massachusetts Correctional Institution at Bridgewater where insane persons charged with crimes and defective delinquents were committed, was enjoined from exhibition in a proceeding brought by the state under its "obligation to protect the right of privacy of those committed to its custody." The decision was significant in that it protected the privacy of inmates at a correctional institution, who traditionally have been considered not to have any rights. The film depicted many inmates in situations that would be degrading to one of ordinary mentality and sensitivity. Although to a casual observer most of the inmates portrayed make little or no specific individual impression, others were shown in close-ups, sufficiently clearly exhibited (in some instances naked) to enable acquaintances to identify them. Wiseman contended that no asserted right of privacy may be protected from the publication of the film because the conditions at Bridgewater are matters of continuing public concern. Indeed, it was concern over conditions at Bridgewater that led various public officials a few years earlier to consider showing a documentary film in the hope that it might arouse public interest and lead to improvement. Arguably, the privacy argument was used by the state to prevent exposure of its own malfeasance and nonfeasance. The court said, however, that a presentation to the public of conditions at an institution would not necessitate the inclusion of some episodes shown in the film, nor would it justify, without valid written consents and releases, the depiction of identifiable inmates naked or in other embarrassing situations.[14] Needless to say, the court's ruling made *Titicut Follies* a prized item on the film society circuit and guaranteed Wiseman's fame, and though the ban is no longer in force, Wiseman is still known as the person who documented, in gruesome detail, the conditions at a facility for the criminally insane.

Ownership and Access to Records

The question often arises as to the ownership of the records of the patient and the right to use or inspect them. A physician or hospital may not grant or deny access to records purely on the basis of an alleged personal property right in them, but confidentiality is a consideration. In the absence of a court order or authorization by the patient, the physician or hospital as custodian may be liable for an invasion of privacy by disclosure of confidential information. On the other hand, when the patient has signed a consent for their inspection, the physician or hospital may not deny an insurance company or other third party access to its records.[15]

Oddly enough, while a court demand for information worries psychiatrists most, the demand that affects them most frequently comes from a third party who has some legal or moral right to information. Confidentiality about the patient and accountability of the therapist are entwined, and to some extent at odds. The crucial questions are: What disclosure is necessary and is that disclosure unfair? Is the alleged privacy of the patient a fig leaf covering the naked self-interest of the therapist? Years ago, Dr. Herbert Modlin of the Menninger Foundation wrote, "We should differentiate the privacy of the patient and the privacy of the doctor. Occasionally it might be that our secrets—not the patient's—are threatened by exposure."[16] There is no "black box" in the treating room as there is in an airplane, and physicians have a code of silence about their colleagues that makes the police blue code relatively garrulous. The most frequent type of demand today is from insurance companies who pay for a good part of psychiatric treatment. They use certain ploys, such as the blanket consent form, and withhold payment unless the information is supplied. They also know the patient cannot go to court for redress without jeopardizing his privacy even more.[17]

Those who support the position that the physician or hospital should have the absolute right to deny access to records argue that the patient, except in rare instances, lacks the understanding, competency, or knowledge to evaluate a record properly or even know what is in it. However, as in the case of the testimonial privilege, when there is waiver of the privilege, the physician or hospital cannot refuse.[18]

Medical records of the physician in private practice are considered his property; however, like hospital records, they are subject to a limited property right on the part of the patient with respect to the information they contain. Access to records allows a patient to question procedures (and to obtain information about his health that may worry him). In cases of physical illness, the courts have held that an x-ray film, for example, belongs to the physician (even though the cost is paid by the patient) without a specific agreement to the contrary. The physician must provide the information contained in the x-ray or other medical record, however, if requested to do so by the patient. Having a limited property right, the patient can demand disclosure not only to himself but also, for example, to an insurance company.

Psychiatrists would argue that a different principle is needed for psychotherapy. The non-physiological part of a psychiatric record, unlike an x-ray, is not hard data and might reasonably be said to be the entire work product of the therapist. There is also the pragmatic consideration that psychiatric records can readily be destroyed or may be prepared in a way unintelligible to others. Before malpractice suits became a matter of concern, many therapists, particularly those who were not engaged in research or teaching, kept no or few records of their sessions, except date of appointment, and would rely entirely upon their memory. Some recordkeeping is now prudent, at least until the time set by the statute of limitations has run on a suit for malpractice. In practice, psychiatrists refuse a patient's request to see his own treatment record on the ground that it would be detrimental to his health. Moreover, the patient has no right to demand that records concerning him be destroyed.

One person, whose sexual history was taken when he was a young man by the Kinsey Institute for Sex Research, later became a United States Senator, and not wanting to take any chance of revelation, he wanted his record. The Institute refused to return or expunge it. Wardell B. Pomeroy, a colleague of Kinsey, wrote in his book on the Institute, "It was Kinsey's guarantee of absolute confidence to those who gave histories that made the research possible. … He was acutely conscious of his responsibilities in this respect, and he drilled it into everyone who came to work for him. Everyone had to understand the supreme importance of respecting confidences." Pomeroy added, "I believe that there was something more to this than Kinsey's basic rocklike integrity. I think he liked secrets, that their possession gave him a sense of power. And there was no question that the histories did give him a unique potential power. They included political, social, and business leaders of the first rank, and, with his intimate knowledge of their lives, Kinsey could have figuratively blown up the United States socially and politically."[19]

Until the latter part of the 19th century, hospital and medical records were used almost exclusively for purposes of treatment, teaching, and research. In the 20th century, new uses developed for them—and the old privacy was gone. In former times, a physician and his patient met in complete privacy in office or home, but now there are other people in the picture: specialists and hospitals, technicians and machines, insurance carriers, employers, and unions. Increasingly, team care has replaced individual practice; government is a third party, providing for all or part of the expense.

Various public or private agencies, such as the police, colleges, credit rating organizations, civil service, and employers, as well as insurance companies, request information or recommendations. The request may come from the patient himself with regard to such matters as a college application or employment. Parents or other members of the family may exert pressure for confidential material. Some psychiatrists, when a release has been given by the patient, provide information if it is "for the good of the patient."

The release of information regarding psychiatric treatment of a patient to an insurance company is an issue of increasing importance. If insurance companies are to provide coverage for psychiatric illness, they must be able to obtain sufficient information to assess fairly the costs of their programs. Psychiatrists, however, generally feel that the insurer should accept their work and not expect the same detailed information regarding psychical disorders as in the case of physical disorders. Some employees, rather than have their employers informed that they are seeking psychiatric help, forego company insurance and pay themselves, or else they forego seeing a psychiatrist. In a position statement, the American Psychiatric Association Task Force on Confidentiality as It Relates to Third Parties urged framers of national healthcare proposals to recognize the imperative need for safeguarding the confidentiality of medical records in any national healthcare system.[20]

Right of privacy, too, may conflict with adequacy of treatment. Quality control of care and treatment means review of individual patients and therapists. In *Wyatt v. Stickney*,[21] Judge Johnson in setting out minimum standards for public institutions ordered individualized treatment plans. For review, data must be submitted to the mental health board. Civil libertarians expressed concern that the data would go beyond the board and they contested the identification of patients. Michigan and New York for a time used a code system to conceal the names of patients and therapists, but the system has been dropped. The disturbing consideration is the use of the records for purposes unrelated to treatment. For example, any federal agency can exercise the legal authority given the government to examine records of patients in Veterans Administration hospitals; it is done not only for purposes of treatment or for determination of disability payments, but also even when the patient makes application for any type of federal employment.

The social or behavioral science researcher can present a reasonable claim for information, but he has no legal right to it. For example, a researcher engaged in a study of suicide may wish to examine the records of every patient who has attempted suicide; he relies on the voluntary cooperation of the hospital, and he sometimes obtains it. Much social science research is modeled on a dyadic relationship between the researcher and subject, and the researcher seeks personal information about the respondent, his family, friends, and associates. Kinsey's research is an example of this professional model for social research.

For research in bureaucratic settings, the information that is collected is *aggregate* information rather than *personal* in the way that it is collected and in the sense that the researcher is interested in aggregates rather than particular individuals. Nevertheless, such information may have profoundly personal consequences if an individual's name comes to light or if sources of information are revealed. Moreover, revelations of information may have important consequences for the bureaucracy or organization itself. This model of research is more like journalistic or investigative activities than professional–client relations.

The impact on privacy resulting from the easy access to information contained in computer data banks has evoked much concern. Present technology will permit, within a very small space, the consolidation and storage of data equivalent to a 300-page book on every person in the country. Actually, though, data inside a computer may be safer than data in old-fashioned records. It provides selective access to information because it may be arranged into groups: (1) information without particular medical significance, such as name, address, occupation, and marital status; (2) medical information, but not of a secret nature, such as height and weight, blood group, immunizations, and refraction; and (3) other types of information, based on the interaction between the physician and patient, which would be available only to someone with the correct code number, namely, the patient's personal doctor or the patient, who could then decide whether to allow anyone else to have the information.[22]

The Health Insurance Portability and Accountability Act (HIPAA)

In 1996, the Health Insurance Portability and Accountability Act (HIPAA)[23] was enacted to encourage standardization of the electronic transfer of healthcare data. It sought to improve access to medical information in order to improve the efficiency and effectiveness of healthcare. The protection of privacy was an afterthought. To most people, however, HIPAA is synonymous with privacy because as soon as one enters a physician's office or hospital, a notice of privacy is given to the individual to read and sign.

By the Privacy Rule adopted in 2003, it is provided that "[a] covered entity may not use or disclose protected health information except as permitted or required by the rule."[24] Covered entities are defined to include health plans, healthcare clearinghouses, and healthcare providers who transfer data electronically. Healthcare providers who submit paper claim forms and do not transfer other types of medical information electronically are not subject to the provisions of HIPAA.

Although many states already had laws protecting patient privacy, it was felt there should be a federal standard that would establish a minimum level of protection. State laws that are more stringent than HIPAA in protecting patient's records take precedence over HIPAA.

Protected health information is defined as "individually identifiable health information" that is transferred or stored, either electronically or in any other form. Psychotherapy notes are subject to a more stringent standard of confidentiality than other medical records. Psychotherapy notes are the only part of the files for which patients do not have access. *Psychotherapy notes* are defined as the notes taken by a psychotherapist "documenting or analyzing the contents of a conversation during a private counseling session, or a group, joint, or family counseling session, and that are separated from the rest of the individual's medical record." Psychotherapy notes are the notations kept during therapy sessions that deal with the patient's personal life and the psychiatrist's reactions, rather than with the patient's disorder. These notes must be kept separate from the rest of the medical record (i.e., on a different sheet of paper) if they are to be protected as a separate entity. Otherwise, they must be released with the rest of the record.

Psychotherapy notes do not include references to medication prescribing and monitoring, session start and stop times, modality and frequency of treatment furnished, result of clinical tests, or any summary of diagnosis, symptoms, functional status, treatment plan, progress to date, and prognosis. All of this information is part of the medical record.

"Minimum necessary disclosure" is the rule for all disclosures of patients' individually identifiable information under HIPAA. The minimum necessary requirement does not apply to uses or disclosures by healthcare providers for treatment, it does not apply to disclosure or use by the U.S. Department of Human Health Services (HHS) for enforcement and compliance activities, and it does not apply to uses or disclosures covered by law. When a patient gives authorization for a specific nonroutine disclosure, minimum necessary disclosure does not apply. Revocation of authorization can be done at any time, with one exception: if the authorization was relied upon or was a condition of obtaining healthcare insurance. Authorization is required for fundraising, marketing, employment determinations, preenrollment underwriting, and disclosure of psychotherapy notes. The restriction does not preclude the therapist from obtaining the support of significant others, as when a patient is in a suicidal crisis.

Patients can name a personal representative. HIPAA requires covered entities to regard the personal representative as they would the patient. An exception can be made to this rule if the covered entity suspects the patient has been a victim of abuse, domestic violence, or neglect by the personal representative. If the covered entity believes that it is not in the best interest of the patient to share information with the personal representative, he is not required to do so.

Covered entities must provide privacy training for their workers and must document the privacy education of their workers (including unpaid volunteers). Covered entities must designate a privacy officer who is responsible for developing and implementing privacy practices and procedures.

The HHS Office of Civil Rights enforces the privacy regulations. Anyone may file a complaint of improper disclosure or use of protected healthcare information. A complaint must be filed in writing no later than 180 days after the complainant knew or should have known about the violation. The privacy rule makes it easier to sue or complain to a licensing board because it sets a standard for the protection of patient information. The HIPAA rules provide for imposing civil fines and referral for criminal prosecution. There are civil fines (up to $25,000 for each calendar year for each provision that is violated) and criminal penalties (up to 10 years imprisonment and a $250,000 penalty) for covered entities that misuse personal health information. HIPAA provides only for enforcement of the privacy rule by HHS; there is no private right of action under HIPAA for individuals to enforce the privacy rights. Congressional action would be required to establish a private right of action under HIPAA. However, patients may still be able to bring suit for breach of confidentiality under state law. Given these penalties, it is not surprising that healthcare providers tend not to use discretion. Writing from experience, Pete Earley, author of *Crazy: A Father's Search Through America's Mental Health Madness*, says, "HIPAA frequently prevents loved ones from being informed and involved in treatment."

HIPAA adds another layer of red tape onto a healthcare system already overburdened with paperwork. While the purpose of HIPAA is to streamline healthcare, it is ironic that it results in more mandatory paper forms, disclosures, consents, and authorizations. The cost of implementing HIPAA is a major concern for healthcare entities, and they are puzzled by what is a permissible use or transmission of protected healthcare data. Many providers, especially smaller clinics or practices, have erred on the side of caution and refused to share data for treatment purposes with other healthcare entities (and this sort of information transfer is, of course, permitted by the privacy rules).

Some opinion of healthcare providers may be noted. A nurse says, "HIPAA is more work and takes away from nursing care. I feel like the police." An information manager says, "It's a pain in the neck. It takes up a lot of time with trees being wasted with useless paperwork. It's time consuming and it limits what I can say on the phone." A department director says, "Access has definitely been more difficult for the families of patients. Our clients in general are elderly and most of them have trusting relationships with their children and grandchildren. Their generation is not savvy about 'legal jargon' and many do not understand the need to be so strict about protecting medical records."[25]

HIPAA is applicable to healthcare providers, healthcare plans, and healthcare clearing-houses. Business associates of covered entities are not themselves liable under HIPAA for any improper use or transfer of private information. The rules require covered entities to contract with business associates; the covered entitles are responsible for a business associate's improper use or transfer of protected healthcare information, but only if the covered entity knew there was an improper use or transfer.

So there are gaps in coverage in the privacy laws. If, for example, a healthcare provider transfers protected healthcare information to a medical biller, who sells lists of patients to marketers without authorization, the covered entity is the only party liable under HIPAA, and it is liable only to the extent that it knew or should have known about the improper use or transfer.

The required privacy contracts lead to problems themselves. It may be impractical to expect large healthcare entities that contract with thousands of business associates to police each one of them with regard to the privacy provisions. The privacy contracts required between covered entities and business associates must meet many requirements under the privacy rules and are troublesome for healthcare entities to draft and maintain.

The "minimum necessary requirement" provision of the privacy rules has created some concern. In theory, it sounds reasonable to say that covered entities should reveal only the minimum necessary information to accomplish the purpose of the permitted use or transfer. In practice, this requirement could be onerous. The minimum necessary requirement is that healthcare providers consider eight factors in determining what is the minimum necessary amount of information transfer. The covered entity must consider the amount of information that would be used or disclosed, the extent to which the use or disclosure would be disclosed, the number of individuals who might have access to the information, the importance of the disclosure, the chance that further disclosures might occur, other ways to achieve the same goal without disclosing information, the technology available to limit the scope of the disclosure, and the cost of limiting the exposure, as well as any other pertinent factors. Large healthcare entities (multistate healthcare providers, for example) may make thousands of information use or transfer decisions every day. To subject every one of these decisions to the balancing act that the privacy rules require is not practicable. Ironically, it may have the opposite of the effect intended by HIPAA; it may well slow down data transfer and make necessary use or disclosure of protected health information more difficult rather than less.

The provisions in the privacy rule on preemption are troublesome. The privacy rules state that HIPAA preempts state law, except where state law is more restrictive than HIPAA. The privacy rules do not, therefore, provide one uniform set of rules that covered entities can look to. They still must respond to state law affecting medical information privacy. Covered entities now have to consider additional questions: Is the state law more or less restrictive than HIPAA, and, therefore, does one have to follow the state law, HIPAA, or both? In instances where HIPAA and state laws conflict, and it is not clear which is more restrictive, the preemption provisions place healthcare providers in a quandary. Only states may seek an advisory opinion from HHS regarding preemption of state laws. Covered entities have no ability, under the privacy rules, to seek an advisory opinion from HHS on this matter. The preemption provisions thus defeat HIPAA's purpose of providing one uniform law throughout the United States concerning medical privacy and electronic data transfer.

These are some of the concerns that healthcare providers and others have about the privacy rules of HIPAA. On the other side, privacy advocates have concerns as well. The privacy rules of HIPAA permit access without patient consent by law enforcement officials, public health officials, and researchers under certain circumstances. It has been held that a physician violates HIPAA by discussing a patient's history with an attorney without authorization from the patient.[26] In the past both sides could conduct *ex parte* (by or for one party) communication with treating physicians.

HIPAA sets out exceptions to a patient's right to privacy:

1. Confidentiality does not apply when a patient is considered to be a threat to others, unless hospitalized.
2. Confidentiality does not apply when the law requires mandatory reporting (this includes communicable diseases, child or elder abuse, impaired driving, and any other requirement in a particular jurisdiction).
3. Court-ordered or subpoenaed records can be released without the patient's written authorization.

4. Hospitals and offices may release healthcare information without the patient's written permission for the purpose of treatment, payment, or operations (TPO), such as quality control, peer review, and teaching.

HIPAA specifically states that psychiatric and drug and alcohol information are specially protected, though limited amounts of information on these diagnoses may be shared for the purposes of TPO. Private and governmental insurers commonly request information concerning suicidal intent or attempts, psychotic breaks with reality, drug addiction, alcoholism, sexual problems, and almost without question, a diagnosis. Would a patient with a diagnosis of schizophrenia, manic depressive disorder, dementia, major depressive disorder, panic disorder, or factitious disorder voluntarily allow this information to be made public? Even the name of a prescribed medication can have a pejorative connotation.

Physicians deal with managed care companies and other third party mental health insurers on a daily basis, and the private thoughts and behaviors of patients are not always respected. In a National Public Radio segment on confidentiality, an HMO manager opined, "Information gathered from insured persons regarding diagnosis, history, and treatment is to ensure that patients receive maximal benefits in terms of treatment and to assist in research." If only it were so. In reality, additional information allows managed care auditors to find a reason to deny or delay payment. Moreover, if a patient refuses to sign a release of medical information, no payment for services will be forthcoming.

The Supreme Court dealt with the issue of medical privacy a few years ago in *Ferguson v. City of Charleston*.[27] In this case, pregnant women who came to a Charleston city hospital to give birth gave urine samples after signing a consent to treatment form, and these samples were tested for the presence of cocaine. It was hospital policy that if cocaine was found in urine samples, the hospital notified the police, and criminal charges would be brought against patients with urine positive for cocaine. The majority held that such use of the sample constituted a search that was not covered under the "special needs" provision of the Fourth Amendment. The Court said that where state hospital employees "undertake to obtain such evidence from their patients for the specific purpose of incriminating those patients, they have a special obligation to make sure that the patients are fully informed about their constitutional rights, as standards of knowing waiver require." The Court remanded the case for the lower court to determine if the patient signing the standard consent form had satisfied that standard. Justice Stevens, writing for the majority, stated that "reasonable expectation of privacy enjoyed by the typical patient undergoing diagnostic tests in a hospital is that the result of those tests will not be shared by nonmedical personnel without her consent."

This language is cited in legal challenges made to the unconsented-to transmission of protected healthcare data to law enforcement and public health entities. It remains to be seen how the courts will balance the provisions of the privacy rule, the desire for privacy in one's healthcare information, and the need for access to that information by the healthcare system, and by the larger society.

Problems lie ahead in the process of streamlining and digitizing the flow of healthcare information. HIPAA calls for steps to be taken to standardize healthcare information and ultimately to standardize identifiers of employers, providers, and, most significantly, individuals. Once everyone has a national individual identifier number, once employers and healthcare providers all have such numbers, society will have gone most of the way toward creating a national healthcare information databank. Such a databank is not called for by HIPAA, but HIPAA has taken every step toward that end, but the final one. A national healthcare databank would provide the ultimate access to patient information for healthcare providers and to other entities in society, such as law enforcement and public health officials. On the other hand, the notion of a national healthcare databank provokes alarm among civil libertarians concerned with individual privacy.

In a time when the United States is facing serious threats to national security, the administration has proposed a Total Information Awareness Network that would mandate a massive federal databank for every sort of personal information, including banking transactions, credit card transactions, Internet mailing records, phone records, and healthcare information. The databank would be used for security and intelligence purposes as well as for law enforcement. HIPAA would complement such a scheme by making the nationalization of healthcare information in a central databank possible.

Americans with Disabilities Act

Under the Americans with Disabilities Act, an employer may ask an individual for documentation when an employee requests reasonable accommodation for a disability. The employer is entitled to know that the employee has a covered disability for which reasonable accommodation is needed. In response to a request for reasonable accommodation, the employer cannot ask for documentation that is unrelated to determining the existence of a disability and the need for an accommodation. This means that in most situations an employer cannot request an employee's complete medical records because they are likely to contain information unrelated to the disability at issue and the need for accommodation.

An employer may require that the documentation about the disability and the functional limitations come from an appropriate healthcare or rehabilitation professional. The appropriate professional in any particular situation will depend on the disability and the type of functional limitation it imposes. Appropriate professionals include, but are not limited to, physicians (including psychiatrists), psychologists, nurses, physical therapists, occupational therapists, speech therapists, vocational rehabilitation specialists, and licensed mental health professionals. The individual can be asked to sign a limited release allowing the employer to submit a list of specific questions to the healthcare or vocational professional. The employer is obliged to maintain the confidentiality of all medical information collected during this process, regardless of where the information comes from.

Disclosure to Avoid Harm

It sometimes happens that strict confidentiality may jeopardize the patient or society. There may be danger, for example, of the patient committing suicide. There may be danger in the patient's continuing work, as in the case of an airplane pilot who should be grounded because of severe mental disorder, but who, fearful of losing his job, does not tell his employer. Although the law imposes no duty to come to the aid of third persons, the psychiatrist may properly act in such emergencies. He may reveal a confidence when it becomes necessary in order to protect the welfare of the patient or the community. In such situations, the revelation is made only to avert catastrophe. As he is acting in his role as healer, a psychiatrist is not likely to be liable in damages for invasion of privacy. Thus, in one case, a physician who revealed to the patient's spouse that the patient was suffering from a venereal disease was not held liable.[28]

The general public and persons in therapy alike will not lose trust in the psychiatrist as a keeper of secrets if in cases of emergency he does not adhere to strict and absolute confidentiality. Sooner or later, the patient usually realizes that the psychiatrist has acted in the patient's best interest (which is not the case when an opposing party in litigation compels a psychiatrist to testify). However, situations of real emergencies necessitating disclosure are rare.

In furnishing psychiatric information, the physician's traditional function has been to treat the sick, not to prepare historical reports or explanatory documents. What happens when psychiatric information is furnished? In all areas, could not the recipient of the information do as well, or even better, if he applied his usual method of decision making, uncontaminated by psychiatric data, which he understands poorly? The practice of supplying a label (e.g., schizophrenic) may be especially misleading. Dr. Marc Hollender suggested that the general expectation that the psychiatrist will answer requests stems, in part, from the general practice of medicine. He points out that too little attention has been paid to the social significance of data applied to how a person feels, thinks, and lives, on the one hand, and to how his body functions, on the other. He added: "It may be that psychiatrists have had too great a need to prove their usefulness as members of society. As possessors of special and secret data (much like the possessor of choice bits of gossip), they can gain recognition, and perhaps even power, if they are willing to share their possessions with others who can use them. In my opinion, they have even been seduced to claim that they have the ability to foretell the future in a way that no one else can."[29]

Dr. Arnold Hutschnecker suggested that mental health certificates should be required for political leaders similar to the Wasserman test demanded by states before marriage. He contended that psychological and axiological (value) tests now exist that would pinpoint psychopathology so that mentally unstable individuals would be prevented from attaining jobs of political importance. He cited the mentally disturbed Secretary of Defense James Forrestal, and John Foster Dulles, with his constant brinkmanship, to name only two. More sensibly, he said, testing should be required at a student level, before a person has acquired a position of power.[30]

While strict confidentiality may jeopardize the patient or society, it is always debatable whether a disclosure can be construed as a benefit either to the patient or society. This thorny problem received wide publicity when two employees of the National Security Agency, Vernon F. Mitchell and William H. Martin, defected to the Soviet Union. A psychiatrist, who had seen Mitchell, turned over his records and testified before a secret session of the House Un-American Activities Committee. He expressed his belief that a patient who defects and causes a threat to national security loses his right to confidentiality because the rights of the government far exceed the rights of the individual. The psychiatrist then disclosed the defector's problems of family, religion, and sex. For this, he was taken to task by a number of general practitioners and psychiatrists. The Medical and Chirurgical Faculty of the State of Maryland, where the psychiatrist practiced, investigated the possible breach of medical ethics, but ruled in his favor, concluding that the interest of the nation transcends that of the individual. The faculty said that the psychiatrist acted in an ethical and cooperative manner with public authorities and had given the testimony in secret session to the committee. The public release was through this committee rather than through the psychiatrist.[31]

The Secret Service from time to time has asked psychiatric hospitals and clinics to report patients who have made verbal or written threats against the president. At one time, FBI Director Hoover urged all physicians to report to the Bureau any facts relating to espionage, sabotage, or subversive activity coming to their attention. Psychiatrists generally criticized the American Medical Association for cooperating with the Bureau and for going even further by urging its members to help catch even a petty thief. Guttmacher attacked this suggestion with wry humor: "It is not too fantastic to predict that before long the physician's inner examining room may resemble a rural post office with its walls plastered with the mugs of wanted felons."[32]

The duty to warn or protect, otherwise known as the *Tarasoff* duty, is discussed at length in Chapter 36 on duty to third persons. The issue of confidentiality is also discussed in Chapter 24 on civil commitment.

Examination at Request of Court or Employer

Psychiatrists are not bound by a confidential relationship when they are carrying out an examination at the request of a third party, such as a court, employer, or university. The psychiatrist in these cases is in an examining rather than a treating role. The individual sometimes cooperates, however, believing that there will be respect for confidentiality as in the usual physician–patient relationship. It seems clear that the individual is entitled to confidentiality when the psychiatrist appears to be acting in a treating role and fails to advise otherwise.

It is contrary to medical ethics, as well as against the law, for the police or the district attorney to exploit the relationship of physician and patient in order to obtain a confession from the accused. While some consider this naive, psychiatrists carrying out an examination pursuant to court order should caution the accused that communications are not privileged, notwithstanding the possible resultant loss of valuable information. The statutes of many states provide that communications to a psychiatrist in the course of a court-ordered psychiatric examination are without privilege only on issues involving the person's mental condition; that is, the psychiatrist may testify to the accused's insanity at the time of the offense or at the time of the trial, but he may not report, for example, on the validity of an alibi.

In *Leyra v. Denno*,[33] the accused had been allowed little sleep and was suffering from a sinus condition when the police brought in a psychiatrist, who was identified as a general practitioner. The questioning by the psychiatrist, who was skilled in hypnosis, was a subtle blend of threats and promises of leniency. Working in a room that was wired, the psychiatrist, "by subtle and suggestive questions, simply continued the police effort" to obtain a confession from the accused. The Supreme Court ruled the confession inadmissible in evidence, equating the procedure with mental coercion.[34] In another case, *Oaks v. Colorado*,[35] it was held that a psychiatrist could not testify about the criminal activity of the defendant, whom he examined for the state before charges had been brought, on the ground that he had obtained the information under the guise of a psychiatric examination.

Presentence Reports

The confidentiality of a presentence investigation report of a probation department, diagnostic center, or court probation clinic is a matter that has been receiving considerable attention. These reports to the court often have great influence on the type and length of sentence given. The issue here is not the right of a criminal defendant to have information withheld from the court, but rather the right of the court to withhold information from the defendant or his attorney. The controversy involves the extent to which due process requires disclosure of the contents of the report to the defendant. According to one view, a presentence investigation report should be treated not as a public document, but as a confidential compilation of information for the sole use of the sentencing judge. It is considered that strict adherence to confidentiality has made it possible for the probation officer to give the court a much more accurate picture of the defendant than would be possible if it were known that the contents of the report were going to be divulged to the defendant or others. As one court said, "To strip a presentence investigation report of its confidentiality would be to divest it of its importance and value to the sentencing judge because there might be lacking the frankness and completeness of disclosures made in confidence."[36]

There is a growing body of opinion, however, which supports the view that the defendant and his attorney should be given an opportunity to examine the presentence report. Defense attorneys contend that the right to see a presentence report is a basic and fundamental right, the denial of which will allow hearsay evidence to go unchallenged, thus depriving the defendant of cross-examination and confrontation of witnesses. Three organizations—the American Bar Association in its Standards Relating to Sentencing Alternatives and Procedures, the American Law Institute in its Model Penal Code, and the National Council on Crime and Delinquency in its Model Sentencing Act—have recommended that the report be disclosed to the defense. Making the report available to the defense provides certain safeguards to the defendant, primarily giving him an opportunity to explain matters in the report that may not have been explained as fully as he feels they should have been. Many years ago, in 1944, an Advisory Committee of the Supreme Court recommended full disclosure of the presentence report, but the recommendation was rejected. More recently, though, either by statute or judicial decision, some states have provided that the defense must be given a summary of the presentence report, and others have ruled that the defendant is entitled to full disclosure.[37]

Rule 32(c) of the Federal Rules of Criminal Procedure gives the court full discretion to disclose information contained in the presentence report when the court believes it is necessary to do so. The rule also provides that a presentence report shall not be submitted to the court or its contents disclosed to anyone else unless the defendant has pleaded guilty or has been found guilty. The policy behind the rule is to avoid prejudice on the part of the court. If the purpose of the report is not for sentencing, but is to provide the court with information to assist it in passing upon the advisability of reducing bail, the report is permissible, even though it contains certain presentence factors.[38] As probation and diagnostic services develop, the issue of the extent to which a presentence investigation report ought to be preserved as a confidential document will assume increased importance.

Confidentiality in Corrections

Psychotherapy and group counseling have been introduced in correctional institutions and agencies. Confidentiality is of utmost importance when dealing with individuals distrustful of others. One administrator has said of his prison psychiatrist's obligation of confidentiality: "Giving parole boards access to what is dug up in individual and group therapy would be opening a veritable gold mine to them. But the shaft is sealed to them and to institution administrators and must be sealed."

There is a difference of opinion, however, as to whether a prison psychiatrist is duty bound to report knowledge of new crimes being planned by the patient.[39] The viewpoint supporting confidentiality defends it thus: "It is not the role of the psychiatrist to uncover such information under the guise of therapy, if he expects to expose it to the warden. ... [D]isclosure under these circumstances is a sort of 'psychic entrapment.' The physician ought to either warn his patient beforehand of the reservations he has concerning confidentiality or, having committed himself to secrecy, he should maintain it."[40]

Testing in Schools

The use of psychological testing in schools gives rise to a similar issue on reporting. For sundry reasons, parents may exert pressure on school authorities for disclosure of confidential material. There has been an upsurge of litigation challenging various testing procedures and placements, seeking parental participation in placement procedures and even money damages for inappropriate placement of students. There is usually contained in a student's records a comprehensive dossier of official test scores, extracurricular activities, teacher appraisals of student attitudes and social behavior, and sometimes reports or letters from psychiatrists and special guidance agencies. In a recent New York case, the mother of a girl who was prohibited from attending her junior high school graduation as punishment for "bad citizenship" sought access to the records to determine the nature of her daughter's offense. The State Education Commissioner ruled in favor of the mother, saying, "No one has a greater right to such information than the parent."[41]

Do test results belong in the category of secrets, to be seen only by professional eyes? Or is their proper function best served when they become common knowledge in the school and its community? In some towns, names and scores are listed in the local newspaper, much like the results of an athletic contest. How should a school administrator, teacher, or guidance worker respond when a mother wants to know, for example, her son's IQ? Should the school send aptitude test profiles home with the children? One cartoonist depicted a mother calling the family physician, "It's about Benny, doctor. He's just come from school with an IQ of 104! Should I put him right to bed?"

Arguments against parental access to records stress that the information is not in terms that parents can absorb and use and that teachers and guidance workers, fearing parental displeasure, will be less than candid in making reports. While parents may have the right to know whatever the school knows about the abilities, performance, and problems of their children, mere access to records would simply give the illusion of information and at the same time would undoubtedly discourage teachers and others from entering subjective judgments in a student's record. In current practice, psychiatric reports and personality test results are not made available to the student or parent; they may, however, discuss these matters directly with the teacher, psychiatrist, or psychologist. The right of parents to know about the abilities and performances of their children refers to knowledge in terms they can understand and absorb.[42]

Psychiatrist as Double Agent

When an institution or agency hires a psychiatrist, his allegiance is diffused between the institution and the patient. This is a relatively new position for the physician who, not so long ago, had a strictly personal relationship with his patient. The physician represented no temporal authority, but was the intermediary between the forces of nature and the individual. He had a priest-like function. Rarely did he have to choose between serving the private and the common good.

Szasz calls the psychiatrist who is hired by a third party a double agent. Writing about the college psychiatrist, Szasz says that in the case of the homosexual student, the psychiatrist serves as a disguised medical policeman.[43] Before publishing this accusation, Szasz presented it at the 1967 annual meeting of the American Orthopsychiatric Association, at which time numerous college psychiatrists came up to the podium to deny that confidences were being divulged to the authorities, except when necessary to prevent a suicide.

Actually, it is in the criminal law and the military settings that the psychiatrist is a double agent. The college psychiatrist may make isolated divulgences, but in the context of criminal proceedings (both pretrial and posttrial) the psychiatrist is required in every case to make a report to the authorities. In order to make an adequate report, he invites the confidence of the accused, which cannot be directly divulged but will surely affect the report. Thus, a person charged with writing a bad check, who confides to the psychiatrist that he has brutally killed someone, will surely not be recommended for probation on the bad check charge.

In the military, as in nonmilitary criminal law administration, there is routine reporting in evaluating offenders as well as persons who apply for discharge as conscientious objectors. Clemenceau said that "military justice is to justice as military music is to music." The analogy can be seen in psychiatry as well.

In the university setting, as elsewhere, there may be a waiver of confidentiality. Some university health services quite appropriately notify the student body that exceptions to confidentiality will be made when a student's mental condition is such that immediate action must be taken to protect the student or others from serious consequence of his illness and also when a student is referred for evaluation and an opinion or recommendation is requested. In the first situation, immediate voluntary or involuntary hospitalization may be arranged, and the college administration and parents may be notified as quickly as possible. In cases of the second type, called administrative referrals, the student is informed initially that a report will be made to the referring individual or agency, but the actual content of the interview remains confidential.[44] The Family Educational Rights and Privacy Act (FERPA) enacted in 1974 allows school officials to notify parents in a "health or safety emergency" or when the student is still claimed as a tax deduction by the parents. All too often, making a Holy Grail of confidentiality, therapists at university clinics do not inform parents that their son or daughter may be a suicidal risk, thereby depriving the student of parental support or involving the family in therapy.

FERPA conditions federal funding on educational institutions' keeping student files confidential. Subject to few exceptions, universities under FERPA may not release student records to anyone, including parents or guardians, unless the student consents. The only real exception is "in connection with an emergency." Universities may release records to "appropriate persons if the knowledge of such information is necessary to protect the health or safety of the student or other persons." The notification provision is not mandatory, and although FERPA permits disclosures in emergencies, it leaves to the school complete discretion to determine what constitutes an emergency and who are the appropriate people to notify. Overall, FERPA has made schools wary about reporting mental health issues for fear of losing federal funding, especially since an administrative regulation accompanying the statute requires strict construction of the disclosure exception.[45]

Thus, the prevailing practice as to notification of parents of minors for treatment of mental disorder is, curiously enough, just the opposite of the procedure generally followed and approved by the law in the case of treatment of minors for physical illness. In psychotherapy, notification is made only in emergencies, whereas in treatment for physical illness, lack of notification in emergencies is legally excused, time being of the essence. With venereal disease and drug use now constituting public health emergencies of the first order, legislation has been enacted in a number of states allowing minors over the age of 12 or 15 to give consent to medical examination or treatment without parental consent.[46]

As part of its program of healthcare, a number of large companies have retained psychiatrists to care for the emotional problems of their employees. The Group for the Advancement of Psychiatry in its report on confidentiality said, "If the psychiatrist is administratively tied to the personnel division of a company, the confidential relationship cannot exist, and it behooves him to clarify his position with the employee. We regard failure to do so as a serious abridgement of the physician's ethical responsibility." The report drew special attention to the psychiatrist working for public mental health hospitals, prisons, and law enforcement agencies.[47]

Actually, there is nothing new about psychiatrists working for public health hospitals. In the latter part of the 19th century, the states, beginning in 1890 with Massachusetts passing a law authorizing the establishment of a lunatic institution, took over responsibility for the care of the mentally ill. Between 1840 and 1850 most of the other states did the same. It will be recalled that the first association of psychiatrists was known as the Association of Medical Superintendents of American Institutions for the Insane. During recent decades, however, psychiatrists by and large have abandoned the mental hospital for private practice.

In the 1960s and 1970s, psychiatry was extended beyond the insulated doctor–patient relationship, and the psychiatrist once again found himself not acting in intimate privacy with his patient. His relationship with the patient, in some cases, has become a matter of public concern. He finds himself in a two-faced position that strains his patient's confidence and demands of him the skill and judgment to satisfy interests other than his patient's while maintaining his professional conscience and integrity intact. The administration of his art and practice is shared partially with other essential parties. The legal profession has encased him in a situation that sets him up as a manipulator of his patient's life—both present and future—despite the fact that confidentiality does not grow well in an environment polluted with deceit. The psychiatrist has contributions to make beyond his traditional role, but in such situations it is necessary that he recognize and clarify, to all parties concerned, the precise nature of each of these situations.[48]

Endnotes

1. Almost all states require physicians to make a report when a patient is injured by a gun, knife, or other deadly weapon. Some states (California, Kentucky, New Mexico, New Hampshire, Rhode Island, and Colorado) have mandatory reporting laws that specifically address domestic violence. In Colorado, for example, physicians must report to the police any injuries caused by a firearm, knife, or other sharp instrument or "any other injury which the physician has reason to believe involves a criminal act, including injuries resulting from domestic violence."

   Mandatory reporting would require complete documentation of domestic violence–related injuries in the victim's medical record that could later be used as evidence in prosecuting the batterer. Opponents of the mandatory reporting laws argue that these laws perpetuate the stereotypes of battered women as being "helpless" and "childlike." The portrayal of victims as helpless is evidence in the legislative intent of some of these state statutes. For instance, the legislative findings and purpose of the New Mexico reporting statute indicate that the "legislature recognized that many adults in the state are unable to manage their own affairs or protect themselves from exploitation, abuse or neglect." See J.T.R. Jones, "Kentucky Tort Liability for Failure to Report Family Violence," *No. Ky. U. L. Rev.* 26 (1999): 43; M.M. McFarlane, "Mandatory Reporting of Domestic Violence: An Inappropriate Response for New York Health Care Professionals," *Buff. Public Interest L. J.* 17 (1998/1999): 1.
2. See R. Slovenko, *Psychotherapy and Confidentiality* (Springfield, IL: Thomas, 1998); D.I. Joseph & J. Onek, "Confidentiality in Psychiatry," in S. Bloch, P. Chodoff, & S.A. Green (Eds.), *Psychiatric Ethics* (Oxford, U.K.: Oxford University Press, 3rd ed., 1999), pp.105–140.
3. S.S. Gilder, "How Safe Is a Secret?" *Medical Counterpoint*, May 1970, p. 54.
4. In Garner v. Stone, No. 97A-320250-1 (Ga. DeKalb Cy. Super. Ct., 1999), a jury found that in this case the therapist's duty to protect a patient's confidence outweighed the duty to warn others. The therapist, a psychologist, issued a warning to the police chief that the patient, a police officer, was "burned out and should not be on the street carrying a gun." The day the therapist issued the warning, the patient began therapy with a psychiatrist, who found him fit for duty and posed no threat. See Chapter 36 on duty of therapists to third parties. See also R. Slovenko, *Psychotherapy and Confidentiality* (Springfield, IL: Thomas, 1998).
5. Years ago, psychiatrist John Felber brought a class action suit in federal court against the state of Connecticut on behalf of all physicians in the state, contending that the law infringed upon physicians' rights to privacy and confidentiality with patients and violated physicians' rights of due process of law. In addition, he contended the law fails to provide a definition of the term *drug-dependent*, it conflicts with the state's privileged communications law, and it constitutes "an unreasonable exercise of police power." Ruling against him, the court said that there is no constitutional basis for privilege or confidentiality between physician and patient and that the matter rests entirely in the power of the legislature to enact laws related to these matters. While some matters of privacy have received constitutional protection in Supreme Court decisions, this court ruled that the physician–patient relationship is not so protected; Felber v. Foote, 321 F. Supp. 85 (D.C. Conn. 1970). The constitutionality of the reporting provisions of the New York law was upheld in Roe v. Ingraham, 357 F. Supp. 1217 (S.D. N.Y. 1973).
6. 695 N.Y.S.2d 903 (N.Y. Sup. Ct. 1999).
7. Furness v. Fitchett, [1958] N.Z.L.R. 396. One of the early cases awarding relief based upon the invasion of privacy, although not characterized as such, involved a doctor who brought in a lay assistant to help him in a childbirth situation. The doctor had made no disclosure that the assistant was not a doctor. DeMay v. Roberts, 46 Mich. 160, 9 N.W. 146 (1881). See S.D. Warren & S. Brandeis, "The Right to Privacy," *Harv. L. Rev.* 4 (1890): 193; W.L. Prosser, "Privacy," *Calif. L. Rev.* 48 (1960): 383.
8. Berry v. Moench, 8 Utah 2d 191, 331 P.2d 814 (1958).
9. Carr v. Watkins, 227 Md. 578, 177 A.2d 841 (1962). See also R.B. Little & E.A. Strecker, "Moot Questions in Psychiatric Ethics," *Am. J. Psychiat.* 113 (1956): 455.
10. McGovern followers said the vice presidential fiasco was to blame for the magnitude of McGovern's loss of the election. It is recounted again in a recent obituary. A. Clymer, "Thomas F. Eagleton, 77, a Running Mate for 18 Days, Dies," *New York Times*, March 5, 2007, p. 21. See P.J. Fink & A. Tasman, *Stigma and Mental Illness* (Arlington, VA: American Psychiatric Publishing, 1992); G. Thornicroft, *Shunned: Discrimination Against People With Mental Illness* (New York: Oxford University Press, 2006).
11. See G. Annas, "Candidates Deserve Medical Privacy," *New York Times*, Feb. 1, 2000, p. 25.
12. Dr. Williams recounts the incident in "The Autobiography of William Carlos Williams." See H. Markel, "Patients Are Discovering 'My Doctor, the Author,'" *New York Times*, Aug. 22, 2000, p. D-7.

13. Janna Malamud Smith, a psychotherapist, argues that Freud violated the privacy of his patients and sensationalized his work. She writes, "[Freud] wished to shock the staid members of his audience, to stir things up, to found a movement." J.M. Smith, *Private Matters: In Defense of the Personal Life* (Emeryville, CA: Seal Press, 2003).

14. Commonwealth v. Wiseman, 356 Mass. 251, 249 N.E.2d 610 (1969); noted in *Colum. L. Rev.* 70 (1970): 259; *Harv. L. Rev.* 83 (1970): 1722. In subsequent legislation, Massachusetts specifically stated that patients are to be protected "from commercial exploitation of any kind. No patient shall be photographed, interviewed, or exposed to public view without either his express written consent or that of his legal guardian"; Mass. Gen. Laws chap. 19 §29(f).

15. Beginning December 19, 2006, Michigan health practitioners and licensed health facilities are required by law to retain patient records for a minimum of 7 years, unless another Michigan or federal law requires a longer period or if the standard of practice would require a longer period. Medical records may not be destroyed within the first 7 years of their creation or the records coming into the physician's possession without written authorization from the patient. The new law also contains requirements applicable when a physician closes or sells a practice. When doing so, physicians are required to notify the Michigan Department of Community Health specifying the identity of the person or entity having custody of the medical records and describing how patients may request access to or copies of their medical records. In addition, physicians must either obtain the patients' specific written permission and destroy the records or transfer custody of the medical records to a successor physician taking over the practice, to the patients themselves, or to a professional storage company contracted by the physician. All of the new requirements also apply to the personal representative of a deceased physician. Physicians who do not comply with the new law can be fined up to $10,000 if the failure was the result of gross negligence or willful and wanton misconduct.

16. H.C. Modlin, "How Private is Privacy?" *Psychiatry Digest*, Feb. 1969, p. 13.

17. Correspondence from Dr. Maurice Grossman, Chairman of American Psychiatric Association Task Force on Confidentiality.

18. Clarkson Memorial Hosp. v. Reserve Life Ins. Co., 350 F.2d 1006 (8th Cir. 1965); Wallace v. University Hosp., 170 N.E.2d 261 (Ohio App. 1970). In Gaertner v. State, 385 Mich. 49, 187 N.W.2d 429 (1971), the plaintiff, as guardian of a mentally incompetent minor, sought access to medical records regarding the treatment of his ward when an inpatient in several state institutions. The State Attorney General asserted that there is a statutory duty to keep such records confidential and also argued that access to the records could not be allowed because the hospital physicians might lose their medical licenses through prosecution for violation of various statutory provisions. Pointing out that the privilege of confidentiality was designed for the protection of the patient, the court held that, because a mentally incompetent ward cannot act for himself, the law would allow his guardian to waive the privilege for his benefit and ruled that the lawful representative should have access to all the patient's hospital records. See generally *Brit. Med. J.*, Feb. 26, 1972, p. 577.

19. W.A. Pomeroy, *Dr. Kinsey and the Institute for Sex Research* (New York: Harper & Row, 1972), reprinted in 1982 by Yale University Press.

20. See M. Grossman, "Insurance Reports as a Threat to Confidentiality," *Am. J. Psychiat.* 128 (1971): 64.

21. 344 F. Supp. 373, 387 (M.D. Ala. 1972) .

22. See D. Brin, *The Transparent Society* (Reading, MA: Addison-Wesley, 1998); A. Etzioni, *The Limits of Privacy* (New York: Basic Books, 1999); C.J. Sykes, *The End of Privacy* (New York: St. Martin's Press, 1999); A.F. Westin (Proj. Dir.), *Databanks in a Free Society* (New York: Quadrangle, 1973).

23. 104 P.L. 191, 110 Stat. 1936 (1996).

24. 45 CFR § 164, 502.

25. Personal communications.

26. Moss v. Amira, 356 Ill. App.3d 701, 826 N.E.2d 1001 (2005); see D. Wirtes, R. Lamberth, & J. Gomez, "An Important Consequence of HIPAA: No More *Ex Parte* Communications Between Defense Attorneys and Plaintiff's Treating Physicians," *Am. J. Trial Advoc.* 27 (2003): 1.

27. 532 U.S. 67 (2001).

28. A.B. v. C.D., 7 Fed. 72 (1905), Simonsen v. Swenson, 104 Neb. 244, 177 N.W. 831 (1920). Dr. Karl A. Menninger observed:

> It is true that the physician has a loyalty to his patient and a responsibility for treating the professional relationship with respect and honor. But the doctor also has other responsibilities. He has a responsibility to society, to the hospital, to the rest of the medical profession, and to science. No patient has a right to exploit the confidential relationship offered by the physician to make

the physician a *particeps criminis* [a partaker in the crime]. The physician cannot condone moral and legal irresponsibility on the part of the patient. For example, a patient comes to a VA Hospital with certain psychiatric symptoms, and in the course of his history he confesses that he has been receiving compensation for self-inflicted gunshot wounds, which he had claimed were received in combat. The psychiatrist who receives this information has no right to withhold from the clinical records the fact that the patient has been defrauding the government, even though this confession was made in confidence. Another instance that recently came to my knowledge was one in which a patient was accepted in a VA Hospital for treatment for which he was completely ineligible. Because certain individuals were sympathetic and felt that he needed the hospitalization (and considered that the information concerning his ineligibility was given to them in confidence and could not be betrayed), they joined in concealing this information from the Registrar over a period of nearly 2 years. In effect, this was conspiracy to defraud the government and did irreparable harm to the patient, even though those in charge of him really felt that they were doing the best thing. If a patient tells a doctor in confidence that he has brought a time bomb into the hospital and hidden it under the bed of one of the other patients, it is a strange doctor indeed who would feel that this professional confidence should not be violated.

A Manual for Psychiatric Case Study (New York: Grune & Stratton, 1962), pp. 36–37.

29. M.H. Hollender, "The Psychiatrist and the Release of Patient Information," *Am. J. Psychiat.* 116 (1960): 828. Following the passage of the Civil Rights Act of 1964, the number of employers utilizing objective personnel tests markedly increased. While ostensibly neutral, these tests disqualified a disproportionate number of nonwhites prompting the Supreme Court to proscribe their use unless the employer could prove that they measured aptitudes and skills related to job performance. Griggs v. Duke Power Co., 401 U.S. 424 (1971); discussed in H.N. Bernhardt, "Griggs v. Duke Power Co.: The Implications for Private and Public Employers," *Texas L. Rev.* 50 (1972): 901.

30. In another proposal, Dr. Leopold Bellak, clinical professor psychiatry at Albert Einstein College of Medicine, suggested that candidates for president and vice-president be tested for organic brain problems, such as lesions and tumors that could interfere with memory, problem-solving, attention span, and the ability to think abstractly. T. Andersen, "Psychiatrist Wants Brain Tests for Presidential Candidates," *Gannett Westchester Newspapers*, August 30, 1984, p. 3. Dr. Abraham L. Halpern responded, "I can see much harm and no good that can come from routine psychological testing of candidates for president and vice-president. ... [S]uch testing is not likely to uncover significant mental impairments or characterological deficits not already discernible by the public." A.L. Halpern (ltr.), "Democracy Beats Mental Tests," *Gannett Westchester Newspapers*, Sept. 7, 1984, p. 13. See M.J. Halberstam, "Who's Medically Fit for the White House?" *New York Times Magazine*, Oct. 22, 1972, p. 39; A.A. Hutschnecker, "The Lessons of Eagleton," *New York Times*, Oct. 30, 1972, p. 31. W. Gaylin, "What's Normal?" *New York Times Magazine*, April 11, 1973, p. 14.

31. *Washington Post*, Sept. 22, 1960, p. 1; Dec. 22, 1960, p. 1.

32. M. Guttmacher, *The Mind of the Murderer* (New York: Grove Press, 1960), p. 215.

33. 347 U.S. 556 (1954).

34. The late law professor Joseph D. Grano, my colleague, wrote: "Totally aside from the issue of coercion involuntariness, the use of the psychiatrist in *Leyra* violated the unfair advantage or improper exploitation strand of the due process voluntariness doctrine." *Confessions, Truth, and the Law* (Ann Arbor: University of Michigan Press, 1993), p. 111.

35. 371 P.2d 443 (Colo. 1962).

36. Morgan v. State, 142 So.2d 308 (Fla. App. 1962); see J.B. Parsons, "The Pre-Sentence Investigation Report Must Be Preserved as a Confidential Document," *Fed. Probation* 28 (1964): 3; P. Roche, "The Position for Confidentiality of the Presentence Investigation Report," *Albany L. Rev.* 29 (1965): 206.

37. California and New Jersey provide that when the conviction has been for serious crime, the report must be fully disclosed and counsel must be given an opportunity to rebut its content. Virginia provides that the report must be presented in open court, with the defendant being apprised of its content and having an absolute right to cross-examine the person who prepared it. Connecticut provides that the defendant shall be furnished the report, but the court's discretion determines the limits of the defense's rights to interrogate the investigator. Maryland, Michigan, Minnesota, and North Carolina provide that the substance of the report must be disclosed, but provision is made to safeguard from disclosure the sources of information it contains (the rule suggested in both the ALI's Model Penal Code and the ABA's Project on Minimum Standards for Criminal Justice). See R.H. Kuh, "For a Meaningful Right to Counsel on Sentencing," *A.B.A. J.* 7 (1971): 1096.

38. E.N. Bartin, "Looking at the Law," *Fed. Probation* 28 (1964): 61.
39. A. MacCormick, "A Criminologist Looks at Privilege," *Am. J. Psychiat.* 115 (1959): 1068.
40. N. Fenton, "Group Counseling: A Method for the Treatment of Prisoners and for a New Staff Orientation in the Correctional Institution," in R. Slovenko (Ed.), *Crime, Law and Corrections* (Springfield, IL: Thomas, 1996), p. 605.
41. *New York Times*, March 5, 1972, p. 9; see W. Creech, "Psychological Testing and Constitutional Rights," *Duke L. J.* 1966: 332; J.H. Ricks, "On Telling Parents About Test Results," *Test Service Bull.* No. 54 (New York: Psychological Corp., Dec. 1959); C.W. Sherrer & R.A. Roston, "Some Legal and Psychological Concerns About Personality Testing in the Public Schools," *Fed. Bar. J.* 30 (1971): 111.
42. State Boards of Education usually set out a policy protecting psychiatric reports and personality test results from disclosure.
43. T.S. Szasz, "The Psychiatrist as Double Agent," *Transaction*, Oct. 1967, pp. 6–24.
44. One university newspaper advises about its health service thus: "The students' contacts with our services are strictly confidential. Absolutely no one in the university is notified of a student's visit, nor does it appear on any student's record. An exception would be if one of the deans or other administrative officials referred a student or faculty member to the clinic in order that it might render an opinion concerning that person. One other exception would be where the clinic feels the student is so upset, for instance, that he should leave school; then the clinic might notify the parents, but almost never over the student's objections." Be that as it may, writing anonymously (later revealed as Dr. Miriam Grossman of UCLA), Dr. Anonymous argues that the culture on campus—and in her profession—is so steeped in political correctness that it hamstrings the ability of therapists to help college students. Anonymous, M.D., *Unprotected: A Campus Psychiatrist Reveals How Political Correctness in Her Profession Endangers Every Student* (New York: Sentinel, 2007); reviewed in S. Satel, "'First, Do Harm': How Campus Therapists Sabotage Their Patients," *Weekly Standard*, Feb. 5, 2007, p. 35.
45. See K. Cohen, "Keeping Students Alive: Mandating On-Campus Counseling Saves Suicidal College Students' Lives and Limits Liability," *Fordham L. Rev.* 75 (2007): 3081. In Jain v. State of Iowa, 617 N.W.2d 293 (Iowa 2000), the plaintiff's son committed suicide at the University of Iowa during his freshman year. He had personal, academic, and discipline problems during his first semester. The university was aware of his problems because his girlfriend notified the dorm authorities of an attempted suicide, and, consequently, he met with a student counselor. He refused to allow the counselor to notify his parents of his suicidal tendencies. After he killed himself, his parents alleged that the university was negligent because the suicide could have been prevented if it had notified his parents. However, the Iowa Supreme Court held that there was no special relationship between the student and the university that obligated the university to notify the parents or affirmatively prevent the suicide; 617 N.W.2d at 299–300.

Recently, however, the courts have been more willing to impose liability on universities in wrongful death cases brought by parents of students who committed suicide on campus. For example, in Schieszler v. Ferrum College, 236 F. Supp.2d 602 (W.D. Va. 2002), the court held that although special relationships do not always exist between students and universities, the facts of the case could demonstrate that the university officials had a special relationship with the student that created a duty to prevent his suicide. In this case, the student was a freshman at Ferrum College, and his girlfriend informed university officials of his suicidal tendencies. The officials had the student promise not to hurt himself, but they offered no further support. When the student hanged himself 3 days later, his guardian filed a wrongful death claim alleging that the university was negligent because it failed to take adequate precautions even though it knew that the student would hurt himself if not supervised. Although the case eventually settled, the court found that a special relationship likely existed in this case because the suicide was foreseeable and the officials had a duty to give further assistance; 236 F. Supp.2d at 609–610.

In 2006, the Massachusetts Institute of Technology paid an undisclosed sum to settle a lawsuit by the parents of Elizabeth Shin, whose death in a dorm room fire was ruled a suicide by a medical examiner. The parents alleged that school officials failed to notify them of the emotional deterioration of their daughter. Other lawsuits have challenged schools that required students to leave dorms or campuses after exhibiting suicidal behavior. In another case, the parents of Chuck Mahoney sued Allegheny College for failing to get them involved in the care of their son. He committed suicide. He had signed a policy statement from the counseling center at the college acknowledging that his confidentiality would be maintained except under "important legally mandated exceptions" such as posing an "immediate threat" to himself or others, including suicide. The jury voted 11–1 for the defendants. The case is discussed in a lengthy article by Elizabeth Bernstein, "After a Suicide, Privacy on Trial," *Wall Street Journal*, March 24–25, 2007. See also ltrs., "Student Suicides: Privacy Rules Must Be Tempered by Common Sense," *Wall Street Journal*, April 16, 2007, p. 13. The ordeal of Sue Kayton to obtain information from the Massachusetts Institute of Technology about her missing son, who eventually was found to have committed suicide, is described in E. Bernstein, "A Mother Takes On MIT," *Wall Street Journal*, Sept. 10, 2007, p.1.

The review panel appointed in the wake of the shootings at Virginia Tech University cited failures to communicate about the gunman, Seung Hui Cho, among campus administrators, the counseling center, police, and others. All parties, said the panel, thought that "such communications were prohibited by federal laws governing the privacy of health and education records." The report highlighted the enormous sources of confusion nationwide among counseling centers about what can and cannot be disclosed. Many barriers arise from either unfamiliarity with applicable laws or misinterpretation of laws or court cases. The Cho family had no idea that there was a problem at the university. A. Levin, "Failure to Communicate Played Role in Va. Tech Tragedy," *Psychiatric News*, Oct. 19, 2007, p. 13. (See the discussion of the shootings at Virginia Tech in Chapter 24 on civil commitment.

It is to be noted that when it is ruled that there is a special relationship between students and the university, there is a duty to provide services, and if it is held that there is no special relationship, but nonetheless the university provides services, it has undertaken a duty of care. A leading case in psychiatry and law, *Tarasoff v. Regents of University of California*, involved the duty of a university clinic to warn those threatened by a patient. See Chapter 36 on duty of therapists to third parties.

46. At least 43 states have passed laws to permit physicians to diagnose and treat venereal disease in minors on their own consent. Twenty-five states have extended, to at least certain minors, the right to treatment in such matters as contraception and other pregnancy-related conditions, drug addiction, and sometimes the full range of medical services. The majority of these states, however, limit the broad range of services to what are called emancipated minors—usually those 18 or over, or married, or living away from home and supporting themselves.

47. Group for the Advancement of Psychiatry, *Confidentiality and Privileged Communication in the Practice of Psychiatry*, Report No. 45, p. 106.

48. For additional and extended discussion of confidentiality issues, see R. Slovenko, *Psychotherapy and Confidentiality* (Springfield, IL: Thomas, 1998).

From early childhood many of us learn to fear two classes of people: police (because they carry guns) and physicians (because they intrude our bodies and they give shots). The police are controlled by the law on search and seizure and physicians by the law on consent.

As a legal matter, liability arising out of medical treatment where consent is lacking can rest on one of two theories: battery or negligence. Typically, an action based on battery occurs where the physician obtains the consent of the patient for the performance of a particular procedure, but thereafter performs a different procedure for which consent was not obtained. Without authorization for a procedure, the physician may be held liable in battery even though it is skillfully performed, and is successful.[1]

On the other hand, when consent is given for a procedure, but injury results due to an undisclosed risk, the theory in such a case is usually negligence. Again, it is of no moment that the treatment was skillfully performed. Two landmark cases decided in 1960 within days of each other announced the doctrine of informed consent.[2] Under the doctrine, the patient's mere consent to a procedure became no longer an adequate authorization for treatment. Instead, the consent must be an informed consent—to wit, the physician must inform the patient of the nature and purpose of the proposed procedure, the likelihood of success, the hazards of the procedure, and any alternative forms of treatment. In other words, the duty became not merely to obtain consent, but also to make disclosures.[3]

Throughout history physicians obtained the consent of a patient to a treatment, and information about the treatment was provided, but information was not given that might unduly alarm the patient. The assumption among physicians was that patients did not really want to know what was wrong with them (it would only cause needless anxiety), or that they could not possibly understand. The Hippocratic tradition of benevolent paternalism is now widely regarded as in conflict with the autonomy of patients and their right to be fully informed in making decisions. Physicians are now expected to be facilitators of patient decision making rather than the decision makers. It is no longer assumed that the patient shares the physician's values about anything. Stirred by wider consumer protection and rights movements, patients learned to abandon the role of a child accepting treatment from a paternalistic physician; they began to assume the guise of adults. The doctrine of informed consent is seen as a bulwark against the medical profession's paternalistic domination of patients.[4]

Professor Alexander Capron has argued that the doctrine can serve six salutary functions. It can (1) protect individual autonomy, (2) protect the patient's status as a human being, (3) avoid fraud or duress, (4) encourage physicians to carefully consider their decisions, (5) foster rational decision making by the patient, and (6) involve the public generally in medicine.[5] The doctrine is now reflected in consent forms that healthcare institutions require all patients to sign upon admission and before various procedures are performed, and it has provided the starting point for federal regulations on human experimentation.

In psychotherapy or psychoanalysis, the spelling out of possible risks of therapy tends to be suggestive and so, Freud recommended, preliminary discussions should be kept to a minimum (but, in the course of therapy, Freud often made suggestions).[6] In any event, psychotherapy is marked by surprises, so what can be told, or should be told? Psychoanalytic psychotherapy is a voyage very much like sailing—where one goes depends on the wind, and that is unpredictable. Should a therapist inform a patient that a risk of therapy might be divorce or erotic feelings toward the therapist? Moreover, unlike surgery, psychotherapy is not a one-time event, but a process, and the patient presumably can withdraw at any time during therapy. In recent years the revival of memory of child sexual abuse has prompted proposals to enact legislation that would require a psychotherapist to obtain an elaborate informed consent before embarking on "any treatment method not proved safe and effective."[7]

The doctrine of informed consent is tied to the doctrine of assumption of risk. Informed consent, in effect, is an assumption of the announced risks of therapy. What about an assumption of the risk of malpractice? Exculpatory clauses are closely scrutinized and are not given effect when there is a special legal relationship or overriding public interest as in the case of medical treatment. As a matter of law, a consent form, signed in advance, that absolves a physician or hospital from liability for negligence is not valid as a release. In a California case,[8] the patient was admitted to the hospital on condition that he execute a release absolving the hospital "from any and all liability for the negligent or wrongful acts or omissions of its employees." The California Supreme Court held that although one may, generally speaking, voluntarily assume a risk, a release is not valid when one is compelled to assume a risk to obtain essential medical treatment. In this situation, the court said, the releasing party does not really acquiesce voluntarily in the contractual shifting of the risk, nor does he receive an adequate consideration for the transfer of the risk.

Determining whether a consent for medical care is valid calls for consideration of three elements: competency, disclosure, and voluntariness. While there is consensus about these elements, the tests in determining them are far less settled. For competency, several cognitive abilities are involved. The first is the ability to communicate and sustain a choice; if the patient cannot make a preference known or if he repeatedly changes his mind, his decision-making capacity is impaired. The second is the ability to understand relevant information. The third is the ability to appreciate the situation and its consequences. The fourth and final ability, as proposed by Dr. Paul Appelbaum and Thomas Grisso, is that required to manipulate information rationally. A patient whose logic is faulty is unlikely to have sound judgment.[9] The appointment of a guardian is called for when the patient is deemed incompetent.

The disclosures required of alternative treatments are those generally acknowledged within the professional community as feasible, their risks and consequences and their probability of success. Some courts have held that alternatives should be disclosed even if an alternative is more hazardous, or the physician is not capable of performing it or evaluating its risk.[10] The courts, however, may limit the disclosure requirement by concluding that some alternatives are not legitimate treatment options.[11]

In the event of a Black Box warning on medication, the physician must document that it was reviewed with the patient.

The field of psychiatry is broadly divided into three fields or combinations thereof: psychotherapy, pharmacological therapy, and behavior therapy. The field is marked by an almost chaotic character of divisions that proclaim one approach as authentic and describe others as moribund. Within psychotherapy, a proliferation of approaches came about in the 1960s: gestalt, transactional analysis, bioenergetics, etc. As therapies proliferated, so did psychotherapists, and now it is a bewildering maze. How does a therapist advise about the alternatives?[12]

Impact of the Healthcare System

In practice, consent is transfigured by the healthcare system. As is well known, healthcare is a function of the interplay among the individual patient, the caregiver, the system that organizes the services, the purchasers and payers who preselect the care, and the private and public agencies that provide oversight and compliance with the system.

Healthcare is now mostly *managed care*. Under it, various alternative forms of treatment, as a practical matter, may be unavailable. Managed care organizations have been accused of withholding necessary services through several mechanisms, including restriction of access to specialists, limitations on covered medications, denial of coverage for new forms of technology, administrative review of physicians' decisions, and capitation plans under which the physician is paid more to do less.[13] A gag clause included in one health plan (but no longer) prevented or discouraged physicians from telling their patients about different kinds of treatments.[14] Under managed care, diagnosis, informed consent, and treatment are to be done in the allotted 10 or 15 minutes for an office appointment.

Elements of an Informed Consent Action

A patient suing under the theory of informed consent is obliged to allege and prove (1) defendant physician failed to inform him adequately of a material risk before securing his consent to the proposed treatment, (2) if he had been informed of the risks he would not have consented to the treatment, and (3) the adverse consequences that were not made known did in fact occur and he was injured as a result of undergoing the treatment. As informed consent is a negligence— not intentional—tort action, proof of damages is necessary. A complaint of battery, on the other hand, may be based solely on an insult to bodily integrity.

The concept of informed consent provides a cause of action in cases of unsuccessful or poor outcome even though consent to the procedure has been given and even though negligence in treatment cannot be established. The Oklahoma Supreme Court put it thus, "[T]his requirement, labeled 'informed consent,' is, legally speaking, as essential as a physician's care and skill in the *performance* of the therapy" (emphasis by court).[15] Moreover, as a legal strategy, a plaintiff by expanding the issues in litigation can expand the scope of discovery or the opportunity to employ experts.

Initially the lack of an informed consent (like lack of consent to a procedure) was deemed a battery, but gradually the various state courts held it constituted negligence (malpractice). The medical profession in Texas persuaded the state legislature to enact legislation to that effect.[16] One by one, the various states by court decision or statute have deemed lack of an informed consent to constitute negligence, not battery; however, a number of recent decisions have again called it battery.[17] Under negligence, any judgment would fall under the practitioner's liability policy. On the other hand, insurance policies do not afford protection against judgments for intentional wrongs such as battery. Moreover, judgments attributable to intentional wrongs also are not discharged in bankruptcy.[18] Punitive damages are usually awarded in the case of an intentional tort.

Viewing the failure to provide information for an informed consent as a negligence case, negligence rules would seem to apply. That means not only that there would be insurance coverage, but also that the standard for disclosure would be the standard prevailing in the relevant medical community. In a malpractice action, the complainant would have to present expert testimony about the risks or alternatives of the treatment. A traditional professional standard would focus on what physicians usually tell patients about a procedure under the same or similar circumstances (a matter of medical judgment), but many jurisdictions have changed the test from what the reasonable physician would disclose to what the reasonable patient would like to know.[19]

Involuntary Hospitalization

Over two decades of litigation and regulation on the right of an involuntary hospitalized patient to refuse treatment have left psychiatrists bewildered as to the state of the law. When an individual is civilly committed, the loss of civil or political rights is not theoretically an integral part of the process. However, in hospitalizing, the various states have combined commitment and competency proceedings. As a practical matter, hospital staffs of public hospitals usually require individuals seeking admission to proceed via involuntary commitment so that they cannot refuse treatment. Given the evidence of serious irreversible side effects, some courts became receptive to the argument that patients have a right to refuse psychotropic medication (with court approval) being required for their use.[20]

Tardive Dyskinesia

The timing of information about the risk of tardive dyskinesia (TD) in the use of neuroleptic medication is controversial, as that side effect is not a result of acute treatment, and many clinicians feel that discussion about a possibly permanent side effect at the initiation of treatment could deter initiation of a needed intervention. Dr. Jerrold G. Bernstein advised in his widely used book on drug therapy, "Since tardive dyskinesia does not occur early in the course of antipsychotic treatment, it is probably not appropriate to discuss this complication at the outset of treatment; discussion of this potential complication can be reserved until later in the treatment, after the patient recovers from the acute manifestations of psychosis, and the physician has decided on a course of treatment that may involve a more prolonged period of administration of the neuroleptic."[21] Likewise, Dr. Frank J. Ayd advised that in the initial stages of neuroleptic therapy, especially when it is reasonable to assume that neuroleptic administration will be of short duration, the risk of TD need not be stressed because all the available data (with the exception of one report) on the time of onset substantiate that it rarely appears until after 3 months of neuroleptic therapy, the risk increasing steadily thereafter.[22] However, because patients may change physicians, it is important to have the patient's neuroleptic drug history. Many chronic patients are transient and may have been taking neuroleptics that were prescribed by a number of physicians for some time. In determining causation, the law is interested more in the straw that broke the camel's back than in all the straws already piled on its back. Arguably, it may be said that the last straw was not the proximate cause, but that is a jury question.

Informed Consent as a Ploy

How often is the doctrine of informed consent used as a ploy in litigation to rationalize a desired outcome? Most of the time? A great deal of the time? Some of the time? A survey of cases would indicate that it is most or a great deal of the time. So, what is the significance of research on informed consent that has been funded by millions of dollars—yes, millions of dollars—by various foundations? The publications of articles and books on the topic continues without end in sight.[23]

Social scientists tend to take the law at face value, but as far as the law is concerned, the doctrine of informed consent is very much a ploy, so research on it might just as well be on abracadabra. As historian A. J. P. Taylor said of one research project, "It is 90% true and 100% useless." In the literature, the tactical use of the concept in litigation is rarely mentioned. Its significance as an ethical concern is another matter.

As a legal matter, as we have noted, the liability arising out of a treatment where consent is lacking can rest on one of two theories: battery or negligence. Typically, an action based on battery occurs where the physician performs a particular treatment for which consent was not obtained. An example is the case where a surgeon removed a fibroid tumor in circumstances where the patient had consented to an abdominal examination under anesthesia, but had specifically requested "no operation." "The wrong complained of," the court said in the oft-cited decision in *Schloendorff v. Society of New York Hospital*,[24] "is not merely negligence. It is trespass."

When consent is given for a particular treatment, but injury results due to an undisclosed risk, the theory in such a case is usually negligence. An example is where vertebrae were broken during electroshock treatment. The latter type of case falls under the doctrine of informed consent that developed during the past 30 years. In either case, the elements of consent include the competence of the patient and the voluntariness of the consent. Information about the risk is the additional element under the doctrine of informed consent.

Trying to measure up to the terms of informed consent, and seeking to avoid liability, medical practitioners encumber their practices with forms as they go through the ritual of providing information. Taking the informed consent doctrine literally, and seeking to avoid liability, the medical practitioner resorts to wordy ritualistic disclosures (which patients rarely read or understand). The patient signs not a "consent" form, but rather an "informed consent" form.

The concept of "informed consent" was essentially developed at law to provide another cause of action in cases of poor outcome when negligence in treatment could not be established. In a case of lack of informed consent, as in a case alleging battery, the fact that the treatment was properly performed is immaterial. And it is always a can of worms whether the elements of informed consent are satisfied.[25]

At other times, the doctrine of informed consent is used as a way to bar or express condemnation of a procedure. To this end, it has been used against electroshock therapy or psychosurgery. The psychosurgery case some years ago at Detroit's Lafayette Clinic is illustrative. At a conference at the clinic, chaired by Dr. Elliot Luby and I, the subject of the experiment, Louis Smith (then known as John Doe), was interviewed in the presence of a group of approximately 30 persons, including psychiatrists, a judge, and some staff members of the clinic. While some expressed doubt about the merit of the experiment, they all agreed that there was a valid consent. Smith was above average intelligence with the ability to communicate better than most university students. He was at the time an inmate at the Ionia state facility for sex offenders, but with repeal of Michigan's sexual psychopath law, he would be released in a few months, irrespective of the experiment. Smith sought the experiment, he said, in order to control outbursts of aggression.[26]

Without consulting Smith, Michigan Legal Services lawyer Gabe Kaimowitz, representing himself and certain individual members of the Medical Committee for Human Rights, filed a taxpayers' suit to halt the state-funded experiment. A panel of three judges in Wayne County Circuit Court listened to 3 weeks of testimony. In a 41-page opinion, Judge Horace Gilmore, writing the opinion, ruled that an involuntarily confined individual cannot give a legitimate consent as he is living in "an inherently coercive atmosphere." The court would allow a prisoner to consent only to low-risk, high-benefit procedures. Nothing was said about Smith's pending discharge.[27]

Several years later, upon Judge Gilmore's retirement from the bench, he said in an interview in the *Detroit News*, "I could control your violent behavior, too, by just removing all of your brain. What they wanted to do just wasn't right."[28] It was clear that he opposed psychosurgery to control violence. The doctrine of consent gave a rationale for the decision to bar it. It served as a ploy.[29]

Product Advertising

Prescription drugs (with the exception of oral contraceptives) have long been recognized as an exception to the rule in product liability law that generally mandates that the manufacturer of a product directly warn foreseeable users of known dangers inherent in the product's use. Under the traditional *learned intermediary doctrine*, the physician and not the manufacturer of a prescription drug has the duty to inform the patient of the drug's risks and benefits, on the theory that the physician is in the best position to evaluate the patient's needs. Four reasons are given for the learned intermediary rule:

1. Patients justifiably rely on their physicians' advice, and the physician–patient relationship should not be undermined by transferring liability from physicians to pharmaceutical companies.
2. Physicians' direct contact with patients put them in a better position than drug manufacturers to weigh and communicate to individual patients the risks associated with a particular treatment.
3. Most patients lack the scientific training needed to understand the risks of a prescription drug without the help of their physician.
4. Drug manufacturers generally lack an effective means to communicate with patients because drugs are prescribed through physicians and distributed through physicians and by pharmacies.

For these reasons, the courts concluded that it would be unreasonable to expect drug manufacturers to disclose risks directly to every patient.

Nowadays, however, direct advertising to consumers by pharmaceutical companies arguably negates the learned intermediary doctrine.[30] By advertising in the media, the companies seek to persuade the public to use their product or to alert them to a new development. At present, pharmaceutical advertising is predominate on television. In 2007, pharmaceutical companies reportedly spent $4.5 billion on direct advertising to consumers, or about 400 times more than they spent 20 years ago. Drug company spending on advertising to consumers is increasing twice as fast as spending on promotions to physicians or on the research and development of new drugs.[31]

Concerning one's health, people tend to be more emotional than rational and they often urge their physician to carry out a procedure or prescribe a medication. A patient, for example, may want an antibiotic simply for a sore throat and will be angry unless given it. Physicians aim to please and are often in a quandary as to whether they should disabuse patients of a treatment they seek. When several medications are appropriate, the physician will likely oblige the patient's request for one of them so as to take advantage of the placebo effect. It is said that, at the very least, direct-to-consumer pharmaceutical advertising with its focus on medication has injected an element of skepticism into psychotherapy.

Pharmaceutical makers are not required to submit commercials to the Food and Drug Administration, though many do so voluntarily. The director of the FDA's drug marketing division reports that probably the most common problem is a lack of balance—the presentation of the risk information is not commensurate with the benefits information.[32] In 2000, when the U.S. Supreme Court protected commercial speech no less than noncommercial speech, the "consumer's right to know" (Ralph Nader's great triumph of the 1970s) became the corporation's right to "subtly encourage." There then appeared advertisements, such as Viagra that showed men partying in the street, and Celebrex that showed arthritics dancing in the street.[33]

Then, too, medical information is found on the Internet. Some physicians now say that one third of their patients get health information online, and they complain of the added time these patients often require because of their online-inspired questions and preconceptions. Patients turning to the Internet come to their physician's office with printouts from Web sites detailing the latest drug or medical technology. Physicians must wade through stacks of downloaded data full of irrelevant information and bizarre cures, and must defend their expert opinions against tales derived from the Internet. Also, patients put additional demands on physicians' time with questions sent by e-mail. Physicians who do not respond are likely to lose these patients to physicians who are more accommodating.[34]

The Placebo Prescription

What about a placebo? A placebo, Latin for "I shall please," is typically a sham treatment that a physician uses merely to please or placate anxious or persistent patients. The placebo looks like an active drug, but unknown to the patient it has no pharmacological properties of its own. In years gone by, nearly all of medicine was based on placebo because physicians had little effective medicine to offer. Placebos are "lies that heal," as Dr. Anne Harrington, a historian of science at Harvard University, puts it.[35] Much of this sort of improvement can be attributed to spontaneous remission of an illness or to the fact that some people would have gotten better anyway. Of course, the ethics of informed consent would require a physician to tell the patient what he was giving him, but that would undercut the placebo effect.[36] In a wry comment, philosophy professor Gerald Dworkin says, "If placebos are to be prescribed and the patient's confidence enhanced, we need to have a range of names for these inert substances. I suggest the following: Prevaricaine, Fibusef, Deceptement."[37]

Psychiatry, like the rest of medicine, is no stranger to placebo "cures" and to the efficacy of strongly held belief systems in relieving all sorts of distress. One in three adults in the United States uses complementary therapies, such as chiropractic, acupuncture, homeopathy, herbs, and folk remedies. More than half the country's medical schools now offer courses in alternative medical practices, and patients are looking for physicians familiar with complementary as well as mainstream medicine. In many cases the wisdom of it may be questionable. The late Carl Sagan warned against pacifying a public, which is poorly schooled in scientific principles. Those suffering real illnesses need to know how to tell an effective remedy from a gimmick that catches the public imagination.[38]

Assurances About Treatment

The doctrine of informed consent calls for information about expected outcome, which, in some cases, may seem like an assurance. At times, assurances are made to alleviate anxiety or encourage the undertaking of treatment. Suppose the patient says to the physician, "You've told me about risks, but what I want to know is, how will it come out?" In the event of what is considered an assurance, there may result a contractual action for breach of warranty. One court put it thus: "Generally, a physician undertakes only to utilize his best skill and judgment. When he negligently fails to do so he may have committed a tort. However, a physician may, by express contract, agree to effect a cure or warrant that a particular result will be obtained. In such instances, an action in contract may lie against a physician."[39]

Thus, a plastic surgeon was held liable for breach of contract by telling a patient that he would give her "a nose like Hedy Lamarr's."[40] In another case the court held that the statement that electroconvulsive therapy (ECT) is "perfectly safe" might properly be found to be a warranty, and, hence, summary judgment was not granted.[41] As previously noted, the prescriptive period in a contract action is usually 5 years while a tort action is usually barred after 1 year for intentional wrongdoing, 2 years for malpractice, and 3 years for ordinary negligence. Various states have enacted legislation that requires "an agreement, promise, contract, or warranty of cure relating to medical care or treatment" to be in a signed writing.[42]

Disclosure of Risks of Nontreatment

In the event a patient refuses treatment, it is to be noted there comes into play the concept of "informed refusal," according to which the physician is obliged to inform the patient of the significant risks of inaction. Thus, in an opinion often discussed at medical conferences, *Truman v. Thomas*,[43] a patient declined to take a pap test. The physician was held liable for failing to warn her of the risks involved in declining to take it. The patient died from cancer of the cervix.

Had the patient undergone a pap smear at the time recommended, the cervical tumor probably would have been discovered in time to save her life. She had said she could not afford the cost of the test. The physician offered to defer payment, but she wanted to pay cash, and on another occasion she said "she just didn't feel like it."

To be material, a risk must be one that is not commonly appreciated. In *Truman*, there was no evidence to suggest that the patient was less than competent. The physician claimed that the risk of not undergoing a pap smear would be known to a reasonable person. He also argued that a patient who rejects a physician's advice has the burden of inquiring as to the consequences of this decision. The court said it was for the jury to decide whether it was reasonable for the physician to assume that the patient appreciated the potentially fatal consequences of her conduct.

The question has been asked: Should a physician, to avoid *Truman*-type liability, conjure up horrors as vividly as possible in order to persuade the patient? Must the physician do a "hard sell" in order to avoid the application of the *Truman* rule, manipulating information in order to get the patient to do what the physician thinks is best therapeutically? Assuredly, that practice would work against patient autonomy, the goal of informed consent.

Disclosure of Physician's Conflict of Interest

Beginning in the early 1900s, plaintiffs began to seek an expansion of the disclosure obligations of physicians beyond providing information about a proposed treatment. In one group of cases, patients have contended that physicians have an obligation to disclose any personal interests that may affect their professional judgment. Patients have alleged that the physician denied necessary care as a result of a managed care incentive compensation system and that the physician had an obligation to disclose it. In another group of cases, patients have claimed that physicians were obligated to inform them about risks arising out of the personal characteristics of the physician.

A number of courts have held that the concept of informed consent is broad enough to encompass a physician's research or financial interest as it might affect the physician's professional judgment. The California Supreme Court put it thus: "[W]e hold that a physician who is seeking a patient's consent for a medical procedure must, in order to satisfy his fiduciary duty and to obtain the patient's informed consent, disclose personal interests unrelated to the patient's health, whether research or economic, that may affect his medical judgment."[44] Under managed care, the physician is burdened with a conflict of obligations: an obligation to the patient and an obligation to the health plan. Presumably, the financial arrangements between the health plan and the physician should be disclosed.[45] Under managed care plans, the less the physician does, the more money he makes.

And what about the ethics of gifts by pharmaceutical companies to physicians, or the trips and dinners provided by the companies? After all, as was said in *Don Quixote*, "gifts break rocks." They have an influence, at least unconsciously. Observant patients may see the various objects in the physician's office—pens, clocks, books, stationery, briefcases—all emblazoned with the name of a pharmaceutical company. One patient asked the physician, "Are you in the pocket of the company?" Yet another observed, "My psychopharmacologist has a Lucite Prozac clock, Prozac pen set and Prozac stationery in his office."[46] A number of states (California, Maine, Minnesota, Vermont, West Virginia, and the District of Columbia) have enacted legislation requiring some level of disclosure of drug company marketing efforts.[47]

Disclosure of Skill or Status Risks

Most risks that must be disclosed relate to the therapy or procedure, but some courts have required disclosure of risks relating to the physician and the physician's capacity to perform. Like an accordion, the doctrine of informed consent can be contracted or expanded to fit the needs of the moment. The experience and success rate of the physician are relevant, not to the decision to accept treatment, but to the decision to accept it at the hands of a particular physician. In 1986, the federal government established a National Practitioner Data Bank listing malpractice decisions and disciplinary actions, but contrary to expectations, the data is not available to patients. Hospitals, licensing agencies, and other medical groups are given access to the data and, to protect patients, they are expected to use it in the providing of healthcare.[48] Under Medical Practice Acts, physicians have an obligation to report an impaired colleague.

Increasingly nowadays various publications list the "best doctors" of various specialties in a community. A nearly full-page advertisement in the *New York Times* said about a medical guidebook: "Don't leave one of the most important decisions in your life to chance. With this guide in hand, you're on your way to finding the very best doctor where you live and work."[49] Needless to say, it omits many fine doctors and includes many who are merely well-known. The medical profession itself is increasingly studying and sometimes publishing outcome records. In a respected treatise on health law, it is stated: "Informed consent doctrine can encompass the requirement that a physician disclose differential success rates, forcing physicians to present their 'batting averages.'"[50]

Patients normally expect that physicians acting within the ambit of their professional work will exercise the skill, knowledge, and care normally possessed and exercised by other members of their profession of the same school of practice in the relevant medical community. Similarly, physicians implicitly undertake to meet at least such a standard of care. As long as the physician measures up to the standard of care in carrying out a treatment, what more is relevant? If more is required, what would (or should) physicians reveal about themselves to a patient? What compromises their ability to treat a patient? Must they disclose that they have just had a quarrel with their spouse? Must they disclose that they engage in high-risk adventures (such as mountain climbing) that may result in injury and make them unavailable to continue therapy for possibly a lengthy time? That they have a heart condition? Or that they engage in forensic consultations and may have to interrupt therapy from time to time? More seriously, must a physician reveal that he has AIDS or has a history of alcoholism? Does it present a risk to patients? Where is the line to be drawn between a patient's right to know and a physician's right to privacy about his own health?

The courts are divided over whether physicians must inform patients of their level of skill and experience or impairment as part of the informed consent process. In a New Jersey case, the hospital informed patients that the physician, a plastic surgeon, was afflicted with AIDS. The physician was also a patient at the hospital. He brought suit against the hospital claiming invasion of privacy and breach of confidentiality. As a result of the disclosure, his practice declined. He argued (1) the risk of transmission of HIV from surgeon to patient is too remote to require informed consent, and (2) the law of informed consent does not require disclosure of the condition of the physician. The court ruled that the hospital had not only the right but also the duty to disclose.[51] It said: "It is axiomatic that physicians performing invasive procedures should not knowingly place a patient at risk because of the physician's physical condition."[52] While recognizing that the risk of transmission of the virus from a provider to patient is low, the court saw other risks, such as the risk of extended uncertainty and testing for a patient exposed to a surgical accident involving a surgeon with AIDS.[53]

A physician's failure to disclose his chronic alcohol abuse was held in a Louisiana case, *Hidding v. Williams*,[54] to have vitiated the patient's consent to surgery. There was a poor outcome, but the report of the case does not indicate that the physician was under the influence of alcohol at the time of surgery, or that his hands trembled or that the care fell below acceptable standards. Nonetheless the Louisiana Court of Appeals said: "Because this condition creates a material risk associated with the surgeon's ability to perform, which if disclosed would have obliged the patient to have elected another course of treatment, the fact-finder's conclusion that nondisclosure is a violation of the informed consent doctrine is entirely correct."[55]

During the course of the trial, a member of a medical review panel, asked whether a doctor suffering from alcohol or drug dependency has an affirmative obligation to relay this to the patient, answered: "I certainly think that if a physician or anybody in a position of life and death over someone knows that they're suffering from this condition, they should at least let this person know that they have these problems."[56]

In contrast, the Arizona Court of Appeals declined to allow evidence as to alcoholism of an anesthesiologist as a separate claim of negligence, absent a showing that he was intoxicated or impaired at the time of the surgery.[57] The plaintiff argued that alcoholism necessarily diminishes a physician's capacity to render the proper standard of care. The plaintiff cited legislation regulating the medical profession wherein unprofessional conduct is defined to include habitual intemperance in the use of alcohol. The court recognized that an alcoholic doctor might present a danger to the public if allowed to continue to practice medicine, but that, it said, is a matter for the medical board in deciding whether to revoke a license to practice. In a tort case, on the other hand, the court said, the issue is whether the physician exercised the proper standard of care in treating a particular patient at a particular time.[58]

What about a physician in his senior years who is aware that his skills are diminishing or is unaware of developments in the practice? His success rate is dropping. Should or must he disclose to his patients that he is beginning to suffer the inevitable results of aging? Or that his success rate is declining and is a certain percentage? Institutional peer review is designed to restrict a physician's practice to those procedures he is competent to perform. Hospitals, too, are supposed to screen their staff to reduce the level of risk to their patients, defining risk by a competency/quality definition.

In a Wisconsin case,[59] the plaintiff sued her physician for failure to inform her that he had very little experience in performing an operation on an aneurysm. As result of the physician's inexperience, the plaintiff alleged she was rendered a quadriplegic. It was discovered that the physician had never performed surgery on a large basilar bifurcation aneurysm such as the plaintiff's. The Wisconsin Supreme Court stated that the duty to disclose information that is material to a patient's decision must be decided on a case-by-case basis.[60] A bright-line rule that a physician must always give his qualifications to every patient would be impossible, the court said. The court held that in this particular case, the plaintiff introduced enough evidence that had a reasonable patient in her position been made aware that the physician lacked experience with this surgery, it likely would not have been undergone with him. "A reasonable person in the plaintiff's position would have considered such information material in making an intelligent and informed decision about the surgery."[61]

The New Jersey Supreme Court reached a similar result.[62] It provided the following discussion:

> We recognize that a misrepresentation about a physician's experience is not a perfect fit with the familiar construct of a claim based on lack of informed consent. The difficulty arises because physician experience is not information that directly relates to the procedure itself or one of the other areas of required medical disclosure concerning the procedure, its substantial risks, and alternatives that must be disclosed to avoid a claim based on lack of informed consent. But the possibility of materiality is present. If defendant's true level of experience had the capacity to enhance substantially the risk of paralysis from undergoing a corpectomy, a jury could find that a reasonably prudent patient would not have consented to that procedure had the misrepresentation been revealed. That presumes that plaintiff can prove that the actual level of experience possessed by defendant

had a direct and demonstrable relationship to the harm of paralysis, a substantial risk of the procedure that was disclosed to plaintiff. Put differently, plaintiff must prove that the additional undisclosed risk posed by defendant's true level of qualifications and experience increased plaintiff's risk of paralysis from the corpectomy procedure.[63]

In contrast, the Washington Court of Appeals has held that a surgeon's duty to obtain informed consent did not require him to disclose his lack of experience in performing a particular surgical procedure.[64] In this case, the plaintiff needed to have her gallbladder removed. The plaintiff's physician had never performed a gallbladder removal at the time he obtained the plaintiff's consent. The surgery was delayed, however, and during the delay, the physician performed a gallbladder removal on two patients. During the plaintiff's surgery, the physician misidentified and damaged her bile duct and, as a result, she suffered numerous complications after the surgery.

The Washington Court of Appeals stated that the duty to disclose "material facts" include only those facts that relate to the proposed treatment. The court declined to follow the recent number of cases applying a broader construction of "material fact." Applying the traditional approach, the court held that a physician's lack of experience in performing a surgical procedure is not a material fact for purposes of finding liability predicated on failure to secure an informed consent.[65]

The consensus that a physician does not have to disclose his experience or qualifications to a patient apparently has a major exception. In a situation involving high-risk treatment, such as brain surgery, a patient's right to know the doctor's experience becomes more important than a physician's right to privacy. Although this rule is not a bright-line rule, it does set forth a guideline that physicians should follow. In routine, low-risk procedures, a physician does not have a duty to disclose that he is not experienced with the particular procedure. Yet, in situations where experience may determine life or death, the issue of the doctor's experience is critical. Quite likely, in these high-risk situations, the physician has a duty to disclose the fact that he has not performed the procedure or has less experience than someone else who could perform the procedure. The physician should ask himself, "Would I want to know this information if I were the patient?" If the answer is yes, it seems logical that the physician should disclose the information. The diplomas and citations on the walls of the physician's office as well as the age of the physician would, in some measure, indicate the experience and competency of the physician. Often, hospital patients are unaware that they are being treated by a medical student or resident rather than a fully trained physician.

Clearly, misrepresentation arising out of a query by the patient or otherwise may give rise to a cause of action on one of three theories: the informed consent doctrine, the deceit-based tort of fraud, and some states' consumer protection statutes. The courts differ as to which theory is most appropriate. The New Jersey Supreme Court denied a claim based on fraud, stating that a more appropriate basis for legal action would be the informed consent doctrine.[66] On the other hand, the Pennsylvania Supreme Court refused to allow an informed consent action against a physician misrepresenting his credentials, opting instead to endorse a fraud action. The Pennsylvania Supreme Court said that using the informed consent action to include a physician's experience would necessitate expanding the doctrine to include personal attributes of a physician and would only create a redundant cause of action.[67] A few states allow a deceived patient to bring a claim under the state's consumer protection action.[68] Traditionally, state consumer protection statutes have exemptions for the "learned professions" including both lawyers and physicians.[69]

According to a report of the National Conference of State Legislatures, at least 11 states have enacted laws to make physician profiles available to the public. Physicians have managed to keep similar laws from being passed in eight other states. In 1996, Massachusetts became the first state to publish physician malpractice histories and hospital disciplinary records on the Internet. Under the Physician Profile Act, the state now provides information on a physician's number of malpractice suits and settlements, warnings by the medical board, and hospital disciplinary measures.[70] The Ohio State Medical Board Web site currently lists about 32,000 physicians' ages, educations, medical specialties, official reprimands, and license suspensions and revocations. Proposed legislation would add the following physician information to the site: malpractice settlements and awards, felony and some misdemeanor convictions, and any restrictions on hospital admitting privileges.[71] Of course, information about a physician or hospital may be useless if the patient does not have the freedom to choose a physician or hospital.

Causation Complexities

In litigation, it must be shown that if the physician had made proper disclosure, a reasonable patient would have declined treatment. The patient must prove causation, namely, that a reasonable patient would not have consented to treatment had the information been disclosed.[72] A cause of action predicated on the lack of informed consent requires that the patient's injury be the direct and proximate result of the treatment. This element of proof is difficult when an injury is not immediately identifiable as the direct consequence of the treatment. In a casebook on law and the mental health system, this point is illustrated by the following hypothetical fact situation:

> A patient feels that she is not advancing in her job as her intellectual potential might dictate due to excessive passivity and an inability to direct subordinates. On the therapist's recommendation, the patient agrees to undergo assertiveness training, but is not informed that such training may alter personal relationships. The training is successful to the extent that the patient has become more assertive and better able to cope in the work place; however, her husband is unable to adjust to her new and more assertive personality and tensions in the marriage cause it to break up. Theoretically, the patient could assert that she would not have consented to the therapy had she been informed of the risks. In this situation the patient faces the significant difficulty of proving both that the psychotherapy, in fact, led to the personality change and that this was the proximate cause of the failure of her marriage.[73]

The patient must also prove that the omitted risk materialized and constituted the injury that could have been avoided by an alternative treatment or no treatment. Certainly, an alcoholic surgeon may have an impairment that might seriously affect performance, and thus the success rate. As Law Professor Barry Furrow put it: "The statistical probability that an alcoholic may be impaired more often than a nonalcoholic physician of the same skill and training suggests patients face enhanced risks."[74]

In *Hidding*, the Louisiana Court of Appeals held that failure to disclose a history of alcohol abuse violated the informed consent requirement and constituted fault. But, what about the question of causation because alcoholism may not always impair a physician's performance? Is a plaintiff entitled to argue that he would have escaped injury if the defendant had not treated him at all? Is the defendant entitled to argue that the plaintiff may get an award only if he received treatment inferior to that provided by other physicians?[75]

In these and in other situations, the law on torts is used to accomplish the task of hospital supervision or of medical boards in regulating the practice of medicine. The Public Citizen Health Research Group has noted that fewer than one third of the 10,289 physicians disciplined nationwide were kept from practicing medicine, even temporarily. A spokesman for Public Citizen said: "Consumers should be able to find out if their doctors have a black mark on their records."[76] Yet, worthy as this goal may be, it may undercut programs of treatment of impaired physicians.

Exceptions to Informed Consent Doctrine

As a defense, a physician may claim one of several exceptions to the informed consent doctrine: (1) emergency, (2) therapeutic privilege, or (3) waiver. As these are affirmative defenses, the physician bears the burden of proof.[77]

Emergency

In an emergency, a physician may render treatment without the patient's expressed consent. The rationale for the exception is that the patient's consent is "implied" in an emergency, inasmuch as a reasonable person would consent to treatment in an emergency if able to do so. The term *emergency*, however, is not self-defining. At one extreme, an emergency may be said to exist when the patient is injured to the extent of being unconscious. At the other extreme, an emergency is found to exist merely when "suffering or pain would be alleviated" by treatment.[78] Closely related to the emergency exception is the exception for incompetent patients, who in varying circumstances may be treated without their consent.

Therapeutic Privilege

Under what is known as therapeutic privilege a physician may withhold information for therapeutic reasons. The therapeutic privilege is justified where disclosure would complicate or hinder treatment or pose psychological harm to the patient. Few cases turn on its application. Its parameters are uncertain and it is difficult to justify in operational terms. It cannot be used with third-party authorizers, such as guardians.[79] The doctrine appears to be on the wane. At the same time, it is recognized that a patient has no duty to know or inquire.

Waiver

The exception of waiver comes into play when the patient specifically requests not to be informed about the risks but only wants the physician's final judgment. "Whatever you think best, doctor," is the attitude of many patients. Waiver may be conceptualized as the opposite of therapeutic privilege. In waiver, the patient gives up the right to autonomy; in therapeutic privilege, the physician deprives the patient of that right in the interest of the patient's health.[80]

Autonomy is often surrendered to illness. Do patients want decisional autonomy? A number of commentators have noted that patients want to be informed, but do not actually want to make their own healthcare decisions. In his book, *The Practice of Autonomy: Patients, Doctors, and Medical Decisions*,[81] law professor Carl Schneider examines the law of bioethics by looking at the lives of patients. He argues that bioethics has reached a point of paradox. Bioethicists increasingly seem to think patients have a duty to make their own medical decisions, but it is increasingly clear, he says, that many patients do not want to do so. He also notes significant evidence that "the more severe a patient's illness, the less likely the patient is to want to make medical decisions." He writes:

> To appreciate the … reason patients might reject the leading role in their medical decisions, we should recall the syllogism that lies silent at the heart of the autonomist paradigm: People want to make all decisions that shape their lives. Few decisions matter more than medicine's life-or-death, sickness-or-health, fit-or-fall choices. Therefore, patients want to make their own medical decisions. This syllogism is flawed because some patients conclude they will reach wiser decisions by deferring to the expertise and judgment of someone else. But the syllogism errs in other ways, ways suggested by what Talcott Parsons called the "sick role, with how people feel when they are ill." The autonomy paradigm rests on assumptions about the natural desire of all people to control themselves and their surroundings. These assumptions are overstated even for the population at large. But

sick people differ from healthy people, for they often feel frightened, discouraged, dull-witted, abstracted, uninterested, and weary. These feelings, I suggest, may inhibit them from making medical decisions.

In a debate in bioethics circles, it is argued that a patient may not waive the right to information on the theory that the doctrine of informed consent is designed to enhance the autonomy of the patient. Therefore, it is argued, a right to waive information would involve a right to avoid one's responsibility to act as an autonomous moral agent.[82] As a practical matter, however, a patient cannot be forced to listen to the risks of a treatment, or be required to read an informed consent form, or watch a video that is used for risk disclosure. The other side of the debate is typified by the position of John Stuart Mill, the renowned proponent of liberty, who would not preclude individuals from acting in ways that would result even in their certain deaths.[83]

What about genetic testing, about which nowadays there is much publicity? Patients need a great deal of education to be able to assess the need for and the consequences of genetic testing. Some patients want to know if they have an increased risk of a disease, but it may be unethical to test for a disease that is not curable as it would only arouse anxiety. Then there are implications for the patient's family. In the case of a familial gene, there is a good chance that members of the family have the same problem. Informing them may shatter their world as well. And the patient must decide whether to falsify on the myriad forms and applications that ask for divulgence of certain conditions: life and medical insurance policies, job applications, and so on.[84]

Are people ready to confront information derived from genetic testing? The desire of Adam and Eve to become "as gods" precipitated their exile from the Garden of Eden. God gave them a beautiful garden, but forbade them to eat of the fruit of knowledge. God knew that they were not developed enough to deal with the knowledge that would be revealed by the fruit. The emphasis on "No," combined with the availability of the forbidden, however, was, in legal terms, a "pernicious temptation," unfenced and unguarded, provocative by its very obviousness. Likewise, the snake-like configuration of DNA in humans creates a temptation to experiment that could lead to dire or unexpected results. The writer Richard Powers puts it thus: "Humanity's eternal and well-grounded fear is that our wisdom will fail to pace our expertise. Its eternal hope is that our expertise will somehow scare our wisdom into rising to the occasion. With such knowledge, the Bible warns, comes much grief."[85]

Conclusion

The doctrine of informed consent is commonly regarded as a can of worms—the physician can never be sure what information about what risk must be disclosed. The decisions by the courts tend to favor the patient when an untoward consequence results from treatment even though the treatment measures up to standard of care.

We have come a long way. The Hippocratic Oath makes no mention of an obligation of a physician to speak with a patient. Indeed, the only reference to the issue in the Hippocratic Corpus advises against conversation:

Perform … [these duties] calmly and adroitly, concealing most things from the patient while you are attending to him. Give necessary orders with cheerfulness and serenity, turning his attention away from what is being done to him; sometimes reprove sharply and emphatically, and sometimes comfort with solicitude and attention, revealing nothing of the patient's future or present condition. For many patients through this cause have taken a turn for the worse, I mean by the declaration I have mentioned of what is present, or by a forecast of what is to come.[86]

In ancient Greece, the participation of the patient in decision making was considered undesirable because the physician's primary task was to inspire confidence. In medieval times, discussions between physician and patient were viewed solely as an opportunity for the physician to offer comfort and hope. Medical writing of the time emphasized the need for the physician to be manipulative and even deceitful. In his 1803 work, *Medical Ethics*, the English physician Thomas Percival cautioned physicians against providing patients with any negative information:

> A physician should not … make gloomy prognostications. … For the physician should be the minister of hope and comfort to the sick; that by such cordials to the drooping spirit, he may smooth the bed of death; revive expiring life; and counteract the depressing influence of those maladies, which rob the philosopher of fortitude and the Christian of consolation.[87]

Nearly half a century later in 1847, the American Medical Association's first code of ethics included Percival's mandate of communicating hope, admonishing the physician to adhere to his "sacred duty … to avoid all things that have a tendency to discourage the patient and to depress his spirits." Moreover, the AMA explicitly advised against allowing the patient any voice in diagnosis and treatment, indicating that physicians "should … unite tenderness with firmness, and condescension with authority, [so] as to improve the minds of their patients with gratitude, respect, and confidence."[88] Today, that would likely result in litigation.

Endnotes

1. The oft-cited case of Mohr v. Williams, 95 Minn. 261, 104 N.W. 12 (1905), is but one of many cases in which the plaintiff's consent was not to the act actually performed. In Bang v. Miller Hospital, 88 N.W.2d 186 (Minn. 1958), it was held to be a jury question whether consent for removal of a prostate gland included consent to cut the plaintiff's spermatic cords. See A McCoid, "A Reappraisal of Liability for Unauthorized Medical Treatment," *Minn. L. Rev.* 41 (1957): 381.
2. See Natanson v. Kline, 186 Kan. 393, 350 P.2d 1093 (1960); Mitchell v. Robinson, 334 S.W.2d 11 (Mo. 1960). The term *informed consent* first appeared in Salgo v. Leland Stanford Jr. Univ. Bd. Of Trustees, 154 Cal. App.2d 560, 317 P.2d 170 (1957). See R.R. Faden & T.L. Beauchamp, *A History and Theory of Informed Consent* (New York: Oxford University Press, 1986).
3. In the case of psychotherapy, where there is no bodily contact, there is by definition no cause of action in battery (though there may be a cause of action for "intentional" infliction of mental distress). The form of trespass to the person known as "battery" involves some physical contact with the complainant. There being no touching in the talking therapies, there is no battery. The question of defense (consent or whatever) arises only when the plaintiff has proved that a presumptive tort has been committed. With the advent of the doctrine of informed consent, an action lies in negligence where the lack of informed consent is the wrongdoing and the poor outcome is the harm for which damages are assessed. See R. Slovenko, "Psychotherapy and Informed Consent: A Search in Judicial Regulation," in W.E. Barton & C.J. Sanborn (Eds.), *Law and the Mental Health Professions* (New York: International Universities Press, 1978), pp. 51–70.
4. The principle of self-determination includes the right to a death choice, which manifest itself as refusal of life-sustaining or life-saving treatment. Jehovah's Witnesses refuse blood out of obedience to scripture, which they believe is divinely inspired. Thus, when a Witness admitted in a hospital emergency room after suffering a life-threatening trauma injury explained that his refusal of blood was "between me and Jehovah … I'm willing to take my chances. My faith is that strong … I wish to live, but with no blood transfusions. Now get that straight." The court upheld his refusal. *In re* Osborne, 294 A.2d 372 (D.C. 1972). The patient was managed successfully without blood.
5. A. Capron, "Informed Consent in Catastrophic Disease Research and Treatment," *U. Pa. L. Rev.* 123 (1974): 340. Slaveholders generally intervened in the health affairs of their slaves, particularly in the case of life-threatening illnesses. While some slaveholders sought the consent of their slaves for certain treatments, others did not. Concealing ailments from the owners was one way that slaves could maintain a degree of control over their bodies.
6. Freud advised against "lengthy preliminary discussions before the beginning of the analytic treatment," but he did recommend that patients should be told of the difficulties and sacrifice that analytic treatment involves so the patient would be deprived "of any right to say later on that he had been

inveigled into a treatment whose extent and implications he did not realize." He stated that questions as to the probable duration of a treatment are almost unanswerable because psychoanalysis is always a matter of long periods of time—of half a year, or whole years—of longer periods than the patient expects. J. Strachey (Ed.), *Standard Edition of the Complete Psychological Works of Sigmund Freud* (London: Hogarth Press, 1958), vol. 12, pp. 129–130.

7. Allen Feld, director of continuing education for the False Memory Syndrome Foundation and a retired member of the faculty of the School of Social Work at Marywood University, writes:

> The therapist should explain in lay language his or her theoretical orientation and approach to helping, as well as prior experiences with this therapeutic approach and a summary of published outcome studies. It is reasonable for society to expect a therapist to be familiar with the research that supports his or her chosen theoretical orientation and that describes its effectiveness when used with the patient's problems. This process also allows an opportunity to discuss what the therapist perceives to be the risks, side-effect or anxieties that may be common in therapy in general and known to be associated with the chosen therapeutic approach. This is also a suitable time for a therapist to make the patient aware of the emergency procedures available should they become necessary.

A. Feld, "More Thoughts on Informed Consent," *FMS Foundation Newsletter*, July/August 2000, p. 6. See J. Cannell, J.I. Hudson, & H.G. Pope, "Standards for Informed Consent in Recovered Memory," *J. Am. Acad. Psychiat. & Law* 29 (2001): 138.

8. Tunkl v. Regents of University of California, 60 Cal.2d 92, 32 Cal. Rptr. 33, 383 P.2d 441 (1963).

9. P.S. Appelbaum & T. Grisso, "Assessing Patients' Capacities to Consent to Treatment," *N. Eng. J. Med.* 319 (1988): 1635. See also T.G. Gutheil & H. Bursztjn, "Clinicians' Guidelines for Assessing and Presenting Subtle Forms of Patient Incompetence in Legal Settings," *Am. J. Psychiat.* 143 (1986): 1020.

10. See Gemme v. Goldberg. 626 A.2d 318 (Conn. App. 1993); Holt v. Nelson, 523 P.2d 211 (Wash. App. 1974).

11. Lienhard v. State, 431 N.W.2d 861 (Minn. 1988).

12. See P.R. McHugh, "Psychiatric Misadventures," *Am. Schol.* 61 (1992): 497; "Psychotherapy Awry," *Am. Schol.* 63 (1994): 17; both reprinted in P.R. McHugh, *The Mind Has Mountains* (Baltimore, MD: Johns Hopkins University Press, 2006), pp. 3–17, 18–32. See also P.R. McHugh, *Try to Remember* (Washington, DC: Dana, 2008)

13. See T.H. Boyd, "Cost Containment and the Physician's Fiduciary Duty to the Patient," *DePaul L. Rev.* 39 (1989): 131; D. Orenticher, "Paying Physicians More to Do Less: Financial Incentives to Limit Care," *U. Richmond L. Rev.* 30 (1996): 151.

14. The health plan that had a gag rule on treatment alternatives received extensive negative publicity, and it was discredited. The Congress and various states banned it.

15. Scott v. Bradford, 606 P.2d 554, 556–557 (Okla. 1979).

16. Texas Rev. Civil Stat., Tit. 71, art, 4950i; see W.J. Curran, "Informed Consent, Texas Style: Disclosure and Non-Disclosure by Regulation," *N. Eng. J. Med.*, March 1, 1979: 482.

17. See Hernandez v. Schittek, 305 Ill. App.3d 925, 713 N.E.2d 203 (1999); Dingle v. Belin, 358 Md. 354, 749 A.2d 157 (1999); Duttry v. Patterson, 741 A.2d 199 (Pa. 1999). In Rubino v. Defretias, 638 F. Supp. 182 (D. Ariz. 1986), the court held that the state statute abrogating battery as a basis of an informed consent action is unconstitutional on the ground that the Arizona constitution established a fundamental right to bring an action against a physician based on the common law theory of battery.

18. Negligence and intentionally tortuous behavior are as a factual matter points along a continuum, but legally there is a bright line, with dramatically different consequences. Section 523 (a)(6) of the Bankruptcy Code exempts from discharge any debt "for willful and malicious injury by the debtor to another entity or to the property of another entity." A typical malpractice judgment is not a debt for "willful and malicious injury."

19. The prudent physician standard is followed in Culberston v. Mermitz, 602 N.E.2d 98 (Ind. 1992). Apart from fault (failure to provide information), as herein discussed, the plaintiff patient must also establish causation, to wit, that if he had been informed on the risks he would not have consented to the treatment.

20. The two most discussed decisions in this area, handed down in the early 1980s, are Rogers v. Okin, 478 F. Supp. 1342 (D. Mass. 1979) and Rennie v. Klein, 653 F.2d 836 (3rd Cir. 1981). In a case in Maine, a patient who was involuntarily admitted for mental health treatment claimed that the facility needed her consent to wake her in the morning. She wanted to sleep to 11 a.m. The Maine Supreme Court

ruled that the Commissioner of the Department of Mental Health had properly decided that consent was not required for waking the person because it did not constitute treatment or services, but was instead intended to give her opportunity to participate in treatment, to give clinical staff a chance to observe her, and for smooth hospital operation; Green v. Commissioner of Dept. of Mental Health, 776 A.2d 612 (Me. 2001).

21. J.G. Bernstein, *Handbook of Drug Therapy in Psychiatry* (St. Louis: Mosby, 3rd ed., 1995).

22. F.J. Ayd, "Ethical and Legal Dilemmas Posted by Tardive Dyskinesia," *Int. Drug Therapy Newsl.* 12 (1977): 29; see R. Slovenko, "Update on Legal Issues Associated With Tardive Dyskinesia," *J. Clin. Psychiat.* 61 (2000): 45 (supp. 4).

23. See "Empirical Research on Informed Consent/An Annotated Bibliography," *Hastings Center Report Special Supplement*, Jan.–Feb. 1999; see also E.R. Saks & S.H. Behnke, "Competency to Decide on Treatment and Research: MacArthur and Beyond," *J. Contemp. Legal Issues* 10 (1999): 103.

24. 105 N.E. 92 (N.Y. 1914).

25. In Australia, a physician was found negligent for not warning a patient of a 1:14,000 risk of sympathetic ophthalmia when operating to restore vision in an affected eye, but causing impaired vision in the previously unaffected eye; Rogers v. Whitaker, [1992] 175 CLR 479. Even a speculative risk has been deemed the basis for a successful claim of negligence. In Chapel v. Hart, [1998] 156 ALR 517, a claim of negligence was upheld when an ear, nose, and throat surgeon failed to warn of a risk that was so rare as to be deemed by the court to be speculative in an operation that the court unanimously agreed was performed in a competent and technically satisfactory manner. In his book, *The Silent World of Doctor and Patient* (New York: Viking, 1984), Dr. Jay Katz of Yale University called the doctrine a fairy tale.

26. For this experiment, the principal physician–investigator, whom I had not known previously, asked that I chair an informed consent review committee that was a separate entity from the medical committee set up to oversee the soundness of the experimental design. As I was dependent on the clinic for teaching and research opportunities, the appointment of two independent outsiders to the committee—a priest (a man of God) and an accountant (a man of commerce)—were welcome additions. A few days after the initial meeting of the consent committee, I advised the principal investigator that litigation was pending in Mississippi in connection with psychosurgery performed on young delinquents apparently without consent. I was told that "we will make sure that there is informed consent available from our patient."

I met individually with Louis Smith on six occasions, each session lasting approximately an hour. In addition, he was interviewed in my seminar on law and psychiatry. On this occasion the group consisted of approximately 30 persons including some psychiatrists, a judge, and a few staff members from Lafayette Clinic, in particular, the principal investigator. Following the interview, after Louis Smith left the seminar room, the atmosphere was highly critical of the value of the experiment. I have never been an advocate of psychosurgery to control behavior. As is customary, the subject or patient did not hear the discussion of his case.

No one can be sure of another's motive, or even of one's own motives. Some of the group believed his desire "to do something useful, to atone for my guilt" was a motivating force in his volunteering for the experiment. A few others felt that he was volunteering as a means to obtain release. But there was near unanimity of opinion that his prime motivation was fear; fear that he would explode in the free world as he had done 17 years earlier, when he had strangled a nurse and performed necrophilia. He insisted that he would seek psychosurgery if it were "the only means of helping my physical problem," even if there were other ways to obtain release. He had little faith in his ability to control himself. In a conversation with the Director of the State Department of Mental Health, I was told the subject had been informed that he would be released in a few months, irrespective of the experiment.

Louis Smith was told of the risks, even of the risk of death. There was, actually, a one-page headline in a local paper, "Surgery May Cure—or Kill—Rapist" (*Detroit Free Press*, January 7, 1973). He was given no promises. To summarize my interviews, I asked him to write his answers to the following questions, which he did:

Q. Would you seek psychosurgery if you were not confined in an institution?

A. Yes, if after testing showed that it would be of help.

Q. Do you believe that psychosurgery is the way to obtain your release from the institution?

A. No, but it would be a step in obtaining my release. It is like any other therapies or program to help a person to function again.

Q. Would you seek psychosurgery if there were other ways to obtain your release?

A. Yes, if psychosurgery were the only means of helping my physical problem after a period of testing.

Q. Would you want legal representation to explore whether or not there are ways to obtain your release without psychosurgery?

A. No, because I feel that [the principal investigator and the Director of the State Department of Mental Health] will release me when I have shown I am a capable person.

Q. Are you in favor of newspaper and other publicity surrounding your case?

A. It makes no difference because if the [principal investigator] thinks that by me stating my views in public will be of help to him and the clinic, so be it.

Smith protested the intervention by Michigan Legal Services Lawyer Gabe Kaimowitz, saying to me: "I was in the institution for 17 years and no one showed any concern. Now Kaimowitz speaks out for my 'rights' without even talking to me. The doctors came to the institution, gave me a chance, treated me like a man. I have great faith in [the principal investigator]. He'll check out the best treatment. He'll do the best. I did wrong, and perhaps by this experiment something will be learned to help others. I killed a woman. I can't function as I am. I need some kind of treatment."

Shortly after Kaimowitz filed suit, I received a phone call from Charles Halpern of the Mental Health Law Project in Washington D.C. At the time I was Chairman of the Committee on Legal Approaches to Mental Health of the American Orthopsychiatric Association, which subsequently co-sponsored the Mental Health Law Project. Halpern said that he wanted to join forces with Kaimowitz, but he, for reasons known only to him, chose to go it alone.

As I told Halpern, I felt that the experiment could not be tainted due to lack of consent. But I added, the subject had a great deal of faith in the investigator, the first person in his 17 years of confinement to show any interest in him, and a strong relationship had developed between them. The development of such a relationship, *de facto* though not *de jure*, causes consent not to be really informed. As the "informed consent" concept has developed at law, "sufficient information must be disclosed to the patient so that he can arrive at an intelligent opinion," but by whom is the information to be given? The crucial factor is not the amount of information, or even the contents, but rather *who* provides it.

Obtaining a statement of alternatives from one experimenter or physician is not the same as obtaining opinions from different parties with whom a relationship has developed. Smith was advised of the alternatives by the principal investigator. Not until that relationship was diluted by other health professionals did his view change. (The United Store Workers Union says that it has been able to reduce the amount of surgery performed on its members by having a second doctor review each recommended operation before it is performed.)

De facto, it is neither age nor confinement that puts consent in question. Indeed, Smith, not being under pain or stress, made a more valid consent than does the ordinary ill person who calls upon a doctor. The expectations of a patient and the great dependence on a doctor affect mightily the rationality of decision making. When in distress or pain, one regresses to a childlike state. To put it another way, the child in everyone tends to dominate the personality when one is in great stress or pain. We cannot yet quantitate stress to measure the legality of a consent.

Actually, the consent given by Smith was not before the court. On the first day of trial, the Director of the Department of Mental Health withdrew authorization of the experiment because of adverse public reaction to news reports about it. The court, however, stated that the issues raised were of sufficient public importance to be decided in a declaratory decree. No one, except the State Attorney General, wanted to let go of the case. All of the participating attorneys contended the trial should be continued in order to establish the rights of institutionalized persons.

A panel of three judges listened to 3 weeks of testimony. As there were no factual issues to be resolved, the proceedings took on the air of a seminar. In a 41-page opinion drawing heavily from the briefs submitted by the petitioners, the court concluded that an involuntarily confined individual cannot give a legitimate consent as he is living in "an inherently coercive atmosphere." (The court would allow a prisoner to consent only to low-risk, high-benefits procedures.) The decision did not foreclose "the performance of psychosurgery on such persons once the procedure has advanced to a level where its benefits clearly outweigh its risks." Given the current state of knowledge about how the brain works, the court judged that presently the benefits did not outweigh the risk.

Historically, as we have noted, the informed consent doctrine evolved to facilitate proof of cases and the payment of compensation to injured persons, but in the psychosurgery case, the concept was used not to facilitate proof of the complainant's case, but to bar a modality of practice. In any event, to take informed consent literally is to miss the point. In the case of psychosurgery, there was no rationalization available to the court in its quest to ban psychosurgery in prisons, with the possible exception of the Eighth Amendment prohibition against cruel and unusual punishment.

Informed consent is thus a spurious issue. To apply the time-honored test of consent literally is to expend energy needlessly. Review committees, as they presently look over consent forms, are one example of the waste of time. A more realistic approach would be to provide a subject or patient with different opinions, from different persons over a span of time in which a relationship can develop.

Moreover, the information that is disclosed does not now include after-care. An experimenter sometimes promises a subject that he will receive good care in the event of a poor outcome. Is he able to make good on that promise? To my knowledge there has been no systematic study of the subjects of failed experiments. Society, having high stakes in research, must pay the cost of unpredictable results. At a minimum there should be a "no fault" clinical research insurance plan to provide care for anyone harmed. A guardian *ad experimentem* might be appointed.

27. Kaimowitz v. Department of Mental Health, Cir. Ct. Wayne County, Mich., 2 Prison L. Rptr. 433 (July 10, 1973). For a discussion of the case, see S.I. Shuman, *Psychosurgery and the Medical Control of Violence* (Detroit: Wayne State University Press, 1977).

28. D. Josar, "Judge of 40 Years Never Tires of Career," *Detroit News*, Dec. 29, 1996, p. E1.

29. See Chapter 34 on experimentation.

30. In Johnson & Johnson v. Karl, 2007 WL 188877 (W. Va. 2007), the West Virginia Supreme Court of Appeals rejected the learned intermediary doctrine in its entirety, on the ground that direct-to-consumer advertising made the rule outdated. Some years ago, the New Jersey Supreme Court held that the learned intermediary rule did not protect drug manufacturers when they advertise directly to consumers. Perez v. Wyeth Laboratories, 734 A.2d 1245 (N.J. 1999); J.O. Castagnera & R.R. Gerner, "The Gradual Enfeeblement of the Learned Intermediary Rule and the Argument in Favor of Abandoning It Entirely," *Tort & Ins. L. J.* 36 (2000): 119; T. Hall, "Reimaging the Learned Intermediate Rule for the New Pharmaceutical Marketplace," *Seton Hall L. Rev.* 35 (2004): 193; W.J. Thomas, "Direct-to-Consumer Pharmaceutical Advertising: Catalyst for a Change in the Therapeutic Model in Psychotherapy?" *Conn. L. Rev.* 32 (1999): 209. General warnings, such as "see your doctor," do not give the consumer a sufficient caveat on the risks of a drug. J.D. Hanson & D.A. Kysar, "Taking Behaviorism Seriously: Some Evidence of Market Manipulation," *Harv. L. Rev.* 112 (1999): 1420.

31. "Pharmaceutical companies are increasingly souping up their advertising for prescription drugs in a style more commonly associated with products sold from open shelves in drugstores and supermarkets." M. Freudenheim, "Influencing Doctor's Orders: Ads Help Sales of Prescription Drugs, But at What Cost?" *New York Times*, Nov. 17, 1998, p. C1. See also H.W. Jenkins, "Ads That Make Us Well," *Wall Street Journal*, April 11, 2001, p. 19. According to surveys, many patients get meds they would not otherwise. J. Appleby, "Drug Ads Push Rx Requests Higher," *USA Today*, March 4, 2008, p. 1.

32. See G. Winter, "Search for an Easy Solution Fuels an Industry Rooted in Gullibility," *New York Times*, Oct. 29, 2000, p. 1.

33. See G. Critser, *Generation Rx* (New York: Houghton Mifflin, 2005).

34. "Doctors are being pressured," says Dr. Raymond Woosley, chairman of the pharmacology department at Georgetown University. "People are saying, 'I will go to another doctor if I don't get it from you.'" Quoted in S.G. Stolberg, "Want a New Drug? Plenty to Choose From on TV," *New York Times*, Jan. 23, 2000, p. WK5. A 28-page special section, "Health & Medicine," *Wall Street Journal*, Oct. 19, 1998, discusses the impact of healthcare information available to consumers.

35. Quoted in S. Blakeslee, "Placebos Prove So Powerful Even Experts Are Surprised," *New York Times*, Oct. 13, 1998, p. D8.

36. Stuart Derbyshire, a psychology researcher at the University of Birmingham, says, "It sounds reasonable to say that medicine should harness and improve the placebo effect, but I think it moves the debate in a worrying direction to say that doctors should deliberately be giving patients placebos. This would undermine the trust between society and medicine." Quoted in C. Cookson," Is There an Ethical Way to Fine-Tune the Placebo Effect?" *Financial Times*, March 1–2, 2008, p. 7. See T.S. Jost, "The Globalization of Health Law: The Case of Permissibility of Placebo-Based Research," *Am. J. Law & Med.* 26 (2000): 175; M. Talbot, "The Placebo Prescription," *New York Times Magazine*, Jan. 9, 2000, p. 34.

37. G. Dworkin (ltr.), "The Placebo Prescription," *New York Times Magazine*, Jan. 30, 2000, sec. 6, p. 8. Harms resulting from placebos are known collectively as "nocebo effects." The loss of an opportunity to achieve a better result is actionable. See Fulton v. William Beaumont Hosp., 253 Mich. App. 70, 655 N.W.2d 569 (2002).

38. An estimated 15 million adults in the United States are coupling prescription drugs with herbal remedies or high-dose vitamins, inviting unpredictable interactions. Physicians and patients often do not broach the subject of alternative medicine or herbal supplements, and that could be dangerous. M. Chase, "Patients Need to Keep Their Doctors Informed about Herbal Therapies," *Wall Street Journal*, Nov. 16, 1998, p. B1. A special issue of the *Journal of the American Medical Association* that was devoted to alternative medicine had its genesis in letters from physicians asking the *Journal* for information on some of the treatments their patients were asking About. D. Grady, "To Aid Doctors, *A.M.A. Journal* Devotes Entire Issue to Alternative Medicine," *New York Times*, Nov. 11, 1998, p. 21; G. Kolata, "The Herbal Potions That Make Science Sick," *New York Times*, Nov. 15, 1998, p. WK-4.

39. Kozan v. Comstock, 270 F.2d 839, 845 (5th Cir. 1959). See also Clevenger v. Haling, 394 N.E.2d 1119 (Mass. 1979); Guilmet v. Campbell, 385 Mich. 57, 188 N.W.2d 601 (1971); see A.J. Mioler, "The Contractual Liability of Physicians and Surgeons," *Wash. U. L. Q.* 1953: 413; K. Tierney, "Contractual Aspects of Malpractice," *Wayne L. Rev.* 19 (1973): 1457. The Northeastern Health Alliance advertises: "Stop smoking in just 2½ hours. Money back guarantee. Many times more effective than drugs or traditional hypnosis." Advertisement in *Baltimore Sun*, Nov. 15, 1998, p. 5.

40. Sullivan v. O'Connor, 363 Mass. 579, 296 N.E.2d 183 (1973). In a lawsuit that was settled, Julie Andrews claimed that doctors assured her that surgery to remove noncancerous throat nodules would eliminate her vocal problems, but instead she was left with "profound vocal difficulties, including severe hoarseness." AP news release, Sept. 12, 2000.

41. Johnson v. Rodis, 251 F.2d 917 (D.C. 1958).

42. See, e.g., Mich. Comp. Laws 566.132. Quite often a consent form includes a paragraph that no guarantees are made, such as: "I understand that the practice of medicine and surgery is not an exact science and that diagnosis and treatment may involve risks of injury, or even death. I acknowledge that no guarantees have been made to me as to the result of examination or treatment in this hospital."

    It may be said that linking payment to outcome creates better incentives for providers and reassures patients. Lawyers may be paid on a contingency fee basis. The medical profession, however, has shown virtually no interest in such arrangements. Indeed, the American Medical Association flatly condemns outcome-based payments as unethical. The AMA's Code of Medical Ethics 6.01 (1994) provides, "A physician's fee should not be made contingent on the successful outcome of medical treatment. Such arrangements are unethical because they imply that successful outcomes from treatments are guaranteed, thus creating unrealistic expectations of medicine and false promises to consumers." See D.A. Hyman, "Medicine in the New Millennium: A Self-Help Guide for the Perplexed," *Am. J. Law & Med.* 26 (2000): 143.

43. 27 Cal.3d 285, 611 P.2d 902, 165 Cal. Rptr. 308 (1980).

44. Moore v. Regents of the University of California, 51 Cal. 3d 120, 131–132, 793 P.2d 479, 485, 271 Cal. Rptr. 146, 152 (1990). But cf. Neade v. Portes, 739 N.E.2d 496 (Ill. 2000). See K. Eichwald & G. Kolata, "When Physicians Double as Businessmen," *New York Times*, Nov. 30, 1999, p. 1; S.G. Stolberg, "Financial Ties in Biomedicine Get Close Look," *New York Times*, Feb. 20, 2000, p. 1. To avoid a conflict of interest, Dr. George Nicklin of the NYU School of Medicine says that he does not own any drug stocks. Address at the annual meeting of the American Academy of Psychoanalysis, "Spirituality and Money," on May 13, 2000, in Chicago.

45. R.D. Alarcon, "Culture and Ethics of Managed Care in the United States," in A. Okasha, J. Arboleda-Florez, & N. Sartorius (Eds.), *Ethics, Culture and Psychiatry* (Washington, DC: American Psychiatric Press, 2000); E.H. Moreim, "Economic Disclosure and Economic Advocacy: New Duties in the Medical Standard of Care," *J. Legal Med.* 12 (1991): 275.

46. L. Slater, *Prozac Diary* (New York: Random House, 1998), p. 5. Dr. Bruce Leff of John Hopkins University puts it this way, "There is no free lunch." B. Leff (ltr.), "When Doctors Go for Drug Makers' Gold," *New York Times*, Dec. 30, 2000, p. 30. The increasing number of publications critical of the influence of the pharmaceutical industry on medical practice include M. Angell, *The Truth About Drug Companies* (New York: Random House, 2004); C. Barber, *Comfortably Numb: How Psychiatry Is Medicating a Nation* (New York: Pantheon Books, 2008); S. Brownlee, *Overtreated* (New York: Bloomsbury, 2007); M. Petersen, *Our Daily Meds: How the Pharmaceutical Companies Transformed Themselves into Slick Marketing Machines and Hooked the Nation on Prescription Drugs* (New York: Farrar Straus & Giroux, 2008); C. Elliott, "The Drug Pushers," *Atlantic Monthly*, April 2006, p. 82.

See also C. Adams, "Doctors on the Run Can 'Dine 'n' Dash' in Style in New Orleans," *Wall Street Journal*, May 14, 2000, p. 1; G. Harris, B. Carey, & J. Roberts, "Psychiatrists, Troubled Children and Drug Industry's Role," *New York Times*, May 10, 2007, p. 1; S.G. Stolberg & J. Gerth, "High-Tech Stealth Being Used to Sway Doctor Prescriptions," *New York Times*, Nov. 16, 2000, p. 1; A. Zuger, "Fever Pitch: Getting Doctors to Prescribe Is Big Business," *New York Times*, Jan. 11, 1999, p. 1.

Studies suggest that receiving even cheap pens and modest lunches creates a sense of obligation— and detailers always provide them. Howard Brody, a medical ethicist, has urged physicians not to see drug representatives as their information is not trustworthy. H. Brody, "The Company We Keep: Why Physicians Should Refuse to See Pharmaceutical Representatives," *Ann. Fam. Med.* 3 (2005): 82. The American Medical Association Council on Ethical and Judicial Affairs has developed guidelines entitled "Gifts to Physicians From Industry" that addresses entertainment, gifts, and subsidized Continuing Medical Education (CME) conferences. In sum and substance, if the subsidized gift or activity is of modest value and serves to enhance the educational aspect of a meeting or CME event, it is ethical. One psychiatrist surmises, "Riding the ski train to Winter Park, with a 30-minute presentation given on the train followed by 6 hours of free skiing, may not pass the AMA's guidelines." C. Zilber, "Pharmaceutical Industry Gifts and Integrity," *Colo. Psychiat. Soc. Newsl.*, Sept. 2000, p. 3. See E.G. Campbell et al., "A National Survey of Physician-Industry Relationships," *N. Eng. J. Med.* 356 (April 26, 2007): 1742; J. Pereira, "Gifts to Doctors Are Widespread," *Wall Street Journal*, April 26, 2007, p. 6; see also Randy Cohen's ethicist column on "Conference call," *New York Times Magazine*, Sept. 24, 2000, p. 28. Abigail Zuger, a physician in Manhattan who writes for *Science Times*, says: "Study after study shows that when doctors are plied with free pens and elegant restaurant meals, trips to snow-white beaches and turquoise waters, not to mention cash payments for listening to drug testimonials disguised as educational meetings, they will begin to endorse the products of their benefactors." A. Zuger, "Drug Pitchmen: Actor, Doctor or Pfizer's Option," *New York Times*, March 4, 2008, p. D-6.

47. Minnesota records from 1997 to 2005 indicate that pharmaceutical companies paid more than 5,500 physicians, nurses, and other healthcare workers in the state at least $57 million. Another $40 million went to clinics, research centers, and other organizations. The median payment per consultant was $1,000; more than 100 people received more than $100,000. See G. Harris & J. Roberts, "A State's Files Put Doctors Ties to Drug Makers on Close View," *New York Times*, March 21, 2007, p. 1. In an industry advisory in 2007, the FDA announced new conflict-of-interest rules against physicians who sit on its advisory committees, which recommend whether the FDA should allow pharmaceutical companies to market their new products. The new rules bar any individual from sitting on any committee to evaluate a drug up for approval when that individual has a financial interest exceeding $50,000 in stock ownership, related research, and consulting arrangements. See R.A. Epstein, "Drug Crazy," *Wall Street Journal*, March 26, 2007, p. 14. A number of courts, however, have refused to recognize a claim for breach of fiduciary duty for the failure of a physician to disclose financial ties with pharmaceutical companies. These jurisdictions hold that the breach of fiduciary duty is simply duplicative of a medical malpractice claim. See, e.g., D.A.B. v. Brown, 570 N.W.2d 168 (Minn. App. 1997).

48. M. Fretag, "Tracing Doctors Who Err," *New York Times*, Nov. 5, 1989, p. E4.

49. Advertisement of Castle Connoly Guide, "How to Find the Best Doctors," *New York Times*, Oct. 10, 1998, p. 13. See also Survey, "Detroit's Top Docs," *Hour*, Oct. 2000, p. 79.

50. B.R. Furrow et al., *Health Law* (St. Paul, MN.: West, 2d ed., 2000), p. 317.

51. Behringer Estate v. Princeton Medical Center, 249 N.J. Super. 597, at 649-49, 592 A.2d 1251, at 1277-28 (1992).

52. 592 A.2d at 1277-78.

53. 592 A.2d at 1280. The Maryland Supreme Court has also held that a physician who has tested HIV positive must disclose that fact to the patient before performing an invasive procedure; Faya v. Almaraz, 329 Md. 435, 620 A.2d 327 (1993). Arguably, the risk of AIDS may be the basis for an emotional distress claim. See Marchia v. Long Island R.R. Co., 31 F.3d 1197 (2nd Cir. 1994). The courts that require a physical injury resulting from the tort as a basis for emotional harm recovery may dismiss the case on the ground that no physical injury (or manifestation or objective symptom) has been shown. In such a jurisdiction, the patient exposed to carcinogens may possibly be able to show some actual physical changes at the cellular level, even though those changes are not presently causing any symptoms. In that event, the court could conceivably regard the fear of future harm as parasitic to a claim for physical harm. See Buckley v. Metro-North Commuter R.R., 79 F.3d 1337 (2nd Cir. 1996).

54. 578 So.2d 1192 (La. App. 1991).

55. 578 So.2d at 1196.

56. 578 So.2d at 1197. In a treatise on health law it is stated:

[T]he fact that alcohol abuse might on some occasions create risks for patients does seem at first glance to mandate disclosure. Disclosure creates the risk that a patient will refuse the physician's care because of the status or the addiction, rather than looking at the particular case and the risks posed. The physician will then be stigmatized on the basis of personal information not previously known, and now used against him. On the other hand, alcoholism might be argued as most similar to other risks that a physician might present to a patient, such as a surgeon's wound infection rates or a loss of ability with age. The principle of informed consent, requiring disclosure of all risks material to a patient's decision, appears elastic enough to include these addiction risks.

B.R. Furrow et al., *Health Law* (St. Paul, MN.: West, 2nd ed., 2000), pp. 321–322.

57. Ornelas v. Fry, 151 Ariz. 324, 727 P.2d 819 (1986).

58. In Reaves v. Bergsrud, 982 P.2d 497 (N.M. App. 1999), the New Mexico Court of Appeals cited the Arizona decision in holding that absent proof that a physician's mental impairment contributed to the plaintiffs injuries, the physician's condition is irrelevant. In this case, during discovery, the plaintiff learned that the physician had bipolar disorder and that his medical license had been temporarily suspended some years earlier when he inappropriately quit his psychiatric care and medication. The physician refused to answer the plaintiff's interrogatories regarding his condition and treatment. The plaintiff did not allege that the physician's mental health was the cause of postoperative problems. In fact, she conceded that "she did not claim that the defendant was impaired during the time of treatment of her." Therefore, the court concluded that the physician's mental status at the time of the plaintiff's treatment was irrelevant to the proceedings. Moreover, the court held that the physician–patient privilege applied, barring discovery of the physician's mental health treatment. However, where relevant, discovery of a litigant's medical history, be that of a plaintiff or defendant, has been allowed under the patient–litigant exception to testimonial privilege (see the discussion in Chapter 5 on testimonial privilege). For another holding in accord with the Arizona and New Mexico decisions, see Shamburger v. Behrens, 380 N.W.2d 659 (S.D. 1986).

59. Johnson v. Kokemoor, 545 N.W.2d 495 (Wis. 1996).

60. 545 N.W.2d at 504.

61. See A.D. Twerski & N.B. Cohen, "The Second Revolution in Informed Consent: Comparing Physicians to Each Other," *Nw. U. L. Rev.* 94 (1999): 1.

62. Howard v. University of Medicine & Dentistry of New Jersey, 800 A.2d 73 (N.J. 2002).

63. 800 A.2d at 84–85.

64. Whiteside v. Lukson, 947 P.2d 1263 (Wash. App. 1996).

65. 947 P.2d at 1265. Likewise, in Ditto v. McCurdy, 947 P.2d 952 (Haw. 1997), the Hawaii Supreme Court ruled that a physician does not have an affirmative duty to disclose his qualifications to a patient prior to providing treatment.

66. Howard v. Univ. of Med. & Dentistry of New Jersey, 800 A.2d 73 (N.J. 2002).

67. Duttry v. Patterson, 771 A.2d 1255 (Pa. 2001).

68. See, e.g., Chapman v. Wilson, 826 S.W.2d 214 (Tex. App. 1992).

69. See H.H. Bouknight, "Between the Scalpel and the Lie: Comparing Theories of Physician Accountability for Misrepresentations of Experience and Competence," *Wash. & Lee L. Rev.* 60 (2003): 1515; M.J. Mehlman, "Dishonest Medical Mistakes," *Vand. L. Rev.* 59 (2006): 1137.

70. Massachusetts law provides patients with profiles of all physicians licensed in the state, including disciplinary actions and malpractice payments. James B. Stewart, author of *Blind Eye: How the Medical Establishment Let a Doctor Get Away With Murder* (New York: Simon & Schuster, 2000), urged the House Commerce Committee to put the database on the Internet and also add criminal convictions to the reports of malpractice awards and license suspensions. F. Barringer, "Seeking Access to Data on Doctors," *New York Times*, Sept. 18, 2000, p. 18.

71. Various state bureaus of health services list licensing actions regarding healthcare providers (information listed includes the provider's name, profession, license number, date of birth, address, the nature of the complaint, the licensing action taken, and the effective date of the action). Public Citizen (1600 20th St., N.W., Washington, DC 2009) has published a three-volume set listing 13,012 "questionable doctors."

72. Cases dealing with informed consent present a special problem in regard to causation. How crucial is testimony by the plaintiff patient in order to hurdle the issue if he testified that he would have not undergone the medical procedure if the defendant physician had informed him of the risk? In Hamilton v. Hardy, 37 Colo. App. 375, 549 P.2d 1099 (1976), the plaintiff patient's failure to testify what she would have done if the physician had informed her of the risk of abnormal blood clotting associated with birth control pills did not defeat her claim. The court said the test is what a reasonable

person would have decided if adequately informed. Is that sufficient proof of what the plaintiff would have done? Is the plaintiff's testimony on the issue enough? The courts are reluctant to permit a jury to believe the plaintiff's testimony, and they require that the plaintiff go farther and show that a reasonable person would also have refused it. However, in Scott v. Bradford, 606 P.2d 554 (Okla. 1979), the Oklahoma Supreme Court said that a patient need only testify that he would not have undergone the treatment if he had known of the risk. The jury would determine whether the testimony was credible.

73. C. Slobogin, A. Rai, & R. Reisner (Eds.), *Law and the Mental Health System* (St. Paul, MN: West, 5th ed., 2009).
74. "Quality Control in Healthcare: Developments in the Law of Medical Malpractice," *J. Law, Med. & Ethics* 21 (1993): 173, 178.
75. In a concurring opinion in *Hidding*, Judge Grisbaum wrote (578 So.2d at 1198):

> I agree with the majority and the trial court's analysis … that a doctor's failure to inform his patient that he suffers from an alcohol or any other related substance abuse problem constitutes de facto a breach of the "intent" of the informed consent statute. However, it appears that the majority and the trial court went to great lengths in elaborating upon the fact that (1) in this case there was the existence of a material risk, which was unknown to the patient and that (2) there was a failure to disclose that risk on the part of the physician and that (3) no doubt this want of disclosure would have led a reasonable patient in the plaintiff's position to reject the medical procedure or at least choose a different course of treatment. However, neither the majority nor the trial court addressed the last and most vital inquiry, which is necessary to prove a breach of the Uniform Consent Statute and that is the question of injury. Both the majority and the trial court seem to imply that, if there is a breach of the informed consent statute and a resulting injury, then (automatically) liability attaches. In other words, a cause-in-fact relationship between failure to disclose and injury appears unnecessary. On this conclusion, I disagree. After reviewing this record in its entirely, I am convinced there was a reasonable factual basis to conclude that [the physician], at the time of the operation in question, was a practicing alcoholic. From this factual scenario, I suggest the gut question proposed is simply this: whether a professed and practicing alcoholic can operate upon any patient without breaching his standard of care. In other words, if there is a resulting injury and the doctor performing the operation is a practicing alcoholic and this alcoholism is not disclosed to the patient prior to the surgery, do we have liability? Given this factual scenario and considering the record in its entirety, I say, "Yes." Ergo, this question must be viewed on a case-by-case basis.

76. C. Stevens, "Bad Doctors Keep Eluding State's Discipline," *Detroit News*, Oct. 20, 1993, p.1.
77. See A. Meisel, "The 'Exceptions' to the Informed Consent Doctrine: Striking a Balance Between Competing Values in Medical Decision Making," *Wis. L. Rev.* 1979: 413.
78. Sullivan v. Montgomery, 155 Misc. 448, 279 N.Y.S. 575 (City Ct. 1935).
79. For criticism of therapeutic privilege, see E.G. Patterson, "The Therapeutic Justification of Withholding Medical Information: What You Don't Know Can't Hurt You, or Can It?" *Neb. L. Rev.* 64 (1985): 721; M. Somerville, "Therapeutic Privilege: Variation on the Theme of Informed Consent," *Law, Med. & Healthcare* 12 (1984): 4.
80. E.A. Plaut, "The Ethics of Informed Consent: An Overview," *Psychiat. J. Univ. Ottawa* 14 (1989): 435.
81. New York: Oxford University Press, 1998.
82. D.E. Ost, "The 'Right' Not to Know," *J. Med. & Philos.* 9 (1984): 301.
83. M. Strasser, "Mill and the Right to Remain Uninformed," *J. Med. & Philos.* 11 (1986): 265.
84. S.C. Gwynne, "Living with Lethal Genes: Some Advice," *Time*, Oct. 12, 1998, p. 89. See Comment, "Father and Mother Know Best: Defining the Liability of Physicians for Inadequate Genetic Counseling," *Yale L. J.* 87 (1978): 1488. See also the debate in G. Laurie, "In Defense of Ignorance: Genetic Information and the Right Not to Know," *Eur. J. Health Law* 6 (1999): 199; M.C. Bottis, "Comment on a View Favoring Ignorance of Genetic Information: Confidentiality, Autonomy, Beneficence and the Right Not to Know," *Eur. J. Health Law* 7 (2000): 173.
85. "Too Many Breakthroughs," *New York Times*, Nov. 19, 1998, p. 31.
86. Hippocrates, *Decorum* 2: 297–299 (W.H.S. Jones, trans. 1923).
87. Pages 31–32.
88. Codes of Ethics of American Medical Association, chap. 1, art. 1, §4 (1847).

32

Contributory Fault of the Patient in a Malpractice Action

If assuming medical malpractice, then what about the contributory fault of the patient? Negligence does not result in liability. There must be a causal nexus, a connection with the alleged harm. The following is a discussion of the patient's contributory or comparative negligence or intentional act that breaks the chain of causation in an action against a physician for malpractice.

The plaintiff (the patient) has the burden of persuasion of having suffered an injury that more probably than not was proximately caused by negligence of the defendant (the physician). On the other hand, the defendant has the burden of persuasion that the plaintiff was contributorily or comparatively negligent. In a contributory negligence jurisdiction, any negligence of the plaintiff precludes any monetary recovery, but dissatisfaction with the rule has led nearly all jurisdictions to adopt comparative negligence where the plaintiff's damages are simply reduced in proportion to its fault. By and large, at the time when contributory negligence was the prevailing rule, the courts tended to ignore the plaintiff's contributory negligence, particularly when it was not significant, and would not submit the issue of contributory negligence to the jury.

Informed Consent

What about contributory negligence of a patient in failing to request or obtain information? Is informed consent one-way or two-way? What are the responsibilities, if any, of the patient in obtaining information? Might not the patient pose questions when details about a proposed treatment are unclear? Customarily, patients are asked whether they have any questions about the treatment, or what they might expect of the treatment, but they are never tested on their understanding of the "informed consent" form that they sign. If patients were to have a duty, would it be objective or subjective? Who is the reasonably prudent patient? In *Truman v. Thomas*,[1] a divided California Supreme Court held a physician liable for not telling a patient about the potentially fatal consequences of refusing a suggested Pap test. The trial court did not make findings as to whether the patient had knowledge or should have had knowledge concerning the consequences of her refusal.

Ordinarily, contributory negligence is a defense to an action based on negligence, but it is not responsive to an action in battery or other intentional wrongdoing. When an individual is attacked intentionally, it is no defense that the individual did not get out of the way. Although an action based on lack of informed consent is categorized as negligence, not intentional wrongdoing, the courts nonetheless impose no duty on a patient to ask questions or otherwise obtain information about a proposed treatment. Almost without exception and contrary to theory, the courts are uniform in so holding. As an appellate court in Hawaii said, it is "unfair and illogical" to impose an affirmative duty on a patient to make an inquiry or otherwise affirmatively act with respect to informed consent.[2] Dr. Jerome Groopman of the Harvard Medical School observes that patients who think that a physician possesses a near-divine capacity for healing cause problems for the physician. The patient may assume that the physician knows everything, and the patient, or the family, does not offer information that can be vital to a correct diagnosis or treatment.[3]

In *Brown v. Dibbell*,[4] the Wisconsin Court of Appeals observed that the informed consent doctrine speaks "solely in terms of the *doctor's* duty to disclose and discuss information related to treatment and risks" (emphasis in original). The court said:

> [The doctrine] does not intimate, let alone place upon a patient an affirmative duty to investigate, question, or seek quantification of the information provided by the doctor. Rather, the entire gravamen of the informed consent [doctrine] is that a patient is not in a position to know treatment options and risks and, standing alone and unaided, is unable to make an informed choice. The doctor, who possesses medical knowledge and skills, has the affirmative burden both to comprehend what a reasonable patient in a similar situation would want to know and to provide the relevant information. Moreover, while every individual has a duty of ordinary care for their person, the underpinning of the contributory negligence defense, we perceive defining the dimensions of a patient's duty in an informed consent case to be a virtually impossible task. What degree of knowledge or insight can be demanded of one whom the law recognizes as unqualified to make decisions involving the complexities of medical science without assistance? The concept that a patient can be contributorily negligent, for example, by not asking enough or precisely proper questions, seems contrary to the [doctrinal] scheme and the reason for placing the burden on the doctor.[5]

Some years ago the Washington Supreme Court, quoting from a decision from North Dakota, said:

> On the question of contributory negligence, in such cases as the one at bar, it is the law that "it is not a part of the duties of a patient to distrust his physician, or to set his judgment against that of the expert whom he has employed to treat him, or to appeal to other physicians to ascertain if the physician is performing his duty properly. The very relation assumes trust and confidence on the part of the patient in the capacity and skill of the physician, and it would, indeed, require an unusual state of facts to render a person who is possessed of no medical skill guilty of contributory negligence because he accepts the word of his physician and trusts in the efficacy of the treatment prescribed by him. A patient has the right to rely on the professional skill of his physician, without calling others in to determine whether he really possesses such skill or not. The patient is not bound to call in other physicians, unless he becomes fully aware that the physician has not been, and is not giving proper treatment."[6]

In *Dibbell*, on appeal from the Wisconsin Court of Appeals, the Wisconsin Supreme Court took a unique tack. It agreed with the defendant that a doctor's duty to inform a patient does not obviate a duty of patients to exercise ordinary care for their own health and well-being; rather, a doctor and a patient have a joint responsibility to ensure that informed consent is obtained.[7] The Wisconsin Supreme Court said:

> [P]atients have a duty to exercise ordinary care for their own health and well-being; that contributory negligence may, under certain circumstances, be a defense in an informed consent action because the action is based on negligence. We thus recognize that a patient bringing an informed consent action is not exempt from the duty to exercise ordinary care for his or her own health and well-being. We also agree, however, with the court of appeals that the very patient–doctor relation assumes trust and confidence on the part of the patient and that would require an unusual set of facts to render a patient guilty of contributory negligence when the patient relies on the doctor.[8]

The court concluded that the trial court in this case should have given the jury an instruction on contributory negligence tailored to the patient's duty to exercise ordinary care in providing complete and accurate information to the doctors in response to their questions concerning personal, family, and medical history.[9] In a footnote, the court cautioned, "We do not address whether a patient's duty to exercise ordinary care requires the patient to volunteer information or to spontaneously advise the doctor of material of personal, family, or medical histories that the patient reasonably knows should be disclosed."[10]

Would a physician welcome numerous inquiries by a patient? Would it be an annoyance not easily tolerated? Dr. Ira Ockene of the University of Massachusetts Medical Center commented, "Every so often an appropriately assertive patient and family ask all the right questions, and on such occasions I have commented to the house staff that, if all patients and families were similar, the practice of medicine would grind to a halt."[11] Time pressures do not permit it. "This inadequacy of time allotment has been exacerbated by managed care and by the pressures of modern medicine, but existed long before HMOs ever darkened the horizon."[12] Dr. Jerome Groopman of the Harvard Medical School maintains that the accuracy of a diagnosis would be improved by questions from patients or family or friends, but, he finds, most physicians interrupt a patient 18 seconds after he starts talking. Testing may be necessary, but it is not sufficient for an accurate diagnosis; moreover, the patient's history underscores what tests are needed.[13]

In regarding a lawsuit filed against Lenox Hill Hospital by a woman alleging that its mishandling of a lab test led her to have an unnecessary abortion, Dr. Bertrand Bell, distinguished university professor at Albert Einstein College of Medicine at Yeshiva University, writes, "Perhaps the situation would have been different if all patients had the option of routinely reviewing laboratory, x-ray, and pathology reports. These reports are frequently not definitive, and a patient's interpretations can be useful—sometimes critical."[14]

Failure to Follow Instructions

Surveys indicate that two of every five senior citizens do not follow their physician's instructions, sometimes because of cost, sometimes because they just do not believe they need the medicine prescribed, or they do not take their medicine because of the side effects involved.[15] The courts look at the reasonableness of a patient's conduct and at proximate cause when analyzing the issue of a patient's failure to follow the physician's instructions. In *Shirey v. Schlemmer*,[16] the malpractice action was based on a physician's allegedly negligent setting and treatment of the patient's fractured arm. Evidence was presented that the patient had failed to follow the physician's instructions not to lift heavy objects. The patient had attempted to lift a 50-pound bag with his injured arm. The appellate court upheld the jury finding for the defendant because the plaintiff had been contributorily negligent.[17]

The case of a patient delaying return for treatment is similar to cases of a patient's disregarding a physician's directions. In *Myers v. Estate of Alessi*,[18] the patient claimed that the physician was negligent for not diagnosing the patient's throat condition. The physician claimed that the patient was contributorily negligent because the patient had returned to the physician's office only once in 14 months, although the physician had instructed her to return if her sore throat persisted. The jury was instructed that if an ordinary person in similar circumstances would have sought medical assistance, the patient would be negligent in not returning. The Maryland Court of Appeals agreed with the trial court's jury instruction on contributory negligence and affirmed the jury decision in favor of the defendant.

Furnishing False, Incomplete, or Misleading Information

Failure of the physician to have information is a major cause of medical error.[19] In determining whether a patient is at fault, the courts examine whether the patient has cooperated with the physician. In *Mackey v. Greenview Hospital*,[20] the Kentucky Court of Appeals concluded that the patient knew or should have known of her heart condition and that her misleading the physician about her medical history was a substantial factor in her heart attack during surgery. A patient's contributory negligence in giving a false or misleading history would not have been a bar to recovery if the physician by the exercise of ordinary care would have known of that aspect of the patient's medical history without regard to the actual history related by the patient.[21]

Barriers in communication may result in false, incomplete, or misleading information. In particular, language barriers hinder immigrant patients from adequately informing physicians about their condition or remedies that they still may be using from their native countries and cultures. (These might include elixirs from botanicals, especially among Latinos). In lengthy articles in the *New York Times* and *Newsweek*, it was noted that Elmhurst Hospital Center in New York probably deals with more than 100 languages and dialects. It processes more than 500,000 patient visits a year and roughly half speak so little English that they need some help with translation. Because the group of inhouse translators is relatively small, the hospital relies on freelance interpreters or a contracted phone translation service.[22] Apart from language problems, there are cultural problems. The ideas of the patients concerning their illness varies from culture to culture (some even believe that their symptoms arise from sorcery or from something they did in a previous life).

Patients who have a substance abuse disorder often attempt to hide or legitimize their substance use when they try to procure psychoactive pharmaceuticals from healthcare professionals. Some substance abusing patients are quite creative and ingenious in their efforts to obtain prescriptions (e.g., faking painful medical illnesses in order to obtain pain medications).[23]

Suicide

The professional duty of care encompasses, and is shaped by, the patient's condition. In a number of cases, it has been held that evidence of the patient's self-inflicted injury was sufficient to warrant submission of, or an instruction on, the defense of contributory or comparative negligence or voluntary act that breaks the chain of causation. In *Hobart v. Shin*,[24] a wrongful death action against a physician arising from the decedent's suicide by taking an overdose of a prescribed antidepressant medication, the Illinois Supreme Court affirmed a judgment of the trial court in favor of the physician and held that the evidence supported the trial court's decision to allow the defense of contributory negligence. In the case, the plaintiff pointed out that the physician knew of the decedent's previous suicide attempts and diagnosed her as having suicidal thoughts only a few weeks before her death. The plaintiff argued that those strong suicidal tendencies showed that the decedent was incapable of taking responsibility for her actions. The court, however, observed that when the decedent was released from the hospital prior to her suicide, she was no longer experiencing symptoms of depression. Moreover, the court noted that the last time the physician saw the decedent (more than 2 weeks before her death) the decedent was smiling and upbeat, and spoke positively of her plans for the future. Both the defendant physician and another physician who treated the decedent testified that in light of the decedent's improved condition, they considered her request for increasing her antidepressant prescription strength both natural and rational. Furthermore, on the day of her death, the decedent acted in a premeditated and deliberate fashion: she left home, refused to contact her doctors, and checked into a motel under a fictitious name. Given these facts, the court ruled that the trial court was justified in concluding that the issue of the decedent's contributory negligence was appropriate for the jury's consideration.

The Illinois Supreme Court also rejected the plaintiff's argument that the pattern jury instruction on contributory negligence given by the trial court was inadequate because it failed to take into account the fact that the decedent was being treated for mental illness at the time of her death; she should not have been held to the standards of "ordinary care" and "reasonably careful person" contained in the pattern instruction. The instructions defined *ordinary care* of the decedent's conduct as "the care a reasonably careful person would use under circumstances similar to those shown by the evidence." In light of the evidence that the decedent was competent and rational in the days and weeks immediately preceding her death, the Illinois Supreme Court was unable to say that the trial court erred in concluding that the pattern instructions on contributory negligence were appropriate. The instructions allowed the jury to evaluate the decedent's contributory negligence, if any, based on the particular circumstances of the case.

The Illinois Supreme Court relied on the reasoning of the California Court of Appeals in *DeMartini v. Alexander Sanitarium*.[25] There, it was held that the issue of contributory negligence of a mentally disturbed person is a question of fact unless, of course, the evidence discloses that the person whose actions are being judged is completely devoid of reason. If a person is so mentally ill that he is incapable of being contributorily negligent, he would be entitled to have the jury so instructed. But only in those cases in which the evidence would admit to no other rational conclusion would the plaintiff be entitled to have the issue determined as a matter of law.

In *Bundo v. Christ Community Hospital*,[26] the Illinois Court of Appeals found no error in the trial court's decision to instruct the jury on contributory negligence in an action for medical malpractice in which it was claimed that the decedent was driven to jump or fall out of a hospital window by excessive pain following an operation due to the neglect of the defendant physician. While it was claimed that the decedent was unable to comprehend the danger of his actions and was incapable of contributory negligence, the court stated that whether a mentally disturbed person is capable of contributory negligence is a question of fact for the jury where, as in this case, the decedent was never found mentally ill or incapacitated.

Undue Familiarity

The doctrine of comparative negligence, adopted in most states, allows the court to apportion fault between plaintiff and defendant. Yet, it is rare that any fault is attributed to the patient in cases where undue familiarity on the part of the physician is established. In an exceptional case, one jury found the patient to be 15 percent at fault and reduced the award accordingly.[27]

Patient's Behavior Prior to Seeking Medical Attention

The cases are many in which the physician alleges that the plaintiff was contributorily negligent by virtue of behavior that occurred before the patient sought treatment. In *Bourne v. Seventh Ward General Hospital*,[28] the Louisiana Court of Appeals addressed the argument of the defendant that a young woman was contributorily negligent due to her deliberate, self-inflicted injuries. She had attempted suicide by ingesting pills from two bottles of prescription pain medication. She was hospitalized and began to exhibit bizarre and violent behavior, and she was transferred to a psychiatric facility where she died the next day. Expert witnesses testified that the physician's care of the patient was substandard.

In addressing the element of causation, the court found, "If the action or inaction of the healthcare provider destroyed any substantial possibility of the patient's survival, the trier of fact is warranted in finding that the healthcare provider's conduct was a proximate cause of the patient's death." The court stated that although there was another "cause in fact" of the patient's death—the ingestion of a lethal dose of prescription medication—there can be more than a single cause in fact in a particular case. In this case the medical care provider's negligent acts ensued between the overdose and death, depriving the decedent of an 80 percent chance of survival. The court determined that the defendant's negligence was an intervening force and superseding cause. Thus, the provider's negligence supplanted the suicide attempt as the cause of death. The court held that the plaintiff's suit was not barred by the doctrine of contributory negligence.[29]

Conclusion

In accord with the trend of making it difficult to make out a case of medical malpractice, and with the adoption of comparative negligence, the courts and legislatures are increasingly (but not uniformly) considering the fault of patients in bringing about their injury. This may be the result of increased consumer activism in healthcare issues in recent years. The public is more informed about healthcare as a result of the media, the Internet, and pharmaceutical company advertising. Healthcare consumers are no longer presumed to be totally uninformed and unaware of their healthcare needs. By and large, the courts are more cognizant of heightened consumer awareness of healthcare issues, and as a consequence, it is increasingly considered that the patient's fault may diminish or supersede the fault of the physician.

Endnotes

1. 27 Cal. 3d 285, 165 Cal. Rptr. 308, 611 P.2d 902 (1980).
2. See Keomaka v. Zakaib, 8 Haw. App. 516, 532, 811 P.2d 478, 486 (1991).
3. Quoted in G. Niebuhr, "Believer and Skeptic See Spirituality in Medicine," *New York Times*, Nov. 18, 2000, p. 19.
4. 220 Wis. 2d 200, 582 N.W.2d 134, 137 (Wis. App. 1998).
5. 582 N.W. 2d at 137–138.
6. Kelly v. Carroll, 36 Wash.2d 4872, 501, 219 P.2d 79, 90 (1950), quoting from Halverson v. Zimmerman, 60 N.D. 113, 125, 232 N.W. 754, 759 (1930).
7. Brown v. Dibbell, 227 Wis. 2d 28, 595 N.W.2d 358 (1999).
8. 595 N.W. 2d at 367.
9. 595 N.W. 2d at 369.
10. 595 N.W.2d at 369 n. 13.
11. I.S. Ockene, "Why Hospitals Are Getting Dangerous" (ltr.), *Wall Street Journal*, Dec. 9, 1999, p. 27.
12. *Ibid.* In a consumer guide to hospital stays, *Take This Book to the Hospital With You: A Consumer Guide to Surviving Your Hospital Stay* (New York: St. Martin's Press, 1997), Charles B. Inlander, president of the People's Medical Society of Allentown, Pennsylvania, suggests that patients ask lots of questions. See A. Tang, "Staying on Guard for Medical Errors," *New York Times*, Dec. 5, 1999, p. BU11.
13. J. Groopman, *How Doctors Think* (New York: Houghton Mifflin, 2007); see also N. Shute, "The 18-Second Doctor," *U.S. News & World Report*, March 26, 2007, p. 14.
14. "Read Your Own Chart," *New York Times*, Oct. 5, 1998, p. 22.
15. AP news release, "Many Seniors Don't Follow Doctors' Orders on Prescriptions," *Wall Street Journal*, April 19, 2005, p. D3.
16. 140 Ind. App. 606, 223 N.E.2d 759 (1967), discussed in M.R. Orr, "Defense of Patient's Contribution to Fault in Medical Malpractice Action," *Creighton L. Rev.* 25 (1992): 665.
17. See Annot., 84 A.L.R. 5th 619, 108 A.L.R. 5th 385.
18. 80 Md. App. 124, 560 A.2d 59 (1989).
19. L. Andrews, "Studying Medical Error *In Situ*: Implications for Malpractice Law and Policy," *DePaul L. Rev.* 54 (2005): 357.
20. 587 S.W.2d 249 (Ky. App. 1979).
21. See Annot., 33 A.L.R. 4th 790. According to the Centers for Disease Control and Prevention, the number of emergency room visits in the past decade rose 23% to 110.2 million a year with the result that it has created a difficult challenge for emergency room physicians responsible for distinguishing indigestion from heart attack, influenza from meningitis, bronchitis from pulmonary embolism. With patient loads increasing, misdiagnosis is a growing problem. Misdiagnosed heart attack is among the most common causes of malpractice litigation for emergency medicine physicians. Many patients—out of guilt or fear—do not timely volunteer information on their risk factors (smoking, diabetes, hypertension, bad cholesterol, or a family history of heart disease), factors that could assist physicians in determining how suspicious they should be and, thus, what tests to administer. K. Helliker, "Is It a Heart Attack—or Indigestion? Helping the ER Doctors Get It Right," *Wall Street Journal*, March 29, 2005, p. B1. Yet in a book that has had a wide readership, *Blink: The Power of Thinking Without Thinking* (Boston: Little, Brown, 2005), Malcolm Gladwell maintains that decisions made very quickly can be every bit as good as decisions made cautiously and deliberately. He tells the story of an emergency

room physician at Cook County Hospital in Chicago, an overcrowded and financially strapped institution whose emergency department treats a quarter of a million patients a year. Through an algorithm taking only three factors into account, in addition to an ECG, the physician was able to have a more accurate and less costly method of finding out who was not experiencing cardiac arrest.

22. See N. Bernstein, "Language Gap Called Health Risk in E.R.," *New York Times*, April 21, 2005, p. C20.

23. C. Kilgannon, "Learning Many Ways to Say 'Ah,'" *New York Times*, April 15, 2005, p. C20; A. Underwood & J. Adler, "When Cultures Clash," *Newsweek*, April 25, 2005, p. 68.

24. 185 Ill.2d 283, 235 Ill. Dec. 724, 705 N.E.2d 907 (1998), noted in 108 A.L.R.5th 385.

25. 192 Cal. App.2d 442, 13 Cal. Rptr. 564, 91 A.L.R.2d 383 (1961).

26. 104 Ill. App.3d 670, 60 Ill. Dec. 394, 432 N.E.2d 1293 (1982).

27. Kulick v. Gates, No. 41624 (Mass. Super. Ct. May 21, 1985), referenced in *Am. L. Rep.* 28 (1985): 471. See Chapter 33 on undue familiarity.

28. 546 So.2d 197 (La. App. 1989).

29. A recent case in Michigan gave rise to various opinions by the Justices of the State Supreme Court on a patient's prior behavior. In Shinholster v. Annapolis Hospital, 471 Mich. 540 (2004), the decedent visited the defendant hospital four times complaining of dizziness and was examined by defendant physicians. Her fourth visit was precipitated by a massive stroke, after which she entered a coma for several months and died at the age of 61. Her husband filed suite under the Wrongful Death Act alleging that the hospital and physicians failed to recognize that his wife had been experiencing ministrokes on her three prior visits, and that ministrokes often precede a more full-blown, serious stroke. She failed to regularly take her prescribed blood pressure medication during the year preceding her fatal stroke.

The court addressed the issue of whether, and to what extent, MCL 600.6304 permits a trier of fact in a medical malpractice action to consider the plaintiff's own pretreatment negligence to offset, at least in part, the defendant's fault. According to the Michigan Supreme Court: "MCL 600.6304 generally provides that the trier of fact in a tort action shall determine by percent the comparative negligence of all those who are a proximate cause of the plaintiff's injury and subsequent damages," including the plaintiff. The court said that MCL 600.6304 is unambiguous and "calls for the trier of fact to assess by percentage the total fault of *all* persons that contributed to the death or injury, including the plaintiff, as long as that fault constituted a proximate cause of the plaintiff's injuries and subsequent damages." As to what constitutes proximate cause, the court reiterated the prevailing definition: "The proximate cause of an injury is not necessarily the immediate cause; not necessarily the cause nearest in time, distance or space. Assuming that there is a direct, natural, and continuous sequence between an act and an injury, … the act can be accepted as the proximate cause of the injury without reference to its separation from the injury in point of time or distance."

The question is whether the conduct of the plaintiff merely created the condition that led him or her to seek treatment or whether the plaintiff's conduct constituted a proximate cause of the injury. If it is the latter, evidence may be presented to the trier of fact so damages may be apportioned accordingly, if at all. The court in *Shinholster* provided the following analogy to make the determination: "It is possible to hypothesize situations where a plaintiff's pretreatment negligence will do nothing more than create the condition leading the plaintiff to seek treatment. In such a situation, the negligent practitioner might be found to constitute a superseding cause that produced an injury different in kind. For example, if a person negligently broke her leg and during surgery to set the leg the doctor cut an artery causing her to bleed to death, the decedent's original negligence could be said to have done no more than bring the plaintiff to the operating table. But, if the surgeon merely set the broken leg negligently, such an injury would constitute a natural and foreseeable result of the plaintiff's original negligence"; 471 Mich. at 553 n. 9. Accordingly, it was said, if reasonable minds could conclude that based on evidence presented by defendants that a plaintiff's own negligence was the proximate cause and the foreseeable, natural, and probable consequences of his or her actions or inactions then the conduct of the plaintiff must be considered in the apportionment of fault as stated in MCL 600.6304. Indeed, it was said, the decedent's failure to properly take her medication, in fact, may have constituted a proximate cause of her death; 471 Mich. at 553.

In a dissent, one justice suggested that the patient's conduct before seeking medical treatment is merely a factor the physician should consider in treating the patient. The lead opinion, it was said, in holding that the plaintiff's pretreatment negligence may be considered a proximate cause of the plaintiff's damages for purposes of comparative negligence, abandons the long standing principle of tort law that the defendant takes the plaintiff as he finds her. Another justice dissenting said, "Today, a plurality of this Court makes a mockery of tort law by holding that a jury can consider a plaintiff's pretreatment negligence to determine liability. … Make no mistake, allowing a jury to consider a plaintiff's pretreatment negligence in a medical malpractice action is a sweeping new decision, with no basis in this Court's prior rulings"; 471 Mich. at 597–598.

33

The Boundary Violation of Undue Familiarity

Boundary violations in psychotherapy involve transgressions that may be sexual or nonsexual in nature. Of these transgressions, the most publicized is the sexual exploitation of a patient, or *undue familiarity* in the language of the American Psychiatric Association (APA). In a boundary violation, one cannot as a rule assess the immediate impact to discern whether harm has occurred, but for the boundary violation of undue familiarity, the inevitability of harm or causality is alleged and assumed.

In 1918, at the Fifth Congress of the International Psychoanalytic Association held in Budapest, Freud gave a stern lecture warning of the dangers of the transference relationship. With their patients, Freud said, analysts must avoid affection, friendship, pity—even sharing news like holiday plans. If a patient professes love, the analyst "has no grounds whatever for being proud of such a 'conquest.'" None in the audience except perhaps Sandor Ferenczi, his close friend, knew that Freud at the time was analyzing his own daughter, Anna.[1]

Questions arise: What is the appropriate recourse: a disciplinary proceeding, a malpractice action, or a criminal prosecution? What "fits" the offense? Is the psychotherapist unfairly singled out? Special moral principles, we know, apply to people because of the role that they occupy. This is called role-specific morality.

A sexual relation between a psychotherapist and patient is compared to incest or rape, upon the observation that the patient's ostensible consent is a result of the phenomenon of transference, or the power imbalance that exists between therapist and patient. Dr. Judd Marmor, a former president of the APA, stated: "[S]uch behavior between a patient and therapist has all the elements of incest at an unconscious level and represents an equivalent dereliction of moral responsibilities."[2] Psychiatrist Nanette Gartrell observed, "These patients end up with the same emotional problems you see in incest victims."[3] Laura Brown, a clinical psychologist, testified at a trial:

> The reason sexual involvement with a patient is so harmful is due to the "parent–child" relationship symbolized by the transference. Were a therapist to be sexual with a client, it would be replicating at a symbolic level the situation in which a parent would be sexual with a child. The kinds of harm that can flow from those sorts of violations of trust are very similar.[4]

In a number of speeches and publications, sex therapists William Masters and Virginia Johnson urged that when sexual seduction of a patient can be firmly established by due process, regardless of whether the seduction was initiated by the patient or the therapist, the therapist should be prosecuted for rape.[5] (In Greek, the word *transference* means "metaphor.")

Sexual relations between psychotherapist and patient is a topic that captures the headlines and is sensationalized. Books and journal articles about the issue, written by both patients and therapists, have proliferated in recent years.[6] A review of four books by therapists, all published in the early months of 1990, appeared in an essay aptly titled "Disturbances in the Field."[7]

In a commentary typical of the genre, a writer of a law review article stated: "Therapist-patient sexual exploitation is a significant social problem. … The consequences to victims, who are primarily women, are devastating."[8] Another stated: "The worst misfortune that can befall a vulnerable female psychiatric patient is to superimpose upon her already fragile condition a lascivious psychiatrist and compulsive lecher as a healer."[9] The symptoms usually suffered by patients as a result of the sexual intimacy are said, but not proven at trial, to include a worsening of previously existing psychiatric symptoms, increased difficulty in personal relationships, feelings of guilt, emptiness and suppressed rage, an inability to trust, and an increased risk of suicide.[10] Some reports have suggested that as many as 1% of the patients who become sexually involved with their therapist commit suicide.[11] The studies are not clear on how the patients were located or whether subsequence is mistaken as consequence.

The reports in the literature have become the basis for legislation or for the justification of large awards in litigation with the number of lawsuits dramatically increasing.[12] In recent years, no less than 16 states (Arizona, California, Colorado, Connecticut, Florida, Georgia, Iowa, Maine, Minnesota, New Hampshire, New Mexico, North Dakota, South Dakota, Texas, Utah, Wisconsin) have passed legislation making sexual contact between psychotherapist and patient a criminal act. These laws declare that consent is no defense.[13] Three states (California, Minnesota, Wisconsin) have enacted statutes requiring a therapist to report a former therapist accused by a patient of sexual exploitation to the appropriate licensing authority, or to inform and enable the patient to report the sexual conduct.[14]

The statutes have been challenged, to no avail, on the ground that they are vague. Colorado's statute defines "sexual contact" as:

> [K]nowingly touching ... the victim's intimate parts by the actor, or ... the actor's intimate parts by the victim, or ... knowingly touching ... the clothing covering the immediate area of the victim's or actor's intimate parts if that sexual contact can reasonably be construed as being for the purposes of sexual arousal, gratification, or abuse.[15]

In upholding the constitutionality of the statutory definition, the Colorado Supreme Court noted that the trial court had instructed the jury that the state had to prove beyond a reasonable doubt that the sexual contact was "for the purpose of sexual arousal, gratification, or abuse."[16]

The Minnesota Supreme Court used the same reasoning in upholding the constitutionality of a similar statutory definition of sexual contact.[17] However, shortly thereafter, the Minnesota legislature amended its statute to provide a detailed definition, and to include the "touching of the clothing covering the immediate area of the intimate parts."[18] The statutes of Florida and Maine prohibit the specific sexual acts of intercourse, fellatio, cunnilingus, and sodomy, rather than any contact for sexual gratification.[19]

A civil cause of action for sexual exploitation likewise arises regardless of any actual consent of the patient or former patient, and regardless of whether such acts occurred during any treatment, consultation, assessment, interview, or examination. The legislatures of four states have specifically made sexual contact with a patient malpractice per se.[20] The following is an example of language from a complaint: The defendant "mishandled the transference by not terminating treatment when the plaintiff took her clothes off in front of the defendant"; as a result of the ensuing sexual acts, the plaintiff suffered "physical pain and suffering, emotional pain and suffering, shame, attempted suicide, and expenses for recovery and rehabilitation."[21]

Assuredly, intimacy with patients does them no good, and it will disillusion them because transference is not reality. Frieda Fromm-Reichmann, who was married briefly to her analyst, Erich Fromm, advised therapists, "Don't have sex with your patient. You'll always disappoint them." However, should it be *automatically* assumed that it does *great* harm, as though the patient had actually suffered rape or incest? Should it be *automatically* assumed that the patient is without the capacity to consent? Transference of feelings from the past to the present is not the same as present reality. Transference jargon has beclouded common sense and has gotten juries and judges to accept the existence of *transference dementia*.

Transference—the unconscious assignment to others of feelings and attitudes that were originally associated with important figures in one's early life—is a universal phenomenon occurring in every aspect of one's daily life. In psychoanalytic or insight-oriented psychotherapy, the therapist utilizes this phenomenon as a therapeutic tool to help the patient understand emotional problems and their origins. The transference may be negative (hostile) or positive (affectionate).[22] Questions arise such as: When does transference begin and how can we know it? Does transference interfere with the capacity to make intimate or important personal decisions? When does transference end? Does it end with treatment? If not, how soon after treatment, if ever?

As a rule, intimacy with a patient does not occur with hospitalized or incompetent psychotic patients, but rather with well-functioning or borderline individuals. In psychiatric parlance, a borderline individual is one who is unstable in a variety of areas, including interpersonal relationships, behavior, mood, and self-image.[23] In the vast majority of cases, the patient is not caught up in a psychotic transference. Does the patient, as a result of the sexual relations, suffer a broken marriage, a suicide attempt, or severe deterioration of social function? Why are the patients not hospitalized after such an episode? Indeed, the APA's malpractice insurance policy, like most other policies, does not cover undue familiarity, thereby depriving these patients, who have allegedly suffered great harm, of a source of compensation for their suffering.

In the usual tort case, the plaintiff has the burden of establishing fault, causation, and the extent of damages. In undue familiarity cases, however, the courts today tend to *assume* great harm and a causal nexus linking the defendant's conduct to the injury. In no other area of tort law is professional misconduct or incompetence, standing alone, sufficient to impose liability. Only in the sexual misconduct cases have the courts, for the most part, adopted a *per se* rule that liability is established even in the absence of proof of actual injury. For instance, in a Washington case,[24] a therapist defended a sexual misconduct suit on the grounds that the patient had not been damaged by the affair. The court replied: "The most elementary conceptions of justice and public policy require that the wrongdoer shall bear the risk of the uncertainty [of actual damages], which his own wrong has created."[25] Only exceptionally is proof of damages required.[26]

In a statement that would not be made in the United States, Israeli therapists Rivka Yahav and Sheri Oz contend that a distinction must be made between "those who experienced the sexual interaction as traumatic and those who experienced it as an exciting and happy romance."[27]

In the usual case, the jury, shocked by the reprehensible behavior, punishes the therapist by awarding compensatory damages. If the jurisdiction allows punitive damages, they are added for good measure. The large jury awards establish a basis for substantial settlements in later cases, and for blackmailing: "Pay up, or I'll sue." Insurance carriers have come to consider these cases as indefensible, and most now specifically exclude coverage. Justice James Heiple of the Illinois Supreme Court entered a dissent to lawsuits based on sexual relations with a patient:

> This is not a proper claim for malpractice. It should not be recognized in law. There is no suggestion that the plaintiff in this case was a minor, was mentally retarded or was under any other legal disability. She knew what she was doing and did it.
>
> At the moment the sexual relationship began, the treatment relationship ended. From that time forward, the plaintiff and the defendant were engaged in a frolic, a mutually agreeable detour from any recognized or accepted treatment regimen. To hold the defendant legally liable under such conditions is to countenance a legal form of extortion or blackmail. The law should not permit it. The complaint should be dismissed. Even if such a claim were to be recognized, the attempt to fit this type of claim into a negligence or willful and wanton format is wholly misplaced. There is no allegation that the parties fell off a bed or injured any part of the plaintiff's anatomy. The plaintiff, having willingly engaged in a frolic, now seeks to use the legal system as a toll for a shakedown.[28]

Ordinarily, it is incumbent upon the complainant to establish an exacerbation of symptoms as a result of the behavior of the defendant. However, this burden of proof is notably absent in undue familiarity cases. In reality, the posttraumatic stress disorder (PTSD) claimed by the complainant may only be a secondary gain syndrome, which occurs when patients' symptoms increase when they become aware that they will be awarded damages for the symptoms.[29] One of the more amusing examples in the literature is the Pope and Bouhoutsos elaboration of the "therapist–patient sex syndrome." In their 1986 book, *Sexual Intimacy Between Therapists and Patients*, Pope and Bouhoutsos noted that patients most likely to develop this syndrome (a configuration of symptoms constituting a condition) may be those with borderline and histrionic personality disorders. They also noted that the syndrome itself resembles the borderline and histrionic personality disorder. Hence, this is a syndrome that resembles the way the sufferers were before they developed the syndrome and, in fact, is characterized by the sufferers' premorbid condition. In relation to any other issue, this train of logic would simply be laughable.

Litigation alleging sexual misconduct by a therapist is actually of fairly recent origin. Until the 1970s, such events rarely led to litigation. The landmark cases are *Zipkin v. Freeman*,[30] a decision by the Missouri Supreme Court in 1968, and *Roy v. Hartogs*,[31] a much publicized New York case from the mid-1970s. The impetus to sue can be attributed to the decreased stigma associated with being a psychotherapy patient, the realization that patients who report undue familiarity are probably not fantasizing, and, certainly, media reports of high damage awards and the theory of the case.

In *Zipkin,* a court, for the first time, conceptualized the therapist–patient sexual intimacy in psychodynamic terms of transference and the therapist's handling of that transference. Writing for the majority of the Missouri Supreme Court, Judge Seiler wrote: "[The defendant] mishandled the transference phenomenon, which is a reaction the psychiatrists anticipate and which must be handled properly."[32] In discussing therapist–patient sexual intimacy in terms of the therapist's responsibility to handle the transference appropriately, the opinion indicated that even less extreme expressions of the therapist's attraction to the patient (e.g., swimming, dancing) may constitute malpractice. The jury awarded the plaintiff $17,000. The court, however, reduced the award to $5,000. That was in 1968, when the dollar had much more value than today.

Zipkin did not specifically turn on allegations of sexual contact, although a sexual relationship was at least implied by the testimony, which included allegations of nude swimming parties. The doctor's misconduct consisted of misusing the therapeutic relationship to induce the plaintiff to attend social events with him, to leave her husband, move into a farm owned by the doctor, and to take property from her husband. The plaintiff testified that she fell in love with the defendant and put her faith and trust in him. Experts testified that the defendant's "treatment" of the plaintiff was a distortion of the transference phenomenon, which caused the plaintiff serious, and perhaps permanent, emotional harm.[33]

Prior to *Zipkin*, most of the reported cases were brought by husbands who claimed damages as a result of their wives' sexual relationship with a therapist. In most jurisdictions, these types of cases were barred by so-called "heart balm" statutes that did away with civil liability for alienation of affections, seduction, and criminal conversation. In a California case, the California Court of Appeals held that the therapist owed no duty of care to the patient's husband, and the husband was also held not to be a direct victim despite his attendance at some therapy sessions.[34]

In *Hartogs*, Julie Roy charged Dr. Renatus Hartogs with inducing her to have sexual intercourse as a part of her prescribed therapy. The case, decided in 1976, was chronicled in a book, *Betrayal*, co-authored by the plaintiff and Lucy Freeman.[35] A television film followed. In the film, the doctor orders the timid woman around his office, screams at her, talks incessantly of curing her, and sits behind a large, imposing desk to conduct the noncouch sessions. The advertisements for the film proclaimed, "The true story of a vulnerable woman who turns to a psychiatrist for help. … Instead, he lures her into a sexual relationship!" The book carries the subcaption, "The true story of the first woman to successfully sue her psychiatrist for using sex in the guise of therapy." As it turned out, neither in this case nor in later cases would it be necessary to allege that sex was engaged in under the guise of therapy. It is irrelevant whether the therapist tells the patient at the outset that a sexual relationship is proper therapy, with the patient consenting.

The trial court in *Hartogs* was convinced by the argument of plaintiff's counsel that can be paraphrased as follows: Transference deprives patients of the ability to exercise independent judgment. It negates any free will. It accomplishes the same result as hypnosis or drugs. Therefore, the legislation, in abolishing the common-law cause of action for seduction, should not apply in the case of a psychotherapist.[36]

After a protracted trial, the jury awarded Julie Roy $250,000 in compensatory damages and $100,000 in punitive damages. However, Judge Myers, the trial judge, reduced by $200,000 the jury's compensatory verdict, leaving $50,000 for damages in that category. He allowed the $100,000 in punitive damages to stand. The judge stated that the plaintiff had not proved that permanent emotional damage resulted from Dr. Hartogs' "treatment." In a 23-page opinion, Judge Myers wrote:

> The court has observed this plaintiff during the trial, which lasted almost 2 weeks. She certainly did not appear to be psychotic. She was well poised and well groomed. She spoke coherently and related her case with precision, clarity, excellent memory, and without inhibition. I could not discern the slightest sign of abnormal behavior during the entire trial even under what must have been harrowing cross-examination.[37]

At the same time, Judge Myers described Dr. Hartogs' behavior as "heinous and atrocious." He stated: "When one considers how vital it is both for society at large and, more particularly, for the medical profession that such conduct, as presented here, be eradicated … it cannot be held as a matter of law that the jury's assessment of $100,000 was excessive." He concluded, "A patient must not be fair game for a lecherous doctor."[38]

Dr. Hartogs appealed Judge Myers' decision and later, in September 1975, filed for bankruptcy. In January 1976, the Appellate Term of the Supreme Court of New York cut the compensatory damages from $50,000 to $25,000 and eliminated the punitive damages. The majority opinion stated:

> Plaintiff's condition was of long standing, and began years before she became defendant's patient. There is no evidence to support a permanent worsening of the condition by defendant's acts; nor is there proof demonstrating a permanent impairment of her ability to work in a position comparable to that she had before or during the period she was defendant's patient. Given the fact that she may recover only for the aggravation of her condition by defendant … we conclude that an award of more than $25,000 would be excessive.[39]

The court further ruled that Dr. Hartogs' conduct, while inexcusable, did not warrant punitive damages. In a concurring opinion, Presiding Justice Markowitz commented: "The subject matter of this case was highly sensational forcing the participants to operate in a charged atmosphere rather than the calm almost cloistered climate of the routine civil courtroom."[40]

Justice Riccobono dissented from any award of damages. He pointed out that although the plaintiff was suffering from a number of emotional problems, her competency was never placed in issue, stating, "Is it not fair to infer, therefore, that she was capable of giving a knowing and meaningful consent?"[41] He added, "The relief sought by this plaintiff constitutes the closest approach to a conventional action for seduction, and hence must be treated as such."[42] While

New York and most other jurisdictions have abolished actions for seduction or alienation of affection, for the psychotherapist, and the psychotherapist alone, "malpractice" replaces "seduction" or "alienation of affection" and the action continues.[43]

Justice Riccobono's dissent has not received attention. Since 1976, sexual misconduct has represented 15% of all lawsuits against psychiatrists and has accounted for one third or more of the payout for psychiatric malpractice claims. Judgments in the 6-digit range have not been uncommon.[44] In a California case,[45] the parties agreed to a $2.5 million settlement to avoid an appeal, after an initial $4.7 million award, all compensatory, no punitive damages, was returned by a jury. In a Virginia case,[46] the jury awarded $650,000 in compensatory damages. A claim for punitive damages was dropped because of doubts as to whether defendant's insurance policy would cover or indemnify against punitive damages. Today, as a result of these jury verdicts, merely filing a complaint against a psychotherapist alleging sexual misconduct usually results, on average, in a settlement of $110,000. To avoid the peril of the jury, or a hearing before a medical board, and to avoid publicity, most cases are settled. One might ask, why gamble when the law provides a sure win? A few years ago Joel Klein, then general counsel for the APA, observed:

> Probably the biggest single problem, and the one that's most difficult to address, is the issue of sex between therapist and patient. Insurance companies generally are so concerned about the explosive nature of this problem and the risks involved—sympathetic juries, large damages, punitive damages—that they now refuse to cover it. Very few cases actually go to trial, since most are settled, usually at a high figure, perhaps higher than one would expect. In malpractice terms, the best data we have suggests that during the years when insurance companies were covering this risk, probably a third or more of the payout for malpractice claims was for sex cases.[47]

In a Pennsylvania case,[48] the jury returned a verdict for the plaintiff in the amount of $665,000: $275,000 for compensatory damages exclusive of costs for future psychiatric care, $90,000 for future psychiatric care, and $300,000 for punitive damages. The court disallowed the $90,000 awarded for future psychiatric treatment as "the plaintiff did not demonstrate that it was probable she would undergo future psychiatric care … and could not trust another doctor."[49] In this case, the plaintiff sought treatment from the defendant when she was suffering from a condition called *harried housewife syndrome*.[50] She testified that the defendant "became a God" to her and that she "was dependent on him."[51] In various cases, clinics are also held responsible for negligent supervision.[52]

In the usual case, the analysis is cursory.[53] The fact of sexual intimacy alone clouds the issue of injury. There is a principle in our jurisprudence that injury must be individually established, not presumed based on the class of alleged misconduct. Lawyers say that a classification is no substitute for personalized accounts. In general, however, in therapist sexual relations cases, the court does not closely inquire whether this patient's relations with men have actually worsened, or whether *her* emotional problems have been resolved, but for the therapist's undue familiarity, or even whether there were lost wages or medical bills. The undue familiarity may very well have caused emotional harm, but if so, one would expect the plaintiff, as in other cases alleging emotional distress, to exhibit or prove it. Women who have been raped suffer a "rape trauma syndrome." Do women who are sexually involved with a therapist as a result of the transference phenomenon suffer a similar syndrome? The answer is no. The exception is so rare that it warrants comment in the professional journals.[54]

Nearly all of the reported cases have involved sexual relations between a male doctor and a female patient. It has been said that this is another example of the exploitation of women. In actuality, there have been instances of sexual relations between female doctors and male patients. Surveys show that anywhere from 6 to 10% of male therapists and 3 to 8% of female therapists acknowledge being sexually involved with patients during treatment. However, regardless of the harm, a man even in these litigious times does not think of suing a woman for having had sex with him. The news of a man filing such a suit would be as odd as that of a man biting a dog. To what psychological aberration can we ascribe this failure to file suit? Is it because a man who brings suit on this account would be treated with derision, or are men better able to handle such sexual episodes than women? Does transference turn women, but not men, into helpless waifs?[55]

In past years, a therapist in a gesture of empathy might put his hand on the shoulder of a depressed, weeping mother who had recently lost her son. However, in today's litigious climate he shrinks from doing so, fearing, as one therapist stated, "the witch hunt against consciously or unconsciously experienced sexual intent toward an innocent patient."[56] One of the consequences of the current climate is that depersonalization has taken place between therapists and patients. Therapists sit defensively behind their desks, careful not to spontaneously smile. They conduct themselves in a very prim and proper manner, and dispense their psychotherapeutic or medication products to "consumers," no longer fellow human beings experiencing emotional pain. When Dr. Elissa Benedek, in her capacity as president of the APA, stated that as soon as a therapist experiences an emotion of sexuality toward a patient, the therapist must immediately transfer the patient to another therapist, it was apparent that the leadership in psychiatry had gone overboard.[57]

Some suggest that sexual relations with a former patient are never permissible.[58] Others suggest a waiting period following termination of therapy, during which time even social contact would be precluded.[59] In 1988, the APA amended its ethics code to read: "Sexual involvement with one's former patient generally exploits emotions deriving from treatment and, therefore, almost always is unethical."[60] Dr. Ruth Tiffany Barnhouse entered a protest: "To claim that former patients are forever out of bounds is to say that the wounds cannot be healed and that maturation does not occur. It infantilizes patients by preserving indefinitely the therapist's superior status as one who is more powerful, more mature, and still symbolically in the parental role."[61]

Legislation in California and Minnesota prohibits sexual contact with a former patient for 2 years.[62] The ban is allegedly warranted in order to deal with the risks of impaired decision making, fraud, and exploitation of a fiduciary relationship. Furthermore, even after years of marriage to a therapist, the patient under the theory might, when seeking a divorce, also claim damages for emotional distress—a cause of action arguably not barred by a statute of limitations because the damages were not earlier recognizable.[63] What about freedom of association? Are people who "fall in love" able to exercise any better judgment about the qualities of their companion? The decision-making ability of former patients is said to be impaired by residual transference.

One survey of psychologists, conducted in California, found the perceived harm of sexual relations with a patient during the course of therapy to range from great to none at all. Positive effects were reported in some cases. The 704 psychologists who responded said that 559 of their patients reported having sexual relations with the previous therapist. Female patients were involved with a male therapist in 92% of the cases. One half of the sexual contacts with male patients involved male therapists. When the therapist initiated sexual intimacies, the respondents felt that the patient was adversely affected in 82% of the cases. When the patient initiated sexual intimacies, respondents thought the patient was adversely affected in 39% of the cases. The patients had negative feelings about the relationship in 29% of the cases. And, 16% reported positive effects.[64]

Actually, anyone, male or female, unable to handle sex will be traumatized by it, whether the partner is a doctor, lawyer, or movie star. Every person "in love" is exposed, extended, and fragile; damage may arise from any broken relationship.[65] Judging from the reports, however, the consequences of sexual involvement with a therapist are even more dire than those arising from a rape in the streets. It boggles, or ought to boggle, the imagination.

What about causal connection? Mere simultaneity between an event and an illness does not demonstrate any causal connection between the two events. Indeed, without statistical studies with reasonable confidence limits, one might well conclude that the temporal relationship is simply the result of chance.

Suppose a woman is all at once a patient in psychotherapy, a churchgoer, a law student, and a litigant in a divorce proceeding. The illustration is not far-fetched. How does a sexual affair with her therapist compare with one involving a priest, a lawyer, or law professor? Is she less or more vulnerable in one situation than another?

The transference phenomenon is construed as unique to the psychotherapist–patient relationship, and as validation of emotional injury when sexual relations occur. In *Simmons v. United States*,[66] the Ninth Circuit Court of Appeals explained:

> We note that courts do not routinely impose liability upon physicians in general for sexual contact with patients. … The crucial factor in the therapist–patient relationship, which leads to the imposition of legal liability for conduct that arguably is no more exploitative of a patient than sexual involvement of a lawyer with a client, a priest or minister with a parishioner, or a gynecologist with a patient is that lawyers, ministers, and gynecologists do not offer a course of treatment and counseling predicated upon handling the transference phenomenon.[67]

Physicians other than psychiatrists are allegedly not trained to recognize or deal with the transference phenomenon and, hence, are not held liable for malpractice (though they may be sanctioned by a medical board).[68] As one who in this context would single out psychotherapists, Dr. Spencer Eth says:

> I would distinguish sexual relations with a therapist from sexual activity with other classes of individuals such as attorneys, professors, or employers. Although all of these relationships are asymmetric, only the psychotherapeutic relationship emphasizes self-disclosure and transference. In that context, the capacity for free choice is significantly diminished and the potential for exploitation significantly enhanced.[69]

The ethical provision of the American Psychiatric Association states:

> The requirement that the physician conduct himself/herself with propriety in his/her profession and in all the actions of his/her life is especially important in the case of the psychiatrist because the patient tends to model his/her behavior after that of his/her psychiatrist by identification. Further, the necessary intensity of the treatment relationship may tend to active sexual and other needs and fantasies on the part of both patient and psychiatrist, while weakening the objectivity necessary for control. Additionally, the inherent inequality in the doctor–patient relationship may lead to exploitation of the patient. Sexual activity with a current or former patient is unethical.[70]

To be sure, transference feelings are particularly intense in the psychoanalytic situation. However, most cases of sexual intimacy do not occur with patients in psychoanalysis, but with patients in other forms of therapy where the transference is less intense and quite like that which occurs in other human situations. Under managed care, the prevailing practice in psychiatry is chemotherapy, where the role of transference, it is quipped, is about the same as that with a druggist in a supermarket.

All human relationships are tinged with transference. Nearly everything we do can be traced to earlier experiences. Every relationship is a mixture of a real relationship and transference phenomenon. Additionally, every relationship is asymmetrical, but in courtroom arguments transference becomes something mysterious and powerful. Dr. Martin Bauermeister says, "The suggestion that another human being by coming in clinical contact with us is incapacitated to make decisions about sexual relations is suspect of hubris and of a gross overestimation of our power over other people."[71]

From what I have seen or heard, the patients in the majority of litigated cases became sexually involved with the therapist in the hope of developing a long-term relationship. When the relationship failed to develop, joy turned to rage. The patient once again felt rejected. In these litigious times, such a patient retains a lawyer, for revenge as much as for compensation. It is the termination of the relationship, not the sexual relations, that causes the outrage.[72] In every reported case, the patient apparently sued only when the therapist terminated the relationship. In *Hartogs*,[73] Julie Roy turned to the legal process when, after making increasing demands for more time with Dr. Hartogs, he abruptly ended the relationship and refused to see her any longer. In *The Mourning Bride*, William Congreve wrote: "Heaven has no rage like love to hatred turned, nor hell a fury like a woman scorned."

In many cases, the patients have a history of drug abuse, delinquent behavior, broken homes, and sexual promiscuity. They are manipulative, often outwitting the therapist. In rape cases, the sexual history of the victim is generally inadmissible in assessing credibility.[74] Should the same policy be followed in undue familiarity cases? During the Middle Ages, exorcists knew about the danger of becoming possessed themselves after being closeted alone for long periods of time with demoniacally possessed young ladies who, as a sign of their bewitchment, often acted seductively. Evidence that the Devil also had taken possession of the priests was naturally based on their later developing sexual feelings toward these women while trying to rid them of their demons.[75]

In sexual misconduct cases before medical boards or at a trial, the defense typically claims that a psychiatric disorder led the complainant to make false accusations. Typically, evidence of the sexual histories of the complainant at a trial is inadmissible in assessing credibility.[76] At board hearings, however, where the rules of evidence do not apply, a New York study reports that physicians there are allowed to make reasonable connections between the complainant's psychiatric history and her discounted credibility. South Carolina reports experts testifying on the classification of patients as borderline personalities. Massachusetts reports the introduction of psychiatric evidence that patients were suffering from the types of mental instabilities that would cause them to lie about their experiences with their physicians.[77]

The assumption that women, whether or not in psychotherapy, are helpless victims in sexual relationships bespeaks of ignorance in worldly matters. One of the great themes of literature is the power that women have exercised over men who have fallen for them. In a cover story, *America's Decadent Puritans*, London's *Economist* wrote: "The decadence lies in too readily blaming others for problems, rather than accepting responsibility oneself."[78] Yet, Dr. Thomas Gutheil's suggestion that patients play an observable role in therapist–patient sexual relations brought forth a flurry of letters in protest.[79]

Might the patient be, ever so slightly, to blame? The doctrine of comparative negligence, adopted in most states, allows the court to apportion fault between plaintiff and defendant. Yet, it is rare that any fault is attributed to the patient. In the case of incest, where the participants are both adults, they are both culpable under the law. As previously mentioned, one jury in an undue familiarity case found the patient to be 15% at fault and reduced the award accordingly.[80]

It is observed that "a professional relationship is essentially a fiduciary one and that even women who engage willingly in sex with the fiduciary have the right to consider themselves victims,"[81] but such dictum applies, in practice, only in the case of psychotherapy. The theory of a "fiduciary duty" usually involves financial transactions (as in the relationship between a bank and client).[82] Sexual relations with a therapist, however, have been called *the ultimate betrayal*.[83]

In a theory of malpractice, the tort is negligence rather than a breach of a fiduciary duty, and the fault is placed entirely on the therapist. Steven Bisbing, a psychologist and lawyer who is with the program in psychiatry and law at Georgetown University Medical Center, states: "Both ethically and legally, patient–therapist sex is always the therapist's fault."[84] Dr. Larry Strasburger claims that "responsibility is always with the therapist. If the patient is a masochist and asks to be beaten, the therapist has a duty not to beat the patient."[85]

The theory in a malpractice action is that the psychotherapist, by virtue of his training, is supposed to be able to handle the transference. To accept this as an explanation, however, one must believe that the therapist is diabolically clever and manipulative while reducing the patient to a mere dupe. For one thing, transference usually has little or nothing to do with the behavior. Secondly, the law does not distinguish the transference in intense five-times-a-week psycho-analysis from once-a-month psychotherapy.[86] In many instances, the therapist is the innocent and vulnerable one, especially where the patients are young, attractive, sexy, and malicious. Resistance in therapy takes many forms. One of them is to seduce the therapist out of his pro-fessional distant and objective attachment. Often, both therapist and patient are emotionally deprived, and they short-circuit therapeutic work to gratify their immediate emotional needs. Various religions forbid a man and a woman who are not married to be alone together in a closed space—the risk of a sexual encounter is recognized, especially when the get-togethers are frequent.

Having already been held liable to his patient for damages for mental distress, Dr. Hartogs also lost his bid to have his insurer pay the award or repay him for the cost of his defense. A malpractice insurance contract does not cover intentional torts or acts that are not necessarily related to the rendering of professional services. The court ruled that because the psychiatrist's "therapy" was undertaken for his own personal satisfaction, his actions did not, as between the psychiatrist and his insurer, constitute malpractice within the meaning of the policy.[87] Hence, there was no coverage. The court further held that, in any event, public policy precluded the court from allowing the psychiatrist to recover such expenses. To allow recovery would be "to indemnify immorality and to pay the expenses of prurience."[88]

In later cases, however, a number of courts ruled that because sexual familiarity occurs with some frequency in the course of psychotherapy, it is a risk of the practice, not an intentional tort, but malpractice, and, therefore, comes within malpractice insurance coverage.[89] These courts have ruled that sexual activity is a departure from the standard of care, no different from an improper administration of medication and, therefore, covered by the malpractice insur-ance policy.[90] In a Michigan case, *Vigilant Insurance Co. v. Kambly*,[91] the court upheld coverage for sexual familiarity under the malpractice insurance policy on the rationale that the victim should not be penalized for the acts of the insured—the coverage is as much protection for the victim as it is for the doctor. The court stated, "Coverage does not allow the wrongdoer unjustly to benefit from his wrong. ... It is not the insured who will benefit, but the innocent victim who will be provided compensation for her injuries. ... In this instance, there is great public interest in protecting the interests of the insured party."[92]

In 1985, however, the APA excluded coverage for undue familiarity from its member mal-practice insurance program. The policy still provides cost of legal defense up to $100,000 when sexual involvement is denied. Most members of the APA Board of Trustees thought that drop-ping coverage for unethical sexual behavior would help deter its occurrence. A women's com-mittee took a strong stand, to no avail, in favor of retaining insurance coverage "to compensate victims for their distress."[93] The exclusion reads: "This insurance does not apply to injury due to or caused by any sexual activity by the insured. ... 'Sexual activity' is defined to include the physical touching of any person intended as sexual stimulation." Were the concern primarily about the great harm presumably sustained by patients, one should logically desire a source of compensation for them. Deterrence sounds fine, but other unethical or harmful conduct is not excluded from coverage.[94] To get around the undue familiarity exclusion, attorneys are alleging other theories as a cause of action (e.g., abandonment, breach of fiduciary duty).[95] Tort liability rules do (or should) appreciably depend on the principle of compensatory justice.[96]

In reality, deterrence was not the motive for excluding coverage. With cases multiplying like locusts, the main concerns involved the drain on the APA's liability insurance program and the image of the profession. The insurance program had gone through hard economic times and could not afford to compensate all of these claimants.[97] The program's London reinsurers were willing to continue providing full coverage for sexual misconduct cases only if premiums were raised to a level that would have made malpractice insurance unaffordable for the majority of APA members.[98] With all of the publicity, the reputation of the profession was at stake, including fears of an erosion of public trust in psychiatry. Even Ann Landers, a longtime champion of psychiatry, expressed second thoughts about the ethics of psychiatrists.[99]

Every profession has concern about its image. It is so important that, as Sir Francis Bacon once said: "Every man is a debtor to his profession." When Judge Brigieta Volopichova entered a topless glamour contest in Czechoslovakia, her colleagues were furious, demanding that she be removed from the bench. She brought the judicial profession into disrepute, but to justify a disciplinary hearing, the demand was said to be necessary to protect society: "Young men will be committing crime in the hope of being tried by her. … She may cause the crime rate to rise."[100]

Psychiatry as a profession is especially sensitive about its image. Over a century ago, Sigmund Freud cautioned his followers not to become romantically involved with their patients. Despite his warning, a number of them married former patients or conducted lengthy affairs with them. He warned about the peril to the profession, and he taught his followers that once sexual contact between therapist and patient begins, the therapeutic relationship is destroyed. He believed that no kind of erotic contact, not even an innocent kiss, should be initiated in the therapeutic relationship. Freud feared that sexual contact might confuse the patient and lead to the danger of further erotic intimacy.[101]

Sexual contact with a patient or client, whether or not there is actual harm, jeopardizes the professional relationship and tends to make it a waste of time. When sexual relations begin, therapy ends. In their book, *The Imperial Animal*,[102] anthropologists Lionel Tiger and Robin Fox point out that people are limited in the type of bond or pattern of relationship that is possible with another person. One kind of relationship seems to preclude another. Thus, the nurturing relationship cannot co-exist with a sexual relationship, hence, the incest taboo. When people in a professional relationship enter into a love or courtship relationship, they usually imperil the professional one. One type of relationship is replaced by another or none at all. It is quite another thing to say, however, that harm to the therapy relationship is always accompanied by great harm to the patient.

To be sure, the numerous publications about undue familiarity are not taken by lawyers with a pinch of low-sodium seasoning. They rely on them for litigation purposes, and for large awards. The use by psychotherapists of such terms as *incest, rape, permanent injury, suicidal ideation*, or the myriad diagnostic entities that have been applied to patients who have had sexual relations with their therapist have made them vulnerable to civil and criminal condemnation in the courts. Surely, there is an injunction in the Hippocratic Oath against seducing a patient, and another in the profession's code of ethics. For violations of such injunctions, let therapists suffer the sanctions of the appropriate medical and licensing authorities. However, the therapist alone should not be singled out for condemnation in a tort or criminal action. In so doing, the psychotherapist is denied the equal protection of the laws without reasonable justification.[103] Criminalization plays into the image of a psychiatrist as sex-mad, weirdo, or not like others. As a rule of law the psychotherapist is denied a defense of consent, whereas, for other fiduciaries, consent is a question of fact.

The repeal of laws on seduction and alienation of affections, practically speaking, does not apply to the psychotherapist. He is not home free. Under the rubric of malpractice, the psychotherapist is held liable on the theory because of misuse of transference. Jorgenson and Randles write: "The nature of the psychotherapist–patient relationship grants great power to the psychotherapist."[104] Presumably, through the relationship, the psychotherapist can exercise more magic than a magician. Moreover, on a theory of breach of fiduciary duty, the therapist is held liable, though transference is not involved, when he engages in a sexual relationship with a friend or spouse of the patient. In any event, the condemnation must mirror the offense, and compensation must reflect actual, rather than presumed, harm.

Victim groups want to criminalize the behavior of the therapist, as has been done in a number of states. But these groups fail to appreciate the impact of such criminalization. The trauma of a criminal or even civil process is rarely taken into account. Sanctions imposed by a medical or licensing authority, on the other hand, constructively punish the perpetrator without harming the victim. Rightly or wrongly, however, medical or licensing authorities are perceived as ineffective in disciplining their errant members. Others say that legislation criminalizing sexual contact between therapist and patient is needed in view of the many unlicensed therapists who are not accountable to any authority.[105]

In any event, prosecutions of therapists under the criminal statutes have not occurred and are unlikely. The statutes will not be used to put therapists behind bars, rather they will more likely be used by prosecutors to pressure therapists to resign or take leave from their profession. It will be an end run around a medical board proceeding. It will be less time consuming, but will it provide a fairer result? Furthermore, given that consent is no defense, entrapment by a police agent would also be unavailing as a defense.

Will an angry patient threaten to file a criminal complaint or a complaint with a medical board as a means of extortion? A complaint to a medical board of undue familiarity immediately results in the suspension of a license to practice until the matter is resolved. In 1939, when New York repealed its law on alienation of affections, seduction, and criminal conversation, it explained in the preamble that it was doing so because of the

> grave abuses, causing extreme annoyance, embarrassment, humiliation and pecuniary damage to many persons wholly innocent and free of any wrongdoing, who were merely the victims of circumstances, and such remedies having been exercised by unscrupulous persons for their unjust enrichment, and such remedies … in many cases having resulted in the perpetration of frauds, it is hereby declared as the public policy of the state that the best interests of the people of the state will be served by the abolition of such remedies.[106]

Today, the action for seduction or criminal conversation is viable against psychotherapists under the rubric of malpractice, or as sexual misconduct under the criminal statutes. Calling sexual relations with a therapist incest or rape is hyperbole. Either all love is incestuous and the meaning of incest becomes so broad that it is useless, or we have to draw a line between true incest of father–child and the therapeutic situation.

It is also recognized that a patient may bring an action against a therapist who becomes sexually involved with relatives or companions of that patient. In *Rowe v. Bennett*,[107] a therapist began dating the patient's sexual companion, having learned of the companion through the course of psychotherapy with the patient. In this situation, the cause of action is "negligent infliction of emotional or mental distress." While it is often required that an action for mental distress be accompanied by physical impact or an underlying tort (such as battery), here the court held that because of the nature of the psychotherapist–patient relationship, an action for mental distress may be maintained in their absence. The Maine Supreme Court stated:

> The rationale for requiring an independently actionable tort is that absence of either tactile contact or the usual indicia of harm, no objective evidence exists that the defendant's negligence actually has caused the plaintiff to suffer emotional distress. There is little likelihood, however, that objective evidence of mental distress will be unavailable in a claim by a patient against his psychotherapist. Given the fact that a therapist undertakes the treatment of a patient's mental problems and that the patient is encouraged to divulge his innermost thoughts, the patient is extremely vulnerable to mental harm if the therapist fails to adhere to the standards of care recognized by the profession. Any psychological harm that may result from such negligence is neither speculative nor easily feigned. Unlike evidence of mental distress occurring in other situations, objective proof of the existence *vel non* of a psychological injury in these circumstances should not be difficult to obtain. As this case illustrates, the severity of such an injury can be medically significant and objectively supportable. We, therefore, conclude that the reasons for precluding recovery for mental distress are not cogent here.[108]

Therapist involvement with a relative or companion of a patient may give rise not only to an action for infliction of emotional distress, but also to an action of malpractice. A relationship with a relative or companion of a patient—be it social and especially sexual—would have the strong probability of affecting the therapeutic relationship with the patient. In many cases, it has resulted in total disruption of the therapeutic relationship.[109] The Hippocratic Oath prohibits doctors from having relations with a patient or the patient's household.

Having a social or sexual relationship with a relative or companion of a patient has been depicted in a number of films, including *Prince of Tides*, *Final Analysis*, and *Whispers in the Dark*. In a Woody Allen film, a patient sees his therapist strolling with his (the patient's) girlfriend and is shocked.[110] Barbra Streisand in the film *Prince of Tides*, which she directed, portrayed a psychiatrist having a relationship with the patient's brother and was met with criticism in the press reflecting the views of a number of psychiatrists.[111] *The Principles of Medical Ethics With Annotations Especially Applicable to Psychiatry* do not specifically prohibit such behavior.

In *Mazza v. Huffaker*,[112] a malpractice action by a patient against a therapist who had a sexual relationship with the patient's spouse, the North Carolina Court of Appeals stated, "A psychiatrist who becomes sexually involved with a relative of a patient is not exercising the requisite amount of skill, learning, and ability that a psychiatrist in any community in the United States ought to exercise."[113] In this case, there was a novel argument about contributory negligence. The therapist claimed error in the trial court's refusal to instruct the jury on the issue of contributory negligence. The therapist contended that the patient failed to exercise ordinary care for his own safety in light of foreseeable danger and unreasonable risk. That contention was based on an argument that (1) prior to discovering his wife and psychiatrist in bed together, the patient suspected that the two were having an affair; (2) prior to his breaking down the door of the bedroom occupied by his wife and psychiatrist, the patient was aware of the possibility that the psychiatrist was in the house with the patient's spouse because the patient had seen the psychiatrist's clothing on the floor and the psychiatrist's automobile parked nearby; and (3) the patient was sufficiently informed about his psychological vulnerabilities to have reason to know he would be very distressed if he were to see his wife and his psychiatrist in bed together. Characterizing the psychiatrist's argument as imaginative, the North Carolina Court of Appeals declared that it could hardly perceive of a situation where an issue of contributory negligence would be less appropriate.[114]

What about the action of a nonpatient spouse against a therapist who has been involved sexually with a patient? In times gone by, there were tort actions called *criminal conversation*, which involved adultery and alienation of affections, which involved depriving one spouse of the affection of the other. Damages in these cases included the traditional award for loss of services and society, and also punitive damages. These actions were derisively called *heart balm*. Added to this was the recognition that each spouse was an autonomous human being, that neither was the property of the other, and that a home so easily broken was not worth maintaining. As a consequence, since the 1930s, these actions have generally been abolished.[115] In a case alleging alienation of affections, Chief Justice Charles O'Neill of the Louisiana Supreme Court quipped informally that the plaintiff had not lost anything, but rather, had merely learned something.[116]

In *Richard H. v. Larry D.*,[117] the California Court of Appeals addressed the question of whether the state's antiheart balm statute, which listed no exceptions, applied to therapy sessions. In this case, a husband and wife went to the psychiatrist (defendant) for marital counseling. After the defendant and wife began having an affair, the husband sued for breach of duty. The psychiatrist argued that the husband could not recover because of the antiheart balm statute, which prohibited the bringing a cause of action for (1) alienation of affections, (2) criminal conversation, or (3) seduction of a person over the age of legal consent. The court ruled in favor of the husband, stating: "We do not think the statute was intended to lower the standard of care that psychiatrists owe their patients, nor to permit them to avoid liability for breach of their professional fiduciary responsibilities, or commit fraud."

Thus, it is clear that when both spouses are patients of the therapist, as in *Richard H. v. Larry D.*, the therapist's seduction of one may constitute malpractice or intentional or reckless infliction of mental distress upon the other, in the light of the therapist's undertaking to care for both.[118] Then, to posit the question again. What about a lawsuit brought by a nonpatient spouse or companion? If these lawsuits may be brought, under what legal theory?

By and large, the courts tend to agree that to allow a third-party action by the nonpatient spouse under a theory of malpractice or infliction of mental distress would be to resurrect the actions of criminal conversation or alienation of affections. However, in an area of the law that has developed over the last half-century, a bystander may have a cause of action under the "bystander proximity" doctrine; i.e., the bystander is located near the scene of the wrongdoing (physical proximity), the bystander personally observes the wrongdoing (temporal proximity), and the bystander is closely related to the victim (relational proximity).[119]

The physical proximity of the bystander proximity requirement would rule out the possibility of a cause of action being brought by the bystander (the husband) against the therapist inasmuch as the undue familiarity would not occur in the presence of the husband. Thus, in *Homer v. Long*,[120] the Maryland Court of Appeals denied the plaintiff husband a cause of action against the therapist, as he was not a percipient witness to the sexual behavior. The husband asserted claims for negligence, fraud, negligent misrepresentation, and intentional infliction of mental distress, but to no avail. It was claimed that the therapist's involvement with his wife resulted in the breakup of the marriage. The court distinguished the decision a year earlier by the State Supreme Court where the husband was also a patient of the therapist.

In that case, *Figueiredo-Torres v. Nickel*,[121] the Maryland Supreme Court noted that the nature of the relationship between therapist and patient is unlike one in which the seducer was "'the milkman, the mailman, or the guy next door.' ... The gravamen of [the husband's] claim for intentional infliction of emotional distress is not merely the sexual act or the alienation of his wife's affection. It is the entire course of conduct engaged in by his therapist, with whom he enjoyed a special relationship."[122] The court quoted from an opinion in an Ohio case, *Strock v.*

Pressnell,[123] where a minister had an affair with a woman, while the woman and former husband were seeking marriage counseling.

In *Weisbeck v. Hess*,[124] the South Dakota Supreme Court held that a spouse may bring an action against a therapist who had an affair with his wife, but on the ground of confidentiality, it declined the spouse's request to obtain the names of the therapist's former female patients to bolster his claim that his marriage fell victim to the therapist's (alleged) usual ploy of taking advantage of vulnerable female patients. In this case, the husband had had a few counseling sessions with the therapist.

There is division of opinion in deciding who is and who is not a patient when therapists permit family members to join therapy sessions. In *Smith v. Pust*,[125] the California Court of Appeals noted that "it was clear from [the husband's] own deposition that he was not the therapist's patient." The husband was denied a cause of action on the ground that he was not a patient. He attended two therapy sessions in order to assist in the therapy of his wife. The therapist had sexual intercourse with the wife and the husband sued.

The threshold question in any negligence action is whether the defendant owed a legal duty to the plaintiff. As a general principle, the risk that may result from one's behavior, as reasonably perceived, determines the duty of care as well as to whom the duty is owed. It is an axiom that good medical care involves consideration not only of the patient, but also of others. The duty to others is expressed in legislation imposing various reporting obligations on physicians. However, in determining to whom a duty of care is owed, the courts are mindful of the extent of liability insurance coverage. The courts not only consider the foreseeability of harm, but also assess the competing public policy considerations for or against imposing a duty. One way or another, as the courts say, liability must be controlled by workable and just limits.[126] The issue of duty was highlighted in the most discussed of all torts cases, *Palsgraf v. Long Island R.R. Co.*[127] Judge Benjamin Cardozo, writing for the majority, ruled that negligence must be founded upon the foreseeability of harm to the person in fact injured. The plaintiff must "sue in her own right for a wrong personal to her, and not as the vicarious beneficiary of a breach of duty to another." The law on negligence does not include a concept of "transfer of negligence" (as in the case of transfer of intent in intentional torts).

Policy lines, which are to some extent arbitrary, are drawn to narrow the scope of duty and also actionable causation. These policy lines are confined to civil (tort) liability, and do not involve liability for criminal prosecution or disciplinary action involving the revocation or suspension of a license to practice. For those remedies, anyone (not just the aggrieved party) may file a complaint. In disciplinary actions by the medical board, as it has a duty to protect the public, the standard of proof is much lower than that required in litigation. In contrast, in a tort action, a higher standard of proof is required, and those who are deemed to have a cause of action are limited. In a tort action for malpractice, a number of states do not allow anyone but the patient to sue over negligent treatment, even when the malpractice causes physical injury to others, such as when an infectious disease is improperly treated and is passed on to family members. In Illinois, in a case of this sort, the defendant physician raised the specter of potentially unlimited liability to all those infected by his patient as well as all those whom they infected. The defendant also asserted that allowing the patient's immediate family to sue would constitute an artificial distinction between family members and all others whom his patient or they might infect. The majority of an intermediate appellate court agreed.[128] Justice Freedman, dissenting, would have extended the duty to the patient's immediate family. He said, "I cannot agree that limiting the right to sue ... to a patient's immediate family members, i.e., to those with whom he has special relationships, is an artificial and arbitrary distinction."[129] In this type of situation, other states have not limited a cause of action only to patients.[130]

Conclusion

A patient has a malpractice cause of action against a therapist for undue familiarity, and an action for infliction of mental distress in the event of sexual involvement with a member of the patient's family. The nonpatient spouse's cause of action is, however, very problematical on the ground that professional duties are ordinarily owed only to patients or clients. The nonpatient spouse tends to be regarded not as a "direct victim" but rather as a bystander, which calls into play the requirements of the proximity doctrine. However, the individual who sees the therapist, albeit briefly in consultation for the treatment of the spouse, may be categorized not as a bystander, but as a patient. It is putting form over substance. Should it make a difference whether the individual was seen by the therapist? To safeguard a cause of action in tort, the nonpatient spouse might consult with the therapist in order to be considered a patient.

Endnotes

1. There have been numerous complaints against psychotherapists for many kinds of boundary violations and sanctions against them after investigation. The fundamental ethical issues revolve around providing competent treatment without exploitation. Competent treatment can be provided best when the therapist maintains a clear professional relationship with the patient not influenced by intrusions that would weaken objectivity. Also, a patient enters treatment with the expectation that the therapist is obligated to do what is in the patient's best interest and not what is in the therapist's best interest.

   With the movement away from psychoanalysis to other forms of therapy, a distinction is made now between a boundary crossing and a boundary violation. A half-day course was given at the annual meeting of the American Psychiatric Association May 20, 2007, on "Using Boundary Crossings as Creative Therapy Instead of Slippery Slopes," that teaches "how to (1) recognize the difference between a boundary violation and a boundary crossing and (2) evaluate when the creative use of such actions as nonsexual touching, self-disclosure, and other boundary crossings may be beneficial to a patient." A decade ago Dr. Jeremy Lazarus of the APA Ethics Committee gave examples of common boundary violations that led to ethics complaints: (1) patient gives the therapist an expensive gift; (2) a patient takes the therapist out to lunch; (3) patient gives the therapist insider information about a stock deal; (4) a famous patient invites the therapist to a high social party; (5) a social relationship turns into a professional relationship and the social relationship continues; (6) a patient gives the therapist an expensive piece of medical equipment that will benefit the therapist's patients, but also will provide additional revenue for the therapist; (7) the therapist asks the patient for personal advice in an area in which he or she is an expert; (8) the therapist gives a patient a gift or reduced fee after the patient refers a friend; (9) the therapist solicits funding for the therapist's research project from a wealthy patient; (10) the therapist routinely hugs or holds the patient; (11) the therapist regularly reveals personal information about the therapist to a patient; (12) a grateful patient arranges groups of people to whom the therapist can talk about his innovative treatment; (13) the therapist writes the introduction for a book the patient is about to publish; (14) the patient wants to introduce her daughter to the therapist's son for the purpose of a social relationship; (15) the patient, a restaurant owner, offers the therapist a special, free meal at his restaurant; (16) the therapist attends important social functions of the patient; (17) the therapist meets a patient for treatment sessions outside of the usual place of practice without therapeutic justification; (18) the therapist is in a book discussion group with the patient; (19) the therapist asks his spouse to have the family auto serviced by the patient, an excellent auto mechanic; (20) the therapist consciously or unconsciously lives out his fantasies through his patients; (21) the therapist gives his patient a ride home. J. Lazarus, "More on Boundary Violations," *Psychiatric News*, Nov. 5, 1993, p. 4. See R.S. Epstein, *Keeping Boundaries* (Washington, DC: American Psychiatric Press, 1994); T.G. Gutheil & A. Brodsky, *Preventing Boundary Violations in Clinical Practice* (New York: Guilford Press, 2008); see also G.O. Gabbard, "Boundary Violations," in S. Bloch, P. Chodoff, & S.A. Green (Eds.) *Psychiatric ethics* (Oxford, U.K.: Oxford University Press, 3rd Ed., 1999), pp. 141–160. PRMS, manager of the APA-endorsed Psychiatrists' Professional Liability Insurance Program, advises that a surefire way to increase the risk of a malpractice suit or a board complaint is to allow a patient to pay for services by doing personal tasks, such as mowing the clinician's lawn, washing his or her car, painting the house, and babysitting. *Psychiatric News*, March 2, 2007, p. 32.

Marilyn Monroe became a member of the household of Dr. Ralph Greenson, her psychoanalyst—a totally antianalytic approach to therapy that was highly criticized by psychiatric colleagues when it became known years later. Eleven years after her suicide, Dr. Greenson defended his unorthodox therapeutic procedure in the *Medical Tribune* (Oct. 24, 1973), saying, "It was controversial, I know that. Nevertheless, I have practiced for some 35 years, and I did what I thought best, particularly after other methods of treatment apparently hadn't touched her one iota." But, by making her a quasi-member of his household, he transgressed one of the rules of analysis stated in his own textbook, *The Technique and Practice of Psychoanalysis* (New York: International Universities Press, 1967). In the book, *The Last Days of Marilyn Monroe* (New York: William Morrow, 1998, pp. 383–384), the author Donald H. Wolfe suggest that Dr. Greenson was faced with the dilemma of justifying himself before colleagues, while at the same time not revealing the depth of his knowledge concerning the circumstances of Marilyn Monroe's death, for in doing so he would have to reveal his identity as an agent of the Communist International Party.

The unorthodox approach by Michigan psychiatrist Reuven Bar-Levav led to his death at the hands of one of his patients (who also wounded or killed other patients in group therapy). He violated every boundary rule that therapists are supposed to practice. He took groups of patients on trips, he had lunch or dinner with them, and he also had sex with at least one patient and was accused of assaulting her. His style was often confrontational. He entered the lives of his patients. A number of psychiatrists in the community wrote to him over the years, urging him to practice psychotherapy according to well-developed and well-established rules. Granted, following the rules does not ensure a cure, but it prevents many therapists from going off the deep end. He was completely impervious to criticism and reason. He was his own authority and, therefore, learned nothing from others. He was a clever psychopath (in the view of many psychiatrists) who probably did some good, which has largely been exaggerated by former patients, as their well being depends on their maintaining a positive transference. They do not know or do not care to know that transference is a distortion. D. Zeman, "Therapy's Deadly Dividing Line," *Detroit Free Press*, Sept. 30, 1999, p. 1. See M.T. Singer & J. Lalich, *'Crazy' Therapies* (San Francisco: Jossey-Bass, 1996).

2. See K. Pope, "Research and Laws Regarding Therapist–Patient Sexual Involvement: Implications for Therapists," *Am. J. Psychother.* 49 (1986): 564. Psychoanalyst Richard Chessick says, "It is well known that sexual activity between a patient and a therapist represents a crossing of the incest barrier." "Malignant Eroticized Countertransference," *Am. Acad. Psychoanaly.* 25 (1997): 219; reprinted in R. Chessick, *Psychoanalytic Clinical Practice: Selected Papers* (London: Free Association Book, 2000).

3. See D. Goleman, "New Focus on Presenting Patient-Therapist Sex," *New York Times*, Dec. 20, 1990, p. B21.

4. Simmons v. United States, 805 F. 2d 1363, 1365 (9th Cir. 1986).

5. W. Masters & V. Johnson, "Principles of the New Sex Therapy," *Am. J. Psychiatry* 133 (1976): 548. See also G.C. Hankins, M.I. Vera, G.W. Barnard, & M.J. Herkov, "Patient-Therapist Sexual Involvement: A Review of Clinical and Research Data," *Bull. Am. Acad. Psychiat. & Law* 22 (1994): 113.

6. See S. Baur, *The Intimate Hour* (New York: Houghton Mifflin, 1997); R.S. Epstein, *Keeping Boundaries* (Washington, DC: American Psychiatric Press, 1994); J.C. Gonsiork (Ed.), *Breach of Trust/Sexual Exploitation by Health Care Professionals and Clergy* (Thousand Oaks, CA: Sage, 1995); H.S. Strean, *Therapists Who Have Sex With Their Patients/Treatment and Recovery* (New York: Brunner/Mazel, 1993); P. Trumpi, *Doctors Who Rape/Malpractice and Misogny* (Rochester, VT: Schenkman, 1997). For a bibliography, see H. Lerman, *Sexual Intimacies Between Psychotherapists and Patients, an Annotated Bibliography of Mental Health, Legal and Public Media Literature Including Relevant Legal Cases* (Fullerton, CA: Dept. of Counseling, California State University, 1984).

7. J. Bolker, "Disturbances in the Field," *Readings/A Journal of Reviews and Commentary in Mental Health*, 5 (1990): 8. At the time of the 1985 annual meeting of the APA, an extensive three-part series embarrassing to the profession appeared in the *Dallas Times-Herald*. S. Smith & B. Laker, "Sex & Therapists," *Dallas Times-Herald*, May 20-22, 1985.

8. L. Morin, "Civil Remedies for Therapist–Patient Sexual Exploitation," *Golden Gate U. L. Rev.* 19 (1989): 401, 432.

9. T. Lambert, "Tom on Torts," *Assn. of Trial Law. of Am. L. Rep.* 25 (1982): 98, 99. A full-page drawing depicting the therapist as a wolf accompanies the article by J. Epstein, "The Exploitative Psychotherapist as a Defendant," *Trial*, July 1989, p. 52. See also M. Beck, "Sex and Psychotherapy," *Newsweek*, April 13, 1992, p. 52; E. Goode, "The Ultimate Betrayal," *U. S. News & World Report*, March 12, 1990, p. 63.

10. K. Pope, "Therapist–Patient Sex Syndrome—A Guide for Attorneys and Subsequent Therapists to Assessing Damage," in G.O. Gabbard (Ed.), *Sexual Exploitation in Professional Relationships* (Washington, DC: American Psychiatric Press, 1989), pp. 39–55. One study reports a wide range of uncomfortable and sometimes life-threatening feelings or symptoms experienced by "survivors of sexual exploitation" by medical and mental health professionals and clergy, but, without explanation, notes a few exceptions (e.g., a lesbian who did not feel damaged by her first—and apparently only—sexual relationship with a man). Its data showed that the clients abused in medical contexts experienced the greatest harm, whatever the brevity of the relationship. E. Disch & N. Avery, "Sex in the Consulting Room, the Examining Room, and the Sacristy: Survivors of Sexual Abuse by Professional," *Am. J. Orthopsychiat.* 71 (2001): 204.

11. S. Smith, "The Seduction of the Female Patient," and S.W. Twemlow & G.O. Gabbard, "The Love-Sick Therapist," in G.O. Gabbard (Ed.) *Sexual Exploitation in Professional Relationships* (Washington, DC: American Psychiatric Press, 1989), pp. 57–87; K. Pope & J. Bouhoutsos, *Sexual Intimacy Between Therapists and Patients* (New York: Praeger, 1986).

12. N. Gartrell et al., "Sexual Abuse of Patients by Therapists: Strategies for Offender Management and Rehabilitation," in R. D. Miller (Ed.), *Legal Implications of Hospital Policies and Practices* (San Francisco: Jossey-Bass, 1989); N. Gartrell et al., "Management and Rehabilitation of Sexuality Exploitive Therapists," *Hosp. & Comm. Psychiat.* 39 (1988): 1070.

13. See L.H. Strasburger, "There Oughta Be a Law: Criminalization of Psychotherapist–Patient Sex as a Social Policy Dilemma," in J.D. Bloom, C.C. Nadelson, & M.T. Notman (Eds.), *Physician Sexual Misconduct* (Washington, DC: American Psychiatric Press, 1999), pp. 13–36; L. Jorgenson et al., "The Furor Over Psychotherapist–Patient Sexual Contact: New Solutions to an Old Problem," *Wm. & Mary L. Rev.* 32 (1991): 645; S. Diesenhouse, "Therapists Start to Address Damage Done by Therapists," *New York Times*, Aug. 20, 1989, p. E5.

14. L. Strasburger, L. Jorgenson, & R. Randles, "Mandatory Reporting of Sexually Exploitative Psychotherapists," *Bull. Am. Acad. Psychiat. & Law* 18 (1990): 379. Of 1,423 psychiatrists responding to a national survey, 65% reported treating patients who had been sexually involved with previous therapists, but they reported it in only 8% of cases. The majority favored mandatory reporting of such incidents. N. Gartrell et al., "Reporting Practices of Psychiatrists Who Knew of Sexual Misconduct by Colleagues," *Am. J. Orthopsychiat.* 57 (1987): 287.

15. Colo. Rev. Stat. § 18-3-401(4) (1986).

16. People v. West, 724 P. 2d 623, at 625 (Colo. 1986).

17. State v. Tibbets, 281 N. W. 2d 499 (Minn. 1979); State v. Bicknese, 285 N. W. 2d 684 (Minn. 1979).

18. Minn. Stat. Ann. § 609.341 (11) (IV) (West Supp. 1992), discussed in Jorgenson et al., *supra* note 13.

19. Fla. Stat. Ann. § 491.0112 (West 1991); Me. Rev. Stat. Ann. Tit. 17A, §§ 251(1)(C), 253(2)(1)(West Supp. 1991).

20. Cal. Civ. Code § 43.93(b)(West Supp. 1992); Ill. Ann. Stat. Ch. 70, par. 802 (Smith-Hurd 1989); Minn. Stat. Ann. § 148A.02 (West 1989); Wis. Stat. Ann. § 895.70(2)(West Supp. 1991).

21. Sigmund Freud said of the transference experiences of the patient on the couch: "What are transferences? They are new editions or facsimiles of the impulses and phantasies ... aroused ... during the progress of the analysis ... they replace some earlier person by the person of the physician ... a whole series of psychological experiences are revived, not as belonging to the past, but as applying to the person of the physician at the present moment." S. Freud, "Fragment of an Analysis of a Case of Hysteria" (1905), *Standard Edition* (London: Hogarth, 1953), p. 16. Over the years, Freud enlarged this aspect of transference to make it central to the analytic situation as a process of the patient's living out his infantile relationships via the transference neurosis. S. Freud, "Remembering, Repeating and Working-Through" (1914), *Standard Edition*.

22. Bahry v. Laucher, Washtenaw County, Michigan, No. 89-5191-NM (1990).

23. While a single profile of a victim of sexual misconduct may be impossible, some of the commonalities that the literature and clinical experience have demonstrated to be found repeatedly in this population include dynamics of vulnerability, aspects of borderline personality disorder, previous sexual abuse, and various bonding mechanisms. T. Gutheil, "Patients Involved in Sexual Misconduct With Therapists: Is a Victim Profile Possible?" *Psychiat. Ann.*, Nov. 1991, p. 661.

24. Omer v. Edgren, 38 Wash. App. 376, 685 P. 2d 635 (1984).

25. 685 P. 2d at 638, citing Wenzler & Ward Plumbing & Heating Co. v. Sellen, 330 P. 2d 1068, 1069 (Wash. 1958), and quoting Bigelo v. RKO Radio Pictures, Inc., 327 U. S. 251 (1946). See also Corgan v. Muehling, 167 Ill. App. 3d 1093, 118 Ill. Dec. 698, 522 N. E. 2d 153 (1988).

26. In Carmichael v. Carmichael, 597 A. 2d 1326, 1329 (D.C. App. 1991) (quoting Washington v. Washington Hosp. Ctr., 579 A. 2d 177, 181 (D. C. App. (1990)), the District of Columbia Court of Appeals held that the patient failed to present sufficient evidence that any malpractice had caused her harm, noting that she did not present expert testimony showing "a causal relationship between [the malpractice] and [her] injury." The court found that the expert testimony that her symptoms were of the sort commonly associated with transference abuse was "simply insufficient." 597 A.2d at 1330. The court pointed out that this witness was never asked if in his opinion the patient's injuries were caused to a reasonable medical certainty by the therapist's malpractice, *Ibid.* Furthermore, the testimony that the patient's symptoms were consistent with malpractice was held to be "not enough." On this basis, the judgment on the malpractice claim was reversed. *Ibid.* at 1330–1331. In Iwanski v. Gomes, 611 N.W. 2d 607 (Neb. 2000), the court found that the complainant had not supported her claim, beyond her assertion, that transference had played a role in her sexual involvement with her physician. Other cases requiring that expert testimony on proximate cause in cases of alleged sexual misconduct by a psychiatrist include Singh v. Lyday, 889 N. E. 2d 342 (Ind. App. 2008); Hare v. Wendler, 949 P.2d 1141 (Kan. 1997); Carmichael v. Carmichael, 597 A.2d 1326 (D.C. App. 1991).
27. R. Yahav & S. Oz, "The Relevance of Psychodynamic Psychotherapy to Understanding Therapist–Patient Sexual Abuse and Treatment of Survivors," *J. Am. Acad. Psychoanaly. & Dynam. Psychiat.* 34 (2006): 303.
28. Corgan v. Muehling, 143 Ill. 2d 296, 574 N. E. 2d 602 at 611–612 (1991). In this case, the treatment began in March 1979 and continued until October 1980, and during this period of time, the plaintiff and the defendant repeatedly engaged in "mutually agreeable sexual intercourse. The plaintiff now claims that this sexual relationship disturbed her psychological well being, and she would like the defendant to pay her damages of $3.75 million"; 574 N. E. 2d at 611.
29. This was claimed by the defense in the 1989 malpractice case brought by a Denver woman, Ms. Roberts-Henry, against her former psychiatrist, Dr. Jason Richter, the subject of a 90-minute *Frontline* documentary on PBS. The documentary was reviewed in W. Goodman, "When a Psychiatrist Becomes a Lover," *New York Times*, Nov. 12, 1991, p. C18. Dr. Richter, immediately after terminating psychotherapy, began a sexual affair with the patient. A subsequent psychiatrist, Dr. Martha Gay, helped the patient to complain, and was attacked by Dr. Richter's defense attorneys. Drs. Gay and Richter were both insured by the APA's insurance company, but Dr. Gay complained that Dr. Richter's attorneys were too aggressive, risking harming her and her patient, and that the case manager's handling of herself, Dr. Richter, and their lawyers contained a conflict of interest. The jury found Dr. Richter 82% responsible for the patient's injuries. L. Hartman, "Doctor-Patient Sex and Frontline," *Psychiatric News*, Dec. 6, 1991, p. 1; "APA Responds to Ethical Issues in 'Frontline' Telecast," *Psychiatric News*, Dec. 6, 1991, p. 1.
30. 436 S. W. 2d 753 (Mo. 1968).
31. 366 N. Y. S. 2d 297 (N. Y. Civ. Ct. 1975), *reversed*, 381 N. Y. S. 2d 587 (N. Y. App. Term. 1976).
32. 436 S. W. 2d at 761.
33. 436 S. W. 2d at 759–760.
34. Smith v. Pust, 23 Cal. Rptr. 2d 364 (Cal. App. 1993).
35. (New York: Stein & Day, 1976).
36. 366 N. Y. S. 2d at 299.
37. 366 N. Y. S. 2d at 299.
38. 366 N. Y. S. 2d at 299.
39. 381 N. Y. S. 2d at 589.
40. 381 N. Y. S. 2d at 389.
41. 381 N. Y. S. 2d at 591.
42. *Ibid.* at 592. In Cotton v. Kambly, 300 N. W. 2d 627 (Mich. App. 1980), the plaintiff filed suit claiming that the defendant induced her to engage in sexual intercourse with him as part of her therapy. The defendant argued that the plaintiff's allegations were akin to claims for alienation of affection, criminal conversation, or seduction. Because these causes of action had been abolished by statute, the defendant contended that the plaintiff failed to state an actionable claim. The court disagreed, however, and held that plaintiff had sufficiently pleaded a claim for malpractice. The court reasoned that the essence of her claim was the doctor's departure from proper standards of medical practice. Thus, "while the facts alleged by plaintiff might also state a cause of action for common law seduction, we do not find that seduction was the gist of her malpractice claim." *Ibid.* at 628–29.

43. Seven states still allow lawsuits by people who claim someone stole their wives or husbands: Hawaii, Illinois, Mississippi, New Mexico, North Carolina, South Dakota, and Utah. In a recent Mississippi case, a plumber and a millionaire squared off over a woman. Sandra Fitch, the woman in the case, was married to Johnny Valentine, a plumber, when she was hired by a real estate company owned by Jerry Fitch. Within a year, she and Fitch began an affair. She became pregnant by Fitch, but she told Valentine his suspicions about adultery were unfounded. Soon, though, Valentine had genetic tests done showing he was not the baby's father. He sued for divorce and then he sued Fitch, who was worth $22 million. Fitch initially denied that he was the father of the baby, that he was involved with his employee, or that he was giving her extra money, but he eventually acknowledged his role. A jury awarded Valentine more than $750,000, including $112,000 in punitive damages. M. Sherman (AP news release), "Supreme Court Urged to Limit Damages in Lawsuit Over 'Alienation of Affection,'" *Detroit Legal News*, Oct. 30, 2007, p. 3.

44. R. Simon, *Clinical Psychiatry and the Law* (Washington, DC: American Psychiatric Press, 2nd. ed., 1991), pp. 411–413.

45. Walker v. Parzen, Cal. Super. Ct. July 7, 1981, referenced in *Am. L. Rep.* 24 (1981): 295.

46. Combs v. Silverman, No. LE596 (Va. Cir. Ct., Feb. 5, 1982).

47. J. Talbot, "The Professional Liability Crisis—An Interview With Joel Klein," *Hosp. & Commun. Psychiat.* 37 (1986): 1012.

48. Greenberg v. McCabe, 453 F. Supp. 765 (E. D. Pa. 1978).

49. 453 F. Supp. at 773.

50. 453 F. Supp. at 770.

51. 453 F. Supp. at 771.

52. See, e.g., Nelson v. Gillette, 571 N. W. 2d 332 (N. D. 1997).

53. See, e.g., L.L. v. Medical Protective Co., 362 N. W. 2d 174 (Wis. Ct. App. 1984).

54. R. Goldstein, "Pseudo-Rape Trauma Syndrome," *Am. Acad. Psychiat. & Law Newsl.*, 15 (Sept. 1990): 58–59.

55. G.V. Laury, "When Women Sexually Abuse Psychiatric Patients Under Their Care," *J. Sex Educ. & Ther.* 18 (1992): 111. In Department of Community Health v. Risch, 274 Mich. App. 365, 733 N.W.2d 403 (2007), the respondent's registration to practice as a certified social worker and limited license psychologist were revoked, based on allegations that she engaged in a sexual relationship with a patient, and altered records to hide the fact that the individual was a patient. After reviewing the record, the Michigan Court of Appeals determined that there was sufficient evidence to support the findings that (1) the individual was respondent's patient, and (2) respondent altered records to hide the fact. Therefore, the revocation was affirmed. The Court of Appeals noted that judicial review of administrative orders is whether the order is "authorized by law" and "supported by competent, material, and substantial evidence on the whole record." The necessary evidentiary support is that which "a reasonable person would accept as sufficient to support a conclusion." Findings based on the credibility of the witnesses will generally not be disturbed. Finally, if the evidence supports a finding, a court may not set that finding aside "merely because alternative findings could also have been supported by evidence."

56. Communication from psychiatrist Theodore Pearlman (Oct. 30, 1990). The healing power of touch has a long history. The Scriptures tell of healing by the laying on of hands. In popular custom, parents kiss away a child's "boo-boo." Touching is regarded as alternative medicine. See B.A. Brennan, *Hand of Light: A Guide to Healing Through the Human Energy Field* (New York: Bantam Doubleday, 1988).

57. E. Benedek, Editorial, *Psychiatric News*, Aug. 17, 1990, p. 3. When the patient is referred, will the patient be told the reason for the referral? How will the patient feel? Rejected? In certain cases, consultation with another therapist would be appropriate.

58. C.C. Kleinman, "Crossing the Border: Sexual Relationships Between Therapist and Patients," address at the Carrier Foundation Medical Foundation Education Symposium, Nov. 13, 1991.

59. P. Appelbaum & L. Jorgenson, "Psychotherapist–Patient Sexual Contact After Termination of Treatment: An Analysis and a Proposal," *Am. J. Psychiat.* 148 (1991): 1466. Iowa's statute covers sexual activity with a patient occurring within one year of the termination of therapy; Iowa Code § 709.15 (Supp. 1992). Some laws cover instances in which it can be proven that therapy was "terminated primarily for the purpose of engaging in sexual contact." "Patient–Therapist Sex, Civil Commitment Getting State's Legislative Attention," *Psychiatric News*, Dec. 20, 1991, p. 4.

60. American Psychiatric Association, *Principles of Medical Ethics With Annotations Especially Applicable to Psychiatry* (1989). See R. J. Maurer, "Ohio Psychotherapist Civil Liability for Sexual Relations With Former Patients," *U. Toledo L. Rev.* 26 (1995): 547.

61. R.T. Barnhouse (ltr.), "Sex With Former Patients," *Clinical Psychiatry News*, Oct. 1992, p. 4.

62. Cal. Bus. & Prof. Code § 43.93 (West Supp. 1992); Minn. Stat. Ann. § 148A (West 1989).

63. L. Jorgenson & R. Randles, "Time Out: The Statute of Limitations and Fiduciary Theory in Psychotherapist Sexual Misconduct Cases," *Okla. L. Rev.* 44 (1991): 181. See also D. DeRose, "Adult Incest Survivors and the Statute of Limitations: The Delayed Discovery Rule and Long Term Damages," *Santa Clara L. Rev.* 25 (1985): 191; S. Torry, "Divorce-Malpractice Suit Won by Heiress," *Washington Post*, Oct. 22, 1989, p. B1; C. Allen, "Power to Make Therapists Jittery," *Insight*, Dec. 4, 1989, p. 49.

64. J. Bouhoutsos et al., "Sexual Intimacy Between Psychotherapists and Patients," *Prof. Psychol. Res. & Prac.* 14 (1983): 185.

65. P. Rutter, *Sex in the Forbidden Zone: When Men in Power—Therapists, Doctors, Clergy, Teachers, and Others—Betray Women's Trust* (New York: St. Martin's Press, 1989).

66. 805 F. 3d 1363 (9th Cir. 1986).

67. 805 F. 3d at 1366.

68. By way of illustration: In Odegard v. Finne, 500 N.W.2d (Minn. App. 1993), a sexual relationship developed after Dr. Charles Finne performed 11 surgeries to alleviate the symptoms of Jane Odegard's ulcerative colitis. The doctor proposed that the two divorce their respective spouses and marry each other, but when he decided to return to his wife and child, she sued for medical malpractice. The Minnesota Court of Appeals declined to accept her claim that the doctor had negligently mishandled the transference phenomenon and instead held that "transference is not a recognized component in the medical treatment of physical conditions." The court further said that nonmedical health physician liability would be restricted to situations in which the sexual relationship was commenced "under the guise of treatment." As to the plaintiff's claims, the court found that the relationship was consensual and that her complaint was simply that "she had an unhappy affair with a man who happened to be her doctor … [and] is plainly insufficient to make out a cause of action for professional negligence." The court also held that the plaintiff failed to establish a claim for intentional infliction of emotional distress.

    In Newland v. Azan, 957 S.W.2d 377 (Mo. 1997), Dr. Nohaud Azan performed root canal treatments on Brenda Newland and while she was sitting in the dental chair after receiving several pain-killer shots, the dentist "touched her pubic area, kissed her, caressed her cheek and hand, rubbed his own genital area, and made several suggestive remarks." Following her treatment, she filed a medical malpractice suit and also alleged battery and intentional infliction of emotional distress. The Missouri Court of Appeals affirmed the trial court's summary judgment ruling for the dentist on the medical malpractice claims concluding that "it must be a dental act or service that caused the harm, not an act or service that requires no professional skill." The court also found that there was no evidence that linked the sexual touching to any "course of dental treatment," nor to the existence of a psychologist–patient relationship. The court noted, if a dentist shoots his patient or ties the patient to a chair in the dentist's office, that would not fall within the realm of malpractice.

69. Personal communications.

70. *The Principles of Medical Ethics With Annotations Especially Applicable to Psychiatry*, American Psychiatric Association, 1993, Sec. 2, Annot. 1.

71. "Consent for Sex?" *Psychiatric News*, May 5, 1989, p. 44. A century ago it was considered that even extended eye contact with any predatory male would be sufficient to lead a woman astray. As a consequence, it was suggested that women should neither travel alone nor stare at strangers. In one prosecution, the prosecuting attorney asked the expert witness: "Do you advise nervous women never to travel alone since a man, simply through mental suggestion. …" The expert replied: "Simply through mental suggestion … no, but from a steady gaze, yes." R. Harris, *Murders and Madness* (New York: Oxford University Press, 1989), p. 189.

72. Psychotherapist Carl Goldberg says that the wrong is a breach of a "psychological contract." *Therapeutic Partnership/Ethical Concerns in Psychotherapy* (New York: Springer, 1977). In one case known to me, a psychiatrist upon the death of his wife notified all of his patients that he would not be seeing them for a month. One patient, a middle-aged woman who was seen in therapy triweekly, responded, "I see that you are in grief. Come and stay with me." He declined, but a few days later, she called urging him to come and stay with her. He agreed, while informing her that in doing so she would no longer be his patient. After several moths of staying with her, he moved out. She was incensed, apparently expecting marriage or a long-term relationship. She filed a complaint. He lost his license and membership in the American Psychiatric Association, and she got $110,000. To be sure, he might have sought counseling to help deal with his grief, but was justice done?

73. 366 N. Y. S. 2d 297 (N. Y. Civ. Ct. 1975), *reversed*, 381 N. Y. S. 2d 587 (N. Y. App. Term 1976).

74. Federal Rules of Evidence, Rule 412.

75. See A. Huxley, *The Devils of Loudun* (London: Chatto & Windus, 1952); see also A.M. Ludwig, *How Do We Know Who We Are?* (New York: Oxford University Press, 1997).

76. Department of Professional Regulation v. Wise, 575 So. 2d 713 (Fla. Ct. App. 1991); C. Gentry, "Court Veils Sexual History," *St. Petersburg Times*, Feb. 16, 1991, p. B12.

77. A.L. Hyams, "Expert Psychiatric Evidence in Sexual Misconduct Cases Before State Medical Boards," *Am. J. Law & Med.* 18 (1992): 171.

78. "American's Decadent Puritans," *Economist*, July 28, 1990: 11.

79. T. Gutheil, "Borderline Personality Disorder, Boundary Violations, and Patient-Therapist Sex: Medicolegal Pitfalls," *Am. J. Psychiat.* 146 (1989): 1356, 1518–19; 147 (1990): 129–130, 963, 1258–59, 1391.

80. Kulick v. Gates, No. 41624 (Mass. Super. Ct. May 21, 1985), referenced in *Am. L. Rep.* 28 (1985): 471. See Chapter 32 on contributory negligence.

81. Kulick v. Gates.

82. See Treadt v. Lutheran Church, 237 Mich. App. 567, 603 N. W. 2d 816 (1999).

83. E. Goode, "The Ultimate Betrayal," *U. S. News & World Report*, March 12, 1990, p. 63.

84. D. Goleman, *supra* note 3, at p. 87.

85. Comment at meeting of the American Academy of Psychiatry and Law in Orlando, Florida (Oct. 18, 1991).

86. C. Clements, "The Transference: What's Love Got to Do With It," *Psychiat. Ann.* 17 (1997): 556.

87. Hartogs v. Employers' Mut. Liab. Ins. Co., 391 N. Y. S. 2d 962 (N. Y. Spec. Term 1977).

88. 391 N. Y. S. 2d. at 965. The courts generally hold that a medical malpractice insurance policy does not cover a therapist's sexual contact with a patient. See, e.g., Smith v. St. Paul Fire & Marine Ins. Co., 353 N. W. 2d 130, 132 (Minn. 1984); Standlee v. St. Paul Fire & Marine Ins. Co., 693 P. 2d 1101 (Idaho App. 1984); Hirst v. St. Paul Fire & Marine Ins. Co., 683 P. 2d 440 (Idaho App. 1984). See S. Gunnells, "Patient–Therapist Sexual Relations: Professional Services Rendered? A Case Comment on *Doe v. Swift*," *Law & Psychol. Rev.* 14 (1990): 87.

89. St. Paul Fire & Marine Ins. Co. v. Mitchell, 164 Ga. App. 215, 296 S.E.2d 126 (1982). In two subsequent cases decided on the same day, the Minnesota Supreme Court ruled that a malpractice insurance carrier may be held liable for a therapist's sexual involvement with a patient. In St. Paul Fire & Marine Ins. Co. v. Love, 459 N. W. 2d 698 (Minn. 1990), the Minnesota Supreme Court stated (859 N.W. 2d at 701):

    In determining whether the patient's claim results from professional services provided or which should have been provided, we believe the focus must be on the therapist's entire conduct. The question then becomes whether the sexual aspect of the conduct is inextricably related to the professional services provided or withheld. If the linkage is absent or slight, the patient's claim cannot be said to result from professional services provided or withheld.

    The court concluded: 459 N. W. 2d at 701.

    When ... the transference phenomenon pervades the therapeutic alliance, we believe the sexual conduct between therapist and patient arising from the phenomenon may be viewed as the consequence of a failure to provide proper treatment of the transference. In other words, the patient's claim results from the providing of improper professional services or the withholding of proper services.

    In the other case, St. Paul Fire & Marine Ins. Co. v. D. H. L., 459 N. W. 2d 704 (Minn. 1990), a marriage and family therapist, while counseling a patient for sexual addiction and marital problems, had a sexual relationship with the patient. As in the *Love* case, St. Paul refused to defend the therapist in a suit brought by the patient, arguing the policy was limited to "claims that result from professional services that you provided or should have provided." 459 N. W. 2d at 705.

    Agreeing with St. Paul, the trial court found no coverage. The Minnesota Supreme Court remanded to determine whether transference was involved in the sexual conduct. If transference was involved, there would be coverage. How will the court divine whether the sexual behavior was the result of transference? The Minnesota Supreme Court decided that it would resort to expert testimony to resolve the issue; 459 N. W. 2d at 706. However, what expert can sufficiently distinguish between transference and reality.

90. Cotton v. Kambly, 300 N. W. 2d 627 (Mich. App. 1980).

91. 319 N. W. 2d 382 (Mich. App. 1982).

92. 319 N. W. 2d at 385 (citation omitted).

93. "APA Moves to Discourage Sexual Misconduct in Therapy," *Psychiatric News*, Jan. 4, 1985, p. 17.

94. B. Northrup, "Treating the Mind & Psychotherapy Faces a Stubborn Problem: Abuses by Therapists," *Wall Street Journal*, Oct. 29, 1986: A1.

95. See A.A. Stone & D.C. MacCourt, "Insurance Coverage for Undue Familiarity: Law, Policy, and Economic Reality," in J.D. Bloom, C.C. Nadelson, & M.T. Notman (Eds.), *Physician Sexual Misconduct* (Washington, DC: American Psychiatric Association, 1999), pp. 37–88; L. Jorgenson, S.B. Bisbing, & P.K. Sutherland, "Therapist–Patient Sexual Exploitation and Insurance Liability," *Tort & Ins. L. J.* 27 (1992): 595; R. Slovenko, "Liability Insurance Coverage in Cases of Psychotherapy Sexual Abuse," *J. Psychiat. & Law* 21 (1993): 277.

There is division of opinion whether a clinic where the therapist is on the staff may be held liable for the therapist's sexual abuse of a patient. One of two broad approaches is used: direct and vicarious. Under direct liability, the clinic is held responsible for its own negligence in hiring, retaining, or supervising the therapist. Under vicarious liability, otherwise known as *respondeat superior*, it is not necessary to prove fault on the part of the clinic. Vicarious liability may be imputed to the clinic even though the therapist is not acting in the course of his employment. In Andrews v. United States, 732 F.2d 366 (4th Cir. 1984), the court held that the employer was not liable for the acts of a physician's assistant who "seduced" a patient because the physician's assistant was not furthering the employer's business by seducing the patient. In Marston v. Minneapolis Clinic, 329 N.W.2d 306 (Minn. 1982), the court, applying a "but for" test, held the clinic liable for its employee's sexual misconduct. The court ruled that the jury could weigh the facts and determine that the sexual contact would not have occurred but for the psychologist's employment with the clinic. In the conclusion of a vigorous and lengthy dissent in Doe v. Samaritan Counseling Center, 791 P.2d 344 (Alaska 1990), which held a clinic responsible for the sexual abuse of a patient by a therapist, Justice Moore wrote:

> The motivation for the court's holding is not difficult to find. Therapist–patient sex is a serious problem in the psychotherapeutic community. However, imposing vicarious liability on mental health employers for the sexual misconduct of their employees is not an appropriate response to the problem. … [I]mposing vicarious liability would create incentives to invade the privacy of the therapist–patient relationship that is essential to the psychotherapeutic enterprise. … [P]erhaps most important, spreading the cost of therapist–patient sex to the consumers of mental health services is unfair.

96. G. Schwartz, "The Ethics and the Economics of Tort Liability Insurance," *Cornell L. Rev.* 75 (1990): 313.
97. A.A. Stone, "No Good Deed Goes Unpunished: The Case of Martha Gay, M.D.," *Psychiatric Times*, March 1990, p. 24; see also S. Diesenhouse, "Therapists Start to Address Damage Done by Therapists," *New York Times*, Aug. 20, 1989, p. E5.
98. Letter of October 24, 1994, from Dr. Alan I. Levenson, CEO of Psychiatrists' Purchasing Group, to the newsletter of the Louisiana Psychiatric Medical Association.
99. Interview with Ann Landers, reprinted in *Time*, Aug. 21, 1989, p. 62. Dr. Jules Masserman, one of the preeminent psychiatrists of the 20th century, was accused of drugging a female patient with sodium amobarbital in order to have sexual relations with her in his office. B. Noel, *You Must Be Dreaming* (New York: Poseidon Press, 1992). In response, Dr. Alan Stone commented, "The APA had been terribly battered by two decades of revelations about sexual abuse of patients. Now the finger of accusation had pointed at a former president." A.A. Stone, Book Review, *Psychiatric Times*, April 1993, p. 32.
100. Reuters news release, Aug. 9, 1990.
101. Freud made these comments in response to the practice of Dr. Sandor Ferenczi embracing his patients. In nearly 30 years of practice, it never became erotic intimacy, and he claimed that his technique helped his patients. From all reports, they did improve. Freud was mainly concerned about the reputation of the profession. E. Jones, *The Life and Work of Sigmund Freud* (New York: Basic Books, 1953), vol. 3, p. 163.
102. L. Tiger & R. Fox, *The Imperial Animal* (New York: Holt, Rinehart & Winston, 1971).
103. Of equal protection of the laws, see Williamson v. Lee Optical, 348 U.S. 483, 489 (1955); Briggs v. Kerrigan, 431 F. 2d 967, 969 (1st Cir. 1970); Doe v. Director of Dept of Social Servs., 468 N. W. 2d 862, 870 (Mich. App. 1991), *reversed*, 487 N. W. 2d 166 (Mich. 1992).
104. L. Jorgenson & R. Randles, *supra* note 63, at p. 189.
105. M. Borruso, "Sexual Abuse by Psychotherapists: The Call for a Uniform Criminal Statute," *Am. J. Law & Med.* 17 (1991): 289.
106. T.C.W. (Annot.), "Constitutionality, Construction, and Application of Statutes Abolishing Civil Actions for Alienation of Affections, Criminal Conversation, Seduction, and Breach of Promise to Marry," 158 A. L. R. 617–618 (1945; discussing New York Civil Practice Act, Art. 2A, § 61-a).
107. 514 A.2d 802 (Me. 1986).
108. 514 A.2d at 806–807.

109. Patients have established medical malpractice claims against therapists involved with a relative in a number of cases, including Richards v. Weersing, No. 146282, LC No. 90-001773-NH (Mich. App. 1995); Jackenthal v. Kirsch, N.Y. Cty. S. Ct., No. 18423/90 (1995); Doe v. Wood, 10 PNLR 50 (1995).

110. R. Schickel, *Woody Allen: A Life in Film* (Chicago: Ivan R. Dee, 2003).

111. Cover story, "Sex and Psychotherapy," *Newsweek*, April 13, 1992, pp. 52–58; B. Streisand, "Physicians, Heal Thyselves," *Newsweek*, June 29, 1992, p. 14.

112. 61 N.C. App. 170, 300 S.E.2d 833 (1983).

113. 300 S.E.2d at 838.

114. 300 S.E.2d at 841.

115. See Veeder v. Kennedy, 589 N.W.2d 610 (S.D. 1999); Annot., "Civil Liability of Doctor or Psychologist for Having Sexual Relationship With Patient," 33 ALR 3d 1396.

116. Moulin v. Monteleone, 165 La. 169, 115 So. 447 (1928). A few states still have the alienation of affections law on the books. The alienation of affections case in North Carolina of Dorothy Hutelmyer vs. Margie Cox Hutelmyer attracted much national attention. A jury ordered the second Mrs. Hutelmyer (Margie) to pay the first Mrs. Hutelmyer (Dorothy) $1 million for stealing away her husband. O. Goldsmith, "Vindication, Not Vengeance," *New York Times*, Aug. 14, 1997, p. 15.

117. 198 Cal. App. 3d 591, 243 Cal. Rptr. 807(1988).

118. See also, e.g., Horak v. Biris, 130 Ill. App. 3d 140, 474 N.E.2d 13 (1985). In Destefano v. Grabrian, 763 P.2d 275 (Colo. 1988), a clergyman providing marriage counseling to both spouses and who had sexual intercourse with one of them was held liable to the other for outrageous infliction of distress. In Marlene F. v. Affiliated Psychiatric Med. Clinic, 48 Cal.3d 583, 770 P.2d 278, 257 Cal. Rptr. 98(1989), a therapist treating both mother and son was held liable to the mother for molestation of the son.

119. Dillon v. Legg, 69 Cal. Rptr. 72, 441 P.2d 912 (1968).

120. 90 Md. App. 1, 599 A.2d 1193 (1992).

121. 321 Md. 642, 584 A.2d 69 (1991).

122. 584 A.2d at 75, 77.

123. 38 Ohio St.3d 207, 527 N.E.2d 1235 (Ohio 1988). In Scamardo v. Dunaway, 650 So.2d 417 (La. App. 1996), the husband of a wife sexually involved with the treating physician was allowed to assert claims of negligent and intentional infliction of emotional distress, thus distinguishing these causes of action from statutorily abolished alienation of affections action. The husband and wife consulted with the doctor for treatment for infertility.

124. 524 N.W.2d 363 (S.D. 1994).

125. 19 Cal. App. 4th 263, 23 Cal. Rptr.2d 364 (1993).

126. See Thing v. LaChusa, 48 Cal.3d 644, 771 P.2d 814, 257 Cal. Rptr. 865 (1989); see also R. Slovenko, "Blaming a Book," *J. Psychiat. & Law* 22 (1994): 437.

127. N.Y. 339, 162 N.E.99 (1928).

128. Britton v. Soltes, 205 Ill. App. 3d 943, 150 Ill. Dec. 783, 563 N.E.2d 910 (1990). See also Renslow v. Mennonite Hosp., 67 Ill.2d 348, 10 Ill. Dec. 484, 367 N.E2d 1250 (1977); Soto v. Frankford Hosp,. 478 F. Supp. 1134 (1979). Summary disposition—judgment without the necessity of going to trial—is the appropriate remedy when the court determines the defendant did not owe the plaintiff a duty of care.

129. 563 N.E.2d at 916.

130. See, e.g., DiMarco v. Lynch Homes, 525 Pa. 558, 583 A.2d 422 (1990).

34
Experimentation and Clinical Trials

Standards in experimentations or clinical trials involving human subjects have been a major development of the 20th century, coming about in response to the horrendous experiments carried out by Nazi Germany and also in the United States and elsewhere. Among the best known of the Nuremberg trials that took place after World War II was the Doctors' Trial, also known as the *Medical Case*. It was conducted under U.S. military auspices; those appointed by President Truman to hear the case were all American judges and lawyers. The case was prosecuted by then Supreme Court Justice Robert Jackson and Telford Taylor, a military lawyer.[1]

Physicians, who were ambitious in pursuing a career in research and unencumbered by compassion, found Auschwitz a laboratory without parallel. The Nuremberg tribunal was asked to determine the culpability of 23 high profile German physicians under "the principles of the law of nations as they result from the usages established among civilized peoples, from the laws of humanity, and from the dictates of public conscience." The trial was a murder trial (murder was identified by the tribunal as a crime against humanity), but throughout the trial, the question was presented of what were or should be the universal standards for justifying human experimentation. The alleged lack of a universally accepted principle for carrying out human experimentation was the central issue pressed by the defendant physicians. A few of the ethical arguments presented by the defendants during the trial at Nuremberg as justification for their participation in the experimentation programs were the following:

1. Only people who were doomed to die were used in the experiments.
2. Research is necessary in times of national emergency; extreme circumstances demand extreme action.
3. There were no universal standards of research ethics.
4. The state determined the necessity for the human experimentation—the physicians were merely following orders.
5. Sometimes it is necessary to tolerate a lesser evil, the killing of some, to achieve a greater good, the saving of many.
6. Because there were no statements that the subjects did not consent, it should be assumed that valid consent existed.
7. Participation in research offered expiation to the subjects for their crimes (that is, polluting German society).
8. The Hippocratic Oath was not betrayed as Jews posed a public health problem, a "disease" that contaminated the body politic.

Actually Nazi Germany learned much about eugenics from the United States. At the turn of the 20th century, melting-pot America provided fertile soil for eugenics. (In 1883, Sir Francis Galton, a cousin of Charles Darwin, coined the term *eugenics*, which derives from the Greek word for *well-born*.) The science of eugenics would improve the human stock by giving the more suitable races or strains of blood a better chance of prevailing speedily over the less suitable than they otherwise would. The U.S. eugenics movement was funded by the industrial titans of the country—Andrew Carnegie, John D. Rockefeller, Jr., and Mary Harriman, widow of the railroad magnate Edward Harriman—and was championed by graduates of Harvard, Yale, and other Ivy League universities.[2]

In the United States at the time, white Anglo Saxons were favored over other peoples. Laws or practices segregated blacks, discriminated against Jews, prohibited miscegenation and homo-sexual behavior, carried out risky experiments on captive populations, and sterilized thousands of mentally retarded individuals, not to mention the earlier decimation of the Native American population.[3] In 1927, the U.S. Supreme Court ruled by an 8–1 majority that eugenic steriliza-tion was constitutional.[4] Justice Oliver Wendell Holmes supported the decision by noting that "experience has shown that heredity plays an important part in the transmission of insanity, imbecility, etc." He went on to say, "It is better for all the world, if instead of waiting to execute degenerate offspring for crime, or to let them starve for their imbecility, society can prevent those who are manifestly unfit from continuing their kind." In editorials, the *New York Times* and leading medical journals such as the *New England Journal of Medicine* wrote positively about eugenic sterilization. By 1945, some 45,127 people in the United States had been sterilized, 21,311 of them patients in mental hospitals.

Prior to World War I, eugenics was not nearly as popular in Germany as it was in the United States; sterilization at that time was illegal in Germany. But after Hitler came to power in 1933, Germany passed a comprehensive sterilization bill. The leaders in the German sterilization movement stated repeatedly that their legislation was formulated only after studying experi-ments in the United States. Over the next 6 years, Germany sterilized 375,000 of its citizens. The fervor with which Germany was carrying out sterilization prompted some American eugeni-cists to fret that Hitler was now "beating us at our own game."[5]

In 1935, Hitler signed into law the so-called Nuremberg Laws to further "cleanse" the German population from unwanted elements. The medical profession was at the forefront in carrying out the program and they did so enthusiastically. Medical journals praised the Nuremberg laws. These laws contributed to the expansion of German medical services. Medicine prospered under the Nazis, as Germans under Nazi guidance became increasingly obsessed with racial and phys-ical fitness. Hitler was lauded as the great doctor of the German people. The Nazi state was based on what Hitler's deputy, Rudolf Hess, called *applied biology*. One slogan said, "National Socialism is the political expression of our biological knowledge." In 1933, Hitler asked the German medi-cal profession to move with all its energy into the forefront in the race question; racial hygiene was to be the task of the German physician.[6]

In 1947, the American judges found 15 of the 23 doctors at Nuremberg guilty and sentenced 7 to death by hanging.[7] The two American physicians who testified for the prosecution, physiolo-gist Andrew Ivy and neuropsychiatrist Leo Alexander, contributed to the writing of the 10-point Nuremberg Code for ethical human experimentation. The writing of the code was prompted by the justifications given by the defendants at the trial. At the heart of the code (its first point) was the principle that the interests of science should never take precedence over the rights of the human subject. Research subjects were not to be taken as means to a scientific end, and they needed to always give informed consent. That principle in the code was put in absolute terms: "The voluntary consent of the human subject is *absolutely* essential. This means [the capacity] to exercise free power of choice without the intervention of any element of force, fraud, deceit, duress, overreaching, or other ulterior form of constraint or coercion" (emphasis added). To be sure, a morality code addressed to the medical profession such as the Nuremberg Code is not needed in order to condemn the barbarities of the Nazi doctors.[8]

The doctrine of informed consent was not an invention of American law or ethics. A legal requirement for the informed consent of the subject of human experimentation was earlier made in a ministerial directive issued in Berlin in 1900. The directive came about as the result of the research conducted by Dr. Albert Neisser, best remembered nowadays for giving his name to the organisms that cause gonorrhea and meningitis. In 1898, when a professor of dermatology and venereology at the University of Breslau, he sought to develop an antisyphilis serum by injecting cell-free serum from syphilitic patients into others—mostly prostitutes—without their full knowledge or consent. Some developed syphilis as a result. In 1900, the Royal Disciplinary Court of Prussia fined him an amount representing two-thirds of his annual income. By the late 1920s, there was frequent criticism in the German press of unethical research undertaken by the medical profession. Ironically, Germany was the first country in the world to enact an all-encompassing protection for human research subjects, yet in the Nazi period it became the country that carried out the greatest perversion of medical morality in history.[9]

In the United States the concept of informed consent arose not in cases of experimentation, but rather it originated in the clinical care setting. The first U.S. case to use the term *informed consent* was in 1957 in *Salgo v. Leland Stanford, Jr. University Board of Trustees*.[10] It ruled that patients must not only freely consent, but also be fully informed about treatment options.[11] The legal concept was essentially developed to provide a cause of action in cases of poor outcome when negligence in treatment could not be established, and it later also became a medical ethic.[12] Prior thereto, the question was only whether the patient consented to a procedure, and the failure to obtain that consent constituted a battery.[13] Informed consent became a branch of the law of malpractice that allowed insurance coverage, but required expert testimony and a different (longer) statute of limitations. It became a "bag of worms" whether the patient was informed of the relative risks of treatment and alternatives to the proposed treatment.[14]

Informed consent is now an accepted principle for medical research in the United States, but it is a relatively late development. In 1969, one prominent observer of the relationship between law and medicine, Professor William Curran of Harvard University, wrote: "In the years prior to the current decade, there was little law in the United States concerning medical research. There were no specific federal or state statutes purporting to regulate research organizations or investigators in their research methods, their areas of research, or the use of subjects or patients in such work. There were also no reported court actions involving liability issues or criminal actions against research organizations or personnel."[15]

The United States in conducting the Doctors' Trial presented itself as the country that would insist that science be carried out in a moral manner, but the reality was that gross misuse of humans in research occurred in the United States not only before but also after the formulation of the Nuremberg Code. Journalist Robert Whitaker has noted: "[T]he ink on the Nuremberg Code was barely dry when Paul Hoch, director of research at the New York State Psychiatric Institute, began giving LSD and mescaline to schizophrenics in order to investigate the 'chemistry' of psychosis."[16]

The events described at the Nuremberg trials have not been perceived by researchers or commentators to be directly relevant to the American scene. As a consequence, the Nuremberg Code, as well as the subsequent 1964 World Declaration of the World Medical Association, have had an uneventful reception in the United States in the sense that they are seldom cited by the courts (a LEXIS search reveals only 14 cases citing the code more or less in dicta).[17] They are rarely discussed in the legal literature, with the notable exception of the publications written or edited by George Annas, director of the law, medicine, and ethics program at Boston University.[18] The Secretary of Defense in 1953 did promulgate the Nuremberg Code as a guide to research dealing with atomic, biological, and chemical warfare, but this decision was treated as a state secret, and it was kept classified and released to only key parties.[19] Lawsuits against the government for injuries suffered by military personnel are barred. Thus, the United States Supreme Court has held that a serviceman may not maintain a tort action against the government, even though it secretly administered doses of a hallucinogenic drug as part of an experimental program because his injuries were service-related.[20]

Ultimately, research scandals in the United States provided the political impetus to institute formal protections for research subjects, to complete the work begun with the Nuremberg Code. In 1966, Henry K. Beecher, a professor of research in anesthesia at Harvard Medical School, published a widely discussed article identifying 22 examples of objectionable research.[21] Although the article did not lead to immediate change, it did more in the United States than the Nuremberg Code to sensitize the medical community to the protection of subjects. Only six pages long, it was devastating in its indictment of research ethics. David Rothman, a professor of social medicine at Columbia University, compared its impact to that of Harriet Beecher Stowe's *Uncle Tom's Cabin*, Upton Sinclair's *The Jungle*, and Rachael Carson's *Silent Spring*.[22]

It was a long-running Tuskegee study that finally moved the United States toward a systematic formal regulation of research standards. In 1932, the government had initiated an observational study of syphilis in African-American men that did not end until a journalist brought it to national attention in 1972.[23] The aim of the study was to learn whether syphilis had a different pathological course in black men than in white men. For decades infected subjects were not treated, even though an effective therapy had become widely available. In fact, the researchers actively conspired with physicians in the area to prevent these subjects from obtaining treatment. The repercussions remain to this day, as African-Americans, mindful of the study, are wary of experimentation.[24]

In 1974, Congress approved the National Research Act and established an advisory body, the National Commission for the Protection of Human Subjects of Biomedical and Behavioral Research. It also required that all research funded by the Department of Health, Education, and Welfare receive prior review and approval from local review committees. The National Research Act established the system of Institutional Review Boards (IRBs), local committees that determine whether certain standards of subject protection are met before research may commence. No IRB involvement is required (though it may be utilized) when the research is supported by private funds.[25] Most clinical studies nowadays that bring new drugs to market are financed by pharmaceuticals (and much testing is carried out in countries with little or no regulation).[26] The Food and Drug Administration requires comprehensive reporting on drug trials (but keeps the information confidential to protect manufacturers' interests).

The work of the National Commission also led to the influential 1978 Belmont Report, which identified three main concepts by which to evaluate the ethics of research: (1) respect for persons, (2) beneficence, and (3) justice. Respect for persons stresses the importance of recognizing persons as their own decision makers and protecting those who are unable to make decisions for themselves (researchers must offer potential subjects adequate information about the project, ensure that subjects comprehend the information, and ensure the voluntary nature of participation). The concept of beneficence asserts the importance of protecting the welfare of subjects (it requires researchers to offer a meaningful balance of risks and benefits). And justice requires that no particular group is favored in access to and distribution of research benefits. The IRBs have the responsibility of implementing these concepts as embodied in federal regulations.[27] The nature and scope of oversight remain a matter of continuing debate.[28]

The IRB is supposed to evaluate whether a research project is designed in a way that protects the rights and welfare of its subjects. IRBs are charged to ensure that research participants know that they are involved in research and that they have the right to participate or not. Specifically, the IRB has the duty to ensure that subjects know what kind of research they are involved in, how long it will last, what risks and discomforts it might involve, and what benefits are involved, if any.[29] For medical interventions, the IRB must ensure that researchers disclose to subjects alternatives to participating in the research. The IRB must also ensure that informed consent makes it clear that subjects have the right to withdraw from the study at any time without penalty or loss of benefits they would otherwise have.[30]

The Belmont Report, which served as the foundation for the federal regulations for the protection of human subjects, outlines the boundaries between research and clinical practice. Delineating those boundaries was important because physicians could otherwise cloak research under standard-of-care practices.[31] The Belmont Report states that if any portion of a patient's therapy is experimental, the treatment or strategy must be reviewed for the protection of human subjects.[32] The report explicitly authorized combining research and practice, though it mandated review for the protection of the rights of human subjects for any activity involving research. Medical intervention is typically categorized: *Standard treatment* involves practices designed solely to enhance the well being of an individual patient through diagnosis, preventive treatment, or therapy; *innovative treatment* is a deviation from standard practice, the efficacy or safety of which has not yet been validated; *clinical research* is an activity designed to produce generalizable knowledge through the application of procedures of potential diagnostic or therapeutic value to those involved as patient–subjects; and *experimentation* or *nontherapeutic research* is an activity designed to produce generalizable knowledge through the application of procedures without the intention of directly benefiting those involved as subjects. But arriving at a reasonable degree of precision regarding the meaning of these phrases has been confounding.[33] The Belmont Report notwithstanding, IRBs do not monitor experimental treatment, only experimentation that is not designed for the benefit of the subject.

Of combining research and practice, Beecher warned that the relationship between physician–investigator and patient–subject is one that can easily be manipulated. He pointed out: "If suitably approached, patients will accede, on the basis of trust, to about any request their physicians may make."[34] In the oft-cited decision in *Moore v. Regents of the University of California*,[35] the California Supreme Court appended a fiduciary duty to informed consent.[36] It ruled that the physician not only had to engage in the traditional informed consent procedure of disclosing risks, benefits, and alternatives, but in addition had to disclose his research and economic interest to the patient, even though they were unrelated to the patient's death. The court concluded that a reasonable person would want to know if his physician had an economic interest that might affect his professional judgment in providing treatment.[37] The economic aspects of medical research may also be regulated under federal fraud and abuse laws.[38]

Following World War II, the U.S. Congress made large grants to researchers, medical centers, and universities to conduct clinical research. This development led to an increased interest in academic research. Some physicians were then able to devote a substantial portion of their time to clinical research as opposed to clinical practice. Publications in medical journals resulting from research efforts became increasingly important for academic promotions and tenure, and for financial gain significant for individual researchers. Before long, academic centers realized the support that clinical research could provide. Increased financial opportunity raised the risk of unethical practices. It is questionable whether the IRBs have been able to adequately judge whether a potential conflict of interest exists.

Skepticism abounds as to the efficacy of informed consent as a protective device. Beecher himself believed that a "far more dependable safeguard than consent is the presence of a truly responsible investigator," but he nevertheless agreed that "[consent] remains a goal toward which one must strive for sociologic, ethical, and clear-cut legal reasons." Yet consent in any fully informed sense may not be attainable due to the condition of the subject.[39] Informed consent forms 5 to 10 pages long that are often presented to a subject are, as a practical matter, a ritual designed more to protect the researcher and the IRB than the subject.[40] Can a subject be informed of risks that are unknown? Does the uncertainty of a clinical trial necessarily invalidate a purported consent? Numerous studies have found that the typical procedures used in seeking informed consent leave the participant uninformed.[41] More often than not, the subject of an experiment is unable or does not want to read the consent document.[42] Moreover, research subjects or patients are not tested as to their understanding of what is in the consent form.

Why would any individual agree to seriously jeopardize his health or his life for the sake of science? Dr. Carl Elliott points out that individuals suffering depression simply may not care about the risks of an experiment.[43] In various writings, Dr. Paul Appelbaum and Dr. Jay Katz have noted what Appelbaum and colleagues have called the *therapeutic misconception*, that is to say, many subjects are not likely to readily comprehend that the research in which they are being asked to participate might not be beneficial to them.[44] They have pointed out that this is particularly problematic when the subject's treating physician is the individual making the overture to become a research participant. Appelbaum and colleagues explain their findings as follows:

> Most people have been socialized to believe that physicians (at least ethical ones) always provide personal care. It, therefore, may be very difficult, perhaps nearly impossible, to persuade subjects that *this* encounter is different, particularly if the researcher is also the treating physician, who has previously satisfied the subject's expectations of personal care. Further, insofar as much clinical research involves persons who are acutely ill and in some distress, the well-known tendency of patients to regress and entrust their well-being to an authority figure would undercut any effort to dispel the therapeutic misconception.[45]

Questions remain whether researchers and subjects are in a common-law special relationship, a fiduciary-like relationship, or something altogether different. The view that a researcher's duties are equivalent to those of a treating physician would bring a halt to clinical research. The imposition of a fiduciary duty would go against the goals of research. The goal of research is to test out new medical procedures, drugs, or devices through a small number of research participants that would, in turn, benefit a large number of people. To achieve that goal, the researcher may have to act contrary to the best interest of the research participants. That goal would not be achievable if every time an injury occurred, the researcher was held liable for breaching a fiduciary duty to follow the best interest of the participant.

Recent years have been marked by a spate of litigation against researchers and research institutions, based on a variety of legal theories, including informed consent violations, claims related to the inappropriate enrollment of subjects or the improper monitoring of subjects' health during the course of a study, and theories related to researchers' alleged fraudulent conduct or conflict of interest.[46]

Currently, federal research regulations do not require that institutions, sponsors, or investigators provided any compensation to subjects injured in research. Common-law claims are unlikely to succeed when the risks of physical injury were disclosed in advance, and there is no negligence in carrying out the research. Comprehensive research subject compensation, such as no-fault administrative programs to help subjects with health-related claims, have been the subject of recurring policy debate.[47]

For the most part, at various medical centers, the subjects of experiments are generally poor African Americans who know nothing about science. They engage in the experiment solely for the money, yet this is never openly acknowledged. The longer the study or the more days they must be confined to the center, the more they are paid, but how the dollar amount is determined is a mystery.

The issue of what motivates individuals in a prison to participate in research has been discussed in the medical literature. In a study of prison volunteers, Dr. Frank Ayd listed 11 motivating reasons: (1) financial reward; (2) hope for a reduction in the sentence; (3) direct or indirect seeking of medical or psychiatric help through professional advice or a drug; (4) to escape a lonely, tedious existence; (5) to have something to do and talk about; (6) to participate in what is looked upon as a stimulating, exciting adventure; (7) a desire to prove to himself and to others that he can do something good and admirable; (8) to command and receive respect and accolades; (9) the absence of obligations to others; (10) some form of psychopathology to gratify self-destructive urges; and (11) simple curiosity.[48] Psychoanalyst Anna Freud, daughter of Sigmund Freud, doubted whether there is such a thing as a genuinely altruistic relationship to one's fellows.[49]

The subjects of malaria experiments carried out during World War II were portrayed as heroes, and presumably that prompted volunteering.[50] These volunteers were prisoners, conscientious objectors, and hospital patients. They were knowingly infected with malaria to test an antimalarial drug. The University of Chicago student Nathan Leopold, who was incarcerated for the kidnapping and murder of a 12-year-old boy, participated in the malaria experiments. In his 1958 autobiography, he stated that he "wanted very badly to do my bit [in the war, and] being a malaria volunteer represented by far my best opportunity. … Here was a chance to get in a payment on my debt, an opportunity much more important and favorable than most to expiate some part of my guilt."[51] Be that as it may, for participating in the research he was released from prison. In his autobiography, he states that some of the subjects were motivated by their desire to leave prison. Was he also so motivated? Was his decision to volunteer affected by his confinement? Would he have volunteered had he not been in prison?

There are limits, however, to what people may consent to. Not all apparent exercises of autonomy are tolerated. Consent, for example, is no defense to a charge of murder or to render the infliction of other serious injuries lawful.[52] However, for medical research, human beings may be used within limits as guinea pigs. Public policy accepts the value of research. Without tests on human subjects, progress in medicine would be handicapped or stymied. Much of the medical progress that has benefited humanity would have been impossible without human subject research. This progress was accomplished primarily through clinical drug or device trials, psychological evaluations, studies of environmental hazards, and by many other avenues.[53]

Out of the shadows of the Nazi experiments, concerns over the advancement of science began to take precedence over the integrity or autonomy of the individual. In the section "Basic Principles" of the first official version of the Declaration of Helsinki in 1964, the requirement of consent is not even mentioned. In the 1975 revision, the requirement of informed consent, which had been the centerpiece of the Nuremberg Code, was reintroduced, but as its ninth basic principle. The Rules and Regulations for the Protection of Human Research Subjects set out by the U.S. Department of Health and Human Services provides: "An IRB may approve a consent procedure that does not include, or which alters, some or all of the elements of informed consent … or waive the requirement to obtain informed consent, provided … [t]he research could not practically be carried out without the waiver or alteration; [t]he research involves no more than minimal risks to the subjects; [t]he waiver or alteration will not adversely affect the rights and welfare of the subjects."[54] Henry Beecher and others, though critical of the lack of research ethics, have asserted that adherence to the Nuremberg provision that "voluntary consent … is absolutely essential" would effectively curtail the study of mental illness and children's diseases, as neither population has the legal capacity to give consent.[55]

Does the Hippocratic Oath apply to research or only to treatment? Hippocrates observed, "As to diseases, make a habit of two things: to help, or at least to do no harm," an injunction that has often been simplified as "do no harm" (*primum non nocere*).[56] While noting that the trial of the Nazi doctors was a murder trial, prosecutor Telford Taylor pointed out in his opening statement that this was "no mere murder trial" because the defendants were physicians who had sworn to "do no harm" and to abide by the Hippocratic Oath. In their testimony at the trial, Alexander and Ivy cited Hippocrates in regard to human experimentation. Alexander said: "Every professional relationship between the physician and another human being, irrespective of whether the physician treats the patient, examines him, or performs an experiment upon him with his permission, is bound by the principles laid down in the Hippocratic Oath."[57] However, when defense counsel at the trial asked Ivy to reconcile the Hippocratic Oath forbidding physicians to "administer a poison to anyone even when asked to do so" when conducting potentially lethal experimental interventions on volunteer subjects, Ivy replied, "I believe this Hippocratic commandment refers to the function of the physician as a therapist, not as an experimentalist, and what refers to the Hippocratic Oath is that he must have respect for life and the human rights of his experimental patient."[58] In nontherapeutic research, there is no claim of any benefit for the subject. The risks to the subject are balanced against the benefits to society at large.

The issue of autonomy was presented in a much publicized psychosurgery case in Detroit in the early 1970s. It is apparently the only decision by a United States court to rely on the Nuremberg Code as authority to judge the sufficiency of the consent obtained for proposed experimental brain surgery. The case is discussed in the chapter on informed consent. As a member of the informed-consent review committee established to evaluate the consent given by the subject of the experiment, I felt that the experiment could not be tainted due to lack of consent. The subject had a great deal of faith in the investigator, the first person in his 17 years of confinement to show any interest in him, and a strong relationship had developed between them. The development of such a relationship, *de facto* though not *de jure*, causes consent to be not really informed. As the informed consent concept has developed at law, "sufficient information must be disclosed to the patient so that he can arrive at an intelligent opinion," but *by whom* is the information given? The crucial factor is not the amount of information given, but rather *who* provides it. The concept of informed consent must be redefined to include the source of the information.

In considering consent for experimentation, the court referred to the principles of the Nuremberg Code for guidance and quoted them. The court would allow a prisoner to consent only to low-risk, high-benefit procedures. The decision did not foreclose "the performance of psychosurgery on such persons once the procedure has advanced to a level where its benefits clearly outweigh its risk." Given the current state of knowledge about how the brain works, the court judged that presently the benefits do not outweigh the risk.[59]

In the psychosurgery case, as in others, the informed-consent concept was used as a rationale to bar a procedure. The use of subterfuge, if you will, is as ancient as history itself. Over 2,000 years ago, the Talmud did away with capital punishment, but it could not do so directly, for the world was unprepared for it. And so the sages of the Talmud devised regulations that made it impossible to carry it out. In the case of psychosurgery, there was no rationalization available to the court in its quest to ban psychosurgery in prisons, with the possible exception of the Eighth Amendment's prohibition against cruel and unusual punishment. Those who adhere to the maxim "call a spade a spade" may be fit only to use one. Assuredly this is not the style of the judicial process. Several years after the decision, upon his retirement from the bench, the trial judge let the cat out of the bag when in an interview he said, "I could control your violent behavior, too, by just removing all of your brain. What they wanted to do just wasn't right."[60] It was clear that the judge opposed psychosurgery to control violence. The doctrine of consent gave a rationale for the decision to bar it.[61]

The opinion in the psychosurgery case set the stage for national regulation barring experimentation involving prisoners, which theretofore had been a common practice. Indeed, pharmaceutical companies would underwrite the cost of constructing or operating penal institutions in return for the opportunity to carry out drug testing. Throughout the 1950s, drug companies competed for access to prison populations. In 1969, some 85% of all new drugs were tested in 42 prisons. As late as 1975, at least 3,600 prisoners in the United States were used by drug companies as the first humans on whom the safety of new medication was tested.[62]

Also in the 1970s, the federal government, through the Atomic Energy Commission, funded a decade-long radiation study on inmates in Oregon and Washington State prisons. The experiments were designed to determine how much radiation astronauts could tolerate during space flights. Prisoners who volunteered for the testing received small monetary payments. They were required to undergo radiation exposure to their testicles at rates equivalent to approximately 20 diagnostic x-rays. Test subjects suffered painful, lasting effects.[63]

As a consequence of research abuses, the U.S. Department of Health and Human Services (HHS) regulations now limit inmate participation in clinical investigations to the following: (1) studies of the possible causes, effects, and processes of imprisonment and criminal behavior so long as the research involves only minimal risk and inconvenience to the subject; (2) studies of prisons as institutional entities or of inmates as incarcerated individuals so long as the research involves only minimal risk and inconvenience to the subject; (3) research on particular conditions affecting prisoners as a class so long as the research is approved by the secretary of HHS or an authorized HHS employee; and (4) research involving a treatment likely to benefit the prisoner himself or herself. In addition, the institutional review board assessing the clinical trial must include at least one prisoner or prisoner representative and must certify that a variety of conditions have been met and that a number of precautions have been taken.[64]

In light of history, the concern exists that individuals in a prison setting cannot, under any circumstances, be adequately protected, and that any biomedical experimentation will lead to a violation of the prisoners' legal and moral rights. But, is it wise to exclude inmates from all clinical trials? Has the proverbial pendulum swung too far in the other direction? Denying seriously ill prisoners access to experimental treatments may constitute an equivalent violation of prisoner rights and is similarly problematic in moral and legal terms. Arguably, prisoners have a right to participation under the Eighth Amendment, the Due Process clause, and Equal Protection.[65]

The shadow of the Nazi experiments, though the ideology of that day has waned, continues to hover over experimentation with prisoners. People in captivity, as a matter of law, may not consent to experimentation, for fear that they may be enticed by special treatment or early release, though in reality they may be more competent and informed than those suffering various kinds of mental incapacity for whom voluntary consent is no longer "absolutely" essential.[66] Today there are criminal and tort laws to ensure (except in the military) that those doing research with human beings are using sound scientific designs, have the consent (however imperfect) of their subjects, have no conflict of interest in undertaking or interpreting their findings, and can obtain relevant information about what other researchers are doing in a timely manner. IRBs, whatever their shortcomings, cause researchers to pause and consider the ethics of their experiment, or else go to other countries to carry out their research.

Endnotes

1. *Trials of War Criminals*, vol. 11, p. 181 (1949); 6 F.R.D. 305 (1949).
2. In 1935, Alexis Carrel, a Nobel Prize-winning physician at Rockefeller Institute for Medical Research in New York, wrote in his book *Man Unknown*: "Gigantic sums are now required to maintain prisons and insane asylums and protect the public against gangsters and lunatics. Why do we preserve these useless and harmful beings? The abnormal prevent the development of the normal. This fact must be squarely faced. Why should society not dispose of the criminals and insane in a more economical manner? ... The community must be protected against troublesome and dangerous elements. How can this be done?" Carrel answered his own question: The insane, or at least those who committed any sort of crime, "should be humanely and economically disposed of in small euthanasia institutions supplied with proper gases." A. Carrel, *Man the Unknown* (New York: Harper & Bros., 1935), pp. 318–319.
3. William McDougall, professor of psychology at Harvard, in a book published in 1921, set out the psychological need of black people to be directed or commanded by white people. W. McDougall, *Is America Safe for Democracy?* (New York: Scribner, 1921). Woodrow Wilson as governor of New Jersey, a year before he was sworn in as president, signed legislation that created the Board of Examiners of

Feebleminded, Epileptics, and Other Defectives. Under the law, the state could determine when "procreation is inadvisable" for criminals, prisoners, and children living in poorhouses. "Other Defectives" was a fairly open category. See J. Goldberg, *Liberal Fascism* (New York: Doubleday, 2007), 255.

4. Buck v. Bell, 274 U.S. 205 (1927).

5. D. Kelves, *In the Name of Eugenics* (San Francisco: University of California), 1985), p. 116.

6. See J.M. Glass, *"Life Unworthy of Life": Racial Phobia and Mass Murder in Hitler's Germany* (New York: Basic Books, 1997).

7. See R.J. Lifton, *The Nazi Doctors: Medical Killing and the Psychology of Genocide* (New York: Basic Books, 1986); R.N. Proctor, *Racial Hygiene: Medicine Under the Nazis* (Cambridge, MA: Harvard University Press, 1988). See also R.N. Proctor, "Bitter Pill," *The Sciences*, May/June 1999, pp. 14–19.

8. The most sadistic of the doctors—Josef Mengele, also known as the "Death Angel" of Auschwitz—escaped to Brazil, where he lived until his death in 1979. He never regretted his crimes and died convinced of the superiority of the Aryan race. See E. Black, *War Against the Weak* (New York: Four Walls Eight Windows, 2003); J. Cornwell, *Hitler's Scientists* (New York: Viking, 2003). Years after the collapse of the Nazi regime, Laurence Rees of the BBC was dismayed to find that the Nazis who killed Jews had no regrets about it. They continued to believe it was the right thing to do—they had not been ordered to do it. No one was required to work in the concentration camps. No one was conscripted into the SS. They were not coerced by a few mad people or by crude threats to kill Jews; it was a collective enterprise by millions of people who contributed initiatives in order to facilitate the task of killing human beings and disposing of their bodies. L. Rees, *Auschwitz: A New History* (New York: Public Affairs, 2005).

9. L. Doyal & J.S. Tobias (Eds.), *Informed Consent in Medical Research* (London: BMJ Books, 2001), p. 156; G.S. Stent, *Nazis, Women and Molecular Biology* (Piscataway, NJ: Transaction, 2004).

10. 154 Cal. App. 2d 560, 317 P.2d 170 (1957).

11. See also Natanson v. Kline, 186 Kan. 393, 350 P.2d 1093 (1960). In a medical battery case, the physician performs an unauthorized procedure. It typically occurs when (1) the physician performs a procedure that the patient was unaware the physician was going to perform, or (2) the procedure is performed on a part of the body other than that part explained to the patient. In contrast, a lack of informed consent claim typically occurs when the patient was aware that the procedure was going to be performed, but was unaware of the risk associated with the procedure. In *Natanson*, a patient sustained injuries from excessive doses of radioactive cobalt during radiation therapy. The patient had consented to the radiation treatment, but she alleged that the physician had not informed her of the nature and consequences of the risks posed by the therapy. Thus, the case sounded in negligence rather than battery; 186 Kan. at 400, 350 P.2d at 1100. The court established the standard of care to be exercised by a physician in an informed consent case as "limited to those disclosures that a reasonable medical practitioner would make under the same or similar circumstances"; 186 Kan. at 409, 350 P.2d at 1106.

12. See Chapter 31 on informed consent.

13. See, e.g., Mohr v. Williams, 104 N.W. 12 (Minn. 1905). In a statement that is often quoted, Judge Cardozo in Schloendorff v. Society of New York Hospital, 211 N.Y. 125, 105 N.E. 92 (1914), said, "Every human being of adult years and sound mind has a right to determine what shall be done with his body." At that time patients did not have to be informed of the risks of treatment or treatment options, but only had to consent to the procedure. In *Schloendorff,* the patient consented to an incision and an examination of her stomach under ether, but expressly and emphatically forbade anything more. The surgeon nonetheless went ahead and removed part of her stomach. He was held liable in battery.

14. See, e.g., Truman v. Thomas, 27 Cal. 3d 285, 165 Cal. Rptr. 308, 611 P.2d 902 (1980). In this case, failure to inform about the risk of not following the treatment recommendation resulted in tort liability. Under the old medical battery law, there would have been no cause of action, as there was no improper or nonconsented-to touching. On the vagaries of information that must be provided the patient, see R.A. Epstein, "Medical Malpractice: The Case for Contract," *Am. Bar Found. Res.* 1976: 87–149; P.H. Schuck, "Rethinking Informed Consent," *Yale L. J.* 103 (1994): 899.

15. W.J. Curran, "Governmental Regulation of the Use of Human Subjects in Medical Research: The Approach of Two Federal Agencies," in S.R. Graubard (Ed.), "Ethical Aspects of Experimentation With Human Subjects," *Daedalus* 98 (2): 1969.

16. R. Whitaker, *Mad in America* (Cambridge, MA: Perseus Books, 2002), p. 235.

17. See G.J. Annas, "Mengele's Birthmark: The Nuremberg Code in United States Courts," *J. Contemp. Health Law & Policy* 7 (1991): 17. While the Nuremberg Code is rarely cited in U.S. court opinions, there is a tendency to refer to the Nazi experiments or to Hitler to condemn whatever is disliked. Thus, those who argued against withdrawing food and fluid from Nancy Cruzan, and from others

in the same state of permanent unconsciousness, compared it to the actions of Nazi physicians who engaged in active euthanasia. A.L. Caplan, "The Doctors' Trial and Analogies to the Holocaust in Contemporary Bioethical Debates," in G.J. Annas & M.A. Grodin (Eds.), *The Nazi Doctors and The Nuremberg Code* (New York: Oxford University Press, 1992), pp. 258–275. In an interview in 1997 on CBS's *60 Minutes*, Dr. Harold I. Eist, then president of the American Psychiatric Association, stated that managed care executives should be held accountable for crimes against humanity according to the Nuremberg Code. Patients have experienced dramatic erosion of their autonomy through managed care practices. He repeated the allegation to Ralph Slovenko (personal communication, Dec. 6, 2004). Dr. Marcia Goin, a subsequent president of the American Psychiatric Association, in a keynote address focused on the closing of psychiatric hospitals, the resulting crowding in psychiatric emergency rooms, and the elimination of community mental health resources. They speak to "the abandonment of the country's health and social responsibilities." Some consequences include homelessness, family disintegration, loss of work productivity, and an increase in the mentally ill in jails and prisons. M.K. Goin, "Presidential Paper," *Am. J. Psychiat.* 160 (2003): 1763.

18. G.J. Annas & M.A. Grodin (Eds.), *The Nazi Doctors and the Nuremberg Code: Human Rights in Human Experimentation* (New York: Oxford University Press, 1992); G.J. Annas, L.H. Glantz, & B.F. Katz, *Informed Consent to Human Experimentation: The Subject's Dilemma* (Cambridge, MA: Ballinger, 1977). Professor Annas has said, "It makes absolutely perfect sense to use Nuremberg as a cause of action in U.S. courts. The provisions of the Nuremberg Code were not articulated exclusively as war crimes. They are crimes against humanity." Quoted in J. Washburn, "Informed Consent," *Washington Post*, Dec. 20, 2001.

19. 45 CFR (Code of Federal Regulations) 46, sec. 111.

20. Shortly after the end of World War II, the U.S. Supreme Court held that those who had served on active duty may not recover under the Federal Tort Claims Act for claims arising out of or in the course of activity incident to their service. Feres v. United States, 340 U.S. 135 (1950). Rationales for the doctrine include the need for uniformity of law, the health and welfare benefits provided to service men and their dependents, the absence of private liability in like circumstances, and the potential for disrupting military discipline. The definition of "incident to service" has been exhaustively litigated over the past half-century. See, e.g., United States v. Stanley, 483 U.S. 669 (1987). In that case, a serviceman injured by an LSD experiment conducted by the government without informing him of the risks was precluded from suit because the experiments were "incident to service."

21. H.K. Beecher, "Ethics and Clinical Research," *N. Eng. J. Med.* 274 (1966): 1354–1360.

22. D.J. Rothman, *Strangers at the Bedside* (New York: Basic Books, 1991), p. 15.

23. J.H. Jones, *Bad Blood: The Tuskegee Syphilis Experiment* (New York: Free Press, rev. ed., 1993).

24. H.A. Washington, *Medical Apartheid: The Dark History of Medical Experimentation on Black Americans From Colonial Times to the Present* (New York: Doubleday, 2006); reviewed in D. Grady, "White Doctors, Black Subjects: Abuse Disguised as Research," *New York Times*, Jan. 23, 2007, p. D5. Not long ago, the Detroit Public Library hosted a conference about the Tuskegee experiments. E. Bey, "Local Chapter Flier Teaches About Tuskegee Airmen," *South End* (Wayne State University), Feb. 21, 2005, p. 1. See T.F. Murphy, *Case Studies in Biomedical Research Ethics* (Cambridge, MA: M.I.T. Press, 2004), pp. 3–4.

25. The Belmont Report drew no distinction between the ethical obligations owed to subjects in federally sponsored studies and those owed to people in studies supported by private funds. It simply listed the basics: informed consent, minimization and justification of risk, and IRB review. In 1997, the National Bioethics Advisory Commission took note of the dual standard of protection in the United States: one for subjects in federally regulated research and the other for those in unregulated research. To no avail, it called for a single standard of basic protections and resolved that "no person in the United States should be enrolled in research without the twin protections of informed consent by an authorized person and independent review of the risks and benefits of the research." R.A. Charo, "Human Subjects Have It Worse Than Guinea Pigs," *Chronicle of Higher Education*, June 25, 1999, p. 64.

26. The pharmaceutical industry has exported clinical trials to underdeveloped countries. The number of countries where the research is carried out has increased from 28 to 79 and the number of researchers going abroad has gone from 271 in 1990 to 9,458 in 1999. The pharmaceutical companies finance orphanages and other institutions in return for carrying out research on the residents. Professor David J. Rothman observed, "Until the 1990s, American medical researchers performed most of their experiments on other Americans, frequently choosing subjects who were poor and vulnerable. Now, however, they are increasingly likely to conduct their investigations in third world countries on subjects who are even poorer and more vulnerable. ... Part of the reason ... is the mounting financial and

regulatory burdens of research in the rich nations, which cause investigators, both from universities and drug companies, to go to the poorer countries to test new treatments." D.J. Rothman, "The Shame of Medical Research," *N.Y. Review of Books*, Nov. 30, 2000, p. 60. See S. Shah, *The Body Hunters: Testing New Drugs on the World's Poorest Patients* (New York: New Press, 2007); M. Angell, "The Ethics of Clinical Research in the Third World," *N. Eng. J. Med.* 337 (1997): 847; T. Bodenheimer, "Uneasy Alliance: Clinical Investigators and the Pharmaceutical Industry," *N. Eng. J. Med.* 342 (2000): 1539; P. Lurie & S. Wolfe, "Unethical Trials of Interventions to Reduce Perinatal Transmission of the Human Immunodeficiency Virus in Developing Countries," *N. Eng. J. Med.* 337 (1997): 853; H. Varmus & D. Satcher, "Ethical Complexities of Conducting Research in Developing Countries," *N. Eng. J. Med.* 337 (1997): 1003, 338 (1998): 836; A. Jack, "New Lease on Life?/The Ethics of Offshoring Clinical Trials," *Financial Times*, Jan. 29, 2008, p. 7; J. Stephens, "Where Profits and Lives Hang in the Balance," *Washington Post*, Dec. 17, 2000, p. 1.

27. 45 C.F.R. 46.

28. See L.W. Roberts, "Ethics and Mental Illness Research," *Psychiat. Clin. N. Am.* 25 (2002): 525–545.

29. 45 CFR 46, sec. 416.

30. A number of pharmaceutical companies want the research agency to state in the informed consent that if subjects suffer severe adverse events (such as the need for hospitalization), the pharmaceutical company will pay for their treatment if they do not have insurance, but if they do have insurance, they would be required to use it, even though the cost of their treatment would be applied toward their lifetime cap. At Tulane University, when the IRB disagreed, the pharmaceutical companies threatened to take away their business. The university compromised by putting a statement in the informed consent advising the subject that if they have insurance, the cost of the treatment would be applied to their lifetime cap, and thus their insurance may be used up when they may need it at some future time. Personal communication from Dr. Sally T. Knight of Tulane University (Feb. 21, 2005). See S. Ruberstein, "When Drug Trials Go Wrong, Patients Have Little Recourse," *Wall Street Journal*, Jan. 31, 2008, p. 1.

31. Jay Katz identified "drawing the line between research and accepted practice … [as] the most difficult and complex problem facing the [National Commission for the Protection of Human Subjects of Biomedical and Behavioral Research]." Thomas Chalmers stated, "It is extremely hard to distinguish between clinical research and the practice of good medicine. Because episodes of illness and individual people are so variable, every physician is carrying out a small research project when he diagnoses and treats a patient." Herrmann Blumgart stated, "Every time a physician administers a drug to a patient, he is in a sense performing an experiment." These quotes appear in R.J. Levine, *Ethics and Regulation of Clinical Research* (New Haven, CT: Yale University Press, 2nd ed., 1988), p. 3. Levine observes: "Experimentation is commonly and incorrectly used as a synonym for research. Although some experimentation is research, much of it is not. Experiment means to test something or to try something out. In another sense, an experiment is a tentative procedure, especially one adopted with uncertainty as to whether it will bring about the desired purpose or results. [M]uch of the practice of diagnosis and therapy is experimental in nature. One tries out a drug to see if it brings about the desired result. If it does not, one either increases the dose, changes to another therapy or adds a new therapeutic modality to the first drug. All of this experimentation is done in the interests of enhancing the well-being of the patient. When experimentation is conducted for the purpose of developing generalizable knowledge, it is regarded as research." Levine, p. 10.

32. National Commission, Part A, par. 3.

33. A.M. Capron, "Different Compensation Approaches to Bad Outcomes From Standard Treatment, Innovative Treatment, and Research," in M. Siegler et al. (Eds.), *Medical Innovation and Bad Outcomes: Legal, Social and Ethical Responses* (1987), pp. 145, 149; quoted in J.A. Goldner, "An Overview of Legal Controls on Human Experimentation and the Regulatory Implications of Taking Professor Katz Seriously," *St. Louis U. L. J.* 38 (1993): 63.

34. H. Beecher, *Research and the Individual: Human Studies* (1970), p. 18. See also S. Kaplan & S. Brownlee, "Dying for a Cure," *U.S. News & World Report*, Oct. 11, 1999, p. 34.

35. 51 Cal. 3d 120, 271 Cal. Rptr. 146, 793 P.2d 479 (1990).

36. Typically, the concept of fiduciary responsibility attached to financial decisions about managing assets and property. See Villazon v. Prudential Health Care Plan, 843 So.2d 842 (Fla. 2003).

37. The California Supreme Court stated:

It is important to note that no law prohibits a physician from conducting research in the same area in which he practices. Progress in medicine often depends upon physicians, such as those practicing at the university hospital where Moore received treatment, who conduct research while caring for their patients.

Yet a physician who treats a patient in whom he also has a research interest has potentially conflicting loyalties. This is because medical treatment decisions are made on the basis of proportionality—weighing the benefits *to the patient* against the risks *to the patient*. ... A physician who adds his own research interests to this balance may be tempted to order a scientifically useful procedure or test that offers marginal, or no, benefits to the patient. The possibility that an interest extraneous to the patient's health has affected the physician's judgment is something that a reasonable patient would want to know in deciding whether to consent to a proposed course of treatment. It is material to the patient's decision and, thus, a prerequisite to informed consent. ...

We acknowledge that there is a competing consideration. To require disclosure of research and economic interests may corrupt the patient's own judgment by distracting him from the requirements of his health. But California law does not grant physicians unlimited discretion to decide what to disclose. Instead, "it is the prerogative of the patient, not the physician, to determine for himself the direction in which he believes his interests lie." Unlimited discretion in the physician is irreconcilable with the basic right of the patient to make the ultimate informed decision...

Accordingly, we hold that a physician who is seeking a patient's consent for a medical procedure must, in order to satisfy his fiduciary duty and to obtain the patient's informed consent, disclose personal interests unrelated to the patient's health, whether research or economic, that may affect his medical judgment. 783 P. 2d at.

38. See P.E. Kalb & K.G. Koehler, "Legal Issues in Scientific Research," *JAMA* 287 (2002): 85.
39. See, e.g.., E. DeRenzo, "The Ethics of Involving Psychiatrically Impaired Persons in Research," *IRB: A Rev. Hum. Subj. Res.* 16 (1994): 7–11. The polio vaccine was developed by testing flu vaccines in Ypsilanti State Hospital, a mental institution, on what even a U.S. military medical history Web site describes as "volunteers" (in quotes).
40. Personal communication from Dr. Allen R. Dyer, author with L.W. Roberts of *Concise Guide to Ethics in Mental Health Care* (Arlington, VA: American Psychiatric Publishing, 2004) to Ralph Slovenko (Sept. 30, 2004). See D.B. Resnik, "Liability for Institutional Review Boards," *J. Legal Med.* 24 (2004): 131.
41. When medical battery (treatment without consent) evolved into medical malpractice (treatment without informed consent), perplexities arose as to what must be revealed. Incredibly, some 5,000 articles have been published on informed consent. Many of them have noted that the informed consent process is often flawed as a result of insufficient information and incomplete comprehension, often exacerbated by illness, depression, anxiety, anger, or desperation. See J.W. Berg & P.S. Appelbaum, "Subjects' Capacity to Consent to Neurobiological Research," in H.A. Pincus, J.A. Lieberman, & S. Ferris (Eds.), *Ethics in Psychiatric Research* (Arlington, VA: American Psychiatric Publishing, 1999), pp. 81–106; R.B. Dworkin, "Getting What We Should From Doctors: Rethinking Patient Autonomy and the Doctor–Patient Relationship," *Health Matrix* 13 (2003): 235; C. Elliott, "Caring about Risks: Are Severely Depressed Patients Competent to Consent to Research?" *Arch. Gen. Psychiat.* 54 (1997): 113; S. Hewlett, "Consent to Clinical Research: Adequately Voluntary or Substantially Influenced?" *J. Med. Ethics* 22 (1996): 232; E.G. Laforet, "The Fiction of Informed Consent," *JAMA* 235 (1976): 1579; S. Sollitto et al., "Intrinsic Conflicts of Interest In Clinical Research: A Need for Disclosure," *Kennedy Inst. Ethics J.* 13 (2003): 83; P. Walter, "The Doctrine of Informed Consent: To Inform or Not to Inform?" *St. John's L. Rev.* 71 (1997): 543. The case of Lenahan v. University of Chicago, 348 III. App.3d 155 (2004), is an illustration where a physician sponsor and principal investigator of a clinical trial could be held liable for failing to obtain valid informed consent. The plaintiff must still prove causation of the alleged injuries. Causation cannot be based on general statistical information for a particular clinical trial, the court ruled in Compton v. Pass, 2006 WL 2419187 (Mich. App. 2006).
42. Veteran researcher Dr. Mark W. Ketterer of the Henry Ford Health System in Detroit says that not once in his experience has he encountered a subject who read the consent form. Personal communication to Ralph Slovenko (Jan. 20, 2005).
43. C. Elliott, "Caring About Risks: Are Severely Depressed Patients Competent to Consent to Research?" *Arch. Gen. Psychiat.* 54 (1997): 113.

44. P.S. Appelbaum, L.H. Roth, & C.W. Lidz, "The Therapeutic Misconception: Informed Consent in Psychiatric Research," *Int. J. Law & Psychiat.* 5 (1982): 319; J. Katz, "Human Experimentation and Human Rights," *St. Louis L. J.* 38 (1993): 7. See also J. Katz, *The Silent World of Doctor and Patient* (New York: Free Press, 1984); J. Katz, "Ethics and Clinical Research Revisited," *Hastings Cent. Rpt.* 23 (1993): 31.

45. P.S. Appelbaum, L.H. Roth, C.W. Lidz, P. Benson, & W. Winsdale, "False Hopes and Best Data: Consent to Research and the Therapeutic Misconception," *Hastings Cent. Rpt.* 17 (1987): 20, 23.

46. See C.H. Coleman, "Duties to Subjects in Clinical Research," *Vand. L. Rev.* 58 (2005): 387; S. Hoffman, "Continued Concern: Human Subject Protection, the Institutional Review Board, and Continuing Review," *Tenn. L. Rev.* 68 (2001): 725.

47. See R.S. Saver, "Medical Research and Intangible Harm," *U. Cincinnati L. Rev.* 74 (2006): 941.

48. F. Ayd, "Drug Studies in Prison Volunteers," *So. Med. J.* 65 (1972): 440.

49. A. Freud, *The Ego and the Mechanism of Defence* (London: Hogarth Press, 1961), p. 146.

50. *Life* magazine, June 1945.

51. N. Leopold, *Life Plus 99 Years* (Garden City, NJ: Doubleday, 1958).

52. In a New Mexico case, an individual convicted of aggravated battery had told the victim that if he had a gun he would shoot him. The victim obtained a gun, and gave it to the defendant, saying, "If you want to shoot me, go ahead." The defendant took the gun and shot the victim in the head, seriously wounding him. The court held that the consent was no defense, stating, "Whether or not the victims of crime have so little regard for their own safety as to request injury, the public has a stronger interest in preventing acts such as these." State v. Fransua, 85 N.M. 173, 510 P.2d 106 (1973). See also HMA v. Rutherfords, 1947 J.C. 1; R. v. Donovan [1934] 2 KB 498; R. v. Brown [1993] 2 All E.R. 75.

53. Jessica Berg and Paul Appelbaum write: "Clearly, biomedical research is necessary if we are to find treatments and possibly cures for some of the most devastating illnesses that exist in our society (e.g., schizophrenia and AIDS). Investigators should be allowed, and perhaps even encouraged, to participate. Yet the populations involved in such research are among the most vulnerable in our society. Although we are interested in allowing these individuals the same freedom to make choices as other members of our society, we are concerned about protecting persons whose capacity to make decisions autonomously is impaired. ... Should incompetent subjects be permitted to participate in high-risk/low-direct benefit protocols?" J.W. Berg & P.S. Appelbaum, "Subjects' Capacity to Consent to Neurobiological Research," in H.A. Pincus, J.A. Lieberman, & S. Ferris (Eds.), *Ethics in Psychiatric Research* (Washington, DC: American Psychiatric Assn., 1999), pp. 81–106 at 102.

54. CFR 45(1983): sec. 46.101–46.409.

55. H. Beecher, "Experimentation in Man," *J.A.M.A.* 169 (1959): 461. Law professor Richard Garnett writes: "The [Nuremberg] Code stands tall in memory, but its influence has never lived up to its aims. Seen by many as a product of and reaction to Nazi terror, the Code is often dismissed as a context-bound relic, no longer useful for today's researchers. Pragmatists argue that the Code is simply too demanding, that its standards are too high for necessary research to meet, and that its absolutism cannot compete with the utilitarian and impersonal ethics of modern medicine. ... Today, human experimentation is regulated by a crazy-quilt of hortatory codes and maxims, scattered federal laws and regulations, and most importantly, by Institutional Review Boards, which provide peer review of proposed experiments. "Informed consent" is still the touchstone, but modern regulations and procedures tolerate and expect deviations from this ideal. Thus, when addressing human experimentation—and they rarely do—courts occasionally mention the [Nuremberg] Code, but generally apply and enforce the more flexible informed consent requirements of later regulations." R.W. Garnett, "Why Informed Consent? Human Experimentation and the Ethics of Autonomy," *Cath. Law* 36 (1996): 455.

56. See A.R. Jonsen, "A Map of Informed Consent," *Clin. Res.* 23 (1957): 277.

57. See Military Tribunal, vol. II, pp. 53–56; see also L. Alexander, "Limitations in Experimental Research on Human Beings," *Lex et Scientia* 3 (1966): 8.

58. See E. Shuster, "Fifty Years Later: The Significance of the Nuremberg Code," *N. Eng. J. Med.* 337 (1997): 1436.

59. Civil Action No. 73-19434-A W, Wayne County, Michigan, Cir. Ct. July 10, 1973. The opinion is not officially reported, but available in *2 Prison Law Reporter* 433 (Aug. 1973), and excerpted in *42 U.S. Law Week* 2063 (July 31, 1973). The opinion also appears in G.J. Alexander & A.W. Scheflin, *Law and Mental Disorder* (Durham, NC: Carolina Academic Press, 1998), pp. 970–981; A.D. Brooks, *Law, Psychiatry and the Mental Health System* (Boston: Little, Brown, 1974), pp. 902–924. The issues in the case are extensively explored in "Symposium on Psychosurgery," *B.U.L. Rev.* 54 (1974): 215–353. Given the opaqueness of the court's opinion, it is not surprising that commentators on the decision have

stated that Smith withdrew his previously given consent upon release from custody. It was withdrawn before the court's decision and before his release. See, e.g., G.J. Annas & L.H. Glantz, "Psychosurgery: The Law's Response," *B.U.L. Rev.* 54 (1974): 263.

60. D. Josar, "Judge of 40 Years Never Tires of Career," *Detroit News*, Dec. 29.1996, p. E1.

61. R. Slovenko, "Consent to Psychosurgery," *Hastings Cent. Rpt.* 5 (1975): 19; reprinted in *Reflections* (West Point, PA: Merck, 1976), vol. 11, no. 3, 1976; also in N. Abrams & M. Buckner, *Medical Ethics: A Clinical Textbook and Reference for the Health Care Professions* (Cambridge, MA: M.I.T. Press, 1981). The psychosurgery case is discussed in Chapter 31.

62. See W.T. Reich (Ed.), *Encyclopedia of Bioethics* 4 (rev. ed., 1995): 2056; A.C. Ivy, "The History and Ethics of the Use of Human Subjects in Medical Experiments," *Science* 108 (July 2, 1948): 1.

63. See J.D. Marino, *Undue Risk* (New York: Freeman, 1999); E. Welsom, *The Plutonium Files* (New York: Dial Press, 1999).

64. See 45 C.F.R. 46.301 et seq. (1998).

65. S. Hoffman, "Beneficial and Unusual Punishment: An Argument in Support of Prisoner Participation in Clinical Trials," *Indiana L. Rev.* 33 (2000): 475. See also S.J. Brakel, "Considering Behavioral and Biomedical Research on Detainees in the Mental Health Unit of an Urban Mega-Jail," *N. Eng. J. Crim. & Civ. Confine.*, 22 (1996): 1.

66. See K. Morin, "The Standard of Disclosure in Human Subject Experimentation," *J. Legal Med.* 19 (1998): 157.

35
Suicide

Suicide or attempted suicide is appallingly common. Since the 1950s, the suicide rate in the United States has tripled. More than 32,000 Americans a year commit suicide, or about 11 per 100,000 in the general population; another 750,000 attempt it, including 500,000 whose suicidal attempts are severe enough to bring them to an emergency room. One in five high school students say they seriously considered suicide within the year. According to a 2005 survey by the American College Health Association, 10% of college students said they had "seriously considered suicide." More than 90% of all suicides involve mental illness or the abuse of alcohol, drugs, or an alcohol–drug combination.[1]

Needless to say, the majority of people who commit suicide are profoundly depressed. Sixty percent of suicides occur during a mood disorder episode. When living hurts too much, when hope is lost, suicide is taken as a way out. Most people at high risk for suicide, however, remain undiagnosed and untreated, though there are effective ways to treat the psychiatric illnesses most commonly associated with suicide.[2] The reasons for suicide vary, but a number of common risk factors have been identified.[3]

The rate of suicide attempts in individuals with co-morbid panic disorder tends to be higher than the rate of suicide attempts in individuals with depression alone. The association is strong between suicide attempts and panic disorder. Panic disorder's debilitating symptoms can lead to major depression, as might be expected when being constantly plagued by recurrent unexpected panic attacks where there is intense apprehension, fearfulness, or terror, often associated with feelings of impending doom. The idea of suicide to end the pain becomes attractive.[4]

Suicide is a murder (but suicide or attempted suicide is not now penalized in modern criminal codes). The word *suicide* comes from Latin, meaning self-murder, a violation of an ancient law: "Thou shalt not kill," even thyself. In the German language it is, literally, a murder of the self (*selbstmord*), and, in all the earlier philological equivalents, the idea of murder is implicit. But, it is also a murder *by* the self—it is a death in which one person becomes the murdered and the murderer. Freud's paper, *Mourning and Melancholia*, which describes the dynamics of depression as essentially the turning of an individual's hate against himself, also provides the basis for the psychoanalytic theory of suicide. In Freud's words, "No neurotic harbours thoughts of suicide, which are not murderous impulses against others redirected upon himself."[5]

In many cases, it is a happenstance whether an individual carries out a suicide or homicide, or both. Reports of murder–suicide are commonplace. Danger to self is often the flip side of danger to others. Self-hatred or introject formations may be so tormenting that the individuals may seek release from them by suicide or homicide. In severe depression, the individual may unconsciously direct unacceptable hatred or aggression toward himself or others. The indescribable pain of depression (often as a result of rage turned inward) may prompt suicide. In certain times and places, exorcism would be used to get rid of the introject, or as commonly said, the devil.

Suicide or attempted suicide devastates a family. The person who seriously considers taking his own life places a tremendous burden on others. There are many instances where a child is asked to watch over a potentially suicidal parent, "Call daddy right away at the office if mamma seems real upset"; or "Make sure you watch and go with her if she goes down to the basement."

This enormous burden is transformed to an equally intense guilt if the child fails to give a warning or to stop the suicide.

In *Games People Play*, Eric Berne illustrates that mental illness may be a strategy to gain that which might otherwise be refused. For one thing, a suicide attempt is used to obtain care and attention. The attempted suicide may say or think, "Can't you see how I hurt? I'm bleeding. Take care of me." In *Cactus Flower*, Toni's attempted suicide makes her boyfriend Julian feel like a bastard. A suicide attempt may also be an act of revenge. A suicide, direct or even indirect, often implies, "I'll die and then they will be sorry."

Literature provides pertinent illustrations of suicide as a means of punishing the depriving, frustrating figure. Tom Sawyer, frustrated by his aunt, was comforted by the thought of committing suicide by drowning himself in the Mississippi. He thought to himself how sad his aunt would be when his pale, limp body would be brought into her presence. He imagined her saying, "Oh, if I had only loved him more. How differently I would have treated him if I had only known." Anna Karenina, before throwing herself beneath the wheels of a passing train, contemplated the guilt the suicide would induce in her husband Vronsky, "To die! And he will feel remorse; he will suffer on my account."

After a suicide attempt, a person may say to members of the family, "Are you satisfied?" Saying this to make the family members feel extremely guilty. Attempted suicide, as a means of negotiation, is a manipulation in interpersonal relations, which is unfair and one-sided. And, of course, a successful suicide ends in nothing. In *Carousel*, Joshua, the Heavenly Friend, says to Billy Bigelow, "As long as there is one person who remembers you, it's not over." Suicide or attempted suicide has been described as a selfish act that affects so many people. Paul W. Smith, a radio talk host, put it thus: "In all suicides, there are people, family, and friends who are left behind with tremendous guilt piled on to the usual and expected normal grief. It is not fair to the person suffering from the depression, nor the victim left behind, that society has not yet figured out how to deal with the privacy 'rights' of people too ill to make the right decisions for themselves in seeking and accepting treatment."

Clinicians usually carry a lifelong emotional burden when a patient commits suicide. A malpractice suit adds to the emotional burden.

Suicide, then, is not an act that is isolated in effect. To say that a person may do with his life as he wishes is to ignore the reality that his actions mightily affect others. In John Donne's famous observation, "No man is an Island, entire of itself." To be sure, out of pragmatic considerations, the law imposes no duty to aid another unless a special relationship, such as parent–child exists, or a relationship is undertaken such as patient–physician. Generally speaking, the law imposes liability for misfeasance, not nonfeasance. Society as a whole has the responsibility to render aid to a person unable to care for himself.

Aid that involves deprivation of an individual's liberties, however, is to occur only if absolutely necessary. A general principle espoused by courts is that the "doctor–patient relationship cannot be imposed upon a competent patient without his consent." It is to be noted that the statement is qualified by the term *competent*. Moreover, social policy may override even the competent person's control over his body, as can be seen in compulsory sterilization, smallpox vaccination, and fluoridation.

Involuntary hospitalization is justified in some cases, but assuredly this is a complex problem that cannot be resolved by simple rules. Often commitment may not be in a person's best interest because his problems may be complicated by having to face the additional trauma of the stigma attached to the label *mentally ill*. He might lose his job and his friends because he is mentally ill. Given the opportunity, he may be able to work out his difficulties in the context in which they arise.

Suicide risk assessments surprisingly are rarely conducted, but even when performed, predictions are right only about one in 25 cases. The rarity of suicide is the reason that so many false positives arise in predicting suicide. In any event, psychiatrists who adequately examine for risk factors are much less likely to be held liable for inadequate suicide risk assessment. When a psychiatrist is sued, it is not under the theory of failure to predict suicide, but rather for failing to take ample assessment procedures. The best gauge to determine whether a patient will attempt suicide is whether there have been prior suicide attempts. A strong indicator of seriousness in suicide is the existence of a suicide plan. Another leading risk indicator of suicide is depression or alcohol abuse. The rate of suicide of individuals with bipolar and other mood disorders is 18 times that of the national suicide rate. A personality disorder is another common risk factor. Another consideration is the individual's age and gender. Adults over 65 represent only 13% of the population, but compose 20% of all suicides. Also, males commit 80% of all suicides.

Researchers point out that midlife suicide is rising. Among many people, sadness, ennui, or feeling of emptiness has become more marked. Emile Durkheim in his classic 1897 book attributed suicide foremost to anomie. To quote: "Man is the more vulnerable to self-destruction the more he is detached from any collectivity." Today's scene is that of the impermanence of friendship, greater mobility, and the breakdown of family structure. Increasingly, people live in a cocoon (at home or in an automobile). Robert Putnam in his book *Bowling Alone* (2000) describes the modern-day loss of community. Putnam describes how we have become increasingly disconnected from family, friends, neighbors, and social structures. It is a bleak picture of social isolation and civil disengagement. Depression has struck earlier and much more pervasively in each successive generation. Clinical depression is a prime risk factor for suicide.

Among youths, the strongest risk factors are depression, substance abuse, homosexuality, and suicide contagion. Homosexual youths are two to three times more likely to attempt suicide than other young people, and annually they compose up to 30% of completed youth suicides. Whatever the cause, be it discrimination or sexual conflict, internalized self-loathing is common.[6] Suicide has notably increased among youths with significant conformity problems, which supports the concept of contagion: When they closely identify with those who have committed suicide, and when faced with seemingly impossible problems, suicide may appear an attractive solution.[7]

According to reports, not only those in midlife and the elderly, but more youngsters than ever are depressed. Suicide rates for children and teens have tripled during the past 30 years. Nearly one of 10 youngsters who develop major depression before puberty goes on to commit suicide. Youngsters who develop depression are three to four times more likely than peers to have drug and alcohol problems by their mid 20s. Their parents are more likely to be divorced or in conflict. Studies routinely document that children of divorce have a significantly higher suicide rate than children from intact families. There is often a family history of mental illness, giving rise to a genetic explanation for the depression.[8]

In 2003, the FDA ordered that all antidepressant medications carry a black box warning stating that these medications increased the risk of suicidal thoughts in adolescents; more recently, the FDA extended the warning to include young adults. The black box was implemented after a study found that youngsters taking antidepressant medications reported a greater number of self-harmful thoughts when compared with youngsters taking a placebo. With the publication of the black box warning, primary care physicians have increasingly left the task of medicating depressed youngsters to psychiatrists. As a result, between the years 2003 and 2005, antidepressant prescriptions decreased by 50%. At the same time, the rate of adolescent suicide rose 18%. Psychiatrists generally believe that antidepressants are quite safe and should be feared far less than the condition they are designed to treat.

In this day of genetic research, it is said that there are genes not only for mental illness, but also for impulsivity, aggression, and violence that may lead to heavy risk. Researchers today set out organic causes of suicide along with the social ones. Neurological damage to the fetus, caused by alcohol or cocaine use, may predispose children to mood disorders that lead to suicide; lack of maternal attention may deprive them of early developmental stability; diet may work adversely on their brains.[9]

Malpractice Suits

Suicide is reportedly the leading cause of malpractice suits filed against mental health professionals—about 20% of the total. That number has little to do with the merit of most litigation involving suicide, as it is often based on a mistaken belief that the therapist could have predicted, and intervened to prevent, the suicide, or that hospitalization would have made a difference. The therapist is often made the scapegoat.

The psychiatrist or hospital is required to use reasonable care and skill to detect a patient's tendency to commit suicide or otherwise injure himself. The most common allegations in a complaint for malpractice following a patient's suicide are the following:

1. Failure to predict or diagnose the suicide.
2. Failure to control, supervise, or restrain.
3. Failure to medicate properly.
4. Failure to observe the patient continuously (24 hours) or on a frequent enough basis (e.g., every 15 minutes).
5. Failure to take an adequate history.
6. Inadequate supervision and failure to remove belt or other dangerous objects.
7. Failure to place the patient in a secure room.

Failure to detect suicidal tendency, however, is not malpractice "where there is no proof that generally accepted medical standards required the psychiatrist to conclude that the patient was likely to commit suicide."[10] The psychiatrist or hospital is not an ensurer of the safety of the patient or others. There must be something to give notice that special care is required.[11]

No one is required to guard against or take measures to avert that which, under the circumstances, would not be reasonably anticipated as likely to happen. It is said, though, that some 50 to 70% of patients who subsequently kill themselves communicate their intent in advance, yet for one reason or another, there is a failure to respond to these "clues to suicide." Dr. Robert Simon observes, "The evaluation of suicidal risk is one of the most complex, difficult, and challenging clinical tasks in psychiatry. Patient suicides are all too common in the practice of mental health clinicians. It is even more common in the practice of primary care physicians. Thus, it is extremely important for the practitioner to understand how to conduct a competent suicide-risk assessment."[12]

Suicide is the number one cause of premature death among manic depressives and schizophrenics. Approximately 15% of suicides are people diagnosed as manic depressive or schizophrenic, whereas among individuals in the general population the suicide rate is approximately 1%.[13] Studies have found that a person who buys a handgun is 57 times more likely than a member of the general population to commit suicide within a week of purchasing the weapon and that suicide is the leading cause of death among gun buyers in the first year after the weapon was purchased.

No-Suicide Pact

In recent years the *no-suicide pact* (or *contract for safety*) has made its way into clinical practice as a way to remove the threat of a suicide. Patients are asked to promise (in writing) that they will not engage in suicidal behavior for a set period of time and that they will call for help rather than act out suicidal thoughts or impulses. This approach is designed to solidify the therapeutic alliance, but it may falsely reassure the clinician and it may take the place of adequate suicide assessment.[14] The no-suicide pact was originally conceived as an inpatient management technique, but it subsequently has been used in other settings and situations, often unfortunately, with scant effort to evaluate efficacy. There is no indication that suicide is less likely in the case of a no-suicide pact or that it serves a preventive function.[15] Indeed, the pact may have a negative impact on a patient. Several people close to Marilyn Monroe, because of their concern for her, got her to agree to a no-suicide pact, whereby if she ever seriously thought of killing herself, she would call them. Suicidal individuals have been heard to object to an obligation put on them under the pact. As they say, "Don't lean on me." "The only time you can really rely on a suicide prevention contract is when the patient refuses to sign one," says Dr. Robert Simon. In that case, he says, at least the practitioner will not be misled into a false sense of security.[16]

Determinative Factors in Litigation

Determinative factors in litigation are knowledge or notice that the patient is likely to harm himself and subsequent failure to take reasonable and permissible precautionary measures. If the evidence shows that the patient has had a suicidal proclivity of which the psychiatrist knew or should have been aware, a case of malpractice may be made out against him or the hospital. This is a form of faulty diagnosis, which results in faulty prognosis. As the courts put it, a psychiatrist or hospital has a responsibility to protect a patient from self-inflicted injuries if the possibility of such acts is reasonably predictable. In order for there to be contributory negligence, or an independent intervening cause, which would bar a claim, the patient must be capable of exercising the care of a reasonable man.[17] With the shift in tort law from a concept of contributory negligence, which bars a claim of a plaintiff entirely, to that of comparative negligence, which only lessens that claim, there is a tendency to consider the patient's own behavior resulting in suicide.[18] The issues of foreseeability of self-inflicted injuries and the ability to exercise reasonable care are both questions for the jury.[19]

If the psychiatrist or hospital has been put on guard as to a patient's suicidal tendency and as to the probable method of carrying it out, as in the case where suicides or dangerous escapes have been attempted in a particular way in the past, the duty to protect and prevent is increased correspondingly. Among allegations that are asserted are the following: (1) the psychiatrist did not give proper attention to the patient's history; (2) the psychiatrist failed to give appropriate orders to the hospital staff, or (3) the hospital staff failed to carry out the orders. In the managed care era, the heightened risk of patient suicide arises from premature discharge.

Documentation is important. Indeed, it is said: "What protects you [the psychiatrist] from liability is *not* that you have made the 'right' decision, but your documentation of a process, the process by which you have assessed and responded to the likelihood that your patient would commit suicide. Your documentation should answer three basic questions: What did I do? Why did I do it? On what basis did I reject alternative ways of responding?"[20]

Unlike a hospital, a household tends to be informally organized, unable to watch over a family member who is suicidal, so they bring the individual to a hospital, expecting it to provide the necessary care and attention. Hence, the liability rate of a psychiatrist or hospital is greater in the case of an inpatient suicide than that of an outpatient suicide, where there is less control over a patient, but there may be a duty to seek commitment of a patient.[21] (This issue is discussed in Chapter 25 on failure to treat.

Physician-Induced Suicide

Suicide-inducing characteristics of the psychiatrist or what may be called iatrogenic or physician-induced suicide has rarely been alleged in a legal action, notwithstanding the psychiatric literature on suicide as a possible response to the therapist behavior or to counter-transference attitude. Harry Stack Sullivan pioneered the concept that the therapist influences simply by observing. In law, however, suicide-inducing characteristics are too subtle and difficult to establish.[22]

The question is, can psychotherapy precipitate or contribute to a suicide? The answer is yes (to put it starkly, Jim Jones in Guyana sent hundreds of his followers to their deaths).[23] In the outpatient setting, the issue is not one of control or supervision as in the case of a hospitalized patient, where security is expected, but rather whether the therapist by malignant intervention triggered or precipitated the suicide. Suppose, for example, the therapist dwells on homosexuality in a way that upsets the patient, and he is unable to deal with it and becomes increasingly depressed. Other examples in the outpatient setting where it might be said that the suicide is the fault of the therapist are where the patient is abandoned, or a confidence is breached causing the patient great humiliation. Clearly, returning a gun to a suicidal patient would be hard to explain to a jury.

Failure to Provide a Particular Treatment

What about not providing a particular treatment, such as medication or electroconvulsive therapy (ECT)? Though the patient is suicidal, some psychiatrists, psychologists, and social workers contend that there is no need for chemicals or ECT, and, if anything, they are counterproductive; they would suggest a glass of wine instead. Others take an opposite opinion.

A psychiatrist who testifies against a psychologist whose patient has committed suicide may say that the suicide could have been averted by the use of medication or other somatic therapy that a psychologist or social worker, by the limitation of his license, would be unable to perform. The late Dr. Stanley Leese, psychiatrist and editor of the *American Journal of Psychotherapy*, wrote:

> Those who treat severe depressions should have the broadest possible knowledge of the limitations of various psychotherapeutic techniques. Similarly, they should have an intimate knowledge of the benefits and limitations of the antidepressant drugs. ... Finally, the therapist who does not have facilities for emergency hospitalization at his disposal, should this become necessary, should not treat severely depressed patients, let alone suicidal patients.[24]

> Likewise, says Dr. Mortimer Ostow: "A patient with psychotic or suicidal depression should not be treated by a psychologist, even under supervision."[25] One might say that on the day that Sylvia Plath committed suicide by putting her head in an oven, she might, if she had had ECT, still be alive.[26]

Until fairly recently, medical psychoanalysts themselves avoided psychiatric drug therapy. Even now, those who use it consider it a kind of second-class treatment. Many psychoanalysts, however, continue to withhold drug therapy entirely on the general principle that it might interfere with the treatment, and that it involves the psychoanalyst in direct interference with the patient's life. Others contend that where drug therapy is indicated, withholding it constitutes a far greater interference and can be challenged from an ethical, if not from a legal, point of view.[27]

Those analysts or nonmedical therapists who do not do drug therapy set up a combined treatment in which they provide the psychotherapy and call upon a drug therapist to offer that treatment simultaneously. Although, in many instances, this is the best arrangement that can be made for a given patient, some consider it bad practice. Ostow claims that it is bad practice because to administer drug therapy properly, one needs the data obtained in psychotherapy. Second, Ostow, says that in order to understand what the patient has to say, one must be able to distinguish between the contribution made by the patient and that made by the medication.[28] Others say division of treatment is poor practice because it splits the transference.

The practice of writing prescriptions for a patient, sight unseen, is a violation of the medical code even though done at the request of a psychologist or social worker or other member of a treatment team. In many large state hospitals, as an operational or practical matter, it may not be possible for the doctor to regularly see all patients, or to see them adequately, so he writes a prescription or order and it is carried out over a long period of time by nurses or other aides. As a consequence, patients in hospitals have protested and have claimed a right to refuse treatment. Under the Michigan Medical Practices Act (as others), a physician should not prescribe medication for a patient whom he has not personally seen, nor should the medication be administered and its effect monitored by someone who is not a physician.[29] In these circumstances, malpractice is readily assessed by showing breach of the statutory standard of care.

Police Suicide

Police officers, we all know, are exposed daily to potential assaults and murder on the streets, yet there is another danger lurking within their own ranks: suicide. Line-of-duty deaths grab the public's attention, but police officers more often—perhaps two or three times more often—die by their own hand. Some 400 to 450 officers kill themselves each year, compared with the 150 to 200 that are killed in the line of duty. In thinking of epidemics, we think of diseases such as AIDS, which ravage an entire society, but epidemics can also occur within specific groups of people. Police work is an occupation replete with psychological stress and trauma, danger, and availability of firearms. Under such conditions, an increased risk of suicide can be expected.

Indeed, police officers kill themselves more than they are killed by others. Major epidemiological studies have shown that the police suicide rate is over three times that of the general population, and rates appear to have increased over the past decade. Moreover, many police suicides are purposely misclassified on death certificates as accidents or undetermined deaths. Suicide has an insurance dimension that could foreclose benefits for the family. Also, out of a desire to protect family members and the department from the stigma of suicide, fellow officers at the scene of the suicide withhold information from medical examiners. Thus, the actual number of police suicides may be substantially higher than what is officially reported.

Police suicide can devastate the morale of entire agencies and leave individual officers with intense feelings of guilt, remorse, and disillusionment; many feel they should have done something to prevent the suicide. To dissuade suicide, police departments often view it as a disgraceful rather than a heroic police death, and do not afford police families the support after a suicide that they would ordinarily receive in the case of the death of an officer.

There is an interaction of personality and environment, but there is controversy as to whether personality or occupational elements most influence police suicide. Occupational influences include psychological stress, interpersonal and work relations, availability of firearms, alcohol use, and retirement.[30]

Police officers generally choose police work because, like physicians, they want to help people. The police motto is "to protect and to serve." Psychiatrists generally consider the desire to help people as being partially determined by a need to sublimate one's dependency needs by taking care of others.

Police officers are often found to be immature and to have a need to sublimate conflicts with authority by becoming the authority (police officers are often characterized as bullies), and they are often macho (with need to prove their masculinity and adequacy). By and large, police officers walk a very narrow line between power and authority. There is an inverse relationship between authority and power—power is used when there is a failure of authority. In the words of one police officer complaining of burnout, "It seems like no one has any respect for the uniform anymore." Another stressed out police officer described police work as the "human garbage collectors for the city." Another said, "We protect the rich from the poor."

A spate of police suicides in France set off uncommon news coverage and embarrassed the government. A prominent Paris lawyer commented, "The cops are scorned by the public and badly treated by their superiors. No wonder they feel bad." To a number of young people, *les flics* (as the police are known in France) are walking emblems of the state, who are fun to taunt, insult, and, when possible, bombard with bottles and stones. Some days, police officers say they feel surrounded by hostility. They feel they get no support or understanding from their superiors. During the days of the Soviet Union, police suicide there was a very infrequent event. The police had unchallenged authority.

What about professional help for the police? Approximately 80% of suicides have communicated their intent by speaking of their plans or of "when I won't be around anymore." Psychiatrists find a pattern of early suicide predictors among these individuals: They become overly aggressive, they use alcohol to treat sleep problems, they buy a better and more powerful pistol, they put their family in the background in favor of their drinking buddies, they cause damage to people's property, they kill animals, and they withdraw, watching progressively more violent films.

There is a relationship between suicide and the reluctance of police officers to see a psychiatrist. Police officers tend not to be introspective, and they often internalize their frustrations and negative emotions. On psychological testing, an increased risk of suicide has been found in persons with high hostility scores. Police officers are expected to use as little force as possible, and to always be "pleasant" regardless of what others did or said to them. Even though their authority is challenged, they are expected to contain their rage. Suggestions for police suicide prevention include intervention programs and suicide awareness training. Organizational support and confidential psychological services that officers feel they can trust are important in reducing suicide. Training in suicide awareness may also help officers to understand their own feelings and to cope with emotional adversities. The first and most important step is to recognize that the problem exists. Police suicide is a fact not to be ignored.[31] In recent years, most police departments have instituted mandatory counseling for all officers who have shot someone, as a way of helping these officers cope with the stresses that arise from such an act.

Certifying the Cause of Death

Insurance coverage for accidental death or injury usually includes exclusionary language for self-inflicted injuries that occur within a certain period of time but, by and large, the courts have tempered the exclusion by reading into it an intent requirement. A suicide is defined in the Random House Dictionary as "a person who *intentionally* takes his or her own life" (emphasis added). Mental illness may undercut intent as in the test of criminal responsibility.[32] Social and judicial attitudes regarding suicide have gradually turned away from assessing guilt and toward protecting suicidal persons and their beneficiaries.[33]

In the absence of policy language proving that the exclusion applies whether the insured was sane or insane, the courts have allowed recovery when the deceased was not able "to form a conscious intention to kill himself and to carry out that act, realizing its physical and moral consequences." This standard calls for psychiatric testimony that addresses the mental state of the insured at the time of his death. In a minority of jurisdictions, courts construing policies that contain the additional exclusionary language that it applied whether the death by the insured's own hand occurred while sane or insane have held that the language does not apply when the insured was so mentally disordered as not to understand that his act would result in death or that the act was committed under an insane impulse.[34]

Penal statutes against suicide or a suicide attempt have been repealed, or they are unenforced. Relatives of those who commit suicide, feeling not only bereaved but stigmatized, often try to persuade the certifying authority against the certification of suicide on the death certificate. The death certificate is *prima facie* evidence of the cause of death.

To be sure, there is a broad borderline area between clear-cut suicide and other modes of death that are equivocal, and there is tremendous variability in the information about the personality and behavior of the deceased. Unless there is a suicide note, it is not easy to evaluate the intention of a dead person: did the person die of natural causes, by accident, by suicide, or was he murdered?[35] It is often difficult, for example, to decide whether a person dying in an automobile collision was an accident or suicide. Addicts are disturbed persons on the edge of deliberate suicide, but there is the possibility of accident in the course of the barbiturate habit. Males who enact masturbation fantasies of being tied up and abused, with partial hanging as part of the fantasy, may accidentally be asphyxiated.[36] Those who engage in repeated acts of self-injury do not wish to kill themselves, but use their self-injury to relieve pain, while suicidal persons seek to terminate unendurable pain by ending their lives.[37]

One of the important roles of the coroner or medical examiner is to classify the manner of death among the categories of natural, accident, suicide, and homicide. Is the coroner or medical examiner up to the task? Most coroners are elected (many are funeral directors); few pathologists are medical examiners. In more than 80% of cases, manner of death is readily and unambiguously assigned to one of these four categories on the basis of scene investigation, witness interviews, autopsy findings, and toxicology results. In some cases, however, manner of death is not so readily established and will be listed as pending until further investigation, analysis, or consultation is completed.

Manner of death determinations have important legal implications in homicide prosecutions, denial of life insurance coverage as we have noted under a suicide or self-inflicted injury exclusion, establishment of liability for accidental deaths, and other contexts. Manner of death determinations may also have important emotional implications for survivors of the decedent and may affect the reputational interests of the decedent and those associated with the decedent.

During the latter half of the 20th century, coroners and medical examiners began to turn to psychiatrists, psychologists, and criminologists for assisting in determining manner of death in equivocal cases, resulting in the development of the approaches known as psychological autopsy, psychiatric autopsy, and behavioral reconstruction. Apparently, however, no coroner or medical examiner office has a psychiatrist on its staff. The *Daubert* ruling on scientific evidence has apparently not been held to apply to psychological testimony on manner of death.[38]

Suicide—Why Not?

Dostoevsky pondered why more people do not commit suicide. Why do not all of us commit suicide, as many philosophers have advised? Freud's theory of the death instinct postulates a great impulse toward death in all of us. Moreover, it has long been taught that toil and suffering in this life will lead to an afterlife in heaven, so why waste time on earth? (Protestants have no proscription against suicide.) To what extent, if any, does belief in a life hereafter affect the way one lives in this life? The "suicide bomber" believes that his enemy will go to hell and he will go to heaven. So many Muslims are eager to turn themselves into bombs; the Koran makes this activity seem like a career activity. The bomber becomes a martyr and his family is honored. In the Koran, God says, "Those who are slain in the cause of God, He will not allow their works to perish. He will vouchsafe them guidance and ennoble their state. He will admit them to the Paradise."[39]

In the Russian film *Lilya4*Ever* (2002), a youngster finds life miserable and wants to die. In heaven, he says, "I will play basketball all day." Andrea Yates drowned her children believing they would go to heaven. Facing a possible death sentence, convicted murderer Marvin Charles Gabrion II told jurors at his sentencing hearing that he does not care whether he lives or dies. He said, regardless of their decision, "I am returning to heaven, which can be likened to a continuous, happy, erotic dream that I can control."[40]

Behold the joy in heaven: no traffic jams. Sun Myung Moon's *The Completed Testament Age and the Ideal Kingdom* assures us,

When one walks on earth to get somewhere, you have to walk continuously, but in the spirit world, because location changes according to one's thinking, walking has a different meaning. One can ride in a car wherever and whenever one desires it.[41]

Summary

In a study of suicide in a state hospital setting, Dr. M. J. Kahne found that 25% of the psychiatrists whom he interviewed had experienced a consummated suicide by a patient in treatment. These psychiatrists, however, did not differ in any significant respect as to personality, sex, marital status, or counter-transference attitudes from their more fortunate colleagues. In looking over this 25%, which numbered 79 psychiatrists, Kahne found that the foreign-born or foreign-educated psychiatrist was more likely to have a patient suicide. Language and cultural barriers are impediments to good psychiatric care. The most vulnerable psychiatrists also tended to have the largest caseloads and received a minimum of advisory and consultative support.[42]

Dr. Seymour Halleck suggests that the detriments of authorizing malpractice litigation for suicide may outweigh any social benefit. Speaking as a teacher at a medical school, Halleck noted, "I usually work with residents and I don't want them to get sued. So, we do a lot of things that I don't think are in the best interest of the patient."[43] Halleck, however, does not call for complete immunity from liability, recognizing that there are times when therapists are grossly negligent with suicidal patients.[44] The following case illustration points out the considerations in suicide litigation.

SUICIDE IN MALPRACTICE LITIGATION: CASE ILLUSTRATION

An action was brought by a widow for the death of her husband, Louis R. Genovese, who committed suicide by jumping from a window of the Veterans Administration hospital in New Orleans after having cut the window screen with a pocket knife in his possession. There were no threats of suicide or previous attempts. She alleged that failure to detect the suicidal intent of the deceased and remove him to the psychiatric ward to take other measures for his security constituted negligence on the part of the hospital and its agents.

Genovese at an earlier time was admitted to the hospital complaining of "vague abdominal pains, intermittent shortness of breath, swelling of the feet and ankles, dizzy spells, orthopnea, and stiffness of the fingers." His medical history shows that he suffered from ulcerative colitis and he had undergone surgery for this condition 2 years earlier. Various examinations and clinical tests were made. Dr. George Adcock examined the patient and wrote the following order: "Consult psychiatry in the A.M. 48-year-old white male postoperative colectomy for ulcerative colitis. Has lost all interest in caring for self and exhibits marked intermittent periods of hostility and feelings of persecution. Would you evaluate? Thanks." The consultation was not obtained, however, as the patient left the hospital 3 days later against medical advice.

Approximately 4 months later, the patient was again admitted to the hospital, complaining of mild pain and discharge from his rectal stump. Various tests were made in contemplation of possible additional surgery. A routine psychiatric consultation was ordered by Dr. Mohammad Atik and Dr. Richard S. Cohen, with the notation: "Psychiatric consults. Patient—ulcerative colitis. Past history psychosis. Please evaluate." The request was received by Dr. Richard Stone, staff psychiatrist, but the consultation was not made prior to the patient's death. Five days after the consult request, however, the patient was presented by a senior medical student to Dr. Henry Colomb, psychiatrist and professor of psychiatry at Louisiana State University (LSU) Medical School, in connection with a demonstration form of clinical teaching. Student notes made as a result of this demonstration showed, "Patient presented this A.M. to Dr. Colomb. Diagnosis of anxiety with some degree of depression was arrived at." Three days later the patient jumped to his death.

Numerous members of the Veterans Administration hospital staff and other physicians who had occasion to examine or observe the patient testified that there had been no indication that would justify placing the patient in a neuropsychiatric ward. Expert witnesses were called by the plaintiff and the defendant.

Dr. William Sorum, a psychiatrist, testified as an expert on behalf of the plaintiff. His testimony follows.

Direct Examination by Plaintiff Attorney

Q. Have you had experience in determining the presence of suicidal intent in hospitalized patients?

A. Yes. Every psychiatrist has.

Q. Have you treated such patients?

A. Yes.

[The doctor's qualifications are set out to qualify him.]

Q. Dr. Sorum, is suicidal intent discoverable in a patient?

A. I think to a greater or lesser degree you can. You can usually find leads that you look for in a patient if they truly have suicidal intent, but of course in some patients it would be what we consider obscure. I mean, there is no such thing as saying this one will and this one won't; it's an individual thing that you have to look for with the aid of guide posts, which are set up by the patient as a rule.

Q. But there are factors and leads that are discoverable in patients with that intent, are there not, Doctor?

A. Yes, they are often discoverable, at least in retrospect; a lot of leads can be found after it is all over. There are a lot of suicides that take place in general hospitals. At Charity Hospital, we used to have similar incidents to this every year, just by people jumping out of windows, in surgical wards and in other wards besides that.

Q. Is the medical profession becoming more aware of this problem?

A. Yes, it is. I believe it is considered around the fourth leading cause of deaths. …

Q. Is there a movement on to increase security measures to prevent this, Doctor?

A. Well, yes, and for other reasons. There is no doubt that the presence of psychiatric wards in general hospitals is increasing, and in the private hospitals I am associated with, there is general agreement for the need for increasing security measures. For example, when a patient displays a certain behavior pattern whereby we would suspect the possibility of something like that, the patient is transferred to the psychiatric ward if at all possible.

Q. And by transferring this patient to a psychiatric ward, what security measures would actually be put in force, Doctor?

A. Well, he would come under closer control and increased supervision, for one thing, and he would be kept from just wandering through the hospital corridors or anything like that, and objects are taken from him that he could use to hurt himself or somebody else. …

By the Court

… I want to know what you would look for in a patient to make [the determination that he has suicidal tendencies].

A. Well, first, what he has been saying about it, if anything, if he has ever talked about committing suicide, or had any past history of any attempt at suicide, or any recent signs of change in his behavior pattern, if he appeared to be vague, or impulsive in his actions, whether he has been showing any depression, or loss of weight, or loss of appetite, some of the cardinal signs of anorexia, waking up early in the morning, expressions of hopelessness, any changes in personal habits, and things of that sort. ... The general appearance of the patient is of course an important indication as to whether or not he has any emotional problems or any mental illness that needs attention. ... You have to correlate all of your findings. ...

By Plaintiff Attorney

Q. Dr. Sorum, aren't there several places in this record where there are entries denoting anxiety reaction on the part of the patient?

A. This is one here. ...

Q. Doctor, doesn't this student admit note give the history of the patient, and doesn't it list as an impression "anxiety reaction"? Doesn't it say that, Doctor?

A. Yes. ...

Q. This is the consultation sheet, isn't it, Doctor?

A. Yes, sir.

Q. Now, isn't there a diagnosis of anxiety reaction appearing on the clinical record signed by Dr. Adcock? I am referring to the narrative summary, signed by Dr. Adcock, stating, "Initial impression was anxiety reaction, possible underlying psychosis"?

A. Yes, that's what it says. ...

Q. Would anxiety that was present to the degree that a physician would make a note of it in the medical record indicate that it was to a greater degree than, let's say, most of us would be considered to possibly have?

A. Yes, I would say so. ...

By the Court

Q. Does it sound like a man who was about to commit suicide from your experience?

A. Well, just from reading these entries, it would sound like somebody who was disturbed and depressed. Losing all interest in self is a sign of depression. It would appear, just from that, that here was a person who could have been unconsciously asking for help. You can't say that one or any of these things would be an indication that a man was about to take his life, but it does show that he was very disturbed and upset, and, of course, it is significant that a behavior pattern of that nature would interfere with his care, and that probably should be taken into consideration in all respects.

By Plaintiff Attorney

Q. I show you an entry. "Patient has lost all interest in caring for self," and again that is dated May 24, and it is signed by Dr. Adcock. What does that indicate to you, Doctor?

A. That is often a sign of depression and would suggest some deterioration in his character, perhaps. ...

Q. The diagnosis is, "Probable manic depressive psychosis," and it's signed by Dr. Toups. What does that mean, Doctor, probable manic depressive psychosis?

A. Well, that's a diagnosis that usually indicates mood swings, instability, and temperament, which approaches a very pathologic trend. It's more beyond the average swing, I would say.

Q. I show you another entry, Doctor, and it is dated October 6, 1962, and was signed by Dr. M. Belanger, "Very quiet and withdrawn." Now, the fact that a patient is withdrawn, does this perhaps indicate one of the signposts you previously discussed?

A. It may or may not indicate the presence of depression in a patient. I mean, you couldn't make a decision on that from just that entry.

Q. But would that be part of a cumulative effect?

A. Yes. ...

Q. Dr. Sorum, taking the cumulative effects of the various entries that we have covered, does the medical record of Mr. Genovese indicate to you that he had suicidal tendencies, and if that is so agreed, that the patient's security should have been indicated?

A. Well, this is certainly in retrospect, but certainly he had suicidal tendencies, because he did take his own life. Now, what you are asking me is to tell you from the record whether they should have been aware of his disturbed condition during his different admissions to the hospital, and whether during his last admission he showed signs that should have put them on guard to the extent that security measures would have been taken; is that what you are asking me?

Q. Yes, sir.

A. I note that a psychiatric consult was ordered, according to this record, so we can certainly assume this man was depressed. It is also evident from the record that he was largely uncooperative and that he was quite careless with his person and apparently was hostile at points, and also withdrawn, so I think that we can say, judging from this entire history of his treatment and his behavior pattern in the hospital, that he was disturbed grossly.

Of course, when you attempt to predict what a patient may or may not do, it is difficult. Some persons can enter a hospital for treatment and display many of the symptoms and be quite harmless to themselves or others, and, of course, the reverse could also be true, but taking this record in its entirety, I think you can safely say that this was a situation that warranted, as you say, security measures.

Q. Doctor, from this record that you have reviewed, would you consider his death by suicide probable or not?

A. I think you would have to consider it possible, yes.

Q. Would you say it was a distinct possibility?

A. As a possibility, yes. Of course, I feel that I would be in a much better position to answer your questions had I been there and seen and talked to this patient. There's no better way to learn a person, to really find out about his attitudes and temperament and his condition than being right there and studying him firsthand. That's the best way to evaluate a patient. There's no better substitute than personal contact with the patient.
...

Q. ... the position of the hospital record indicates that there was no psychiatric consult held; isn't that right, Doctor?

A. Yes, there was no formal consultation, at least, not from what I can observe here. ...

Q. Doctor, would the ordinary standard of care indicate that if a formal psychiatric consultation was held that there would be a formal report or some report in the record, that there was a formal psychiatric consultation?

A. Well, I'm not familiar with the procedural aspect of the VA hospital.

Q. Doctor, what would a delay of some 8 days between the time of a request for a psychiatric consult and the psychiatric consultation itself, what would that indicate to you? Wouldn't that be undue delay?

A. Well, again, I don't know what the situation is in the VA hospital, what problems they may have, or the procedure, but we often have consultations that are delayed for various reasons, so that's something I wouldn't be qualified to answer.

Q. Considering the record of this individual, his medical record, with which you are familiar, would you say an 8-day delay was an undue delay, Doctor?

A. It's really hard to answer that question, since, as I said, I am unfamiliar with the conditions there. On the surface one would wonder about that, but again that is a qualified statement. I don't know what the situation was.

Q. Well, would it be more desirable to have it sooner, Doctor?

A. Yes, you could say that, certainly, the sooner the better. I guess in retrospect, we can say that easily. ...

Q. Would an entry by a physician in the medical record, that he was awaiting the results of the psychiatric consult, would that express his concern over the delay?

A. Perhaps.

Q. Dr. Sorum, in view of the medical record that was present at the time, in view of the pending delay of the psychiatric consultation, would the ordinary standard of care indicate that you should take, or that the physician should take, some minimum security measures, such as removing knives?

A. I would say this: In a really depressed patient, it might be a good idea if he appears to be that depressed. It all would depend on his behavior pattern at the time.

Q. Would it include removing the availability of easy access to windows in a high building?

A. Well, of course, that's one of the chief ways that this happens in general hospitals. ... I would say that's one of the chief things you have to look for. In fact, that's one of the two most acute situations you have to watch for, that and a gun.

Cross-Examination by Defense Attorney

Q. Doctor, whom do you consider to be expert in the field of suicide in the United States?

A. Dr. Shneidman, Dr. Farberow, and others. Those two men in particular are well-known authorities in the field, and they have written books on the subject.

Q. Are you familiar with the books, *Clues to Suicide*, and *The Cry for Help?*

A. Yes, sir, I am and if I had known that Dr. Shneidman was going to be here, I would have brought one down for him to autograph. ...

Q. Doctor, as far as you know from your own knowledge of the medical record in this case, the notations that were made by the various doctors were not made by psychiatrists, but by medical doctors; isn't that correct?

A. I don't believe there were any notations by psychiatrists. ...

Q. Doctor, isn't it true that approximately 8 out of 10 people who commit suicide have given definite prior warnings of their suicidal intentions, namely either having attempted suicide or threatened to commit suicide?

A. I am sure it's something like that. I mean, that's the one, big thing. Of course, you have people who do talk about it and threaten to do it and who do not do it, so there's just no 100% answer to that. I will say that usually people who have committed suicide have given some leads. The difficulty is ascertaining what the leads are and whether they are sufficient to justify a psychiatric consultation or psychiatric care.

Q. So, in other words, Doctor, would you say that prior attempts at suicide or threats to commit suicide, that those cases would be considered the more probable suicidal risks; isn't that true?

A. Yes, those are the best signs. Of course. There are other signs—pressure, depression, that sort of thing, but as I say, those are good signs and should be watched for. ...

Q. Now, Doctor, you used the word *retrospectively* in your direct examination in connection with this man's suicidal intentions.

A. Yes, that's right, and he must have had then because he did end his life. It's easy to look back retrospectively after something has already happened.

Q. In other words, that was after the fact; the man did commit suicide. I think we can all agree now that he had plenty of signs, such as depression and signs of waking at an early hour, and trailing feces, and things of that sort. Also, you can say retrospectively that he was probably thinking in terms of being unable to get a job afterwards, and being put on charity, and things of that sort, but, again, that's conjecture, just my opinion.

I also think you testified, if I understood you correctly, that depression in and of itself is not evidence of a person who is going to commit suicide. Is that correct, Doctor?

A. There are many depressed people who do not commit suicide to everyone that does, but there is no doubt that this is becoming an increasing problem that does come up over and over again.

By the Court

Q. Are there more suicides per capita now than there were, say, 25 years ago?

A. I believe so, but Dr. Shneidman can probably give you later facts on that.

Q. Life is more complicated, now, isn't it?

A. Much more, yes, sir.

Q. Do you think, based on what you have seen in this hospital chart, that there should have been an indication that a treating physician should have transferred him to a neuropsychiatric ward to prevent him from doing just this sort of thing?

A. Well, I don't know how crowded this ward might have been at the time that they would have transferred him to it, and I don't know what the setup and the rules are at the VA hospital, although I know it is a good hospital. I can say that I think now they should have transferred him, but what I would have thought then, before this happened, since I wasn't at the hospital and am not familiar with their procedures there, I just couldn't say. I hadn't seen the man. My thought now is that he either should have been transferred or proper precautions taken to prevent this sort of thing. I wish they had, but it may actually have been that they didn't have sufficient psychiatric help to take care of the situation. I just don't know. When you're sitting in this vantage point, you can look back and second-guess what could have been done to prevent this, but as to just what action I would have advocated prior to this suicide, I couldn't say at this time. ...

Redirect Examination by Plaintiff Attorney

Q. Doctor, forgetting the problem of whether or not this hospital had enough psychiatric help available to provide for the consultation requested, wouldn't it have been favorable and desirable to have this consultation earlier than 8 days in any event?

A. I would think it would be desirable.

Q. Would not the ordinary standard of care in the community dictate that this patient should have had a psychiatric consultation earlier than eight days?

A. Yes, I would think so. ...

Q. And concerning these signs, which are noted in this record, would not the ordinary standard of care dictate that pending a psychiatric workup, weapons, for example, would be removed from the patient?

A. Weapons?

Q. A penknife.

A. Oh, I would think so. However, we have used a lot of open-ward care with certain types of patients, even if they have depression. I mean, sometimes we take what would be considered, I suppose, calculated risks, and I have at times ordered people to be allowed to retain certain things in their possession because it gives them a sense of identity, of being themselves.

By the Court

Q. Razors?

A. Yes, sir, exactly. Of course, sometimes that doesn't work out so well. Even psychiatrists are not infallible. ...

Dr. Edwin S. Shneidman, co-director and founder of the Suicide Prevention Center in Los Angeles, testified as an expert on behalf of the defendant. His testimony follows.

Direct Examination by Defense Attorney

Q. Dr. Shneidman, will you give us your full name and present position, please?

A. My name is Edwin S. Shneidman, and I will indicate my three main positions.

I am co-director and founder of the Suicide Prevention Center, which is a unit supported by a 7-year grant of which I am the principal recipient, with Dr. Norman Farberow, from the National Institute of Mental Health of the United States Public Health Service; secondly, I am co-principal investigator for the Veterans Administration Central Research Unit, for the study of unpredicted deaths. These two facilities work hand and hand in their overall study of suicide and its cause. Third, I am currently clinical professor of psychiatry and psychology of the University of Southern California School of Medicine.

Those are my three main positions. In addition I serve as consultant to the State Hospitals in California, and on their editorial boards, and so on ...

Q. Have you published any books or any other professional articles in the field of suicide and suicide prevention?

A. Yes, sir, specifically in the field of suicide. I have coauthored with Dr. Farberow two texts, one called *Clues to Suicide*, and the other is called *The Cry for Help*, both published by McGraw-Hill, the first in 1957, and the second in 1961. ...

By Defense Attorney

... Your Honor ... we tender him at this time as an expert witness in the field of suicides.

The Court

All right. [Plaintiff attorney] may cross-examine.

Cross-Examination by Plaintiff Attorney

Q. Doctor, I take it from your testimony here today that you are not a psychiatrist?

A. That's true, sir.

Q. You have had no medical training?

A. That's right.

Q. In other words, you are not a doctor of medicine?

A. That's true.

Q. Is Dr. Farberow a physician?

A. No, we are both clinical psychologists, and we are practitioners, and we do research in the field of psychology. ...

Q. Have you ever testified as an expert witness before in court?

A. Yes, sir.

Q. For the Veterans Administration?

A. No, sir, but Dr. Farberow has done that. ...

By the Court

Q. Doctor, I am just a little interested in this subject from perhaps another viewpoint. I am a former legislator, and this question of people practicing medicine who have not obtained a medical license has been brought up a number of times.

Do the physicians in California where you practice consider that you are practicing medicine?

A. Oh, no, sir. I am not practicing medicine. ...

Q. ... Do you have to be licensed to do what you are doing by the State of California?

A. Yes, sir. I am licensed. Would you like to see the license?

Q. No, I am just trying to find out if there is any comparison in the status of a psychologist in California as compared to Louisiana, and particularly where a question of medical treatment is concerned. ...

A. As a matter of fact, Your Honor, I am not licensed; I am certified.

Q. Certified?

A. Certified by the American Board of Medical Examiners. Here's the certification. No person in California can call himself a psychologist without that certificate. It's awarded as a result of examinations.

By the Court

I think the Doctor's qualifications are acceptable. ... You may proceed.

By Defense Attorney

Q. Doctor, will you tell us about your position in the Veterans Administration in the Central Research Unit for the Study of Unpredicted Deaths and at the Suicide Prevention Center?

A Yes, sir. First, there are two separate units actually, and I will deal with them separately, if you don't mind, and I will deal with them, if I may, historically.

For a number of years, we in the VA family have been interested in this problem of suicide and its many and varied causes, and as a result of work already done in that field, we had completed a book and perhaps a dozen or so articles, and that's the way it began. Then, as a result of joint discussions on the subject, it was decided to establish a central research unit, which was to serve Veterans Administration Hospitals throughout the country, and all records of all individuals who committed suicide, while wards of the VA hospitals in patient status, were to be sent to this central research unit in Los Angeles. The next folder to the suicide folder in the case was to be sent along also as a nonsuicide control folder, so that we would have at this repository a clinical correspondence folder very much like the present one, and likewise a folder that had been next to the suicide folder, which as I said, was labeled a nonsuicide control folder. The purpose was to analyze and compare the two folders, the suicide and the nonsuicide, in an effort to ascertain the motivating factors that might have brought about the suicide in question, and to try and ascertain the signs or indications or any possible tip-offs that a person might be contemplating taking his own life.

In a sense, our main responsibility might be labeled as a searching for clues to attempted suicides and as trying to ascertain, from a comparison of these two records, the type of behavior patterns that should be looked for in patients, particularly with regard to any symptoms of despair or despondency and things of that sort. There are many clues to be looked for in connection with a patient's mental behavior or pattern while being treated in a hospital, so that could be called the primary purpose of this study and of the records in individual cases.

By the Court

Q. Can this study be applied to the problem of preventing suicides as well as finding out what may have caused the suicide after it has happened?

A. Oh, yes, Your Honor, that's what we are actually trying to do in this study of these records. We hope, by going through them and analyzing them and comparing them, to take a case of suicide, for example, out of the realm of unpredicted deaths into the realm of predictable suicides, the results of which might through proper application prevent suicide in many cases; it might keep them from reaching fruition.

Of course, our biggest problems, as you might expect, are sudden unexpected deaths where there have been no indications that they were going to take place, and that's why we get in these records and go over them minutely, looking for clues that might well serve as signposts in the future dealing with patients. That's our principal mission, as I said, at the Central Research Unit, and as a result of our studies along that line, we have published three medical bulletins. ... I have copies of all these here, if they would be of any interest to you. ...

By Defense Attorney

Q. Doctor, could you tell us a little bit more about these suicidal folders and the nonsuicidal control folders, what you do with them, and what you try to find out from them in your work at the Central Research Unit?

A. Yes. These suicide and nonsuicide folders are sent into the VA from hospitals throughout the country. I get the folders as a matter of routine at the center in Los Angeles in due time. Now, those are the suicide folders. The other folders are simply folders of veterans, some dead and some alive, who did not commit suicide. ... We have a procedure that we have initiated, which we have labeled "Psychological autopsy."

... [We] discuss the case, and then each of us will indicate whether we think the case was a suicide or a control folder, where no suicide occurred. ...

By the Court

Q. Do the majority of you agree or disagree in advance of finding out what actually happened?

A. Well, at the beginning we found that we were in disagreement more often than not, I guess you would say; but after a couple of years ... it got so we independently found that we were agreeing more than at the beginning. Through the benefit of the discussions, we found that we were refining the clues, the distilled notions, we call them, and it got to be a rare event when we couldn't agree from the facts as presented in the record on a diagnosis of the particular psychological autopsy. After a couple of years, it got so we would have a pretty good notion of what was going on, and we rarely disagreed after that. ...

By Defense Attorney

Q. Doctor, do you receive many calls at the Suicide Prevention Center from people, for one reason or another, who are in some kind of emotional condition where suicide could be considered a possibility?

A. Yes, we are listed in the telephone book, and we receive calls from around the community every day and every night. We are always receiving calls from people who are in distress in the local community. ...

Q. Doctor, would you tell us about suicides in Veterans Administration hospitals in comparison with other hospitals and hospital systems?

A. Yes. ... Of all the statistics on deaths in Veterans Administration hospitals, suicides account for 0.3 of 1% of all deaths. Now, this is not very different from other suicidal death statistics in other hospital systems. In fact, it's lower than some others. For example, state hospital systems have a slightly higher suicidal rate than the Veterans Administration hospitals ...

Q. Dr. Shneidman, how many clinical folders have you reviewed approximately in this type of system you are talking about, the control cases and the suicide cases?

A. If you would permit me to say it loosely, I will say hundreds. That would not be an exact answer, of course, but I don't know how many—a great many.

Q. Doctor, at my request did you examine the clinical folder of the patient, Louis R. Genovese?

A. Yes, sir, I did.

Q. After having reviewed that folder, Doctor, would you tell us your judgment—in the light of having examined and studied many other folders of veterans who did and did not commit suicide?

A. I am sure the Court will not, nor anyone else in the courtroom, misunderstand my remark when I begin saying that it was an extremely interesting folder, I mean, in the sense that it's a cryptic folder and a kind of mysterious folder in a way, at least to me, who looked at it.

For one thing, I knew that it was a folder of suicide, so I was not obliged to make a blind analysis in this case without knowing the outcome. I knew he had committed suicide.

If I can deal with an analysis rather than a technicality, in a suicide, it can be thought of as a kind of internal debate, a debate within the individual. It's when the forces of life and the forces of death are in concert. We call this a debate, internal ambivalence. Rarely do we find a case where the individual is unambivalent about taking his own life.

Now, the evidence of internal debate in this case is not actually visible in the record. There are certain symptoms, but nevertheless I want to say that I would have called this a control case; in other words, I would have classified this as a nonsuicide control case.

If I may use the word *perturbation*, which is just a general English word meaning "the state of being upset," the evidences of perturbation are there, but hospital patients generally are perturbed.

There are evidences here of anxiety, but anxiety is a normal concomitant of hospitalization. Those are some of the reasons why I say that if I had made a blind diagnosis of this case, without knowing the result, I would have said this would have been in the category of a nonsuicide.

By the Court

Q. If you had used the blind autopsy that you spoke of, you would have held that this was not a suicide?

A. Yes, sir, I would have. Of course, I know now that the man did commit suicide, so I would have been wrong, but from all the evidence set forth in these records, I would have felt otherwise.

Q. You would have put this death in the nonsuicide category?

A. Yes, I certainly would, Your Honor, I would have put this case in the nonsuicide group.

Now, if I may elaborate a bit on some of these symptoms that are noted in the record and their possible significance, I would like to do so.

By Defense Attorney

Q. Go right ahead.

A. These are things that can have significance, but sometimes only for the person who is doing the performing, so to speak, and if I am getting out of order in this discussion, you will please so rule me.

Q. You may proceed.

A. ... I take the position theoretically that most people who kill themselves—and incidentally suicide, we must understand, is an occurrence that is comparatively infrequent.

Just for the record, I will say that suicide across the board is about the tenth leading cause of death, so you would have to say that it occurs relatively infrequently. Now, of course, in some age groups and some occupations that will vary. In fact, in some occupations it would be listed as the third cause of death possibly, and in others maybe eleventh, depending on the many factors necessarily involved, but as I say, in general, suicides are listed as about the tenth leading cause of death ...

Also, in hospital care, one must treat the entire patient. It's something like a fire, a conflagration. I think one ought to be alert to fires, but you don't turn the hospital upside down in the terms of fire prevention.

There is something else I might point out in connection with any determination that is made as to whether to put a psychiatric label on a patient; relatives and friends do not generally take kindly to placing the patient in a psychiatric ward, so something like that has to be considered very seriously before such action is taken. The presence of anxiety or depression in a patient is something that has to be assessed as to the total picture.

By the Court

Q. Do people consider that a disease or illness of this sort has a stigma attached to it?

A. Oh, yes sir. ... We are ever mindful of the terrific taboo on suicidal deaths. It is factual, I believe, that in our society there are only two kinds of death that are understandable and expected, and those are natural deaths and deaths due to accidents. Other deaths, particularly suicides, fall into another category, and suicides are the worst kind of thing because they leave such a question mark, particularly from the viewpoint of family and friends. The question involves possible emotional problems, possible physical impairment, or both, and it is, regardless of how we would have it, a stigma in our society today. No one wants to go through with anything like that. ... Well, this patient did not communicate in anything like a discernible way his own private suicidal intentions; that is, in theory persons who are bent on self-destruction will generally let other people know about it, either in clearly stated language, such as, "I am going to kill myself," and "I am going to commit suicide." Or, they will let people know this in a somewhat coded, or elliptical, or guarded language. If I should say in this court, for example, "This is the last time in my life I will ever be in New Orleans."

Physicians and psychiatrists and psychologists in this courtroom would not from the mere uttering of that sentence arrive at any meaning such as that I was contemplating suicide, unless there were other substantiating clues or signs that they had previously observed, whether it be depression or despondency or other type of irregular mental disturbance. … You have to have something to go on more than just a statement. You have to notice irregularities or recall clues of various kinds in a patient's behavior pattern before the groundwork is laid for any such assumption. An example of that would be if a patient shows a tendency to give away things, like, "Here, have my box of cigars," or "Take my watch," things of that sort. Those are all clues that we have to look for in any patient, regardless of whether they are in a psychiatric ward or not.

The only clues of any significance that I have noted in this record with respect to that sort of thing, were those stated by the widow, and they are very cryptic. One would have needed literally the wisdom of Solomon and the genius and intuition of Freud to have caught them in this case.

Now, whether these clues were given by the individual deliberately, or whether those things just happened, we don't know. We know that in some cases a patient who ultimately ends up taking his life will give guarded signs of his intention. They may even give these unconsciously, but in other cases there have unfortunately been absolutely no signposts to indicate that something was going to happen of that nature. It just happens all of a sudden, and that's it.

Sometimes a person will write something that obviously gives away, so to speak, his suicidal intent; for example, something to the effect that no one is to see it until after he is dead, and he may leave it in a place where it can obviously be found. This happens all the time.

I have looked in vain in this record for such signals. I was not impressed by the patient's sleep record, for example. Sometimes that is a signal, the way a patient will display sleeplessness in various ways, such as sitting on the side of his bed or walking through the corridors during the night, or making a disturbance of some sort during the early morning hours, displaying evidence of insomnia in some fashion, but none of that is listed in this record.

I used the word *code* a few moments ago. One of the things we are continually trying to do in connection with a patient's behavior pattern is what we call to *break the code*, which means simply to unravel all the clues we do uncover, or that the patient voluntarily discloses, or perhaps accidentally, so we are principally engaged in watching for typical clues in persons who are under observation.

Q. What are some examples of some of these typical clues?

A. Well, Your Honor, like someone going on vacation, and Mr. Jones, for example, might say, "I won't be here when you come back," or something like that. Now, of course, you can't take a simple statement like that, as I said before, and arrive at a definite diagnosis of his condition, but that is one of the clues we do take into consideration in evaluating a patient's behavior, both emotional and physical; and if there are enough clues, we can arrive at an evaluation and then determine what is the next step to be taken.

In summary, behavioral clues are clues of behavior such as would give rise to the indication in any way that a person may be contemplating suicide, and as I said, these clues would include giving away things, making arrangements of one sort or another which could be interpreted as some kind of signal, or remarks made in conversation to those about him, which may or may not be couched in language that would alert someone to his intentions.

A typical suicide is a person who has made some kind of threats or, of course, attempts on his life, so as to put the universe on the alert so that they will come around to treating his pain or anguish or loneliness, or putting him in this state of perhaps despondency and anxiety.

Now, we do have cases that present a clinical story of a person shooting himself or throwing himself out of a window, and that being the first overt suicidal act on his part that has been indicated. That would come more under the nature of an impulsive category, and there would be hardly any clues or signals given in advance of the act.

Q. Do you think that some of these acts or signals, as you call them, result from a desire to arouse sympathy?

A. Well, that could be in some cases, Your Honor, but in the case where a person does end his life, it is a very profound and deep thing which is done rather than a desire to arouse sympathy, I would think. It may start out as what we would call a cry for help, or something of that nature, and, if there is no help, then perhaps it gets into another category where there is no turning back, at least in the mind of the potential suicide.

By Defense Attorney

Q. Dr. Shneidman … In general hospitals, what is the appropriate use of a neuropsychiatric ward in the prevention of suicide?

A. To give him sanctuary, that is, to put him at a place where he can't hurt himself.

Q. … When is a neuropsychiatric ward used for a patient in a medical hospital?

A. … I would say when a patient shows acute and gross emotional disturbance, when he really becomes a management problem, and I am referring particularly to his impact on other patients. He may not be a problem to himself actually, but he may just be a problem to the others about him, in which case a change would be desirable, but that's a management problem more than it would be an individual one. Now, if he shows signs of delusions, or anxiety, or hallucinations, or something such as that, he would be better cared for in terms of that specialty, so that would be another reason for him to be transferred to the neuropsychiatric ward.

Q. Doctor, in your opinion, from reviewing this clinical record and from reviewing the other clinical information furnished you in regard to this patient, do you think that this patient should have been placed in a neuropsychiatric ward?

A. No, I don't think so. I have voiced that opinion after reviewing all the records I have had available in this case, and it is based on my knowledge and experience in this field. I think there would have been protests all around if this had been done in this case.

By the Court

Q. Protests by whom?

A. By him.

Q. By the patient?

A. Yes, sir.

By Plaintiff Attorney

If the Court please, I am going to object to any further questions along this line. I don't think this man is a medical expert in any sense of the word, from his own admission, nor is he an expert on admissions to hospitals. I have waited a long time to make the objection, but I think we are getting far afield now.

By the Court

Well, I don't think the question of being admitted to the hospital is a medical problem or that it requires the action of a medical doctor. Actually that was my question of the Doctor because I want to get the whole picture before me. I am going to have to decide this case. The Doctor certainly is a prominent expert in the field of suicides and comparing records, one record with another. and making autopsies about suicides. The objection is overruled. You will have an opportunity to cross-examine him, and I will weigh his testimony in the light of the qualifications that the Doctor has given me. The objection will be overruled because I feel that I must have his entire opinion based on his experience and his training and his qualifications.

By the Court

Q. Doctor, I don't know whether you answered my question or not. I had asked you by whom protest would have been made, in your opinion, had he been moved to the neuropsychiatric ward.

A. I thought I answered that question, Your Honor—by him.

Q. You mean by the patient himself?

A. Yes, sir.

Q. Now, in the light of the objection that has been made by [the plaintiff attorney], I would like for you to go into the question of why you feel that you are qualified to answer this question, if you will, Doctor.

A. Yes, sir. Based on my experience as a person who has worked in general medical and surgical hospitals and who has examined hundreds and hundreds and hundreds of these records, about which I have already testified, together with my work in the Suicide Prevention Center in Los Angeles, and the fact that I have made a study of this particular matter for years and years, and that I have authored or coauthored several books on the subject, and my vast experience with the Veterans Administration in connection with these many hospitals and hospital records.

Q. Have you actually worked with MDs in hospitals in connection with your work in this field?

A. Oh, yes, sir, very often. I don't want to sound immodest, but I think Dr. Farberow and I occupy a somewhat unusual position in current American psychology, that is, in the new specialty, which is called *suicidology*.

By Defense Attorney

Q. Now, Doctor, in your examination of the records in this case, did you find indications that, in your opinion, would have called for emergency action?

A. No, sir, I did not.

Q. Doctor, can you say something about the relationship between a condition like depression and suicide?

A. Well, depression has classically been related to suicide, and it is accurate to say that if one were limited to one single symptom, the best answer to suicide would be depression, but now most depressives are not suicidal, and many suicidals are not depressives. It's kind of an overlapping ellipsis ... the two are not synonymous. They are far from being synonymous.

Q. Would you say something about the relationships between psychotics and suicides?

A. Well, there again the same answer would hold true. Most psychotics, or I would say over 99%, do not commit suicide. On the other hand, psychosis and suicide do overlap.

Q. Doctor, after having examined this particular folder in this particular case, in the light of your psychological autopsy that you have described in your testimony and your general background in this field, how would you have assessed this case, as a suicide or nonsuicide?

A. Well, I can only repeat, of course, what I have said before. I would have assessed this case as nonsuicidal.

Q. Will you give us your reasons for that opinion, Doctor?

A. Yes. From my examination of the record, based on my experience in going over many hundreds of similar type folders, you might say, I would have seen his psychological symptoms in the normal range of perturbation for a person who is hospitalized. I would have noted that he had some changes in mood, but I simply would have felt that these were explainable in terms of what was going on in his life.

For me to holler "fire" (and I am not hollering "fire"), but for me to say "suicide" would have meant that I would have had to have some visible clues which weren't apparent from what I could ascertain from these records.

Q. Doctor, do you feel that any special action on the part of the VA staff was called for prior to the time of this veteran's death in relation to suicidal risk?

A. No.

Cross-Examination by Plaintiff Attorney

Q. Doctor, for the record, you would say that you never saw Mr. Genovese, wouldn't you?

A. Yes, sir, I never saw him.

Q. Would you give us some of the signposts that you look for in these records, Doctor, some tip-offs that would be likely to be found in these clinical records?

A. Yes, sir.

By the Court

Do you mean tip-offs in the records when the patients committed suicide?

By Plaintiff Attorney

Yes, Your Honor.

By the Court

Very well.

By Plaintiff Attorney

Q. Would you give us some of the signposts and guides, so to speak, that you would be likely to find in clinical records of patients who take their own lives?

A. Yes, sir. First, we look for a history of a previous suicidal intent, like a cutting of the wrist, an injection or pills, an attempted hanging, and so forth, any history that might be in the record pertaining to that sort of thing.

Q. Well, those things that you just mentioned fit in one category, a previous attempt at suicide, do they not?

A. Yes, sir. I might point out at this time that we consider the most critical sign to be the history of the patient and a continuous, growing concern on the part of others of its general downward course. I mean history of eating disturbances, sleeping disturbances, and behaviors of sorts. And that might well include a history of impulsive self-destructive behavior. That history would also include things that wouldn't look like suicide intent, such as accidents, some sorts of mutilation, and getting hurt in different ways. Unless supported by other symptoms, these would seem to be purely accidental for the most part. We try to keep all of those possibilities in constant focus in our diagnosis and treatment of these patients.

Q. How about leaving the hospital against medical advice? … Isn't that included in this record, Doctor?

A. Yes, it is.

Q. Isn't that a sort of tip-off of possible suicidal tendencies, Doctor? …

A. No, that would be more of a tip-off, I think, to difficulties in caring for him. I would look to see what preceded this, as to what motivated him to leave, and as to what he did when he left. I don't think that in itself would be consistent with suicidal behavior.

Q. Let me phrase that a different way, Doctor. Would you be more likely to expect suicide from a patient who had left the hospital without medical advice than from one who hadn't?

A. As a statistics case, I think so, yes.

Q. Well, any kind of case; isn't that right?

A. Yes, that's right. …

Q. And this is not completely unlike a tendency to self-destruction, is it?

A. I must distinguish, if you will permit me, in my own mind between the mere fact of being upset and an indication or tendency of being upset to the point where suicide might be contemplated. Of course, in this case we know that it was a suicidal record.

Q. Doctor, we are not asking you now to tell us whether this was a suicidal record. You have already told us that, and you have already said that you would vote the other way, and that you would have made a mistake on that because he was a suicide; isn't that right?

A. True.

Q. So we know that already. We are trying now to get for the benefit of the Court all these facts, so that the Court can weigh all factors, and we are entitled to explore these things with you. Would you agree to that?

A. Absolutely.

Q. I think you want to be fair to these litigants in the determination of this case, do you not, sir?

A. Yes, I do.

Q. Now, getting back to my question. A person who leaves a hospital against medical advice is somebody who is mentally disturbed, at least to some extent; wouldn't that be true?

A. Yes, it would.

Q. Most suicides are mentally disturbed, aren't they, Doctor?

A. Yes. …

Q. I believe you stated that it would take Solomon and Freud to find enough clues in this record to be able to anticipate suicide, as far as this patient was concerned.

A. No, I didn't say that. My previous statement was that it would have taken Solomon and Freud to determine that this was a suicide record. Now, they are indicia of suicide in this sense in practically every record; I mean, far as finding peculiar behavior patterns on the part of the patient, but you have to get the complete workup on the patient before trying to analyze what's wrong with him. Until you get all the factors in place, it's more or less an educated guess, as far as the true picture is concerned.

Q. Does it help you, when you're trying to make this educated guess, if you call in a psychiatric consultant and thereby get the benefit of his notes about that?

A. Yes.

Q. Would it be fair to say that that would have helped a great deal in this case?

A. Yes, sir. …

Q. Wouldn't a psychiatrist have been in a better position to judge whether this man was a potential suicide if he did a complete psychiatric consultation than you did from this record?

A. It would depend, sir. I don't know how to answer that question. I will have to say in this field I am not an ordinary psychologist. I have had years of experience in this field, as I stated at the beginning. …Well, it's a curious thing, but what's going through my mind right now is that it has been my experience that very often psychiatrists who conduct a consult will have to go to the record and look it over to recall what the true situation was.
…

Q. Doctor, is character change one of the tip-offs you look for?

A. Yes, sir.

Q. Character change is reflected in this record, is it not, Doctor?

A. Yes, sir….

Q. Would a feeling or demonstration of a feeling of hopelessness be one of the things you would look for?

A. Oh, yes.

Q. That's in this record, too, isn't it?

A. I'm not sure, sir.

Q. Isn't there an indicium of that in this record? … Would an entry that reads, "Has lost all interest in caring for self," be a tip-off, Doctor?

A. Of suicide, sir?

Q. Yes, sir.

A. It could be in the context of other things.

Q. Including such things as character change, depression, loss of sleep, mutilating surgery; is that right, Doctor?

A. Well, obviously I am thinking of, and I think we are both talking about a total picture, a cumulative effect, a gestalt of the many items involved, and in all candor I have to say that I would have had to put this case in the background, just from going over it and considering its many aspects.

Q. Would it be fair to say, Doctor, that most records that you see do have the benefit of psychiatric work-ups? … Do you see many records where there is an entry made months before about requesting a psychiatric consult and no consult, and then another entry in a later admission to the hospital requesting a psychiatric consult, and then a delay of 8 days is allowed to take place? Do you see any records like that?

A. No, sir. …

Q. Do you have any impression that you could give as to whether or not that would be an unusual thing?

A. Oh, it would be on the side, yes.

Q. It's on the long side?

A. Yes, sir.

Q. And if there had been a psychiatric workup, Doctor, two things might have occurred, would they not? Number one, treatment might have helped this man, and number two, it might have produced some information on which to make a better judgment on whether he was suicidal; isn't that correct? …

A. Could I state, sir, that I was impressed by the fact that he was seen by a psychiatrist, who, I was told, was a professor of psychiatry at LSU on the Saturday before; and I can't believe that had that person noted suicidal tendencies, he would not have been alerted to the fact, and he would have done something, noted it in the record or something. That transgresses my imagination.

Now, as to your question, had there been a psychiatric consult, and had the results indicated that the patient was a potential suicide, I am sure then that the psychiatrist would have put down some appropriate entry, and medical steps would have been taken.

Q. Doctor, being seen by a psychiatrist the Saturday before, as you stated, would not be the same thing as having a psychiatric consult, would it?

A. No, it wouldn't, but I can only repeat what I said before, which was that if the psychiatrist had examined him (and if he was a qualified psychiatrist, which I understand he was), then I can't believe that if he had found trends that would indicate that the man was a potential suicide, that he would not have done something about it. I just can't believe that.

Q. Doctor, considering the state of this record, would you agree, perhaps in the light of several tip-offs that were present, that some minimum security might have been put into effect, such as, for example, removing a knife from the patient?

A. From the record, no, sir.

Q. You don't think that would have been advisable?

A. Not from the record.

Q. Do you mean to say, Doctor, that these signposts and the several tip-offs that we talked about were not significant enough in this record to justify this kind of action in your judgment?

A. That's true, sir; they would not have been.

Q. You mentioned some sort of tip-off, such as giving a box of cigars away, is that right, Doctor?

A. Yes, that is considered one of the tip-offs that we look for, and like telling the nurse goodbye on the floor, things of that sort. Those are all things that we look for, but as I said before, they are not of necessity in themselves indicia that the man, or that anybody, is contemplating taking his life.

Q. Saying goodbye to the nurse, that would be one of the tip-offs?

A. Yes, that's the kind of thing that you would consider to be a tip-off, but not necessarily of itself. There has to be other substantiating evidence if such is the case.

Q. Do you put entries in the hospital record, such as telling the nurse goodbye, or anything like that?

A. Yes, ordinarily, that is put in if it has any special significance. Of course, if it's just on somebody leaving the hospital, then it has no significance, so it's not put in. … A lot depends on the circumstances of such an incident, of course, whether we place any significance to it. …

In a lot of cases like that, the nurse on duty will use her own judgment as to whether to include it in her notes, the same as any of the hospital personnel and physicians. Although that is common phraseology, it can be significant of a diseased mind. We call that sort of thing suicidal ideation, talking as though well, he was going away, things like that. Now, once the staff is alerted, then, of course, that generates a lot more information because then a closer surveillance is kept on the patient's activities and demeanor, and particularly on anything he might say that would fall into the phraseology. …

Q. In a case where there has been no alert made, Doctor, you wouldn't ordinarily find entries such as saying goodbye to the nurse, would you?

A. No, that's true.

Q. Or giving away boxes of cigars?

A. No, you wouldn't find that ordinarily.

Q. But you might find that kind of entry if there had been a complete psychiatric consult, might you not, Doctor?

A. Yes, sir. It wouldn't be in the typical language of a psychiatric consult perhaps, but it might. ...

Q. Doctor, I think in one of your books or papers, you wrote that in a study made at random of 12 cases, 11 of them were jumps out of windows, isn't that right?

A. Yes, sir.

Q. Don't you think it would be a good idea to build all VA hospitals with similar protections for the patients?

A. I'm not sure about that. I have had debates with myself over that over the years, and I'm not sure of my position.

Q. Patients wouldn't jump if these stops were on all the windows, would they?

A. No, but it's more complicated than that. There are cases where definite harm can result from putting these stops on the windows, just like putting certain persons behind bars, and things like that. You just can't adopt the same method for everybody. At least, that's my thought on it.

Q. Well, Doctor, a suicide in a hospital could not take place without the availability of a method of doing so; isn't that correct?

A. No, that's not correct, sir. We have cases where individuals will get up from a chair and run across a hall and smash their skulls against the other wall.

Q. Well, that type of suicide is rare in hospitals, is it not, Doctor?

A. Oh, very, yes, sir.

Q. You wouldn't take a person whom you think might be a suicidal risk and put him on a window ledge just to find out if he would take a jump, would you?

A. No, not I. ...

Q. And you wouldn't give him a weapon, would you, sir?

A. No, I wouldn't give him a weapon. Now, are you referring to a knife?

Q. Yes, any weapon.

A. Well, I need to modify that statement, which I stated too quickly. Although I wouldn't give him a weapon, if that means that I wouldn't permit him to eat with a knife and fork or permit him to shave himself, then that would be something else. It would depend upon the state of the patient in his own mind, his own stature.

Now, I certainly wouldn't give him a loaded gun, not would I put him in a room in seclusion. It is the general psychiatric consensus, with which I happen to concur, that isolation of a patient can be injurious. We believe that putting a person in seclusion is not only not the best treatment for a potential suicide but is one of the worst.

Q. Is a psychiatrist likely to be more apt or able to predict traits of a potential suicide than a layman?

A. Oh, yes, sir.

Q. Would he be more likely to detect those traits in a hospital where he had him under observation than in a nonhospital situation?

A. Yes.

Q. The likelihood would increase in both situations; is that right, Doctor?

A. Yes, sir. ... Well, I am reflecting, and in response to your question, often the first important tips come from nursing personnel, and psychiatric aides, and aides on the ward; that is to say, it doesn't take a psychiatric consultation to see these clues if they are visible enough.

Q. Well, the kind of prompt, suitable treatment that we are talking about, or that you referred to in your text, is treatment by a professional psychiatrist, or someone like you; isn't that true?

A. Yes, sir. If a person is determined to be suicidal or to have suicidal tendencies, there should be prompt treatment.

Q. Would you recommend, or would you not, Doctor, that some security measures be taken for many patients where you may not be ready to make a diagnosis that he is suicidal, but it is suspected? Don't you recommend conservative treatment in that kind of situation?

A. No, sir. My record indicates that I actually recommend the open-door policy, and part of the total treatment is reintegration with the community and reunion with the family.

Q. I don't think I made my question clear.

A. I'm sorry, sir.

Q. Let's assume that you have a patient who had signs that may not be sufficient for you to determine that he is definitely suicidal, but you suspect it. Would you not treat that patient different from a patient, let's say, where you did not suspect it?

A. If I suspected he was suicidal?

Q. Yes.

A. Yes, I would. ...

Q. Could we use as an analogy a situation where often a physician will treat someone for a disease that may necessarily not occur or exist, but where they have a suspicion of it?

A. I'm not sure I follow your reasoning on that question, sir.

Q. I am thinking of a situation for example, if I may enlarge upon the question, Doctor, of a childhood disease that the child is treated for, but which he isn't necessarily going to contract, for instance, tetanus, for which he is given antitoxin.

A. Well, I am one who likes to use analogies, and I know some of the pitfalls of using them. People have pointed this out to me, but giving a shot in relation to tetanus is different, I think, in our society, from putting a person in a neuropsychiatric ward, or in suicide status.

I think it would be possible to put every person who shows any sign of psychiatric impairment in wards and throw a net over the whole ward, indeed, over the whole hospital, but that's something I would not agree with.

Q. What about protection on the windows, instead of a net over the whole hospital, Doctor?

A. I can say in all honesty, and I am speaking in all honesty when I say that I am not sure. For one thing, it's a minor inconvenience to many people in terms of ventilation and this kind of thing, but if it's a question of serving to accomplish its set purpose, that's the big question, of course. ...

By the Court

Q. How many suicides occur a year in VA hospitals?

A. A couple of hundred, sir.

Q. A couple of hundred a year?

A. Yes, sir.

By Plaintiff Attorney

Q. Would it be fair to say, Doctor, that this record contains most of the symptoms you look for, except threats of suicide and previous attempts?

A. Yes, sir, it contains many of them. ...

Q. Do most of your control records have ... repeated requests for a psychiatric consult?

A. Many of them show requests for psychiatric consult. ...

Q. Doctor, are there any signposts or tip-offs missing here from this record except a previous attempt and threats of suicide?

A. Yes, sir.

Q. What is that, Doctor?

A. The wholeness or the gestalt of it; the fact that no one sensed it was going to happen, none of the hospital staff, no doctors, nobody said, "Suicide." That's what's missing—no relative, nobody. It came as a complete surprise.

Redirect Examination by Defense Attorney

Q. Doctor, a number of factors were discussed by you on cross-examination as to whether there were suicide signposts.

A. Yes, sir.

Q. Isn't it really a question of degree?

A. Well, I would rather say it would be a qualitative difference, in that each signpost would depend somewhat on the other, and that's why I mentioned a few minutes ago that you have to take the gestalt, or the whole picture, in order to arrive at an opinion.

Q. Now, Doctor, on direct examination you gave an expert opinion. Do you wish to change that opinion now?

A. What opinion is that?

Q. That from your experience, from looking at that clinical folder involving this patient, that you were of the opinion that it was a nonsuicide case.

A. No, sir, I don't wish to change that.

Re-Cross-Examination by Plaintiff Attorney

Q. Doctor, in considering all the signposts and all the testimony and the whole record that we discussed, would it be fair to say that it would all add up to the slightest suspicion of suicide?

A. Yes, in this sense, no suspicion to an absolute certainty, but in this sense, one can have some suspicion of suicide about everybody—me, you, everybody—and in that sense I will say yes. As I said at the beginning of my testimony, I don't want to holler "fire" unless there's something to alert me to it. It's not good practice, either, to call everyone suicidal. So, to answer your question, I would not have suspected it in this case. I would have guessed wrong on this case.

Q. You would have guessed wrong.

A. Yes, sir.

Dr. William C. Super, psychiatrist, and Director of Psychiatry at Charity Hospital in New Orleans, testified as an expert on behalf of the defendant. His testimony follows.

Direct Examination by Defense Attorney

Q. Dr. Super, would you state your full name and occupation, please?

A. Dr. William C. Super. I am a psychiatrist.

Q. Doctor, would you give us a brief history of your background and education and the various Boards to which you belong?

A. I received my medical degree from Tulane University in 1949. I had a year of internship at the Walter Reed General Hospital in 1949 and 1950. I received my psychiatric training at the Menninger Foundation Hospital from 1950 to 1953. I served as chief of the mental installation at Fort Hood, Texas, from 1953 to 1955, and since that time I have been director of psychiatry at Charity Hospital.

I am certified by the American Board of Psychiatry and Neurology, I am a Fellow in the American Psychiatric Association, and I am on the staff of the Tulane and LSU Medical Schools.

Q. Do you have any connection with any other hospitals beside Charity Hospital?

A. I am on the staff of DePaul, and I was formerly on the staff of Touro Infirmary.

Q. Approximately how long have you been director of psychiatry at Charity Hospital?

A. Since 1955.

Q. During that time, Doctor, did you have any occasion to come into contact with patients in which suicide was a possibility?

A. Yes.

Q. Approximately how often, how many patients would you say that would have been?

A. That's difficult to say, but I would estimate that approximately of all the patients I examined, perhaps suicide was a question in at least 10 a month, so that I would say probably several thousand patients in which suicide has been a question.

By Defense Attorney

I tender the Doctor as an expert in the field of suicide.

By Plaintiff Attorney

I have no questions.

By the Court

All right, proceed. Your qualifications are accepted.

By Defense Attorney

Q. Doctor, I am going to ask you some questions, but I would ask that you don't go into them in great detail, but answer them fully, if you please. Are you familiar with the standard of care in the community as regards psychiatric patients in psychiatric wards?

A. Yes.

Q. Would you tell us something about that, please? What is the standard of care; how are they handled?

A. I am familiar in general with the standard of care as we know it, but, of course, there will be variations in what I have to say with regard to that because different conditions exist in different hospitals and with regard to different patients, but generally there are some facets that I can discuss. Do you want me to refer specifically to depressed patients or suicidal patients?

Q. Well, just take a psychiatric patient in general, just how are they handled in a psychiatric ward? Are they locked up, or what? That's what I want to know.

A. Oh, I see. As I said now, there is a great variation in this. Some of the severely ill psychiatric patients for the most part are placed in closed wards where they are protected from themselves and from their environment, and this is the case in a general hospital, such as Charity, VA, or Touro, or in specific psychiatric hospitals, such as DePaul, or one of the state mental hospitals.

Some patients, who are less severely ill, are placed in open psychiatric units and are cared for there. Other patients in general hospitals remain on the general hospital wards, medical wards, that is, if their condition is not considered dangerous and if they have come in with physical complaints that are to be treated there.

Then many, of course, are treated as outpatients, either in clinics run by the state or by private psychiatric offices or doctors.

Q. Doctor, would you tell us briefly how you would handle a psychiatric patient with suicidal intent in contrast with psychiatric patients with no suicidal intent?

A. Well, if suicide is a question and one considers that to be so after an evaluation of the situation, that this patient would be a serious risk, the patient is placed immediately in a closed ward and precautions are taken; and this is certainly so at Charity Hospital, to see that he doesn't injure himself or anyone else. Precautions are instituted immediately, and we even go beyond simply putting the patient in a closed ward; it involves the patient being constantly observed, and, with patients of this sort, we remove shaving equipment or knives or pens, even spectacles, and also belts, anything with which a patient might harm himself; and we place him at that time in a room in which there is nothing except a bed and a mattress, but no other items, and the room is a safe room. There is no way to get out of it. It has safety screens.

Now, these precautions are taken until such time as the psychiatrists treating him are convinced that he is no longer a suicidal risk or until it is discovered that the initial impression was a mistaken one and that he really wasn't a suicidal risk in the first place.

Q. How do you care for other medical patients with emotional problems?

A. Well, of course, that varies a great deal. It depends on the severity of the mental problem, and if it is considered severe enough to recommend that the patient be transferred to the psychiatric unit, then that is done. The patient is transferred; however, sometimes he is transferred to the open unit, in fact, more commonly to that one than the closed one. And then at other times, he is left on the medical ward where he is, of course, more easily treated, and it is decided later what disposition is to be made.

Q. What are the signs that indicate to you that a patient has suicidal tendencies or is a suicidal risk?

A. Well, one becomes concerned about the risk of suicide when there are sufficient signs that point in that direction. No one particular item is generally enough to make a diagnosis that a person is a suicidal risk, but given enough items, you are able then to decide whether or not he comes in that category. I think with enough observation of a patient … and after gathering all the information you can about him, including his demeanor and habits and complaints, if any, and so forth, you can be about 95% or 99% sure whether he is a suicidal risk or not. Of course, first off we try to find out everything we can about the patient because the more we know, the more we can either corroborate our suspicions that he is a suicidal risk or determine that he is not. For instance, his age, sex, marital status, anything that we can find out about him. Given enough clues and piecing them all together, you can come up with a pretty good diagnosis of his mental problem, if there is one. If you arrive at a diagnosis of a manic-depressive type, that will make you quite concerned, and if you have a schizophrenic reaction with depression, you are concerned. And even if you have alcoholism with depression, then one is concerned. Those are some of the diagnoses.

Now, if a person or patient talks in terms of feeling very despondent, saying things to the effect that life isn't worthwhile, or that he doesn't want to go on, or that it's hopeless, or that he has nothing to live for, or if patients talk in terms of what should be done with their belongings and this kind of thing, or if they have a great deal of preoccupation with death, or as to the time they are going to go, then you would have concern.

We run into all those symptoms, such as a patient saying he would be better off dead, and things like that. Other things we look for are symptoms of severe insomnia, lack of appetite, weight loss, and so forth.

Q. How about prior attempts at suicide, Doctor?

A. Well, of course, any attempt or prior attempt at suicide, you have to take that into consideration, certainly.

Q. Doctor, is depression synonymous with suicidal risk?

A. No.

Q. What are the different kinds of depression?

A. Well, there are different types of diagnoses in which depression is an important aspect. You have the psychotic depressive reaction, the manic depressive, the neurotic depressive reaction, or just ordinary depressive reaction. You can have obsessive compulsive reaction, with depression, and so forth. In other words, the depression is the primary thing.

Q. What would be the difference between neurotic depression and psychotic depression?

A. Well, psychotic depression presents the type of person that I was referring to, the severe depressive type who is often profoundly changed in that he has suddenly lost appetite, lost weight, and has feelings of persecution, and unworthiness, and uselessness, things of that sort. He may even have delusions of guilt and may even be dangerous to himself or others.

Now, neurotic depression is something that most of us have experienced at times when we feel depressed. That's what the term neurotic depression means. It's something denoting anxiety and brings on crying spells usually, but ordinarily it produces hope for the future and the individual wants to go on with life.

Q. There is quite a difference, then, isn't there, Doctor?

A. Yes, there is.

Q. Doctor, is there any way of telling whether a person is a probable suicidal risk?

A. Well, yes, when you take the whole thing. You have got to make a complete study, and learn all you can about him before you can make such a judgment.

Q. Doctor, at my request, have you examined the complete medical record of the deceased Louis R. Genovese?

A. Yes.

Q. Doctor, based on the hospital records, do you have an opinion as to whether or not the treatment rendered to the deceased was equal to the standard of care in the community?

A. Yes, I will say it was up to the standard of care in the community.

Q. What would be the reason for your opinion, Doctor?

A. Well, it was handled pretty much the way most patients would be with the kind of findings that were apparent in the chart, and I think the hospital staff acted in what would be ordinary medical practice.

Q. Doctor, from your complete survey of this chart, is it your opinion that this man has a psychosis prior to the time he committed suicide?

A. It is my opinion that there is insufficient evidence to indicate that he did have this psychosis. I don't know if he had that psychosis. I don't know that.

Q. Doctor, I show this clinical record, dated 10/8, and this is a notation by Dr. Cohen, and I ask you to read that, please.

A. Right here?

Q. Yes.

A. "Blood pressure four times a day and record. Psychiatric consult. Patient with ulcerative colitis. Past history psychosis. Please evaluate."

Q. In your opinion, Doctor, did this man have a record of a past history of psychosis?

A. As far as I know, I saw no evidence of such degree of disturbance to warrant such a diagnosis.

Q. And that would be in your field more than Dr. Cohen's, who is a general M.D.; is that right?

A. Yes.

Q. Doctor, I show you from the clinical record a notation on 5/24/62, and I will ask you to read that, please.

A. Consult psychiatry—I can't make this out. "Forty-eight-year-old white male, postoperative. Colectomy for ulcerative colitis. Has lost all interest in caring for self and exhibits marked intermittent periods of hostility and feeling of persecution. Would you evaluate?" That's May 24, 1962.

Q. That's right. Now, doctor, in your opinion, would that be sufficient in itself to conclude that this man had a psychosis?

A. Well, one would have to consider that there is a possibility, particularly with this phrase about having lost all interest because that is one of the classic symptoms. If someone has lost interest in caring for himself, that can be a sign of severe depression reaction, or it can be a sign of schizophrenic reaction. Hostility would indicate possibly a serious mental disturbance, and certainly feeling of persecution would point toward a possible paranoid type of psychosis.

Q. Doctor, if the language appears in the record that this man had a possible underlying psychosis, would that in itself connote that this man was an actual psychotic?

A. No.

Q. Would that be more or less to evaluate and to rule out that possibility?

A. Yes.

Q. Doctor, based on the hospital record of the deceased, do you have an opinion as to whether or not this man could have been considered a suicidal risk?

A. Based on the record prior to the suicide, the actual suicide, there was insufficient evidence to indicate that he was a suicidal risk.

Q. Doctor, what are the reasons for your opinion?

A. I thought there was a lack of sufficient evidence.

Q. A lack of sufficient evidence to anticipate an attempt to commit suicide?

A. That's right.

Q. Doctor, do you have an opinion as to whether this man should have been removed to a neuropsychiatric ward?

A. Well, surely he should have been because he ultimately did commit suicide, but based on the record, there was insufficient data to warrant such a judgment that one would need to remove him to a locked ward.

Q. Doctor, the evidence in the case shows that Dr. Colomb, a noted psychiatrist, examined the deceased some 3 days prior to his death and did not find that this man was a suicidal risk in all probability. Would your opinion have been the same?

By Plaintiff Attorney

I object to that question, if the Court please. That's a misstatement of fact. There's no evidence in the record to that effect.

By the Court

Well, I will let him answer. He can say whether he would agree or not. He's an expert.

By Defense Attorney

Q. What is your answer, Doctor?

A. I would agree.

By the Court

Q. What do you base that answer on, Doctor?

A. Well, I know Dr. Colomb, and I respect him and his knowledge and ability, but, of course, I would make my own evaluation of the patient's condition.

If a psychiatrist says to me that a patient that I am going to get one way or the other is a suicidal risk, or even that he is not a suicidal risk, I am not going to accept that at its face value because I always make my own evaluation and judgment. After I do that, I either agree totally with what they have said, or I do not.

By the Court

Q. Is this testimony your own independent judgment of the situation, then?

A. Yes, sir.

Q. The fact that Dr. Colomb, the psychiatrist, makes his finding does not have control over what your evaluation is?

A. Certainly not, sir.

By the Court

That's what I thought. I could have almost answered that for you.

Cross-Examination by Plaintiff Attorney

Q. If Dr. Colomb interviewed this man and was of the opinion that he was not a suicidal risk, would the hospital be correct in relying on that evaluation, the VA hospital?

A. Well, yes, that's right. Certainly they would be right to rely on his recommendations since he is a qualified psychiatrist.

By Plaintiff Attorney

Q. Doctor, would it have been helpful to you if you had examined this patient while he was still alive, if you had seen him before making your determination?

A. Oh, yes.

Q. The best way to determine whether a patient has suicidal tendencies is to have a psychiatrist do a full work-up on him, isn't that true?

A. Yes, I would say so. A five-minute interview with a patient is worth several hours of reports from other people. Just to see someone for a few minutes to me is worth so much more.

Q. I suppose it would be more helpful to have a formal psychiatric consult, a full-length one, than have a five-minute interview, too; wouldn't you say that is correct?

A. Yes.

Q. You don't do psychiatric consultations in five minutes, do you, Doctor?

A. No.

Q. Would you agree that with a depressed patient psychiatric consultation is therapeutic in itself?

A. Yes.

Q. If a surgeon—a physician not a psychiatrist—referred a patient to you with the notation that he had a past history of psychosis, would you be more likely to schedule a patient for an early consultation than if you didn't have that notation?

A. Well, simply to take a past history of psychosis in itself does not say too much because certainly there are patients who are psychotic for years and out in the community. If I had a patient who was psychotic, I would try to ascertain whether it was really an emergency situation. For instance, if the patient was acutely psychotic or had acute paranoid schizophrenia or a manic-depressive reaction, then I would certainly try to see him as soon as possible.

Q. Doctor, I realize that there are signals which you can get that are more significant than others, and there has been some reference to that in this case; but is it fair to say that you would consider a reference note of a past history of psychosis as a significant reference, particularly if you did not ever see the patient, which is true in this case?

A. Yes, I would have to take it in the terms in which it was presented, if I didn't see the patient. I would consider it a fairly serious case if that's all I had to go on.

Q. And you would accept the reference at its face value if that's all you knew about the patient; is that right?

A. Yes, I would.

Q. Do you sometimes place patients in psychiatric wards, pending psychiatric work-up, if you can't get to them right away?

A. Well, I do if it's an acute problem such as widely disturbed patients, very paranoid patients, or possibly dangerous or violent depressed patients. In fact, where you had a marked depressed patient, you would more than likely admit him to the closed unit pending a thorough evaluation because if you didn't, you might be too late.

Q. Is it fair to say, Doctor, that the ordinary standard of care in the community would dictate that a patient who is awaiting a psychiatric consultation, and who has some emotional problem, ought to be watched more closely than the patient who doesn't?

A. No, I don't think so. Simply the fact that one is awaiting consultation doesn't mean the patient would bear more close watching than any other patient. Usually patients who are awaiting psychiatric consultation are no real management problem on a ward. Of course, if they did display any type of violence, or if we considered them dangerous, we would put them in a closed ward.

Q. What about the patient about whom the observation has been made that he has lost all interest in himself? Would that kind of patient bear more watching than one about whom that observation is made?

A. You mean that the physician may be requesting this of the nursing staff?

Q. In terms of total hospital care.

A. Well, he might request this, but I would have to know more about whom the notation was being addressed to. I think normally it is up to the judgment of the physician to decide if the patient needs more observation, but, as I say, I don't think that notation by itself means anything in particular, I don't think that that necessarily implies any emergency. I think rather that that must be for the benefit of the nursing staff or the personnel who had the care of this patient.

Q. Let me put it differently, Doctor. If you had a patient and you had noted that the patient had lost all interest in the care of himself, that he exhibited marked intermittent periods of hostility and feelings of persecution, would you make the suggestion to the staff that he be watched a little more carefully than a patient about whom those entries were not made?

A. I would, yes.

Q. Would you consider, in the ordinary standard of care among physicians and psychiatrists in the community, that there would be something that ought to be done?

A. Well, putting it in the terms that you do, yes.

Q. Is that a signpost to a possible suicide attempt, that a patient has lost interest in caring for himself, or no longer takes care of himself?

A. Yes, that's one of the possible indications, but, as I said before, that in itself is not diagnostic. Any one thing can mean many things. You have to take the whole picture.

Q. Is this one of the things that could be included in that picture, Doctor?

A. Yes.

Q. If a patient appears to be withdrawn or unusual, is that a signpost?

A. It might be, yes. Now, some of these things you are referring to were present in his previous admittance, as I recall, not in the current one.

Q. Well, Doctor, let me say that we are looking at the whole gestalt, as Dr. Shneidman put it, and if we did that, we would take not only the present signposts, but the ones with references to his previous admission; wouldn't that be correct?

A. Not so much the first visit. I think we would be more concerned with the current picture rather than the earlier one. I mean, in the terms of immediate management, one would be concerned with how the patient appeared and acted at the time of his current admission, not when it was present at the previous admission. For instance, if he was depressed about something on the first admission, and it had more or less worked itself out, then he would be over that. In that light, I think these would be comparatively new symptoms that we would be concerned with.

Q. However, these current symptoms that we have been discussing could be regarded as signposts to possible suicide; would that be a correct statement?

A. Yes, but with these depressed conditions, they do get over them, and this patient could have been depressed over something or some condition that existed or developed following his previous visit to the hospital. That's what I mean.

Q. Well, Doctor, I don't want to quibble, but I am just asking if, in evaluating a man's emotional condition, we shouldn't take in his entire history and background to further aid the evaluation?

A. Yes, we always take the history.

Q. And you consider the background of what prior troubles he may have had in evaluating his entire condition, don't you, Doctor?

A. Yes, you do that. What I am getting at is that we are more concerned with current problems as a rule than in something that he might successfully have gotten over.

Q. Would you consider it significant that in the course of a couple of days in the hospital, two doctors don't see anything significant that would call for a psychiatric consultation, and then in the course of 2 days two other doctors decide that the patient ought to have a consultation? Would you conclude that something had occurred to make them reach that conclusion?

By Defense Attorney

That's an unfair statement, if the Court please. We object to it.

By the Court

… I think you ought to be more specific with that question. Suppose you tell him who did what and ask him what he thinks about it, and for what reason.

Plaintiff Attorney

Q. What I am getting at, Doctor, is—let's assume that it is a fact, according to the record, that Dr. Valle, who admitted the patient, and Dr. Toups, who examined him the same day, that neither one of them saw any necessity for a psychiatric consultation; and then within the course of 2 days, Dr. Colomb and, I believe, Dr. Atik decided that one was necessary. Would you consider that to be significant, that there was some change in the patient that brought that about?

A. It could be that, or it could be that these were different doctors with a different view of the thing, and that they saw things the previous doctors hadn't seen. They might have made a more thorough examination, and they might have simply, in the course of evaluating his illness of ulcerative colitis, determined that he should have a psychiatric workup or consultation. It's not uncommon to obtain a psychiatric consultation when one is indicated. It doesn't have to be an emergency or anything like that.

Q. Doctor, if you were referred to a patient for a psychiatric consultation with an entry on the referral note of past history of psychosis, would you try to see that patient sooner than within 8 days?

A. Well, I try to see any patient as soon as I can.

By Defense Attorney

If Your Honor please, is he talking about a general situation or this specific patient?

By the Court

I think he's asking a general question.

By Defense Attorney

All right, thank you.

By Plaintiff Attorney

Q. Would you answer the question, Doctor?

A. Well, generally speaking, I attempt to see them as soon as I can. Now, if I have direct communication with the physician, I will ask him if this is an emergency or can this patient wait, and, of course, then my next step depends on what he says. Sometimes, therefore, when it would contain a past history of psychosis, I would be inclined to handle it in a routine manner, to answer your question.

Q. You wouldn't put that patient ahead of one on whom there was no such note on the referral slip?

A. No, not just on that alone. As I said before, I would not be so much interested in a past history of psychosis as I would be in whether he currently was psychotic.

Q. Is character change one of the signposts you would look for in a possible suicide?

A. Well, no, it's not particularly direct in itself. It's not one of the cardinal signs of suicide. More often when you see a person with a character change, it could well be a brain tumor or brain damage of some sort, rather than an indication that the person is going to commit suicide.

Q. What about previous mutilating surgery; is that significant?

A. Previous mutilating surgery?

Q. Yes.

A. Well, you would have to consider that this might tend to make a person depressed in itself, but it is not common enough to be one of the cardinal signs of suicide in general; but it would make you wonder if the person was not depressed as a result of this, yes. Now, certainly just on the face of it, a man who has the kind of surgery that Mr. Genovese had has to be somewhat depressed; anyone is with this.

Q. Would you say, Doctor, that a person who is hospitalized and who is a potential suicide is more likely to be detected than one who is not hospitalized?

A. Not necessarily. Generally speaking, many suicides, successful suicides, communicate their intent to someone, and often this includes physicians who miss the boat and don't pick it up.

Q. What about psychiatrists, aren't they more capable of ascertaining that possible development through these various signposts we have been discussing?

A. Well, psychiatrists ought to be able to pick it up. Certainly they should be more apt to pick up these indications, these potential suicides.

Q. Does psychiatric treatment help depression?

A. Yes. That's one of the things we can cure.

By the Court

Q. Is that done by drugs, or how?

A. The best treatment for a severe depressive is still electroconvulsive therapy, which is shock treatment. That will snap them out of it.

Q. Shock therapy sometimes also has unpleasant side effects, doesn't it?

A. Yes, sir.

Q. Are depressives the most common type of suicide?

A. Yes, sir, depressives commit suicide more often than patients with other categories of illness or disease that we know about.

By the Court

Very well.

The court ruled for the defendant. It found that foreseeability of harm, an essential element to actionable negligence, was not established by the plaintiff. Frederic v. United States, 246 F. Supp. 368 (E.D.La. 1965).

Endnotes

1. One psychiatrist says: "Half of my patients seen every day have attempted suicide, and I am not talking of 'gestures.' One-quarter have tried to kill themselves in the last 12 months. Suicidality is the norm in the practice of psychiatry. So, how to deal with all this, especially in a managed care environment? If I focus on their imminent death, I would usually fail them, as hospitalization of a few days would yield only another failure." Personal communication.

2. B. Bongar et al. (Eds.), *Risk Management With Suicidal Patients* (New York: Guilford Press, 1998).

3. R.I. Simon, *Assessing and Managing Suicide Risk* (Arlington, VA: American Psychiatric Publishing, 2004); R.I. Simon & R.E. Hales (Eds.), *Textbook of Suicide Assessment and Management* (Arlington, VA: American Psychiatric Publishing, 2006). Dr. John Chiles and Kirk Strosahl, PhD, in a study of hospitals and suicidal behavior point out that there is little conclusive evidence to suggest that being placed on a psychiatric unit reduces the chance of suicide in either the short or the long term, and indeed, they say it may exacerbate the chance of suicide. The study is counter-intuitive and it would undercut malpractice suits for failure to hospitalize. See J.A. Chiles & K.D. Strosahl, *Clinical Manual for Assessment and Treatment of Suicidal Patients* (Arlington, VA: American Psychiatric Publishing, 2004), p. 203. A 1997 study reported in the American Psychiatric Association's *Psychiatric News* states that "the long-term clinical risk suicide decreased from 40% at admission to 30% at discharge"; www.psych.org/pnews. Follow-up of patients is crucial to suicide prevention, but quite often it is not done. In following up on its discharged patients, the Henry Ford Department of Psychiatry claims that it

has reduced the suicide rate among its patients by 75%, to 22 per 100,000 patients, compared with the expected rate in the literature of 1,000 per 100,000. C.E. Coffey, "Pursuing Perfect Depression Care," *Psychiat. Serv.* 57 (2006): 1524.

4. F.J. Ayd & C. Daileader, "The Correlation Between Suicide and Panic Disorder," *Psychiatric Times*, Sept. 2000, p. 37.

5. Murder–suicide is commonly the result of self-hatred turned outward and then turned inward. It is exemplified in the 1999 attack on Columbine High School by two of its students, Eric Harris (aged 18) and Dylan Klebold (aged 17), resulting in 15 dead and 24 wounded, and their suicides. In their diaries they wrote that they hated the world, and themselves. See D.J. West, *Murder Followed by Suicide* (London: Heinemann, 1965). The classic sociological study of suicide is E. Durkheim, *Suicide* (New York: Free Press, 1951). The book has stood the test of time. Durkheim talked of alienation, a disconnection of a sort.

6. Despair and self-loathing drive untold numbers of homosexuals and African Americans to end their lives. See A.F. Poussaint & A. Alexander, *Lay My Burden Down* (Boston: Beacon Press, 2000); G. Remafedi, "Suicide and Sexual Orientation," *Arch. Gen. Psychiat.* 56 (1999): 885.

7. J. Leo, "Could Suicide Be Contagious?" *Time*, Feb. 24, 1986, p. 59. The songs of the rock group "Dead Dolphins" in Russia were invariably about death and suicide. Not long ago a member of the group, Sergie Zolotyuna, the son of a famous actor, committed suicide. The day before, in the presence of his father, he broke furniture. He was the son of the second marriage of his thrice-married father. It is speculated that the songs of the group influence many youngsters to commit suicide. A. Velugehsnun, "Son of Valerie Zolotyuna—A Victim of Cult of Death," *Komsomolyskaya Pravda*, July 6–12, 2007, pp. 16–17.

8. See J. Barron, "Youth Suicides: Are Their Lives Harder to Live?" *New York Times*, April 15, 1987, p. 13; M. Elias, "Kids and Depression: Are Drugs the Answer?" *USA Today*, Nov. 30, 1999, p. 1.

9. See K.R. Jamison, *Night Falls Fast: Understanding Suicide* (New York: Knopf, 1999). See also H.L.P. Resnik (Ed.), *Suicidal Behaviors: Diagnosis and Management* (Boston: Little, Brown, 1968).

10. See Fernandez v. Baruch, 52 N.J. 127, 244 A.2d 109 (1968); Johnson v. Grant Hospital, 286 N.E.2d 308 (Ohio App. 1972). See Special Section, "Suicide," *Am. J. Psychiat.* 130 (1973): 450.

11. For an extensive annotation of cases, see P.C. Kussman, "Liability of Doctor, Psychiatrist, or Psychologist for Failure to Take Steps to Prevent Patient's Suicide," 81 *A.L.R.* 5th 167 (2000).

12. R.I. Simon, "The Suicidal Patient" in L.E. Lifson & R.I. Simon (Eds.), *The Mental Health Practitioner and the Law* (Cambridge, MA: Harvard University Press, 1998), p. 166.

13. See E.F. Torrey, *Surviving Schizophrenia* (New York: HarperCollins, 4th ed., 2001).

14. R.I. Simon, "The Suicide Prevention Contract: Clinical, Legal, and Risk Management Issues," *J. A. Acad. Psychiat. & Law* 27 (1999): 445.

15. See J.A. Chiles & K.D. Strosahl, *The Suicidal Patient: Principles of Assessment, Treatment, and Case Management* (Arlington, VA: American Psychiatric Publishing, 1995).

16. R.I. Simon, 445. See also J. Kroll, "No-Suicide Contracts as a Suicide Prevention Strategy," *Psychiatric Times*, July 2007, p. 60; D.A. Lott, "Risk Management With the Suicidal Patient," *Psychiatric Times*, August 2000, p. 9.

17. See Chapter 32 on contributing fault. In Weathers v. Pilkinton, 754 S.W.2d 75 (Tenn. 1988), the Tennessee Supreme Court held that suicide of a patient is an independent intervening cause that will relieve a physician of liability unless the patient "did not have willful and intelligent purpose to accomplish this." It is generally held, however, liability may attach even if the patient "knew and understood the nature of his or her act." They impose an affirmative duty on the therapist "to see that the patient does not do harm to himself or others."

In Cowan v. Doering, 215 N.J. Super. 484, 522 A.2d 444 (1987), the New Jersey court said:

We find no sound reason to adopt the sterile and unrealistic approach that if a disabled plaintiff is not totally incompetent, he is fully legally accountable for his own negligence. In view of the present state of medical knowledge, it is possible and practical to evaluate the degrees of mental acuity and correlate them with legal responsibility. In our view, a patient known to harbor suicidal tendencies whose judgment has been blunted by a mental disability should not have his conduct measured by external standards applicable to a normal adult. Where it is reasonably foreseeable that a patient by reason of his mental or emotional illness may attempt to injure himself, those in charge of his care owe a duty to safeguard him from his self-damaging potential. This duty contemplates the reasonably foreseeable occurrence of self-inflicted injury regardless of whether it is the product of the patient's volitional or negligent act.

See P.S. Appelbaum, "Patients' Responsibility for Their Suicidal Behavior," *Psychiat. Serv.* 51 (Jan. 2000): 15; S.H. Behnke, "Suicide, Contributor Negligence, and the Idea of Individual Autonomy," *J. Am. Acad. Psychiat. & Law* 28 (2000): 64. See Chapter 20 on duty to mitigate damages.

18. In Sheron v. Lutheran Medical Center, 2000, CJ C.A.R., 4416, the Colorado Court of Appeals said, "[A]lthough there is some contrary authority in other jurisdictions, we hold that a patient who is treated by healthcare providers for suicidal ideations, and who later commits suicide, may be found comparatively negligent or at fault in a subsequent wrongful death action based upon that treatment."

19. Hunt v. King County, 481 P.2d 593 (Wash. 1971). A number of cases are cited in Annot., "Civil Liability for Death by Suicide," 11 A.L.R. 2d 751, 782-92 (1950). See H.J. Zee, "Blindspots in Recognizing Serious Suicidal Intentions," *Bull. Menninger Clin.* 36 (1972): 551.

20. At trial, in the case of an institutionalized patient, the argument that is made is that precautions were inadequate in view of the suicidal tendency; and there are many cases holding hospitals and psychiatrists responsible for the death. Liability for the suicide of a hospitalized patient turns on the foreseeability of suicidal tendency and upon the duty owed by the physician and hospital to provide reasonable precautions to protect the patient from himself. Vistica v. Presbyterian Hosp. & Medical Center, 67 Cal.2d 465, 62 Cal. Rptr. 577, 432 Cal. 2d 193 (1967). See A. Holder, "Liability for Patient's Suicide," *J. Am. Med. Assn.* 215 (1971): 1879; I. Perr, "Liability of Hospital and Psychiatrist in Suicide," *Am. J. Psychiat.* 122 (1965): 631; H. Waltzer, "Malpractice Liability in a Patient's Suicide," *Am. J. Psychother.* 34 (1980): 89.

Expert testimony is needed in suicide cases. Payne v. Milwaukee Sanitarium Foundation, 260 N.W.2d 386 (Wis. 1977). Problems of suicide are examined in Surprenant v. State, 46 Misc.2d 190, 259 N.Y.S.2d 306 (Ct. Cl. 1965). The plaintiff was a mentally retarded patient given to temper tantrums during which he would break glass; also during a tantrum, the plaintiff drove his hand through a window. See Collins v. State, 23 App, Div. 2d 898, 258 N.Y.S.2d 938 (1965). The patient had a history of suicide attempts, yet the mental hospital assigned him to a general ward and he hanged himself. See also Lawrence v. State, 44 Misc.2d 756, 255 N.Y.S.2d 129 (Ct. Cl. 1964). The patient with known suicidal tendencies was placed in a room on the second floor of a state mental hospital without proper gates or bars on the windows and with inadequate supervision; this was constituted actionable negligence, which was the proximate cause of the death of the patient who jumped from a window. See Benjamin v. Havens, 60 Wash.2d 196, 373 P.2d 109 (1962). The psychiatrist was sued for failure to select a suitable hospital and failure to prescribe necessary restraints, and the hospital was sued for failure to supervise or restrain the patient properly. See Tissinger v. Wooley, 77 Ga. 886, 50 S.E.2d 122 (1948). The psychiatrist was sued for selecting hospital unsuitable for a suicidal patient, and the hospital was sued for not guarding the patient. See Stallman v. Robinson, 364 Mo. 275, 260 S.W.2d 88 (Mo. 1960). The patient pushed his way through the door as the psychiatrist was leaving the closed ward and leaped out of an unbarred window.

Hospitals have been held liable for allowing a patient to commit suicide in sundry ways, as in Daley v. State, 273 App. Div. 552, 78 N.Y.S.2d 584 (1948); this suicide was by drowning in a vat of boiling soap. In Browner v. Bussell, 50 Ga. App. 840, 179 S.E. 228 (1935), suicide was by slashing wrist and throat. In Hunt v. King County, 481 P.2d 593 (Wash. 1971) and in Spivey v. St. Thomas Hosp., 31 Tenn. App. 12, 211 S.W.2d 450 (1947), the patient jumped from a window. In Broz v. Omaha Maternity and Gen. Hosp. Ass., 96 Neb. 648, 148 N.W. 575 (1914), suicide was by taking poison; in Dow v. State, 183 Misc. 674, 50 N.Y.S.2d 342 (1944), suicide was by hanging.

Liability is also imposed where negligently allowed escape terminates in a patient's death, as in Burtman v. State, 188 Misc. 153, 67 N.Y.S.2d 271 (1947)—exposure to inclement weather. In Arlington Heights Sanitarium v. Deaderick, 272 S.W.497 (Tex. Civ. App. 1925), the patient escaped and was killed by a train; in Phillips v. St. Louis & S.F. Ry., 211 Mo. 419, 111 S.W. 109 (1908), by a streetcar; in Hawthorne v. Blythewood, 118 Conn. 617, 174 Atl. 81 (1934), by drowning.

21. In Bellah v. Greenson, 81 Cal. App.3d 614, 146 Cal. Rptr. 535 (1978), the court pointed out the duty of care owed to a hospitalized patient differs from that of treatment of an outpatient, but there is a duty as well in the outpatient setting "to see that the patient does not do harm to himself or others." See S.H. Behnke & J.T. Hilliard, *The Essentials of Massachusetts Mental Health Law* (New York: Norton, 1998), p. 144.

22. V.E. Schwartz, "Civil Liability for Causing Suicide: A Synthesis of Law and Psychiatry," *Vand. L. Rev.* 24 (1971): 217; A. Stone, "Suicide Precipitated by Psychotherapy," *Am. J. Psychother.* 25 (1971): 18. It has been suggested that Freud out of rivalry drove Victor Tausk, one of his most brilliant students, to suicide. Freud arranged for Tausk to go into analysis with Helene Deutsch while she was in analysis with Freud, and he allegedly got at Tausk via Deutsch. P. Roazen, *Brother Animal: The Story of Freud*

and Tausk (Middlesex, U.K.: Penguin Press, 1970). Psychoanalysts say that a poor termination of an analysis may ruin a "good analysis" and, in some cases, result in catastrophe such as a serious physical illness or even suicide. See, e.g., J. Novick & K.K. Novick, *Good goodbyes* (Lanham, MD.: Rowman & Littlefield, 2006).

23. The same question has been asked about medication. The development of new onset suicidal ideation or violent behavior has been linked to medication. See J. Cornwell, *The Power to Harm* (New York: Viking, 1966); C.M. Vale, "The Rise and Fall of Prozac: Products Liability Cases and 'The Prozac' Defense in Criminal Litigation," *St. Louis U. Pub. L. Rev.* 12 (1993): 525.

24. S. Lesse, "Editorial Comment," *Am. J. Psychother.* 19 (1965): 105.

25. Personal communication from Dr. Mortimer Ostow.

26. R.G. Arnot (ltr)., "Electroshock Therapy," *Atlantic*, March 1980, p. 31.

27. Communication from Dr. Mortimer Ostow.

28. See M. Ostow (Ed.), *The Psychodynamic Approach to Drug Therapy* (New York: Mental Health Materials Center, 1979); M. Ostow, "Is It Useful to Combine Drug Therapy With Psychotherapy?" *Psychomatics* 20 (1979): 731. See also M. Clark, "Drugs and Psychiatry: A New Era," *Newsweek*, Nov. 12, 1979, p. 98.

29. Mich. Comp. Law § 333.1801 *et seq.* But see Mich. Stat. § 17074(3) (physician's assistant prescribing drugs).

30. It is estimated that 300 to 400 physicians in the United States each year commit suicide, or roughly one a day. Dr. Paula Clayton, a psychiatrist and medical director for the American Foundation for Suicide Prevention, says, "Physicians have the means and the knowledge and access to a way to kill themselves.... We don't have any data that says any particular specialty has any higher rates of suicide." J. Anderson, "Physician Suicide Rates Suggest Lack of Treatment," *Clinical Psychiatry News*, July 2008, p. 1. See also D. Noonan, "Doctors Who Kill Themselves," *Newsweek*, April 2008. Depression among medical residents has been reported to be as high as 25 to 30 percent. B. Rogers, "Depression and Its Consequences Among Physicians in Training," *New Physician*, Sept. 2008, 57(6). Psychiatrist Andrew McFarland, following his treatment of E.T.W. Packard, resolved to treat only men, then committed suicide. B. Sapinsley, *The Private War of Mrs. Packard* (New York: Paragon House, 1991). See Chapter 24 on civil commitment. Workers' compensation law does not provide benefits for an injury caused "by the employee's willful intent to injure the employee's self." See, e.g., Iowa Code § 85.16(1). A claimant must show that the job caused the mental injury and the mental injury was caused by stress of a greater magnitude than the day-to-day experienced by workers in the same or similar jobs. See Humboldt Community Schools v. Fleming, 603 N.W.2d 759 (Iowa 1999).

31. See J.M. Violanti, *Police Suicide: Epidemic in Blue* (Springfield, IL: Thomas, 2nd ed., 2007); A.L. Cowan, "Police Struggle With a Threat Deadlier Than a Criminal's Gun: Suicide," *New York Times*, April 8, 2008, p. C-18.

32. See State Farm Fire & Cas. Co. v. Wicka, 474 N.W.2d 324 (Minn. 1991); Comment, "Mental Incapacity and Liability Insurance Exclusionary Clauses: The Effect of Insanity Upon Intent," *Cal. L. Rev.* 78 (1990): 1027.

33. There is in law a presumption against suicide. Thus, when violent death is shown to have occurred and the evidence is not controlling as to whether it was due to suicide or accident, it is presumed that the death was not by suicide. See, e.g., Dick v. New York Life Ins. Co., 359 U.S. 437 (1959). The reasons: There is the human revulsion against suicide, and a social policy that inclines toward the fruition rather than the frustration of plans for family protection through insurance.

34. The California Supreme Court stated, "If the insured did not understand the physical nature and consequences of the act, whether he was sane or insane, then he did not intentionally kill himself"; Searle v. Allstate Life Ins. Co., 38 Cal.3d 425, 439 (1985). See G. Schuman, "Suicide and the Life Insurance Contract: Was the Insured Sane or Insane? That Is the Question or Is It?" *Tort. & Ins. L. J.* 28 (1993): 745. To determine the manner of death, coroners do not routinely secure psychological data. Only a few self-inflicted gunshot head wound cases are referred for a psychological autopsy, and those were instances where members of the decedent's family contested the manner of death. Thus, nearly all cases of self-inflicted gunshots to the head are classified as suicide without the benefit of a psychological autopsy. L.E. Weinberger et al., "Psychological Factors in the Determination of Suicide in Self-Inflicted Gunshot Head Wounds," *J. For. Sci.* 45 (2000): 815.

35. An expert is permitted to testify on cause of death because the testimony would be helpful to the jury as it may not be able to differentiate between a self-inflicted wound and one inflicted by another; State v. Bradford, 618 N.W.2d 782 (Minn. 2000). The expert need not offer a definitive answer as to the cause of death for the testimony to be admissible. Jahn v. Equine Servs., PSC, 233 F.3d 382 (6th Cir. 2000).

See R.I. Simon, "Murder Masquerading as Suicide: Post-Mortem Assessment of Suicide Risk Factors at the Time of Death," *J. Foren. Sci.* 43 (1998): 1129; R.I. Simon, "You Only Die Once—But Did You Intend It? Psychiatric Assessment of Suicide Intent in Insurance Litigation," *Tort & Ins. L. J.* 25 (1990): 650. "Suicide by cop" is particularly common among African Americans. See V.B. Lord, *Suicide by Cop: Inducing Officers to Shoot* (Flushing, NY: Looseleaf, 2004); A.F. Poussaint & A. Alexander, *Lay My Burden Down* (Boston: Beacon Press, 2000); E.F. Wilson, J.H. Davis, J.D. Bloom, P.J. Batten, & S.G. Kamara, "Homicide or Suicide: The Killing of Suicidal Persons by Law Enforcement Officers," *J. For. Sci.* 43 (1998): 46.

36. R.E. Litman, "Psychological–Psychiatric Aspects in Certifying Modes of Death," *J. Foren. Sci.* 13 (1968): 47.

37. B.S. Yasgur, "Self-Mutilating Patients Generally Aren't Suicidal," *Clinical Psychiatry News*, August 2000, p. 36. Freud postulated a death instinct, a theme taken up by Dr. Karl A. Menninger in his books *Man Against Himself* (New York: Harcourt, Brace, 1938) and *Love Against Hate* (New York: Harcourt, Brace, 1942). Many people choose slow destruction by alcohol or drugs or by smoking. See M.V. Llosa, "A Languid Sort of Suicide," *New York Times*, Sept. 1, 2000, p. 25.

38. See generally M. Baden, *Unnatural Death: Confessions of a Medical Examiner* (New York: Random House, 1993); W. Spitz (Ed.), *Medicolegal Investigation of Death: Guidelines for the Application of Pathology to Crime Investigation* (Springfield, IL: Thomas, 1993).

39. Suicide in the Western mind is invariably associated with despair, depression, or a disordered mind. On the other hand, those with significant mental illness are usually excluded from involvement in terrorist groups or as a suicide bomber because they do not tolerate the rigors of training, preparation, planning, or teamwork that is required. In interviews with would-be suicide bombers (or suicide killers as they are sometimes called), they reveal the view that they will go to paradise where they will have 72 virgins (apparently heaven will not run out of virgins). They are sexually repressed and they look forward to life in paradise. Incredibly, when carrying out a suicide attack, they protect their penis.

These suicide bombers are regarded as martyrs. They are honored by their parents as well as by their society. Once a person has pledged himself or herself to a suicide mission, groups such as Hamas and Islamic Jihad cement that commitment by thenceforth referring to the member as "the living martyr." Women, far more than men, tend to choose self-sacrifice as an exit from personal despair. Like male suicide bombers, these women often are promised a special place in paradise for their martyrdom. See S. Harris, *The End of Faith* (New York: W.W. Norton, 2004); see also A.M. Dershowitz, "Worshipers of Death," *Wall Street Journal*, March 3, 2008, p. 17. Death is not death—it is life in another and better place. See, in general, E. Becker, *The Denial of Death* (New York: Free Press, 1972). Pierre Rehov's documentary film "Suicide Killers" (2007) has interviews of would-be suicide bombers and jailed terrorists who set up suicide bombings. See also A. Klein, *Schmoozing With Terrorists* (Los Angeles: WND Books, 2007), pp. 54–57.

40. J. Prichard, "Killer Says It Doesn't Matter If He Dies," *Detroit Free Press*, March 16, 2002, p. 3.

41. S.M. Moon, *The Completed Testament Age and The Ideal Kingdom* (New York: The Holy Spirit Association for the Unification of World Christianity, 1997), p. 601.

42. M.J. Kahne, "Suicide Among Patients in Mental Hospitals—A Study of the Psychiatrists Who Conducted Their Therapy," *Psychiatry* 31 (1968): 32.

43. Quoted in J.L. Kelley, *Psychiatric Malpractice* (New Brunswick, NJ: Rutgers University Press, 1996), p. 67. See also J.I. Klein & S.I. Glover "Psychiatric Malpractice," *Int. L. Law & Psychiat.* 6 (1983): 141.

44. Quoted in J.L. Kelley, *op. cit. supra* note 43, p. 68.

36

Duty of Therapists to Third Parties

The law is in controversy as to when therapists owe a duty to persons other than their patients. The general principle is elastic; to wit, the risk that may result from one's behavior, as reasonably perceived, determines the duty of care to be obeyed as well as to whom the duty is owed. Third-party liability cases are subject to a variety of doctrinal descriptions. The courts may find as a threshold matter that the party owes no duty to the injured person or that the party's action was not the proximate cause of the injury. Establishing duty is a matter of surviving summary judgment and getting the case before a jury. If a duty is found, then the question is whether there has been a breach of that duty. *Duty* and *breach* are the touchstones of liability.

The issue of duty was highlighted in the most celebrated of all torts cases, *Palsgraf v. Long Island R. R. Co.*[1] A late-arriving passenger rushing to catch the defendant's train was pushed by a train porter as he was about to board and a package was dislodged from his grasp, and fell upon the rails. The package contained fireworks, it exploded, and the concussion overturned a weight scale a distance away on the platform, injuring Mrs. Helen Palsgraf, the plaintiff, who was waiting for a train to take her and her young daughter to the beach.

Judge Cardozo, for the majority, held that though there was physical injury, there was no liability because there was no negligence toward the plaintiff. Negligence, he noted, must be founded upon the foreseeability of harm, hence duty, to the person in fact injured. The defendant's conduct was not a wrong toward the plaintiff merely because there was negligence toward someone else. The plaintiff, Judge Cardozo said, must "sue in her own right for a wrong personal to her, and not as the vicarious beneficiary of a breach of duty to another." The train porter's behavior was reasonably foreseeable to cause injury to the passenger, but not to Mrs. Palsgraf standing a distance away on the platform. Given the circumstances, the train porter owed a duty to the passenger boarding the train, but not to Mrs. Palsgraf.

The fact that the porter's action led to Mrs. Palsgraf's injury, albeit physical, made no difference. The conduct of the porter involved "no hazard [to Mrs. Palsgraf that] was apparent to the eye of ordinary vigilance," said Judge Cardozo. His theory, now the prevailing view in various jurisdictions, ended the case. There being no duty as to Mrs. Palsgraf, there was no need to discuss causation or harm. The young daughter, witnessing the injury to her mother, and suffering emotional distress, was likewise outside the ambit of duty.

In dissent, Judge Andrews rejected Cardozo's theory that a defendant owed a duty of care only to foreseeable plaintiffs. Andrews argued that a person's duty to act reasonably is owed to society at large, not simply to particular persons. All persons injured by negligent conduct were wronged, Andrews argued, not just those as to whom harm was foreseeable. The crucial question for Andrews involved the issue of causation that Cardozo said the court did not have to face. Andrews understood that the law does not impose liability for all injuries that were caused by a defendant's negligence in the sense that they would not have occurred but for that conduct. The injury must have been proximately caused by that conduct. Andrews argued that the term *proximate cause* meant that "because of convenience, of public policy, of a rough sense of justice, the law arbitrarily declines to trace a series of events beyond a certain point." Andrews argued that foreseeability was a more malleable concept than Cardozo believed, and that the question whether the defendant's negligence was a proximate cause of the plaintiff's injury was properly the jury.

The opinions thus disagreed on two grounds: (1) whether the issue was duty or proximate cause and (2) whether the issue (whichever it was) should go to the jury. Cardozo thought that Mrs. Palsgraf was an unforeseeable plaintiff as a matter of law, whereas Andrews did not. Cardozo's view, limiting duty to foreseeable plaintiffs, limits the extent of liability. Cardozo's view was adopted in the *Restatement of Torts*.

In the event a duty of care is owed to the plaintiff, by whatever theory, that of Cardozo or Andrews, then the question arises as to whether the type of harm (or damage) is compensable. In a view that has changed, courts have ruled that emotional distress, without physical injury or physical impact, is not compensable.

The question arises: Can therapy of a patient result in a foreseeable risk of harm to a third party? The answer is yes. One result of malpsychotherapy may be a patient's acting out in an unlawful manner. Clearly, to take an extreme example, one who hypnotizes a patient and suggests the commission of a crime is a wrongdoer.[2]

In preventing physical injury, mental hospitals, we know, have a duty to protect third parties. They are obliged to exercise reasonable care in preventing escapes and in deciding on releases. In numerous cases, hospitals or staff members have been held liable for breach of this duty. Thus, as one court put it, a state mental hospital "has a duty to protect the community from acts of insane persons under its care."[3]

Hence, in jurisdictions where there is no charitable or governmental immunity, the courts have placed on mental hospitals a duty owing to the general public to exercise reasonable care in escape prevention or release decisions. In these cases, the courts, for the most part, have not distinguished between foreseeable and unforeseeable victims. The cases, for the most part, involved rather obvious diagnostic, administrative, or communication errors.[4]

The courts are mindful of the extent of liability insurance coverage, although this is not mentioned in determining to whom a duty of care is owed. Liability insurance policies are drawn to narrow the scope of liability coverage. There is a miscegenational union of insurance and liability. The courts not only consider the foreseeability of harm, but they also assess the competing public policy considerations for or against imposing liability. As one court expressed it, "Liability must be controlled by workable and just limits."[5]

Jurisdictions on essentially identical facts reach different conclusions in carrying out the formula that the risk as reasonably perceived determines the duty to be obeyed. Apart from hospital discharge cases, a number of jurisdictions (or various courts within a jurisdiction) allow only the patient to sue over negligent treatment, even when that malpractice causes physical injury to others—as occurs when tuberculosis is improperly treated and consequently passed on to family members. In an Illinois case of this sort, the defendant physician raised the specter of potentially unlimited liability to all those infected by his patient as well as all those whom they infect. The defendant physician also asserted that allowing the patient's immediate family to sue would constitute an artificial distinction between family members and all others whom his patient or his patient's family might infect. The majority of an intermediate appellate court agreed.[6] Justice Charles Freeman, however, dissented and would have extended the duty to the patient's immediate family. He said, "I cannot agree that limiting the right to sue ... to a patient's immediate family members, i.e., to those with whom he has special relationships, is an artificial and arbitrary distinction."[7]

In this type of situation, on the other hand, many jurisdictions have not limited a cause of action only to the patient. In a case decided by the Pennsylvania Supreme Court, a physician negligently advised a patient exposed to hepatitis that she could be confident she had not contracted the disease and was not contagious if she remained symptom-free for 6 weeks. However, the correct waiting period is 6 months. The patient refrained from sexual intercourse for 8 weeks after the exposure and then resumed sexual intercourse with the plaintiff. Both patient and plaintiff were later diagnosed with hepatitis. The court held that the plaintiff had a cause of action against the physician.[8]

For negligent infliction of emotional distress (as distinguished from physical injury), many jurisdictions restrict liability in the absence of a preexisting relationship between the plaintiff and the tort feasor. In a 1980 California case, *Molien v. Kaiser Foundation Hospital*,[9] the California Supreme Court relaxed the rule to permit recovery by plaintiffs who meet a direct victim test. The direct victim question is said to be a matter of duty. In all cases, judges decide the question as to whom a duty is owed, whereas causation is usually a jury determination.

In *Molien* a physician incorrectly and negligently informed a patient that she had an infectious type of syphilis, and she was advised to tell her husband. The misdiagnosis allegedly caused her to become "upset and suspicious that [her husband] had engaged in extramarital sexual activities; tension and hostility arose between the two, causing a breakup of their marriage and the initiation of dissolution proceedings." The husband sued the hospital and the diagnosing physician for the emotional distress that he suffered and for the loss of consortium. The California Supreme Court, in holding that the complaint stated a cause of action, said that the husband was a direct victim of the physician's alleged negligent act.

The California Supreme Court reaffirmed the basic principle underlying *Molien* in 1992 in *Burgess v. Superior Court*.[10] In *Burgess*, the plaintiff was a pregnant woman who went into labor and, because of the physician's malpractice, delivered a child with brain damage. She filed suit in her own behalf against the physician on a theory of negligent infliction of emotional distress. In upholding a judgment in favor of the plaintiff, the court reviewed the dimensions of the doctrine of negligent infliction of emotional distress because the use of the direct victim designation has tended to obscure rather than illuminate the relevant inquiry.

In a unique fashion, the court made a distinction between *bystander* cases and *direct victim* cases. Bystander liability is premised upon a defendant's violation of a duty not to negligently cause emotional distress to people who observe conduct that causes harm to another. Because in such cases the class of potential plaintiffs could be limitless (resulting in the imposition of liability out of all proportion to the culpability of the defendant), the courts have circumscribed the class of bystanders (nearby family members) to whom a defendant owes a duty to avoid negligently inflicting emotional distress.[11] In contrast, the label *direct victim* was used by the court to distinguish cases in which damages for serious emotional distress are sought as a result of a breach of duty owed the plaintiff that is "assumed by the defendant or imposed on the defendant as a matter of law, or that arises out of a relationship between the two."

Duty to Warn or Protect Under *Tarasoff*

Social changes have increased the likelihood that therapists will care for potentially dangerous patients who are not under custodial control. No decision caused more concern in the psychiatric community than the decision by the California Supreme Court in *Tarasoff v. Regents of University of California*.[12] Among psychiatrists, the name of the case has become a household word. Decided in the mid-1970s, it continues to be discussed at numerous psychiatric meetings and in countless publications.[13]

Nonetheless, psychiatrists, by and large, seem not to realize that it was a case based on the pleadings, that is, to resolve the question whether the law imposes a duty owing to third parties as a result of a danger posed by a patient in an outpatient setting. Duty is essentially a question of whether the law will impose a legal obligation on one party for the benefit of another. While foreseeability of the harm is an important consideration in determining whether a duty exists, the courts must also assess the competing public policy considerations for and against recognizing the asserted duty in any individual case. In the event that the court determines that no duty exists, summary disposition for failure to state a claim is the appropriate remedy.

In *Tarasoff*, the trial court had sustained a demurrer to the complaint. (A demurrer declares that even if everything stated in the complaint were true, it does not state facts sufficient to constitute a cause of action. It is, in effect, a legal shrugging of the shoulder. "So what?" In modern procedure, a motion to dismiss or summary judgment replaces the demurrer, and, if denied, the case simply proceeds to trial on the merits.) The California Supreme Court, in reversing the trial court, imposed a duty on psychiatrists or other psychotherapists to protect third parties from potential harm by their patients. In so doing, the court made the therapist a proper party defendant whenever a patient causes injury to another. In the course of discovery, when it is learned that the offender was or is in therapy, the therapist is named as defendant, jointly or singly.

In jurisdictions following *Tarasoff*, it is no longer possible for therapists to get out of the case by summary disposition on the ground that they owe no duty in law to the injured party. Under *Tarasoff*, there is a duty, and it is a matter for the jury to decide on the basis of the facts of the particular case whether reasonable care was exercised. The outcome then becomes, many have said, a lottery. "It must be borne in mind," the U. S. Supreme Court once observed, "negligence cannot be established by direct, precise evidence such as can be used to show that a piece of ground is or is not an acre. Surveyors can measure an acre, but measuring negligence is different."[14]

The *Tarasoff* litigation did not go to trial on the merits, that is, on the basis of the facts involved, it having been settled. The importance of the case is that it imposed a legal duty on therapists to third persons irrespective of the standard of care in treating the patient, or whether there was any treatment. When a case may go to a jury, insurers and others tend to settle. *Tarasoff* involved physical injury to a third person.

In *Tarasoff*, Prosenjit Poddar, a 25-year-old graduate student from India at the University of California, had met weekly with Dr. Lawrence Moore, a clinical psychologist at the outpatient department of the university hospital, for a total of eight sessions. He revealed his fantasies of harming, even killing, a young woman who had rejected him (Figure 36.1). He distrusted Dr. Moore, for he believed that Dr. Moore might betray him.

Dr. Moore, with the concurrence of a colleague at the clinic, concluded that Poddar should be committed for observation under a 72-hour emergency psychiatric detention provision of the California commitment law. He notified the campus police both orally and in writing that Poddar was dangerous and should be committed.[15] The campus police went to Poddar's apartment, brought him to the station for questioning, and they also talked to other people familiar with him. They warned him to stay away from the girl. They concluded that commitment was not necessary. Poddar did not return to the clinic. Two months later, when the young woman, Tatiana Tarasoff, returned from vacation, he stabbed her to death. She was 19, immature, and unaware of what her sexuality was doing to Poddar.

The chief of the clinic was outraged that Dr. Moore would break confidentiality and report Poddar to the police. He scolded Dr. Moore, "You realize, don't you, that by betraying his trust, you destroyed whatever chance you had of helping him?" "It was past that point," replied Dr. Moore. "And, besides, I think he wanted me to break confidentiality. His telling me of his intentions was his way of saying, 'Look, I'm out of control. I'm going to kill this girl unless you stop me. Won't you please stop me.'"

What if the *Tarasoff* case had gone to trial? What would the plaintiff have had to prove at trial? How could the plaintiff establish that the patient divulged a threat to the therapist or otherwise posed a danger if records may be protected from discovery under the therapist–patient privilege?[16] How should the warning have been made and to whom should it have been made? It may have been held that the therapist, in fact, discharged the duty mandated by the court because he had notified the campus police, and the victim's brother also had notice of the threat

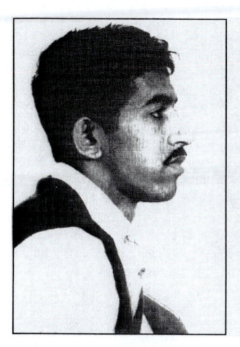 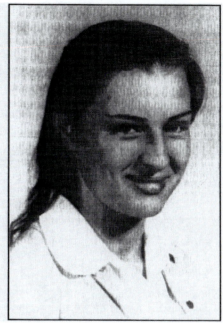

Figure 36.1 Prosenjit Poddar and Tatiana Tarasoff

as the police spoke to Poddar in the brother's presence. Given these facts, it could be said that the therapist discharged his duty of care as outlined by the court.

However, one might ask, was the therapy below standard of care? The *Tarasoff* case might have been litigated, purely and simply, as one of malpsychotherapy, like malchemotherapy, resulting in the patient harming others. One colleague at the clinic had suggested that the treatment of Poddar may have been beyond the ability of Dr. Moore. Was Dr. Moore able to handle the case? Not long before, events in Dr. Moore's life—a suicide attempt by his wife and her attempted murder of their child—had traumatized him. Following the death of Tatiana, he was dismissed from the clinic (that would not have been admissible at trial as the law of evidence excludes "subsequent remedial repairs").

The case might have been litigated or decided on the basis of negligent treatment rather than on the formulation of a special duty to third persons. That approach was not taken because of the difficulty in establishing standard of care in psychotherapy. The attorney for the Tarasoff family decided not to argue that malpractice in psychotherapy resulted in the killing because of the difficulty or impossibility, he perceived, in establishing standard of care in psychotherapy.[17] When the treatment of the patient is negligent and results in a foreseeable injury to a third person, there is no need to establish a "special relationship" as liability would follow under the principle set out in *Palsgraf*. Instead of arguing negligence in treatment, the attorney in *Tarasoff* argued that as a result of the special relationship between physician and patient, there is also a special relationship to those who might be injured by the patient. It was a novel argument. In the circumstances of the case, the defendants contended no duty of care was owed to Tatiana or her parents and that, in the absence of such a duty, they were free to act in disregard of Tatiana's life and safety.

The California Supreme Court during the 1970s was "a progressive court" that wanted to expand theories of law. The court did so in this case and others, and the court's ruling was followed in other jurisdictions. The argument by the attorney for the Tarasoff family prevailed. The court held that by virtue of the special relationship that a therapist has with a patient, there is a duty of care owing to third parties who might be injured by the patient. It is immaterial whether the treatment of the patient falls below the standard of care or whether there is a causal nexus between the treatment or the lack of it and the injury to the third person. Under the rule of the case, the duty is imposed even when there is no treatment whatever, only simply being seen in an interview. The court noted:

> Although under the common law, as a general rule, one person owed no duty to control the conduct of another, nor to warn those endangered by such conduct, the courts have carved out an exception to this rule in cases in which the defendant stands in some special relationship to either the person whose conduct needs to be controlled or in a relationship to the foreseeable victim of that conduct.[18]

The court went on to say that the special relationship with the patient also creates a special relationship with a victim of the patient. The common law did not impose an obligation to aid or protect another, even if the other is in danger of losing his life. In a classic example, an accomplished swimmer, with a boat and rope at hand, who sees another drowning, but did not put him in that peril, is not required to do anything at all about it.[19] The common law imposed a duty on a person to render aid only when that person created the peril or when there is a special relation between the parties. Thus, because of a special relation, a carrier is required to take reasonable affirmative steps to aid a passenger in peril, an innkeeper to aid a guest, or a physician to aid a patient. There are other relations calling for a duty to render aid. Unless there is a special relation between the parties, a duty arises only by virtue of misfeasance that foreseeably will cause injury to the plaintiff; that is, the risk reasonably to be perceived determines the duty to be obeyed.

Under the *Tarasoff* innovation, a special relation between A and B creates a special relation with C who is hurt by B even though A is not negligent toward B. Under the common law, a special relation between A and B did not create a special relation between A and C who may be injured by B. *Tarasoff* and its progeny represents an evolution of the law from no duty, to a duty to those in a special relation, and now to those who might be harmed by one to whom a duty is owed.[20] The court said:

> Although plaintiffs' pleadings assert no special relation between Tatiana and defendant therapists, they establish as between Poddar and defendant therapists the special relation that arises between a patient and his doctor or psychotherapist. Such a relationship may support affirmative duties for the benefit of third persons. ... Although the California decisions that recognize this duty have involved cases in which the defendant stood in a special relationship *both* to the victim and to the person whose conduct created the danger, we do not think that the duty should logically be constricted to such situations (emphasis by court).[21]

Under the ruling, when it is fairly known or knowable that a patient poses a danger, the therapist is obliged to use reasonable care to protect potential victims. What care is reasonable, the court ruled, is not limited to the issuance of a warning. The court set out various courses of action, to wit, warning the victim or someone likely to tell the victim of the danger, notifying the police, or taking other steps reasonably necessary under the circumstances. What is reasonable, the court said, can be determined only on a case-by-case basis.[22]

In Louisiana, it has been held that a *Tarasoff*-type lawsuit is not one of malpractice, or professional negligence, but ordinary negligence, inasmuch as the plaintiff is not a patient but a third party; hence, the therapist is not covered under the Medical Malpractice Act that Louisiana enacted to limit liability for physicians who enroll in the plan. The act was enacted in 1975 in response to a perceived medical malpractice insurance crisis. To circumvent its limitations, injured third parties argued that the *Tarasoff*-type case is one of ordinary negligence, and the Louisiana Supreme Court held accordingly. The court ruled, "The act applies solely to claims 'arising from medical malpractice.'" Furthermore, as the act limits liability in derogation of the general rights of tort victims, any ambiguities in the act must be strictly construed against coverage.[23]

Identity of Potential Victim in a Tarasoff-Type Case

Is the identity of the victim a matter of consequence in a *Tarasoff*-type case? Legally, should identity matter? Should it matter whether danger is to person or property?[24] Logically, what difference should the identity of the victim or type of harm make? Logically, the test would be: Is the threat serious, and is the potential harm imminent and serious? The patient says he plans to poison the water supply, blow up a building, or kill the first person that crosses his path. Is there not a *prima facie* absurdity to limiting the duty of care to the situation when the victim is identifiable? The scope of harm is potentially greater when the general populace is threatened. The answer, of course, lies not in logic but in law—the legal consequences of the distinction are enormous. If the therapist's duty is to protect society, every victim can sue. If the duty is owed only to an identifiable victim, only that victim has a cause of action. Under a duty to protect society, one and all in a crowd of people harmed by the patient could maintain a suit against the therapist. The potential of liability could be withering (save the practice of limiting liability to insurance limits).

The potential victim in the *Tarasoff* case was readily identifiable. In the years since *Tarasoff*, the courts in various states have responded either by narrowing its range of applicability to a specific individual or by broadening it to include unidentifiable individuals.[25] The U. S. District Court in Connecticut expanded its range of applicability from an identifiable individual to a class of victims. In the Connecticut case, a duty was imposed on a psychiatric resident's psychoanalyst for not notifying that resident's medical school that the resident was a pedophile. The court noted that the analyst had feasible and not unreasonably burdensome mechanisms for control available.[26] Apart from *Tarasoff*, legislation mandates that physicians and others report child abuse when there is suspicion of it; the degree of proof is minimal.

In the *Tarasoff* scenario, to safeguard themselves and to make sure of their legal duty, psychiatrists in various states have lobbied for legislation to provide that issuance of a warning alone discharges their duty. A number of states have enacted such legislation (sometimes known as a *Tarasoff-limiting statute*) that makes it possible for the psychiatrist to obtain summary disposition by having given a warning. Such legislation encourages psychiatrists to take that route, though it is formalistic and not likely to be helpful. While these statutes do not exclude other options, they do establish warnings as the easy and simple route to take. Ironically, a legal concern for patients and victims has produced a response in which formalism—not clinical judgment—has become the rule of the day.[27]

The Ohio Supreme Court ruled that the *readily identifiable victim* rule is applicable only in the context of failure to warn, but there is a duty to protect when the victim is not identifiable. The court, citing authority, stated,

> Unlike a duty to warn case, in which the therapist needs to know the identity of the victim in order to adequately act, the therapist in a duty to commit case need only know that the patient is dangerous generally in order to adequately commit him. As a practical matter, the victim's identity is irrelevant to whether the doctor can adequately act. By committing the patient, the therapist is able to protect all possible victims.
>
> The court does not believe that it is wise to limit any duty to commit according to the victim. Arguably, the patient who will kill wildly (rather than specifically identifiable

victims) is the one *most* in need of confinement. In negligent release cases, a defendant's duty generally has not been limited to readily identifiable victims, and the court believes a similar rule is appropriate here. Citizens outside of the "readily identifiable" sphere, but still within the "foreseeable zone of danger," are potential victims a therapist should consider if he has a duty to them and a means of adequately protecting them.[28]

In 1998, the South Carolina Supreme Court stated: "South Carolina law does not recognize a general duty to warn of the dangerous propensities of others. … However, when a defendant has the ability to monitor, supervise, and control an individual's conduct, a special relationship exists between the defendant and the individual, and the defendant may have a common law duty to warn potential victims of the individual's dangerous conduct. … This duty to warn arises when the individual has made a specific threat of harm directed at a special individual."[29]

Rejecting Tarasoff

In recent years, when confronted with the scenario of a patient posing a danger, appellate courts in Florida, Mississippi, Texas, and Virginia have rejected imposing a duty under *Tarasoff*.[30] The Florida Court of Appeals stated:

> If our society has progressed (or regressed) to such a point that there should now be recognized new causes of action where none have existed before, we conclude that it is the better part of judicial wisdom to await the establishment of such causes of action by legislative action after input as to all the variables from competing elements of society. We are unprepared and unwilling as jurists to declare that such a cause of action exists because we now conclude, with the more limited fact-finding resources at our disposal, that there is presently a sufficient societal interest to protect that requires judicial activism.[31]

In *Tarasoff*, Chief Justice Mathew Tobriner wrote, "In this risk-infested society, we can hardly tolerate the further exposure to danger that would result from concealed knowledge of the therapist that his patient was lethal." In contrast, in 1999, the Texas Supreme Court said, "Mental health professionals make disclosures at their peril." The court noted that while those who report child abuse in good faith are immune from civil and criminal liability, mental health professionals are not shielded from civil liability for disclosing threats in good faith.[32]

Consequences of Tarasoff

When the *Tarasoff* decision was handed down, many therapists offered fatalistic predictions of harm to the psychotherapeutic relationship. According to a study by Dr. Renee Binder and Dale NcNiel, the impact of *Tarasoff* on the relationship has been minimal. The study examined the effects of *Tarasoff*-like decisions upon the therapist–patient relationship, and also how potential victims fared in light of the decisions. All second-, third-, and fourth-year psychiatric residents (N = 46) in a university-based psychiatric residency program in San Francisco were interviewed about their experiences related to issuing a *Tarasoff* warning. Almost half of the residents (N = 22) reported having issued a *Tarasoff* warning. Most warnings were issued for patients seen in inpatient units and emergency rooms. In almost half the cases, the resident was unable to contact the intended victim, but did report the threat to a law enforcement agency. The most common reaction among those warned was anxiety mixed with thankfulness; most expressed an intent to modify their behavior to increase safety. The second most common reaction was denial that the patient would ever hurt them. The clinicians reported that in most cases issuing the warning had a minimal or positive effect on the psychotherapeutic relationship.[33]

What happens when the police are notified of a threat? It did not safeguard Tatiana Tarasoff. Psychiatrists Richard Balon and Rizwan Mufti of Detroit randomly called three police departments in southeastern Michigan, introduced themselves as physicians, and asked about the disposition of a physician's or psychotherapist's notifications of dangerousness. They were unable to find any procedure for handling these notifications or any established guidelines, and they were unsure if notification was ever registered or acted upon. They pondered, "[O]ne has to question the rationale of mandating the notification of authorities when no guidelines have been established to handle these notifications as well as when it is possible that no action will be taken."[34]

HIV/AIDS

The treatment of a patient with HIV/AIDS involves issues of guilt, shame, fear of contagion, and association with sexually transmitted disease, and especially for the latter reason, therapy places a burden of responsibility on both patient and therapist to prevent its spread. At the same time, they must be mindful that the stigma associated with it drastically affects an individual's personal and social life, occupation, and means of livelihood. All states require that cases be reported to public health authorities, while only some require that the patient's name be reported. Some states also require reporting cases or names of individuals who test positive for HIV. Over 30 states variously require, allow, or forbid healthcare workers (including mental health professionals) to warn patients' sexual contacts of the risk of exposure to sexually transmitted diseases, including HIV/AIDS.[35]

Genetic Disease

The duty of a physician to warn relatives of a patient of the presence of a genetic disease in the family has rarely been addressed, statutory attention to the issue is even more rare, and policy development is embryonic. Theoretically, analogy may be made to the duty to report infectious disease, though infectious diseases are contagious while genetic diseases are not. In *Olson v. Children's Home Society of California*,[36] the California Court of Appeals held that having knowledge of a genetic condition does not create a duty to disclose it to genetic relatives. In this case, Barbara Olson had the defendant adoption agency, Children's Home Society of California (CHS), arrange for her son's adoption. Thirteen years later she, then married, gave birth to another child. This child died of the genetically transmitted disease, combined severe immune deficiency (CSID). She contacted CHS to inquire about the health of the son she had put up for adoption and was informed that he also had CSID, but was alive. The plaintiff and her husband filed suit against CHS for the wrongful death of their child, intentional infliction of emotional distress, and fraud. Claiming that CHS had a duty to warn them that their child had a genetic disease, the plaintiffs alleged that, if warned of the danger, they would have either not conceived the child or received medical treatment to save his life. The trial court dismissed the complaint on the ground that the plaintiffs "failed to allege any legal duty." Affirming, the court of appeals rejected the plaintiff wife's argument that there was a special relationship between her and CHS that imposed a duty on CHS to notify her of the 50% risk of having another affected male child, stating that "special relationship situations generally involve some kind of dependency or reliance." The court distinguished *Tarasoff* by noting that in that case there was a "nexus between the impending peril and the specific duties undertaken by the defendants in those special relationships."[37]

Is *Tarasoff* applicable in respect to genetic information? The harm, genetic disease, has already been done. At best then, a healthcare professional can only prevent a relative from losing a chance of therapy or survival if disclosure is made in circumstances when therapy or a cure are available. In that event, does the healthcare professional have a duty to the genetic relatives of his patients? The New Jersey Supreme Court said, "The foreseeability of injury to members of a family other than one immediately injured by the wrongdoing of another must be viewed in light of the legal relationships among family members. A family is woven of the fibers of life; if one strand is damaged, the whole structure may suffer. The filaments of family life, although individually spun, create a web of interconnected legal interests."[38]

More recently, the New Jersey Superior Court held that a direct duty existed between a health-care professional and the children of a patient who was suffering from retroperitoneal cancer with multiple polyposis of the colon to warn the children of the immediate risk to their own health. "Although an overly broad and general application of the physician's duty to warn might lead to confusion, conflict, or unfairness in many types of circumstances, we are confident that the duty to warn of avertable risk from genetic causes, by definition a matter of familial con-cern, is sufficiently narrow to serve the interests of justice."[39] The relevance of the nature of the information was key to the foundation of the duty. The strong hereditary influence of multiple polyposis alerted the healthcare professional to a specific and easily identifiable class of persons who were at increased risk. Moreover, that class of persons was restricted (blood relatives of the patient) and so to allow the action did not raise the prospect of opening liability to an unlim-ited group of potential litigants. Thus, the nature of the information delineated the duty and its scope. The trial court in the case had found that genetically transmissible diseases differed from contagious or infectious diseases or threats of harm because the "harm is already present within the nonpatient child, as opposed to being introduced by a patient who was not warned to stay away. The patient is taking no action to cause the child harm."[40]

Recovered Memory Cases

In revival of memory of childhood sexual abuse, the harm that is the matter of litigation is alleg-edly created by the therapist. In *Tarasoff*, on the other hand, the danger is posed by the patient. The controversy surrounding newly recovered memories of childhood sexual abuse revolves around their accuracy, and that involves questions about memory:

1. Can memories of childhood sexual abuse, be it a single incident or chronic abuse, be repressed completely?
2. If so, can those memories be recovered?
3. If recovered, how is their accuracy determined?
4. To what extent does the present transform the past?[41]

The debate on reports and recollections of child sexual abuse goes back to at least 1896, when Freud argued that repression of early childhood seduction (sexual molestation) had etiological significance for adult hysteria. He later recanted, saying that he was wrong about the repression of actual experiences of child sexual abuse and that it was fantasies (of sexual contact with par-ents or other adults) that drove the hysteria.

In response to the controversy over the concept of repression, the fourth edition of the American Psychiatric Association's *Diagnostic and Statistical Manual of Mental Disorders* (*DSM–IV*), in its discussion of dissociative identity disorder and other dissociative disorders, shifted from the term *repression* to *dissociative amnesia*. The theory is that trauma, especially childhood trauma, creates a brain process leading to a dissociative episode, in which explicit memories of the trauma are lost. Though the name of the mechanism has changed, the approach to the buried memories remains the same. According to theorists and clinicians, the original memories can be retrieved through the use of recovered memory therapy (RMT), especially if the clinician pays attention to the emerging implicit memories that take the form of bodily sen-sations (often called *body memories*), repetitive memories, flashbacks, and so on.[42] The looking at bodily sensations is another version of the lie detector that is likewise a matter of controversy.[43]

The question arises: Do family members who are hurt by recovered memory therapists have a right to react in the legal setting? They suffer emotional distress. Clearly the patient has a basis for a malpractice action against the therapist; a number of patients who have recanted memories of sexual abuse have reunited with their families and then brought suit against the therapist for malpractice.[44] But what about a claim against a therapist filed by one other than the patient?

Parents conceivably may proceed (1) on a theory as in *Molien* that the parents are direct victims of the therapist's negligence, or (2) on a theory as in *Tarasoff* that the special relationship with the patient creates a special relationship with the victim who is harmed by the patient.

When adults in therapy claim recovery of repressed memories of childhood sexual abuse, the abuse supposedly is repressed until, with the help of a therapist, it is remembered. Treatment programs use a variety of techniques to help patients recover memories of sexual abuse, many of them guided by the book *The Courage to Heal*,[45] which contains statements such as: "If you are unable to remember any specific instances … but still have a feeling that something abusive happened to you, it probably did" and "If you think you were abused and your life shows the symptoms, then you were."

The book encourages revenge, anger, and deathbed confrontations. (It is quite possible that therapists who encourage their patients to "act out" may themselves be acting out vicariously.) The veracity of the patient's recovered memories is apparently never questioned. The book advised, "You are not responsible for proving that you were abused." Various treatment centers advertised, "Remembering incest and childhood abuse is the first step to healing."[46]

A number of therapists arrange for their patients to confront the alleged perpetrator in the therapist's office, with the therapist present to provide support and validation for the survivor. The therapists say that when people hold onto anger, they are at risk for developing a variety of physical illnesses. Some therapists have regular behavioral rehearsals, using an *empty chair* model, whereby the patient yells and screams at the empty chair. Allegedly, the expression of anger and confrontation is empowering.

Psychologist Carol Tavris debunks the approach in these words: "[T]he major side-effect of the ventilationist approach has been to raise the general noise level of our lives, not to lessen our problems. I notice that the people who are most prone to give vent to their rages get angrier, not less angry. I observe a lot of hurt feelings among the recipients of rage."[47] Robert Hughes, astute observer of the culture, writes, "The ether is now jammed with confessional shows in which a parade of citizens and their role-models, from LaToya Jackson to Roseanne Barr, rise to denounce the sins of their parents, real or imagined."[48]

Patients, once convinced that they have been abused, are furious at their parents and blame them for their troubles. They take such actions as suing the parents, refusing to let them see their grandchildren, or ruining their reputations by informing friends and acquaintances about the newly discovered memories.[49] In apparently no case of "revival of memory" has there been any objective or corroborating evidence to support a claim of abuse.[50] What evidence warrants an interpretation by the therapists? Is any needed? The prominent psychoanalyst Dale Boesky commented in an address to a psychoanalytic group: "As the first century of psychoanalysis draws to a close, we confront an ironic paradox. We are elaborating new theoretic models with pluralistic enthusiasm, but we are still unable to reach a consensus about how to evaluate whether even a single interpretation is useful or not."[51]

Dr. Paul McHugh, Chairman of the Department of Psychiatry at John Hopkins University and a member of the Scientific and Professional Advisory Board of the False Memory Syndrome Foundation, says, "To treat for repressed memories without any effort at external validation is malpractice pure and simple."[52] Moreover, he added, to refuse to provide information about the patient to clinicians working with the parents raises the question of absence of "good faith."[53]

In many cases, the memory hurts the psychological well-being of not only the patient but— through false accusations of incest and sexual abuse—other members of the patient's family.

Families, distressed and furious, retaliated with lawsuits and a campaign to deal with revival of memory therapists.[54]

National news weeklies *Time* and *Newsweek*, in the same week in November 1993, both had cover stories on hidden memories.[55] *Time* wrote, "Repressed memory therapy is harming patients, devastating families, and intensifying a backlash against mental health professionals." Earlier that year, *Insight*, another national news weekly, had a cover story, "Malignant Memories: Therapists as Coaches."[56] Also, at about the same time, the *New Yorker* ran a two-part article, "Remembering Satan."[57]

The American Medical Association has twice warned against the use of "memory enhancement" techniques in eliciting accounts of childhood sexual abuse. The wording of its last resolution, in August 1993, was especially harsh. It stated: "The AMA considers recovered memories of childhood sexual abuse to be of uncertain authenticity, which should be subject to external verification. The use of recovered memories is fraught with problems of potential misapplication." The American Psychiatric Association has issued similar warnings.[58] In no uncertain terms, McHugh said, "[Recovery of memory] is the biggest story in psychiatry in a decade. It is disaster for orthodox psychotherapists who are doing good work."[59] Professors Richard Ofshe and Ethan Watters describe memory recovery therapy as a new form of quackery.[60] Psychiatrists have long been called the Rodney Dangerfields of the medical profession—they get no respect— and controversies such as revival of memory make it even more difficult to include mental health under insurance coverage.

Safe from the backlash, enjoying governmental immunity, were prosecutors who brought charges of sexual abuse against parents or others on the basis of little more than the flimsy evidence of a revived memory. Some feminist prosecutors used the occasion to voice rage against sexual abuse. Then, with the backlash, judicial opinion turned against evidence derived from repressed memory. In 1997, Judge Mansfield of the Texas Court of Criminal Appeals said, "I believe that any testimony relating to so-called 'repressed memory syndrome' is inherently suspect and should not be admissible in Texas courtrooms."[61] Health insurers have been urged to act as regulators of healthcare providers by not providing reimbursement to therapists who engage in revival of memory of child sexual abuse.[62]

In California in the early 1990s, Gary Ramona sued a medical center and a pair of psychotherapists who he claimed created false memories in his daughter of his sexually abusing her as a child.[63] His lawsuit alleging malpractice sought damages for emotional suffering from the breakup of his family, and for harm to his career and reputation. He could theoretically have elected to sue on a theory of defamation, but California law grants a conditional privilege to therapists.[64]

Gary Ramona succeeded in getting his complaint put to the jury. It will be remembered that, as Cardozo put it, the court—not the jury—determines whether a duty of care is owed the plaintiff. The trial court rejected a defense motion for summary judgment. The court held that the therapists owed a duty of care not only to the patient, but also to the patient's parents.[65] With the case going to the jury, he was awarded $500,000, but it was consumed by legal expenses. At the time, no attorney would take the case on a contingency fee basis. The jury award was for "pain and suffering"; there were no economic damages; though he lost his managerial job at a wine company, he obtained another position.

The court's holding that a duty of care is owed was by itself a victory for aggrieved parents whatever the outcome at trial. When a defendant is said to owe a duty to the plaintiff, as we have noted, the defendant cannot avoid a trial by summary judgment. It allows litigation, and the possibility of it may discourage irresponsible therapy. Win or lose at trial may be secondary. A legal strategy is to torment one's adversaries until they cease their behavior. Some do, some don't, but most come away largely ruined, financially (if there's no insurance) or emotionally.[66]

Does the decision in *Ramona* open the door to any litigation by a person aggrieved by an interpretation made by a therapist to a patient? In an address at the 1994 annual meeting of the American Psychiatric Association, Dr. Judith Herman, author of *Trauma and Recovery*, said about the *Ramona* decision, "The fact that a third party was given standing to speak on malpractice because he was not happy with the treatment of his daughter really opens the door to permit anyone who is dissatisfied with our treatment of any patient to lay claim against us." Of course, the court did not say that the public at large may bring a claim against the therapist. She acknowledged at the time of her address that she did not have access to the transcripts in the case.

Dr. Thomas Gutheil, who testified on behalf of the defense in *Ramona*, asked: "Whose therapy was this anyway? Should the father have been called in to approve each interpretation as it occurred to the therapist? Should the father's consent to the therapy have been sought, even though the patient was not a minor? Should the patient herself have been warned, in some caricature of the warning needed in a forensic context, that her therapy might conceivably be harmful to her father's peace of mind?"[67]

Gutheil posed a hypothetical scenario: "Let's say a young man comes to treatment to work on trouble with relationships. A few years into psychotherapy, without any prompting by the therapist, the patient decides that the problem has been his failure to acknowledge that he is gay. Working this issue through, he feels much better, until he tells his parents, who are homophobic and become outraged at this news. They decide to sue the therapist for implanting foreign ideas or brainwashing or whatever."

The scenario is what law professors call a "parade of horribles" or "slippery slope" in which it is argued (without proof) that one action will unleash a host of unpleasant consequences. In *Ramona*, the therapists operated on the basis of unsupported theories and they urged the patient to blame someone else for her problems. The trial judge in *Ramona* relied on *Molien* where the patient was advised to inform her husband that she had syphilis. In a special verdict answering questions put to them, the jury concluded: (1) the defendants were negligent in providing healthcare to Holly Ramona by implanting or reinforcing false memories that the plaintiff had molested her as a child, (2) the defendants caused the plaintiff to be personally confronted with the accusation that he had molested Holly Ramona, (3) and the plaintiff suffered damages that were caused by the negligence of the defendants. The court found that the therapists assumed a duty of care to the parent when they encouraged the daughter to confront him with accusations of abuse. The jury foreperson explained that the jury felt the therapist "had reinforced the memories by suggestions and by sending her [the patient] to a therapy group for eating disorders that was filled with sex abuse victims."

In an article in the *American Journal of Psychiatry*, Dr. Paul Appelbaum and law professor Rose Zolteck-Jick cautioned that aggrieved third parties would have the power to bring effective treatment to a halt by filing suit or threatening to do so. Appelbaum and Zolteck-Jick concluded that, although concern about therapeutic practices related to memories of childhood abuse may be warranted, allowing nonpatients to sue would be ill-advised, as it would have therapists unclear regarding how to avoid duties to third parties.[68] In the *Harvard Law Review*, law professors Cynthia Grant Bowman and Elizabeth Mertz wrote that the imposition of third-party liability against therapists would compromise the interest of sexual abuse survivors.[69]

A number of courts have heeded their message. The Minnesota Court of Appeals, citing the Harvard article, declined "to extend the law to recognize a duty to third-party nonpatients when there is no contractual relationship, duty to warn, or duty to control."[70] The Illinois Supreme Court also declined to impose a duty in this type of case.[71] It said:

A number of considerations relevant to the duty analysis strongly militate against imposition of duty here. … Approval of the plaintiff's cause of action … would mean that therapists generally, as well as other types of counselors, could be subject to suit by any nonpatient third party who is adversely affected by personal decisions perceived to be made by a patient in response to counseling. This result would, we believe, place therapists in a difficult position. ... Concern about how a course of treatment might affect third parties could easily influence the way in which therapists treat their patients. Under a rule imposing a duty of care to third parties, therapists would feel compelled to consider the possible effects of treatment choices on third parties and would have an incentive to compromise their treatment because of the threatened liability. This would be fundamentally inconsistent with that therapist's obligation to the patient. ... Hoping to avoid liability to third parties ... a therapist might instead find it necessary to deviate from the treatment the therapist would normally provide, to the patient's ultimate detriment. This would exact an intolerably high price from the patient–therapist relationship and would be destructive of that relationship.[72]

In a dissent, Justice Moses Harrison said, "My colleagues expound at length about the need to protect medical providers from liability to some indeterminate class of nonpatient third parties. ... Plaintiff here was not a chance bystander or random member of the general public. He was a relative of the therapist's patient, he was the alleged cause of the patient's psychological difficulties, and, according to the complaint, the therapist specifically arranged to have him participate in the patient's therapy sessions as part of the patient's treatment program."[73]

Unless such claims are allowed, the third party argued, negligent and harmful treatment may well continue unchecked because the patient is too emotionally altered to recognize the harm that has taken place. In another case, the Iowa Supreme Court rejected this paternalistic approach. The court said, "It assumes that competent adults who voluntarily undergo mental health treatment cannot decide for themselves whether the treatment is beneficial, an assumption we believe is unjustified."[74]

Similarly, in California, in 1999 in *Trear v. Sills*,[75] the California Court of Appeals rendered a decision at variance with *Ramona*. The California Court of Appeals observed, "Out-of-state cases that have allowed such suits to go forward, and commentators who favor tort liability, however, have invariably not come to grips with the impossibility of verification and the conflicts of interest that a duty to a possible abuser creates." In this case, unlike in *Ramona*, the therapist had not seen the parent, but if courts were to hold that therapists only face the possibility of liability upon meeting with a third party, therapists would become reluctant to meet with a parent whose child may be an abuse victim, and would dampen family therapy. In light of the decision of the Court of Appeals in *Trear*, the trial court's decision in *Ramona* might have been reversed if it had been appealed.

In 1994, in the same year as the decision in *Ramona*, the California Court of Appeals carried out a review of every case decided in California after *Moline*. In *Bro v. Glaser*,[76] the California Court of Appeals noted that plaintiffs in California usually lose the argument that they are direct victims. It said that to be a direct victim, the plaintiff must show (1) a preexisting consensual relationship between the plaintiff and the defendant, and (2) that the defendant's conduct was sufficiently outrageous to trigger, as a matter of public policy, an obligation to compensate the plaintiff.

Again in California, and in the same year, the direct victim issue again arose. In *Underwood v. Croy*,[77] the wife, who had been seeing a therapist, abandoned her husband and two minor children. The husband discovered that the wife and therapist were having an affair and claimed that the affair was the reason the wife walked out. The California Court of Appeals held that the husband and minor children were not direct victims and, hence, had no cause of action against the therapist. The trial judge had observed:

The bottom line is that the question of duty, as a matter of law, is an issue of public policy. Our appellate courts may wish to extend public policy to find a duty of care is owed by a marriage counselor to his patient's various relatives when his sexual exploitation of the patient destroys the marriage, which he was retained to help preserve. Such is not the law under existing authority.

The Pennsylvania Supreme Court, though earlier ruling that a third party who contracted hepatitis as a result of a negligent diagnosis of the patient had a cause of action against the physician, recently said that a psychiatrist owed no duty to a minor patient's parents that extended beyond the confidential confines of the psychiatrist–patient relationship. The court overturned a lower court verdict in which psychiatrist Judith Cohen and the University of Pittsburgh's Western Psychiatric Institute and Clinic were ordered to pay $272,232 in damages. As time went on in therapy, the patient had memories of her parents sexually abusing her. The allegations were reported, and the father was arrested three times and her mother twice. The court said that a psychiatrist treating a minor for sexual abuse has no duty of care to the child's parents. Justice Ronald Castille, writing for the majority, said, "To hold otherwise would create an unworkable conflict of interest for the treating therapist, … which would necessarily hinder effective treatment of the child."[78]

A Different View

To be sure, there is conflict of authority.[79] In *Hungerford v. Jones*,[80] the New Hampshire Supreme Court in 1998 allowed a cause of action to parents for the malpractice of their adult children's therapist. The defendant, Susan Jones, was a social worker whose only training in diagnosing and treating repressed memories of childhood sexual abuse was her attendance at a weekend seminar. Nonetheless, she took on the treatment of the patient. During the course of the therapy, the defendant led the patient to believe that her anxiety and nightmares were caused by "body memories" of past abuse. She led the patient into a trance to employ a recovery technique she referred to as *visualization* or *imagery*. Through this, the patient claimed to have recalled five specific episodes of sexual assault by her father, the first beginning when she was 5 years old, with the last ending only two days before her wedding. At the defendant's insistence and direction, she confronted her father, Joel Hungerford. When he denied the allegation of abuse, the defendant directed the patient to file a complaint for aggravated felonious sexual assault with the police. The defendant came to the police station to validate the truth of the allegations and to encourage prosecution as a means of empowering the patient. Criminal charges were brought against the father, but were subsequently dropped when the court determined the recovered memories were inadmissible for lack of scientific reliability. Thereafter, the father filed suit against the therapist for malpractice in the care of his daughter.

The New Hampshire Supreme Court was certified to address two issues upon appeal of the defendant's motion to dismiss. First, does a mental healthcare provider owe a duty of care to the parent of an adult patient when identified as the perpetrator of sexual abuse in the course of the patient's therapy? Second, to what extent is any such duty owed? The court found four elements that need to be met to establish third-party liability: (1) The accused is the patient's parent, (2) the therapist lacks appropriate experience and qualifications, (3) the therapist uses a psychological phenomenon or technique not generally accepted by the mental health community, and (4) the accusations are made public. The court clarified that although it was extending the duty of care to parents in such cases, the court was imposing "no more than what a therapist is already bound to provide—a competent and carefully considered professional judgment." The court said:

> Imposing a duty of care on therapists who elect to publicize accusations of sexual abuse against parents, or who encourage patients to do so, should not unreasonably inhibit sexual

abuse diagnosis or therapy. Recognizing such a duty where parents are implicated, however, should result in greater protection for parents and families from unqualified or unaccepted therapeutic diagnoses. While imposition of this duty may impair societal efforts to bring some sexual abusers to justice, we recognize its need due to the increased foreseeability and devastating consequences of publicized false accusations against parents.

Accordingly, in response to the district court's questions, we hold that a therapist owes an accused parent a duty of care in the diagnosis and treatment of an adult patient for sexual abuse where the therapist or the patient, acting on the encouragement, recommendation, or instruction of the therapist, takes public action concerning the accusation. In such instances, the social utility of detecting and punishing sexual abusers and maintaining the breadth of treatment choices for patients is outweighed by the substantial risk of severe harm to falsely accused parents, the family unit, and society. The duty of care to the accused parent is breached by the therapist when the publicized misdiagnosis results from (1) use of psychological phenomena or techniques not generally accepted in the mental health community, or (2) lack of professional qualification.[81]

The Wisconsin Supreme Court in 1999 addressed the duty of therapists to third parties and, over a dissent, said that it agreed with the reasoning of the New Hampshire Supreme Court. In *Sawyer v. Midelfort*,[82] parents brought suit against their daughter's longtime therapists, a psychiatrist and an unlicensed social worker, for implanting false memories of abuse. The daughter had confronted her parents with allegations of physical abuse by both parents and childhood sexual abuse by the father. She filed a lawsuit against her parents alleging that her father had impregnated her at age 13 and that her mother had arranged for an abortion. That lawsuit died for lack of progress. In the lawsuit by the parents against the therapists, the court noted that it had extended third-party liability in professional malpractice cases against architects, attorneys, and accountants. But, most importantly, the court noted, it had extended a psychiatrist's duties to warn patients of side effects of medications to protect third parties from injury.[83]

The Wisconsin Supreme Court then engaged in a six-prong analysis to determine whether public policy precluded imposing third-party liability. The court determined that (1) the injury sustained by the parents was not too remote from the alleged negligence, (2) the injury was not too wholly out of proportion to the culpability of the negligent tortfeasor, (3) in retrospect it did not appear too highly extraordinary that the negligence should have brought about harm, (4) allowance of recovery would not place too unreasonable a burden on the negligent tortfeasor, (5) allowance of the recovery would not be too likely to open the way for fraudulent claims, and (6) allowance of recovery would not enter a field that has no sensible or just stopping point. However, the court indicated that such an analysis is fact specific.

The court pointed out that the only reason that the parents were able to bring their lawsuit was because they had obtained their daughter's records. The court, in dicta, observed that confidentiality and testimonial privilege may prevent other lawsuits, but, as other courts have noted, when the patient confronts a parent in a therapy session, as occurred in this case, privilege is waived.[84] Moreover, waiver of privilege applies when a patient is named as a party defendant. Otherwise, in jurisdictions that allow a third-party suit against a therapist for malpsychotherapy, the problem arises. How does the third party obtain evidence of what occurred in therapy, given the privilege that shields confidential communications between therapist and patient? In *Ramona*, the court held that privilege was waived because the patient filed a lawsuit against her father, and the therapist had seen the father on an occasion or two.[85] In *Tarasoff*-type cases, a third-party injured by a patient is given access to records to establish that the therapists should have given a warning of the danger posed by the patient.

Psychotherapists have long resisted the notion that they prove the value of what they do—and they claim confidentiality. They point out that, under the laws in the various states, they are not free even to identify whether a person is in therapy with them, as this would constitute a violation of the patient's confidentiality.[86] The California Board of Behavioral Science states: "If a therapist is incompetent or grossly negligent in treating a client, the board can investigate the particulars of that situation. However, it is virtually impossible for the board to conduct such an investigation without the consent and cooperation of the actual client. The confidentiality of psychotherapeutic communication is protected by law and therapeutic treatment records cannot be obtained without a written release from the client, if the client is an adult."[87] When a patient sues a therapist, the privilege of confidentiality is waived, but when a patient does not waive the privilege, a third-party faces obstacles in obtaining information as to what went on in therapy.

An Ideology of Blaming the Parent

The history of psychoanalysis is marked by blaming the parent—a tendency exacerbated during the tumultuous 1960s when trust was not to be placed in anyone over the age of 30. Then, patients' troubles were frequently attributed to childhood sexual abuse.[88] In *Trear*,[89] the California Court of Appeals observed, "[B]y the late 1970s and 1980s, there was a resurgence of Freud's initial view that childhood sexual abuse was at the root of many if not most psychological ills." The court went on, "Granting the early-Freudian assumption (as distinct from the later-Freudian assumption) that abuse is widespread and the root cause of most dysfunction, it is simply not outrageous for a therapist to act on that premise." Of course, Freud abandoned his blind faith in the idea that alleged memories of abuse are always what they purport to be. However, he found that from the perspective of therapy, the reality of abuse or seduction was irrelevant. Thus, in therapy, it does not matter whether the mind is reacting to trauma, coping with everyday turmoil, or just imagining.

Under this view, the therapist works not with the past, but with the patient's story of the past. The past is immutable, so why any interest by the therapist in the past? Dr. Herbert Spiegel said:

> If the disease is biological or of recent psychosocial origin, a reductionist search for causation is a useful approach. The focus is on signs and symptoms that can be contained or neutralized by various medications. But if the syndrome is dominated by illness behavior, the patient's personal history is most effective as a narrative used within the context of a psychotherapeutic strategy. The therapeutic goal is to free the patient from a preoccupation with causation from the past and, instead, to focus more attention on meaning and direction for the present and the future.[90]

In the early years of psychoanalysis, therapists said very little, sometimes remaining silent throughout the session, or they would say, "Can you tell me more about that?" More and more, however, therapists have turned from listening and exploring with the patient to making interpretations about the cause of symptoms, though without objective evidence in support of those interpretations. Psychotherapy moved from old ideals of neutrality to treatments based on empathy and even advocacy for patients. In his book, *The Unknown Murderer*,[91] Theodor Reik cautioned that psychoanalysis had no contribution to make to evidence of guilt, as psychoanalysis is concerned with mental or inner reality rather than material or outer reality.

Actions against revival of memory therapists could be measured by the harm suffered by the plaintiff, the moral blame attached to the defendant's conduct, and the policy of preventing future harm.[92]

Interference with Family Relations

Another doctrinal approach in law is the old action in tort for *interference with family relations*. As a result of the estrangement of a family following revival of memory of childhood sexual abuse, reunification of families, even after a retraction, has not taken place for most families. In any event, the tort for interference with family relations is rather ragged in form.[93] It developed initially as an offshoot of the action for enticing away a servant and depriving the master of the quasi-proprietary interest in his services. Also, under the early common law, the status of a wife as well as that of minor children was that of more or less valuable servants of the husband and father, and that action was extended to include the deprivation of their services. The loss of such services was the gist of the action.

In comparatively recent years, there as been a gradual shift of emphasis away from services and toward a recognition of more intangible elements in domestic relations, such as companionship and affection. In a widely publicized case in the late 1970s in Boulder, Colorado, a mother whose 25-year-old son sued her for "parental malpractice," filed her own suit against the son's psychiatrist, Dr. Jeffrey Anker. The doctor had encouraged the son to sue her for therapeutic reasons. (The demise of family immunity barring suits between family members began with automobile accident cases and in these cases the insurance company is the defendant as a practical matter.) The son was described as a hippie who was suspended from high school for selling marijuana, who chose to live with friends on a beach in Hawaii, and who refused to find work. In her suit, the mother said the parental malpractice action against her caused her "great grief, sorrow, and even anger" and she claimed that she had been subjected to widespread "ridicule and embarrassment." The case was apparently settled.[94]

Then, too, at one time the law recognized an action for alienation of affections. Thus, in a 1966 case in Washington, an action for alienation of affections was allowed when a pastor counseled a woman to leave her husband who was "full of the devil."[95] That has changed. The courts in various states have held that a husband has no cause of action against a therapist who had a sexual relationship with the wife who was a patient. In a California case, *Smith v. Pust*,[96] the patient's husband was held not to be a "direct victim," and the husband was also held not to be a patient notwithstanding his attendance at some therapy sessions.

To Sum Up

The law on duty to third parties has its twists and turns. The law of torts is evolving on the responsibility of psychiatrists not only to their patients but also to third parties reasonably foreseeable as victims of harm caused by their patients. In many circumstances, the duty of the therapist runs not only to the patient, but also to others.

Endnotes

1. 48 N.Y. 339, 162 N.E. 99 (1928). The opinion is reproduced in every torts coursebook. See G.T. Schwartz, "Cardozo as Tort Lawmaker," *DePaul L. Rev.* 49 (1999): 305; see also A.L Kaufman, *Cardozo* (Cambridge, MA: Harvard University Press, 1998).
2. Under the influence of Jim Jones, members of the People's Temple in Jonestown murdered Congressman Leo J. Ryan and then committed suicide en masse. United States v. Layton, 549 F.2d 903 (N. D. Cal. 1982). See I. Mancinelli et al., "Mass Suicide: Historical and Psychodynamic Considerations," *Suicide Life Threat. Behav.* 32 (2002): 91.
3. Jones v. State of New York, 267 App. Div. 254, 45 N.Y.S. 2d 404 (1943). A hospital breaches its duty of care by failing to provide adequate security in view of a patient's known violent tendencies. See Fair v. United States, 234 F.2d 288 (5th Cir. 1956).
4. See, e.g., Merchants National Bank & Trust Co. of Fargo v. United States, 272 F. Supp. 409 (D. N.D. 1967); Homere v. State, 79 Misc. 2d 972, 361 N. Y. S. 2d 820 (1974).
5. Iancona v. Schrupp, 521 N.W. 2d 70 (Minn. App. 1994).

6. Britton v. Soltes, 205 Ill. App. 3d 943, 563 N.E. 2d 910 (1990). In Ellis v. Peter, 211 A.D.2d 353 (1995), the New York Supreme Court declined to recognize a duty on the part of a healthcare professional to the spouse of a patient who had contracted tuberculosis (but who had been wrongly diagnosed) because "a physician's duty of care is ordinarily one owed to his or her patient and does not extend to the community at large; the wife may also be considered to be in that class of persons whom the defendant knew or reasonably should have known were relying on him for a duty of care to his patient, but defendant's duty of care will not be so extended, since there is no indication of the point where that duty would end."

7. 563 N.E.2d at 916.

8. DeMarco v. Lynch Homes, 525 Pa. 558, 583 A.2d 422 (1990).

9. 27 Cal. 3d 916, 616 P.2d 813, 167 Cal. Rptr. 831 (1980).

10. 2 Cal. 4th 1064, 9 Cal. Rptr. 2d 615, 831 P.2d 1197 (1992).

11. See Thing v. LaChusa, 48 Cal. Rptr. 3d 644, 257 Cal. Rptr. 865, 771 P.2d 814 (1989).

12. The case was actually heard twice. *Tarasoff I*, 118 Cal. Rptr. 129, 529 P. 2d 553 (1974), *vacated*, *Tarasoff II*, 17 Cal. 3d 425, 121 Cal. Rptr. 14, 551 P. 2d 334 (1976).

13. See F. Buckner & M. Firestone, "'Where the Public Peril Begins': 25 Years after *Tarasoff*," *J. Legal Med.* 21 (2000): 187; A.R. Felthous, "The Clinician's Duty to Protect Third Parties," *Psychiat. Clin. N. Am.*, (Philadelphia: Saunders, 1999), vol. 22, no. 1, p. 49; D. Truscott, "The Psychotherapist's Duty to Protect: An Annotated Bibliography," *J. Psychiat. & Law* 21 (1993): 221. The *Tarasoff* case provoked discussion not only concerning the duty to warn or protect but also concerning confidentiality and prediction of dangerousness. In March 2006, on *Tarasoff*'s 30th anniversary, a full-day symposium on the case, organized by Dr. Douglas Mossman, was held at the University of Cincinnati College of Law. The symposium appears in the *University of Cincinnati Law Review*, 75 (2006): 429–661. See also C.P. Ewing & J.T. McCann, *Minds on Trial: Great Cases in Law and Psychology* (New York: Oxford University Press, 2006), pp. 57–67.

14. Schulz v. Pennsylvania Railroad Co., 350 U. S. 523, 525 (1956).

15. In *Tarasoff*, Dr. Moore wrote: "At times he appears to be quite rational, at other times he appears to be quite psychotic. … [C]urrently, the appropriate diagnosis for him is paranoid schizophrenic reaction, acute and severe. He is at this point a danger to the welfare of other people and himself. That is, he has been threatening to kill an unnamed girl who he feels has betrayed him and has violated his honor. He has told a friend of his … that he intends to go to San Francisco to buy a gun and that he plans to kill the girl. He has been somewhat more cryptic with me, but he has alluded strongly to the compulsion to 'get even with,' and 'hurt' the girl."

16. See discussion in Chapter 5 on testimonial privilege.

17. Personal communication.

18. 551 P.2d at 334.

19. Osterlind v. Hill, 263 Mass. 73, 160 N.E. 301 (1928).

20. Compare the Restatement (Second) Torts § 315, which provides: "There is no duty to control the conduct of a third person as to prevent him from causing physical harm to another unless (a) a special relationship exists between the actor and the third person, which imposes a duty upon the actor to control the third person's conduct, or (b) a special relationship exists between the actor and the other, which gives to the other the right to protection."

21. 551 P.2d at 334.

22. In a Maryland case, Shaw v. Glickman, 45 Md. App. 718, 145 A.2d 625 (1980), the plaintiff, a dentist, was in group therapy conducted by the defendant psychiatrist and his wife, a psychiatric nurse. In the group were Mr. and Mrs. Billian. Unknown to Mr. Billian, an amorous relationship developed between Mrs. Billian and the dentist. One of the group therapists, upon learning of the extramarital affair, disclosed it to Mr. Billian in an individual therapy session. Some days later, Mr. Billian broke into the dentist's home, and finding his wife in bed with him, shot him. The dentist filed an action for damages, naming as defendants both Mr. Billian and the psychiatric team that had been conducting the group therapy sessions. The complaint charged that the defendant therapists had failed to warn him of Mr. Billian's unstable and violent condition and the foreseeable and immediate danger that it presented to the plaintiff. The Maryland Court of Appeals held that unlike in *Tarasoff*, there was no threat revealed to the group therapists by Mr. Billian to kill or injure the dentist, and there was no confiding of any animosity or hatred toward the dentist. Although Mr. Billian was known by the therapists to tote a gun, the court held that that fact does not give rise to the inference that Mr. Billian did so for the purpose of harming the dentist. Anyhow, we must say, the dentist ought to have known of the danger. As the court put it, Mr. Billian invoked "the old Solon law and [shot] his wife's lover."

23. Hutchinson v. Patel, 637 So. 2d 415 (La. 1994). See A.L. Almason, "Personal Liability Implications of the Duty to Warn Are Hard Pills to Swallow: From *Tarasoff* to *Hutchinson v. Patel* and Beyond," *J. Contemp. Health Law & Policy* 13 (1997): 471; P.D. Liuzza, "*Hutchinson v. Patel*, Louisiana Supreme Court's First Response to *Tarasoff* Duty to Warn: Broadens Recovery but Narrows Liability," *Loy. L. Rev.* 40 (1995): 1011.

24. In a Vermont case, the court held the duty to protect included a situation where the patient set fire to the family barn, located 130 feet from their home. At the time the patient was a voluntary outpatient under the care of a counselor in a community mental health clinic. He told the counselor that he "wanted to get back at his father." Peck v. Counseling Service of Addison County, 146 Vt. 61, 499 A. 2d 422 (1985). *Query*: What would the therapist have had to do if the patient had threatened to damage his father's car or kill his father's dog? In *Peck*, the therapist allegedly honestly believed that the patient would not burn his father's barn, but the law of negligence does not have a "good faith" exception; such an exception would likely spawn falsification of what the therapist in fact believed. The decision was based on a finding that the therapist should have had better procedures, which might have enabled him to make a better assessment of the risk.

25. See Jablonski v. United States, 712 F.2d 391 (9th Cir. 1983); Brady v. Hopper, 570 F. Supp. 1333 (D.C. Colo. 1983); Hamman v. County of Maricopa, 161 Ariz. 58, 775 P.2d 1122 (1989); Eckhardt v. Kirts, 179 Ill. App. 3d 863, 534 N.E.2d 1339 (1989).

26. Almonte v. New York Medical College, 851 F. Supp. 34 (D. Conn. 1994); discussed in F. Bruni, "Jury Finds Psychiatrist Negligent in Case of Pedophile Patient," *New York Times*, Oct. 9, 1998, p. 27; L. McCullough, "A Training Analyst's Dilemma: The Limits of Confidentiality," *Psychiatric News*, Sept. 4, 1998, p. 2. The court compared Doe v. British Universities North American Club, 786 F. Supp. 1286 (D. Conn. 1992), finding no duty to warn about a counselor's sexual orientation because sexual molestation is not a foreseeable risk of homosexuality; 851 F. Supp. at 41.

27. R. Slovenko, "The *Tarasoff* Progeny," in R.I. Simon (Ed.), *Review of Clinical Psychiatry and the Law* (Washington, DC: American Psychiatric Press, 1990), vol. 1, ch. 8, p. 177; R. Weinstock, G. Vari, G.B., Leong, & J.A. Silva, "Back to the Past in California: A Temporary Retreat to a *Tarasoff* Duty to Warn," *J. Am. Acad. Psychiat. & Law* 34 (2006): 523.

28. Estates of Morgan v. Fairfield Family Counseling Center, 77 Ohio St. 3d 284, 673 N. E. 2d 1311, 1331 (1997).

29. Bishop v. So. Car. Dept. of Mental Health, 331 S. C. 79, 502 S.E.3d 78 (1998). See also Valentine v. On Target, 353 Md. 544, 727 A.2d 947 (Md. 1999).

30. Green v. Ross, 691 So.2d 542 (Fla. App. 1997); Boynton v. Burglass, 590 So.2d 446 (Fla. App. 1999); Thapar v. Zezulka, 42 Tex. 824, 994 S.W.2d 635 (1999); See also Nasser v. Parker, 455 S.E.2d 502 (Va. 1995). A federal district court in Mississippi stated, "While *Tarasoff* may be the law in California, plaintiff has cited no authority showing that this decision represents the law in Mississippi." Evans v. United States, 833 F. Supp. 124 (S. D. 1995). The Hawaii Supreme Court limited *Tarasoff* to cases involving potential victims of violent assault, thereby declining to extend it to risks of self-inflicted harm or property damage. Lee v. Corregedore, 925 P.2d 324 (Haw. 1996); c.f. Pate v. Threlkel, 661 So.2d 278 (Fla. 1995), noted hereinafter in regard to genetic disease.

31. Green v. Ross, 691 So.2d 542 (Fla. App. 1997).

32. Thapar v. Zezulka, 42 Tex. 824, 994 S.W.2d 635 (1999). Clinicians are required to warn in Arizona, California, Colorado, Delaware, Idaho, Indiana, Kentucky, Louisiana, Maryland, Massachusetts, Michigan, Minnesota, Missouri, Montana, Nebraska, New Hampshire, New Jersey, Ohio, Oklahoma, Pennsylvania, South Carolina, Tennessee, Utah, Vermont, Washington, and Wisconsin. Clinicians are allowed to warn potential victims, but do not require it in Alaska, Connecticut, District of Columbia, Florida, Illinois, New York, Oregon, Rhode Island, and West Virginia. There is no definitive law on a clinician's duty to warn and protect in Alabama, Arkansas, Georgia, Hawaii, Iowa, Kansas, Maine, Nevada, New Mexico, North Carolina, North Dakota, South Dakota, and Wyoming.

    Even the statutes that are similar are often interpreted differently by courts within the same state. A table of statutes and an analysis of their application appears in C. Kachigian & A.R. Felthous, "Court Responses to 'Tarasoff' Statutes," *J. Am. Acad. Psychiat. & Law* 32 (2004): 263. See also A.R. Felthous, "Warning a Potential Victim of a Person's Dangerousness: Clinician's Duty or Victim's Right?" *J. Am. Acad. Psychiat. & Law* 34 (2006): 338; P.B. Herbert & K.A. Young, "Tarasoff at Twenty-Five," *J. Am. Acad. Psychiat. & Law* 30 (2002): 275. The Texas Supreme Court declined to adopt a duty to warn, reasoning that the confidentiality statute governing mental health professionals in Texas makes it unwise to recognize such a duty. The court found that the Texas Legislature had chosen to guard a patient's communication with a mental health professional. In 1979, 3 years after *Tarasoff* was decided in California, the

Texas Legislature enacted a statute that classifies communications between mental health professionals and their patients as confidential and prohibits mental health professionals from disclosing them to third parties unless an exception applies. No exception in the statute provides for disclosure to third parties threatened by the patient; Thapar v. Zezulka, 42 Tex. 824, 994 S.W.2d 635 (1999).

Without immunity, mental health professionals are faced with a dilemma. If they do not report, they may face a wrongful death suit in the event of a killing of a third person, as in *Tarasoff*, and, on the other hand, if they do report, they may face a suit for breach of confidentiality. In a case in Georgia featured in the *New York Times*, a psychologist warned the police captain that a patient, a police officer, threatened to harm him. The officer was adversely affected by the report and he sued the psychologist. The jury awarded him $280,000, which was settled with the insurance company for $230,000. D.T. Max, "The Cop and the Therapist," *New York Times Magazine*, Dec. 3, 2000, p. 94.

33. R. L. Binder & D. E. McNiel, "Application of the Tarasoff Ruling and Its Effect on the Victim and the Therapist Relationship," *Psychiatric Services* 47 (1996): 1212.

34. R. Balon & R. Mufti (ltr.), "*Tarasoff* Ruling and Reporting to the Authorities," *Am. J. Psychiat.* 154 (1997): 1321.

35. B. Bernstein, "Solving the Physician's Dilemma: An HIV Partner-Notification Plan," *Stan. L. & Policy Rev.* 6: 2 (1995): 127); L.S. Gruman, "AIDS and the Physician's Duty to Warn," *Med. & Law* 10 (1991): 415, 455; L.O. Gostin & J.G. Hodge, "Piercing the Veil of Secrecy in HIV/AIDS and Other Sexually Transmitted Diseases: Theories of Privacy and Disclosure in Partner Notification," *Duke J. Gender Law & Policy* 5 (1998): 9.

36. 252 Cal. Rptr. 11 (Cal. App. 1988).

37. 252 Cal. Rptr. at 13. In Pate v. Threlkel, 661 So. 2d 278 (Fla. 1995), the Florida Supreme Court was asked to decide whether a physician has a legal duty to warn a patient's children of the genetically transferable nature of the condition for which the physician is treating the patient. Though Florida had rejected *Tarasoff*, the Florida Supreme Court in *Pate* held that the physician's alleged duty to warn extended to the children of the patient even though the children were not in the role of patient. The duty, the court said, would be satisfied by warning the patient. There were two reasons for this: (1) confidentiality prohibited the physician from revealing confidential communications in most instances absent the patient's consent, and (2) to require the physician to seek out and warn various members of the patient's family would often be difficult or impractical and would place too heavy a burden upon the physician; 661 So.2d at 282. For a discussion of the issue, see E.W. Clayton, "What Should the Law Say About Disclosure of Genetic Information to Relatives?" *J. Health Care Law & Policy* 1 (1998): 373; L.J. Deftos, "Genomic Torts: The Law of the Future—the Duty of Physicians to Disclose the Presence of a Genetic Disease to the Relatives of Their Patients With the Disease," *U. San Francisco L. Rev.* 32 (1997): 105.

38. Schroeder v. Perkel, 87 N.J. Super. 53, 432 A.2d 834 (1981).

39. Safer v. Estate of Pack, 291 N.J. Super. 619, 677 A. 2d 1188 (1996).

40. See G.T. Laurie, "Protecting and Promoting Privacy in an Uncertain World: Further Defences of Ignorance and the Right Not to Know," *Eur. J. Health Law* 7 (2000): 185.

41. See N.M. Bradburn, L.J. Rips, & S.K. Shevell, "Answering Autobiographical Questions: The Impact of Memory and Inference on Surveys," *Science* 236 (April 10, 1987): 157; J.F. Kihlstrom, "The Cognitive Unconscious," *Science* 237 (Sept. 18, 1987): 1445; L.M. Williams, "Recall of Childhood Trauma: A Prospective Study of Women's Memories of Child Sexual Abuse," *J. Consul. & Clin. Psychol.* 62 (1994): 1167; response, E.F. Loftus, M. Garry, & J. Feldman, "Forgetting Sexual Trauma: What Does It Mean When 38% Forget?" *J. Consul. & Clin. Psychol.* 62 (1994): 1177.

42. See J.R. Noblitt & P.S. Perskin, *Cult and Ritual Abuse* (Westport, CT: Praeger, 2000); K.S. Pope & L.S. Brown, *Recovered Memories of Abuse* (Washington, DC: American Psychological Association, 1996).

43. For a critical view of recovered memory therapy, see H.I. Lief & J.M. Fetkewicz, "Casualties of Recovered Memory Therapy: The Impact of False Allegations of Incest on Accused Fathers," in R.C. Friedman & J.I. Downey (Eds.), *Review of Psychiatry* (Washington, DC: American Psychiatric Association), vol. 18, no. 5, chap. 5, pp. 115–141.

44. Joyce-Couch v. DeSilva, 77 Ohio App. 3d 278, 602 N. E. 2d 286 (1991); see H. I. Lief & J. Fetkewicz, "Retractors of False Memories: The Evolution of Pseudomemories," *J. Psychiat, & Law* 23 (1995): 411.

45. E. Bass & L. Davis, *Courage to Heal* (New York: Harper & Row, 1988).

46. Variations of the theme are commonplace in psychotherapy. Psychoanalyst Michael Miletic, for example, reports a hockey player able to play again when in the course of therapy, a repressed memory is unblocked. Through a lot of work, he said, what was reconstructed was that the act of standing at the blue line with a puck and with a forward potentially charging at him brought back traumatic memories

of when he was beaten as a youngster by his father. R. Lipsyte, "Outside the Norm: The Psychology of Athletes," *New York Times*, Feb. 6, 2000, p. S-1. That notion is exemplified in Alfred Hitchcock's *Spellbound* starring Gregory Peck and Ingrid Bergman. Freud at one time believed this, but it is an oversimplification and ignores the role of narrative and suggestion in psychotherapy. Did the psychoanalyst get any objective evidence that the father beat the player? The question is rhetorical.

47. C. Tavris, *Anger: The Misunderstood Emotion* (New York: Simon & Schuster, rev. ed., 1989), p. 129.

48. R. Hughes, *Culture of Complaint* (New York: Oxford University Press, 1993), p. 7.

49. R. Slovenko, "The 'Revival of Memory' of Childhood Sexual Abuse: Is the Tolling of Statute of Limitations Justified?" *J. Psychiat. & Law* 21 (1993): 7; H. Wakefield & R. Underwager, "Recovered Memories of Alleged Sexual Abuse: Lawsuits Against Parents," *Behav. Sci. & Law* 10 (1992): 483. Leading forensic psychiatrists have written: "On clinical grounds and in the patient's interests, such issues are best resolved in the therapeutic context: working through the past experience, dealing with the troubling symptoms, and going on with one's life. Litigation, however, precludes such an approach by shifting the venue to an adversarial setting that may well prevent, for example, such constructive approaches as working with the family in therapy together." T.G. Gutheil, H. Bursztajn, A. Brodsky, & L.H. Strasburger, "Preventing 'Critigenic' Harms: Minimizing Emotional Injury From Civil Litigation," *J. Psychiat. & Law* 28 (2000): 5. See D. Brown, A.W. Schifrin, & D.C. Hammond, *Memory Trauma Treatment and the Law* (New York: W.W. Norton, 1998); R. Moore, *The Creation of Reality in Psychoanalysis* (Mahwah, NJ: Analytic Press, 1999); R. Ofshe & E. Watters, *Making Monsters: False Memories, Psychotherapy, and Sexual Hysteria* (New York: Scribner's, 1994); R.I. Simon & D.W. Shuman (Eds.), *Predicting the Past: The Retrospective Assessment of Mental States in Civil and Criminal Litigation* (Washington, DC: American Psychiatric Press, 2000).

50. See A. Piper, H.G. Pope, & J.J. Borowiecki, "Custer's Last Stand: Brown, Scheflin, and Whitfield's Latest Attempt to Salvage 'Dissociative Amnesia,'" *J. Psychiat. & Law* 28 (2000): 149.

51. D. Boesky, "Correspondence Criteria and Clinical Evidence in Psychoanalysis," address on Jan. 13, 2000, at meeting of the Michigan Psychoanalytic Society. To what extent, if any, must there be historical truth as the basis for an interpretation? Clinicians say that they are concerned with clinical utility. They lift resistance to memories that are used in treatment if they have efficacy, regardless of their historical accuracy, but historical accuracy is essential in a courtroom. It is also important when third parties will be affected as they are in the case of allegations of sexual abuse. See R. Slovenko, *Psychotherapy and Confidentiality* (Springfield, IL: Thomas, 1998), pp. 523–544; D.P. Spence, *Narrative Truth and Historical Truth: Meaning and Interpretation in Psychoanalysis* (New York: Norton, 1982). In a series of cartoon case histories by Sarah Boxer, a reporter for *New York Times*, the psychoanalyst is "more Freudian than Freud, willing to build an interpretation on the slimmest evidence." S. Boxer, *In the Floyd Archives: A Psycho-Bestiary* (New York: Pantheon, 2001).

52. P. McHugh, "To Treat," *FMS Found. Newsl.*, Oct. 1, 1993, p. 1.

53. P. McHugh, "Procedures in the Diagnosis of Incest in Recovered Memory Cases," *FMS Found. Newsl.*, May 3, 1993, p. 3.

54. The False Memory Syndrome (FMS) Foundation was formed in 1992, and within a year it had a membership of over 4,600. Over 12,000 families have contacted it. The Foundation disseminates information about the nature of memory and about how to deal with "revival of memory" therapists. See T.W. Campbell, *Smoke and Mirrors: The Devastating Effect of False Sexual Abuse Claims* (New York: Plenum, 1998); S. Taub (Ed.), *Recovered Memories of Child Sexual Abuse* (Springfield, IL: Thomas, 1999); H.I. Lief & J.M. Fetkewicz, "Casualties of Recovered Memory Therapy: The Impact of False Allegations of Incest on Accused Fathers," in R.C. Friedman & J.I. Downey (Eds.), *Review of Psychiatry* (Washington, DC: American Psychiatric Press), vol. 18, no. 5, chap. 5, pp. 115–141; J.M. Whitesell, "Ridicule or Recourse: Parents Falsely Accused of Past Sexual Abuse Fight Back," *J. Law & Health* 11 (1996–97): 303.

55. Nov. 29, 1993.

56. May 24, 1993.

57. The two-part article appears in expanded form in L. Wright, *Remembering Satan* (New York: Knopf, 1994); reviewed in M. Kakutani, "A Family Is Destroyed by a Sexual Chimera," *New York Times*, April 29, 1994, p. B7.

58. "APA Stakes Out Positions on Controversial Therapies," *Psychiatric News*, April 21, 2000, p. 45; cited in Chapter 28 on psychiatric malpractice.

59. Quoted in S. Salter, "Recalling Abuse in the Mind's Eye," *San Francisco Chronicle*, April 4, 1993, p. 9. See P.R. McHugh, "The Contemporary Witch-Craze: Remembered Sexual Abuse," *Hopkins Medical News*, Spring 1994, p. 56. For a defense of "recovered memory," see A. Scheflin, D. Brown, & C. Hammon, *Memory, Trauma Treatment and the Law* (New York: W.W. Norton, 1998). A special issue

of the *Journal of Psychiatry & Law*, 27 (1999): 367–705, edited by Daniel Brown and Alan W. Scheflin, focuses on the interrelationship between factitious behavior, dissociative disorders and the law. See also D. Brown, A.W. Scheflin, & C.L. Whitfield, "Recovered Memories: The Current Weight of the Evidence in Science and in the Courts," *J. Psychiat. & Law* 27 (1999): 5. For a response, see A. Piper, G.G. Pople, & J.J. Borowiecki, "Custer's Last Stand: Brown, Scheflin, and Whitfield's Latest Attempt to Salvage 'Dissociative Amnesia,'" *J. Psychiat. & Law* 282 (2000): 149.

60. R. Ofshe & E. Watters, *Making Monsters: False Memories, Psychotherapy, and Sexual Hysteria* (New York: Scribner, 1994). See also E. Watters & R. Ofshe, *Therapy's Delusions* (New York: Scribner, 1999).

61. Schultz v. State, 957 S.W.2d 52 at 77 (Tex. Cr. App. 1997; concurring opinion).

62. In response, some insurers now exclude coverage for revival of memory therapy, which raises the question of its definition—the exclusion in the policy is not defined. To be sure, all therapy involves memory but revival of memory is distinguished from continuous memory. Some define revival of memory therapy as the "persistent encouragement to recall past events." Others define it as an extreme focus on recovering memories of abuse, pressure to remember, stockpile memory, or the pursuit of memory work in a persistently suggestive manner. Retractors of recovered memory report that the search for memories became the cornerstone of therapy while the therapist played an increasingly dominant role in the life of the patient. See F.H. Frankel, "Adult Reconstruction of Childhood Events in the Multiple Personality Literature," *Am. J. Psychiat.* 150 (1993): 954.

63. Ramona v. Isabella, Rose & Western Medical Center, No. Civ. 61898 (Supp. Ct. Napa County, 1994): discussed in M. Johnston, *Spectral Evidence* (New York: Houghton Mifflin, 1997); C.P. Ewing & J.T. McCann, *Minds on Trial: Great Cases in Law and Psychology* (New York: Oxford University Press, 2006), pp. 165–175. See also J. Acocella, *Creating Hysteria* (San Francisco: Jossey-Bass, 1999).

64. California Civil Code §47.

65. In a decision handed down in 1994, the trial judge said:

> This lawsuit is a compelling one, and it's a compelling one because it not only has the novelty of new and current legal issues, but also because it has a salient emotionalism to it. ... [T]he most interesting and compelling and difficult [issue] in this case ... is the question of whether a father may maintain a lawsuit against the therapists or other healthcare providers of his daughter alleging that he was damaged by their negligent treatment of her. ... I have found that a duty did exist to him by reason of the circumstances of the case under [California] Supreme Court law. ... What's going on in a lawsuit of this sort is the conflict of policies. On the one hand, the defendants argue, if you allow nonpatients to sue healthcare providers, it will have a terrible, chilling effect upon the ability of any healthcare provider to do what his or patient needs to provide the kinds of care that his or her patient needs to receive. How, they ask, is a healthcare provider to know what to do when presented with a patient who recalls or thinks he or she is recalling the sorts of things that are presented by this lawsuit. That's a big concern. That's an argument that has significant social implications attendant to it.
>
> Of equal significance, however, and with equal social implications, is the question of what is somebody who, for the sake of this point we will presume to be factually innocent of having engaged in misconduct with respect to his daughter, to do if confronted with the unfounded and incorrect accusation of having molested her that results in his loss of everything?
>
> It's as unpalatable to some to have healthcare providers put in the impossible situation of dealing with a patient presenting real problems, but knowing that the healthcare providers might be subjected to liability as it is to others to have a falsely accused parent to lose everything and have no recourse in court.
>
> Those are the kinds of policy issues that the courts are called upon to resolve, because in the area of tort law, and this a tort action, there's very little law created by the legislature that creates norms. ... And the purposes of tort law are twofold: to provide redress for people who are injured in some way or another, and to mediate, to control, to direct the conduct of other people. ...
>
> [I]n this case the rules are, from my point of view, fairly clear. They were made clear by the California Supreme Court in *Molien v. Kaiser Foundation Hospital* in which the plaintiff had a cause of action and could sue Kaiser Hospital for the emotional distress he suffered as a result of the negligent treatment of his wife, or the negligent diagnosis—misdiagnosis of syphilis.
>
> The defense lawyers have argued vigorously, and with good reason, that in the 10 or 12 years since the *Molien* case was decided, the Supreme Court has been narrowing its application. There's no question but that it has. That case, at the time it was presented to the Supreme Court, had the same kind of conflicts attending to it, the same kind of important policy issues that are present in this case.

The defense lawyers have argued that I should view the *Molien* case as being history; that the Supreme Court has whittled away at it so far that it no longer exists. ... I think that the *Molien* case is still the law because the Supreme Court has had numerous opportunities and has been asked on numerous occasions to simply say it is no longer the law ... even as recently as late last year the Supreme Court was asked to do that, and they stressed that the instruction to his wife to go home and tell him about the diagnosis of her.

Well, think how similar that is to the allegation that the plaintiff is seeking to prove in this case, which is that he was not only—not only did somebody tell the patient, go home and tell the patient, go home and tell your father, but in fact, the father was summoned to the meeting and the confrontation and presentation of the charge occurred.

66. *Ramona* alerted lawyers to the possibility that psychotherapy negligence suits were winnable. Lawsuits resulting in multimillion dollar awards followed, and publicity escalated and led to ever more lawsuits. See E.F. Loftus, "Therapeutic Recollection of Childhood Abuse: When May a Memory Not Be a Memory?" *Champion*, March 1994, p. 5; Editorial, "No Standards," *Wall Street Journal*, May 10, 1994, p. 18.

67. T.G. Gutheil, "True Recollections of a False Memory Case," *Psychiatric Times*, July 1994, p. 28. In a *Murphy Brown* television program, the husband is told by his therapist that his wife is the cause of all of his problems and he is urged not to be passive but act aggressively. He takes out his anger on his wife. The wife complains to the therapist, "Where do you get off telling my husband that I'm the cause of all his problems?"

68. P. Appelbaum & R. Zolteck-Jick, "Psychotherapists' Duties to Third Parties: Ramona and Beyond," *Am. J. Psychiat.* 153 (1996): 457.

69. C.G. Bowman & E. Mertz, "A Dangerous Direction: Legal Intervention in Sexual Abuse Survivor Therapy," *Harv. L. Rev.* 109 (1996): 549.

70. Strom v. C. C., 1997 Minn. App. LEXIS 327.

71. Doe v. McKay, 183 Ill.2d 272, 700 N.E.2d 1018 (1998).

72. 700 N.E.2d at 1023.

73. 700 N.E.2d at 1026.

74. J. A. H. v. Wadle & Associates, 589 N. W. 2d 256 (Iowa 1999).

75. 69 Cal. App. 4th 1341, 82 Cal Rptr.2d 281 (1999).

76. 27 Cal. Rptr.2d 894, 22 Cal. App. 4th 1398 (1994).

77. 30 Cal. Rptr.2d 504 (Ct. App. 1994; unpublished opinion).

78. Althaus v. Cohen & University of Pittsburgh Western Psychiatric Institute & Clinic, Nos. 70 & 71 W.D. Appeal Docket 1998, J-32-1999. C.f. DeMarco v. Lynch Homes, cited *supra* note 8.

79. The cases are noted in A. Lipton, "Recovered Memories in the Courts," in S. Taub (Ed.), *Recovered Memories of Child Sexual Abuse* (Springfield, IL: Thomas, 1999).

80. 143 N.H. 208, 722 A.2d 478 (1998).

81. 722 A.2d at 482.

82. 227 Wis.2d 124, 595 N.W.2d 423 (1999).

83. See Schuster v. Altenberg, 114 Wis.2d 233, 424 N.W.2d 159 (1988).

84. See Truman v. Genesis Associates, 935 F. Supp. 1375 (E. D. Pa. 1996).

85. See Chapter 5 on testimonial privilege.

86. See, e.g., K.S. Pope & L.S. Brown, *Recovered Memories of Abuse* (Washington, DC: American Psychological Association, 1996), p. 203.

87. Quoted in *FMS Foundation Newsletter*, May 3, 1994, p. 7.

88. N.G. Hale, *The Rise and Crisis of Psychoanalysis in the United States: Freud and the Americans* (New York: Oxford University Press, 1995).

89. The case is cited *supra* note 75.

90. H. Spiegel, "Silver Lining in the Clouds of War: A Five-Decade Retrospective," in R.W. Menninger & J.C. Nemiah (Eds.), *American Psychiat. after World War II* (Washington, DC: American Psychiatric Press, 2000).

91. (New York: International Universities Press, 1995).

92. Bastian v. County of San Luis Obispo, 199 Cal. App. 3d 520 (1988).

93. W.P. Keeton (Ed.), *Prosser and Keeton on the Law of Torts* (St. Paul, MN: West, 5th ed., 1984), p. 915.

94. AP news release, "Sued Mom Turns Law on Psychiatrist," May 17, 1979.

95. Carrieri v. Bush, 69 Wash.2d 536, 419 P.2d 132 (1966).

96. 23 Cal. Rptr.2d 264 (Cal. App. 1993).

37

Regulation of the Practice of Psychotherapy

Psychotherapy is generally defined as the noninvasive treatment of emotional states that are understood to be pathological or maladaptive. It may be used independently of or in addition to somatic procedures and psychopharmacology. The tradition of an interpersonal, physically noninvasive psychotherapy, however, has long roots. An important psychological element has always been present in all medicine—therapies that explicitly address the mind were a novelty or reflection, in part, of the decline in religion. The sacrament of confession within the Catholic Church may be seen as the practice of psychotherapy. The Gospels present the image of Christ as physician.

Psychotherapy, in the broad sense of the term, thus existed long before there was a name for it. If it is defined as any procedure or process that changes or influences an individual, then its roots reach back to the dawn of man. The word *psychotherapy*, however, has a medical origin. Its first use is attributed to J. C. Reil in a paper published in 1803, "Rhapsodies in the Application of Psychic Methods in the Treatment of Mental Disturbances."[1]

Since then, the term has acquired a vague and general meaning. It has been used to describe everything from the mystical healing rites of the priest-physicians of ancient Greece, drum-beating and *vaudou* (voodoo) practices of certain modern Caribbean and Brazilian peoples of African descent, classes in rhythmic dancing in a modern psychiatric hospital, forced labor in an old prison asylum, and lectures on ideas of healthy living, to the more subtle and sophisticated psychoanalytic techniques.[2] Thomas Szasz has pointed out that if psychoanalysis had not been discovered by physicians working with hysterical patients, the nature of the analytic process would have been formulated differently.[3] Breuer and Freud were physicians and Anna, an hysteric, took the patient role, and so the psychoanalytic situation was defined as a therapeutic one.

Freud himself was actually embittered by the opposition to psychoanalysis on the part of the medical profession in Vienna, and he, with his early followers, banded together against the hostile medical world. He argued with great passion that psychoanalysts should be broadly trained in the arts and humanities. He welcomed suitable people from all professions, realizing that the discoveries he had made and the theoretical basis established in respect to them had a general and extremely wide bearing. He had no desire to see the potentialities of psychoanalysis limited by regarding it as nothing more than a branch of medical practice. In retrospect, Freud felt that he wasted his youth in the physiological laboratory, although he achieved discipline through it.[4]

Following the death of Freud, the medical profession laid claim to the practice of psychotherapy and to the use of the term. While psychiatrists, with more conviction than proof, insist that a degree in medicine is essential to the rendering of any form of psychotherapy, psychologists and others point out that, in the vast majority of instances, emotional disturbances are entirely beyond the perimeter of traditional medical concerns. The opposition of the medical profession in the United States to the lay use of psychotherapy, in part, can be attributed to the struggle of the medical profession to secure the respect and recognition for its members who had expert knowledge and training in the field and, in part, to the notion of the unity of mind and body (psychosomatic medicine).[5] In the United States, lay psychoanalysis did not come on the scene, with some exception (notably, Erik Erikson), until the 1990s.[6]

The joint official position of the American Medical Association, American Psychiatric Association, and American Psychoanalytic Association, which was set out in 1954 in a "resolution on the Relations of Medicine and Psychology," is that "psychotherapy is a form of medical treatment and does not form the basis for a separate profession."

The Law Department of the American Medical Association has always considered psychotherapy to be a part of the practice of medicine and has never attempted to further specify grades of psychotherapy. It is of the opinion that the term *psychotherapy* covers activities ranging from marriage counseling to electroshock.[7] News magazines also cover psychiatry in their sections on medicine. Likewise, the Association of American Law Schools (AALS) in its directory puts courses in psychiatry and law under the heading "Law and Medicine." However, at the 1972 annual meeting of the AALS, the Law and Medicine Section voted to exclude from its scope matters related to law and psychiatry and to organize a separate section on law and psychiatry. In 1969, *Time* magazine ceased to include psychiatric news items under its section on medicine and inaugurated a new section called "Behavior."

Does any distinction exist between psychotherapy and such clearly nonmedical processes as advice, conversation, and reassurance? In its broader sense, psychotherapy is clearly not a medical discipline; it is obviously the common professional function also of the clergy, teachers, social workers, and psychologists. A question arises, however, if a more cogent definition is used, such as "psychotherapy is a planned technique of altering the maladaptive behavior of an individual (or group) toward more effective adaptation. The essential ingredient of psychotherapy is the utilization of the therapist's personality interacting with the patient's personality."[8]

Szasz, although he always identifies himself as an M.D. and apparently has never urged that his Department of Psychiatry separate from the medical school, argues in support of nonmedical psychotherapists. He contends that attempts to distinguish between the aforementioned processes are based on the institutional treatment of a process that can only be understood in instrumental terms. Any instrumental definition is bound to include so many diverse processes that not only is it impossible to restrict psychotherapy to medicine, but it is equally impossible to limit it to any other one profession.[9]

The supporters of nonmedical psychotherapy point out that the ever-increasing demand for psychotherapists (at low cost) is far from being met. There is a wide gulf, it is said, between supply and demand. There is one psychiatrist for approximately every 10,000 persons in the United States. Over the past decade, the number of U.S. medical graduates choosing psychiatric training has declined by about 50% (many of the residency training slots are filled by international medical graduates who are supported by U.S. federal funding).[10] There is social class and also geographical imbalance in the distribution of psychiatrists. They are disproportionately distributed among the middle and upper classes, leaving large segments of the population without any. More than half practice in 15 of the largest cities in the United States, and 10 states have fewer than 50 each. At one time, one psychiatrist in 10 had formal psychoanalytic training, but the number is far less today.

The Joint Commission on Mental Illness and Health in its final report of 1961 recommended that nonmedical mental health workers with proper training and experience be permitted to do general, short-term psychotherapy, and that "deep psychotherapy" be practiced only by those with special training, experience, and competence.[11] The latter group would include those professional persons who lack a medical education, but have an aptitude for, adequate training, and demonstrable competence in such techniques of psychotherapy. The training and education required to qualify as a nonmedical psychotherapist has been subject to a great deal of disagreement.[12]

This is not to say that the training and education of the medical psychotherapist is beyond reproach. The qualification of the psychiatrist in doing psychotherapy has been challenged. Psychologists in Illinois at one time sought enactment of legislation, which would have precluded psychiatrists from engaging in psychotherapy; they contended that the psychiatric residency program does not provide adequate training in the dynamics of human behavior and in the practice of psychotherapy. Increasingly, psychiatry residency programs devote less attention to psychotherapy and focus on medication. At one time, as it is said, psychiatry was "mind without a brain," now it is, "brain without a mind."

Of course, of all medical disciplines, psychiatry most focuses on psychotherapy. One prominent psychiatrist (who shall remain anonymous) suggests that any restrictive legislation on psychotherapy be aimed primarily at the general medical practitioner. In many medical schools, the only training a student acquires about psychological problems amounts to about 40 hours of class lectures over a 4-year period. Quite often, the general medical practitioner or other physician is unable to handle adequately a patient in a psychotherapeutic situation. Be that as it may, the general practitioner is at the forefront in dispensing psychiatric medication.

The explanation for many cures lies in various circumstances, particularly the transference relationship described by Freud. Patients frequently use the term *father confessor* to describe the functions of the medical practitioner to whom they confide their troubles. The successful physician is almost always a father or God-like figure. Some physicians object to the socialization of medicine because, as one English psychiatrist put it, "One of the most certain guarantees of the future decline of medicine is the fact that you cannot make a father figure from a subordinate official of the civil service." However, even young interns serving on the staffs of city hospitals seem to function very well as father figures.

Medical treatment throughout the ages has consisted, in important part, of the placebo effect; rational therapy based on scientific knowledge of chemistry and physiology is fairly recent. *Placebo*, in Latin, means "I shall please." Even with specific knowledge about drugs today, the psychological factors underlying placebo continue to play an important role. A limited view of placebo is that it consists of inert or inactive drugs, but a broader view would include any drug or procedure that has a placebo effect. Most placebo responses are involuntary responses. If the physician believes in the efficacy of a drug or procedure, his belief increases the likelihood of a placebo response, so placebos are usually an interactive process or component given deliberately to produce a pleasant or soothing effect.

Physicians have been prescribing placebos for hundreds of years, but curiously the role of placebos has increased in the age of technology. A physician who directs a famous medical center says, "There is nothing organically wrong with 70% of the patients who come to us, but if a sugar pill helps them to feel better, isn't it really medicine?" Prominent psychiatrist Jerome Frank years ago suggested in a classic book that the placebo effect might be the primary factor underlying all psychiatric remedies.[13] The latest research supports Frank's finding: Psychiatrists, psychologists, and other scientific healers are really exploiting the power of human belief, just as shamans and witch doctors do.[14] Can they do it as effectively? In a 1933 lecture, Freud remarked, "I do not think our successes can compete with those of Lourdes. There are so many more people who believe in the miracles of the Blessed Virgin than in the existence of the unconscious."

Regulation of Professions

The regulation of professions may be formal or informal. Institutional policies and customs (i.e., those of hospitals, mental health centers, HMOs, insurance) may allocate the functions and responsibilities of the various categories of mental health professionals.[15] Private clinics set out rules for their staff, professional or otherwise, regarding the treatment of patients (e.g., how much time is to be spent with a patient or the type of medication to be used). In some instances, the functions or responsibilities are mandated by law (e.g., psychiatrists are the only category of mental health professionals who are legally authorized to prescribe medication or administer electroshock, except that a number of states have recently allowed psychologists to prescribe medication). Increasingly, the policies and laws that bestow a privilege or monopoly to one or another of the mental health professionals have been the subject of challenge by competing professional groups.

In a very practical sense, insurance coverage of healthcare or malpractice insurance regulates the scope of the practitioner's activity. The practitioner will not likely carry out a treatment not covered by health insurance or by malpractice insurance. Litigation or the threat of it has proven to be a prime regulator of psychotherapy. It has dampened, for example, the practice of "revival of memory" of childhood abuse. Thus, a psychiatrist at the risk of litigation would not treat a patient for a sore throat as that would not be covered by liability coverage for the treatment of mental illness. After a few years out of medical school, the psychiatrist becomes inept at treating physical disorders and he becomes almost on a par with nonmedical therapists, treating only mental disorders.

The regulation and control of certain professions through the use of legislation is not a modern phenomenon. The forerunner of such legislation existed as common law. The medieval guilds, whose organization was at first informal, exercised control over their membership and were entirely self-regulatory. Ultimately, this self-regulation came to be sanctioned by the church and state. Although ecclesiastical control of medical licensure seems strange today, it was logical enough at the time because, until the Renaissance, physicians were usually clergymen. Episcopal authority in effect provided a national system. By the end of the Middle Ages, ideas about state examination had reached northern Europe, and the medical groups all sought official authority to carry out these procedures for their respective personnel.[16]

In the United States, the possibilities of using licensing legislation as an administrative device for the control of the professions were not recognized until a late date. Since 1870, when licensing legislation was first used on a state level, it has become an increasingly important regulatory device, particularly since the 1940s, when laws were enacted ostensibly to protect the public, but in actuality, to protect turf. At the present time, licensing or certification of practitioners of the various professions is quite common and readily accepted. There is legislation, for example, regulating architects, dentists, physicians, psychologists, social workers, and to some degree, marriage counselors.[17]

Such legislation has not always been so readily acceptable. Considering the history of the country, it is not surprising that at one time the validity of any and all licensing was contested. (Georgia actually passed a law forbidding the authorities to interfere with quacks.) The most frequent contention was that in a democracy a person possessed an inalienable right to pursue his chosen profession or to meet with and seek assistance from whomever he should choose. It was contended that interference with such a right was a violation of the Fourth Amendment of the Constitution. It was also claimed that it violated freedom of speech guaranteed under the First Amendment. Clergymen pointed out that Jesus spread the word although he was not ordained. It is safe to say that today, however, any regulatory provision, which is based on a social need and is not arbitrary or unreasonable, will be upheld in the courts.[18]

Although some professions were controlled by legislation long before others, the history of the professions and the legislation controlling them shows a remarkable parallel. At first, each profession was an informal organization that had evolved around the specialized skills common to its members. Each group would attempt to limit its membership to those who had attained such skills and applied them in an ethical manner. As soon as conditions permitted, each group urged legislation that would test those who wished to be admitted to the profession. Initially, a grandfather's clause, a provision for the automatic registration of those who had been engaged in practice for a specified time, was usually included in such legislation. Gradually, the educational requirements were raised and the entrance examination became increasingly more difficult.[19]

All licensing or certification legislation is based on two sometimes-contradictory ideas. Such legislation seems to be initiated by the group on the inside that wishes to eliminate competition, but its passage is always urged on the ground that the public must be protected from unfair practices. The profession's public prestige and status is enhanced while the number of persons able to perform these services is limited. Licensing results in an increased cost of the services, but is considered economically justified if the burden of higher prices is less than the social cost that would arise from damages to the public health or safety that would occur in the absence of licensing.[20] Regardless of the justification, such acts aim at regulation by general formal denial of a right, which is then made individually available by an administrative act of approval, certification, consent, or permit.[21]

Licensure and certification acts are the two types of legislation most often used to regulate the professions. A licensing act defines the function of the profession and prohibits practice by anyone who is not licensed under the act.[22] A certification act (sometimes called title licensing) does not define the function of the profession; it only prohibits the use of a title by those who do not meet the requirements of the act.[23] Thus, a licensing law covers the particular practice, no matter what the person calls himself, while a certification statute covers the particular practice only when the person wishes to identify himself by the use of a certain title. The actual words used in the laws do not necessarily indicate the nature of the law; several of the licensing laws are really certification laws in that the use of the title is the controlling factor.

Both types of acts have advantages and disadvantages. There seems to be little doubt that licensing provides the greater protection for the public. If properly enforced, it can control quackery, whereas certification in itself cannot. A prerequisite for enactment of a licensing act, however, is a definition of the function that is to be regulated. In the case of psychotherapy, there is no general agreement on a definition. The same problem arose in regard to psychology. In 1955, because of the interprofessional climate at the time and the difficulty in legally defining the practice of psychology, the American Psychological Association recommended that legislation take the form of certification.

Regulation by means of a certification statute, however, may easily be circumvented. Because the certification statute does not prohibit the function or practice of any particular profession, all that a charlatan has to do is change his title. As sometimes expressed, "the rat goes to a new sewer." Thus, if the certification statute prohibited the use of the title *marriage counselor*, a quack could simply change his title to family counselor and continue with the same work he was doing previously. David Mace, past president and then executive director of the American Association of Family and Marriage Counselors (AAFMC), however, argued that certification can be effective because it would be very difficult for a quack to attract clients when he used an unfamiliar title.[24] New York law, for example, protects only the titles *psychologist* and *social worker*. There are no legal restrictions on the use of such titles as *psychotherapist, group therapist,* and *psychoanalyst*.[25] (New York in 2006 required licensure for the practice of psychoanalysis or use of the title *licensed psychoanalyst* or the title *psychoanalyst* or any other derivatives.) The New York classified telephone directory lists, among others, metaphysicians, astrologers, and yoga instructors.

The executive director of the AAFMC at one time expressed the opinion that without appropriate guidelines provided by the state, the public has little or no means of determining who is or who is not qualified to do counseling and psychotherapy.[26] Since then, the AAFMC has continued to favor, as the best solution to the problem of state licensing of marriage counselors, a broad framework of legislation for the proper control of all counseling service offered to the public in the fields of mental health and family regulations, minimum standards in each field to be established by appropriate authorities within the respective professional groups concerned.

Without a workable legal definition of the function of a profession, a licensing statute would appear to be one of certification. It may be noted that many statutes that were first passed certifying psychologists have been repealed and replaced by licensing statutes.[27] Unless a regulatory statute is drawn in terms that are so definite and clear that a person can reasonably ascertain whether he is within the areas of conduct proscribed by the statute, the statute will be considered a denial of due process of law and consequently void.[28] However, the Missouri Supreme Court has upheld a statute making the practice of medicine without a license a misdemeanor, although the term *practice of medicine* is not given a legislative definition.[29] The court held that the test is whether the language conveys a sufficiently definite warning as to the proscribed conduct as measured by common understanding and practice.

In some parts of the United States and in a number of European countries, individuals with a degree in philosophy advertise (without violating the law) that they are available for philosophical consultation, discussing such issues as the meaning of life, the definition of virtue, and so on. From a movement that began in Germany in the 1980s, a small but growing number of philosophers in the United States have opened private practices as philosopher practitioners, offering a therapy based on the idea that solutions to many personal, moral, and ethical problems can be found not in psychotherapy or Prozac, but in philosophical disclosure. They are the modern-day versions of Socrates.[30] A philosopher says, "Physicians [would] do well to send patients more often to the library than to the pharmacy, since philosophy has traditionally provided us with soothing and inspirational homilies."[31] Philosophy, after all, is about getting your bearings in life. New York is the first state to consider licensing philosophers. At the turn of the 20th century, the American Philosophical Association was founded as a split from the American Psychological Association.

Psychotherapy has become so complex and fragmented that no single approach can be understood as primary. With the rise of psychopharmacological treatments, many of the forms of psychotherapy have been adapted as supportive psychotherapy both within and beyond the clinical setting. Psychotherapy today is extraordinarily diverse and holds an important position within both medical and nonmedical aspects of culture. Indeed, it seems today that just about everyone—schoolteachers, housewives, ministers, lawyers, etc.—is playing therapist. With training or without, are they helpful, or harmful? In one study, eight college-educated housewives were given part-time training over a 2-year period to provide psychotherapy. Their performance was judged comparable to that of more highly trained therapists.[32]

Housewives, however, do not constitute a profession. Indispensable to any would-be profession is a body of esoteric knowledge, mastery of which is the necessary qualification for practice of the profession. In classical sociological theory, professional knowledge becomes social by dint of the professionalization process. Dedication entitles professionals to claim immunity to crass motives or self-interest. It is commonly quipped that professionals practice while others work; however, actually, the idea of practice is an expectation of a dedication to improving one's skills. To profess was, in its earliest use, the public declaration of one's religion, and it signified a commitment to a particular way of life. Prostitution is frequently called the oldest profession, but it is not an honored one.[33]

Through the years the concept of a *learned profession* has been distinguished from that of a trade or business.[34] The traditional concept of professionalism posits that the complexity of professional knowledge and service means that professionals should not be subject to lay control, whether exercised through bureaucratic or market mechanisms. As a corollary to this proposition, licensure by the state should be sufficient to shield professionals from attempts at control by others. The codes of ethics of the profession highlight the fiduciary feature of professional life. They stress the trust that their members should provide those seeking their help. They take a vow of service, so for many years the antitrust or antimonopoly laws were not applied to them.

From 1890, when the Sherman antitrust act was enacted, until 1975, the courts held that the learned professions were exempt from the antitrust laws. Few antitrust claims were asserted against professionals of any sort until the mid-1970s. Then, in 1975, the U.S. Supreme Court held that a Virginia state bar rule requiring lawyers to charge minimum prices for specified services was not immune from antitrust challenge.[35] The Court rejected the lawyers' claim that professional ethics protected their mandatory minimum fees against a price-fixing challenge. The Court, however, noted that the "public service aspect, and other features of the professions, may require that a particular practice, which could properly be viewed as a violation of the Sherman Act in another context, be treated differently."[36] With that decision, the Court ended the exemption of the learned professions from the antitrust laws.[37]

The entrepreneurial aspect of professionalism prompted George Bernard Shaw's claim that the professions are "a conspiracy against the laity." By 1975, it was not uncommon to refer to healthcare as an industry. Soon to go as self-serving would be the traditional restriction of medical societies and other professional organizations against the dissemination of price information and advertising. In 1982, by a decision in favor of the Federal Trade Commission, the Supreme Court inaugurated the era of advertising by physicians and other professionals. The FTC had filed suit against the American Medical Association, holding that it was in restraint of trade because of its code of ethics prohibiting advertising. The FTC did, however, allow the AMA to adopt guidelines prohibiting unsubstantiated, false, and deceptive representations by its members.[38]

Particular Categories of Mental Health Professionals

Psychiatry

The title "psychiatry" is not as such the subject of regulatory legislation as of usage. In Greek, *psyche* means soul and *iatros* means healer. It is commonly assumed that psychiatrists are also physicians, who are the subject of regulation. The *American Psychiatric Glossary* defines a psychiatrist as "[a] licensed physician who specializes in the diagnosis, treatment, and prevention of mental and emotional disorders."[39]

As a matter of custom, it is rare to find a non-M.D. psychotherapist who uses the title "psychiatrist." When the problem arises, it is usually in the case of the foreign medical school graduate who is without a medical license. While there is no legal protection of the titles "analyst," "psychoanalyst" (except in New York), or "psychotherapist," as shall be noted, there is some measure of protection for the term *psychiatrist* under medical practice acts in that it is commonly accepted as a medical specialty and a non-M.D. using the title would likely be ordered to cease and desist.

Psychiatry is singled out in legislation on commitment procedures and sometimes on school personnel. Apart from these special areas, the assumption is that the profession shares with the rest of medicine with regard to regulatory statutes. In the regulation of physicians, most states by the turn of the 20th century had passed laws and established state boards of medical examiners. Many of the early laws were permissive, merely prohibiting unlicensed persons from using the title "doctor of medicine," and did not extend to practice. They were more concerned with protecting the title than with protecting the public health. Between 1910 and 1930, following the Flexner Report on medical education and the establishment of the AMA's Council on Medical Education, the licensing laws assumed their present general form and content. That is, unlicensed persons were specifically prohibited from practicing medicine or the healing arts, but the scope of the prohibition was disputed. The statutory definition usually contained language to the effect that any person who advertises or announces to the public a readiness to heal, refers to himself as a doctor, or prescribes for or treats a person's suffering, is practicing medicine or a healing art.

There have developed within the medical profession optional subdivisions in the form of specialties that deal with distinctive portions of the body, such as dermatology; and specialties dealing with forms of treatment, such as surgery. These specialties are recognized by certifying boards within the profession itself. In this manner, the American Board of Psychiatry and Neurology is, like other medical specialty boards, a voluntary, nonprofit, nongovernmental organization established under the sponsorship of the American Medical Association. Training programs are accredited on request and their graduates are examined by the board if they so desire.

A psychiatrist, thus, may opt to take the examination given by the American Board of Psychiatry and Neurology and thereby represent himself as a board-certified psychiatrist. The American Board of Psychiatry and Neurology certifies approximately half of the membership of the American Psychiatric Association, which now totals some 40,000. In other words, about half of the nation's psychiatrists practice without certification. The certification examination, however, while it measures something about the psychiatrist's understanding of theory, history, and his diagnostic ability, tells practically nothing about his ability to relate to other people or to treat them. An effort, though limited, is made during the examination to get a "feel" for the way the candidate interacts with patients.

Many general practitioners who work in mental hospitals call themselves psychiatrists although they have had no formal training in psychiatry. While there is no legal requirement of certification or licensure, board certification is required by many private hospitals as a condition to use of its facilities. In the law of torts, one who holds himself out as a specialist in a specific area of practice is held to a higher standard of knowledge and skill. In or out of the mental hospital, psychiatric medication is mostly prescribed by the general practitioner.

With the development of medication, insurance, and managed care limitations, and competition with nonmedical mental health professionals, psychiatrists are less engaged in psychotherapy or psychoanalysis. Until the 1960s, psychiatric training was predominantly psychoanalytic. Psychiatrists were taught to look for the (unconscious) cause of the patient's difficulties—the theory being that interpreting these hidden meanings would take care of the difficulties. Then in the 1960s there came a proliferation of psychotherapy approaches: gestalt, transactional analysis, bioenergetics, and so on. As therapies proliferated, so did psychotherapists.

The growth of managed care has also affected the market for mental health services. Psychiatrists have found themselves at a competitive disadvantage because, on a per-unit-of-service basis, their fees are generally higher than those of other mental health professionals and, as a group, they are more reluctant to embrace managed care principles. Moreover, managed care systems tend to compartmentalize the roles of various mental health professionals. Thus, psychiatrists are often restricted to providing medical management or pharmacotherapy for patients, whereas psychologists, social workers, and other caregivers who are perceived as less expensive are used to provide verbal therapies. The vast majority of articles in the *American Journal of Psychiatry* are now on pharmacotherapy, not on psychodynamics. Training programs in psychiatry provide less and less attention to psychotherapy. The psychiatrist is now called the "hydraulic doctor"—one who raises and lowers the dosage. Biopsychiatrists believe that all serious emotional problems have a physiological cause and can (and should) be treated with medication, perhaps also with psychotherapy as supportive therapy.[40]

Psychoanalysis

Psychoanalysis is the "talk therapy" devised by Sigmund Freud. It is based on free association, dream interpretation, and interpretation of resistance and transference manifestations. In 50-minute sessions three to five times a week for a number of years, the analysand lies on a couch with the analyst sitting behind and from time to time, making an interpretation. For decades it has been the butt of jokes, cartoons, and movie spoofs, much to the detriment of its reputation. To this day, just about every issue of the *New Yorker* has a cartoon or two about psychoanalysis.

It is commonly thought that a person who goes to a psychoanalyst several times a week for several years must be very sick. In actuality, it takes a rather healthy person to withstand the requirement of frequent free association without coming apart. So, why do such people undertake the rigors, demands, and expense of psychoanalysis? Because, as Socrates would say, self-knowledge is a source of strength and wisdom. Many prominent individuals, such as Judge David Bazelon, have acknowledged that they were in analysis.[41] In some places, it is considered fashionable to be in analysis. Auditors at the Internal Revenue Service are often perplexed that the taxpayer looks healthy yet claims large medical deductions.

It is commonly believed that the field of psychoanalysis is governed by licensing or certification laws, as is the case with psychiatry, but in fact it is not (with the recent exception of New York). There are, moreover, no official accrediting agencies for psychoanalysis. The American Psychoanalytic Association approves training institutes, while a newer group, the American Academy of Psychoanalysis, which proclaims a constructive coexistence, does not technically approve training institutes, but admits individual members deemed qualified and *de facto* accepts graduates of a number of institutes. The association, at one time, tried to develop a subspecialty certifying board within the American Board of Psychiatry and Neurology, but this was defeated initially within the association and then by the American Boards when the academy protested. This issue crops up periodically as a possibility.

The association's position has been that only those who are trained in its approved institutes are qualified psychoanalysts. The academy's position has been that qualified persons wherever trained should be permitted, if they so desire, to join both organizations. As things stood, a number of analysts trained in association-approved institutes were also members of the academy, but the association excluded those not trained at its approved institutes. Some of the leading training centers that were not recognized by the association included the American Institute of Psychoanalysis, the William Alanson White Institute of Psychiatry, the Psychoanalytic Institute of the New York Medical College, and the psychoanalytic training program of the Tulane University School of Medicine, Department of Psychiatry and Neurology.

The Tulane program was an offshoot of Columbia University. As a result of the efforts of the late Dr. Sandor Rado and other psychoanalysts from the New York Psychoanalytic Institute, who were convinced that psychoanalysis was and should continue to be a medical discipline, the Psychoanalytic Clinic for Training and Research was established in 1944 as part of the Department of Psychiatry of the College of Physicians and Surgeons at Columbia, where the faculty developed a graduate psychoanalytic curriculum, which was approved by the association. Shortly after World War II, in 1949, a group of Columbia University–trained psychoanalysts headed by Dr. Robert G. Heath and including Drs. Harold I. Lief, Irwin Marcus, Russell Monroe, and Norman Rucker arrived at Tulane and, in setting up its department of psychiatry, which to this day is combined with neurology, integrated psychoanalytic training into its residency program.

The development of the Tulane program was viewed initially as a threat to the existence of nonuniversity-affiliated training institutes. Communications were sent to the president of Tulane that urged against the development. Some members of the Tulane group were ostracized by the association. Heath was at first granted and then refused admission in an extraordinary session; Monroe's application was not approved because he was participating in an unapproved training institute. A few years later, Marcus and Rucker, when they left Tulane, became members of the association, playing a leading role in that organization. Lief, who later became director of the Division of Family Study of the University of Pennsylvania Department of Psychiatry, never applied to the association for membership, but in 1999, the association invited him to join, and he accepted (without having to pay dues).

The excommunicated and other members at Tulane, along with a number of members of the association regarded as analytic pioneers (such as Franz Alexander, Jules Masserman, Sandor Rado, and Clara Thompson) formed the academy, which reached a membership of 706 in 1974 (declining to 639 in 1999). The membership consists of Fellows who are physicians and now nonphysicians, and another category—scientific associates—who make up approximately 15% of the membership and who may or may not be physicians. The scientific associates include nonpsychoanalytically trained psychiatrists, many of whom are chairmen of departments, and a number of behavioral scientists. The association, which has double the academy's membership, consists of psychiatrists and a number of psychologists, all psychoanalytically trained in its approved institutes.

Since the development of the Tulane program, a number of psychoanalytic programs have come under the aegis of universities and medical schools. Apart from the program at New York Medical College, a number of the training institutes of the Association itself have close ties with medical schools and universities, such as at Case Western Reserve, New York Downstate Medical Center, Pittsburgh, and from the early date, Columbia. Such relationships tend to arrest the isolation of psychoanalysis from the mainstream of medical thought. They tend to explore the connection between behavior and biology.

Psychoanalysis, as well as psychiatry generally, but less so, is characterized by (1) fewer patient referrals, (2) lower fees per visit, (3) shorter inpatient and outpatient time to treat a patient, and (4) alternatives including social workers, psychologists, and B.A.-level or below mental health professionals. Enrollment in psychoanalytic training institutes, which peaked at 1,194 trainees in 1980, dropped to 909 by 1989.[42] In 1988, in response to the restraint of trade suit by psychologists, a settlement agreement overturned the American Psychoanalytic Association's longstanding policy of restricting analytic training to candidates with medical degrees, opening the field to lay analysis. In 1995, the Michigan Psychoanalytic Institute, so bereft of candidates, opened its doors to attorneys to become psychoanalysts. A frequent topic at meetings of psychoanalytic institutes is: "Does Psychoanalysis Have A Future?"

Psychoanalysis at one time was considered the gold standard of psychotherapy. Eric Kandel, winner of the Nobel Prize in physiology, writes: "It is difficult to capture today the fascination that psychoanalysis held for young people in the 1950s. Psychoanalysis had developed a theory of mind that gave me my first appreciation of the complexity of human behavior and of the motivations that underlie it. ... Psychoanalysis held the promise of self-understanding and even of therapeutic change based on an analysis of the unconscious motivations and defenses underlying individual actions." And he added, "What made psychoanalysis so compelling to me while I was in college was that it was at once imaginative, comprehensive, and empirically grounded—or so it appeared to my naive mind. No other views of mental life approached psychoanalysis in scope or subtlety. Earlier psychologies were either highly speculative or very narrow."[43]

Psychoanalysis was used in the treatment of neurosis, personality disorders, psychosomatic disorders, sexual disorders, and sexual dysfunction, and also to enhance creativity or productivity. Many of these areas have been taken over by medication or cognitive or behavior therapy. The reasons are several. The work done by the anti-Freudian skeptics has taken hold of the popular imagination. The climate of opinion about psychoanalysis has changed, resulting in the declining prestige of psychoanalysis. It was not always effective and now there is a changing economic climate, calling for proof of efficacy and for briefer therapy. Except for electroshock and psychosurgery, psychoanalysis was the only available treatment, but that too has changed.

In the years following World War II the Menninger Foundation in Topeka, Kansas, was the world-renowned institution for the training of psychoanalysts and psychiatrists and the treatment of patients by psychoanalysis and psychoanalytic psychotherapy, but in the latter part of the 20th century, due mainly to cuts in managed care and an increased use of drugs instead of therapy to treat mental illness, it has moved to Houston to become a partner with the Baylor College of Medicine and Methodist Healthcare System.

At the 2001 annual meeting of the American Academy of Psychoanalysis members voted to expand the academy's name to The American Academy of Psychoanalysis and Dynamic Psychiatry. The new level of support for the name change was explained: "We are finding a growing interest in our programs among psychiatrists who are informed by dynamic teaching but not formally trained and certified as analysts." One member dissented to the name change thus: "I want to remind you of the law of unintended consequences. I think we are giving a message to the public that we are done with psychoanalysis. I am not one of the people who thinks psychoanalysis is dead."

Though psychoanalysis may be on the wane as a treatment modality, most of its concepts permeate treatment programs and in developmental and social uses. Freud's theories left their mark on many endeavors outside psychiatry, and nowhere more so than in the United States (or Argentina). The terms we use, such as *neurotic* and *hysteric*, are part of the common language that is heard on the streets, in soap operas, and in the movies.[44] As a result of the influence of psychoanalysis, particularly around mid-20th century, 80% of undergraduate college students in the United States studied psychology, either as a major or minor.

Psychology

In 1954 the American Psychoanalytic Association and the American Psychiatric Association jointly condemned the practice of psychotherapy by any but trained physicians, but nevertheless the number of psychotherapists who were not physicians, mostly psychologists, continued to grow rapidly; many of them were graduates of new clinical psychology programs set up with funding from the National Institute of Mental Health (NIMH) or the Veterans Administration.

As of a number of years ago, the American Board of Examiners in Professional Psychology offers a Diplomate in Clinical Psychology. Minimal requirements are 5 years of post-PhD experience and successful completion of oral and written examinations. Most states regulate the practice of psychology, some by licensure and some by certification by state boards.[45]

A number of state statutes license or certify psychologists according to level or specialty. However, the Committee on Legislation of the American Psychological Association does not favor legislation that permits differentiation of specialists within psychology, regardless of whether these specialties are defined by the functions carried out or by the locale where the work is done. It is believed that these matters are best dealt with by intraprofessional controls.[46] The American Psychological Association, now represents more than 159,000 clinicians, researchers, and educators. In 1975, there were an estimated 15,000 clinical psychologists.

Many acts regulating the practice of psychology include a correlating section that specifically states that nothing in the statute shall be construed as permitting a psychologist, certified or licensed under the statute, to administer or prescribe drugs or in any manner to engage in the practice of medicine. The American Psychological Association Committee on Legislation contends that because psychologists do not represent themselves as being anything other than psychologists, a disclaimer clause on the right to practice other professions is inappropriate. The same might be argued regarding any possible enactment regulating the practice of psychotherapy, but it does allay other professions' fears of encroachment.

While psychologists over the years have generally berated the use of pharmacological treatment, increased competition among caregivers has prompted some psychologists as well as nurse clinicians to seek prescription privileges. They have argued that the knowledge and experience base needed to provide competent pharmacological treatment can be obtained without a medical school education or psychiatric residency training.[47] The American Medical Association, the American Psychiatric Association, and other professional associations have voiced strong opposition, and, thus far, psychologists have obtained prescribing privileges in only a few states. A number of states, moreover, permit prescribing by nurse clinicians, albeit within a limited formulary and with medical oversight. In 1999, the Florida Psychological Association failed in an effort to obtain legislative approval to change the name of psychologists to *psychological physicians*. In previous years, it unsuccessfully sought to limit psychological testing to their profession and also to obtain prescribing privileges and independent hospital privileges.[48] Quite often, when medication is considered necessary, psychologists refer the patient to a primary care physician for it (rather than to a psychiatrist to avoid the perceived stigma of seeing a psychiatrist).

Arguing that medical training is not essential to the practice of psychoanalysis, psychologists brought antitrust litigation that forced the American Psychoanalytic Association to allow them (and social workers) into their association. They also challenged insurance practices that excluded them (and other nonmedical mental health professionals) and won the right to compete with physicians as psychotherapy providers.[49]

Social Work

The practice of social work as a certified social worker is defined in regulatory legislation as engaging, under such title, in social casework, social group work, community organization, administration of a social work program, social work education, social work research, or any combination of these in accordance with social work principles and methods. The New York legislation states that "the practice of social work is for the purpose of helping individuals, families, groups, and communities to prevent or to resolve problems caused by social or emotional stress." The Academy of Certified Social Workers issues certificates to qualified social workers who have completed at least 2 years of supervised experience beyond the MSW (Master of Social Work) requirement. The MSW is the usual degree requirement representing at least 2 years of graduate course study, one of which normally consists of supervised field experience. Schools of social work offer bachelor's (BSW), master's (MSW), and doctoral (DSW) degrees. The Council on Social Work sets national standards for social work accreditation. State licensing and certification requirements vary.

In the early part of the 20th century the Boston Psychopathic Children's Clinic, the Juvenile Psychopathic Institute in Chicago, and the Henry Phipps Psychiatric Clinic in Baltimore introduced social workers to assist people to get help that E.E. Southard, a psychiatrist, and Mary C. Jarrett, a social worker, described in its broadest sense to mean "restoration of capacity for normal living or provision for the greatest possible comfort." The social worker was originally called a friendly visitor. It was World War I and the impact on existing treatment facilities of the returning psychiatric casualties—the shell-shocked veterans—which gave impetus to formal training for increased numbers of practitioners of what henceforth was to be known as psychiatric social work, i.e., social work practiced in collaboration with psychiatry.

Psychiatric social work has grown in prominence with the increasing acceptance of both managed care and community-based public sector service and in political strength as the number of its practitioners increases. According to the Bureau of Labor Statistics, the United States now employs over 170,000 social workers in one capacity or another. Social workers provide a large share of the psychotherapy for poor patients. Programs for drug addicts rely heavily on social workers. The growing effort to move mental patients out of long-time hospitalization in state institutions depends on social workers to supervise outpatient cases in the community.[50]

Marriage and Family Counseling

The field of marriage and family counselors has shown the most explosive growth of all. While before 1964 no state recognized them, and today apparently no more than nine do, there are now by some estimates more than 50,000 marriage and family counselors, up from 7,000 in 1979. Their exact number is not known because in most states, they are not licensed, although they are generally free to practice nevertheless.

According to the American Association for Marriage and Family Therapy (AAMFT), 2.2 million individuals are seeking marriage and family counseling, as are 863,000 couples and 549,000 families. Several national trade organizations representing social workers, psychologists, and family and marriage counselors do not have statistics on the number of lawsuits or administrative complaints filed annually against therapists, but is said that suits and complaints against therapists with state licensing boards have increased significantly in recent years, particularly in the area of family law.[51]

Many charlatans in the mental health field practice under the aegis of the title marriage counselor or family counselor. Some years ago, to test the competency of marriage counseling, investigators, either alone or accompanied by their pretended wives, who visited marriage counselors chosen at random in six cities, found that most of the counselors' performances fell below commonsense standards, and that the credentials displayed on their office walls were fraudulent.[52]

Qualified marriage counselors have sought to improve counseling techniques by training more competent practitioners. In the 1930s, they set up the AAMFT, which has established educational criteria and qualification standards. In past years, proposed state legislation outlining qualifications and licensing procedures for counselors has come and gone, usually disappearing in some committee. But the AAFMC is a national accrediting body for the specialty of marriage counseling, an organization composed of interprofessional membership, divided somewhat equally among psychologists, social workers, psychiatrists, family-life educators, and pastoral counselors. The basic membership requirement is that the person has a doctorate and a few years' experience in one of these fields. An exception to the requirement of a doctorate is made in the field of social work, where an MSW plus experience is accepted. The organization also requires a minimum of 2 years of specialization in marriage counseling with at least one of the years at an internship center.

Professional Licensed Counselor

About two decades ago, various states provided for the licensing of professional counselors. Licensure as a professional counselor requires a master's or doctoral degree in counseling or student personnel work from an approved program and at least 2 years of counseling experience under the supervision of a licensed professional counselor.[53]

In the battle over turf, psychologists were more opposed to the legislation than were psychiatrists. Like the psychologists, professional counselors are precluded from prescribing medication and, thus, are more in competition with psychologists. Professional counselors joined with psychiatrists in persuading legislatures not to grant prescribing privileges to psychologists. That would have given psychologists an advantage over the counselors.

Encounter and Other Groups

There is no legislation or requirement of professional standards for leaders of encounter or sensitivity training groups. They have a variety of backgrounds, no common fund of knowledge or experience, and no common set of professional ethics. The issue of control was raised when the New York weekly paper, *The Village Voice*, refused to advertise groups whose claims implied therapy. The paper said that advertising therapy was against professional standards and, in general, unethical. The sponsors of encounters argued that they did not conduct therapy or aim at changing the psychological state of participants in a fundamental way. Encounter groups propose by intensive group experiences to reduce man's alienation from other persons, from nature, and from genuine emotion.

There is always the hazard of a psychotic breakdown when a person moves from a structured into an unstructured society. The emphasis in encounter or sensitivity groups is on impulse or primary process behavior. Kurt W. Back in *Beyond Words: The Story of Sensitivity Training and the Encounter Movement* and Jane Howard in *Please Touch* point out the almost casual acceptance by encounter group leaders of possible breakdowns and other effects commonly considered as detrimental. Fritz Perls in his book on Gestalt therapy states, "Sir, if you want to go crazy, commit suicide, improve, get turned on, or get an experience that would change your life, that is up to you. You came here out of your own free will." Some encounter group leaders believe that breakdown or disintegration of personality is essential to a redevelopment of personality. "Breakdown" is a "breakthrough."

Some sensitivity groups, which are not of an intensive nature, are coming more and more to approximate religious retreats, yoga centers, halfway houses, and singles' weekends at mountain and beach resorts. Apart from sensitivity groups, the Manhattan telephone directory lists over 60 entries of sundry groups, including a number of anonymous-titled organizations (the label was first used in 1937 by Alcoholics Anonymous), such as Overeaters Anonymous, Gamblers Anonymous, Neurotics Anonymous, Parents Anonymous. Also in the parental field is the 7,000-member Parents Without Partners organization. Many of these organizations have developed into big businesses. In many of these groups, psychiatrists are looked upon with disdain (though some members are in psychiatric treatment concurrently with their group meetings).

The cultural phenomenon of the increasing number of groups in recent years reflects the fact that many of the old sources of intimacy and emotional support—notably the family—have been dispersed. The license and freedom of the group atmosphere also contribute to its appeal. The open expression of feelings discouraged in an increasingly impersonal world are encouraged in the intimacy of the group. The group thus contributes to alleviating human distress, but its commercial aspects tend to vulgarize the encounter.[54]

Pastoral Counseling

As elsewhere, many persons in the United States, before the decline of religion, turned to members of the clergy for counseling and guidance. Surveys show that American young people today put the profession of the clergy near the bottom of the list of occupations they would like to enter. With contemporary psychiatry or psychology now the standard, pastoral counseling is widely regarded as inept. A survey of 1,045 pastors reveals that 24% had not received any training in counseling. Although 64% reported taking one or more courses in pastoral care, pastoral psychology, or pastoral counseling, only 10% reported any kind of clinical training involving actual counseling experience under supervision. Furthermore, only 24% reported having any counseling or therapy experiences of their own.[55]

Many religious denominations have now established training programs in pastoral counseling and psychology in their seminaries. In the early 1960s, the Menninger Foundation established a pastoral counseling program for clergymen, exposing them to the basic principles of psychiatry. A generation before this, Rev. Anton Boisen of Elgin State Hospital founded the Council on Clinical Training with active programs for ministers. In recent years, there has been an upsurge of strong fundamentalist religious beliefs to which more and more people are attaching themselves. Freud, though, very much like Marx, believed that religion is an opiate.

Over the past half-century, the number of mental health personnel increased by almost the number of decline of clergy. Churches are turned into restaurants or psychotherapy centers.

In considerable measure, psychiatry has replaced religion in America, although polls indicate that most Americans consider themselves religious to some degree, if not particularly devout or observant. The public hears far more about human behavior from psychologists and psychiatrists than from clergy. U.S. Supreme Court Justice Antonin Scalia expressed his bewilderment, "When is it, one must wonder, that the psychotherapist came to play such an indispensable role in the maintenance of the citizenry's mental health?"[56]

Sex Therapy

Sex therapy is probably the most successful of all the psychological therapies. It deals only with sexual problems so it cannot be regarded as a mainstream psychotherapy. The boom time for sex therapy began in the early 1970s, following the work of researchers Dr. William H. Masters and Mrs. Virginia Johnson of the Reproductive Biology Research Foundation in St. Louis, Missouri. Pioneers in psychiatry such as Havelock Ellis, Krafft-Ebbing, and Freud focused broadly on human sexuality, but the research by Masters and Johnson has been more specific on physiological responses to sexual stimulation and a treatment method to deal with specific sexual complaints. They were accused of mechanizing and dehumanizing sex, of ignoring love and psychology, and of prostituting the most intimate expression to exercises in technique. Even more controversial were some of the methods they developed to treat heretofore incurable cases of male sexual inadequacy through the use of surrogate wives—otherwise known as *in-bed therapists*. They said that "there is no such thing as an uninvolved partner in any marriage in which there is some form of sexual inadequacy," hence, a marital unit was seen together, but a surrogate was used in cases of men without partners. Stemming from one of these cases was an alienation-of-affection suit brought by one George E. Calvert against Dr. Masters and several "John Doe" defendants, alleging that without his knowledge or consent his wife was persuaded by Dr. Masters to serve as a surrogate partner, being paid $500 for the first time and $250 for each subsequent sexual service. An out-of-court settlement was reached.

The issue of treatment of symptoms versus treatment of underlying causes of a disorder finds expression in the controversy over techniques employed in sex clinics. Critics argue that sexual expression is not separate but a part of the person; that sexual physiology reflects the psychological, but has little to offer in itself; and that sexual problems, unless they are caused by simple ignorance, which is rare, are likely to require long psychological and, not always successful, treatment.

In the wake of Masters and Johnson, numerous sex clinics of this type sprang up around the country. The use of surrogate sexual partners, because of the lawsuit and adverse publicity, was discontinued at the St. Louis clinic. Masters and Johnson emphasized, however, the need to understand first the fundamental mechanics of sex. (Some observers say that Americans seem to be the only people in the world who feel a need for instructions on how to copulate.) Masters and Johnson reported an overall success rate of 80% in the varieties of sexual disorders that they treated. Their style of therapy was behavior therapy, or conditioning therapy, as it was once called.

The opinion that the effects of behavior therapy are superficial and do not remove the basic neurosis, and that relapse and symptom substitution are to be expected, presupposes as dogma the psychoanalytic view of neurosis and its treatment method. Traditional psychotherapy may have overemphasized the subjective antecedents of behavior. Behavior therapists deny recurrence of symptoms, relapse, and symptom substitution. They suggest that changes in thoughts and feelings may be effected by changing the way that one acts, rather than vice versa. In behavior therapy, nonadaptive habits are weakened and eliminated; adaptive habits are initiated and strengthened.

Anyone can call himself a sexologist, or an expert in human sexuality. A malpractice lawsuit by an injured client is not likely because, apart from the difficulty of establishing causation, it would probably involve embarrassing testimony of impotency. As that deterrent, thus, is not available, a licensing law to regulate the practice has been recommended by a number of persons in the field, notably Masters and Johnson. The popular Dr. Ruth Westheimer (a.k.a. Dr. Ruth) offers sex advice in a syndicated column and on radio and television.[57] Nowadays, to deal with their sex problems, more people turn to Viagra rather than to psychotherapy.

Counseling by Lay Persons

Some efforts have been made to utilize lay persons in counseling work. One pilot program trained "mental health counselors."[58] The assumption underlying this experiment was that, in general, short-term psychotherapy could effectively be done by nonmedical mental health workers. The group chosen to be trained consisted of middle-aged women, experienced in child rearing and family living, who were looking for constructive activity outside the home. On the whole, their efforts achieved good results, but they suffered from the inability to raise the expectations of their patients. The magic element, it was found, is diminished when the therapist does not stand out as different, apart from the great mass of people. North Dakota has experimented with bartenders and beauticians as licensed therapists and counselors.

Comments

Just as a country's artistic and social institutions usually reflect its particular outlook on life, the kind of psychotherapy practiced there often expresses its characteristic philosophy. The increasing Westernization of so-called underdeveloped countries may make their own therapies decreasingly effective. Contrariwise, some Oriental practices now in vogue among certain elements in the United States are not sustained by the dominant culture and can hardly be expected to be effective or to endure. A cartoon depicts a wealthy businessman, with briefcase, sitting in a chauffeured limousine chanting, "Krishna, Krishna, Hare Hare." Such out-of-the-ordinariness provokes laughter.

Various programs are indicative of the growing awareness that the treatment for many mental illnesses must meet the cultural expectations of the patient and that virtually every culture has given rise to healers who are as effective in dealing with mental problems among their own people as are psychiatrists in Western society. The National Institute of Mental Health, in one of its projects to improve the delivery of psychiatric services, employed some Navajo medicine men on a reservation in Arizona to teach young Native Americans the elaborate ancient chants that often cure the mental ailments of Navajos.

Psychiatrists may dislike such jocular sobriquets as faith-healer, headshrinker, or medicine man, but there may be more truth than metaphorical cleverness in the terms. (A headshrinker is a witchdoctor whose knowledge of the occult constitutes a powerful magic that justifies the reestablishment of infantile dependency.) Among others, it is the thesis of Dr. E. Fuller Torrey, then of the NIMH's International Activities Branch, that "witchdoctors and psychiatrists perform essentially the same function in their respective cultures." He made a study of indigenous psychotherapists in several parts of the world and learned from the so-called witchdoctors that he, as a psychiatrist, was using the same mechanisms for curing his patients as they were and getting about the same results. (In many cultures, however, the therapist can collect his fee only if the patient gets well.) In the Western scientific world, psychiatrists plaster their office with diplomas (often in Latin), while a witchdoctor achieves the same effect by rattling a sacred gourd.

Torrey cites four basic components of curing used by psychotherapists all over the world. The first is naming the affliction (a step that removes the frightening element of the unknown); the second is the effect of their own personal qualities (successful healers have accurate empathy, nonpossessive warmth, and genuineness); the third is the patient's expectation (the great importance of patients' expectations is clearly seen in the use of placebos, the pilgrimage, and the building used for the healing); the fourth comprises the techniques of therapy (some cultures favor one technique over others, but the same techniques are used all over the world).[59]

Under most statutes, even when cause has been established, suspension or revocation of a license is not mandatory on the board. The statutes provide that a license may be revoked or invalidated. Throughout the country, a license is virtually a blank check; once a license is granted it is virtually permanent, subject only to the payment of a periodic fee. Self-regulation tends to provide not regulation, but protectionism. In 1961, the Board of Trustees of the American Medical Association, alarmed by the growing problems of discipline within the medical profession with the resultant increasing public apprehension and lack of confidence, appointed a Medical Disciplinary Committee, which concluded: "Medicine's efforts have largely ceased with the discharge of the licensing function. All too seldom are licensed physicians called to task by boards, societies, or colleagues."

Other Legislation Controlling the Practice of Psychotherapy

The medical practice acts, which define medical practice and require practitioners to possess a physician's license, usually apply expressly to the treatment of both mental and physical afflictions and, therefore, may include psychotherapy within their scope.[60] A few of the physicians' licensure acts, however, do not appear to regulate the practice of psychotherapy at all. For example, the Oklahoma act regards a person as practicing medicine when he treats disease, injury, or deformity of persons by any drugs, surgery, and manual or mechanical treatment.[61] The South Dakota statute defines the practice of medicine as prescribing any drug, medicine, apparatus, or other agency for the cure, relief, or palliation of any ailment or disease.[62] North Carolina and Minnesota specifically omit persons who endeavor to prevent or cure disease or suffering by mental or spiritual means.[63] Tennessee and Ohio define the practice of medicine as treatment of physical ailments or physical injuries.[64]

Opinions of a number of state legal officers have stated that the practice of psychotherapy is not restricted to physicians. In 1959, the New York State Education Department, which is responsible for administering the laws governing all professions in New York, ruled that the use of the title "psychotherapist" was not restricted to physicians by the Medical Practices Act. This ruling was arrived at following extensive hearings, at which representatives of the several professions active in the mental health field were heard. Earlier, in 1956, the Attorney General of Michigan rendered an opinion on the question of whether the practice of psychotherapeutics by psychologists constituted the practice of medicine within the meaning of the state's Medical Practices Act. It was concluded, "Therapy as such is not prohibited by the Medical Practices Act, which covers only therapy medical in nature." Psychologists and others are not in violation of this act unless they "purport or attempt to cure any physical ailment by the laying on of hands, by magnetic suggestion, or other form of medical or surgical treatment." In 1967, after considerable study of the issue of nonmedical psychotherapy, the Attorney General of California reversed his own previous opinion and ruled that psychologists could perform psychotherapy.

Technically speaking, however, in those jurisdictions where the practice of medicine expressly or by implication includes the care of mental afflictions, it is possible that a non-M.D. psychotherapist, when he treats the emotionally distressed, impinges upon the practice of medicine. The courts, however, are unlikely to say that a non-M.D. psychotherapist who treats cases of extreme mental disturbance is illegally practicing medicine.

The California Psychology Licensing Law provides that any person who holds himself out to the public by any title or description incorporating the words *psychology, psychological, psychologist psychometry,* or *psychometrist, psychotherapy, psychotherapist, psychoanalysis,* or *psychoanalyst,* is representing himself to be a psychologist.[65] The statute defines psychotherapy as "the use of psychological methods in a professional relationship to assist a person or persons to acquire greater human effectiveness or to modify feelings, conditions, attitudes, and behavior that are emotionally, intellectually, or socially ineffectual or maladjustive." The California

Attorney General expressed the opinion that marriage, family, or child counselors might use some psychotherapeutic measure in connection with their work, and while the use of the term *psychotherapist* by a counselor is not proscribed by any statutory provision, the misuse of the term might bring one within the prohibitions in the Psychology Licensing Law and become the basis for disciplinary action.[66]

Informal Regulation of Psychotherapy

Informal or indirect control may have greater impact or at least is as important in influencing a practice as is formal or direct control by licensing or certification. Indeed, explicit regulation of practice is exceedingly difficult. Some have despaired to the extent that support is given only to certification laws that regulate the use of a title rather than to licensing laws that would attempt to regulate a practice.

Indirect controls include taxation, insurance, institutional employment opportunities, tort liability for malpractice, and telephone listings. In particular, tax and insurance considerations may determine whether a practice will prosper or perish. Scientology found it expedient to call itself a church, thereby obtaining benefits accorded religious bodies.

Under the Internal Revenue Code, payments to a psychiatrist, psychologist, Christian Science practitioner, or psychopathist, among others, qualify as a medical tax deduction. (The definition of psychopathist is open to speculation.) Payments are allowed as a deduction under the code for "diagnosis, cure, mitigation, treatment, or prevention of disease or for the purpose of affecting any structure or function of the body." In checking with one internal revenue office, I was told that payments to social workers do not qualify because "they [social workers] turn you off rather than on with their attitudes."

Insurance plans usually cover only limited inpatient treatment. Many policies specifically exclude "mental illness or emotional or personality disorder except as an inpatient in a general hospital not specializing in the treatment of mental illness." Even insurers that offer contracts that cover the diagnosis and treatment of mental and nervous disorders in a number of instances have refused to reimburse patients for psychologists' services unless these services were under medical referral or supervision. Medicare, Medicaid, and Workers' Compensation present a similar picture. A Social Security amendment that would have enabled licensed psychologists to provide mental healthcare to Medicare recipients without a physician's prior approval and outside a physician's plan of treatment was turned down in 1972 by the Senate. One senator noted that patients would be better off with physicians who can prescribe drugs on a one-stop basis because psychologists are not allowed to prescribe drugs. Most states now accept qualified psychologists as independent providers of services.

Institutional employment opportunity is another factor influencing a practice and the development of training and education programs. Here may be noted the decision of the Veterans Administration after World War II to employ large numbers of clinical psychologists, thus creating a market demand. It resulted in pressure for the development of the so-called School of Professional Psychology. Distribution of training grants from the NIMH, while providing important support for psychology as well as social work, has been directed primarily toward the training of psychiatrists.

The acceptance of the psychologist by the courts as an expert witness on the diagnosis and treatment of mental disorders on a par with psychiatrists has generated support for the professional autonomy of psychologists.[67] More recent developments in the area of right to treatment can be interpreted as sanctioning increased utilization and independence for psychologists and other qualified mental health professionals. In the private or quasi-public sector is the question of the role of the non-M.D. in the hospital. Some general hospitals have granted staff privileges to psychologists. At present, psychology is not formally a member of the Joint Commission on

Accreditation of Healthcare Organizations' Council on psychiatric facilities, although it is on the Joint Commission on the Accreditation of Healthcare Organizations' (JCAHO's) council on facilities for the mentally retarded.

Regulatory statutes affect malpractice law to the extent that violations may be admissible as evidence of negligence, but even apart from such statutes, negligence may be established and as a result may deter a practice. The threat of suit for malpractice is probably the most effective regulator of the practice of medicine. In like fashion, the risk of a malpractice suit would tend to control the activities of persons who present themselves as psychotherapists. Thus, a marriage counselor would hesitate to conduct psychotherapy with a suicidal person if he were held responsible for the suicide.

Another important type of control is the telephone directory. Probably the principal way that a professional representation is made known to the public is the listing in the telephone directory. Indeed, listing is so vital to one in business that negligent omission in publishing a name has given rise to legal actions for damages in six figures. The telephone company offers or approves the various headings that appear in its directory, one consideration being the amount of advertising that will appear under the heading, but thereafter apparently exercises little supervision over names published under a particular heading. Telephone companies usually have no policy on checking the credentials of professional listings in directories. One telephone business office simplistically advises: "Normally our customers are honest. The subscriber knows what listing he should be under, and he is not going to mislead because it is to his benefit to be under the right heading. A person who is a plumber would not want to be listed as a physician." In some states, an advertising agency publishes the directory, the telephone company having no voice in the matter other than that the subscriber be a customer.

The New York Telephone Company, after prodding by the State Attorney General's office, agreed to start checking the professional qualifications and licenses of persons listed as physicians or psychologists in telephone books throughout the state. The phone company's action came after a partial survey by the Attorney General's Bureau of Consumer Fraud and Protection disclosed that nearly 10% of the listings under those titles in Manhattan, Brooklyn, and Nassau counties were of unlicensed persons. The Attorney General acted following complaints from the state's Psychological Association and Medical Society that the phone company had refused to determine whether applicants for listing under the two categories were duly licensed to practice as required by law. The Psychological Association, in its complaint, said that "upwards of 50 persons who are not licensed as psychologists are listed in the current Yellow Pages across the state under that heading." The Medical Society's complaint also charged that a cursory examination of the white and yellow pages of directories under the heading Physicians had revealed the names of "chiropractors, family counselors, and other unlicensed persons."[68]

Need for Establishing Statutory Control for Psychotherapy

Concerned about the variance of the legal status of psychotherapists among the different states, the American Orthopsychiatric Association in 1967 formed a committee to formulate a model statute for the practice of psychotherapy, regardless of professional discipline.[69] Initially, the committee addressed itself to defining the underlying objectives of such a statute. This entailed exploration of the existing situation that such action was intended to ameliorate. Most of the substantive advice given the committee focused on the disadvantages of the proposed model statute, stimulating the committee to consider the possible undesirable consequences of a legislative approach.

As a result of these efforts, the committee concluded that psychotherapy, as a function of several different professions, did not require statutory control. As a separate and distinct profession, psychotherapists did not impress the committee, at that time, as being sufficient in numbers or organizational maturity to warrant legislation. It was the committee's opinion that legislation controlling the profession of psychotherapists (distinguished from psychotherapy practiced as one of the functions of another profession, e.g., medicine, psychology, social work.) would be premature. It seemed untimely to run the risk of legislatively freezing the current situation just as nontraditional mental health workers are becoming more active. The traditional professions do not appear to require additional protection, therefore, the possibility of inhibiting innovation should be avoided. The extent to which the public is hurt by quackery advertised under the rubric of psychotherapy appeared to be minimal. Although the shortage of data as to who helps and who harms people presents difficulties, the committee nevertheless concluded that there was scant evidence of the title "psychotherapist" being abused.

However, in 1972, following a 6-month investigation into the practices of unlicensed mental health therapists, New York Attorney General Louis J. Lefkowitz reported evidence of widespread quackery, sexual misconduct, and the deception of clients through the use of phony academic credentials and titles. A public hearing was held to expose these practices by unlicensed therapists and others purporting to practice as psychotherapists, psychoanalysts, hypnotists, and marriage counselors.[70]

Four months later, a bill was introduced in the New York Assembly seeking to define the practice of psychological testing and to limit work in the field to persons working under the supervision of a licensed psychologist, physician, registered nurse, or social worker. Strong opposition to the bill was mounted by mental health workers outside the established associations who charged that the proposal would grant a monopoly of the mental health field to a few professionals with advanced degrees, would stifle innovation in the treatment of mental problems, and would put both mental care and career opportunities in the field beyond the reach of poor people.[71] An editorial in the *New York Times*, pointing to the "irreparable harm that has undoubtedly been done to many troubled people whose need for help was compounded by incompetence or outright exploitation," endorsed the bill, but at the same time noted that "unhappy experiences with overly academic and theoretical licensing criteria in education ought to serve as a caution in the mental health field, with its divergent practical and clinical missions and problems."[72] The bill was rejected.[73]

In the latter part of the 20th century, out of the controversy over repressed memories of child sexual abuse came proposals, as we noted in Chapter 30, for a new law, the Truth and Responsibility in Mental Health Practices Act. Indiana has enacted a new law on therapeutic practices and informed consent and several other states are reexamining their laws. In his report on mental health, Surgeon General David Satcher said that the public should be able to expect therapy that is safe and effective. The report recommended the implementation of specific treatment methods, referred to as "evidence-based practices," that have proven to be effective in the treatment of mental illness.[74] Continuing education programs have been established, but one may wonder what they have accomplished apart from creating a market for speakers. Licensing boards tend to accept credentials at face value in the admission of an applicant to a profession and are more preoccupied with disciplinary matters.

In the 1980s, as we noted, adults began suing their parents and others for sexual abuse that had allegedly occurred decades before, but had been remembered only recently, usually in the course of psychotherapy. The 1980s saw a wave of shocking allegations that young children were being sexually abused in bizarre and hideous ways. The testimony of children—often coached by well-meaning, but badly trained therapists and pushed by zealous prosecutors—sent a number of innocent people to jail, as depicted in the film *The Jaundiced Eye* (the film's title comes from a poem by Alexander Pope, suggesting that those who are determined to see the world in a certain way will find all the evidence they need to support their views).[75]

Finding that professional organizations and licensing boards were of little or no assistance in dealing with malpsychotherapy, as we have noted in Chapter 28 on malpractice, educational psychologist Dr. Pamela Freyd in 1992 brought about the False Memory Syndrome Foundation. The inability of the states' disciplinary process to control highly unconventional therapies was earlier highlighted by the widely publicized case involving the suicide of Paul Lozano, a Harvard medical student, who was treated by a Harvard psychiatrist, Dr. Margaret Bean-Bayog. The therapy, which Dr. Bean-Bayog herself acknowledged as "somewhat unconventional," involved her playing the role of a nonabusive mom. The nature of the therapy, called regressive therapy, came to light when Lozano consulted another psychiatrist, who complained to the Massachusetts Board of Registration in Medicine, but no action was taken.[76] A wrongful death lawsuit brought about suspension of the doctor's license.

A series of successful lawsuits by retractors and parents against therapists using "recovered memory" therapy also had a number of consequences. Studies of memory were stimulated.[77] The late Dr. Martin Orne, who helped found the FMS Foundation, showed that adults under hypnosis are not literally reliving their early childhoods, but presenting them through the prisms of adulthood.[78] In 1993, and again in 2000, the American Psychiatric Association cautioned its members that memories obtained by recovered memory techniques are often not true and that memories obtained under hypnosis may be unreliable. The legal liability associated with recovered memory therapy and hypnosis prompted insurance malpractice carriers to exclude or otherwise limit coverage involving the use of hypnosis in therapy.[79] Many psychiatric clinics specializing in the treatment of dissociative disorders have closed.

In the popular novel, *False Memory*, Dean Koontz wrote, "A therapist without finesse can easily, unwittingly implant false memories. Any hypnotized subject is vulnerable. And if the therapist has an agenda and isn't ethical. ..."[80] Koontz's psychiatrist is an utterly evil character with no sympathetic qualities whatsoever. Koontz clearly wished to portray him as a modern Satan (and he signals that at the outset by naming him Dr. Ahriman, the name of the Zoroastrian devil). He is the most frightening villain in any of Koontz's novels. But the problem is not utterly evil characters, they are found out. Much more difficult are the legions of well-intentioned therapists who unwittingly create the environments that foster false memories or other inept psychotherapy. In response, Koontz said:

> Indeed, there is need to set standards for those who want to use the title "psychotherapist." But there should also be meaningful peer review and discipline for those erring practitioners who then meet the standards. Of course, the peer review and policing in the medical profession is all but an abject failure, so I'm not sure there is an easy solution. My feeling is that society needs to be weaned away from the dependency and blind trust in "experts" of all kinds, and that the average person needs to be better educated and then encouraged to trust more in his commonsense.[81]

In 1910 Freud published a paper attacking what he called "wild analysis." He expressed concern that use of psychoanalytic theories by those untrained in psychoanalysis would cause harm. Coincidently, also in 1910, there appeared the report by Abraham Flexner calling for standards in medical education in order to deal with the pervasive quackery in the practice of medicine. As recently as the end of the 19th century, medical education in the United States was in a deplorable state. Hundreds of medical schools were little more than academically anemic apprenticeships. A revolution in medical education resulted from the Flexner report. Medical schools were overhauled, many were closed and the curriculum became science-based. Several contemporary observers have made the analogy between medical education at the end of the 19th century and professional education of psychotherapists today. Considering the current scene, Freud's "On 'Wild' Analysis" proved prescient. There are increasing calls for another Flexner report to deal with standards in psychotherapy.[82] And what about cyberpsych practice on the Internet? In an address at the 2002 annual meeting of the Association of American Law Schools titled "The Illusory Regulation of Psychology: The Teletherapy Example," Professor George J. Alexander of the Santa Clara Law School observed, "Aside from prohibiting unlicensed persons from practicing psychology. Despite this fact, the practice of cyberpsych is a booming industry on the Internet. There is a dearth of enforcement of state regulation of interstate practice, and effective enforcement is unlikely in the future."

Conclusion

The legal regulation of psychotherapy revolves around the controversy about the medical model and its appropriateness as an approach to the problems of mental illness. Developments in the neurosciences are increasingly expected to inform about the appropriate type of treatment in a given case.[83] In any event, if psychotherapy is indeed a form of education and not part of any medical system, then the legal regulation of psychotherapy becomes similar to the legal regulation of education.[84] In a sense, the process of psychotherapy is to impose order out of chaos. In the course of therapy, the poet Anne Sexton said that the analyst "gives pattern and meaning to what the person sees as only incoherent experience."[85] The task of psychotherapy is to offer the individual a more satisfactory life story or help the individual to move on in the story he already has. Mostly, people enter therapy when they are stuck in a certain chapter of their lives and do not know what they want to do next or do not like what they see ahead. The dreams of one in psychoanalysis are often a symbol of a journey. A successful therapeutic experience helps reestablish the narrative flow, reawaken a sense of meaning in one's life, and restore personal control.[86]

Unfortunately, even the best of therapy does not always succeed. In spite of (or because of) therapy, Anne Sexton committed suicide.

Endnotes

1. J.S. Handler, "Psychotherapy and Medical Responsibility," *Arch. Gen. Psychiat.* 1 (1959): 464.
2. L.S. Kubie, "The General Nature of Non-Technical Psychotherapy," L.S. Kubie (Ed.), *Practical and Theoretical Aspects of Psychoanalysis* (New York: International Universities Press, 1950), p. 21.
3. T.S. Szasz, "Psychoanalytic Treatment as Education," *Arch. Gen. Psychiat.* 9 (1963): 46.
4. See K.R. Eissler, *Medical Orthodoxy and the Future of Psychoanalysis* (New York: International Universities Press, 1965); E. Jones, *The Life and Work of Sigmund Freud* (New York: Basic Books, 1957).
5. *Ibid.* Edward Shorter, professor in the history of medicine, suggests that European physicians were more tolerant of lay analysis because they stood less in awe of themselves generally. In Central Europe, a whole host of titles, such as Herr Hofrat, Herr Geheimrat, Herr Professor, and Herr General were in usage before "Herr Doktor," whereas in the United States MDs were at the top of the pecking order. E. Shorter, *A History of Psychiatry* (New York: John Wiley & Sons, 1997), p. 371.
6. See R.S. Wallerstein, *Lay Analysis/Life Inside the Controversy* (Mahwah, NJ: Analytic Press, 1998).
7. Correspondence of March 8, 1968, from George E. Hall, member of the Law Division of the American Medical Association.
8. J.S. Handler, *supra* note 1. See also G.D. Goldman & D.S. Milman, D.S. (Eds.), *Innovations in Psychotherapy* (Springfield, IL: Thomas, 1972), p. 235. Dr. Robert Michels notes that psychotherapy has been called the "talking cure," and he suggests that it might better be called the "listening cure." Fundamental to listening is thinking, and it is what makes psychotherapy different from simple friendship. R. Michels, "Thinking While Listening," address at the annual meeting of the American Psychiatric Association on May 16, 2000, in Chicago.
9. T.S. Szasz, "Psychiatry, Psychotherapy, and Psychology," *Arch. Gen. Psychiat.* 5 (1959): 455. See also A. Fischer, "Non-Medical Psychotherapists," *Arch. Gen. Psychiat.* 5 (1961): 7; P.E. Huston, "The Relations of Psychiatry and Psychotherapy," *Am. J. Psychiat.* 110 (1954): 814.

10. S.M. Mirin, "Predictions About the Financing and Delivery of Care," in S. Weissman, M. Sabshin, & H. Eist (Eds.), *Psychiatry in the New Millennium* (Washington, DC: American Psychiatric Press, 1999), p. 321.

11. Final Report of Joint Commission on Mental Illness and Health, *Action for Mental Health* (1961).

12. R.R. Holt (Ed.), *New Horizon for Psychotherapy: Autonomy as a Profession* (New York: International Universities Press, 1971); L.S. Kubie, "Need for a New Sub Discipline in the Medical Profession," *Arch. Neur. & Psychiat.* 78 (1957): 283; Symposium, "Qualifications for Psychotherapy," *Am. J. Orthopsychiat.* 26 (1956): 35.

13. J.D. Frank, *Persuasion and Healing: A Comparative Study of Psychotherapy* (Baltimore, MD: Johns Hopkins University Press, 1961).

14. S. Blakeslee, "Placebos Prove So Powerful Even Experts Are Surprised," *New York Times*, Oct. 13, 1998, p. D1; J. Horhan, "Placebo Nation," *New York Times*, March 21, 1999, p. WK15.

15. See D.C. Pate & R.F. Corrigan (Eds.), *Regulation of Healthcare Professionals: A Casebook Approach* (Durham, NC: Carolina Academic Press, 2002).

16. See R. Shyrock, *Medical Licensing in America, 1950–1965* (Baltimore, MD: Johns Hopkins Press, 1967); F. Auman, "The Growth and Regulation of the Licensing Process in Ohio," *J. Can. L. Rev.* 21 (1931): 97.

17. Overall, the level of licensing regulation has risen precipitously in recent years, with more than 20% of the workforce now required to have a license—up from 4.5% in the 1950s. More than 1,000 occupations now control entry. Some professional licensing is a defensive outgrowth of the lawsuit culture, but most is pushed by the age-old reason of restricting competition. Licensing constitutes domestic protectionism. Editorial, "Licensed to Kill," *Wall Street Journal*, Sept. 10, 2007, p. 14.

18. The right of the states to regulate the practice of medicine or other regulation is based on constitutional grounds and traditional interpretations of states' rights. As the power to regulate the health professions was not specifically entrusted to Congress, the Tenth Amendment reserves the power to the states and the people. Critics charge that cumbersome licensure processes unfairly restrict the mobility of competent professionals. Balancing the interests of access to care and public protection has now come to the fore in regard interstate telemedicine licensure and cybermedicine. See R.D. Silverman, "Regulating Medical Practice in the Cyber Age: Issues and Challenges for State Medical Boards," *Am. J. Law & Med.* 26 (2000): 255; see also B. Shartel & M.L. Plant, *The Law of Medical Practice* (Springfield, IL: Thomas, 1959), p. 195.

19. See W. Graves, "Professional and Occupational Restrictions," *Temp. L. Q.* 13 (1939): 334.

20. J. Baron, "Business and Professional Licensing—California, A Representative Example," *Stan. L. Rev.* 18 (1966): 640.

21. See D.B. Hogan, *The Regulation of Psychotherapists* (Cambridge: Bollinger, 1979); J.S. Lloyd & D.G. Langsley (Eds.), *Evaluating the Skills of Medical Specialists* (Evanston, IL: American Board of Medical Specialties, 1983); S. Rottenberg (Ed.), *Occupational Licensure and Regulation* (Washington, DC: American Enterprise Institute for Public Policy Research, 1980).

22. See, e.g., Fla. Stat. Ann.§§ 458.305 440.003. The use of the word *therapy* by a hearing aid dealer in a newspaper ad containing the statement "hearing and speech therapy" indicated the dealer "held himself out" as being able to perform or treat matters embraced within the definition of the practice of medicine; Op. Atty. Gen., 064-115 (Aug. 10, 1964). The state board of medical examiners is authorized to prevent unlicensed medical practice of "psychosomatic therapy" and "medical hypnosis" where such treatment invades the field of medical practice; Op. Atty. Gen., 056-12 (Jan. 13, 1956).

23. See D.G. Langsley (Ed.), *Legal Aspects of Certification and Accreditation* (Evanston, IL: American Board of Medical Specialties, 1983); Abramson v. Gonzalez, 949 F.2d 1567 (11th Cir. 1992).

24. American Association of Marriage Counselors. Report on Conference on the State Regulation of Marriage Counselors, Sept. 1964, p. 5; commonly referred to as the AAMC 1964 Report.

25. Florida expressly regulates the use of the title *psychotherapist*; Fla Code § 490.012.

26. Personal communication (May 7, 1968) from Edward J. Rydman.

27. See, e.g., Calif. Bus. & Prof. Code 6.6:2900.

28. For example, United States v. Cardiff, 344 U.S. 174 (1952); Connally v. General Const. Co., 269 U.S. 385 (1926).

29. State v. Errington, 355 S.W.2d 952 (Mo. 1962).

30. J. Sharkey, "Philosophers Ponder a Therapy Gold Mine," *New York Times*, March 8, 1988, sec. 4, p. 1.

31. P. Koestenbaum, *The New Image of the Person: The Theory and Practice of Clinical Philosophy* (Westport, CT: Greenwood Press, 1978); L. Marinoff, *Plato, Not Prozac! Applying Philosophy to Everyday Problems* (New York: Harper Collins, 1999); see also A. de Botton, *The Consolations of Philosophy* (New York:

Pantheon, 2000). Socrates has been called the first psychotherapist, given the self-examination inherent in the Socratic "Know thyself." R. Chessick, "Socrates: First Psychotherapist," *Am. J. Psychoanaly.* 42 (1982): 71.

32. *Pilot Project Intraining Mental Health Counselors*, Public Health Service Publication No. 125 (1965); "Mothers Good Candidates as Counselors," *Clinical Psychiatry News*, Oct. 1979, p. 32.

33. See, e.g., R. Cohen, "The Oldest Profession Seeks New Market in West Europe," *New York Times*, Sept. 19, 2000, p. 1.

34. See A. Abbott, *The System of Professions: An Essay on the Division of Expert Labor* (Chicago: University of Chicago Press, 1988); S.B. Benatar, "The Meaning of Professionalism in Medicine," *S. Afr. Med. J.* 87 (1997): 427; J. Goldstein, "Foucault Among the Sociologists: The 'Disciplines' and the History of Professions," *Hist. & Theory* 23 (1984): 170.

35. Goldfarb v. Virginia State Bar, 421 U.S. 773 (1975).

36. 421 U.S. at 788 n. 17.

37. R.E. Lee, "Application of Antitrust Laws to the Professions," *J. Legal Med.* 1 (1979): 143.

38. American Medical Assn. v. Federal Trade Commission, 638 F.2d 443 (2d Cir. 1980), *aff'd,* 455 U.S. 676 (1982); L. Greenhouse, "Justices Uphold Right of Doctors to Solicit Trade," *New York Times*, March 24, 1982, p. 10.

39. (Washington, DC: American Psychiatric Press, 7th ed., 1994), p. 170. On the development of the profession of psychiatry, see F.G. Alexander & S.T. Selesnick, *The History of Psychiatry: An Evaluation of Psychiatric Thought and Practice From Prehistoric Times to the Present* (New York: Harper & Row, 1966).

40. See S. Weissman, M. Sabshin, & H. Eist (Eds.), *Psychiatry in the New Millennium* (Washington, DC: American Psychiatric Press, 1999); M. Reiser, "Are Psychiatric Educators Losing Their Mind?" *Am. J. Psychiat.* 145 (1988): 148.

41. See L. Freeman, *Celebrities on the Couch: Personal Adventures of Famous People in Psychoanalysis* (Los Angeles: Ravena Books, no date).

42. See N. Hale, *The Rise and Crisis of Psychoanalysis in the United States* (New York: Oxford University Press, 1995); J. Lear, *Open Minded* (Cambridge, MA: Harvard University Press, 1998).

43. E.R. Kandel, *In Search of Memory* (New York: W.W. Norton, 2006), pp. 39–40.

44. The theory or practice of psychoanalysis has its fervent supporters (see the Introduction) and it has its detractors. Paul Valery was suspicious of it. James Joyce called it "neither more nor less than blackmail." Vladimir Nabokov, author of *Lolita*, was disdainful of Freudian doctrine, calling its founder the "Viennese quack," and characterized psychoanalysis as little more than using classic myths to cover up private parts, referring to "the oneiromancy and mythology of psychoanalysis." He detested what he took to be Freud's crude use of symbolism, with every symbol having a sexual meaning. Quoted in J. Epstein, "Master and Shrink," *Weekly Standard*, Oct. 22, 2007, p. 37. The Peruvian novelist Mario Vargas Llosa says he is not in favor of psychoanalysis, "It's too close to fiction, and I don't need more fiction in my life." Quoted in D. Solomon, "The Storyteller," *New York Times Magazine*, Oct. 7, 2007, p. 15. See, in general, P.D. Kramer, *Freud: Inventor of the Modern Mind* (New York: HarperCollins, 2006); R.M. Restak, "Psychiatry in America," *Wilson Q.* 7 (Autumn, 1983): 95.

45. See Calif. Bus. & Prof. Code 6.6:2903; Mich. Comp. Laws § 18001. Tables enumerating the states having psychology regulatory statutes and the scope of the various statutes are provided in *The Psychologist and Voluntary Health Insurance* (Washington, DC: American Psychological Association, 1968).

46. Four types of licenses are granted by the Michigan Board of Psychology, three of which fall under categories of limited licensure.

47. See P. Coleman & R.A. Shellow, "Prescribing Privileges for Psychologists: Should Only 'Medicine Men' Control the Medicine Cabinet?" *J. Psychiat. & Law* 18 (1990): 269; R.B. Karel, "Psychologists Press Harder to Prescribe," *Psychiatric News*, August 5, 1994, pp. 1, 25; T. Svensson, "Prescribing for Psychologists," *Clinical Psychiatry News*, Jan. 1998, p. 18.

48. C. Lehmann, "Psychologists' Bid to Be 'Physicians' Comes to Dead End in Florida," *Clinical Psychiatric News*, May 21, 1999, p. 4.

49. Virginia Academy of Clinical Psychologists v. Blue Shield of Virginia, 624 F.2d 476 (4th Cir. 1980). In California Association of Psychology Providers v. Rank, 51 Cal. 3d 1, 270 Cal. Rptr. 796, 793, P.2d 2 (1990), the court construed a state statute to require that psychologists be accorded hospital admission privileges equal to those of psychiatrists.

50. D. Goleman, "Social Workers Vault Into a Leading Role in Psychotherapy," *New York Times*, April 30, 1985, p. C1.

51. A. Gribbon, "Shoddy Counseling," *National Observer*, Oct. 30, 1971, p. 1.

52. See T. Baldas, "After Counseling Fails, Many Sue," *Med. Malpract. Law & Strat.*, Oct. 2006: 24.

53. The Michigan licensing law was enacted by Act 369 of 1978. See MCL §333.18105.

54. See L.P. Bradford et al. (Eds.), *T-Group Theory and Laboratory Method* (New York: John Wiley & Sons, 1964); A. Burton (Ed.), *Encounter: Theory and Practice of Encounter Groups* (San Francisco: Jossey-Bass, 1969).

55. The First Amendment's prohibition against judicial review of ecclesiastical disputes does not bar a claim against a pastoral counselor for malpractice or breach of fiduciary duty. A minister who holds himself out as a professional marriage counselor is judged by a professional, rather than religious, standard of care; Sanders v. Casa View Baptist Church, 134 F.3d 331 (5th Cir. 1998).

56. Jaffee v. Redmond, 527 U.S. 123 (1999).

57. See R.K. Westheimer, *All in a Lifetime* (New York: Warner Books, 2001); see, generally, V.L. Bullough, *Science in the Bedroom: A History of Sex Research* (New York: Basic Books, 1994).

58. M.J. Rioch et al., "National Institute of Mental Health Pilot Study in Training Mental Health Counselors," *Am. J. Orthopsychiat.* 33 (1963): 678. See also Report, *Utilization of Paraprofessionals in Three Mental Health Settings* (New York: Institute for Child Mental Health, 1972).

59. E.F. Torrey, *The Mind Game: Witchdoctors and Psychiatrists* (New York: Emerson Hall, 1972); condensed version, "What Western Psychotherapists Can Learn From Witchdoctors," *Am. J. Orthopsychiat.* 42 (1972): 69. In an interesting case at the Tulane University Department of Psychiatry and Neurology, which the author observed, a young woman who had been treated in psychotherapy without much result was suddenly and dramatically healed by a faith healer who cast out demons from within her. After the healing, which included five exorcism sessions over a period of a month, the health of the patient was remarkably improved, her symptoms had disappeared, and she began to function with mature self-confidence. This individual had grown up in a hyper moralistic environment and previously had never been able to resolve many conflicted feelings. She now knew, she reported, that God loved her. The faith healer, who worked with her, had a group who sings, chants, and prays in the background as he performs the exorcism. He addresses each devil by name (e.g., Jeremiah) and carries on a heated conversation with each one. The situation builds up to fever-pitch excitement. "Come out, Jeremiah, I know you're in there! Come out! Come out, Jeremiah! Come on out!" The bedeviled has explosive coughs. As each devil is coughed out, the healer expels him across the ocean to Israel. The devils, several in number, are thus defeated (although they might return). In this concrete manner, devils are blamed for the individual's past wrongdoings, real or imagined, and they are exorcized, freeing the possessed from bondage. This faith healer feels that exorcism and psychotherapy have many similarities, the only real difference being the extent to which the patient is directed and the means by which the psychic problems are symbolically represented. The techniques of exorcism, especially as represented in this case history, support the contention that faith healing, hypnotic suggestion, thought reform, and psychotherapy have some similarities. See J.A. Knight, *Conscience and Guilt* (New York: Appleton-Century-Crofts, 1969), p. 59.

60. Note, "Regulation of Psychological Counseling and Psychotherapy," *Colum. L. Rev.* 51 (1951): 474.

61. Okla. Rev. Stat. 59-492 (West 1989).

62. S.D. Laws, ch. 106-14.

63. N.C. Gen. Stat. Ann., sec. 90-18 (West 1999); Minn. Stat. Ann., sec. 147.081 (West 1999).

64. Tenn. Code Ann., sec. 63-6-204; Ohio Code Ann., sec. 4731.34 (West 1999).

65. Calif. Bus. & Prof. Code 6.6:2902 (Deering's 1999).

66. Op. Calif. Atty. Gen. 49:104.

67. In a landmark decision, Jenkins v. United States, 307 F.2d 637 (D.C. 1962), the District of Columbia Court of Appeals held that a psychologist is not barred as a matter of law from giving expert testimony about mental illness. Following *Jenkins*, most states have provided by statute or case law that doctoral level clinical psychologists may offer opinions on insanity as well as on other issues concerning the mentally disordered. See R. Gass, "The Psychologist as Expert Witness: Science in the Courtroom," *Md. L. Rev.* 38 (1979): 539. See also G. Dix & N. Poythress, "Propriety of Medical Dominance of Forensic Mental Health Practice: The Empirical Evidence," *Ariz. L. Rev.* 23 (1981): 961.

68. *New York Times*, Nov. 28, 1972, p. 55.

69. The author was a member of the committee.

70. I. Peterson, "State Finds Quacks in Mental Therapy," *New York Times*, Dec. 7, 1972, p. 1.

71. *New York Times*, April 11, 1973, p. 32.

72. April 11, 1973, p. 32.

73. *New York Times*, April 13, 1973, p. 52; April 24, p. 38.

74. D. Satcher, "Mental Health: A Report of the Surgeon General," U.S. Public Health Service, 1999.

75. The film is reviewed in A.O. Scott, "Two Lives Torn by a Child Abuse Case," *New York Times*, March 3, 2000, p. B25.

76. *New York Times*, April 12, 1992, p. 22.

77. Papers presented in 1994 at an FMS Foundation conference entitled "Memory and Reality: Reconciliation; Scientific, Clinical and Legal Issues of False Memory Syndrome," appear in *J. Psychiat. & Law* 23 (1995): 347–484. See also J. Acocella, *Creating Hysteria* (San Francisco: Jossey-Bass, 1999), excerpted in "The Politics of Hysteria," *New Yorker*, April 6, 1998, p. 64; M. Johnston, *Spectral Evidence: The Ramona Case* (New York: Houghton Mifflin, 1997); S. Taub (Ed.), *Recovered Memories of Child Sexual Abuse* (Springfield, IL: Thomas, 1999); E. Loftus, "Memory Distortion and False Memory Creation," *Bull. Am. Acad. Psychiat. & Law* 24 (1996): 281. In support of recovered memories, see D. Brown, A.W. Scheflin, & C.L. Whitfield, "Recovered Memories: The Current Weight of the Evidence in Science and in the Courts," *J. Psychiat. & Law* 27 (1999): 5.

78. Dr. Orne's research on memory and undue suggestion has been cited by the U.S. Supreme Court and more than 30 state supreme courts. His expertise in hypnosis played a key role in the trial of Kenneth Bianchi, the former security guard who confessed to killing five women in the Hillside Strangler case. The defense argued that Bianchi suffered from multiple personalities.

79. Bert Peterson of Rockport Insurance Associates advises: "Our Professional liability policy is not being offered to those practitioners who *intentionally* set out to recover failed or repressed memories through hypnotherapy [emphasis by Peterson]. We are aware that, as a result of hypnotherapy, the possibility does exist that such an event may occur. The use of hypnotherapy is not specifically excluded from the policy." Letter to Ralph Slovenko of June 13, 1996.

80. D. Koontz, *False Memory* (New York: Bantam, 1999), p. 384.

81. Personal communication.

82. See E.R. Kandel, "A New Intellectual Framework for Psychiatry," *Am. J. Psychiat.* 155 (1998): 457; P. McHugh, "Psychiatry Awry," *Am. Schol.* 63 (1994): 17.

83. E.R. Kandel, "Biology and the Future of Psychoanalysis: A New Intellectual Framework for Psychiatry Revisited," *Am. J. Psychiat.* 156 (1999): 505.

84. Dr. Jerome D. Frank points out that although persons come to psychotherapy for relief of specific symptoms or disabilities, their primary reason for seeking help is that they are more or less demoralized and the effect of psychotherapy is to restore morale. The effectiveness of any form of psychotherapy, hence, depends on its ability to restore the individual's morale. Psychotherapy may help combat the individual's sense of isolation, inspire his hopes for relief, reduce his confusion, and teach him more effective ways of coping with his feelings and the external world, thereby increasing his sense of self-control and mastery. The hypothesis implies that the major determinants of outcome are not therapeutic procedures *per se*, but rather personal qualities of therapist and patient and the degree of concordance between the patient's belief as to what will help him and the therapeutic method. This depends primarily on the source to which he attributes his symptoms, in turn a function of his education and cultural status and the views of the therapist he happens to encounter. Thus, highly structured concrete procedures, such as crisis management and behavior therapies, may be especially suited to less highly educated patients, while interview therapies appeal to the verbally skilled, who attribute their symptoms and abilities to inner conflicts. J.D. Frank, *Persuasion and Healing. A Comparative Study of Psychotherapy* (Baltimore, MD: Johns Hopkins University Press, 1991). See also W. Gaylin, *Talk Is Not Enough: How Psychotherapy Really Works* (Boston: Little, Brown, 2000). As education, psychotherapy can last a lifetime, and it sometimes does (as Woody Allen made famous). See R.A. Friedman, "How to Figure Out When Therapy Is Over," *New York Times*, Oct. 30, 2007, p. D6.

85. See D. Middlebrook, *Anne Sexton: A Biography* (Boston: Houghton Mifflin , 1991), p. 64.

86. See A.M. Ludwig, *How Do We Know Who We Are? A Biography of the Self* (New York: Oxford University Press, 1997); D.P. Spence, *Narrative Truth and Historical Truth: Meaning and Interpretation in Psychoanalysis* (New York: Norton, 1982).

INDICES

Case Index

Y

Z

Name Index

Subject Index

Acknowledgments

Once again, I am pleased to acknowledge my gratitude to Dr. Abraham L. Halpern, prominent forensic psychiatrist and past president of the American Academy of Psychiatry and the Law, who provided helpful suggestions. Dr. Halpern was always encouraging, and I am most grateful to him. I want also to take the opportunity to thank the many people for interesting discussions over the years, and for their supportive and sustaining friendship. I can only mention a few: Dr. Ramon Bhavsar, Dr. Elliott Luby, Dr. George Mendelson, Dr. Emanuel Tanay, Dr. Gene L. Usdin, and Dr. Tuviah Zabow, and the late Dr. Maurice Grossman, Dr. James A. Knight, Dr. Harold I. Lief, Dr. Karl A. Menninger, and also, of blessed memory, Dr. Daniel Sprehe, and Dr. C.B. Scrignar. I thank Matthew Moussiaux and Salma Safiedine, students at the Wayne State University Law School, for assistance in the preparation of the indices. I thank Georgia Clark and Anne Cottongim of the Wayne State University Law Library for their assistance in obtaining materials, and Charlotte Davis for her word processing assistance.

About the Author

Ralph Slovenko is Professor of Law and Psychiatry at Wayne State University in Michigan. He received B.E., LL.B., M.A., and Ph.D. degrees from Tulane University. He was editor-in-chief of the *Tulane Law Review* and a varsity sports letterman at Tulane University. He served as law clerk to the Louisiana Supreme Court and as senior assistant district attorney under Jim Garrison in New Orleans. He was a Fulbright scholar to France. A tenured professor of law at Tulane University from 1954 to 1964, he was also a member of the faculty of the Tulane University Department of Psychiatry and Neurology. At the invitation of the late Dr. Robert G. Heath, chairman of the Tulane University Department of Psychiatry and Neurology, he did a residency in psychiatry, one of two persons to do so without a medical degree.

He held a joint appointment, from 1965 to 1968, at the Menninger Foundation and the University of Kansas School of Law. Since then, he has been at Wayne State University. He has lectured widely in the United States and also in Australia, Canada, France, Israel, Japan, Russia (Soviet Union), and South Africa. He was visiting professor in South Africa in 1976 and 1989, and he occupied the Rood Eminent Scholar Chair in 1991 at the University of Florida College of Law. He has been a frequent visitor to Lithuania, Mexico, Poland, Russia, and South Africa and has written extensively about them. He has frequently served as an expert witness.

He is a member of the American, Kansas, Louisiana, and Michigan Bar Associations; scientific associate of the American Academy of Psychoanalysis; and amicus of the American Academy of Psychiatry and Law. He is the author of numerous books and articles. His book *Psychiatry and Law* (Boston: Little, Brown, 1973) received the Manfred Guttmacher award of the American Psychiatric Association and was a selection of the Behavioral Science Book Club. He collaborated with Dr. Karl A. Menninger on the book *The Crime of Punishment* (New York: Viking Press, 1966). From 1978 to 2007, he wrote a lengthy commentary in each issue of the quarterly *Journal of Psychiatry and Law* and is currently editor of the American Series in Behavioral Science and Law. He is on the board of editors of the *International Journal of Offender Therapy and Comparative Criminology, Journal of the American Academy of Psychiatry and Law*, and *Medicine and Law*. For years he wrote a weekly column in the *Detroit Legal News*. His articles have appeared in the *New York Times, Wall Street Journal*, and other publications. His writings have been quoted on several occasions by the U.S. Supreme Court, and in over 150 state and lower federal court cases.